Dedication

This text is first and foremost dedicated to medical students as they embark on their surgical clerkships and attempt to assimilate the enormous and ever-increasing body of knowledge required for today's surgeons. We would be remiss if we failed to acknowledge our families, particularly our wives, Christine Becker and Angela Stucchi, who have supported us in this effort and throughout our careers.

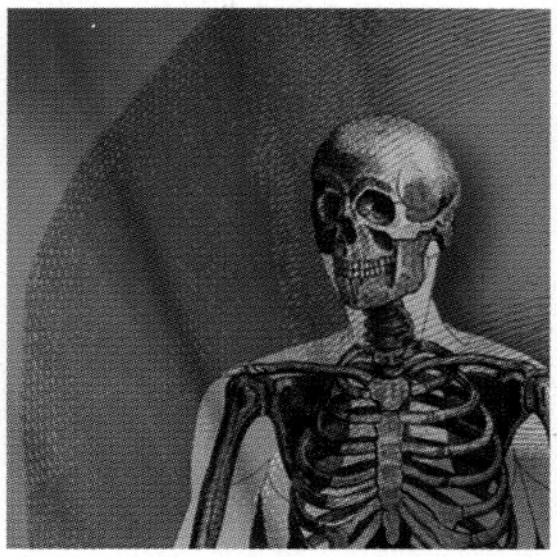

Essentials of Surgery

Essentials of Surgery

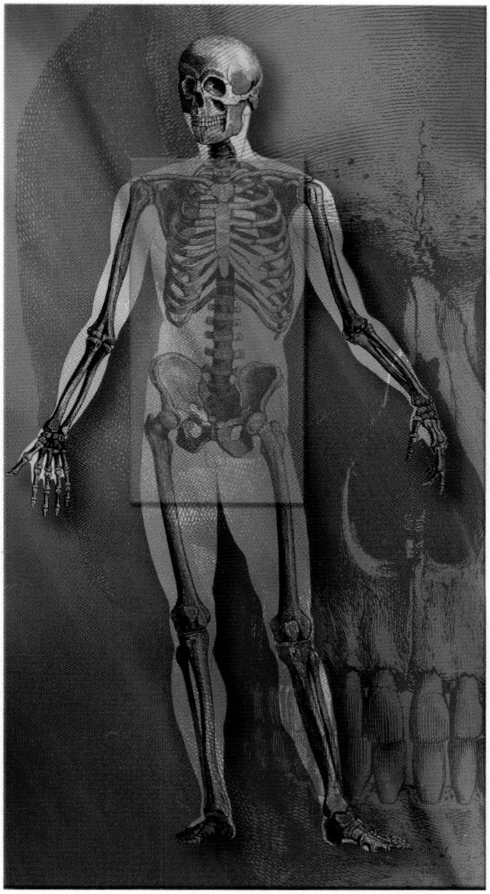

James M. Becker, MD, FACS
James Utley Professor and Chairman
Department of Surgery
Boston University School of Medicine
Surgeon-in-Chief
Boston University Medical Center
Boston, Massachusetts

Arthur F. Stucchi, PhD
Associate Professor
Departments of Surgery, Pathology, and Laboratory Medicine
Boston University School of Medicine
Boston, Massachusetts

SAUNDERS
ELSEVIER

SAUNDERS
ELSEVIER
An Imprint of Elsevier

1600 John F. Kennedy Boulevard
Suite 1800
Philadelphia, Pennsylvania 19103

ESSENTIALS OF SURGERY

ISBN-13 978-0-7216-8186-3
ISBN-10 0-7216-8186-7

NOTICE

Knowledge and best practice in this field are constantly changing. As new research and experience broaden our knowledge, changes in practice, treatment and drug therapy may become necessary or appropriate. Readers are advised to check the most current information provided (i) on procedures featured or (ii) by the manufacturer of each product to be administered, to verify the recommended dosing or formula, the method and duration of administration, and contraindications. It is the responsibility of the practitioner, relying on their own experience and knowledge of the patient, to make diagnoses, to determine dosages and the best treatment for each individual patient, and to take all appropriate safety precautions. To the fullest extent of the law, neither the Publisher nor the Editors assume any liability for any injury and/or damage to persons or property arising out of or related to any use of the material contained in this book.

Library of Congress Cataloging-in-Publication Data
Essentials of surgery/[edited by] James M. Becker, Arthur F. Stucchi.
p. ; cm.
Includes bibliographical references.
ISBN 0-7216-8186-7
1. Surgery. 2. Surgery, Operative. I. Becker, James M. II. Stucchi, Arthur F.
[DNLM: 1. Surgical Procedures, Operative WO 500 E7829 2006]
RD31.E87 2006
617′.91--dc22

Acquisitions Editor: William Schmitt
Developmental Editor: Jacqueline Mahon
Publishing Services Manager: Joan Sinclair
Design direction: Ellen Zanolle

Printed in the United States of America
Last digit is the print number: 9 8 7 6 5 4 3 2 1

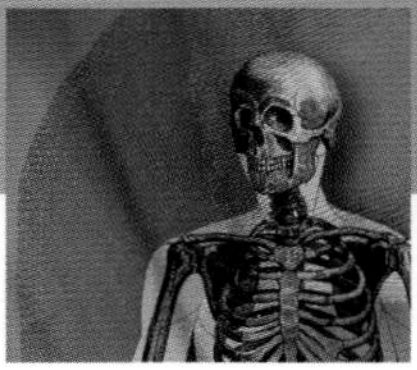

CONTRIBUTORS

Rie Aihara, MD, FACS
Trauma Surgeon/Surgical Critical Care Specialist
Department of Surgery
Lee Memorial Hospital
Fort Myers, Florida

Stanley W. Ashley, MD
Frank R. Sawyer Professor of Surgery
Harvard Medical School
Vice-Chair, Department of Surgery
The Brigham and Women's Hospital
Boston, Massachusetts

Timothy J. Babineau, MD, MBA, FACS
Associate Professor of Surgery
Chief, Sections of Gastrointestinal and Minimally Invasive Surgery
Boston University Medical Center
Boston, Massachusetts

Maryann Barry, RN, FNP
Vascular Nurse Practitioner
Department of Vascular Surgery
Boston University Medical Center
Boston, Massachusetts

Robert M. Beazley, MD
Emeritus Professor of Surgery
Emeritus Chief
Section of Surgical Oncology and Endocrine Surgery
Boston University Medical Center
Boston, Massachusetts

James M. Becker, MD, FACS
James Utley Professor and Chairman
Department of Surgery
Boston University School of Medicine
Surgeon-in-Chief
Boston University Medical Center
Boston, Massachusetts

Erica A. Brotschi, MD
Associate Professor of Surgery
Surgical Clerkship Director
Boston University Medical Center
Staff Surgeon
Boston VA Healthcare System
Boston, Massachusetts

Neil E. Brown, MD
Attending Physician
Department of Otolaryngology–Head and Neck Surgery
Franciscan Skemp Healthcare
Mayo Health System
LaCrosse, Wisconsin

Riad Cachecho, MD
Director, Trauma and Critical Care
Department of Surgery
Crozer Chester Medical Center
Chester, Pennsylvania

Nancy L. Cantelmo, MD, FACS
Associate Professor of Surgery
Boston University Medical Center
Vascular Surgeon
Boston VA Healthcare System
Boston, Massachusetts

Sang I. Cho, MD
Professor of Surgery
Chief of Transplant Surgery
Boston University Medical Center
Boston, Massachusetts

Raymond L. Comenzo, MD
Director, Cytotherapy Laboratory
Hematology Service
Memorial Sloan-Kettering Cancer Center
New York, New York

Michael S. Cookson, MD
Associate Professor
Department of Urologic Surgery
Vanderbilt University School of Medicine
Attending Physician and Surgeon
Department of Urologic Surgery
Vanderbilt University Medical Center
Nashville, Tennessee

Matthew J. D'Alessio, MD
Fellow
Department of Surgical Oncology
University of Pittsburgh
University of Pittsburgh Hospital
Pittsburgh, Pennsylvania

Merril T. Dayton, MD, FACS
Professor and Chair
Department of Surgery

State University of New York
Chief of Surgery
Kaleida Health System
Buffalo, New York

Richard C. Dennis, MD, FACS
Associate Professor of Surgery and Anesthesiology
Boston University Medical Center
Director
Surgical Intensive Care Units
VA Medical Center
Boston, Massachusetts

Anand K. Devaiah, MD
Assistant Professor
Departments of Otolaryngology—Head and Neck Surgery and Neurological Surgery
Attending Physician
Departments of Otolaryngology—Head and Neck Surgery and Neurological Surgery
Boston University Medical Center
Boston, Massachusetts

Peter Dewire, MD
Assistant Professor
Department of Orthopedic Surgery
Quincy Medical Center
Quincy, Massachusetts

Anthony DiScipio, MD
Assistant Professor of Surgery
Dartmouth Medical School
Department of Cardiothoracic Surgery Dartmouth-Hitchcock Medical Center
Lebanon, New Hampshire

Elof Eriksson, MD, PhD
Joseph E. Murray Professor of Plastic and Reconstructive Surgery
Harvard Medical School
Chief of Plastic Surgery
The Brigham and Women's Hospital
Chief of Plastic Surgery
Children's Hospital
Boston, Massachusetts

Marina I. Feldman, MD, MBA
Medical Student
Tufts University School of Medicine
Boston, Massachusetts

Stephen J. Ferzoco, MD
Assistant Professor of Surgery
Harvard Medical School
Associate Surgeon
Department of Surgery
Brigham and Women's Hospital
Boston, Massachusetts

Jonathan F. Finks, MD
Clinical Assistant Professor of Surgery
University of Michigan Health Systems
Ann Arbor, Michigan

Thomas M. Fishbein, MD
Chief
Intestinal and Pediatric Liver Transplantation
Children's National Medical Center
Director
Small Bowel and Pediatric Liver Transplantation
Transplant Institute
Georgetown University Hospital
Associate Professor of Surgery and Pediatrics
Georgetown University School of Medicine
Washington, DC

R. Armour Forse, MD, PhD, FRCS(C), FACS, FCCM
Lempka Professor and Chairman
Department of Surgery
Creighton University
Chief of Surgical Services
Creighton University Medical Center
Omaha, Nebraska

Gene A. Grindlinger, MD, FACS
Clinical Professor of Surgery
University of Vermont College of Medicine
Burlington, Vermont
Director of Surgical Critical Care
Maine Medical Center
Portland, Maine

Kenneth M. Grundfast, MD
Professor and Chair
Department of Otolaryngology–Head and Neck Surgery
Chief of Otolaryngology–Head and Neck Surgery
Boston University Medical Center
Boston, Massachusetts

Fady Haddad, MD
Department of Surgery
American University of Beirut-Medical Center
Beirut, Lebanon

Valerie J. Halpin, MD
Assistant Professor of Surgery
Washington University School of Medicine
St. Louis, Missouri

Roger Hartl, MD
Assistant Professor
Department of Neurological Surgery
Weill Cornell Medical College
Assistant Attending
Department of Neurological Surgery
New York Presbyterian Hospital
New York, New York
Neurosurgeon
St. Barnabas Hospital
Bronx, New York

John G. Hunter, MD, FACS
Mackenzie Professor and Chair
Department of Surgery
Oregon Health and Science University
Portland, Oregon

Tamara J. Intner, MD
Resident
Department of Emergency Medicine
Johns Hopkins Hospital
Baltimore, Maryland

Scharukh Jalisi, MD
Assistant Professor
Department of Otolaryngology—Head and Neck Surgery
Boston University Medical Center
Boston, Massachusetts

C. Starck Johnson, MD

Willard C. Johnson, MD
Professor (Retired)
Department of Surgery
Boston University Medical Center
Boston, Massachusetts
Vascular Surgeon
Veterans Affairs Pacific Islands Healthcare System
Kailua-Kona, Hawaii

Maureen T. Kavanah, MD
Associate Professor of Surgery
Section of Surgical Oncology
Department of Surgery
Boston University Medical Center
Boston, Massachusetts

R. James Koness, MD
Clinical Assistant Professor of Surgery
Brown University School of Medicine
Oncology Surgeon
Roger Williams Medical Center
Providence, Rhode Island

Cathy Korn, RN, MPH, CIC
Nurse Epidemiologist
Department of Hospital Epidemiology
Boston University Medical Center
Boston, Massachusetts

Harold L. Lazar, MD
Professor of Cardiothoracic Surgery
Director, Cardiothoracic Research
Boston University Medical Center
Attending Cardiothoracic Surgeon
Boston, Massachusetts

Dennis Lee, MD
Assistant Clinical Professor of Dermatology
Tufts University
Assistant Clinical Professor of Dermatology
New England Medical Center
Boston, Massachusetts

Keith P. Lewis, MD
Associate Professor
Division of Anesthesiology
Chair
Department of Anesthesiology
Boston University Medical Center
Boston, Massachusetts

David C. Longcope, MD
Clinical Assistant Professor
Department of Surgery
Tulane University College of Medicine
Department of Colon and Rectal Surgery
Memorial Medical Center
New Orleans, Louisiana

James A. Madura, II, MD, FACS
Assistant Professor of Surgery
Rush University
Attending Surgeon
Rush University Medical Center
The John Stroger Jr. Hospital of Cook County
Chicago, Illinois

Elizabeth J. Mahoney, MD
Resident
Department of Otolaryngology
Boston University Medical Center
Boston, Massachusetts

Brian J. Marien, MD, RVT, FACS
Vascular Surgeon
Wilkes-Barre General Hospital
Wilkes-Barre, Pennsylvania

David McAneny, MD, FACS
Associate Professor of Surgery
Staff Surgeon
Section of Surgical Oncology and Endocrinology
Boston University Medical Center
Boston, Massachusetts

Pushkar Mehra, BDS, DMD
Assistant Professor
Department of Oral and Maxillofacial Surgery
Director
Department of Dentistry and Oral and Maxillofacial Surgery
Boston University Medical Center
Boston, Massachusetts

James O. Menzoian, MD
Professor of Surgery
University of Connecticut School of Medicine
Professor of Surgery
University of Connecticut Health Center
Medical Director
Collaborative Center for Clinical Care Improvement, John Dempsey Hospital
Farmington, Connecticut

Frederick H. Millham, MD, MBA
Associate Clinical Professor
Department of Surgery
Harvard Medical School
Surgeon
Massachusetts General Hospital
Boston, Massachusetts
Chair
Department of Surgery
Newton-Wellesley Hospital
Newton, Massachusetts

Steven L. Moulton, MD
Associate Professor of Surgery and Pediatrics
Chief
Pediatric Surgery
Division of Surgery
Boston University Medical Center
Boston, Massachusetts

Thomas A. Mustoe, MD
Professor and Chief
Division of Plastic Surgery
Northwestern University Feinberg School of Medicine
Chief of Plastic Surgery
Northwestern Memorial Hospital
Chicago, Illinois

Donna M. Pacicca, MD
Assistant Professor of Orthopaedic Surgery
University of Missouri–Kansas City School of Medicine
Attending Surgeon
Children's Mercy Hospital
Kansas City, Missouri

Haroon I. Patel, MD
Pediatric Surgeon
Driscoll Children's Hospital
Corpus Christi, Texas

John H. Pemberton, MD
Professor
Department of Colon and Rectal Surgery
Mayo Clinic College of Medicine
Consultant
Colon and Rectal Surgery
Mayo Clinic and Mayo Foundation
Rochester, Minnesota

James G. Petros, MD, MPH, FACS
Consultant in Graduate Medical Education
Surgical Staff
Department of Surgery
Boston University Medical Center
Boston, Massachusetts

Paul K. Pietrow, MD
Hudson Valley Urology
Poughkeepsie, New York

James J. Pomposelli, MD, PhD, FACS
Assistant Professor of Surgery
Division of Hepatobiliary Surgery and Liver Transplantation
Tufts University Medical School
Boston, Massachusetts
Senior Staff Surgeon
Lahey Clinic Medical Center
Burlington, Massachusetts

Laura M. Prager, MD
Assistant Professor
Department of Psychiatry
Harvard Medical School
Director
Child and Adolescent Emergency Services
Massachusetts General Hospital
Boston, Massachusetts

Richard A. Prinz, MD
Helen Shedd Keith Professor and Chair
Department of General Surgery

Rush University
Attending Surgeon and Chair
Department of General Surgery
Rush University Medical Center
Chicago, Illinois

Elizabeth Renaud, MD
Surgical Resident
Boston University Medical Center
Boston, Massachusetts

Harry M. Richter, III, MD
Associate Professor of Surgery
Rush University
Attending Surgeon
The John Stroger Jr. Hospital of Cook County
Chicago, Illinois

Gary S. Rogers, MD
Director
Dermatologic Surgery and Oncology
Tufts University School of Medicine
Chief
Surgical Division
Department of Dermatology
Tufts–New England Medical Center
Boston, Massachusetts

Alexander S. Rosemurgy, II, MD, FACS
Professor of Surgery and Medicine
The Reeves/Culverhouse Chair for Digestive Disorders and Pancreatic Cancer
University of South Florida College of Medicine
Chief
General Surgery Section
Director
Surgical Digestive Disorders
Tampa General Hospital
Tampa, Florida

John J. Ryan, MD, FRCSI, FACS
Professor of Surgery
University of South Dakota School of Medicine
Sioux Falls, South Dakota

Jeffrey R. Saffle, MD, FACS
Professor of Surgery
University of Utah School of Medicine
Director
Intermountain Burn Center
University of Utah Health Sciences Center
Salt Lake City, Utah

Francesco M. Serafini, MD
Assistant Professor of Surgery
Universita Cattolica del Sacro Cuore
Rome, Italy

Oz M. Shapira, MD
Associate Professor of Cardiothoracic Surgery
Clinical Director
Department of Cardiac Surgery
Boston University Medical Center
Boston, Massachusetts

Richard J. Shemin, MD
Professor and Chair
Department of Cardiothoracic Surgery
Chief
Cardiothoracic Surgery
Vice Chair
Department of Surgery
Codirector
Cardiothoracic Center
Boston University Medical Center
Boston, Massachusetts

Daniel K. Smith, MD
Otolaryngologist
Colorado Center for Otolaryngology
Colorado Springs, Colorado

Joseph A. Smith, Jr., MD
Professor and Chair
Department of Urologic Surgery
Vanderbilt University School of Medicine
Attending Physician
Vanderbilt University Medical Center
Nashville, Tennessee

Ryan R. Snyder, MD
Resident
Department of Orthopaedic Surgery
University of Missouri–Kansas City School of Medicine
Kansas City, Missouri

Nathaniel J. Soper, MD, FACS
James R. Hines Professor of Surgery
Northwestern University Feinberg School of Medicine
Chief of Gastrointestinal/Endocrine Surgery
Vice-Chair of Clinical Affairs
Director of Minimally Invasive Surgery
Department of Surgery
Northwestern Memorial Hospital
Chicago, Illinois

Jeffrey H. Spiegel, MD, FACS
Associate Professor and Director
Division of Facial Plastic and Reconstructive Surgery
Department of Otolaryngology–Head and Neck Surgery
Chief of Facial Plastic and Reconstructive Surgery
Boston University Medical Center
Boston, Massachusetts

Glynne D. Stanley, MBChB, FRCA
Assistant Professor
Department of Anesthesiology
Director of Residency Education
Boston University Medical Center
Boston, Massachusetts

Andrew B. Stein, MD
Assistant Professor of Orthopaedic Surgery
Department of Orthopaedic Surgery
Boston University Medical Center
Boston, Massachusetts

Philip E. Stieg, MD, PhD
Professor and Chair
Department of Neurological Surgery
Weill Medical College of Cornell University
Neurosurgeon-in-Chief
New York Presbyterian Hospital
Memorial Sloan-Kettering Cancer Center
Hospital for Special Surgery
New York, New York

Mark E. Stoker, MD, FACS
Assistant Professor
Department of Surgery
University of Massachusetts Medical School
Chief
Department of General and Vascular Surgery
Fallon Clinic
Division Director
Department of General Surgery
St. Vincent Hospital
Worcester, Massachusetts

Arthur F. Stucchi, PhD
Associate Professor
Departments of Surgery, Pathology, and Laboratory Medicine
Boston University School of Medicine
Boston, Massachusetts

Ann T. Sweeney, MD
Assistant Professor of Medicine
Tufts University School of Medicine
Staff Endocrinologist
Caritas St. Elizabeth's Medical Center
Boston, Massachusetts

Gordon L. Telford, MD, FACS
Professor of Surgery
Medical College of Wisconsin
Attending Surgeon
Froedtert Memorial Lutheran Hospital
Zablocki VA Medical Center
Milwaukee, Wisconsin

Michael P. Vezeridis, MD
Professor of Surgery
Brown University School of Medicine
Chief of Surgical Services
VA Medical Center
Providence, Rhode Island

Harold J. Wanebo, MD
Professor of Surgery
Boston University Medical Center
Boston, Massachusetts
Adjunct Professor of Surgery
Brown University School of Medicine
Chief
Division of Surgical Oncology
Roger Williams Medical Center
Providence, Rhode Island

Michael T. Watkins, MD
Associate Professor of Surgery
Harvard Medical School
Associate Visiting Surgeon
Division of Vascular and Endovascular Surgery
Director of the Vascular Surgery Research Laboratory
Massachusetts General Hospital
Boston, Massachusetts

Edward E. Whang, MD
Assistant Professor in Surgery
Harvard Medical School
Associate Surgeon
Brigham and Women's Hospital
Boston, Massachusetts

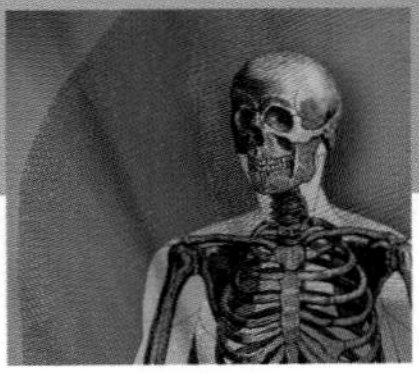

PREFACE

Essentials of Surgery is dedicated to teaching medical students and junior surgical residents the essentials of the entire field of surgery, including general surgery and the surgical specialties. Chapters focus on surgical disease, providing only need-to-know information on molecular genetics and other basic science topics. The authors are academic surgeons focused on medical student education; all are recognized experts in their fields. Discussions of surgical management include emphasis on minimal-access surgery and ambulatory surgery. Surgery is considered within the armamentarium of therapeutic options. Critical information is condensed in the form of "Pearls for the OR" and "Pearls for Rounds," and original full-color artwork created especially for this book complements the text.

Our goal was to continue the tradition of excellence of Drs. Sabiston and Lyerly but to offer a completely new contribution to the surgical literature. *Essentials of Surgery* has been designed and written to provide medical students and junior residents the critical information that they will need in caring for surgical patients of all types.

James M. Becker, MD, FACS
Arthur F. Stucchi, PhD

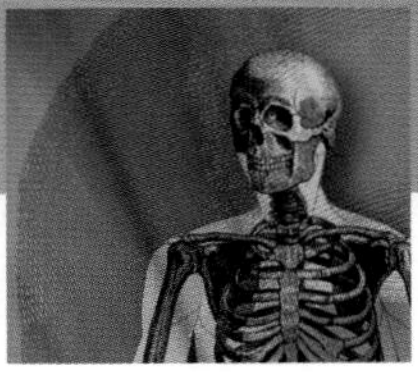

ACKNOWLEDGMENTS

Dr. Stucchi and I would like to acknowledge the enormous contributions of all of the authors of this textbook. Each author was selected for his or her recognized expertise in one or more of the various fields of surgery and for a commitment to surgical education. Each has served as a devoted and effective mentor for medical students, surgical residents, and young practicing physicians. We are delighted that this text will expose students and residents to these many committed mentors.

It is clear to me who the most influential mentors were early in my career. My father, Dr. Norman Becker, instilled in me the desire to become a top-level clinician and surgeon. He showed me that general surgeons are in many ways the "last of the real doctors." I certainly appreciated the importance of mentors in other disciplines during medical school. Perhaps the most important of these was Dr. Edward Chester at Case Western Reserve University, who, as an internist, taught me the importance of physical diagnosis and clinical acumen. Although my father was in the private practice of general and noncardiac thoracic surgery, he encouraged me to pursue a career in academic surgery from the very beginning. One of his most cherished positions was to serve as the secretary of the Wisconsin Surgical Travel Club. This gave him the opportunity to scout out surgical residency programs throughout the country. In this capacity, he visited the program that Dr. Frank Moody was developing at the University of Utah. He strongly encouraged me to seriously consider this program. It was clear when I visited Utah that something special was happening there and that an environment that would provide the best possible training for someone interested in a career in academic gastrointestinal surgery had been created. I cannot imagine a chairman being more stimulating and supportive of medical students and inspiring young surgeons. Not only did Dr. Moody help train me clinically, but he also stimulated me to pursue basic research and scholarly activity. He served as an important role model for how a chairman could create an environment that would allow the nurturing and development of future surgical leaders in a relatively short period of time. It is now well recognized that, during the golden 10 years that Frank Moody was chairman at Utah, probably as many, or more, future chairmen and leaders in academic surgery were trained than in any other program in the country.

After my surgical residency, I had the opportunity to work as a research fellow with Dr. Keith Kelly at the Mayo Clinic in Rochester, Minnesota. Dr. Kelly is the epitome of a surgical scientist. He further nurtured my interest in basic research, scholarly excellence, and the importance of teaching. Through his mentoring, I developed a clinical interest in inflammatory bowel disease, which I have maintained for 25 years.

I moved to Washington University in St. Louis in early 1987 to serve as chief of gastrointestinal surgery in Dr. Samuel Wells's department. His style of leadership and mentoring were quite different from those of Drs. Moody and Kelly, but I found it to be remarkably effective. Certainly, Dr. Wells put together a blockbuster department and was a very powerful leader at Washington University nationally, and also internationally. My final mentor was Dr. John Mannick at the Brigham and Women's Hospital. I joined his faculty at the Brigham and at Harvard Medical School in 1989. I was always impressed that Dr. Mannick was a master clinical surgeon as well as an active investigator. He has had continuous NIH funding for decades. He was very supportive of my activities and helped expand my administrative responsibilities and skills. He also allowed me to direct the Surgical Education Program for Harvard medical students at the Brigham and Women's Hospital. Dr. Mannick had served as chairman of the Department of Surgery at Boston University prior to taking the job at the Brigham. Thus, when I was being recruited for my current position, he was very encouraging about it and helped a great deal in my negotiations to make it an optimal position. Having been chairman of surgery at Boston University for the past 11 years, I have had the opportunity and privilege of teaching and mentoring many classes of Boston University medical students and surgical residents. It is my hope that future students and trainees in surgery will benefit from the textual mentoring provided in *Essentials of Surgery*.

I would like to thank the editors and production team at Elsevier who resurrected this project after taking over the rights to the textbook several years ago. I would particularly like to thank Jacqueline Mahon, senior developmental editor, and Bill Schmitt, publishing director, who pushed and supported all of us involved in the text to complete it in a timely fashion. In addition, I would like to thank my academic and administrative assistant, Maureen Burke, who contributed countless hours of her time to this text. Finally, I would like to particularly thank my coeditor, Dr. Arthur Stucchi, without whose diligence this book never would have materialized.

James M. Becker, MD, FACS

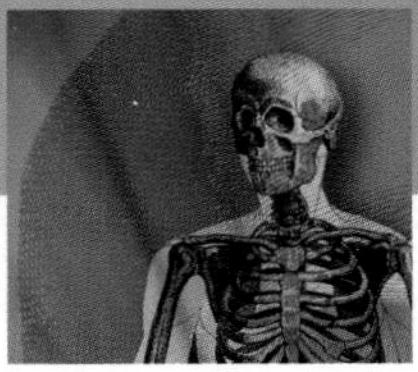

CONTENTS

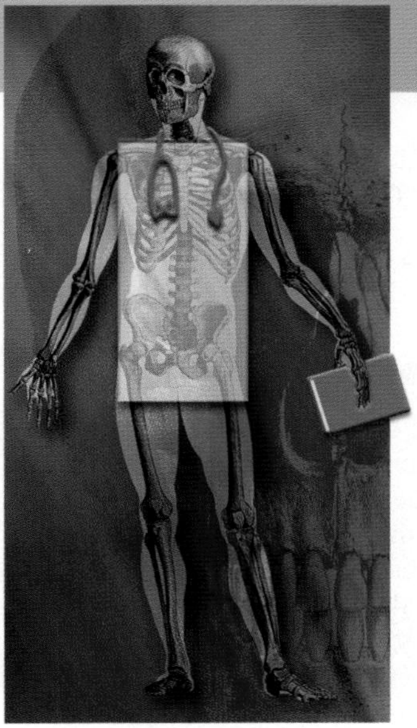

SECTION I

STUDENT-SPECIFIC ISSUES

Chapter 1

Conquering Your Surgical Clerkship

ERICA A. BROTSCHI, MD, and NANCY L. CANTELMO, MD

If you are starting your first experience on a surgical service, this chapter is for you. Surgery may seem overwhelming at the beginning because of the long hours, the amount of medical knowledge involved, and the need to adapt to the surgical "culture" and way of doing things. But if you participate actively on a surgical service, you will learn a great deal about medical disease and management of medical problems, as well as about surgical disease. Some of you will enjoy the surgical approach to problem solving and the pleasure of working with your hands and will want to consider surgery as a career. Many others will use this clerkship to learn more about diseases that surgeons treat and when to refer patients. We hope that whether or not you end as a surgeon, the knowledge you gain on the surgical service will help you throughout your career.

TIPS

DO Prepare to enjoy an exciting experience in a demanding but interesting field.

DON'T Be discouraged if it takes a week or two to "catch on" to the routines and pace of your new service. Just keep trying, and show your interest.

Organization of a Surgical Service

As a student on surgery, you will be expected to follow the instructions of your residents and attending surgeons. A chief or senior resident usually supervises a surgical team, with junior residents and interns managing patients under his or her direction. Attending or staff surgeons supervise the chief resident and are legally responsible for the conduct of surgery and the outcome of the patients. The chief resident will usually make most decisions in the day-to-day management of patients and tell the junior residents and students what needs to be done. If difficult management problems or decisions involve when or whether to operate, the chief resident will ask the attending surgeons for help and advice.

When you are on the surgical team, you will notice the hierarchical structure that underlies the culture of surgery. The respect for seniority probably arises because surgery is both a body of medical knowledge and a set of skills and judgments that are heavily based on experience. Choosing the best approach to a given disease is often dependent more on having seen and treated the disease many times before, than on having read the most recent literature about it. Because of the respect for experience and seniority in surgery, decisions are made and orders given in a "top-down" style that is somewhat different from those of other medical disciplines.

Students usually learn the most when they work closely with an intern, junior resident, or physician's assistant, who can guide them through the daily details of patient care.

TIPS

DO Try to identify a friendly resident or other member of the team whom you can "shadow" in daily activities and on-call periods. You can help your mentor with notes and procedures, and that person can teach you in return.

What you are asked to do to help the team. On a good surgical service, everyone works together for the good of the patients and the team. Teamwork is one of the highest values in surgery.

Show your respect for the knowledge and experience of the residents and attendings, and avoid public disagreement. Help your residents look good.

DON'T Criticize the decisions of people with more experience. That runs counter to the culture of surgery.

Argue or make other team members look bad, including your fellow students.

Daily Routine of a Surgical Service

Surgeons tend to work long hours because their schedules involve operating room (OR) and clinic responsibilities as well as patient care on the wards. Certain areas of surgery also have many emergency cases that keep the team working at night. The key to getting everything done is good teamwork.

Typically, surgical ward services start with morning rounds for the entire team at about 6 or 6:30 AM. Before the start of rounds, students and residents "pre-round" by visiting the patients' wards to obtain vital signs and data of intake and output recorded overnight. They determine whether any important events have occurred in the patients' course. The entire team reviews this information and walks through the hospital wards to visit each patient and write the orders for the day. By 7:30 or 8 AM, rounds must be finished so residents can go to the OR to assist with the day's surgeries. Residents who were on call overnight can usually leave after rounds. Some residents may stay on the wards to write daily progress notes and care for the patients, and some may go to clinic. At the end of the day, when the OR cases are finished, the entire team gathers again for evening rounds. The course and events for the day are reviewed for each patient, and the team goes to see some or all of the patients. The members of the team who are not on call can then leave.

Students are usually assigned by the chief resident to follow up specific patients on the service, collect their data, write the notes, and assist the residents with care. Students should go to the OR to assist with their patients' surgeries and to improve exposure of the operative field. The chief resident should let the students know what their responsibilities will be each day, and if the instructions are unclear, the students should ask the junior residents for clarification.

TIPS

DO If you are not assigned specific patients, volunteer to follow up and care for two or three patients at a time, so that you get the experience of providing patient care. When you are following a patient, ask to write the progress notes and orders. See the patient before rounds to get the data and find out how the person is feeling. Try to get any laboratory and imaging results for rounds. Let the team know they can count on you.

When you are assigned a patient, you should make a brief summary of the patient's history and physical examination on a file card that you can carry with you. Each day you can record the vital signs, intake and output, laboratory values, and other important numbers on the card, so you have the information handy.

DON'T Come late or miss rounds without very good reason.

How to Become a Member of the Surgical Team

Surgical teams value students because of their interest and enthusiasm, as well as their help in patient care. Students can become trusted members of the team by showing up reliably and on time, showing enthusiasm and eagerness to help, and conscientiously performing duties assigned to them. Most surgeons and surgical residents like their work and will gladly volunteer to do what is required to help a patient. A similar degree of eagerness and interest is highly valued in students, so step forward and offer to observe and help the residents. As you become more familiar with the team, you will be able to take more responsibility in writing notes and orders, checking laboratory tests, doing patient workups, and doing procedures such as IVs and Foley catheters.

TIPS

DO Look interested, and volunteer to help. If a resident is called to see a patient, ask if you can come along, and ask what you can do.

DON'T If you want to make a good impression, try not to complain about long hours, hunger, or fatigue to your residents. Surgeons consider that part of the job and appreciate a "can do" attitude.

Introduction to the Operating Room

Surgeons enjoy being in the OR, and you may find that you do too. The OR is a carefully organized exercise in teamwork, where each person has a role. Your major role as a student during the case will probably be to retract tissue and help expose the area where the surgeon is working. Most OR teams consist of four or more people:

- An anesthesiologist, sometimes assisted by a nurse anesthetist or a resident
- A surgeon and often an assistant surgeon
- A nurse or operating technician who scrubs to pass instruments
- A "circulating" nurse who is not scrubbed, who obtains what the operating team needs and performs documentation

Before entering the OR, you will change into surgical scrubs and put on a hat that covers all your hair, a mask, and shoe covers. When you first go into the OR, you should introduce yourself to the circulating nurse. You can ask the nurse if it is all right for you to watch or "scrub in." If the surgeon does not know you, you should also introduce yourself to the surgeon. If you are going to scrub, the nurse will ask for your glove size, which you will soon figure out.

If you are going into the OR to observe, keep your hands and arms close to your body and move carefully to avoid touching sterile drapes and equipment. The nurses can tell you where to stand so you can see the field. If you are going to scrub for the case, do it first with someone who can explain the sequence: soaping hands, soaping arms, careful scrubbing of hands and nails, and rinsing from hands downward. Once you have scrubbed, keep your hands at chest level. The scrub nurse will hand you a towel and assist you in getting into gown and gloves. Then fold your gloved hands over your chest until the field is draped. You can then place your hands on the draped patient. It is easy to contaminate yourself by touching or brushing against nonsterile objects

During the case, the surgeons will tell you what they want you to do. Usual student responsibilities are holding retractors and cutting sutures after knots are tied.

TIPS

DO Always introduce yourself, and be friendly and courteous to the OR staff.

Consider yourself a guest in their OR, and they will make you welcome.

If you do not know the patient, read the history in the chart so you know why the operation is being done. If possible, read about the planned operation beforehand in a textbook or atlas.

Try to meet the patient before the operation, and do a brief physical examination. That preparation will help you if the surgeon asks you questions during the operation.

If you are holding a retractor and the surgeon reaches for it, let go of it immediately. Don't get into a wrestling match with the surgeon.

If the surgeon gives you the scissors to cut a suture, hold the scissors in your thumb and ring finger, and cut with the tips.

Ask a resident to show you how to tie knots, and practice at home. Then if you are given the opportunity, you will be able to suture and tie.

DON'T Argue with the nurses if they tell you to get a different hat or change your gown or gloves. The circulating nurse is in charge of sterile technique.

Ever touch any table where the scrub nurse has instruments. Even the attending surgeons are not supposed to do that.

Caring for Patients Having Surgery

Patients who will have surgery with sedation or anesthesia need to have a preoperative workup to identify any medical problems that may increase their surgical risk. The preoperative workup starts with a complete history and physical examination. This may be done on admission but is often done at a separate outpatient visit. Preoperative evaluation also includes standard laboratory tests: complete blood count (CBC), coagulation studies, electrolytes, blood urea nitrogen (BUN), creatinine, liver function tests, and urinalysis. Patients older than 40 years usually must have electrocardiograms (ECGs), and some hospitals obtain preoperative chest radiographs on all patients. If transfusion may be required during surgery, blood should be requested, and a clot sent to the blood bank for typing. In addition, all patients undergoing anesthesia must be seen preoperatively by an anesthesiologist. Patients with multiple medical problems may need more extensive evaluation by internists, cardiologists, or other specialists.

Before surgery, documentation in the patient record should include the surgical consent, the history and physical, as well as a "preoperative note" including the results of the preoperative tests and stating the planned procedure. Immediately after the surgery, someone from the surgical team enters an "operative note" describing the case. The attending surgeon or a designated assistant also dictates a detailed report.

The evening before surgery, the patient is examined, and a "postoperative note" is written. Important issues to evaluate at this time include the vital signs, the patient's level of alertness, the patient's pain or other complaints, and whether the patient has an adequate urine output. A brief physical examination should evaluate the patient's respiratory function, and the wound or dressing should be examined. Any postoperative laboratory tests or radiographs should be checked and documented. Each day after surgery when the patient is in the hospital, write a progress note addressing these issues, as well as evidence of returning gastrointestinal function and any other events of importance in the patient's course.

TIPS

DO If you order a laboratory test on a patient, always be sure someone checks the result promptly. Abnormal results that are not identified result in poor patient care and have serious medicolegal consequences.

Be obsessive about checking urine output. Hypovolemia is a major cause of complications (renal failure, myocardial infarction, bowel ischemia) in postoperative patients. Normally patients should make at least 40 mL urine per hour in the postoperative period, as evidence that intravascular volume is adequate. If the patient is not making 40 mL urine per hour, or has not voided by an appropriate time after surgery, *tell your resident!*

BOX 1–1 Surgical Notes

Preoperative Note	Brief Operative Note	Postoperative Note
Preoperative diagnosis Planned procedure Consent Labs Radiographs ECG Blood bank Anesthesia note Special preop orders	Preoperative diagnosis Postoperative diagnosis Operation Surgeon Assistant surgeon(s) Anesthesia Operative findings Estimated blood loss (EBL) Fluids (given in OR) Specimen Drains Complications Condition (e.g. stable and extubated to recovery room)	S/P (status post) type of operation Subjective assessment: patient complaints, degree of pain Objective findings: • Brief physical examination (vital signs, mental status, listen to chest, check wound site or dressing, check extremities for perfusion) • Intake and output (always check and document urine output and any surgical drains) • Postop labs • Postop radiographs Impression Plan

BOX 1–2 Admission Orders

Mnemonic ADCA-VAN-DIDIL

Admit to surgical service (you may add the ward or attending surgeon's name)
Diagnosis
Condition
Allergies
Vital signs
Activity
Nursing
Diet
Intake and output
Drugs
IV
Labs, radiographs, etc.

Writing Notes and Orders

Each surgical service will have its own routines for writing notes and orders that you can learn from your residents. Here are some common formats that you can use for writing preoperative notes, brief operative notes, postoperative notes, and admission and postoperative orders, to show you what is usually included (Boxes 1-1, 1-2, and 1-3). Students should write these formats on a card to carry in their pocket until they have memorized them.

BOX 1–3 Postoperative Orders

Mnemonic ADCA-VAN-DIDIL

Admit to recovery room
Diagnosis (s/p type of operation)
Condition
Allergies (so you look it up before you write the med orders!)
Vital signs: per recovery room routine, then q 4 hours on ward (or q 1 hour in ICU). Give call parameters, e.g., "Call HO for T >102, HR >110, BP <100."
Activity: usually "up with assistance" the evening of surgery, and "ambulate qid starting in AM." If the operation is on the leg, check with the resident or surgeon.
Nursing: respiratory care (incentive spirometer, cough, and deep breath), dressing changes if required
Diet: often NPO after general anesthesia
I&O*: If patient has a Foley catheter, "Urine output q 1hour, call HO for urine <40 mL/hr." If patient does not have a Foley catheter, "Call HO if no void by 5 PM " or pick a time several hours after the end of the case. You must write an order for every tube in the patient, or you will get called (e.g., NG to low wall suction, measure JP drain output q shift, etc).
Drugs: check with the resident which preop meds should be continued. Remember to add pain medication, antibiotics if required, steroids if required.
IVs: Check with the resident. The most common order is D5 0.5 NS at 150 mL/ hr.
Labs, radiographs rays: Check with the resident. Many patients will not need any laboratory tests after surgery, and some will need laboratory values checked immediately. The most common routine is to check a CBC, electrolytes, glucose, BUN, and creatinine the morning after surgery.

HO, house officer; I&O, intake and output.
*This is critically important in postop patients.

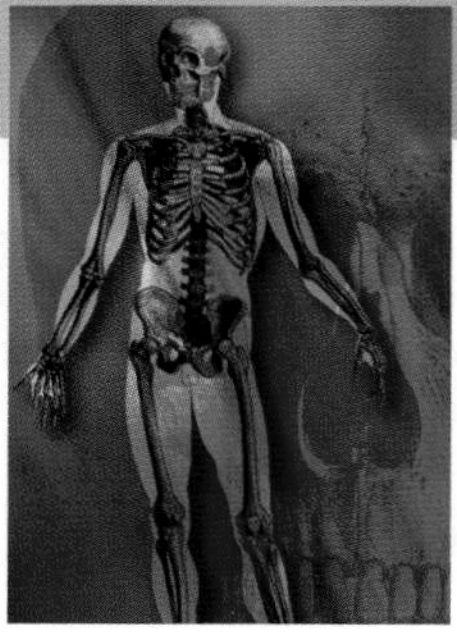

Chapter 2

Interpersonal and Communication Skills and Professionalism*

ERICA A. BROTSCHI, MD

Even if you have good social skills, interpersonal communication in the world of medicine will bring challenges. Medical work is stressful, and medical personnel must work closely as a team in situations that may be loaded with time pressure, anxiety, frustration, or grief. Medical personnel also must learn to interact with patients in a way that eases anxiety and promotes trust and communication. As you continue your medical career, you will develop your own style of interaction, but this section will give you suggestions to get you started. First, a few general rules will help you succeed with communication in the medical workplace throughout your career:

TIPS

DO Go out of your way to treat each person you meet with courtesy and respect.

Try to see the staff and patients you interact with as individuals, and be friendly to people at all levels in the medical system.

Remember that in the end, your patients and colleagues will judge you as much on your kindness and courtesy as on your medical knowledge.

DON'T Ever lose your temper or say anything disparaging to another person publicly, even if it seems justified. It will almost always turn out to be the wrong thing to have done.

Communicating on the Surgical Team

Good communication helps a medical or surgical team function well. At the level of the ward team, it is important that each person understand what is required of him or her. On a surgical service, the structure of the team is a clear hierarchy, in which each level (student, resident, or staff) receives orders and guidance from the levels above. You are expected to do what the people above you on the team ask of you. This hierarchical structure may be frustrating to you as a student, if you like to exercise independent judgment; but it is part of the tradition of surgery. It also is an efficient approach that allows a rapid and coordinated response to emergencies. You will learn how more experienced doctors handle situations, and you will not be asked to make decisions you do not have the knowledge to make.

The main responsibility for assigning duties usually falls on the senior or chief resident, but you should ask your intern for advice and help. If you feel uncertain about what to do for a patient, you should ask someone else on the team, rather than guess.

TIPS

DO If you are not sure what the chief resident is asking you to do, or how to get information, ask your intern or resident to explain. Show that you are interested in doing your best, and be as reliable as possible in doing what is asked of you.

You may be asked to do something for the team, like obtaining food. This does not show disrespect for your knowledge. You are being asked to contribute to the welfare of the group. Do it graciously.

DON'T Argue when someone above you on the team asks you to do something.

Guess at what you are expected to do for a patient. Ask!

Communicating with Other Services

When multiple services are involved in caring for a patient, the groups of doctors must communicate with each other. The medical record is useful to give straightforward recommendations, but when controversy exists about the best course of action, those issues should be resolved by direct conversation and not argued in the medical record. When a patient comes to a surgeon for care, it is extremely important that the surgeon communicate with the patient's primary care providers to let them know about the patient's course. That allows providers who know the

*All material in this chapter is in the public domain, with the exception of any borrowed figures or tables.

patient to feel involved in care and promotes a sense of teamwork that encourages good patient care as well as further referrals.

TIPS

DO Be friendly when you interact with consulting services. Show your appreciation for their help. They may be referring patients to you some day.

DON'T Record a diagnosis or plan of action in the chart unless you are sure of it. Never write anything negative about a patient or a provider in a chart. Even exclamation points can be damaging. Remember that the medical record is a legal document, and patients have the right to review it.

Communicating with Nurses and Other Staff

Hospitals and clinics are complex social structures where many people have to work closely together. Each job is important, whether it is providing care as a doctor or nurse, or cleaning, answering phones, or arranging long-term care. It is important that you communicate by friendliness and courtesy that you appreciate the contributions of the personnel around you.

In the hospital, doctors have frequent interaction with nurses on matters of patient care. Ideally, doctors and nurses work as a cooperative team. Nurses have their own hierarchy in the hospital and their own standards for performance. Although doctors have the job of writing orders for patient care, doctors should not order nurses around or criticize how nurses do their job. It is important for physicians to establish a two-way communication with the nurses caring for their patients. The doctor can ensure that the nurses understand what the patient's medical issues are, and what the nurses should be watching for, and the nurses can communicate concerns that the physician may have missed.

Experienced nurses often know more about the appropriate treatment for a patient than an inexperienced physician does, so doctors should listen to their suggestions. Nurses also pick up physician errors, so if a nurse questions your order, carefully review it. Within the operating room (OR), the circulating nurse (the nurse who is not scrubbed) is the person responsible for sterile technique for the room.

TIPS

DO Be friendly and helpful with nurses who are caring for your patients. Ask them if they have concerns about a patient.

If nurses in the OR instruct you about sterile technique and OR manners, thank them and do what they say.

DON'T Ever show anger at a nurse who questions your orders. Someday you probably will make a big mistake that a nurse may pick up. Check your order or have a more senior person on the team confirm it.

Communication Pitfalls in the Surgical Workplace

The surgical team functions most smoothly when all members are enthusiastic and willing to help. The interest and eagerness of students helps create a pleasant work climate for the residents and faculty. Most residents and faculty really enjoy having students on their service. Despite this, some residents and attending surgeons may seem brusque or even unfriendly to students at times. Most of the time, this reflects the stress that the senior members of the team are feeling, as well as a tradition in Surgery of honesty and blunt speaking. It is important for you as a student not to take these brusque communications as directed against you personally, because they are seldom intended that way. If you feel you are being criticized because a senior person thinks you did something wrong, the best course is usually to wait for a quiet time when the stress of the situation has subsided and then ask a resident if you should have done something differently.

Humor is often used on surgical teams to diffuse tension and raise morale. Teasing is common, and students may be subject to it at times. The intent is usually friendly, as a way to indicate that the student is becoming a real member of the team.

Remember that the hospital and clinics are a work setting, rather than a place for social or romantic interaction. This is particularly important in a hierarchical group, where social advances can be construed as (or become) sexual harassment. Close-knit groups like surgical teams function best without romantic undertones or active flirting. Any socializing should occur away from the hospital. If you feel that someone on the service is pressuring you for closer social interaction than you want, it is appropriate to tell that person that you are not interested, and that you want a purely professional relationship. If the person does not back off, you should communicate your discomfort to the clerkship or residency director. Otherwise you could end up in a situation in which a disgruntled colleague could affect your evaluations. Sexual harassment (sexual or gender-based comments or activities that create a negative workplace environment) is illegal; it also is looked on very unfavorably in Surgery, because it destroys team morale and is considered unethical behavior.

TIPS

DO Accept that blunt or direct comments are common in communication among surgeons, and try not to take comments personally. If you are teased, the best response is to laugh.

DON'T Flirt or dress provocatively if you want to be taken seriously in a work setting.

Make sexual comments and inappropriate physical contact.

Tolerate sexual harassment. It is not part of surgical culture.

Communication with Patients

Although we go into medicine to help our patients, the training we receive in medical school often decreases our ability to communicate with them. We effectively spend years learning a different language that is Latin or Greek to our patients. Students often communicate with patients better than residents do, because patients sense the students' real and personal concern about their problems. However, good doctor-patient communication requires that students learn new nonverbal and verbal skills.

Nonverbal communication is often more important than verbal communication between patient and doctor. As a doctor, you must evaluate how the patient looks, to determine whether the person is seriously ill or in pain. You also should assess the patient's emotional state, particularly whether the person is excessively frightened or depressed about health issues. Often simple reassurance can greatly relieve a patient's anxiety, if the doctor recognizes the patient's fear.

The doctor also must be aware how he or she is communicating in a nonverbal way. Medical providers should be neatly and conservatively dressed, to show that they take their role seriously, and to inspire the patients' trust. Many clinical areas strongly discourage wearing scrubs during clinic, because doctors wear dress clothes as a mark of respect for the patient. However, in some clinic settings, patients see surgical scrubs as a sort of uniform, and clean scrubs are acceptable; check with your residents or do as they do.

For many patients, the most important communication they want to receive from their provider is that you care about them and their health issues. The doctor should use both nonverbal and verbal means to demonstrate respect and concern for each patient. This is done with eye contact, and greeting the patient as "Mr." or "Ms." The doctor should introduce himself or herself, shake hands, and then sit down, to avoid hovering over the patient. Even if the provider is in a hurry, he or she should spend some time listening to the patient with full attention and eye contact; the patient should have an opportunity to ask questions. The doctor communicates respect and caring during the physical examination by washing hands before the examination, explaining what will be done, and avoiding roughness or unnecessary discomfort to the patient.

If you must examine a personal part of the body on someone of the opposite sex, it is wise to have a chaperone or third person present. With any patient, if you sense that either you or the patient is uncomfortable with the examination, do not hesitate to ask a nurse or other medical provider to observe or to hold the patient's hand.

To communicate meaningfully with patients about their medical problems, avoid the use of medical jargon. This is difficult, but you should develop a set of simple synonyms for medical words: "tube" for catheter, "blood vessel" for artery, "bile tube" for common duct, "soreness" for inflammation. The ordinary language is not as precise as the medical terms it replaces, but patients have a chance of understanding it. If the patient wants a more sophisticated description with medical language, he or she will usually ask or use some medical words to show familiarity with the terms.

An ethical and legal standard of care requires that the doctor communicate clearly with the patient. The doctor should tell the patient as much about the illness as the patient needs to know to make appropriate decisions about care. At a minimum, consent for surgery or treatment should include the reason for the procedure; an understandable description of what will be done, and why; what the common complications and risks are; and how the patient's life may be different after surgery.

TIPS

DO Wear neat and conservative dress clothes.

Always make eye contact, introduce yourself, and address the patient (if an adult) by last name.

Give the patient a chance to tell you about the problem.

Wash your hands before and after the physical examination.

Describe to the patient what you will be doing, particularly if it is uncomfortable.

Have a chaperone or third person in the room if you examine a personal part of the body on someone of the opposite sex.

DON'T Wear clothes that make you look sexually attractive. That can make patients uncomfortable during examinations.

Use medical terms that the patient will not understand. Do use the simplest possible plain English to describe the medical problem.

Privacy of Health Information

Patient health information in a hospital or other healthcare setting is protected from disclosure by traditional medical ethics and also by new federal regulations under HIPAA (Health Insurance Portability and Accountability Act, 2002). What this means in practice is that you can give health information to the patient, to providers who are part of the treatment team, and to family and others only if the patient gives explicit consent. Release of any information to an employer, outside healthcare provider, and so on, requires a release document signed by the patient. Certain information that is particularly sensitive, such as alcohol or drug use, psychiatric diagnoses, or human immunodeficiency virus (HIV) status, cannot be released unless the patient signs a document that specifies that information on those topics will be released. Patient identifiers should be omitted from presentations, and you also must be careful to protect written information such as charts, notes, or conference material from unauthorized view.

TIPS

DO Maintain patient privacy at all times by closing examination room doors and concealing records and computer screens.

Ask patients before disclosing their medical information to family members.

DON'T Discuss patient issues in elevators, hallways, and other public places.

Release medical information to employers, hospitals, or other facilities without written consent from the patient.

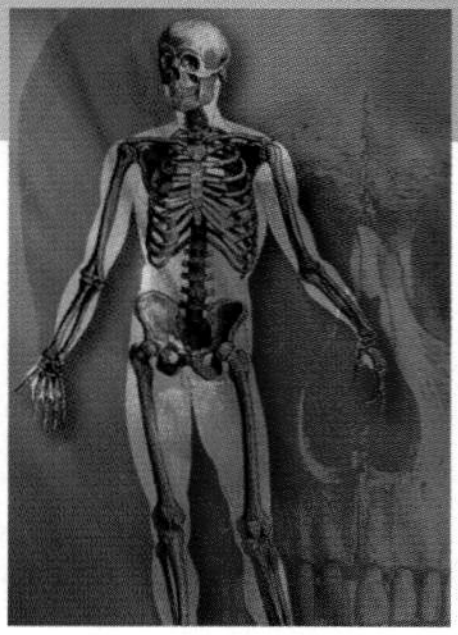

Chapter 3

Health and Safety

DAVID McANENY, MD, and CATHY KORN, RN, MPH

Acquired Immunodeficiency Syndrome

A thorough review of the human immunodeficiency virus (HIV) and of acquired immunodeficiency syndrome (AIDS) is beyond the practical scope of this chapter. Moreover, it would be presumptuous to summarize HIV in a few paragraphs when volumes are devoted to it. However, HIV has certainly affected surgical diseases, the conduct of surgery, and the surgical team. Therefore the impact of HIV on surgical practice merits consideration. (The effects of HIV and AIDS on specific organ systems, such as anorectal disorders and immune thrombocytic purpura, are discussed in the respective chapters of this text.)

HIV and AIDS have afflicted millions of individuals worldwide. It is estimated that the seroprevalence of HIV among hospitalized patients in the United States ranges from 0.2% to 14.2%, depending on geography, specialty, and the nature of the practice. A 20% incidence of HIV infection has been recorded among victims of penetrating trauma in metropolitan emergency rooms. Thus nearly all surgeons will treat patients with HIV, wittingly or not.

Accidental blood exposures are unfortunately a relatively common event in surgery. One study in San Francisco documented 5.6 exposures per 1000 operating room hours, the risk being greater with longer operations, blood loss greater than 300 mL, and vascular or other major operations. Most reported exposures involve direct skin contact, whereas fewer than 10% are percutaneous injuries. Another study reckoned that for every 100 hours in the operating room, surgeons have 12 blood exposures, of which one is percutaneous. Nevertheless, no surgeon has contracted a *documented* HIV infection from a patient. Six cases of surgeons with HIV infections were possibly from occupational exposures. These surgeons had no other identifiable risk factors, but none had documented occupational exposures before HIV seroconversion.

The nature of the blood exposure dictates the risk of seroconversion. Skin-surface contact is an unusual route of contamination. A Centers for Disease Control (CDC) surveillance program reports no cases of seroconversion among more than 2,700 healthcare workers who had blood exposure to intact skin. The risk after exposure to nonintact skin has not been quantified but is estimated to be less than the risk for mucous membrane exposures, which is 0.09%. Whereas percutaneous injuries are the most likely to cause HIV seroconversion among healthcare workers, the risk is remarkable low in comparison with that of hepatitis: 0.2% to 0.5% for HIV, 6% to 30% for hepatitis B virus (HBV), and 0% to 7% for hepatitis C virus (HCV). The actual risk is established by the depth of the cutaneous penetration; the amount of blood on or within the scalpel, suture, or needle (especially if hollow); direct contact of the instrument with the patient's vasculature; and an infected patient whose late-stage disease rapidly escalates to death.

The potential risk of a surgeon infecting a patient has received much publicity and garnered a good deal of unnecessary fear among laymen. The testing of sera from 3420 orthopedic surgeons revealed a 0.06% incidence of HIV infection. (Both of the infected surgeons had non-occupational risks for HIV.) Flum estimated that the risk of transmission of HIV from any surgeon to a patient is one chance per 21 million hours of surgery. Even if the surgeon were known to be infected with HIV, the risk might still be one per 83,000 hours of surgery. When a surgeon contracts HIV, it is wise to convene an expert review panel to determine practice restrictions and the obligation to notify patients of the unusual situation. At this time, the likelihood of patients becoming infected with HIV from healthcare workers is exceedingly remote.

Routine HIV screening of patients and surgeons alike has stirred controversy and warrants deliberate attention to the available data. One analysis considered the frequency of percutaneous injury in the operating room, the risk of HIV transmission, and the prevalence of HIV to estimate that the likelihood of any given patient infecting a surgeon with HIV would be one in 450,000 to 1,300,000. Among patients known to have HIV, the risk might be one in 130,000. Moreover, the fallibility of HIV testing must be factored into the analysis. For example, false-positive tests could wrongly implicate between 130,000 and 1,300,000 people as having HIV for each surgeon protected. This argument even presumes that knowing a positive HIV status will alter injury rates in the operating room, although it has never been proven to do so. Conversely, false-negative tests might impart a certain careless bravado or diminished vigilance in the operating room. This attitude also neglects the more infectious viruses that convey hepatitis B and C. Finally, cases of delayed seroconversion would elude preoperative detection. Therefore no current justification exists for mandatory preoperative HIV screening, for patients or for surgeons.

Standard (or universal) precautions have been instituted to diminish the risks of blood exposures to healthcare workers. These routine precautions are applied with the philosophy that all patients are potential carriers of HIV or other infectious viruses, such as hepatitis B or C. Personnel protective equipment such as "double-gloves," eye and face protection, and impermeable gowns should be routinely worn to prevent exposure. Some investigators contend that double gloving can reduce the viral inoculum as the needle passes through two gloves. Perhaps the greatest benefit of double-gloving is that one pair serves as a secondary barrier when an occult perforation is present in the other glove. Conversely, double gloving compromises manual dexterity and tactile senses.

Percutaneous injury by scalpel blades and suture needles is a regrettably common occurrence in the operating room. Recent technologic advances and implementation of certain practices may reduce the likelihood of exposure. The following devices and techniques should be considered: retractable, rounded-tip, and disposable scalpel blades; blunt suture needles; and the creation of a "neutral zone" that facilitates hands-free transfer of sharp items across the surgical field. Consistent use of these safety products and compliance with standard precautions is variable, likely because of doubts about their efficacy and their general inconvenience. Ongoing education of medical staffs is clearly indicated, including how to respond to potential HIV exposure.

When an exposure to HIV occurs, the healthcare worker should immediately cleanse the site with soap and water (or flush with water in the case of a mucous membrane exposure). If this involves a percutaneous injury, blood may be expressed from the wound in hopes of reducing the viral inoculum; an antiseptic agent (e.g., povidine-iodine) also can be applied, although no scientific data support these maneuvers. Each healthcare facility should have a standard protocol for dealing with such incidents and for notifying the proper authorities, as mandated by the Occupational Safety and Health Administration and by individual state laws. Appropriate clinicians are to be available to determine the risk of HIV infection and to counsel regarding the relative risks and benefits of expeditious postexposure prophylactic systemic therapy. Data are gathered about the circumstances of the exposure. These include the wounding instrument used, the depth of penetration (into both the patient and the worker), the type and volume of material introduced, the duration of exposure, the integrity of the worker's skin, and the HIV status of the patient (e.g., HIV risk factors, HIV test result, viral load, CD4 count, stage of disease, history of responses to antiretroviral therapy, other viral infections). Blood should be obtained from the patient and from the injured party, with informed consent for HIV and hepatitis B and C testing. The healthcare worker should have additional tests for HIV antibodies at intervals of 6 weeks, 12 weeks, and 6 months, as practically all seroconversions will manifest within the first 12 weeks. The worker also is evaluated regarding past medical history, renal or hepatic dysfunction, pregnancy, and lactation.

The role and extent of chemoprophylaxis after HIV exposure has evolved, but the efficacy of antiretroviral medications for postexposure prophylaxis in humans has not been well studied, partially because of the low rate of seroconversion. A retrospective, case–control study conducted by the CDC revealed an 81% reduction in the risk of HIV infection after postexposure prophylaxis with zidovudine, although the study was limited. A comprehensive review of exposure data, of postexposure prophylaxis, and of follow-up serologic data suggests that the administration of antiretroviral drugs at the time of exposure to HIV decreases the risk of virus transmission. Data on primary HIV infection indicate that systemic infection does not occur immediately. This provides a window of opportunity during which treatment might modify or prevent virus replication.

The United States Public Health Service's current guidelines recommend two- and three-drug regimens. Treatment algorithms are based on Exposure Codes that consider the severity of contamination and the HIV Status Codes of the source patient, as documented in the Public Health Service guidelines. The treating physician uses these factors to determine the likelihood of HIV transmission and the advisability and extent of prophylaxis. It seems that the immediate (within a few hours of exposure) administration of antiretroviral therapy confers the greatest likelihood of success. Combivir (zidovudine and lamivudine) is the most common basic regimen used. Treatment may be expanded to include medications such as Indinavir, Nelfinavir, Efavirenz, and Abacirin in the event of a more severe percutaneous exposure. Empiric prophylaxis is suspended if the source patient's HIV test is negative and if the clinical scenario does not suggest a delayed seroconversion "window." Most blood and fluid exposures do not result in HIV infection, so the potential benefit of prophylactic therapy must be weighed against the toxicity, particularly when the efficacy and safety of these new agents are still being studied.

The American College of Surgeons has issued a "Statement on the Surgeon and HIV Infection" that acknowledges the medical, political, social, and economic implications of HIV on the practice of surgery. The College affirms the surgeon's ethical obligation to care for patients with HIV, and it advocates the highest standards of infection control. The College avers that HIV-infected surgeons may practice surgery, but only if the surgeon's physician or an expert review panel believes that this will not pose a significant risk of transmission of HIV to patients. Finally, the College

PEARLS FOR THE OR

Risks of seroconversion after percutaneous exposure: human immunodeficiency virus, 0.2%–0.5%; hepatitis B virus, 6%–30%; hepatitis C virus, 0%–7%.

Standard (universal) precautions presume that all patients potentially carry HIV or other viral infections.

The risks of HIV exposure in the operating room increase with longer operations, blood loss greater than 300 mL, and vascular or other major operations.

The risk of transmission of HIV from any patient to a surgeon in the operating room is estimated to be one in 450,000 to 1,300,000.

The risk of transmission of HIV from any surgeon to a patient is estimated to be one chance per 21 million hours of surgery.

expresses a commitment to the care of patients with HIV and to HIV-infected surgeons and their families.

Hepatitis B and C

HBV and HCV infections are well-recognized risks for healthcare workers, and they are related primarily to the extent of exposure to blood or other potentially infectious body fluids. The presence of hepatitis B "e" antigen increases the degree of infectivity. The rate of HBV infection in healthcare workers has decreased dramatically with HBV vaccination and with postexposure prophylaxis using immune globulin. The risk of HCV transmission is less than that of HBV, which is fortunate because no HCV vaccine is available, and prophylaxis with immune globulin has not been effective. Avoidance of accidental exposure is the best means of prevention.

Prions

Creutzfeldt-Jakob disease (CJD) is a rare degenerative neurologic condition caused by a prion, a proteinaceous infectious particle. Iatrogenic CJD has been linked to contaminated medical equipment, use of extracted pituitary hormones or gonadotropin, and the implantation of contaminated dura mater and cornea grafts. No evidence exists of occupational transmission of CJD. Standard precautions must be used when caring for patients with CJD, and instruments must be properly sterilized or disposed.

Hand Hygiene

Attempts at increasing awareness of the importance of hand hygiene date to 1847, when Ignaz Semmelweis was ridiculed for postulating that maternal mortality was associated with

PEARLS FOR ROUNDS

Combivir (zidovudine and lamivudine) is the first line of prophylactic therapy after HIV exposure.

Hand hygiene consistently performed by healthcare workers reduces the risk of iatrogenic infections.

The seroprevalence of HIV among hospitalized patients in the United States ranges from 0.2% to 14.2%.

The risk of HIV infection from a percutaneous injury is established by the depth of cutaneous penetration; the amount of blood on or within the scalpel, suture, or needle (especially if hollow); direct contact of the instrument with the patient's vasculature; and an infected patient whose late-stage disease rapidly escalates to death.

No surgeon has contracted a *documented* HIV infection from a patient. (Six cases of surgeons with HIV infections were possibly from occupational exposures. These surgeons had no other identifiable risk factors, but none had documented occupational exposures before HIV seroconversion.)

inadequate hand sanitation. Semmelweis observed that women whose babies were delivered by medical students and physicians had a higher rate of mortality than did those who were attended by midwives. (Students and physicians went from performing autopsies to delivering babies without sanitizing, whereas the midwives cleansed their hands.) After chlorine was incorporated into a hand-washing protocol, maternal mortality rates decreased significantly. Noncompliance with proper hand hygiene is still a problem. Reports indicate that physicians and nurses wash their hands only 30% as often as they should.

The CDC estimates that nearly 2 million patients in the United States acquire infections in hospitals. Healthcare-associated infections contribute to increased patient morbidity, mortality, and cost of care. In October 2003, the CDC recommended the use of an alcohol-based waterless hand rub before and after all patient contacts. These rubs are less time consuming, more easily accessible, and less drying than regular soap. The hope is that these factors will increase compliance with hand hygiene and decrease both the incidence of healthcare-associated infections and the transmission of resistant organisms.

Suggested Reading

American College of Surgeons: Statement on the surgeon and HIV infection. Bull Am Coll Surg 89:27–29, 2004.

American College of Surgeons: Statement on the surgeon and hepatitis. Bull Am Coll Surg 89:35–39, 2004.

Centers for Disease Control and Prevention: HIV/AIDS surveillance report. MMWR 12(No.1):1–41, 2000.

Centers for Disease Control and Prevention: Updated U.S. Public Health Service guidelines for the management of occupational exposures to HBV, HCV and HIV and recommendations for postexposure prophylaxis. MMWR 50(No. RR-11):1–56, 2001.

Centers for Disease Control and Prevention: Guideline for hand hygiene in health-care settings: Recommendations of the healthcare infection control practices advisory committee and the HICPAC/SHEA/APIC/IDSA hand hygiene task force. MMWR 51(RR16):1–44, 2002.

Flum DR, Wallack MK: The surgeon's database for AIDS: A collective review. J Am Coll Surg 184:403–412, 1997.

Gerberding JL: Occupational exposure to HIV in health care setting. N Engl J Med 348:826–833, 2003.

Website

Centers for Disease Control, National Center for HIV, STD, and TB Prevention: HIV/AIDS Surveillance Reports, 2002. (Also see at this site Most Recent Issues of MMWR.) ***(http://www.cdc.gov/hiv/stats/hasrlink.htm)***

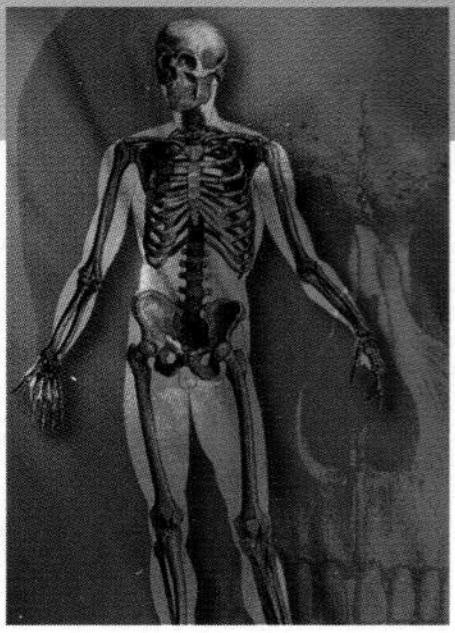

Chapter 4

The Core Competencies

JAMES G. PETROS, MD, MPH

Today's U.S. healthcare market is characterized by total expenditures of approximately $1.7 trillion per year, with costs increasing 4% to 9% annually. This represents about 17% of our gross domestic product. For every dollar spent on defense in the United States, approximately $4 is spent on health care. In such a healthcare market, tremendous pressure exists to control increasing costs while increasing healthcare quality. In other words, healthcare providers (hospitals, physicians) must deliver value for the healthcare dollar. Healthcare payers (Medicare, Medicaid, managed care organizations, insurers) are increasingly in the market to purchase patient outcomes from providers, not necessarily products or services. Patient outcomes can be in the form of declining mortality rates, better disease control, improving symptoms, or better physical functioning.

For providers to compete successfully in today's healthcare market, they must harness their competencies to enable them to deliver value. A competency is a unique resource of an organization or the organization's ability to channel the resource for a purpose. If the organization does not possess unique resources, then it may have a unique ability to manage common resources. The ability to use one's competencies is important not only in large medical centers but also in private physician practices as well. Delivering value for the healthcare dollar will attract payers and patients alike. To provide improving patient outcomes, providers must constantly make changes in the way they provide health care. In the long run, these changes are initiated and sustained by physicians trained in the competencies of high-quality patient care.

Providers have come to realize that three components make up the value-based healthcare system. The first component is cost reduction. Overall healthcare system costs must be reduced. More efficiently using healthcare resources while achieving better patient outcomes can reduce costs. Quality improvement is the second component. Quality cannot be taken for granted. It must be measured and constantly improved for a value-based healthcare system to work. Physicians have been skeptical about methods to increase health care quality. Many physicians believe that quality-improvement programs harass them and rarely result in better patient care. Outcomes are frequently difficult to measure and are influenced by the underlying severity of illness and not just by the quality of care that patients receive. In addition, many physicians think that quality-improvement efforts are, in reality, cost-containment or marketing strategies rather than efforts to improve patient care. Despite these impressions, quality improvement in health care is here to stay, and future physicians must learn to monitor how well caregivers and healthcare institutions are performing. Physicians and other healthcare professionals must constantly review the structure (system used to create healthcare services), process (actual delivery of services), and outcomes of their respective institutions to ensure that quality is constantly improving.

The third component is customer satisfaction. Our patients are our customers and their satisfaction must be measured to determine the effectiveness of medical treatment and the appropriate level of customer service. Payers will continue to collect patient-satisfaction and clinical-performance data to judge the quality of health care offered by providers. They will use this information to make value-based purchasing decisions. By using the Internet and information supplied by payers, patients will make better-informed decisions when choosing their healthcare plans, providers, and services. By increasing available product information, competition in the healthcare system will increase resulting in greater quality and cost control.

In the value-based healthcare system, it is not sufficient for physicians to be just clinicians. To remain major players in the future of health care, physicians must become proactive managers and make total quality improvement their mantra. Physician-managers must respond to the needs of busy, well-informed patients. In turn, physician-educators must ensure that medical schools and residency programs produce the kinds of physicians that are aware of the competencies that lead to better health care. In pursuing these ends, medical school and residency program curricula must be integrated with the core competencies of high-performing healthcare providers. These competencies include communication, information management, leadership, collaboration, assessment, planning, evaluation, and promoting health and preventing disease. Learning the core competencies of high-performing healthcare providers will enable physicians to be active in building great healthcare organizations as well as in training great healthcare professionals.

Residency Training

Physicians have been receiving much bad press lately: poor customer service, geographic variations in medical and surgical care with no medically appropriate reasons, allegations of supplier-induced demand, and the Institute of Medicine report, which claims approximately 98,000 deaths per year secondary to medical errors. Physician educators appear to be teaching as much from newspapers as from the medical literature. One must wonder if a better way to train a physician exists.

To ensure healthcare quality in the future, educational quality must be pursued in the present. More than 7000 graduate medical education programs are training more than 100,000 residents in the United States. To remain accredited, residency training programs have tried to satisfy minimal standards of educational quality in terms of didactic and clinical experience. Accreditation agencies have relied on the site visit as the primary way to measure quality in a residency program. During site visits, inspection as well as minimal standards of structure, process, and outcome are used to evaluate the educational quality of the particular residency program. However, reliance on inspection and discipline as agents of change has commonly added cost and delayed quality improvement in education. Such an evaluation system creates fear in those being measured and can result in gaming of the system. Today, residency programs spend a huge amount of time building defenses against accreditation site visits. A more productive way to use this time would be to understand better a particular residency program's deficiencies and take steps to create a culture that is wedded to quality improvement in physician education. As physicians, we must take an active part in avoiding minimal standards of educational quality.

The Core Competencies

The Accreditation Council of Graduate Medical Education (ACGME) and its various Residency Review Committees are responsible for accrediting the residency and fellowship programs in the United States. Starting in 1998, the ACGME began to endorse educational outcomes to enhance residency education. Since then, measurement tools of educational quality that represent the common values of high-performing healthcare providers, the public, and the residency programs themselves have been in development. The core competencies of residency education represent such a direction. Borrowing from the competencies of healthcare providers, the ACGME has endorsed educational outcomes measures and has developed a list of six core (general) competencies of residency education. Designing curricula to teach the competencies as well as assessing resident progress in learning the competencies are still in their early stages and have been left primarily to the individual programs to develop and implement. The core competencies of residency education presently include instruction and assessment in patient care, medical knowledge, practice-based learning, communication skills, professionalism, and systems-based practice. Since July 2002, residency programs should have been able to provide evidence of learning the competencies. By 2011, residency programs must show evidence of full integration of the competencies into their curricula. The first and second of these competencies have been part of traditional residency training. However, the remaining four competencies have often been assumed rather than actually being included in residency program curricula. Assessment of education in the competencies can be accomplished with a number of methods including observation, in-training examinations, standardized patients, medical record review, structured clinical examinations, and 360-degree evaluations.

The first competency to be discussed is **patient care**, which is defined by the ACGME as "compassionate, appropriate, and effective for the treatment of health problems and promotion of health." This competency includes diagnostic assessment and the use of clinical principles to treat healthcare problems. This is done after consultation with the patient and family members. Residency programs have traditionally used a progressive clinical experience, under supervision, along with lines of accountability from core faculty and senior residents to teach this competency. The constantly changing healthcare-delivery system with its emphasis on outpatient management can threaten education in this competency. Therefore physician-educators must constantly adapt their curricula to ensure that education in this competency remains intact.

The competency of **medical knowledge** is defined by the ACGME as "established and evolving biomedical, clinical, and cognate (epidemiologic, sociobehavioral) sciences and their application to patient care." When teaching this competency, physician-educators have constantly stressed the development of an adequate fund of clinical knowledge through clinical activity, didactics, and reading. The educational goals and objectives of each residency program guide the accumulation of knowledge and methods of assessment in this competency.

One of the foundations of a career in medicine is lifelong learning and professional development. No longer can physicians be content with the knowledge acquired in medical school and residency. The time to professional obsolescence has never been shorter. Habits, which continually maintain and build a knowledge base through continuing medical education, must be instilled during residency for the newly minted physician to be professionally successful. To ensure the public safety, the medical profession requires certification and recertification. This is one of several ways the medical profession regulates itself.

Practice-based learning has been described as "investigation, evaluation, and improvement in patient care, appraisal, and assimilation of scientific evidence." Residency programs teach evidence-based decision making as the basis of practice-based learning. Residents must learn to appraise the current medical literature and make this an integral part of the continuous expansion of one's fund of knowledge. The result will be optimal care for one's patients.

Effective information exchange and collaboration with patients, families, and other healthcare professionals are the basis of **interpersonal and communication skills.** Instruction in communication skills must be offered in medical schools and residency programs. Communication skills must be assessed objectively by observing residents in history taking, consulting, rounding, as well as dealing with peers, allied health care professionals, and core faculty. In addition, the ability to establish relationships with patients and families, effective listening skills, and discussion of therapeutic options must be assessed. This requires time on the faculty's part. Time is becoming an increasingly precious commodity in today's managed care era. As in teaching patient care**,** opportunities to interview patients are becoming less and less available in this era of managed care. Patient follow-up has shifted to clinics and faculty offices. Even these encounters are brief. Physician-educators must be resourceful in providing residents and medical students with supervised ambulatory experiences in clinics and offices where resident behavior can be assessed. Keep in mind that most malpractice litigation is due to the breakdown in communication between physician and patient.

Another aspect of **interpersonal communication** is collaboration. Physicians have to be collaborators in this era of multidisciplinary treatment. Residents and medical students must be able to develop adequate relationships with other healthcare professionals. Without such skills, they will not be able to manage the often-complex demands of patient care. For residents and medical students to become collaborators, they must be given the opportunity to interact with faculty who are role models. Deficiencies in collaborative skills can be identified early in residency training and remediation performed on an individual basis.

The competency of **professionalism** is described as the "commitment to carrying out professional responsibilities, adherence to ethical principles, and sensitivity to a diverse patient population." As in teaching communication, physician-educators must be role models to teach residents concerning professionalism. Physician-educators have a great deal of influence on medical students and residents. This trust must not be compromised. Teaching by example can be accomplished by the core faculty. The result will be residents and medical students regarding their teachers as mentors.

The competency of **systems-based practice** has traditionally received little attention in training programs. It is defined as "actions demonstrating awareness and responsiveness to the larger context of health care, the ability to call on system resources to provide care of optimal value." At no time has it been more important for residents and medical students to acquire knowledge of the healthcare system beyond the walls of their teaching hospitals. The utilization of scarce healthcare resources, the relationship between payers and providers, healthcare financing, managed care organizations, and the use of computer technology to aid clinical activities must be taught to make physicians proactive in the healthcare fields of the future. Time management should be included in this competency to ensure a balance between clinical and home life. Many physicians have experienced compromised professional lives because of unstable lives outside the hospital or office.

PEARLS FOR ROUNDS

More than $1.7 trillion is spent by the United States on health care each year. This figure increases by about 4% to 9% annually.

Healthcare quality is based on (1) structure, (2) process, and (3) patient outcomes.

Measurable patient outcomes include mortality rates, disease control, improving symptoms, and better physical functioning.

The core competencies of resident training are (1) patient care, (2) medical knowledge, (3) interpersonal communication, (4) professionalism, (5) practice-based learning, and (6) systems-based practice.

Cost reduction, quality improvement, and customer (patient) satisfaction are the components of value in health care.

Future Challenges

The present graduate medical education system must continue to integrate the core competencies into their curricula to create great physicians who then go on to create great healthcare institutions. Such physicians will eventually build value into our healthcare system, resulting in greater cost-effectiveness. The structure, processes, and outcomes of healthcare delivery must be better understood so even better systems can be designed. A commitment to value has to exist at all levels of healthcare organizations. This applies as much to the single physician as to the chief executive officer of a large academic medical center.

Industry has used competencies and measurable outcomes since the 1980s. Companies have spent a considerable amount of time stamping out variance in production processes, thus increasing quality and reducing costs. As physicians, we can use competencies and outcomes to decrease inappropriate variations in healthcare services, which do not make clinical sense. However, variance among future healthcare professionals must be fostered. Physicians from diverse backgrounds trained in the competencies of value-based health care will continue to be the source of new, innovative ideas for increasing healthcare quality. Preventing disease and promoting health is regarded as a core competency of healthcare providers. Medical students and residents must be regarded as the core competency of our graduate medical education system.

Suggested Reading

Halpern R, Lee MY, Boulter PR, Phillips RR: A synthesis of nine major reports on physicians' competencies for the emerging practice environment. Acad Med 76:606–615, 2001.

Itani K: A positive approach to core competencies and benchmarks for graduate medical education. Am J Surg 184:196–203, 2002.

Langdale LA, Schaad D, Wipf J, et al: Preparing graduates for the first year of residency: Are medical schools meeting the need? Acad Med 78:39–44, 2003.

Strauss RW: The quiet revolution in postgraduate training. Acad Emerg Med 9:1222–1225, 2002.

Swing SR: Assessing the ACGME general competencies: General considerations and assessment methods. Acad Emerg Med 9:1278–1286, 2002.

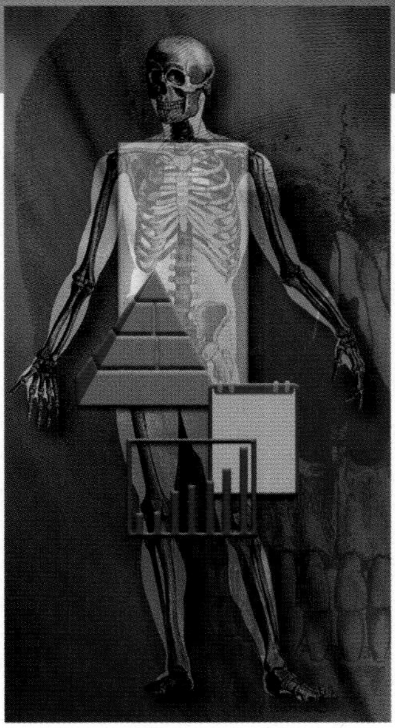

SECTION II

HOMEOSTASIS IN SURGICAL PATIENTS

Chapter 5

Principles of Preoperative Care and Risk Assessment

MICHAEL T. WATKINS, MD

Over the past decade, routine preoperative evaluations and consultations that used to take place during inpatient hospitalizations are now completed in the outpatient setting. Immediate preoperative preparations are instituted in the patient's home. Fewer preoperative opportunities allow surgeons to become aware of conditions that might affect the outcome of elective or urgent surgical interventions. A thorough evaluation of the patient's overall medical condition is essential *before* surgical procedures. These preoperative evaluations are best coordinated with the patient's primary care provider or medical specialists or both before surgery, but the ultimate responsibility to identify and address these problems before surgery remains the responsibility of the surgeon.

The decision to proceed with an operative procedure depends on analysis of the risk-benefit ratio, which in turn is dependent on the history, physical examination, and laboratory tests. A specific review of systems with particular consideration of how a patient might respond to the stress of surgery is required. Willingness to communicate with the patient is essential in the preoperative period; in instances in which the patient is either quite young or elderly, communication with the family may be indicated to coordinate postoperative care. Information must be provided to the patient preoperatively regarding the operative procedure, duration of hospitalization, extent of postoperative disability, need for postoperative follow-up, postoperative medications, and detailed discharge planning.

This chapter reviews the principles of preoperative evaluation of patients undergoing a variety of surgical procedures; specific recommendations for many different organ systems are provided. Mastery of the art and science of surgery will allow competent surgeons to determine the appropriate focus for their patients and circumstances.

Cardiac Risk Assessment

Incidence

Cardiovascular disease remains the most widespread major medical complication in the United States. Over the next 30-year period, patients (older than 65 years) requiring surgical procedures are predicted to have a 25–35% increase in the incidence of cardiovascular disease. This is the same group that has the highest number of surgical procedures overall. Based on the history, physical findings, and a few simple laboratory studies, efforts have been made to quantify surgical risk. The more commonly used system, the Dripps-American Society of Anesthesiology Classification (i.e., ASA class), categorizes patients into five groups (Box 5-1). This system offers little guidance, however, for identifying patients who are at risk for postoperative myocardial ischemia.

The purpose of a preoperative cardiac evaluation is to identify patients with high, medium, and low risk. These risks vary with both the underlying disease and the procedure performed. Appropriate interventions can be pursued preoperatively in patients with high and medium risks for perioperative cardiac problems. Patients with documented prior myocardial infarction (MI) have acute MI at a rate of 6.6% as compared with patients with no

BOX 5–1 Dripps-American Society of Anesthesia Classification

Class I	Healthy patient: limited procedure
Class II	Mild to moderate systemic disturbance
Class III	Severe systemic disturbance
Class IV	Life-threatening disturbance
Class V	Not expected to survive, with or without surgery

history of MI (0.13%). The patient who is scheduled to undergo elective surgery should be questioned carefully about the nature, severity, and location of chest pain. Additional historic issues include a history of dyspnea on exertion and dates of MIs (suspected or confirmed). Other clues to the existence of coexisting heart disease include syncope, palpitations, and arrhythmia. Patients with a history of rheumatic heart disease require prophylactic antibiotic therapy to prevent endocarditis, even for minor procedures.

In 1977, Goldman and colleagues published a validated model to predict cardiac complications in a general surgical population. Initially, patients with angina were excluded from their review. They defined a cardiac risk index for cardiac death and life-threatening complications of MI, pulmonary edema, and ventricular tachycardia in four risk classes. Modifications of the original cardiac risk index included angina pectoris, remote MI, CHF, aortic stenosis, and emergency surgery. A task force of the American College of Cardiology in conjunction with the American Heart Association undertook the development of guidelines for the perioperative cardiovascular evaluation of patients before noncardiac surgery. This effort resulted in the establishment of a set of clinical predictors of increased perioperative cardiovascular risk and stratified cardiac risk for noncardiac procedures. This task force reviewed the literature, incorporated the opinions of leaders in the field, and established a group of clinical predictors of increased perioperative cardiovascular risk and stratified the risk into major, moderate, and minor categories. Major risk factors include unstable coronary syndromes, recent MI, severe valvular disease, and ventricular arrhythmias. Intermediate risk factors include asymptomatic MI, diabetes mellitus, and compensated CHF. Minor risk factors include history of stroke and uncontrolled hypertension.

Although risk prediction is a useful tool based on strong statistical inferences and a large number of studies, it is important to consider new data as they become available. Early studies suggested dramatic increases in the risk of reinfarction until after 3 and 6 months after infarction; however, recent data do not support this increased risk. New data suggest that the risk of reinfarction is limited to those patients with myocardium at risk of ischemia due to coronary artery lesions, and most patients can be operated on safely with proper hemodynamic monitoring within 4 to 6 weeks of infarction.

Laboratory Assessment for Cardiac Diseases

The aim of noninvasive testing is to provide objective measure of functional capacity, to estimate perioperative cardiac risk, and to identify the presence of significant life-threatening or treatable myocardial ischemia. Untreated, significant life-threatening myocardial ischemia may adversely affect surgical outcome.

The tests commonly available include resting left ventricular function, ambulatory ECG monitoring, exercise stress testing, and nonexercise stress testing by using either myocardial perfusion imaging or dobutamine stress echocardiography. Resting ventricular function can be evaluated with echocardiography or radionuclide angiography. Although patients with an ejection fraction less than 35% are at greatest risk for complications, resting left ventricular function measured by either angiography or echocardiography has not been a reliable predictor of perioperative ischemic events. Patients with poorly controlled CHF should have an objective assessment of left ventricular function. Ischemia characterized by ST-segment depression can be identified by ambulatory ECG monitoring in patients at high risk for perioperative ischemic outcomes. Unfortunately, a substantial number of patients cannot be reliably evaluated with this method because of baseline ECG abnormalities. The largest prospective study of this testing modality failed to show benefit for screening with this technique; therefore it should not be used as the only diagnostic criterion to trigger referral of patients for invasive cardiovascular evaluation.

Exercise stress testing is widely available, relatively inexpensive, and of moderate specificity (68%) and sensitivity (77%). Unfortunately, 30–70% of patients with peripheral vascular disease cannot attain target heart rates and thus have nondiagnostic exercise stress test results. Infusing small-vessel vasodilators dipyridamole or adenosine followed by thallium imaging can induce increases in myocardial perfusion. Areas of myocardium supplied by fixed coronary stenoses have small-vessel vasodilation at rest, and therefore have diminished hyperemic response when compared with normally perfused myocardium. Fixed defects continue to show decreased flow over time, but reversible defects reveal improved flow over time (i.e., redistribution). Two prospective randomized trials found a negative predictive value of 95% by using dipyridamole-thallium imaging. Boucher et al. defined a 30% risk of perioperative ischemic events in patients with redistribution on thallium scans. Although both the sensitivity and specificity of dipyridamole-thallium imaging are high, the low risk of MI or death after noncardiac surgery results in a low positive predictive value (23%). In this setting, broad screening of patients at low clinical risk should be avoided.

Dobutamine stress echocardiography has been studied in a prospective blinded fashion and found to have a negative predictive value of 93% to 100% and a positive predictive value ranging from 7% to 30%. Dobutamine should not be used in patients with a history of serious tachyarrhythmias or severe hypertension or hypotension. In summary, patients undergoing high-risk surgical procedures or patients who are at intermediate risk should be considered for noninvasive testing for further risk stratification. Patients at high risk should be considered for angiography, and patients at low risk should receive no further testing. Indications for preoperative coronary angiography are similar to those in the nonoperative setting and include those patients with suspected left main disease or triple-vessel coronary occlusive disease or patients with unstable coronary syndromes.

Preoperative Treatment for Cardiac Diseases

Identification of factors that can be modified to reduce risk provides an opportunity for perioperative intervention that may improve outcome. Several large retrospective studies have demonstrated that coronary artery bypass grafting before a planned elective general surgery procedure has immediate and long-term benefit. Several studies support the use of surgery in severe multivessel or critical lesion coronary artery disease in patients with coexisting peripheral vascular disease. The role of prophylactic coronary artery bypass remains controversial because of the absence of large prospective randomized clinical trials. The role for prophylactic coronary angioplasty is similarly unclear, because it has been associated with a perioperative MI rate of 5.6% and mortality of 1.9% in high-risk patients treated before elective surgery.

Intensive medical therapy for coronary artery disease has been offered as an alternative to surgical revascularization. The use of β-blockers, calcium channel blockers, and nitrates plays a significant role in ensuring that the myocardial oxygen demand does not exceed supply. Sudden withdrawal of β-blockade should be avoided to prevent sudden excess in catecholamine effects. Immediate use of β-blockers before surgery has been shown to decrease frequency of ST-segment depression to 2% versus 28% for untreated patients. The incidence of perioperative MI in patients treated with β-blockers immediately before and after surgery was decreased from 18% to 3%. In a randomized prospective trial, Poldermans et al. provided additional strong evidence to suggest that medical intervention with a selective β-blocker reduced the risk of short-term cardiac complications associated with vascular surgery. In this study, β-blockade reduced the perioperative incidence of both deaths from MI and nonfatal MI in high-risk patients undergoing major vascular surgery by 10-fold. The observed differences could not be attributed to differences between the two groups with respect to clinical characteristics, surgical procedures, anesthetic or analgesic technique, duration of hospitalization, or results of dobutamine echocardiography. It has been recommended that, in the absence of major contraindications, therapeutic dosages of β-adrenergic antagonists should be given to patients with an intermediate or high risk of cardiac complications. Patients who are not regularly taking β-blockers should be started on this therapy perioperatively. The drug may cause complications such as fatigue or impotence; these side effects should be tolerated during the perioperative period.

Perioperative Management of Cardiac Risk Factors

Specific surgical approaches to a particular procedure do not appear to influence cardiac complications. Although laparoscopic surgery is associated with serious changes in hemodynamics, the reduced surgical stress associated with this approach may reduce the risk of cardiac complications.

With respect to cardiac complications, the length of time the anesthetic is used rather than the route or type of agent contributes significantly to perioperative cardiac risk. Regional anesthesia appears to have no cardiac benefit over general anesthesia but may reduce the need for reoperation in patients undergoing peripheral vascular surgery.

The role of the pulmonary artery catheter and hemodynamic monitoring in reducing cardiac perioperative complications remains controversial. Preoperative invasive monitoring in an ICU may optimize oxygen delivery in patients at high risk. It has been proposed that indexes derived from the pulmonary artery catheter and invasive blood pressure measurement can be used to maximize oxygen delivery, which should lead to reduction in organ dysfunction. A prospective randomized assessment found that when MI or nonarrhythmogenic cardiac death was used as outcome, preoperative pulmonary catheterization and cardiac optimization provided no significant benefit in patients who were either (1) monitored overnight before surgery, (2) monitored 3 hours preoperatively by the anesthesia team, or (3) monitored intraoperatively based solely on clinical indications.

The patient population in this study (a high preponderance of renal failure and multisystem organ failure) was not relevant to the majority of high-risk patients undergoing surgical procedures. In several meta-analyses, the preponderance of evidence points to improved outcome in patients who achieve high-output and high-oxygen-delivery states. When this can be achieved by using only volume and hemoglobin, a positive impact is noted on decreased cardiac complications.

The use of inotropic support to achieve improved output or high oxygen state or both is less clear. The diagnostic importance of the pulmonary artery catheter may reside primarily in its sensitivity in determination of the patient's volume status. Preoperative risk of patients with underlying cardiac disease is determined largely by the balance of CHF, adequacy of cardiac output, and perfusion of vital organs, which is often influenced by volume status and degree of diuretic therapy. Therefore should any doubt exist regarding the volume status of a patient with underlying cardiac disease, placement of a pulmonary artery catheter should be considered. The ideal cardiac filling pressures must be individualized for each patient, based on cardiac output and urine output. Some patients may require increased filling pressures to maintain adequate cardiac output, whereas other individuals may require gentle diuresis.

Pulmonary Assessment

Incidence

Postoperative pulmonary complications have been found to be as common as or more common than cardiac complications in 17 of 25 studies of postoperative complications. Pulmonary complications are the most common form of postoperative morbidity experienced by patients who undergo general surgical abdominal procedures and thoracotomy. In addition to pneumonia, massive lobar collapse due to mucus plugging, pneumonitis, atelectasis, and a combination of one or more of these problems can result in postoperative respiratory insufficiency. Most postoperative pulmonary complications develop as a result of changes in lung volume that occur in response to dysfunction of muscles of respiration and other changes in chest-wall mechanics.

Abdominal and thoracic surgical procedures cause large reductions in vital capacity and smaller but crucial reductions in functional residual capacity (FRC). FRC decreases in lower abdominal operations by 10% to 15%, after upper abdominal operations by 30%, and after thoracotomy/lung resection by 35%. Patients undergoing nonabdominal or nonthoracic surgery do not have consistent changes in FRC. FRC is decreased by the supine position, obesity, sepsis, ascites, and the development of peritonitis. The other important factor in the etiology of postoperative pulmonary complications is the closing volume (CV). The CV is the volume at which the flow from the dependent portion of the lungs stops during expiration because of airway closure. Factors that promote an increase in CV include advanced age, tobacco use, fluid overload, bronchospasm, and the presence of airway secretions. Under stable baseline conditions, FRC is about 50%, and CV is approximately 30% of total lung capacity. When FRC is reduced or CV is increased, portions of the lung are subject to premature airway closure and atelectasis. This condition results in a ventilation-perfusion mismatch, resulting in hypoxemia, and promotes trapping of secretions, which promotes pneumonitis and causes respiratory insufficiency.

Patient-related risk factors that may contribute to the risk of postoperative pulmonary complications include smoking, poor general health status, older age, obesity, chronic obstructive pulmonary disease (COPD), and asthma. Smoking increases risk among those without chronic lung disease. Relative risk of pulmonary complications among smokers as compared with nonsmokers ranges from 1.4 to 4.3. This risk can be reversed by cessation of smoking at least 8 weeks before surgery. Patients with COPD have increased risk of postoperative complications. Preoperative clinical factors associated with pulmonary complications include abnormal lung examination or chest radiography, the Goldman cardiac risk index, and overall comorbid disease burden.

Preoperative Laboratory Assessment for Pulmonary Disease

The accurate preoperative prediction of pulmonary risk has been somewhat elusive. A consensus exists that all candidates for lung resection should undergo preoperative pulmonary function testing. The use of spirometry to assess which patients are at greatest risk for pulmonary complications after other surgical procedures has enjoyed widespread popularity, but its predictive value remains unproven, despite its substantial cost. Neither individual spirometric variables nor degree of obstructive lung disease (as indicated by spirometry) was associated with complications on univariate or multivariate analysis in patients undergoing abdominal surgery.

Pre- and Postoperative Management of Pulmonary Disease

Elective surgery should be deferred in patients who have an acute exacerbation of their underlying COPD. Aggressive treatment should be provided to patients with COPD who do not have optimal reduction in symptoms or optimal exercise capacity, or who have evidence of airflow obstruction on physical examination. The treatments for these patients are no different from those for patients who are not about to have an operation. Combinations of bronchodilators, physical therapy, antibiotics, smoking cessation, and corticosteroids reduce the risk of postoperative pulmonary complications. Preoperative education in lung-expansion maneuvers reduces pulmonary complications to a greater degree than does instruction that begins after surgery. Lung-expansion maneuvers are the mainstay of postoperative prevention and include deep-breathing exercises, which are a component of chest physical therapy, and incentive spirometry; these have been studied most extensively. These maneuvers consistently reduced the relative risks of pulmonary complications by 50%; however, no convincing difference exists between the beneficial effect of incentive spirometry and that of deep-breathing exercises.

Nutritional Assessment

Impact of Surgery on Nutritional State

Surgical procedures place additional nutritional demands on patients because (1) patients are usually required not to take any food because of the surgical procedure; (2) patients are underfed for additional periods because of anorexia or nausea, and (3) the surgical procedure itself causes an injury response that is associated with protein catabolism, negative nitrogen balance, and increased energy expenditure. In uncomplicated situations (usually limited to postoperative days 5–7), these additional nutritional demands are negligible. A well-nourished person should have a 7- to 10-day energy and protein reserve such that starvation alone over this period should be well tolerated. If perioperative complications develop, negative nitrogen balance may be severe, prolonged, and exacerbate complications. In this setting, it is important to identify preoperative clinical indicators of malnutrition.

Indicators of Nutritional Deficiency

Patients with diminished oral intake related to their primary surgical illness might be at increased risk for suboptimal nutrition. Loss of 10% to 15% of preillness weight within 6 months is a significant indication of compromised nutrition. Evidence of muscle wasting, development of edema or ascites, history of weight loss, or a combination of these suggest malnutrition. On physical examination, muscle wasting in the temporalis, thenar, or hypothenar muscles is highly suggestive of malnutrition. Glossitis, loss of ruggae on the tongue, cheilosis, or scaling or cracking of the vermilion border suggests vitamin B or vitamin B-complex deficiency. Laboratory markers such as albumin, total lymphocyte count, prealbumin, transferrin, retinal binding protein, and carnitine have been used to estimate nutritional deficiency.

Anthropomorphic measurements to assess body reserves (e.g., triceps skinfold thickness for body fat) or estimates of body cell mass (e.g., midarm muscle circumference, creatinine height index) also have been used for nutritional assessment. No single measurement has proved to be more useful than a careful history and physical examination. Hypoalbuminemia has been associated with increased mortality and morbidity rates in hospitalized patients. In a recent study, serum albumin level was found to be a strong predictor of perioperative mortality and morbidity independent of the effects of a large diverse set of prospectively determined patient risk variables. For mortality and morbidity, albumin level was the best outcomes predictor, with ASA class and hematocrit ranking second and third. Albumin levels alone discriminated between survivors and nonsurvivors 78% of the time.

Perioperative Management of Nutritional Deficiency

Although controversial, preoperative nutritional supplementations have been shown to benefit some surgical patients. Patients undergoing gastrointestinal or pancreatic surgery that received preoperative total parenteral nutrition (TPN) had a twofold decrease in major postoperative complications and a fourfold decrease in mortality. Patients receiving preoperative TPN were compared with controls treated with intravenous fluids resuscitation and regular hospital diet. Interestingly, when one half of the TPN calories were administered as lipids, the complication and postoperative mortality rates were similar to those in control subjects. These results were interpreted as meaning that the lipids might have an immunosuppressive effect, thereby eliminating all benefits from the supplementation. In a VA Cooperative study, patients receiving TPN had a higher percentage of infectious complications compared with unfed controls (14.1% vs. 6.4%). Patients who were mildly malnourished had no demonstrable benefits from TPN. Only a subset of severely malnourished patients had fewer complications related to infections, wound healing, and maintaining normal organ function.

Preoperative enteral nutrition, in contrast to TPN, has been shown to reduce postoperative morbidity and mortality without added infectious complications. At present, it seems reasonable to delay surgical intervention for only the most severely malnourished individuals, and to provide nutritional support via enteral routes whenever possible. Clinical risk factors for perioperative malnutrition are listed in Box 5-2.

BOX 5-2 Preoperative Indicators of Malnutrition

- Anorexia, dysphagia
- Recent weight loss
- Recurrent nausea, vomiting, or diarrhea
- Malignancy (renal, liver, lung)
- Gastrointestinal disorders (inflammatory bowel disease, pancreatitis, fistulas)
- Drug dependency (i.e., alcoholism, illegal or prescription drugs)
- Dental difficulties
- Impoverished social status (homeless, disabled, or elderly individuals living alone)

Hematologic Considerations

Incidence and Risk of Thrombotic Complications

Deep venous thrombosis (DVT) may be a clinically silent disease with relatively high prevalence among hospitalized patients. Both DVT and pulmonary embolus (PE) may have few specific symptoms, and their clinical diagnosis is often insensitive and unreliable. The first manifestation of the disease may be fatal PE. Unrecognized and untreated DVT may lead to complications of postphlebitic syndrome and predispose patients to future episodes of recurrent DVT. Because of these serious life-threatening and debilitating complications of DVT and PE, prophylaxis for DVT has been steadfastly advocated for surgical patients. Application of effective prophylaxis depends on knowledge of specific clinical risk factors (Box 5-3) in individual patients.

Patients may be classified into low, moderate, and high risk for the development of DVT and PE. Low-risk patients may be older than 40 years, without history of paralysis, obesity, and estrogen use, undergoing uncomplicated minor surgery. This group has a 2% risk of calf vein DVT, a 0.4% risk of proximal vein DVT, and a 0.002% risk of fatal PE if prophylaxis is not used. Moderate-risk patients are older

BOX 5–3 Clinical Risk Factors for Perioperative Deep Vein Thrombosis

Younger than 40 years
Prolonged immobility/paralysis
Prior DVT
Cancer
Major surgery (pelvic, abdomen)
Obesity
Varicose veins
Congestive heart failure
Myocardial infarction
Stroke
Fractures of the pelvis, leg, hip
Indwelling femoral vein catheters
Inflammatory bowel disease
Nephrotic syndrome
Estrogen use
Hypercoagulable states

than 40 years, are having major surgery, but have no prolonged immobilization, paralysis, malignancy, obesity, varicose veins, or use of estrogen preparations. In the absence of prophylaxis, this group has a 10% to 20% risk of calf vein DVT, a 2% to 4% risk of proximal calf vein thrombosis, and a 0.1% to 0.4% risk of fatal PE.

High-risk patients comprise individuals with multiple risk factors, which result in an additive effect. Immobile elderly patients after major orthopedic procedures are among the most susceptible patients for fatal PE. This group has a 20% to 40% risk of calf vein thrombosis, a 4% to 8% risk of proximal vein clot, and a 0.4% to 1% risk of fatal PE if prophylaxis is not used. Congenital and acquired aberrations in hemostatic mechanisms exacerbate the risk of DVT in hospitalized patients undergoing surgical procedures. Hemostatic abnormalities that may predispose patients to DVT/PE include activated protein C resistance; antithrombin III deficiency; protein C/S deficiency; disorders of plasminogen and plasminogen activation; antiphospholipid antibodies and lupus anticoagulant; heparin-induced thrombocytopenia; hyperhomocystinemia; myeloproliferative disorders; dysfibrinogenemia; heparin-induced thrombocytopenia; and hyperviscosity syndromes.

Management of Perioperative Thrombotic Risks

Among antithrombotic drugs, low-dose unfractionated heparin (LDUH) and low-molecular-weight heparin (LMWH) are the most effective in reducing DVT, as assessed with labeled fibrinogen uptake. LDUH was the first antithrombotic agent investigated in large randomized trials, which confirmed its efficacy in reducing proximal DVT and PE. The regimen of DVT prophylaxis with LDUH is as follows: subcutaneous heparin (5000 U) started 2 hours before operation and continued every 8 or 12 hours after surgery until the patient is either fully ambulatory or discharged from the hospital. LDUH therapy reduced the incidence of DVT diagnosed by fibrinogen-uptake confirmation by phlebography from 25% to 8%. Pooled data from meta-analyses show that LDUH reduced the more serious end points of proximal DVT, clinically diagnosed PE, and fatal PE diagnosed at autopsy. These studies showed a 50% reduction in fatal PE with LDUH prophylaxis.

The advantages and disadvantages of LMWH in general surgery patients have been clarified by a number of large trials, as well as meta-analyses. LMWH and LDUH are equally efficacious in preventing DVT in general surgery patients. Doses of LMWH larger than 3500 units/day are associated with more bleeding. Lower doses of LMWH are equivalent to LDUH in preventing DVT and the extent of bleeding complications in moderate-risk patients. Higher doses of LMWH may be superior to LDUH in preventing DVT in high-risk patients. Advantages of LMWH include a once-a-day administration schedule and less likelihood to cause heparin-induced thrombocytopenia when compared with standard heparin preparations. In patients undergoing general surgery procedures, LMWH is usually administered 2 hours before an operation. When higher doses (>3400 U) are used in high-risk general surgery patients, the drug is administered 10 to 12 hours before operation to avoid excessive intraoperative bleeding. In orthopedic patients, this drug is usually administered 12 to 24 hours after operation because of fear of bleeding. LMWH prophylaxis does not require laboratory monitoring of the intensity of anticoagulation or dose adjustment. Recent reports brought attention to patients in whom epidural or spinal hematomas developed with concurrent use of LMWH prophylaxis and regional (spinal or epidural) anesthesia. The majority of these cases occurred in patients receiving regional anesthesia or analgesia for major orthopedic surgery of the leg. The following recommendations have been suggested for patients receiving a preoperative LMWH dose:

- Regional anesthesia should be avoided in patients with an abnormal clinical bleeding history or in patients receiving other drugs that affect hemostasis (e.g., aspirin or nonsteroidal anti-inflammatory drugs, platelet inhibitors, or other anticoagulants).
- Insertion of the spinal needle should be delayed for 10 to 12 hours after the initial LMWH prophylaxis dose.
- A single-dose spinal anesthetic is preferable to continuous epidural anesthetic.
- For patients receiving continuous anesthesia, the epidural catheter should be left indwelling overnight and removed the following day.

Intermittent pneumatic compression (IPC) is an attractive mechanical method of DVT prophylaxis because no risk of hemorrhagic complications occurs. These devices provide rhythmic external compression, thereby decreasing stasis in the lower extremities and stimulating endogenous fibrinolytic mechanisms. Recent literature also suggests that IPC inhibits the primary initiating mechanisms of blood coagulation by increasing plasma tissue factor pathway inhibitor. IPC is effective in reducing leg DVT in most general surgery patients and in high-risk surgical patients with malignant disease. In trials comparing IPC with LDUH, both agents were equivalent in reducing leg DVT.

Graded compression stockings reduce the incidence of DVT, but no convincing data confirm a reduction in proximal DVT and PE. Dextran, a polysaccharide of 40,000 or 70,000 daltons, is not as effective as LDUH or LMWH in reducing DVT, but it has been shown to reduce the incidence of PE. Dextran has not been popular because it is relatively expensive, must be administered intravenously, and is associated with rare anaphylactic reactions. Moreover, dextran is contraindicated in patients with renal insufficiency and limited cardiac reserve. Aspirin has not been found effective in preventing DVT or PE in general surgery patients.

Warfarin, given as a fixed dose (1 mg/day) or adjusted dose to prolong the prothrombin time appears mildly effective in preventing leg DVT. This method is cumbersome, requires monitoring, and may predispose to patients to bleeding complications. Because alternate therapy is readily available, little rationale exists to use warfarin in most general surgery patients. Because of the high risk of perioperative thromboembolic events in patients undergoing elective total hip or total knee replacements, adjusted dose oral most orthopedic surgeons in North America have adopted anticoagulation. In a comparison of LMWH with warfarin in these high-risk patients, the cumulative incidence of venous thromboembolism was 3.6% versus 3.7%, respectively. The specific "in hospital" incidence of venous thromboembolism was 0.7% in patients treated with LMWH and 1.1% for those treated with warfarin ($P = .00083$). No statistical difference was found in the incidence of bleeding complications or fatal PE in these patients. The choice of adjusted-dose warfarin vs. LMWH must be tailored to the individual patient, based on postoperative thrombotic risks, perioperative bleeding risks, and convenience.

Anemia/Dyscrasias

Anemia a very common problem in the perioperative period. Information gleaned from Jehovah's Witnesses who underwent surgery shows that comorbid disease and expected operative blood loss are important covariables determining morbidity and mortality. The level of hemoglobin itself serves as only a rough guide to the adequacy of oxygenation because oxygen delivery is dependent on additional factors such as cardiac output, pulmonary gas exchange, blood volume, blood viscosity, and oxygen affinity for hemoglobin. Substantial discussion has occurred about optimal hemoglobin levels for surgical patients, and a National Institutes of Health consensus panel suggested that a hemoglobin level of 10 g/dL has been accepted as a "safe" level.

Preoperative evaluation of anemia starts with a careful preoperative history and physical examination. Personal or family history of anemia, bleeding, ethnic background, medication, alcohol use, toxin exposure, recent illness, or constitutional symptoms should be sought. Physical findings of jaundice, skin/mucous membrane abnormalities, adenopathy, organomegaly, neurologic dysfunction, and occult blood loss in stool or urine should be noted.

Laboratory evaluation should include the reticulocyte count (i.e., low counts indicate inadequate marrow production, whereas high counts [indicative of excessive red blood cell loss] suggest bleeding or hemolysis). In the event of a low reticulocyte count, the mean corpuscular volume and peripheral blood smear should be examined to determine whether the anemia is microcytic, normocytic, or macrocytic. Microcytic anemia is almost always due to iron deficiency or thalassemia. Macrocytic anemia is often due to alcoholism, liver disease, vitamin B_{12} or folate deficiency, or primary marrow dysfunction. Normocytic anemia is often due to chronic inflammation, infections, neoplasms, uremia, acute blood loss, or bone marrow suppression from drugs or radiation exposure. When the procedure is elective, it seems prudent to delay surgery, complete the evaluation, and treat the underlying problem to avoid problems of transfusion.

Reversal of correctable anemias may take weeks, making transfusion the only recourse for urgent surgery. Patients with uncorrectable anemias also may require transfusion if surgery is urgently needed. The circumstance under which transfusion seems reasonable and for which no further justification is needed is called the transfusion trigger. Prior to the 1980s, surgical patients were considered optimally treated if their hemoglobin level and hematocrit remained greater than 10g/dL and 30%, respectively. Animal studies seem to suggest that oxygen delivery peaks at a hematocrit of 30%, and oxygen transport and survival is maximized between 30% and 40%. Concern for transmission of human immunodeficiency virus forced a re-examination of indications for transfusions, with a conclusion that an absolute number was insufficient for justifying transfusions in all patients. Furthermore, the risk of transmitting hepatitis through transfusions may be as high as 10%, as most cases are not apparent clinically. Hepatitis C accounts for 90% of the cases of transmission-associated hepatitis.

Conversely, in high-risk patients, anemia (Hct <28) may lead to the development of perioperative myocardial ischemia. Results from the National VA Surgical Risk Study revealed that anemia ranked third behind albumin and ASA class as a strong, statistically significant predictor of 30-day mortality and morbidity. The patients' individual risk factors and type of surgery must be taken into consideration when transfusion is contemplated. Transfusions should be given, if possible, at least 24 hours before operation, allowing adequate time for the body to reaccumulate normal levels of 2,3-diphosphoglycerate.

Sickle cell anemia is associated with significant surgical morbidity. Exchange transfusion to reduce hemoglobin S levels to less than 30% and preoperative oxygen administration are advised. Acidosis, dehydration, hypothermia, and infection are to be avoided to prevent the development of sickle cell crisis.

Patients with polycythemia vera have an increased risk of perioperative complications from hemorrhage. It is recommended that phlebotomy and myelosuppressive agents be used to maintain the hematocrit at less than 52% in these patients for several months before elective procedures. Patients with leukemia and platelet counts less that 50,000 may be supplemented with immediate preoperative transfusions of platelets. When surgery is contemplated in patients with granulocytopenia (usually associated with leukemia), antibiotics should be used prophylactically.

Perioperative Management of Patients Given Anticoagulation for Medical Conditions

No consensus is found on the appropriate perioperative management of anticoagulation for patients who have been receiving long-term warfarin therapy. The most common indications for warfarin therapy are atrial fibrillation, presence of a mechanical heart valve, and venous thromboembolism. Management of patients with significant risks for thromboembolism in the perioperative period requires consideration of risks of both thromboembolism and anticoagulant therapy. After warfarin therapy is stopped, it takes approximately 4 days for the international normalized ratio (INR) to reach 1.5, a level at which most surgery can be performed safely. After warfarin therapy is restarted, it takes about 3 days for the INR to reach 2.0. The temporary discontinuation of warfarin exposes the patient to about 1 day of risk for thromboembolism because of the gradual decrease in the INR. Although biochemical evidence suggests a rebound hypercoagulable state caused by the discontinuation of warfarin, the phenomenon has yet to be seen clinically. The risk of recurrent thromboembolic event after an acute venous thromboembolism is greatest during the first 3 months. If surgery is needed within the first 2 weeks after a venous thromboembolic event, insertion of a caval filter should be considered. Six percent of recurrent episodes of venous thromboembolism are expected to be fatal.

Heparin therapy, if started immediately postoperatively will be associated with a marked increase in the risk of major bleeding. The magnitude of this increase is uncertain, but one study reported an 11% incidence of bleeding during the first 5 days of intravenous heparin therapy in the immediate postoperative period. Approximately 3% of the postoperative bleeding episodes are fatal. These risks of bleeding must be balanced with the risks of thromboembolic events. Because surgery is associated with a 100-fold increase in risk of venous thromboembolism, postoperative anticoagulation is recommended. Because the consequences of venous thromboembolism are usually more severe than the risks of bleeding, the uses of postoperative intravenous heparin will produce a small net decrease in morbidity. In patients who are more than 3 months after an acute episode of venous thromboembolism, postoperative heparin can be expected to cause as many episodes of major bleeding as it will prevent major thromboembolism.

Prophylactic measures that are associated with a lower risk of bleeding than intravenous heparin (i.e., LMWH, given with or without graduated compression stockings or intermittent pneumatic compression) are likely to be a safer alternative for such patients. In contrast to recurrent venous thromboembolism, the consequences of arterial thromboembolism are much more serious; approximately 20% of these episodes are fatal, and 40% result in serious permanent disability. Because of the risks of recurrent arterial thromboembolic events, preoperative intravenous heparin therapy is indicated. Because surgery is not known

PEARLS FOR THE OR

The American Society of Anesthesiology classes are
- Class I Healthy patient: limited procedure
- Class II Mild to moderate systemic disturbance
- Class III Severe systemic disturbance
- Class IV Life-threatening disturbance
- Class V Not expected to survive, with or without surgery

Predictors of cardiac risk in surgical patients include the following:

Major predictors
- Unstable coronary syndromes
- Recent myocardial infarction with evidence of important ischemic risk by clinical symptoms or noninvasive study
- Unstable or severe angina
- Decompensated congestive heart failure
- Significant arrhythmias
- High-grade atrioventricular block
- Symptomatic ventricular arrhythmias in the presence of underlying heart disease
- Supraventricular arrhythmias with uncontrolled ventricular rate
- Severe valvular disease

Intermediate predictors
- Mild angina pectoris (Canadian class I or II)
- Prior myocardial infarction by history or pathologic Q waves
- Compensated or prior congestive heart failure
- Diabetes mellitus

Minor predictors
- Advanced age, abnormal ECG (left ventricular hypertrophy, left bundle-branch block, ST-T abnormalities), rhythm other than sinus (e.g., atrial fibrillation), loss functional capacity (e.g., inability to climb one flight of stairs with a bag of groceries)
- History of stroke
- Uncontrolled systemic hypertension

to increase the incidence of arterial thromboembolism, postoperative heparin therapy is not absolutely indicated. Postoperative heparin therapy should be used only after minor surgical procedures, where the risk of bleeding is low.

In conditions associated with lesser risk of arterial thromboembolism (atrial fibrillation, mechanical heart valve), analysis suggests that postoperative heparin therapy may be associated with increases rather than decreases in serious morbidity. This is because the risk of postoperative bleeding is greater than the risk of postoperative arterial thromboembolism. LMWH may be given to patients with history of arterial thromboembolic disease when warfarin is stopped in the preoperative period, but a clear-cut benefit or risk reduction has not been evaluated in a clinical trial.

Fluid and Electrolyte Abnormalities

Patients tolerate operations best when they are properly hydrated. This is not a problem in patients without evidence of peripheral edema, with normal vital signs, adequate urine output, good skin turgor, moist mucous membranes, and normal serum electrolytes. Those patients with varying degrees of dehydration or overhydration will not tolerate operation well. Dehydration with accompanying salt loss is the most frequent disorder encountered in the preoperative patient. Conditions that give rise to this condition include intestinal obstruction, pyloric outlet obstruction, diarrhea, various enterocutaneous fistulas, and sequestration of extracellular fluid into injured tissues. Fluid losses secondary to vomiting and diarrhea are apparent and are reflected as weight losses. Derangements in fluid balance may be iatrogenically created through the use of cathartics and enemas in preparation for bowel surgery. Prolonged fluid restriction in preparation for various radiologic examinations or other diagnostic procedures can contribute to preoperative volume depletion.

Third-space or internal losses are often not appreciated and may reach massive proportions despite minimal weight losses. Third-space losses may result from fluid sequestration in obstructed bowel loops, underneath burns, in soft tissue subjected to massive trauma, and by loss of ascitic fluid caused by cirrhosis of the liver or peritonitis. The degree of volume deficit must be based on a detailed history of the patient's disease coupled with a careful evaluation of physical signs. Clinically significant volume depletion usually does not become manifest until loss of approximately 5% of the body weight has occurred. Under these circumstances, skin turgor is depressed, mucous membranes have lost their moistness, and urine volume is decreased and hyperconcentrated.

Under no circumstances should all losses be replaced in a single 24-hour period. Rapid replacement of estimated losses may actually impose a greater risk than the primary illness, particularly in elderly patients. The type of fluid replaced will depend in most cases on the serum electrolyte profile. If electrolytes are relatively normal in the face of obvious volume depletion, losses can be assumed to be iso-osmotic with plasma and should be replaced with a balanced salt solution, such as Ringer's lactate. If chloride losses exceed sodium losses, as occurs with vomiting, isotonic saline or one half normal saline is generally the preferred replacement fluid. In hypernatremic states, as may occur with patients receiving tube feedings, water alone as 5% dextrose in water is used for replacement. Hyponatremia, conversely, responds in most instances to water restriction but may require the use of hypertonic saline for correction. If hypertonic saline is required, extreme care must be exercised to prevent fluid overload, compromised cardiac function, and possible pulmonary edema. Usually, administration of isotonic saline will be adequate to replace most volume deficits.

Potassium losses may often accompany salt and water deficits, particularly in the setting of vomiting and diarrheal states. Because a serum potassium concentration less than 4 mEq/L may be associated with cardiac arrhythmias, replacement of substantial potassium losses should be accompanied by frequent reevaluations of serum potassium levels. If emergency surgery is anticipated, more rapid replacement can be administered cautiously with electrocardiographic monitoring. At no time should potassium infusions exceed 15 mEq/hour to avoid a potentially lethal hyperkalemia.

States of overhydration also are seen in the preoperative patient and may usually be managed with volume restriction and gentle removal of excess fluid by mild diuretics in most cases. Pure water excess, which has been observed in patients with central nervous system lesions and burns, is thought to be due to an inappropriate secretion of antidiuretic hormone. Cessation of all water administration coupled with the use of solute diuretics (i.e., mannitol) is the treatment of choice. If these measures fail, cautious administration of hypertonic saline may be used to assist in the diuresis of the excess water.

Infectious Considerations

Although postoperative infections may not be likely, they remain a major component of surgical morbidity and mortality. In between 4% and 5% of all patients currently admitted to acute care hospitals in the United States, a nosocomial infection develops. Of those in whom such infections develop, approximately 1% die as a direct result; overall infection contributes to the death of another 2.5%. Much can be done to protect patients from infection during the preoperative period. Assessment of risk, correction of predisposing factors, precise timing of operation, judicious use of antibiotics and containment of contamination must be instituted in the preoperative period. Factors that are known to contribute to increased infection in surgical patients include malnutrition, advanced age, immuno-

PEARLS FOR ROUNDS

Preoperative indicators for malnutrition:
- Anorexia, dysphagia
- Recent weight loss
- Recurrent nausea, vomiting, or diarrhea
- Malignancy (renal, liver, lung)
- Gastrointestinal disorders (inflammatory bowel disease, pancreatitis, fistulas)
- Drug dependency (i.e., alcoholism, illegal or prescription drugs)
- Dental difficulties
- Impoverished social status (homeless, disabled or elderly individuals living alone)

Clinical risk factors for perioperative deep vein thrombosis:
- Older than 40 years
- Prolonged immobility/paralysis
- Prior DVT
- Cancer
- Major surgery (pelvic, abdomen)
- Obesity
- Varicose veins
- Congestive heart failure
- Myocardial infarction
- Stroke
- Fractures of the pelvis, leg, hip
- Indwelling femoral vein catheters
- Inflammatory bowel disease
- Nephrotic syndrome
- Estrogen use
- Hypercoagulable states

suppressive drugs, prolonged hospitalization, recent antibiotic therapy, anergy to skin test, severity of underlying disease, obesity, indwelling catheters, poor tissue perfusion, glucocorticoid medications, and radiation therapy.

The most common and important acquired immune deficiency found in surgical patients is caused by malnutrition. Immunologic abnormalities, which accompany malnutrition, are both cellular and humoral. High-risk surgical patients have been found to have alterations in neutrophil chemotaxis and opsonic function. Many patients with trauma and a variety of advanced chronic diseases also have circulating inhibitors of chemotaxis and lymphocyte activation. Crude measurements of the nutritional status include albumin and transferrin levels; however, skin testing for delayed hypersensitivity antigens will further identify high-risk patients (that is, those with complete or relative anergy). Preoperative enteral nutrition should be instituted for 2 to 3 weeks before surgery if malnutrition appears to be a risk factor for development of infection.

Preoperative showering with hexachlorophene soap may decrease wound infection. Judicious use of prophylactic antibiotics significantly reduces the incidence of postoperative infections. Conversely, their use may be harmful because of toxic reactions, allergic responses, interference with normal immune defense mechanisms, and overgrowth of resistant organisms in the individual patient. Systemic prophylactic antibiotics are of most value in operations in which significant bacterial contamination can be anticipated. The adverse complications of systemic antibiotics outweigh their potential benefits when the expected incidence of infection is or should be less than 2%. This includes nearly all-clean operations, and some clean contaminated operations such as upper urinary tract or bladder operations without infected urine, elective cholecystectomy in patients younger than 70 years, gastrectomy for peptic ulcer, and abdominal hysterectomy. Exceptions to this rule include placement of intravascular prostheses or major joint replacement because of the grave consequences of infections after such operations and for operations on individuals with recent or existing infections who are known to be carriers of pathogenic bacteria. Prophylactic antibiotics are contraindicated for the prevention of infections associated with indwelling intravascular or urinary catheters, intubation of the trachea, and open wounds, because prophylactic treatment in these situations often leads to superinfection with resistant microorganisms. The principal guidelines for the use of prophylactic systemic antibiotics in surgery are

- The duration of contamination must be limited to brief periods, usually within the operative procedure.
- The anticipated degree of contamination should be sufficiently great to result in an expected incidence of infection greater than 2%.

Systemic antibiotics are valuable in preventing wound infection only when they are started before or very shortly after bacterial contamination. The best results are obtained when antibiotics are first given before operation. Prophylactic antibiotics are most effectively administered intravenously and should not be administered for more than 48 to 72 hours. Removal of hair from the operative field should be done with electric clippers immediately before the operation. Depilatories to remove hair may be used in preference to shaving. Preoperative bowel preparation reduces the risk of postoperative infection. It has evolved from a traditional, labor-intensive enema cathartic to an oral intestinal lavage preparation. Because of recent efforts to reduce the cost of medical care, many preoperative bowel preparations may be performed on outpatients.

Metabolic Abnormalities

Diabetes, hepatic dysfunction, adrenal insufficiency, and hyperthyroidism may alter the surgical approach to the patient or may require extra preoperative preparation. These situations are discussed in the following sections.

Diabetes

The stress of surgery leads to metabolic changes that worsen glycemic control, regardless of whether patients have diabetes. Surgical incisions result in increased stress hormone levels and relative insulin deficiency and resistance. Catecholamines, growth hormone, glucagon, adrenocorticotropic hormone, and cortisol levels have been documented to increase in the operative period for several days. These changes result in increased catabolism via glycogenolysis, lipolysis, and proteolysis, with a net increase in the production of glucose, free fatty acids, and ketone bodies. The anabolic action of insulin is blunted during the perioperative period, thereby decreasing the uptake and utilization of glucose by the liver and skeletal muscle.

In addition to surgery, inhalational anesthetics also induce a similar stress hormone release, even before the first incision is made. These combined factors result in hyperglycemia in the postoperative patient. Hyperglycemia adversely affects important clinical outcomes of surgery. Decreased wound healing has been documented in hyperglycemic animal models. Hyperglycemic patients have been found to have decreased neutrophil function and increased postoperative wound infections.

Gastroparesis, secondary to autonomic neuropathy caused by diabetes, can increase the likelihood of aspiration. Tachycardia, believed to be secondary to autonomic cardiac neuropathy, may be associated with orthostatic hypotension in the perioperative setting. The surgical patient should be evaluated for the duration of diabetes, current diet, last insulin administration, and peripheral symptoms. The feet should be examined for evidence of minor injuries, evidence of poor hygiene, and inadequate blood supply.

The goal of therapy is to maintain satisfactory glucose control in all patients with diabetes in the perioperative period. Patients who have diabetes that was previously controlled by diet or oral agents may require insulin in the perioperative period. Conversely, administration of insulin does increase the risk of hypoglycemia in a setting in which classic signs and symptoms may be masked by anesthesia and pain medications. Keeping the blood glucose between 150 to 200 mg/dL minimizes the adverse effect of hyperglycemia on wound healing and infection. Patients with poorly controlled diabetes and blood glucose greater than 250 mg/dL should have their care intensified in the perioperative period to achieve the target blood glucose levels.

The perioperative management of patients with diabetes is approached as follows:

1. Patients who are instructed not to eat or drink after midnight in preparation for an operation the next morning should reduce their AM insulin dose by one-half the usual dose of intermediate- or regular-acting insulin.
2. The patient should receive a continuous infusion of 5% dextrose to provide 10 g of glucose per hour. Intraoperatively, glucose levels should be assessed by fingerstick, and postoperatively, at least every 6 hours. A sliding scale of regular insulin should be administered based on the q6-hour fingerstick glucose levels. In brittle diabetic patients, continuous intravenous infusion of 1 to 3 units of insulin/hr may be preferable.

Diabetic ketoacidosis can be inadvertently overlooked in postoperative patients because it often occurs with nausea, vomiting, abdominal distention, or polyuria; therefore an assessment of urinary ketone levels should be monitored by dipstick.

Hepatic Dysfunction

Patients with liver disease undergoing surgery have significantly increased morbidity and mortality, particularly if overt disease is present preoperatively. Because liver disease is often asymptomatic, it is important to evaluate patients for preoperative risk factors and evidence of a liver disorder. Inquiry should be made about risk factors for chronic liver disease and the presence of symptoms attributable to liver disease. Specific helpful information includes a family history of jaundice, anemia, or liver disease; travel history; occupational history or exposure to hepatotoxins; alcohol or other drug exposure; and the use of prescription or over-the-counter medications. If signs of liver disease are present, elective surgery should be postponed until the cause and degree of hepatic dysfunction can be defined with biochemical testing. Most surgical procedures performed under general or regional anesthesia are followed by transient elevations of liver function tests (serum aminotransferases, alkaline phosphatase or bilirubin levels), which are minor and of questionable significance.

In patients with established hepatic dysfunction in the preoperative period, the additional stress of surgery may precipitate hepatic decompensation, resulting in increased mortality and morbidity. As the liver is a major site of drug metabolism, alterations in hepatic function may result in a prolonged duration of action of agents that are predominantly metabolized there. Drugs such as sedatives or narcotic analgesics that affect the central nervous system may cause a prolonged depression of consciousness or encephalopathy if administered to patients with severe liver disease. Agents such as methoxyflurane and halothane should be avoided in patients with known hepatic dysfunction.

Specific complications of liver disease including coagulopathy, malnutrition, or ascites may influence the outcome of surgical procedures. Coagulopathy may be present because of a vitamin K deficiency associated with cholestasis or impaired hepatic synthesis of vitamin K–dependent factors (factors II, V, VII, and X). Significant hepatocellular damage is necessary before inadequate clotting-factor synthesis results in prolongation of the prothrombin time. Hypoalbuminemia (<3.5 mg/dL) suggests significant hepatocellular insufficiency or starvation. Patients with cholestatic jaundice are at risk for postoperative renal failure.

The most commonly used approach for the prediction of perioperative risks in patients with hepatic dysfunction is based on the Child-Turcotte classification to predict mortality after portocaval shunt surgery; however, this system has never been prospectively validated in patients undergoing other types of surgery. A modification proposed by Pugh and associates replaced nutritional status with prothrombin time in the assessment of patients undergoing esophageal transection. The Child-Pugh score has been shown to correlate with perioperative mortality in the assessment of patients undergoing nonshunt surgery and in cirrhotic patients undergoing abdominal procedures. Serum albumin level, leukocytosis, and increased prothrombin time were the most sensitive indicators of perioperative mortality independent of the Child-Pugh Score. In their study, patients with Child class A, B, and C cirrhosis had mortality rates of 10%, 31%, and 76%, respectively.

Preoperative correction of coagulopathy is essential, even in urgent situations. It may be difficult to differentiate between vitamin K deficiency due to poor nutrition, malabsorption due to cholestasis, or impaired hepatic synthetic function. Both vitamin K (10 mg intramuscularly) and fresh frozen plasma are administered. Some patients may not correct their coagulopathy with this regimen and will require cryoprecipitate (10 U intravenously preoperatively), which contains large amounts of fibrinogen and von Willebrand factor. 1-Deamino-8-D-arginine vasopressin (DDAVP), 0.3 μg/kg intravenously, also causes the release of large amounts of endogenous von Willebrand factor. Prophylactic platelet transfusions may be considered for thrombocytopenia (platelet count, $<20 \times 10^9$/L).

Prevention of renal dysfunction is particularly important in the presence of jaundice. Anemia should be corrected preoperatively. Careful attention to volume status is critical. Nephrotoxic agents such as aminoglycosides or nonsteroidal anti-inflammatory drugs also should be avoided. Urine output should be monitored perioperatively with a Foley catheter. The use of lactulose to reduce endotoxemia may be useful in preserving renal function. Low-dose dopamine has been used to improve renal perfusion. Patients with cirrhosis often have hypokalemia and alkalosis, which should be corrected preoperatively to minimize the risk of cardiac arrhythmias and to diminish encephalopathy. Protein restriction also has been recommended for patients who respond to lactulose treatment, but excessive protein restriction can contribute to malnutrition.

The presence of ascites may influence respiratory mechanics and increase the risk of abdominal wound dehiscence. Ascites should be controlled preoperatively with paracentesis. Dietary sodium restriction is necessary, and reaccumulation of ascites is common with administration of intravenous fluids. Careful attention is essential to avoid excessive use of intravenous saline solutions and medications containing sodium, and the use of albumin or blood products or fresh frozen plasma. Diuretic therapy plays a crucial role in controlling ascites and requires close monitoring of electrolytes levels and renal function. If hyponatremia exists, fluid restriction may be necessary.

Adrenal Insufficiency

Prolonged use of steroids for a variety of inflammatory disorders (such as asthma, rheumatoid arthritis, inflammatory bowel disease) can cause suppression of the hypothalamic release of corticotropin-releasing hormone and the pituitary release of corticotropin, also known as adrenocorticotropic hormone. This leads to a decrease in adrenal production of cortisol, particularly if exogenous steroids are suddenly removed or reduced before surgical procedures. Any outpatient dose greater than the equivalent of 30 mg of hydrocortisone or 7.5 mg of prednisone exceeds the body's daily basal requirements and places the patient at risk of adrenal suppression. Intranasal, inhalational, and topical steroids reduce but do not eliminate the risk of adrenal suppression. A person who discontinues oral steroids after a year or more may still have partial adrenal insufficiency for as long as 9 months. Short courses of oral steroids for a week of less generally do not cause clinically significant suppression of the hypothalamic-pituitary-adrenal axis. Patients with adrenal insufficiency may be asymptomatic, have mild nonspecific complaints, or be in obtunded, hypotensive states. An intravenous drip of hydrocortisone at 10 mg/hr or doses of 100 mg every 8 hours provide adequate replacement for patients undergoing major operative procedures. Replacement therapy is tapered by approximately 20% per day once operative stress is resolved.

Hyperthyroidism

Hyperthyroidism may develop into thyroid storm, precipitated by stresses such as infection, iodine exposure, or surgery. Thyroid storm is a medical emergency with significant morbidity and mortality. Antithyroid drugs should be started immediately. Propylthiouracil is the thiourea drug of choice and is given as a single 1-g oral dose followed by 100 to 300 mg every 8 hours by mouth or nasogastric tube. This helps decrease thyroid hormone synthesis and prevents peripheral conversion of T_4 into the more biologically active T_3. Steroids, given as hydrocortisone, 100 mg intravenously every 8 hours, also help decrease peripheral conversion of T_4 to T_3. Iodide should be given 1 hour after the thiourea agent, as it prevents T_4 release. Hyperadrenergic symptoms and high-output heart failure are best controlled with β-blockers in a monitored setting. General supportive measures include controlling fever and vomiting status. Aspirin should be avoided, because salicylates may precipitate increased circulating levels of free thyroid hormone. Acetaminophen and cooling blankets are preferred to control temperature.

Alcohol Abuse

During recent years, several studies have shown a threefold increase in the postoperative morbidity in alcohol misusers who drink at least five drinks (>60 g ethanol) per day. Alcohol withdrawal, characterized by *delirium tremens,* is one of the most common complications that the addicted patient may experience on hospitalization. The mild symptoms of restlessness and anxiety associated with mild alcohol-withdrawal states can progress to hallucinations, fever, disorientation, and rarely death. Treatment with sedatives, usually benzodiazepines, is indicated. To prevent Wernicke encephalopathy and Korsakoff syndrome, patients should routinely receive 100 mg thiamine parenterally for at least the first day of hospitalization, and it should be administered before glucose administration. Oral thiamine should be avoided because of its decreased absorption in the presence of alcohol. Glucose in the thiamine-deficient patient may further exhaust the body's reserve of thiamine and precipitate Wernicke encephalopathy. These patients should also routinely receive multivitamin supplementation because deficiencies of folate and fat-soluble vitamins are common.

Suggested Reading

Jacobs LG, Nusbaum N: Perioperative management and reversal of antithrombotic therapy. Clin Geriatric Med 17:189–202, ix, 2001.

Kehlet H, Wilmore DW: Multimodal strategies to improve surgical outcome. Am J Surg 183:630–641, 2002.

Liu LL, Wiener-Kronish JP: Preoperative cardiac evaluation of women for noncardiac surgery. Card Clin 16:59–66, 1998.

Park KW: Critical review of the ACC/AHA algorithm for stratifying cardiac patients for noncardiac surgery. Int Anesth Clin 39:81–92, 2001.

Shaw M, Mandell BF: Perioperative management of selected problems in patients with rheumatic diseases. Rheum Dis Clin North Am 25:623–638, ix, 1999.

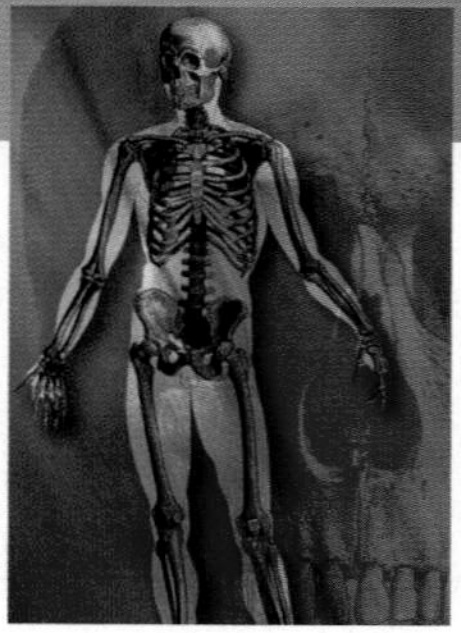

Chapter 6

Fluid and Electrolyte Management

GENE A. GRINDLINGER, MD

The prevention and treatment of fluid and electrolyte disturbances are integral parts of surgical care. To achieve homeostasis, the body maintains strict control of water and electrolyte distribution and of acid-base balance. This control is a function of the complex interplay of cellular membrane forces, specific organ activities, and systemic and local hormonal influences. These components of the metabolic machinery are intimately interconnected, and acute and chronic diseases, trauma, surgery, and the use of medications can adversely affect their interactions.

Total Body Water and Composition

Total Body Water

Total body water accounts for 60% or more of body weight. The percentage varies with age, sex, and proportion of body fat. Water is contained primarily in skeletal muscle. Because mature adipose tissue is nearly water-free, the amount of total body water decreases with obesity.

Fluid Compartments

Water is partitioned into intracellular and extracellular compartments. **Intracellular water** composes approximately two thirds of total body water, and **extracellular water** composes the remainder. Extracellular water is further divided into interstitial and intravascular compartments. **Interstitial water** accounts for 75% of extracellular water or 15% body weight (Table 6-1). **Intravascular water,** or plasma water, constitutes 25% of extracellular water volume or 4% to 7% of body weight. The intravascular, interstitial, and intravascular fluid compartments exist in dynamic equilibrium.

TABLE 6–1 Fluid Compartment

	Volume (L)*	% Total Body Water	% Body Weight
Plasma	3.5	8	4–7
Interstitium	10.5	25	15
Intracellular	28	67	40

*Based on a 70-kg adult.

The fluid compartments are separated by a semipermeable membrane. This membrane and its energy-dependent activities are required to maintain the differences in ionic and protein concentration gradients, which permit the chemical processes that define cellular life to proceed.

Electrolytes and Proteins in Fluid Compartments

Within each fluid compartment, the balance of the concentration of cations and anions maintains electrical neutrality (Table 6-2). In the **intracellular compartment,** potassium is the dominant cation. Most of the intracellular anions are in the form of inorganic and organic phosphates and polyvalent proteins. In the **interstitial and intravascular compartments,** sodium is the dominant cation. Electrical neutrality is maintained by a balanced amount of chloride and bicarbonate anions. Approximately 7% of plasma is in the form of protein, mostly anionic albumin, which cannot permeate the membrane. These proteins are critically important to maintaining intravascular volume. To maintain electrical neutrality, the negative charge on plasma albumin requires an increase in plasma cations, mostly sodium. The redistribution of ions across the semipermeable membrane is called the **Donnan effect.** The forces governing the redistribution are expressed as the **Gibbs-Donnan equation,** which holds that the product of any two cation and anion pairs on one side of the membrane will equal the product of the same two cation and anion pairs on the other side of the membrane:

$$([Na^+]_o \times [Cl^-]_o = [Na^+]_i \times [Cl^-]_i)$$

Osmolarity

Osmotic forces are the prime determinants of water distribution in the body. Osmolarity refers to the number of particles dissolved in a solution. Physiologic concentrations of osmotically active particles are measured in milliosmoles (mOsm). Osmolarity is independent of the chemical activity or ionic strength of the particles. For nonpolar substances like glucose, one mole of glucose added to 1 L of pure water would increase the osmolarity from 0 to 1 Osm/L. For ionic substances that dissociate into two ions (such as saline), one mole added would

TABLE 6–2 Electrolyte Composition in Extracellular and Intracellular Fluid

	Plasma (mEq/L)	Interstitium (mEq/L)	Plasma Water (mEq/L)	Intracellular* (mEq/L)
Cations				
Na^+	140	145.5	151	12
K^+	4.5	4.8	5	160
Ca^{2+}	5.0	3.0	5.5	—
Mg^{2+}	1.5	1.0	2	34
Anions				
Cl^-	104	117	112	2
HCO_3^-	24	27	26	10
SO_4^{2-}	1	1	1	—
HPO_4^{2-}	2	2	2	140
Protein	15	2	16	54
Organic anions	5	6	5	—

* In skeletal muscle.
Data from Carroll H, Oh M: Water, Electrolytes and Acid-Base Metabolism. Philadelphia, Lippincott, 1978, p 9.

produce 2 Osm/L. In plasma, the major determinants of osmolarity are sodium and its accompanying anions, urea and glucose. Normal serum osmolarity is 285 mOsm/L. The terms *osmolarity* and *osmolality* are often confused. Both terms refer to the concentration of osmotically active particles, but they express this concentration in different terms. **Osmolarity** expresses the concentration in terms of osmoles of solute per liter of solution (Osm/L). In contrast, **osmolality** expresses the concentration in terms of osmoles of solute per kilogram of solvent (Osm/kg). The laboratory osmometer measures osmolality, not osmolarity. At the solute concentration of normal body fluids, the osmolality and osmolarity are nearly equivalent. The major determinants of the osmotic activity of plasma are sodium, glucose, and urea. Therefore the osmolarity can be estimated by the simple equation:

$$\text{mOsm/L} = 2[\text{Na}^+] + \text{Glu}/18 + \text{BUN}/2.8$$

By convention, laboratories report glucose (Glu) and blood urea nitrogen (BUN) measurements in terms of milligrams per deciliter. The corrections in this equation for glucose and urea merely convert milligrams per deciliter into millimoles per liter. Because water is freely diffusible across the semipermeable membrane, the osmolarity of the intracellular fluid will be the same as that of the extracellular fluid.

Tonicity. Tonicity, or **effective osmolarity,** determines the movement of water across the cellular membrane. Tonicity is calculated by considering only the concentration of the impermeable solutes in solution. Urea freely crosses cellular membranes almost as fast as water does. This means that urea does not contribute to tonicity. Normal effective osmolarity of body fluids is 280 mOsm/kg. A reduction in effective osmolarity implies a relative water excess, whereas an increase in effective osmolarity implies relative dehydration.

Regulation of Volume. The kidneys exert the greatest influence on the regulation of intravascular volume. **Osmoreceptors** in the posterior pituitary detect small changes in serum osmolarity, which then regulates the release of antidiuretic hormones (ADH). **Baroreceptors** in the kidney, carotid, and elsewhere detect small changes in pressure. Ordinarily, baroreceptors play only a small role in the control of volume homeostasis.

The other key regulator of volume homeostasis is the **renin-angiotensin-aldosterone system.** Renin is an enzyme released from the juxtaglomerular cells of the afferent arteriole in response to a decrease in arterial blood pressure, a decrease in circulating volume, a reduction in sodium delivered to the macula densa (hyponatremia), and increases in β-adrenergic activity. Renin converts angiotensinogen to angiotensin-1 which, in turn, is converted to angiotensin-2 in the pulmonary circulation by angiotensin-converting enzyme (ACE). Angiotensin releases aldosterone from the adrenal cortex. Aldosterone, in turn, acts on the distal tubules and collecting tubules to increase sodium reabsorption and potassium excretion. Angiotensin also increases sympathetic activity as well as cardiac output and peripheral resistance.

Fluid Homeostasis

Fluid homeostasis is maintained under neuroendocrine and renal control. In steady state, water losses are balanced by gains. Normally, an adult ingests 2 to 3 L of water per day. Two thirds of the water intake is liquid, and one third is from ingested solids. In addition, 400 to 500 mL of water is gained by oxidative metabolism of fats and protein.

TABLE 6–3 Composition of Intravenous Therapy Solutions

Solution	Na^+ (mEq/L)	K^+ (mEq/L)	Ca^{2+} (mEq/L)	Mg^{2+} (mEq/L)	Cl^- (mEq/L)	HCO_3^- (mEq/L)	Glu (g/L)	Osm (mOsm/L)
0.9% NaCl (NS: normal saline)	154	—	—	—	154	—	—	308
D5/0.9% NaCl	154	—	—	—	154	—	50	560
0.45% NaCl (1/2 NS)	77	—	—	—	77	—	—	154
D5/0.45% NaCl	77	—	—	—	77	—	50	406
0.225% NaCl (1/4 NS)	38.5	—	—	—	38.5	—	—	77
D5/0.225% NaCl	38.5	—	—	—	38.5	—	50	329
Lactated Ringer's (LR)	130	4	3	—	109	28	—	273
3.0% NaCl (hypertonic)	513	—	—	—	513	—	—	1026

Water losses include those in urine (800–1500 mL/day) and feces (250 mL/day). Urinary losses of water are regulated by renal mechanisms, with 300 mL/day the minimal volume required to allow solute excretion. Water losses also are due to insensible mechanisms, mostly as evaporative water loss from the skin. Insensible loss through the lungs depends on ambient temperature, humidity, and respiratory rate. An average adult loses 600 to 900 mL of insensible water from the skin and lungs or 8 to 12 mL/kg/day. This insensible loss increases by 10% for each 1°C increase in body temperature.

Volume Deficits

Volume deficits may occur from chronic or acute losses.

Evaluation

Chronic volume depletion is manifested by oliguria, loss of skin turgor, orthostatic hypotension, low urine sodium concentration and a BUN/creatinine ratio that exceeds 15:1. The hematocrit will be elevated 5% to 6% per liter of volume deficit.

Acute volume losses are manifested by hypotension, tachycardia, and tachypnea. Signs of end-organ hypoperfusion may be present and include oliguria and altered mentation. In cases of severe volume deficits, skin mottling and acidosis are present.

The purpose of **fluid and electrolyte therapy** is to ensure homeostasis of total body water and its constituent solutes. The assessment of patient needs must account for existing deficits, ongoing losses, and maintenance requirements. Commercially prepared solutions (Table 6-3) can be supplemented with specific electrolytes to correct existing deficits and replace ongoing losses.

The total volume of fluid deficit is best approximated by the volume required to restore physiologic parameters to normal. A urinary output greater than 0.5 mL/kg is desirable. An isotonic solution, such as lactated Ringer's solution, is highly effective in restoring circulating volume. Normal saline (0.9% NaCl) solution also is commonly used.

Blood shed during surgery may require rapid replacement in the immediate postoperative period. In addition, evaporative water losses during a lengthy abdominal operation are considerable since the peritoneal surface is as much as 50% of the body surface area. During laparotomy, the estimated evaporative fluid loss is 10 mL/kg/hr.

Supplemental fluids and electrolytes must be administered to account for ongoing losses. In surgical patients, these losses are most commonly due to nasogastric output and to fistula and diarrheal losses. In addition, considerable fluid may be sequestered at the operative site ("third space"). The quantity of losses should be recorded daily, and the electrolyte content of the losses estimated according to the site of loss (Table 6-4). Third-space losses are replaced with isotonic saline.

Under normal ambient conditions, an average-sized adult requires 2500 mL of maintenance fluid per day. To this is added maintenance amounts of sodium (average, 1.0–2.0 mEq/kg/day) and potassium (average, 0.5–1.0 mEq/kg/day). Calcium, magnesium, and phosphorus supplements are not required for short-term therapy unless the patient is critically ill. If the patient is febrile, maintenance fluid must be increased by 10% for each degree above 37.2°C.

Sodium Homeostasis

Normal dietary salt intake is 6 to 15 g/day (100–250 mEq of sodium per day). A balanced amount of sodium is excreted in urine, stool, and sweat. Urinary losses are

TABLE 6–4 Electrolyte Composition of Gastrointestinal Secretions

	Na^+ mEq/L	K^+ mEq/L	Cl^- mEq/L	HCO_3^- mEq/L	H^+ mEq/L	L/day Volume
Gastric	60	10	140	—	90	1.5
Bile	135	5	105	35	—	0.5
Pancreatic	135	5	65	95	—	1.0
Jejunal	130	5	105	35	—	1.0
Ileal	140	10	70	50	—	3.0
Colon	60	70	15	30	—	—

tightly regulated by renal mechanisms. Ordinarily, 50 to 90 mEq of sodium is excreted each day in the urine. However, urinary losses can be reduced to 1 mEq/day during states of maximal sodium conservation. Conversely, they can exceed 5000 mEq/day.

Sodium Abnormalities

Hypernatremia

Hypernatremia is defined as a serum sodium concentration that exceeds 150 mEq/L. Hypernatremia is always accompanied by hyperosmolarity. Hypernatremia may occur with volume depletion, volume excess, or euvolemia.

Etiology

Hypernatremia may be due to excessive salt intake, excessive water loss, reduced salt excretion, or reduced water intake. Because water is freely permeable to the cell membrane, there is continuous equality of extracellular fluid and intracellular fluid osmolarity. Any net gain in sodium will increase the extracellular fluid and trigger transmembrane water shifts. These transcellular water shifts occur at the expense of intracellular volume leading to cellular dehydration. Ordinarily, the hyperosmolar state will drive thirst and ADH release. A failed thirst mechanism or lack of access to water will render an individual susceptible to hypernatremia.

Abnormalities of ADH synthesis (central diabetes insipidus) or activity (nephrogenic diabetes insipidus) may cause massive free-water losses. Central DI occurs in trauma patients with severe head injuries. Nephrogenic DI is usually a side effect of medication, most commonly lithium. Other causes include postobstructive uropathy and interstitial nephritis. In surgical patients, hypernatremia may result from the administration of loop diuretics, which lead to free water depletion, and from gastrointestinal losses.

Evaluation

Evaluation of the hypernatremic patient begins with a history, physical examination, and assessment of volume status. The degree of hypernatremia is dependent on the adequacy of the thirst mechanism and uninhibited access to water. The very young and the very old and debilitated are the most vulnerable

The principal target organ of hypernatremia is the central nervous system. Symptoms include malaise, lethargy, vomiting, generalized seizures, and coma. Rapid increases in sodium do not allow time for osmoequilibration, so rapid cerebral dehydration results. In the most severe cases, bridging intracranial veins can rupture, causing intracerebral and pericerebral hemorrhage. In chronic hypernatremia states, more time is available for cerebral adaptation by the intracellular accumulation of organic osmolites (mostly amino acids). This is called cerebral osmoregulation. The brain is the only organ that has this adaptation potential.

Treatment

Therapy for hypernatremia is directed first at restoring circulating volume with isotonic saline solution. Once intravascular volume is restored, hypernatremia is corrected by administration of free water in the form of D_5W. The free-water deficit may be calculated by beginning with the following formula:

$$\text{NTBW} \times 140\ \text{mEq/L} = \text{CTBW} \times \text{current}\ [\text{Na}^+]$$

where NTBW is the normal total body water, and CTBW is the current total body water. The free-water deficit is the difference between the NTBW and the CTBW.

Example: Assuming a 70-kg man with a serum sodium concentration of 160 mEq/L:

$$\text{NTBW} = 70 \times 0.6 = 42\ \text{L}.$$
$$42 \times 140\ \text{mEq/L} = \text{CTBW} \times 160\ \text{mEq/L}$$
$$\text{CTBW} = 36.75.$$

The free water deficit is 5.25 L.

Hyponatremia

Hyponatremia is defined as a serum sodium concentration that is less than 135 mEq/L.

Etiology, Classification, and Evaluation

Hyponatremia may be caused by excessive water intake, impaired renal water excretion, and loss of renal diluting capacity.

Symptoms of hyponatremia are mostly neurologic and are due to cellular swelling induced by extracellular fluid (ECF) hypo-osmolality. Cerebral swelling causes lethargy, confusion, vomiting, seizures, and coma. The symptoms rarely occur until serum sodium concentration decreases to less than 120 mEq/L, and then their severity is related to the rate of decrease. Thus rapidly occurring hyponatremia provokes symptoms at higher plasma sodium concentrations.

Hyponatremia may occur with volume excess, euvolemia, or volume depletion.

Hypervolemic Hyponatremia

Patients in this group often have edema. Causes include renal failure, congestive heart failure, chronic obstructive pulmonary disease with hypercarbia, and severe liver disease.

As renal impairment progresses and GFR decreases, the ability of tubules to excrete the normal filtered water load is reduced, resulting in hyponatremia. In heart failure and cirrhosis, although the total body water is increased, effective circulating volume is reduced because of low cardiac output and hypoproteinemia, thereby stimulating renal water reabsorption.

Normovolemic Hyponatremia

The most common cause of normovolemic hyponatremia is the syndrome of inappropriate secretion of ADH

PEARLS FOR THE OR

The most common cause of metabolic alkalosis in surgical patients is nasogastric losses or vomiting.
The peritoneal surfaces represent 50% of body surface area.
During laparotomy, the expected evaporative fluid loss from the exposed peritoneum is 10 mL/kg/hr.
Hyperphosphatemia may result from rhabdomyolysis due to muscle ischemia or crush injury.
The stress response to surgery results in the release of glucagon, aldosterone, cortisol, and antidiuretic hormone.

(SIADH). In this condition, hyponatremia occurs with a large urinary sodium output and an inappropriately high urinary osmolarity, despite the depressed plasma osmolarity. Plasma volume is normal or slightly increased. SIADH is seen in patients with central nervous system pathology such as stroke or injury and in pulmonary conditions including tuberculosis and cancer.

Hypovolemic Hyponatremia

Patients with hypovolemic hyponatremia have renal or extrarenal losses of sodium that exceed water losses.

Urinary electrolytes can help classify these disorders. A urinary sodium level greater than 20 mEq/L indicates renal losses, such as those associated with diuretic use, aldosterone deficiency, salt-losing nephritis, renal failure, and subarachnoid hemorrhage. Urinary sodium of less then 10 mEq/L indicates a normal tubular responsiveness to hyponatremia. Extrarenal losses of sodium include those due to vomiting, fistula, or diarrheal losses.

Pseudohyponatremia

A low plasma sodium concentration is misleading in two situations. In patients with hyperlipidemia or hyperproteinemia, the apparent hyponatremia is the consequence of the measurement technique. In plasma water, the sodium concentration is normal, and the measured osmolality also is normal. However, in whole plasma, the sodium concentration is low, owing to displacement of the water volume by protein or lipid. Calculated osmolarity is low because of factitiously low measured plasma sodium; measured osmolality is normal.

Osmotically active glucose will cause a dilutional hyponatremia. Each 100 mg/dL increase in the serum glucose concentration above normal will depress the serum sodium by 1.6 mEq/L. Correction of the hyperglycemia (with insulin) drives glucose and water into the cells and restores serum sodium concentration to normal.

Treatment

In hypervolemic patients, treatment includes volume restriction and loop diuretics. Patients with renal failure may require dialysis. Patients with SIADH usually respond to fluid restriction. In hypovolemic patients, treatment includes salt and water replacement. If hyponatremia is due to specific endocrine deficiencies, treatment with hormonal replacement is indicated.

In asymptomatic patients, hyponatremia should be treated slowly. Isotonic saline is the preferred fluid in those who require volume therapy. Addition of a loop diuretic may hasten water excretion, provided plasma volume is restored. Fluid restriction, a loop diuretic, and treatment of the underlying condition will suffice in those with normovolemic or hypervolemic states.

Symptomatic hyponatremia that is associated with seizures or coma requires more aggressive treatment. A danger of further neurologic damage exists if the sodium concentration is increased too rapidly. Myelin sheath damage primarily located in the pons (central pontine myelinolysis) has been shown to occur with rapid correction of hyponatremia. Current recommendations are to increase the serum sodium concentration no faster than 0.5 mEq/L/hr. The ultimate goal of therapy is to restore serum sodium concentration to normal. However, a concentration of 120 mEq/L appears safe. Once the serum sodium reaches 120 mEq/L and symptoms have abated, sodium correction should occur at a slower rate still.

The total sodium deficit (TSD) can be estimated from the following formula:

$$\text{TSD} = 0.6 \times \text{weight in kg} \times (140 - \text{measured } [\text{Na}^+])$$

This formula provides only an estimate of the sodium in milliequivalents needed to restore serum sodium concentration to normal. The actual amount of sodium required for correction will depend not only on the deficit but also on the ability of the kidneys to excrete dilute, sodium-depleted urine. Frequent monitoring of serum sodium concentration is essential.

In patients with stupor, coma, or other severe neurologic symptoms, hypertonic saline (3% NaCl) solution is used. Each liter of 3% saline contains 513 mEq of sodium and 513 mEq of chloride for an osmolarity of 1026 mOsm/L. The objective of hypertonic saline therapy is to restore serum sodium rapidly to 120 mEq/L at a rate of correction no greater than 0.5 mEq/L/hr. Thereafter, correction may proceed at a slower pace with isotonic saline.

Potassium Homeostasis

Potassium is the principal intracellular cation of the body. The quantity of potassium of the average-sized adult is 3800 mEq or 55 mEq/kg. Most of the potassium is located in skeletal muscle, where the concentration is 155 mEq/L, or more than 30 times the concentration outside of the cell. This concentration gradient is essential for cellular integrity and paramount for the function of excitable tissue such as muscle and nerve. The gradient is maintained by a membrane-bound sodium-potassium adenosine triphosphatase (ATPase). The energy cost of this electrolyte pump is estimated to be 15% to 20% of total body energy expenditure.

The normal plasma potassium concentration is 3.5 to 5 mEq/L. The normal potassium balance is maintained by external and internal mechanisms. The usual daily dietary intake of potassium is 1 to 1.5 mEq/kg. About 90% of the ingested potassium is eliminated by renal excretion. The remaining 10% appears in the stool. Healthy kidneys are capable of excreting 5 times the normal amount, or 6 mEq/kg/day, without an increase in plasma potassium above 6 mEq/L. Internal factors responsible for potassium balance include the effects of insulin, aldosterone, catecholamines, and acid-base balance.

PEARLS FOR ROUNDS

Tonicity rather than osmolarity determines water movement.

Sodium determines volume, osmolarity, and tonicity of extracellular fluid.

Rapid correction of hyponatremia may cause central pontine myelinolysis.

Hypomagnesemia may cause hypokalemia, hypophosphatemia, and hypocalcemia.

A very low urinary chloride concentration is a good indicator of extracellular fluid contraction from vomiting or nasogastric losses.

Potassium Abnormalities

Hyperkalemia

Hyperkalemia is defined as a serum potassium concentration greater than 5.5 mEq/L.

Etiology

Hyperkalemia can result from renal or adrenal insufficiency, metabolic acidosis, or iatrogenic causes. In patients with acute renal failure, a short-term reduction in the GFR leads to hyperkalemia. However, in those who have chronic renal disease, but intact distal sodium delivery, the body's adaptation mechanisms prevent hyperkalemia from developing until the GFR decreases to less than 10 mL/min. These adaptation mechanisms include an increase in the fractional excretion of potassium and an increase in colonic excretion (≤20–30 mEq/day).

Hyperkalemia occurs with metabolic acidosis due to transcellular exchange of K^+ and H^+. For each 0.1 decline in pH, serum potassium concentration increases by 0.6 mEq/L. Other extrarenal causes of hyperkalemia are intravascular hemolysis, rhabdomyolysis, seizures, and severe GI bleeding. Iatrogenic causes of hyperkalemia include medications (such as nonsteroidal anti-inflammatory drugs and ACE inhibitors) and excessive administration of potassium.

Pseudohyperkalemia

Spurious elevation of serum potassium occurs in a variety of situations. Examples include in vitro hemolysis due to excessive agitation of the specimen before its arrival in the laboratory and prolonged tourniquet time and fist clenching during blood drawing. This latter cause may elevate serum potassium by 1.6 mEq/L. Thrombocytosis (platelet count >1 million) and severe leukocytosis (white blood cells [WBC] >50,000) also falsely elevates serum potassium, presumably because of cellular release of potassium during in vitro clotting. True potassium levels are determined by measuring plasma rather than serum potassium.

Evaluation

The myocardial effects of severe hyperkalemia overshadow all other manifestations in importance. On the electrocardiogram, myocardial toxicity can be detected when the serum potassium concentration increases to more than 6 mEq/L. The earliest abnormality is peaking of the T wave. As plasma potassium increases, the PR interval becomes prolonged, and the RR interval increases. Further increases in the potassium concentration are associated with loss of P waves and widening of the QRS complex. Finally, complete heart block, ventricular tachycardia, and cardiac standstill occur. Extracardiac symptoms of hyperkalemia include paresthesias, flaccid paralysis, and ileus.

Treatment

Prompt reversal of cardiac toxicity is essential to avoid cardiac arrest. Even in the absence of electrocardiographic changes, a true elevation of the serum potassium above 7 mEq/L will require prompt and aggressive intervention.

Because calcium will antagonize the effect of hyperkalemia on cardiac conduction, 10 to 20 mL of 10% calcium gluconate should be administered. The response to calcium salt therapy occurs in 1 to 5 minutes and lasts 30 minutes. Concurrent treatment with insulin or sodium bicarbonate moves potassium into the cells. Administering 100 mEq of sodium bicarbonate is effective in the setting of metabolic acidosis. Its onset is immediate, but the duration of effect is short. Administering 10 units of insulin in 50 mL of a 50% dextrose solution (D_{50}) will elicit a response in 15 to 45 minutes that lasts 4 to 6 hours. None of these treatments will remove potassium from the body.

Potassium can be removed by treatment with the cation-exchange resin kayexalate (50–100 g as enema), or 40 g orally with sorbitol. Each gram of drug removes approximately 0.5 to 1.0 mEq of potassium. The onset of action is slow, and the effect lasts 4 to 6 hours. The most effective method of removing potassium is hemodialysis.

Hypokalemia

Hypokalemia is defined as a serum potassium concentration that is less than 3.5 mEq/L.

Etiology

Hypokalemia is a common problem in surgical patients and is usually caused by GI losses from vomiting, diarrhea, or fistula and by the use of diuretics.

Evaluation

Metabolic alkalosis often coexists with hypokalemia. Metabolic alkalosis decreases renal potassium conservation and so exacerbates hypokalemia.

Clinical manifestations of hypokalemia are often mild and include generalized weakness and fatigue. The electrocardiogram may show T-wave flattening or inversion, a diminished QRS voltage, and U waves. Unlike the findings in hyperkalemia, these changes do not correlate well with the changes in serum potassium concentration. In patients taking digoxin, however, hypokalemia can provoke life-threatening arrhythmias.

Treatment

The therapeutic goal is to increase the serum potassium concentration above 3.5 mEq/L while avoiding overtreatment. Wherever possible, the underlying defect should be corrected. Potassium should be given orally unless the hypokalemia is severe (<2.5 mEq/L), the patient is symptomatic, or the enteral route is contraindicated. Oral potassium supplements (60–80 mEq/day) coupled with normal dietary intake should correct a low serum potassium concentration in a few days. If more rapid oral therapy is required or aggressive intravenous therapy must be started, electrocardiographic monitoring and frequent assessment of serum potassium concentration are required.

Calcium Homeostasis

Calcium homeostasis involves an elaborate interplay of GI, renal, and hormonal influences. The body contains approximately 1400 g of calcium, of which 99% is located in bone, and only 0.07% is present in plasma. Calcium exists in three forms in plasma: 40% is bound to protein (mostly to albumin); 10% is a diffusible nonionized form that is bound to anion; and the remainder is a biologically active ionized form. Of the 1000 mg of calcium that is ingested in a normal diet, 200 mg is absorbed from the GI tract, and an equivalent amount is excreted by the kidneys.

The serum ionized calcium concentration is maintained within a narrow range of 4.4 to 5.3 mg/dL (1.1–1.3 mmol/L). A reduction in this concentration stimulates the release of parathyroid hormone (PTH) which increases calcium reabsorption from bone. PTH enhances calcium reabsorption from the distal convoluted tubule and stimulates the formation of the active metabolite of vitamin D that increases gut absorption of elemental calcium and facilitates the PTH effect on bone resorption. An elevation in serum concentration of ionized calcium causes the steps to take place in reverse.

Calcium Abnormalities

Hypercalcemia

Hypercalcemia is defined as an ionized calcium concentration that exceeds 5.3 mg/dL (1.3 mmol/L).

Etiology

Although hypercalcemia is most frequently associated with hyperparathyroidism in surgical patients, it also is commonly associated with cancer. Both cause excessive bone resorption and overwhelm the renal excretory capacity. Other causes of enhanced bone resorption include Paget's disease, pheochromocytoma, hyperthyroidism, and use of thiazide diuretics.

Evaluation

Patients with mild to moderate hypercalcemia (ionized calcium between 5.3 and 6.5 mg/dL (1.3–1.6 mmol/L) tend to be asymptomatic or complain only of malaise. Conversely, those with severe hypercalcemia (serum ionized calcium in excess of 6.5 mg/dL; 1.6 mmol/L) have a variety of neurologic, cardiovascular, renal, and GI symptoms, some of which are life threatening. Neurologic symptoms begin with lethargy and progress to stupor and coma as calcium levels increase. Cardiovascular manifestations include arrhythmias and a shortened QT interval. GI effects are anorexia, constipation, pancreatitis, and hyperacidity. The most common renal defect is polyuria.

Treatment

Patients with severe hypercalcemia (serum ionized calcium >6.5 mg/dL; 1.6mmol/L) require immediate therapy. If hyperparathyroidism is the cause of hypercalcemia, the best treatment is surgery. Initial supportive therapy includes saline diuresis and furosamide to increase calcium excretion. Calcitonin reduces bone resorption and has an immediate effect. The effect lasts only for 48 hours. Prolongation of calcitonin effect may occur with concomitant corticosteroid treatment. Biphosphonates are highly effective inhibitors of osteoclast activity but have a delayed onset of 2 to 3 days. Mithramycin has a more rapid onset of action, but it is associated with hepatic and renal toxicity. Dialysis may be required in patients with cardiac or renal failure.

Hypocalcemia

Hypocalcemia is defined as an ionized calcium concentration is less than 4.4 mg/dL (<1.1 mmol/L).

Etiology

Hypocalcemia in the surgical patient may occur after parathyroid or thyroid surgery. The onset may be immediate (hours) or delayed (1–2 days). Hypocalcemia also is seen in association with severe pancreatitis, magnesium deficiency, and after massive blood transfusion.

Evaluation

Patients with mild or moderate hypocalcemia, characterized by an ionized calcium concentration between 3.2 and 4.4 mg/dL (0.8–1.1 mmol/L) are usually asymptomatic.

Patients with severe hypocalcemia (serum ionized calcium <3.2 mg/dL; 0.8 mmol/L) usually have neuromuscular and cardiovascular manifestations. Neuromuscular findings include paresthesia, muscular spasm, seizures, tetany, and weakness. Rarely, laryngospasm or bronchospasm occurs. A Trousseau or Chvostek sign can be elicited on physical examination. Cardiovascular symptoms include arrhythmias, heart block, bradycardia, and refractory hypotension. Electrocardiographic findings include prolongation of the QT interval and T-wave inversion.

Treatment

Therapy is directed at treating the underlying disorder. In patients with asymptomatic hypocalcemia, calcium supplementation is usually not required. In patients with symptomatic or severe hypocalcemia, intravenous calcium therapy is indicated. Initially, 100 mg of elemental calcium is given over a 5- to 10-minute period. Subsequently, a calcium infusion of 0.5 to 2 mg/kg/hr is given. The calcium concentration must be monitored. Once the calcium concentration is corrected, enteral therapy with elemental calcium is begun at a dosage of 1 to 4 g/day.

Magnesium Homeostasis

Magnesium is the second most plentiful intracellular cation. The adult body contains about 2000 mEq (21–28 g) of magnesium. About 50% of this amount is found in bone, and the remainder is found principally in skeletal muscle, liver, and other nonmuscular soft tissue. The magnesium concentration is maintained within a tight concentration range of 1.6 to 2.1 mEq/L. Adults ingest approximately 25 mEq of magnesium daily. Approximately one third of magnesium is excreted in the stool, and the remainder is renally excreted.

Magnesium Abnormalities

Hypermagnesemia

Hypermagnesemia is defined as a serum magnesium concentration that exceeds 2.1 mEq/L.

Etiology

As the GFR decreases to less than 10 to 30 mL/min, so, too, does renal excretion of magnesium. Magnesium intake, including magnesium-rich antacids, must be curtailed in patients with acute or chronic renal failure. Hypermagnesemia also occurs in patients with Addison's disease.

Evaluation

Symptoms are usually not seen until the plasma magnesium concentration exceeds 4 mEq/L. Neuromuscular sequelae include loss of deep tendon reflexes, somnolence, and impaired respiratory drive or apnea. Cardiac effects include bradycardia and heart block. Cardiac arrest can occur with profound elevations.

Treatment

In symptomatic patients, therapy consists of antagonizing the physiologic effects of magnesium with calcium infusion (5–10 mEq of calcium), followed by immediate dialysis. If renal function is intact, prompt saline diuresis should be initiated. Long-term therapy consists of removing all exogenous magnesium intake.

Hypomagnesemia

Hypomagnesemia is defined as a serum magnesium concentration less than 1.6 mEq/L.

Etiology

Hypomagnesemia is a common electrolyte disorder in surgical patients and has a variety of causes. It occurs as a result of GI losses, reduced absorption (short bowel syndrome), and excessive urinary losses from alcoholism, primary aldosteronism, and use of diuretics or aminoglycosides.

Hypomagnesemia is associated with other electrolyte disorders. A low serum magnesium level promotes renal potassium wasting (hypokalemia) and diminished renal tubular phosphate absorption (hypophosphatemia). Hypocalcemia occurs as the result of a hypomagnesemia-induced reduction in PTH release (hypoparathyroidism) and diminished renal PTH response (pseudohypoparathyroidism).

Evaluation

Symptoms occur when the serum magnesium concentration decreases to less than 1 mEq/L. Neuromuscular manifestations of magnesium deficiency are tremor, ataxia, carpopedal spasm, and tetany. Cardiotoxicity is exhibited by prolongation of the QT interval, which may lead to ventricular tachycardia (torsades de pointes).

Treatment

Symptomatic magnesium deficiency is treated with a magnesium infusion (8–16 mEq of magnesium over a 5- to 10-minute period, followed by 48 mEq/day). If treatment is not urgent, magnesium supplements can be given orally.

Phosphate Homeostasis

Dietary intake of phosphorus is 800 to 1200 mg/day. Under the control of vitamin D_3 and its metabolites, 80% of ingested phosphorus is reabsorbed, principally in the jejunum. Of the 700 to 800 g of phosphorus that is present in the average adult, 85% is found in bone. However, mobilization of phosphate from bone contributes very little to maintenance of serum phosphate concentration. By varying its resorption of phosphate, the kidney acts as the principal regulator of phosphate homeostasis. Both PTH and vitamin D_3 decrease the renal reabsorption of phosphate, and dietary phosphate deprivation markedly increases renal phosphate reabsorption. The normal serum phosphate concentration is 2.5 to 4.5 mg/dL (0.8–1.5 mmol/L).

Almost all plasma phosphorus exists as phosphate anion. Phosphate is the principal intracellular anion. Phosphorus is an essential element of the phospholipid cell membranes, of nucleic acids, and phosphoproteins. Intracellular phosphate regulates glycolysis, ammonia production, and red blood cell synthesis of 2,3 diphosphoglycerate (2,3-DPG). Phosphorus is the source of the high-energy bonds of ATP.

Phosphate Abnormalities

Hyperphosphatemia

Hyperphosphatemia is defined as a serum phosphate concentration that exceeds 4.5 mg/dL (1.5 mmol/L).

Etiology

The most common cause of hyperphosphatemia is renal insufficiency. It is most severe in those patients with acute renal failure caused by rhabdomyolysis or tumor cell lysis. Other causes of hyperphosphatemia include thyrotoxicosis, malignant hyperthermia, and hypoparathyroidism.

Evaluation

Few symptoms are associated with elevation of the serum phosphate concentration. The electrolyte disorder is discovered most commonly by laboratory testing. The major complication of hyperphosphatemia is hypocalcemia. In chronic hyperphosphatemia, elevated phosphate concentrations may cause metastatic calcifications and even arterial obstruction (calciphylaxis).

Treatment

The best way to manage hyperphosphatemia is to treat the underlying renal failure. In chronic hyperphosphatemia, phosphate-binding antacids are effective. In those with acute hyperphosphatemia or end-stage renal disease, dialysis is required.

Hypophosphatemia

Hypophosphatemia is defined as a serum phosphate concentration less than 2.5 mg/dL (0.8 mmol/L).

Etiology

Hypophosphatemia is commonly seen as a consequence of many disease processes. The reduction in serum phosphate concentration is attributable to transcellular shifts, excessive urinary losses, decreased dietary intake, or decreased intestinal absorption. More than one of these mechanisms is usually operative in a given patient.

Mild to moderate hypophosphatemia may be caused by diuretic use, hyperparathyroidism, malabsorption, hypomagnesemia, and vitamin D deficiency.

Severe hypophosphatemia, with phosphorus concentration less than 1 mg/dL (0.5 mmol/L), may be caused by chronic respiratory alkalosis, chronic alcoholism, severe burns, and treatment of diabetic ketoacidosis.

Evaluation

Mild to moderate reduction in serum phosphate concentration rarely causes symptoms. The earliest signs of severe hypophosphatemia are myalgias and muscle weakness. If the hypophosphatemia is allowed to persist, rhabdomyolysis may result. Progressive muscular dysfunction may precipitate congestive heart failure and respiratory insufficiency. The reduction in red blood cell 2,3-DPG will increase the hemoglobin affinity for oxygen and thereby lead to tissue hypoxia.

Treatment

Treatment of hypophosphatemia consists of oral or parenteral phosphate repletion and correction of the underlying disorder.

Acid-base Balance

Acid-base balance is critically necessary for cellular homeostasis. For biochemical processes to proceed normally, the hydrogen ion concentration must be maintained within a narrow concentration range. Unlike that of other electrolytes, the intake of hydrogen ions is not dietary. Instead, the hydrogen ions are a by-product of normal cellular metabolism.

Approximately 60 mEq of the fixed acids (citric, pyruvic, sulfuric, phosphoric, and acetoacetic acids) are produced daily by normal cellular activity. Because the acids ionize at physiologic pH, 60 mEq of hydrogen ion is liberated daily. This production is matched by an equivalent daily excretion of 60 mEq. Extracellular fluid has a pH of 7.40 and a hydrogen ion concentration of 40 nEq/L. Because the average adult has 17 L of extracellular fluid, a total of 700 nEq of hydrogen ion is present in the extracellular fluid. Because the daily production of hydrogen ion is 100,000 times the entire extracellular reservoir, a simple scheme of production on the one hand and renal excretion on the other would be inadequate. Thus the need for buffers. Bicarbonate and hemoglobin are the main buffers of the body, and they account for 88% of the total buffering capacity.

A parallel source of acid production is the result of the generation of CO_2 by oxidative metabolism. Approximately 200 mL of CO_2 is produced each minute. In body fluids, CO_2 combines with water to form carbonic acid, especially if stimulated by the enzyme carbonic anhydrase.

$$CO_2 + H_2O = H_2CO_3 = H^+ + HCO_3^-$$

If all of the CO_2 produced were converted to hydrogen ion, 13,000 mEq/day would result. This, of course, does not occur. Most of the CO_2 produced is either dissolved in water or bound to hemoglobin, and only 1 in 800 molecules becomes carbonic acid, itself a very weakly dissociating acid. Nonetheless, the hydrogen ion produced from this source is huge. Because carbonic acid is eliminated as a gas, it is referred to as a volatile acid. Volatile acids also are buffered by bicarbonate. The relation is expressed in the Henderson-Hesselbalch equation as follows:

$$pH = pK_a + \log HCO_3^-/H_2CO_3$$

The pK_a of the reaction is 6.1, and the ratio of the buffer pair is maintained at 20:1. This equation is mathematically identical to the following:

$$H^+ = 24 \times Pco_2/HCO_3^-$$

To use this formula, clinicians must convert pH to hydrogen ion concentration (Table 6-5).

The Henderson-Hesselbalch equation is useful because it provides much information about hydrogen ion homeostasis, renal and lung hydrogen elimination, and fixed and volatile hydrogen ion production. In addition to bicarbonate buffer, other buffers also participate. The ways in which the lungs and kidneys handle hydrogen ion are fundamentally different. The lungs are capable of responding instantly to sudden increases in acid production. Healthy lungs can increase CO_2 excretion by a factor of 10 (as in severe exercise). They do so at a cost though, the loss of buffer. The kidney regenerates the buffer by bicarbonate reabsorption and ammonia production. The renal response is slow, however, and maximal adaptation takes days.

TABLE 6–5 Conversion of pH to H^+ Ion Concentration*

pH	H^+ (mEq/L)
7.0	100
7.1	80
7.2	64
7.3	50
7.4	40
7.5	32
7.6	25
7.7	20

*Note that for each 0.1 increase in pH, the hydrogen ion concentration decreases by a factor of 0.8 times the preceding concentration.

Acid-base Imbalances

Metabolic Acidosis

Metabolic acidosis is present when the pH is less than 7.35 and the plasma bicarbonate concentration is less than 22 mEq/L. The increase in hydrogen ion concentration is due to either a reduction in buffer base or an increase in fixed acids. In spontaneously breathing patients, the increase in hydrogen ion concentration should stimulate a compensatory increase in the ventilatory rate, thereby decreasing the Pco_2 (about a 1.3 mmHg decrease in Pco_2 for each 1 mEq/L decrease in HCO_3^-).

Etiology and Classification

The presence or absence of an anion gap helps to categorize metabolic acidoses. The **anion gap** is calculated as the difference between the concentration of the major extracellular cation sodium and the major anions chloride plus bicarbonate. A normal anion gap is 8 to12 mEq/L and corresponds to the "unmeasured anions," primarily plasma protein, and a small amount of fixed acids.

Anion Gap Metabolic Acidosis

The causes of anion gap acidosis (Box 6-1) can be remembered by the mnemonic "DR. MAPLES." In surgical patients, the most important causes are lactic acidosis (which occurs secondary to hypoperfusion, and blood loss), diabetic ketoacidosis, renal failure, and ethanol ingestion. With the exception of renal failure, all of the other causes of anion gap acidosis are clinical states in which the daily production of fixed acids and thus the daily liberation of hydrogen ion exceeds 60 mEq/day.

In trauma patients, metabolic acidosis must be assumed to be due to blood loss (hypoperfusion, and tissue hypoxia) until proven otherwise. Poor perfusion from hypovolemia or other causes results in anaerobic metabolism and an increase in lactic acid production. In some cases, lactic acidosis occurs in conditions unassociated with hypo-

BOX 6-1 Causes of Anion Gap Acidosis

Mnemonic **"DR. MAPLES"**

Diabetic ketoacidosis
Renal failure
Methanol
Alcohol
Paraldehyde
Lactic acidosis
Ethylene glycol
Salicylates

perfusion or tissue hypoxia. These disorders include diabetic ketoacidosis, cirrhosis, leukemia and certain solid malignancies, severe infection, and short gut syndrome.

Non–Anion Gap Metabolic Acidosis

This type of metabolic acidosis is characterized by loss of buffer base. Common causes include GI tract losses (especially biliary and pancreatic losses), renal tubular acidosis, Addison's disease, total parenteral nutrition, and use of carbonic anhydrase inhibitors (Box 6-2).

Evaluation

Metabolic acidosis has obvious detrimental effects on body homeostasis including myocardial depression, hypotension, arrhythmias, hyperkalemia, hyperventilation, insulin resistance, obtundation, and coma. Acidosis reduces hepatic utilization of lactate, and it may stimulate hepatic lactic acid production, thereby worsening acidosis.

Treatment and Complications

Treatment of metabolic acidosis is specific to the etiology. In trauma patients, restoration of the circulating volume with blood and fluids normally will correct the disorder. In patients with diabetic ketoacidosis, management includes administering insulin, restoring the circulating volume, and searching for systemic infection.

Therapy with sodium bicarbonate is reserved for those with severe acidosis (pH <7.2) and in those patients with life-threatening ventricular arrhythmias, hemodynamic instability, inadequate compensatory response, or delay in correction of the underlying disorders. If bicarbonate is used, the goal of therapy is the partial restoration, rather than the complete restoration, of pH. Based on the volume of distribution of bicarbonate (0.5) and the patient's weight (in kilograms), the following formula can be used to calculate the amount of bicarbonate (in milliequivalents) that will be needed:

$$\text{Base deficit} = 0.5 \times (\text{weight in kg}) \times (\text{desired } HCO_3^- - \text{current } HCO_3^-)$$

The buffering of hydrogen with bicarbonate releases CO_2 and increases Pco_2, which may be problematic in patients with limited respiratory reserve. Sodium bicarbonate therapy is associated with other risks including hypernatremia, hyperosmolarity, and volume overload.

BOX 6–2 Causes of Non–Anion Gap Acidosis

- Gastrointestinal tract losses
  - Pancreatic/biliary
  - Diarrhea
- Renal tubular acidosis
- Addison's disease
- Excessive administration of normal saline
- Posthypocapneic
- Use of carbonic anhydrous inhibitors
- Hyperalimentation

Metabolic Alkalosis

Given the enormous rate of acid production by the body, it is a paradox that alkalosis occurs at all. Alkalosis is explained by the inability of the kidney to excrete excess bicarbonate or to retain hydrogen ion. Metabolic alkalosis is accompanied usually by respiratory compensation. Pco_2 increases 5 to 7 mm Hg for each 10 mEq/L of increase in plasma bicarbonate concentration.

Etiology and Evaluation

Causes of metabolic alkalosis can be divided into those that are responsive to chloride and those that are unresponsive (Table 6-6). Patients with **chloride-responsive metabolic alkalosis** usually have a contracted extracellular volume and chloride deficit, and a urinary chloride that is less than 10 mEq/L. Vomiting and high nasogastric outputs are common causes. The volume deficit stimulates sodium retention. The passively absorbed sodium in the proximal tubule requires an accompanying anion. Because a deficit of chloride exists, the anion available to meet this need is bicarbonate. In late stages of severe contraction alkalosis, hydrogen is exchanged for sodium, despite plasma alkalemia (paradoxical aciduria).

Patients with **chloride-unresponsive metabolic alkaloses** are normovolemic or hypervolemic and have a urinary chloride concentration that exceeds 10 mEq/L. Examples include Cushing's syndrome, hyperaldosteronism, and Bartter's syndrome.

Severe metabolic alkalosis (with a pH >7.60 and an HCO_3^- concentration >35 mEq/L) is associated with cerebral hypoperfusion, a leftward shift of the oxyhemoglobin dissociation curve, and hypokalemia. Respiratory symptoms include hypoventilation and hypoxemia.

Treatment

Therapy is directed at the underlying deficit. Patients with a contraction alkalosis are treated effectively with saline. Patients with chloride-unresponsive metabolic alkalosis may require treatment with the carbonic anhydrase inhibitor, acetazolamide. If enteral administration is not

TABLE 6–6 Metabolic Alkalosis

Chloride Responsive	Chloride Resistant
Nasogastric losses	Mineralocortical excess
Vomiting	Aldosteronism
Past use of diuretics	Renal artery stenosis
Volume contraction	Renin-secreting tumor
Posthypercapneic	Cushing's syndrome
	Bartter's syndrome

possible, severe alkalemia can be treated with an infusion of 0.1N HCl. The source of mineralocorticoid excess, if possible, should be corrected.

Respiratory Acidosis

Respiratory acidosis is present when the pH is low and the P_{CO_2} is elevated. Respiratory acidosis may be acute or chronic, depending on the etiology, time of evolution of the disorder, and degree of renal compensation.

Etiology

Respiratory acidosis is due to ineffective alveolar ventilation. Causes include decompensation of preexisting respiratory disease, asthma, neuromuscular disorders, central nervous system depression, and airway obstruction.

Evaluation

Plasma bicarbonate concentrations do not increase substantially in acute respiratory acidosis. The expected response is only a 1 mEq increase in HCO_3^- for each 10-mm Hg increase in P_{CO_2}. However, in chronic respiratory acidosis, renal adaptation is substantial. Plasma bicarbonate concentrations increase 3 to 4 mEq/L for each 10-mm Hg increase in P_{CO_2}. Renal compensation never restores pH to normal levels.

Treatment

Treatment of respiratory acidosis is directed toward improving alveolar ventilation. This may require intubation and mechanical ventilation. In chronic respiratory acidosis, the goal of therapy is restoration of a compensated steady state because the underlying defect is usually uncorrectable.

Respiratory Alkalosis

Respiratory alkalosis is present when the pH is high and the P_{CO_2} is low. The condition may be acute or chronic.

Etiology

Respiratory alkalosis is caused by alveolar hyperventilation. In surgical patients, this may be due to hypoxia, central nervous system lesions, pain, hepatic encephalopathy and mechanical ventilation.

Evaluation

In acute respiratory alkalosis, renal compensation is minimal. In contrast, in chronic respiratory alkalosis, the kidney responds by decreasing the excretion of hydrogen ion. The serum bicarbonate concentration is expected to decrease by 4 to 5 mEq/L for each 10-mm Hg decrease in P_{CO_2}.

Most patients with respiratory alkalosis are asymptomatic. Those with severe alkalosis may have carpopedal spasm, circumoral numbness, cramps, and confusional states. Hyperventilation is particularly dangerous in patients with subarachnoid hemorrhage because it exacerbates vasospasm.

Treatment

Treatment of respiratory alkalosis is directed toward correcting the underlying problem.

Suggested Reading

Adrogue H, Madias N: Management of life-threatening acid-base disorders. N Engl J Med 338:26–34, 1998.

Gennari F: Serum osmolality. N Engl J Med 310:102–105, 1984.

Halperin M, Goldstein M: Fluid, Electrolyte, and Acid-base Physiology, Vol III. Philadelphia, WB Saunders, 1999, pp 386–409.

Kobrin S, Goldfarb S: Hypocalcemia and hypercalcemia. In Adrogue H (ed): Acid-base and Electrolyte Disorders. New York, Churchill Livingstone, 1991, pp 69–96.

Oh M, Corroll H: Disorders of sodium metabolism: Hypernatremia and hyponatremia. Crit Care Med 20:94–103, 1992.

Pestana C: Fluids and Electrolytes in the Surgical Patient, 2nd ed. Baltimore, Williams & Wilkins, 1981, pp 101–144.

Rutecki G, Whittier F: Life-threatening phosphate imbalance: When to suspect, how to treat. J Crit Illness 12:699–704, 1997.

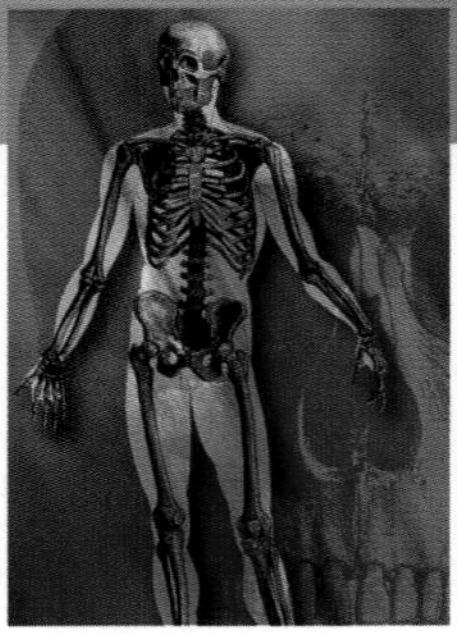

Chapter 7

Nutrition in Surgical Patients

R. ARMOUR FORSE, MD, PhD

Nutritional support is adjuvant therapy used to support the surgical patients until they are able to sustain themselves with adequate spontaneous nutrition by mouth. Nutritional support can be provided in many forms from oral supplements to total parenteral nutrition (TPN). The enteral approach to feeding is optimal, and the objective of nutritional support is to transition to the enteral route and a normal diet as soon as possible. The principles of nutritional support are to reduce the degree of malnutrition and to support or modulate or both the pathophysiology associated with the patients underlying disease. The latter is nutritional pharmacology, an evolving area with some exciting prospects.

Patients require nutritional support because either they are already malnourished or they will become malnourished because of our surgical therapy. This latter individual is typically the person who will not eat for 5 to 7 days because of the surgical disease (i.e., pancreatitis), or because of the surgery. The postsurgery period of receiving minimal or no nutrition is quite varied. Some surgeons leave patients with nothing by mouth (NPO) until evidence of a functional gastrointestinal tract is found, whereas others start oral fluids on postoperative day (POD) 1. This is dependent on the magnitude of the surgery, but also on surgeon bias.

Despite the growing awareness of the importance of nutrition in health and disease, the malnourished patient continues to go unrecognized throughout the medical community. Surveys indicate that up to 40% of hospitalized patients on both the medical and surgical wards are malnourished and are not receiving adequate nutritional support.

The metabolic response to surgery produces both calorie and protein malnutrition, termed *marasmus*. Injury from either surgery, trauma, or complications such as sepsis produces a well-defined metabolic change in the host. The characteristics of the phenotypic change include (1) mobilization of glucose and the development of peripheral insulin resistance; (2) protein catabolism with mobilization of peripheral protein to support the increased protein requirements and to support hepatic gluconeogenesis; (3) hypermetabolism with an increased energy expenditure; and (4) salt and water retention with an expanding third space. Early phases of the response are the ebb phase, when the changes are evolving, and the flow phase, when this response is established. Once the patient recovers from the injury, he or she undergoes a turning point with downregulation of the response and enters convalescence. The complete response can be minimal, occurring over a matter of hours, such as with a hernia repair, or can be quite extensive, extending over weeks, such as with a severe burn that becomes infected. The extent of the convalescence period is directly proportional to the extent of the metabolic response and particularly the protein mobilization. No protein stores exist in the human body, with protein being structural or functional. Any protein lost must be replaced for the patient to return to the preinjury condition.

Nutritional therapy is dynamic and must change and be adjusted to the surgical patient's clinical condition. Nutritional therapy should support the patient and his or her clinical situation and should not be designed to match any one nutritional therapy or delivery system.

Nutritional Assessment

The surgical patient who receives nutritional support is the individual who is malnourished or in whom malnutrition will develop as part of the surgical therapy. The two forms of malnutrition are protein malnutrition, or kwashiorkor, and protein-calorie malnutrition, or marasmus. An example of patients with protein malnutrition are the elderly. Patients with combined malnutrition are those with cancer cachexia. The assessment of the nutritional state of the patient is based on a clinical or a laboratory evaluation or both. The former approaches are more user friendly and clinically applicable. The latter are used to evaluate nutritional therapies and, although they are more accurate, they are not clinically applicable.

Clinical Assessment

This assessment is done in a traditional manner: history, physical examination, and basic laboratory values with a dose of "good clinical judgment." This combination of clinical variables is very effective.

In taking the history, one inquires about the patient's general condition, any fatigue, and the ability to work and carry out daily activities. A key element is a history of altered or poor oral intake, looking for both poor macronutrient and micronutrient consumption. Patients with gastrointestinal symptoms such as anorexia, nausea, vomiting, or diarrhea for more than a 2-week period will often have associated malnutrition. A history of poor wound healing is a concern. Recent unexpected weight loss is very important, and a weight loss of 10% or greater represents malnutrition. On examination, the patient may have temporal and interdigital wasting. The presence of ascites and ankle edema is seen with malnutrition, particularly protein malnutrition. The physical examination must include the anthropometric parameters of weight, height, and body mass index (BMI) and can also include midarm circumference, triceps skinfold, and the creatinine/height index. The weight and height can be used to determine the patient's ideal body weight for comparison. The other anthropometric parameters are used to determine the patient's nutritional assessment against available standards.

Laboratory

Biochemical

The basic laboratory value that is used to determine the nutritional state is the serum albumin. In patients who have only malnutrition and no stress, the albumin is a relatively reliable nutritional marker. With surgical patients, both the disease and the surgical procedure decrease the albumin because of leaking of albumin from the vascular space and relative decreases in albumin production, making the serum albumin an unreliable nutritional measure. The long half-life of albumin of 18 to 21 days makes changes in this protein not a reflection of acute nutritional or metabolic changes. Other biochemical markers include transferrin (half-life of 7–8 days) and prealbumin (half-life of 2 days); however, despite their relative short half-life, disease and recent surgical-injury response makes them unreliable markers.

Body Composition

Body composition is based on water and electrolytes, with potassium being the predominant intracellular anion and sodium the extracellular one. Isotopes are used to measure the concentration of these ions and body water, and thus to calculate the intracellular space or body cell mass, the extracellular space or extracellular mass, and the body fat. Bioelectrical impedance uses the resistance of the body to a very low energy electrical current to assess body composition. The resistance of the body is proportional to its water and electrolyte composition, and from the results, the lean body mass and the body fat are calculated. All of these composition measurements are a problem in the surgical patient, in whom water and electrolytes are altered by the surgical disease and surgical stress (Box 7-1). Although these measurements can be more accurate, they are not clinically practical.

BOX 7-1 Characteristics of Surgical Stress

Hypermetabolism
Protein catabolism
Insulin resistance
Salt and water sequestration

Nitrogen Balance

Nitrogen balance is based on the difference between the nitrogen intake and the nitrogen output over a 24-hour period. Although it is easy to determine, the balance must include estimates of body losses and is accurate only in the patient nutritionally stable for 3 days. Balance studies have intrinsic errors including nitrogen losses, which are always an underestimate, and nitrogen intake, which is always an overestimate. These errors are additive, being carried from day to day, and are in the opposite direction. Consequently, balances of more than 1 one day in the clinical setting only add to the unreliability of the study. To calculate the nitrogen balance, divide the protein intake by 6.25 to obtain the amount of nitrogen. The urinary nitrogen is measured in the urine, and 4 is added to the balance for other losses.

$$\text{Nitrogen balance} = (\text{Nitrogen intake}) - (\text{Urine nitrogen} + 4)$$

In moderate surgical stress, the balance may be 4 to 6 grams negative, and with severe stress, 10 grams negative.

Immunologic Assessment

The immune state is affected by malnutrition, as both micro- and macronutrient deficiencies will cause immune dysfunction. Thus an assessment of immunity can determine the degree and impact of malnutrition on the surgical patient. As the altered immune state is due not only to malnutrition but also to the pathophysiology of the disease and the surgical injury, it is not reliable for the individual patient. An example of this is recall skin antigens used to measure the cellular immunity. Surgical patients have an anergic state (no response to recall antigens) that does not change with changes in body composition until the surgical disease is corrected. This does not distract from the important concept that the malnourished surgical patient has depressed immunity and increased susceptibility to infection.

Requirements

Feeding Weight

An area of controversy is what weight to use in calculating the patient's nutritional requirements (Table 7-1). Usually the patient reports his or her actual weight (ABW) with the ideal weight being (IBW) calculated based on the patient's height. In the patient who is malnourished and who has an ABW less than the IBW, the ABW should be used to

TABLE 7–1 Nutritional Requirements

Component	Requirement
Access	Support is enteral and parenteral using transition to enteral
Fluid	Restriction to 30mL/kg/day
Sodium	Limited to 1.5 mEq/kg/day
Potassium	1.0 mEq/kg/day
Protein	1.5–2.0 g/ kg/day arginine, glutamine for selected patients
Calories	Limited to 20–25 kcal/kg/day
Carbohydrate	4 mg/kg/min. Avoid blood sugar >220 mg/L
Lipid	Not >20% calories or 0.11 g/kg/hr. Continuous source, consider MCT and omega 3
Vitamins	RDA (additional vitamins C and E)
Trace elements	Selenium, copper, magnesium, zinc

MCT, medium-chain triglyceride; RDA, recommended daily allowance.

calculate the nutritional requirements. In the patient who is obese with an ABW greater than the IBW, an estimated body weight (EBW) should be used to try to estimate the lean body mass. The rationale for using the EBW is to avoid nutritional support that will increase the body fat. The EBW is calculated by taking one fourth of the difference between the ABW and the IBW and adding it to the IBW. This is based on the observation that one fourth of fat tissue is actually the lean tissue to support that adipose tissue.

$$\text{EBW} = \text{IBW} + ([\text{ABW} - \text{IBW}]/4)$$

Total Energy

The calculation of the total calories required also is an area for debate. Although one could measure the resting energy expenditure (REE), this is not easy or reliable in the clinical setting. For the critically ill surgical patient, the measurement of the REE is very difficult (Table 7-2). Consequently the REE for the patient is usually calculated by using a formula. A patient requiring nutritional support for prolonged time or who has complicated nutritional support or both should have the REE measured to avoid overfeeding. The recommended number of calories to start with is 25 kcal/kg/day. If overfeeding is a concern, then start with 20 kcal/kg/day and carefully add calories as tolerated. It is always better to underfeed initially than to overfeed your patient.

The REE is calculated by using the Harris Benedict equations, with correction for injury and activity.

$$\text{Caloric requirements} = \text{Harris Benedict} \times \text{Injury factor} \times \text{Activity factor.}$$

The Harris Benedict equations are as follows.

$$\text{Male} = 66.5 + (13.7 \times \text{weight [kg]}) + (5.0 \times \text{height [cm]}) - (6.8 \times \text{age [yr]})$$

TABLE 7–2 Energy Expenditure

Condition and/or Surgery	Percentage of Normal Energy Expenditure
Starvation	80
Normal healthy	100
Hernia repair	105
Cholecystectomy	110
Colon resection	125
Sepsis	150
Burns	200
Septic burns	240

$$\text{Female} = 655 + (9.6 \times \text{weight [kg]}) + (1.8 \times \text{height [cm]}) - (4.7 \times \text{age [yr]})$$

The injury factors are 1.0 for normal patients and those undergoing minor surgery, 1.2 for long-bone fractures, 1.2 to 1.5 for major surgery, 1.5 for 50% burns, 1.2 to 1.5 for cancer, 1.5 to 2.0 for acute sepsis, and 2.0 for third-degree burns. The activity factor is usually a temperature correction with the addition of 1.12 for each degree above 37°C. Despite the apparent sophistication of the equation approach, it is still an estimate.

Macronutrients

Protein

Protein is actively mobilized to support the surgical stress. Patients completely convalesce from surgery when their body protein is repleted to the preoperative levels. Preserving the protein is important for the patient, as no protein stores exist in the body. All protein is either structural or functional and must be replaced to return the body to the same degree of structure and function. Thus every effort is made to minimize protein depletion. Because of the importance of having protein available to support gluconeogenesis, the mobilization of protein is slowed by exogenous protein but cannot be prevented. Thus the first component to calculate for nutritional support is the amount of protein. Studies of surgical patients have demonstrated that a protein intake from 1.25 to 2.0 mg/kg/day of balanced amino acids is required for the stressed and surgical patient. In a patient with a mild degree of malnutrition or stress, the lower level of 1.25 is used, whereas in the patient with severe pancreatitis, open abdominal dressings due to peritonitis, or the burned patient, the protein should be in the range of 2.0 mg/kg/day. A patient with moderate surgical injury or who is critically ill should receive 1.5 mg/kg/day of protein. During the acute injury stress, whether due to disease or surgery, the majority of the exogenous protein supports gluconeogenesis, and thus the protein should be viewed as calories. Once the acute injury response and the hypermetabolism have resolved, the protein is rerouted to an anabolic state and repletion.

Branched-chain amino acids (BCAAs) are mobilized during injury. They support the mobilization of alanine and glutamine from the peripheral muscle to the liver for gluconeogenesis. The infusion of these amino acids in PN is associated with a reduction in muscle breakdown and improved nitrogen balance in surgical trauma patients. As they are more efficiently used as fuel, they will reduce overall protein body catabolism and muscle breakdown and thus the degree of ureagenesis. One additional advantage with these amino acids is that they correct the serum amino acid imbalance present with liver failure, thus reducing hepatic encephalopathy. Thus the two clinical settings in which BCAA are used are in patients with hepatic encephalopathy and in patients with significant increases in their blood urea nitrogen such as renal failure and the renal failure seen with the systemic inflammatory response syndrome of sepsis.

Glutamine is an abundant amino acid in peripheral muscle and is an essential amino acid with injury. Mobilized from the muscle in large amounts, it supports cells with high rates of proliferation including the enterocyte and bone marrow stem cells. Patients who are ill for prolonged periods deplete the reserves of glutamine. Glutamine has been administered to critically ill patients, resulting in decreased infectious complications and decreased intensive care unit (ICU) and hospital lengths of stay. Its main therapeutic advantage has been in patients after bone marrow transplant for whom the glutamine was added to the PN.

Carbohydrates

The predominant form of carbohydrate used for nutritional support is dextrose. With the injured and surgical patient, dextrose supports the primary fuel of the body, glucose. Carbohydrate stores will dictate the amount of glucose that is immediately available, but usually this is 300 g or about 1080 calories. This is sufficient for about a day, and gluconeogenesis is then the major source of endogenous glucose. Basal glucose is produced at the rate of 2 mg/kg/min by the liver. In the injured and surgical patient, the optimal oxidation of infused dextrose is in the range of 4 to 5 mg/kg/min. When the infusions are increased above this rate, two critical problems occur: hyperglycemia and hepatic lipogenesis and steatosis. Both fructose and sucrose have been studied, but no substantiating evidence has been found of their effectiveness.

Lipids

Lipids can be easily added to the enteral formula. With PN, the lipids are delivered in a micelle called an emulsion. The emulsion is designed to increase lipid solubility and biologic availability. Added to the lipids are phospholipids and lecithin to produce both the solubility and particle characteristics required for infusion. Because of the low tonicity, the infusion of lipids in this form is less injurious to the vein endothelium. It has been observed that the lipid particles of the emulsion do have affinity for other lipid-soluble particles such as platelet activating factor and lipopolysaccharide (LPS). The lipid emulsion can be mixed with the other elements of the PN to produce a formula referred to as a "three-in-one mix." When acid, alkaline, excess calcium or phosphorus, or drugs are added to the PN, then the lipids can not be added because of instability of the micelles.

Both enteral and parenteral formulas of lipids use modified triglyceride preparations. In these lipid formulas, the triglyceride molecule is altered so that the free fatty acid (FFA) added to the glycerol backbone is very specific. By doing so, the mixtures of the FFA are delivered more efficiently. These are referred to as structured lipids and often have a medium-chain FFA in the n-2 or middle position.

Omega-6 polyunsaturated lipids are the principal source of lipids. They are oxidized and used as a fuel, but in excess, they are stored in the liver. They are precursors to a number of signaling molecules. If provided as a bolus, they increase prostaglandins that are immunosuppressive (prostaglandin E_2; PGE_2) and vasoconstrictive (thromboxane; TxB_2). This has been associated with increased pulmonary hypertension and increased ventilation/perfusion mismatching in critically ill patients. In addition, a lipid bolus of omega-6 will cause hyperlipidemia, resulting in overloading of the reticuloendothelium system (RES), and decreased Kupffer cell phagocytosis.

Omega-3 lipids have been studied extensively in surgical patients. Biologically, they replace arachidonic acid in the cell membranes with EPA and DHA, two forms of omega-3. Cell stimulation results in a reduction in the production of omega-6 proinflammatory leukotrienes and immunosuppressive and vasoconstrictive eicosanoids, as the omega-3 eicosanoids are less proinflammatory, immunosuppressive, and vasoconstrictive. Clinical studies of patients with acute respiratory distress syndrome in the ICU, burned patients, trauma patients, and after gastrointestinal surgery have all shown clinical improvement. This includes reductions in the ventilatory needs, the degree of multisystem organ failure, infections, and the ICU and hospital length of stay. Omega-3 lipids are available in enteral mixtures designed for surgical patients or those with specific organ failure such as acute respiratory distress syndrome. In patients undergoing elective oncologic and colorectal procedures, formulas with omega-3 decrease infections. Some work is being conducted on parenteral formulas, but these are not clinically available.

Medium-chain triglycerides (MCTs) are a very efficient fuel. They are rapidly taken up by the mitochondria and oxidized, as they are not carnitine dependent. Given to surgical and injured patients as part of their nutritional support, MCTs are effective in being oxidized and decreasing hepatic steatosis with improved nitrogen balance because of decreased protein catabolism. The sole disadvantage is the increased energy expenditure due to the efficient metabolism. Medium-chain lipids are available in enteral formulas and are a predominant ingredient of many preparations. MCTs

PEARLS FOR ROUNDS

Always perform a nutritional assessment for each patient.

Clinical assessment is the best tool.

Calculate the patient's feeding weight and nutritional requirements.

For the average surgical patient, protein is set at 1.5 g/kg/day; total calories are set at 25 cal/kg/day, carbohydrates are set at 4 mg/kg/min, and lipids are no more than 20% of total calories.

Enteral nutrition access is the best delivery system.

Parenteral nutrition can be used with patients who cannot use the gastrointestinal tract, who are severely malnourished, or have a severe disease or injury resulting in malnutrition and/or a delay in the use of the gastrointestinal tract. Use transitional feeding from parenteral to enteral as soon as possible.

Avoid the refeeding and overfeeding syndromes.

Nutritional support is dynamic. Change it with changes in the patient's clinical state.

The degree of obesity is measured by using the body mass index (BMI).

Patients with a BMI greater than 35 and life-threatening comorbidities and those with a BMI greater than 40 are considered for surgery, only after a complete and complex preoperative workup.

The standard bariatric operation is a gastric bypass. Gastric banding may be considered for lower BMIs, and a biliopancreatic procedure, for greater BMIs.

Long-term close follow-up is required monitoring for nutritional, psychological, and surgical complications.

have been included parenteral formulas, but they are not available in the United States.

Micronutrients

Vitamins are important for the surgical patient. A number of surgical or injured patients have vitamin deficiencies. Classic examples are the alcoholic patient, the patient with inflammatory bowel disease, and the patient with biliary obstruction. Presently some suggestion exists that vitamins in quantities greater than the RDA may benefit surgical patients. This is particularly true in clinical conditions with considerable oxygen metabolite formation. The use of the antioxidant properties of vitamins in the setting of vascular reperfusion and organ transplantation has shown some benefit. Patients with sepsis and multiple organ failure (MOF) secondary to systemic inflammatory response syndrome (SIRS) may also benefit for the same reason. Although no good data support the use of vitamins, little disadvantage appears in the use of increased vitamins. Thus vitamins C and E can be used as oxygen metabolite scavengers. Vitamin E stabilizes membranes and decreases lipid oxidation. The lack of vitamin C results in poor wound healing.

Surgical patients requiring nutritional support may have mineral and electrolyte deficiencies. A disease with classic mineral deficiencies is inflammatory bowel disease (IBD), in which zinc deficiency must be ruled out. The role of various minerals as antioxidants is being studied, and they are being added to the nutritional and metabolic support of patients with sepsis, SIRS, and burn patients. A recent study has shown that the addition of copper, zinc, and selenium has decreased pulmonary infections and organ failure in burn patients.

Hormones

The only well-described hormone to be used with nutritional support is growth hormone. Its use will increase protein anabolism; however, its exogenous administration is associated with hyperglycemia and sodium and water retention, two side effects that add complications to the surgical or ICU patient. A large multinational study on the use of growth hormone in ICU patients showed an increased morbidity and mortality with the administration of the hormone. Other studies using growth hormone in patients beyond the short-term injury response showed improved clinical outcome. Thus the use of this anabolic agent should be reserved for patients with a large protein deficiency, and it must be administered beyond the acute metabolic injury response.

Complications of Nutritional Support

Refeeding Syndrome

This syndrome was described in children who were enterally refed with regular formula after prolonged starvation. While being repleted, a number of the children died. The causes of the death were predominantly congestive heart failure and arrhythmias. This problem can also occur with adults, such as those with severe cancer cachexia, cardiac cachexia, or the geriatric patient with kwashiorkor. It occurs with both enteral nutrition (EN) and PN. The problem is that the severely malnourished patient has significant intracellular depletion of glycogen and glucose, resulting in a very rapid glucose uptake when nutrition is reintroduced. With the intracellular glucose uptake, a massive and rapid shift occurs of the extracellular electrolytes into the cell, repleting the low levels of potassium, phosphorus, magnesium, and manganese. The consequence is serious extracellular electrolyte abnormalities, resulting in arrhythmias and cardiac dysfunction and failure. In addition, the relatively low sodium and accompanying anemia will result in renal retention of fluid and sodium, adding to the syndrome producing congestive heart failure.

Prevention and aggressive therapy are the keys to the management of this syndrome. Initially underfeed the patient, limiting the amount of dextrose, and also limiting the fluid volume and sodium intake. Careful monitoring of the electrolytes is very important with frequent corrections. The risk for both arrhythmia and cardiac failure is high in adults, particularly the elderly.

Overfeeding Syndrome

Another complication with either EN or PN is the overfeeding syndrome. The syndrome produces complications that significantly compromise the surgical patient. The first complication of overfeeding is hyperglycemia. This is related to an overinfusion of glucose, usually at a rate of 4 mg/kg/min or greater. Hyperglycemia produces glycosylation of proteins, an example of which is hemoglobin A1C, used to measure chronic hyperglycemia. Other proteins will be glycosylated and become dysfunctional, such as cell-surface receptors on macrophages, neutrophils, and lymphocytes, and the immunoglobulins. Hyperglycemia, usually greater than 220 mg/dL, results in immunosuppression both at the cellular and humoral level, with a resultant increase in infections. Recent studies suggest that the blood glucose must be kept close to 100 mg/dL. A blood sugar of greater than 180 mg/dL results in diuresis and natriuresis. The second major complication of the overfeeding syndrome is lipid synthesis, as shown by the patient's respiratory quotient being greater than 1.0. A major site of lipid synthesis is the liver, resulting in hepatic steatosis and cholestasis. The side effect of the steatosis is hepatic enlargement and decreased drug detoxification.

Hyperlipidemia can result from overfeeding, as well as pancreatitis. The hyperlipidemia increases lipid uptake by the RES system and decreases bacteria and endotoxin clearance by the RES. The blood viscosity will increase, with microvascular sludging decreasing flow. Increased production of the omega-6 prostaglandins occurs with increased arachidonic acid metabolites such as the immunosuppressive PGE_2 and the vasoconstrictive TxB_2. To avoid these problems, the lipid infusion should be limited to 0.11 mg/kg/day, or no more than 20% of the total calories. Monitoring the serum lipid level is important.

Enteral Nutrition

Indications and Technique

EN can be delivered by the oral route or by a feeding tube. These tubes include the nasogastric tube, the nasojejunal tube, the postpyloric tube, the gastrostomy tube, and the jejunostomy tube. These feeding tubes can be placed by a percutaneous route or surgically. Each tube has its advantages as well as its risks. EN is ideal, as it is the natural and a more physiologic method of delivering nutrition. A number of products are available to meet various nutritional needs and metabolic demands (Table 7-3). The uptake of nutrients from the intestine will allow both the liver and the pancreas to control the levels of glucose and lipids, thus minimizing hyperglycemia and hyperlipidemia. In addition, enteral feeding reduces mucosal atrophy, which is thought to be associated with translocation of bacteria and toxins. Enteral feeding decreases enteral stasis and bacterial overgrowth, decreases biliary stasis and acalculous cholecystitis, and decreases gastric mucosal erosions. In addition, the use of the enteral route promotes intestinal mucosal proliferation, an event that may assist in intestinal anastomotic healing.

TABLE 7–3 Enteral Nutrition

Product	Kcal/mL	Protein g/1000 mL	Nonprotein Calorie to Nitrogen Ratio
Ensure	1.1	35	153:1
Sustacal	1.1	35	153:1
Osmolite	1.1	35	153:1
TraumaCal	1.5	55	91:1
Vivonex	1.0	45	114:1
Vital HN	1.0	42	125:1
Hepatic-Aid	1.2	38	148:1
Nepro	2.0	35	157:1
Pulmocare	1.5	42	125:1
Impact	1.0	56	71:1

Feeding by the gastric route is ideal, as the EN is complete, and all of the advantages of enteral feeding are obtained. Gastric feeding decreases problems with gastric erosions and stimulates the gallbladder, thereby decreasing the incidence of acalculous cholecystitis. Gastric feeding can be intermediate and is less susceptible to problems of osmolarity, temperature, electrolyte imbalance, and bacterial contamination. With gastric ileus, or gastroparesis, the feeding can be directed distal to the pylorus by using either a postpyloric tube or a jejunostomy tube. The postpyloric tube does not decrease the incidence of aspiration pneumonia, as the patient with gastric ileus or gastroparesis or both will still have gastric secretions that do not empty. Pharmacologic therapy for gastric ileus/gastroparesis, such as metoclopramide (Reglan) and erythromycin can be used but do not often work if the ileus is associated with an element of stress from the injury or the surgery. A nasogastric tube, an endoscopically guided percutaneously placed gastrostomy, or a surgically placed gastrostomy can achieve gastric feeding. The latter is done with an open procedure by using either the Stamm or Weitzel technique, or by using a laparoscopic technique with a specially designed gastrostomy tube.

Feeding the postpyloric intestine or the jejunum requires nutrition that is carefully administered to avoid problems such as hyperosmolarity/hypoosmolarity, temperature, electrolyte imbalance, and bacterial contamination, all which result in enteral intolerance, with intestinal bloating,

PEARLS FOR THE OR

Always know the patient's nutritional state going into surgery.

Stop both enteral and parenteral nutritional support when going to surgery. With parenteral nutrition, avoid relative hypoglycemia when stopping the infusion before surgery. Use 10% dextrose to cover the patient.

Decide on the postoperative nutritional strategy before surgery. If you think of it, do something about it.

Consider enteral access and intestinal function. Gastrostomies are practical, but if concerns with aspiration are present, then consider a jejunostomy. Jejunostomy feedings can be started in the postanesthesia recovery room, provided that the patient is hemodynamically stable. Always use a low rate such as 10 mL/hr.

Malnourishment will affect the surgical approach, including wound closure. Secure both gastrostomies and jejunostomies to the abdominal wall. With ascites, avoid gastrostomies and jejunostomies, and consider using a nasoduodenal or nasojejunal feeding tube if the need is for the short term.

Restart PN when the patient is hemodynamically stable, and monitor for the surgical stress–induced hyperglycemia.

Gastric banding places an adjustable band around the stomach just below the esophagogastric junction, creating a small gastric pouch.

Gastric bypass creates a small isolated gastric pouch, which is anastomosed to a limb of jejunum, either a short limb of 100 cm or a long limb of 150 cm or greater. The biliopancreatic limb is anastomosed at this point to create the Roux-en-Y.

The biliopancreatic operation with a duodenal switch creates a sleeve gastric pouch of 250 mL anastomosed after the pylorus to a long alimentary limb. The biliopancreatic limb is anastomosed to the alimentary limb, leaving a common channel or limb of 100 to 150 cm before the ileocecal valve.

pain, and diarrhea. Medications and nutrients must be adjusted for intestinal feeding. Jejunal feedings are optimal for patients with any proximal GI surgery (esophageal, gastric, biliary, or pancreatic) and for patients with biliary or pancreatic problems or both. The "jejunal brake" is the ligament of Trietz, and feeding below this brake results in only a 10% stimulation of the pancreas. The postpyloric tube can be placed by extending a nasogastric tube or gastrostomy tube. A jejunostomy must be placed surgically.

Complications

Mechanical complications of enteral feeding include hoarseness and nasal and pharyngeal erosions. The tube can be misplaced or become displaced, resulting in aspiration or perforation of the bowel. It is very important to assure placement of the tubes, particularly in patients who are not alert, cooperative, or ventilated. Frequently tubes can become obstructed. Prevention is very important and includes appropriate tube flushing, avoiding use of the tube for medications, and not using the tube for long periods. If the tube is blocked, it can be flushed with warm water, flat cola, a meat tenderizer, or an enzyme preparation. Tube changes may be required and can be done at the bedside (nasogastric, gastrostomy), with gastroscopy (postpyloric, nasojeujnal), or may require interventional radiology (jejunostomy).

Intolerance of enteral feeding is manifested in several ways. The patient may have nausea, vomiting, high residuals, fullness, distention, bloating, or diarrhea. With problems of high residuals and symptoms suggestive of fullness, the rate should be decreased and subsequently increased at a slower pace. The presence of gastroparesis and intestinal obstruction must be ruled out. With diarrhea, one must consider lactose intolerance, intolerance to osmolarity, too much fat, or the effect of medications (i.e., sorbitol). The diarrhea may be infectious, such as that due to *Clostridium difficile* colitis or the disease itself (i.e., IBD). Adjustments in rate, osmolarity, and lipid content can help (using MCTs), but if the diarrhea persists, then consider stopping the enteral feeds until the diarrhea is controlled.

Metabolic complications occur with enteral feeding and can seriously compromise the surgical patient. Overhydration requires decreasing the rate of enteral feeding or use of a more-concentrated formula. Dehydration, a frequent enteral problem, is treated by dilution of the formula or by adding a water bolus or both. Hyperglycemic hyperosmolar nonketosis responds to decreasing the feedings, with hydration of the patient, and insulin to control the blood sugar. With hyperglycemia, the glucose intake is decreased and insulin coverage augmented. Hypoglycemia responds to increasing the glucose or decreasing the insulin coverage or both. Hyponatremia and hypernatremia require adjustments in the fluid and sodium being administered, and hyperkalemia and hypokalemia require adjustment in the potassium being administered while determining if any major acid/base problems exist. Finally, if hyperuremia is found, consider decreasing the protein administered.

The patient receiving EN is susceptible to both the refeeding and overfeeding syndromes, as outlined in detail earlier.

Infectious complications for EN are very specific. Aspiration pneumonia is the result of high residuals with gastric feeding, or a misplaced tube, and is a devastating complication. Prevention requires feeding the patient in an upright position and monitoring of residuals. Treatment is usually appropriate antibiotics but may require intubation and ventilation. Otitis media, sinusitis, and parotiditis are the result of a prolonged period with a nasal tube or a tube that is too rigid or too large. The treatment is repositioning of the tube and antibiotics. Necrotizing enterocolitis is a very severe complication often seen in patients who are critically ill. The patient is often started on enteral feeding while hemodynamically unstable or requiring vasopressive agents or both. The pathophysiology is uncertain, but it appears to be related to the combined effect of the osmolarity of the feeding in the lumen and the poor intestinal circulation. The consequence is bowel necrosis and perforation. Prevention is the key, as the mortality of the complication is high. Enteral feeding should be stopped in patients in whom hemodynamic instability is developing.

Parenteral Nutrition

Indications

PN is used when the patient cannot or will not eat or the GI system cannot be used. Examples of patients who cannot eat or whose GI tract cannot be used are those with bowel obstruction, ileus, pancreatitis, or the SIRS associated with overwhelming sepsis. Postoperative patients who are not expected to have adequate enteral intake within 7 days also are included in this group. Also included are those with severe emesis secondary to either chemotherapy or pregnancy. The patients who will not eat are usually those with anorexia nervosa or other psychiatric problems. The patients described earlier with associated malnutrition have compromised organ and immune systems, and their ability to recover from their disease or respond to their therapy is enhanced with PN.

Patients with GI obstruction may benefit from PN. If the intestinal obstruction develops, and the patients are malnourished, PN should be started immediately to prevent further malnutrition (which may play a role in any associated ileus). If the patient is well nourished, he or she can wait for up to 5 days before aggressive nutritional therapy must be started.

Another group of patients who will benefit from the use of PN are those with IBD. With an exacerbation of the disease, the intestine is put to rest, and thus nutrition must be by the venous route. The urgency of starting the support is related to the degree of malnutrition and associated systemic sepsis. Another type of bowel inflammation, radiation enteritis, also can require periods of intestinal rest that would require PN support.

Patients with GI fistulae have been treated with PN. Often these fistulae will close with bowel rest, good electrolyte management, and nutritional support in the form of PN.

Other patients who can greatly benefit from the use of PN are those with pancreatitis. These patients have the combined problems of severe pancreatic inflammation and the inability to use their intestine. PN can be used until these problems are resolved. If the patient requires a laparotomy for severe pancreatitis, necrosis, or an abscess, then the patient should have a feeding jejunostomy placed for transition to EN.

Patients in the ICU with a critical illness, such as sepsis, severe trauma, and burns, may require PN early in their hospital course while they recover from the ileus or the multiple organ failure that accompanies this degree of illness.

In all cases of PN, the nutrition must be carefully monitored, and a plan should be made to transition the patient to enteral feeding. Transition feeding is very important and requires a careful plan that is tailored to each patient. The objective is to determine the overall nutritional needs of the patient. The patient is then transitioned by turning down the PN system and increasing the EN. The result is neither overfeeding nor underfeeding. Such an approach can assure the patient good nutrition and has been associated with decreased infectious complications and both ICU and hospital lengths of stay. Overall, evidence suggests that PN will not influence the mortality of surgical patients but can reduce complications in the malnourished patient.

Venous Access

PN is delivered through a venous access catheter. Because of the tonicity of parenteral solutions, it is delivered through a catheter, which ends in a central vein. Solutions with limited concentrations of amino acids, with or without lipids, may be delivered through a peripheral vein. Often the line will only last a few days, and this nutrition system requires a large volume to be administered. Otherwise the line requires central access. The choice of lines is dependent on the patient's clinical situation. A subclavian line is most frequently used because of the ease of placing it (usually from the left side); the line is easy to care for and is comfortable for the patient. The internal jugular is used next often, with a decreased risk of pulmonary injury, but it is more difficult to take care of and more uncomfortable for the patient. An increasing use of percutaneously placed central lines or a PIC line is found. The advantages of these lines are that they are placed peripherally with minimal risk to the patient and can be performed by a nurse or venous access team. Patients are usually comfortable with the line, but one must avoid the antecubital fossa because of problems with line occlusion. The debate continues as to whether these lines are more prone to venous thrombosis and infection.

A line to be used for PN ideally should not have been used for any other therapy. When the line has been used, four choices exist in terms of starting the PN.

1. Use the line, and monitor for infections.
2. Use the line after it is flushed with vancomycin and urokinase.
3. Change the line over a wire.
4. Use the line, and change only if problems develop.

No strong evidence indicates that any of these is the best, but the institution policy should be followed, while the overall line sepsis rate is monitored.

Complications

Line sepsis is a complication often rationalized as a reason to avoid using PN. One of the problems is that the patient receiving PN is often "sicker" and thus more susceptible to infectious complications. The major infectious risk is line sepsis, which, if not properly diagnosed and treated, can lead to septic phlebitis and bacterial endocarditis. It is often difficult to obtain an accurate diagnosis of line sepsis because of the need to have several components present to make the diagnosis. For the diagnosis to be complete, the patient must have clinical signs of an infection with central and peripheral blood cultures, as well as the line-tip culture positive with the same organism. If this is the case, the line is changed to a new site, and antibiotics are administered for up to 14 days. If line sepsis is suspected and the blood cultures are suggestive, then the line should be changed over a wire. If the line tip is negative, the new line can be left; however, if the tip is positive, a new line site should be obtained.

Line thrombosis can limit the length of a course of PN. It depends on whether the access line is in a proximal or distal central vein as to the incidence and severity of the complication. In addition, the incidence is higher in patients who are hypercoagulable because of their disease (i.e., pancreatitis, tumors). Complications of central vein thrombosis include limb and possible head edema and pulmonary embolus, a life-threatening condition. Again, the incidence is more frequent with leg thrombosis than with arm thrombosis. A serious complication of inferior vena cava thrombosis is renal vein thrombosis, resulting in renal failure. To avoid these complications, the parenteral formulations should have a low osmolarity and a low concentration of irritating medications, such as potassium; the end of the catheter should be central; leg veins should not be used for PN; and anticoagulation with low-dose heparin of 10,000 to 12,000 units per day or coumadin adjusted for an INR of 1.5 times should be used.

Metabolic complications of enteral feeding can occur with PN. In both situations, the patient must be monitored, and these complications are best avoided. Besides the ones listed with EN support, the following are more often seen with PN. Carbon dioxide overproduction is a problem with patients receiving PN and who are carbon dioxide retainers. This is treated by decreasing the infusion of glucose calories and increasing the lipid calories to keep the respiratory quotient around 0.85. Hepatic toxicity is diagnosed by increasing liver-function tests and is often due to overfeeding, but can be due to parenteral glucose in a patient with ongoing stress or sepsis. Decreasing the glucose calories and use of a hypocaloric feed will help to control this problem. Rebound hypoglycemia occurs if the parenteral solution contains high amounts of dextrose and is stopped abruptly. This problem is avoided by tapering the PN and using 10% dextrose. Patients receiving PN are susceptible to the metabolic problems of refeeding, overfeeding, and hyperlipidemia, as outlined earlier.

Specific Clinical Conditions

Liver Disease

Usually liver failure patients with malnutrition can be treated with EN, often by using oral supplements. In the situation of acute hepatitis and or in the patient with severe liver failure, significant malnutrition, ascites, and complications such as encephalopathy or spontaneous primary peritonitis, benefit can be obtained from a course of PN. The degree of malnutrition can be quite severe, and these patients are prone to both vitamin and mineral deficiencies. Patients with encephalopathy will benefit from the addition of BCAAs to their PN, as these amino acids will decrease serum levels of aromatic amino acids thought to be part of the etiology of the encephalopathy. PN in liver-failure patients must be configured to reduce salt and water retention and is delivered in a very limited volume. Patients with liver disease, who have undergone hepatic resection and who were supported with PN with BCAAs, had an improved surgical outcome, with fewer complications and a reduced length of stay. The use of lipids should be reduced with active liver failure to reduce any degree of compromise of the reticuloendothelial system.

Pancreatitis

These patients can have a disease that ranges from very mild, resolving in a few days, or one in which 50% will die with necrotizing pancreatitis and multiple organ failure. Patients with the severe forms of the disease need very aggressive metabolic and nutritional support. Much as in the burn patient, the intra-abdominal inflammation associated with pancreatitis is very hypermetabolic and catabolic. Patients with chronic pancreatitis can be malnourished because of protein depletion and malabsorption of lipids with vitamin deficiencies. Obviously the pancreatitis patient is very susceptible to the metabolic and hyperglycemic complications of PN. Usually these patients will require PN early to decrease the degree of malnutrition, particularly protein depletion. Careful administration of glucose is important with the background of insulin resistance and decreased insulin production. These patients can be fed enterally with good evidence that feeding below the "jejunal brake" or the ligament of Trietz is well tolerated. Gaining access to this region can be very difficult, and a feeding jejunostomy must always be considered if the patient is operated on. The enteral feeding should be adjusted to limit the lipids because of the associated pancreatic insufficiency. The use of MCTs is good in these patients if they have significant steatorrhea. The use of enzyme replacement is very effective in treating any degree of exocrine dysfunction.

Renal Failure

Patients with renal failure are usually quite hypermetabolic and catabolic. The catabolism is worse because of the protein loss with either hemodialysis or peritoneal dialysis.

When this clinical problem is a complication of an underlying medical condition, the nutritional problems are compounded. Conceptually it is important to remember that the complications of renal failure, including metabolic acidosis, hyperkalemia, increased creatinine, and increased urea, are worse with catabolism. Consequently it is important to diagnose and treat the nutritional problems of the renal failure patient expectantly. The PN must be carefully administered, with daily adjustments to avoid any of the standard complications as well as the problem of fluid overload.

Cardiac Failure

The patient with severe cardiac failure may be first seen with cardiac cachexia. Enteral support can be difficult with cardiac failure, and thus PN is started. One must also be concerned about using EN in the cardiac patient who is unstable or has a high need for pressors. The physician must be careful to avoid the refeeding syndrome and, in particular, the problems of electrolyte imbalance and fluid overload. The failing heart is in need of glucose and calcium, and it is important to deliver the nutritional support in a low total fluid volume. Some evidence indicates that a combination of glucose, insulin, and potassium can improve the myocardium if administered during infarction.

Sepsis

Patients with sepsis often have MOF and the syndrome associated with it, SIRS. It is important not to allow malnutrition, particularly protein, to complicate the serious illness of these patients. Septic patients with the SIRS are hypermetabolic, usually in the range of 50% above basal REE. They are catabolic, with urinary nitrogen losses of up to 10 g/day. Although the optimal nutrition is enteral, if associated ileus is present, enteral feedings are not tolerated. If the enteral route is not tolerated or delayed, then aggressive PN support is needed. Aggressive PN can help with the metabolic complications associated with SIRS and help to decrease the malnutrition, particularly the protein depletion. Nutritional support, either parenteral or enteral, should be considered only after the patient is adequately resuscitated and hemodynamically stable. These patients may benefit from the use of MCTs and omega-3 lipids, which are available for PN in Europe and Asia. Omega-3 has reduced the incidence of infectious complications and the overall length of stay in these patients, but the work has been predominantly based on enteral formulation. It is important in these patients to avoid overfeeding with resulting hyperglycemia and hepatic cholestasis.

Inflammatory Bowel Disease

These patients can demonstrate a spectrum of disease that has a wide variation in the nutritional state. In the worse forms, the patients can have very significant malnutrition with large weight loss and life-threatening electrolyte abnormalities associated with diarrhea. The PN is set up initially to deal with the dehydration and electrolyte issues while avoiding the refeeding syndrome. Eventually these patients can tolerate larger volume, and they are left on the PN until adequate oral intake is established, to help replete the depleted state. Often these patients are taking steroids and have associated complications, including fluid retention, hypokalemia, hypocalcemia, and hyperglycemia. The nutrition must be adjusted for these issues. Another problem for these patients is zinc deficiency.

Pregnancy Emesis

This can be a very debilitating condition. The patient often has electrolyte derangements secondary to vomiting and nutritional concerns not only for herself but also for her fetus. The patient must be aggressively treated with a pharmacologic approach to the emesis, but if the patient is nutritionally depleted (>10% weight loss), then PN is initiated. If she is not depleted, then a few days of emesis therapy while the fluid and electrolytes are corrected is reasonable. A central line can be a concern, so a PIC line is used. Be sure that the patient is receiving adequate vitamins and minerals. It is important that the patient be consuming adequate calories by mouth before the PN is terminated.

Oncology Patients

Often these patients can be very malnourished, and whether they undergo surgery, chemotherapy, or radiation therapy, the addition of malnutrition will make the therapy less successful. The side effects of radiation therapy and chemotherapy can leave patients very ill for weeks. The accompanying neutropenia makes them more susceptible to infections, including line sepsis. In patients receiving bone marrow transplants, the addition of glutamine to the PN has decreased the septic complications and improved their overall success, with decreased hospital length of stay. Carefully tailored diets and eating habits will help with the oncology patient. Speculation and concern that the nutrition also is feeding the malignancy is not a reason to avoid or decrease the nutritional support. Although it is inevitably true, starving the patient with its complications does little for the overall cause.

Intestinal Dyskinesia and Short-Gut Syndrome

This appears to be a growing diagnosis and one with multiple etiologies. Often these are patients who receive home TPN. Patients with short gut can have a variety of intestinal resections and anastomoses, but they are not all doomed to a life on TPN. Intestinal dyskinesia is an increasingly recognized syndrome of intestinal dysfunction with decreased motility. These patients have a clinical picture of an ileus that can involve the small and large bowel and produces pain, nausea, vomiting, and abdominal distention. The problem can develop with chronic laxative and narcotic abuse, but also can be idiopathic. During the acute illness, the patient is given PN to treat the associated fluid and electrolyte problems as well as the protein and calorie malnutrition. Often the patient may only have protein malnutrition, evidenced by a low serum albumin. These patients are very difficult to advance to EN feeding, and the PN must be maintained to treat the malnutrition and also to prevent any further malnutrition as a possible reason for the dyskinesia. Patients who cannot be converted to the enteral route are then candidates for home PN.

The short-gut syndrome is due to massive intestinal resection secondary to bowel necrosis resulting from a low-flow state, mesenteric artery embolus, mesenteric vein thrombosis, volvulus, Crohn's disease, and extensive intestinal damage from intestinal lysis. The patients are often initially very ill but can recover quickly, then developing extensive diarrhea. They will need fluid and electrolytes (Na, K, Cl, Ca, and P) for the deficiencies and nutritional support for the protein and calorie depletion. Once they have recovered from the acute illness, they can then be carefully advanced to EN support, while maintaining the PN. If this fails, a program of intestinal rehabilitation is started. This program uses a combination of glutamine, growth hormone, and fiber, such as pectin. If all fails, then these patients are committed to a life receiving PN. In this situation, the patient is truly receiving TPN, although he or she is not totally NPO. They will often eat despite their short gut producing serious diarrhea, which results in difficult fluid electrolyte and pharmacologic problems.

Surgical Patients

Patients who undergo surgery and have a preoperative diagnosis of malnutrition should have the malnutrition treated before the operation. Although not practical in the hospital setting because of cost, the nutrition can be administered as either EN or PN, either in a nonacute hospital setting or even at home. The best examples of this are patients with esophageal carcinoma, in which the pathophysiology of the disease includes serious protein and calorie malnutrition. How long to administer the preoperative nutrition has been a much-debated question. Currently the optimal plan would call for the repletion of the glycogen stores, stopping the protein catabolism and beginning anabolism, and repletion of the mineral and vitamin stores, all of which require 2 to 3 weeks. To reverse the protein depletion would require months and is not practical. Postoperatively, patients with preexisting malnutrition should be treated aggressively. Patients who cannot or do not eat within 5 days of their surgery should have nutritional support. If the enteral route is not available, then PN is used. In the postoperative patient, the key is to minimize the protein depletion and to correct and prevent any electrolyte and metabolic abnormalities. In terms of calories, minimal dextrose is used to prevent aggravating the hyperglycemia of injury, and lipids are supplied continuously, with some being MCTs, and possibly omega-3 polyunsaturated FA. The ideal route of administration of the nutrition is enteral. This should be kept in mind during surgery, and every effort should be made to obtain access to the GI tract (i.e., either gastrostomy or jejunostomy) in cases of complex abdominal surgery.

Trauma Patients

Trauma patients are treated very similar to the surgical patients. If preexisting malnutrition is present, nutritional support is started early in the treatment. Otherwise, they can be observed for up to 5 days before instituting nutritional support. In cases in which the injuries are severe and it is clear that the patient will not eat for a prolonged time, nutritional support is started earlier. EN is ideal and can be delivered via gastric or intestinal feeding. The patients can be started on PN and transitioned to EN as they improve.

Transplantation Patients

These patients are often complex. Malnutrition adds to their morbidity and mortality. It is best if the malnutrition is treated preoperatively; however, this is often difficult, as with the patient in hepatic failure. Postoperatively they are supported with nutritional therapy and special diets with immune-enhancing nutrients such as omega-3 lipids, which can reduce infection and septic complications. Such diets also have been associated with reduced episodes of rejection with kidney transplants.

Home TPN

The patient who is placed on TPN for the home is usually a patient requiring long-term PN. It is often truly TPN, in that many of these patients will obtain their total nutritional support from the PN. The life expectancy for these patients is in the range of 15 to 20 years. Septic complications and liver failure most frequently cause their eventual death. These patients must be carefully monitored to assure that the calories and protein are adequate. After the acute illness, they will require less protein, and the calories must be gauged to their activity. Although the basic PN formula will work in these patients, some data support using MCT lipids as part of the calorie mixture. Electrolyte and metabolic problems must be monitored, particularly in the active patient (who engages in swimming, bicycling, or hiking) A home TPN patient can be involved with any number of physical activities, and the nutrition must be adjusted. The PN is administered through a long-term line often referred to as a Hickman or Broviac line. These lines are tunneled under the skin, and the exit is in a convenient place for the patient to use. To reduce the incidence of infections, they may have a Teflon cuff added to the line, which will rest just under the skin. A number of antimicrobial-treated lines are on the market; however, the data are not clear as to their use. Because of the serious nature of venous thrombosis in these patients, it is imperative that they be reasonable anticoagulants. Line infections are best avoided, and thus the proper care of these lines is extremely important, particularly when these patients are admitted to an acute care facility. Often these line infections can be treated with a course of urokinase and vancomycin for gram-positive bacteria and gentamicin for gram-negative bacteria. If the infection is suppressed, the patient will require a long course of about 8 weeks.

Areas of controversy include the use of home TPN for terminally ill patients such as those with metastatic carcinoma or AIDS. If the therapy allows the patient to be free of institutions, it is reasonable to consider, particularly if it will keep the individual independent. If the patient is very debilitated and the life expectancy is very short, then the home TPN is of little benefit.

Nutritional Strategy

The key strategic principles are to assess the patients and to determine the degree of malnutrition and nutritional requirements. If no malnutrition exists, the patients can be observed for 5 days unless the disease or surgery precludes them from returning to PO nutritional support after 5 days. In these cases and in those with malnutrition, nutritional support should be initiated. If the nutritional support is to be aggressive, then the patient is provided PN with the objective of transitioning to EN as soon as possible. Whereas this may occur over time in some patients, the therapeutic approach to nutrition should include EN from the beginning. While the PN is being started, enteral access is obtained by using feeding tubes, and therapy to control emesis or diarrhea is started.

Using both forms of nutrition simultaneously seems intuitively correct, yet it also is associated with increased opportunities for complications. The answer is that nutritional therapy, like all other therapies, must be done correctly with careful monitoring and appropriate adjustments. The therapy must be tailored to the changing clinical course of the patient. Studies of burn patients who were provided with combined nutritional therapy initiated from the day of their admission and who were appropriately transitioned from PN to EN show that they had a reduced morbidity, particularly infections, and decreased the hospital length of stay by 20 days. The key to such success was the vigilant nutritional care these patients received and the fact that they had adequate nutrition from early in their disease. By using the combined approach, investigators were able to keep the patients from significant malnutrition and its associated complications. Although a tendency exists for nutrition to be directed toward hypocaloric feeding, this study indicated the importance of preventing malnutrition from becoming an additional complication. Other situations like this are seen with patients who undergo surgery for GI tumors and who have significant preoperative weight loss. The immediate postoperative nutritional needs are often treated with PN, while the enteral therapy is slowly advanced. The objective is to have the combination of the PN and EN equal the nutritional requirements for the patient. By not exceeding the calculated nutritional requirements, one avoids the overfeeding complication and its significant morbidity.

Remember that the first part of setting up the nutritional therapy is to determine the nutritional requirements for the patient. Once set, the combined therapy is directed toward providing the total nutritional package. Although considerable changes may occur in the formula for either PN of EN, or the relative proportions of both, the total assessment or requirement is not changed. This will require that the physician or the nutritional support team make frequent assessments of the patient's clinical course, adjusting the nutrition to the clinical state.

Obesity Surgery

A growing problem in the United States and the world is obesity. Now considered the number one nutritional problem of the world by the World Health Organization, it affects 30% of Americans. Although the main focus of therapy is prevention, such lifestyle changes are slow to occur. The foundation for treatment of the established disease is caloric reduction, achieved through diet and increased activity. Resistance to this approach can be treated with the use of drugs that affect appetite or reduce the ability to absorb calories. Patients for whom these therapies continue to fail and who achieve a certain degree of obesity known as morbid obesity or complications of the obesity should be considered for surgical treatment of their obesity. The BMI is currently used to determine the degree of obesity (BMI = [weight in kilograms] divided by the height in meters squared). The waist/hip ratio can be used to identify a patient with peripheral or gynecoid distribution from the central or android presentation, which is medically worse, with greater comorbidities and mortality.

The surgery for obesity can be divided into three groups: restrictive, malabsorptive, and combination. With restrictive surgery, the idea is to reduce physically the intake of food such as by wiring the jaws closed or by making the stomach smaller. Jaw wiring failed because when the wires were removed, the patients regained their weight. A smaller stomach can be achieved by a band around the stomach or by stapling the stomach and creating a small pouch. These procedures are referred to as either gastric banding or gastroplasty.

The malabsorptive procedure is intestinal bypass or jejunoileal bypass. A fixed length of proximal jejunum was attached to the side of the distal ileum. These operations were associated with serious complications and death from hepatic failure and thus are no longer done.

The third group of operations is the combined procedure, using a gastric pouch for restriction and bypassing a length of bowel for malabsorption. Examples of these procedures are gastric bypass and biliopancreatic diversion. Gastric bypass is the operation of choice, with gastric banding and biliopancreatic diversion a possibility for selected patient populations.

The overwhelming increase in obesity in the United States has spawned an entirely new field: bariatric surgery. The number of GI operations performed annually for severe obesity increased from about 16,000 in the early 1990s to about 103,000 in 2003 (Fig. 7-1). The indications for bariatric surgery were outlined by a National Institutes of Health consensus conference. These include a patient between the ages of 21 to 55 years, with either a BMI of 40 or a BMI greater than 35 with life-threatening comorbidities, and for whom supervised weight-reducing programs have failed. Such patients have intractable morbid obesity, and as their life expectancy is greatly reduced, they should consider surgery as a treatment option. Currently for such patients, surgery is the only therapy that provides sufficient and persistent weight loss.

In preparing patients for surgery, perform a dietary assessment, including their eating behavior, a psychological assessment, and a medical assessment, with emphasis on their GI, cardiovascular, and pulmonary systems. The patient should be screened for cholelithiasis as well as tumors including endometrial and breast. Encourage him or her to increase daily activity, stop smoking, and lose some weight.

Although various bariatric operations exist, two dominate surgical practice in the United States. With the normal anatomy of the stomach and small intestine in mind (Fig. 7-2*A*), the Roux-en-Y gastric bypass uses a series of staples to separate a small pouch of 1 to 2 ounces from the rest of the stomach (Fig. 7-2*B*). The small bowel is divided about 30 to 50 cm from the ligament of Treitz and then reanastomosed at 100 cm from the distal end for morbidly obese or 150 cm (or more) for the superobese. The end of the distal bowel is placed either in front of the colon (antecolic) or behind the colon (retrocolic) and anastomosed to the gastric pouch by either a suturing or a stapling technique. Weight loss with this operation is around 70% of the patient's excess weight.

An option to the Roux-en-Y gastric bypass is the adjustable gastric band (Fig. 7-2*C*). The gastric band is placed around the stomach just below the esophagogastric junction, providing for a small 1- to 2-ounce pouch. The band is connected to a reservoir, providing the opportunity to adjust the size of the band. Weight loss is around 40% of the patient's excess weight.

The biliopancreatic procedure is now frequently performed with a duodenal switch. This operation creates a long gastric pouch by excising a tube of stomach along the greater curve of the stomach. The bowel is divided about 250 cm from the ligament of Treitz and then reanastomosed with a common channel of bowel of 100–150 cm from the anastomosis to the cecum. The duodenum is detached from the pylorus, and the other end of the divided small bowel is anastomosed to the pylorus. This very complex operation does provide significant weight loss, which can be 70% or greater, but also provides greater complications, particularly metabolic, such as protein malnutrition and bone reabsorption.

The operating suite must be able to accommodate a morbidly obese patient. The surgery can be conducted by either the laparoscopic or the open route. Currently the operations are more often done laparoscopically, as the surgeon becomes more proficient. The surgery done this way reduces the hospital length of stay and the disability time. It also has decreased the incidence of wound complications including infections and incisional hernias.

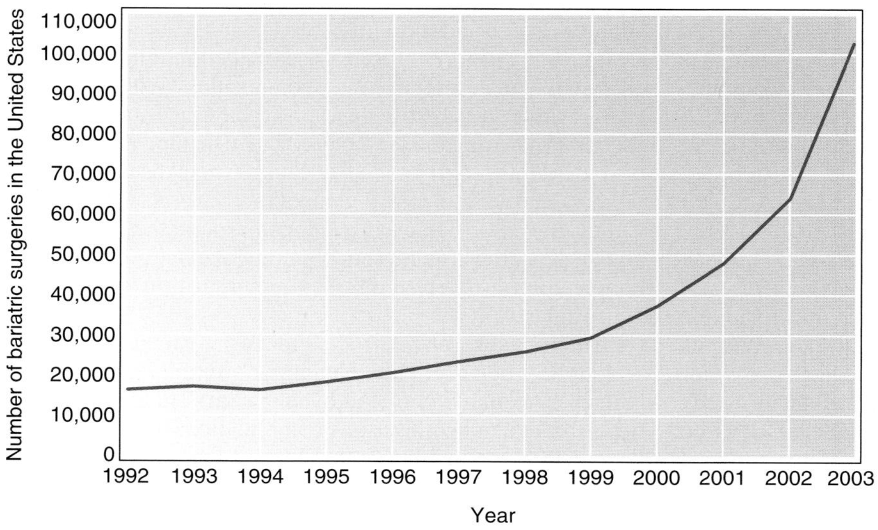

FIGURE 7–1 Estimated number of bariatric operations performed in the United States, 1992–2003. Data from the American Society for Bariatric Surgery.

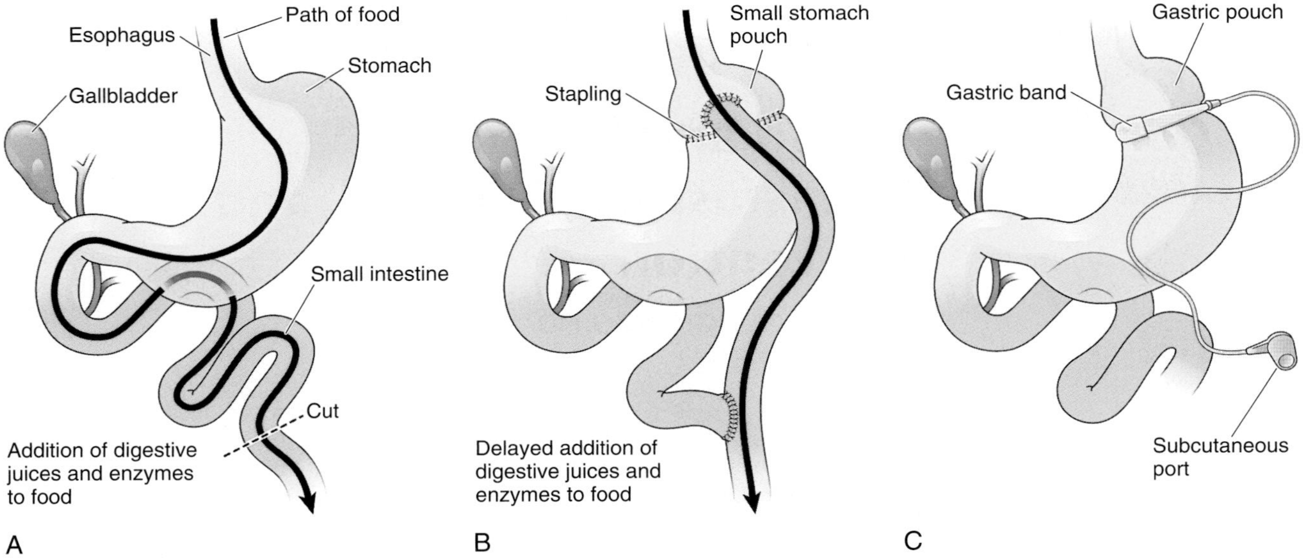

FIGURE 7–2 Commonly used bariatric surgical procedures. *A*, Normal anatomy of the stomach and small intestine, showing key surgical landmarks. *B*, The Roux-en-Y gastric bypass, in which a small proximal gastric pouch is connected to a Y-shaped loop of the small intestine. The proximal stomach is separated from the remaining part of the stomach with staples. *C*, The gastric banding procedure. The band, which can be adjusted by the infusion of saline, is placed around the stomach near its upper end, creating a small pouch and a restricted passage to the larger remaining part of the stomach. The gastric pouch is generally less than 30 mL in total volume for both procedures.

For the morbidly obese patient with a BMI of 40 to 50, the gastric bypass is the operation of choice; with patients with a lower BMI or a younger age, consideration for gastric banding should be entertained, although a limited experience with the band is available in North America. Patients with a BMI greater than 50 are referred to as super-obese, and they should have a gastric bypass with a longer limb of bowel in the Roux-en-Y to increase malabsorption. They also should be considered for the biliopancreatic procedure, although this procedure is associated with increased metabolic complications including vitamin and mineral deficiencies and osteomalacia. Patients who undergo this surgery need careful and close follow-up with frequent visits, monitoring for surgical, nutritional, metabolic, and psychological complications. Such follow-up must be intense early after the surgery and continue for a lifetime, with diminishing visit frequencies as the patient becomes more independent and adjusted to life after bariatric surgery. Important nutritional complications include anemia (iron and B_{12} based), calcium deficiency, electrolyte deficiencies, dehydration, and protein malnutrition. Surgical complications are predominantly wound complications of infections and hernias, anastomotic stenosis, marginal ulcers, and small bowel obstruction.

Suggested Reading

Brolin RE: Bariatric surgery and long-term control of morbid obesity. JAMA 288:2793–2796, 2002.
Bruun LI, Bosaeus I, Bergstad I, Nygaard K: Prevalence of malnutrition in surgical patients: Evaluation of nutritional support and documentation. Clin Nutr 18:141–147, 1999.
Heyland DK, Montalvo M, MacDonald S, et al: Total parenteral nutrition in the surgical patient: A meta-analysis. Can J Surg 44:101–111, 2001.
Maxfield D, Geehan D, Van Way CW: Perioperative nutritional support. Nutri Clin Pract 16:69–73, 2001.
Steinbrook R: Surgery for severe obesity. N Engl J Med 350:1075–1079, 2004.
Torosian MH: Perioperative nutrition support for patients undergoing gastrointestinal surgery: Critical analysis and recommendation. World J Surg 23:565–569, 1999.

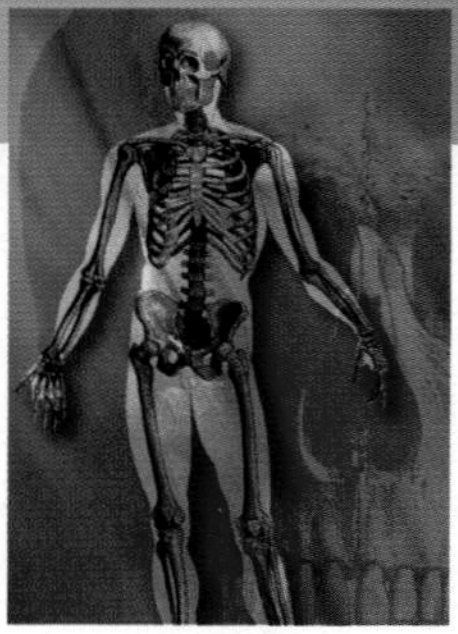

Chapter 8

Blood and Bleeding: Transfusions, Control, and Prevention

RAYMOND L. COMENZO, MD

Hemostasis

Hemostasis is the physiologic process that exists to maintain vascular and tissue integrity and functional blood flow in the face of normal growth and activity and despite injury and disease. The components of hemostasis are shown in Figure 8-1. Hemostatic function is dependent on blood flow, pH, and temperature; anatomic factors such as the subendothelium and endothelium of the vasculature; the cellular elements of blood, particularly platelets and red blood cells; and the soluble and membrane-bound pro- and anticoagulant proteins, enzymes and glycoproteins, and calcium.

Defects of hemostasis may be anatomic due to traumatic injuries, penetrating wounds, surgical interventions, or congenital abnormalities such as arteriovenous malformations. They may also be hematologic, due to congenital or acquired functional abnormalities of platelets or of the soluble pro- or anticoagulant factors, or to severe anemia or thrombocytopenia. Von Willebrand's disease is the most common congenital abnormality of platelets and causes a platelet-function defect that can result in bleeding.

Primary hemostasis refers to the immediate response to vascular injury that involves vasoconstriction and platelet adhesion and aggregation. Secondary hemostasis refers to the processes involved in the generation and regulation of thrombin and fibrin clot formation at the site of vascular injury. Coagulation tests assess the integrity of the soluble factors that control thrombin generation and fibrin formation and dissolution.

The international normalized ratio (INR) measures primarily the function of fibrinogen (factor I), prothrombin (factor II), and factors V, VII, and X and is used to follow patients taking the anticoagulant warfarin (Coumadin; vitamin K inhibitor). The partial thromboplastin time (PTT) measures the function of those factors as well as factors VIII thru XII. Mild factor VIII, IX, or XI deficiencies (e.g., 40% of normal levels), as well as deficiencies of factor XIII, are not usually identified by these tests.

The best measures of platelet function include the patient history, the patient's medications, and the platelet count. The bleeding time does not predict risk of bleeding and is a test of limited utility. Specific historical questions regarding nosebleeds, gingival bleeding, blood loss, and need for transfusions during or after tooth extractions, childbirth, or prior surgeries, are useful in eliciting a risk profile for surgical bleeding. Medications such as aspirin, vitamin E (>800 U/day), nonsteroidal anti-inflammatory drugs, nitrates, and calcium-channel blockers can diminish platelet function. Many over-the-counter (OTC) medications contain aspirin. The risk of bleeding is inversely related to the platelet count and begins to increase as the count decreases to less than 100,000/μL. The risk accelerates as the count decreases to less than 50,000/μL and becomes excessively high when the count is less than 5000/μL. If a disorder of platelet function or number may be present, hematology consultation is often useful.

Other relevant tests include specific laboratory evaluations for liver disease and kidney disease. The soluble coagulation factors are produced in the liver, and important activated anticoagulant proteins are cleared from the blood by the liver. As the synthetic capacity of the liver wanes and liver cells are injured, production of coagulation factors and clearance of anticoagulant proteins decrease. The presence of a hepatic coagulopathy significantly increases the risk of surgical bleeding. In patients with liver disease, further tests for the fibrinogen level, D dimer level, and for plasmin activation or fibrinolysis (the euglobulin lysis time) may be useful. Renal failure also may increase the risk of bleeding by diminishing platelet function. Management of patients with complex coagulopathies due to organ failure requires consultation with hematology and other appropriate services.

Clinical preoperative assessment for the risk of bleeding with moderate- to high-risk surgical procedures includes a patient history with questions regarding transfusions with prior procedures; a medication history that includes OTC drugs; and examination and laboratory evidence of liver or kidney disease. Surgical procedures with a moderate to high risk of bleeding include laparotomy, thoracotomy, mastectomy, neurosurgery, cardiopulmonary bypass, and oral, ophthalmic, plastic, or prostatic surgery. Rarely, dietary history can be relevant, particularly in elderly patients who have diets deficient in green leafy vegetables (vitamin K

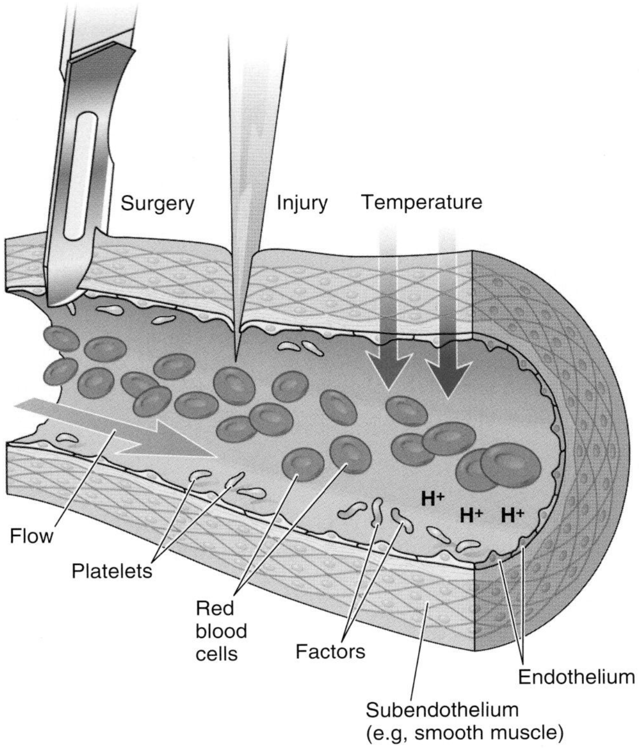

FIGURE 8–1 The components of hemostasis include generic ones such as blood flow and maintenance of temperature and pH, aberrations of which can cause platelet dysfunction. Specific components of hemostasis include the subendothelium, which contains tissue factor (which forms a complex with factor VII), and smooth muscle cells that constrict in the event of injury to limit blood loss, and the endothelium of the vascular wall, an active tissue that has on its surface anticoagulant molecules such as heparans and contains within its Weibel-Palade bodies procoagulant substances such von Willebrand's factor (vWF). vWF helps platelets to adhere to endothelium despite shearing stresses. Blood also contains the procoagulant soluble factors fibrinogen (factor I), prothrombin (factor II), and factors VII, IX, and X, which with prothrombin are vitamin K dependent, and the anticoagulant or profibrinolytic factors plasminogen, protein C, protein S, tissue inhibitor of activated factor VII, and antithrombin III. The formed elements of blood, particularly red blood cells and platelets, are critical components of hemostasis. Transfusion products can replace the soluble and cellular components in blood. Cryoprecipitate replaces fibrinogen, whereas fresh-frozen plasma contains pro- and anticoagulant factors. Packed red blood cells and pooled or apheresis platelet products replace cellular losses.

deficiency) or in citrus fruits (vitamin C deficiency). The only clinically relevant acquired defect of the subendothelium that can cause excessive bleeding is scurvy, a nutritional disorder due to lack of vitamin C. Physical examination findings suggestive of scurvy include perifollicular purpura and entrapped corkscrew hairs.

Transfusion Components

The most commonly used blood components include packed red blood cells, platelets, fresh-frozen plasma (FFP), and cryoprecipitate. Every effort should be made, especially in the setting of massive blood loss, to provide a sample of the patient's blood to the blood bank promptly so that the most specific compatible components can be used (Table 8-1).

At all hospital blood banks, however, red blood cells and other components are available to go on an emergency release basis by physician order and signature. Therefore, unless an absolute shortage of blood components exists at your institution, a need to wait unnecessarily for blood components in an emergency never occurs, because red blood cells that are O^- or O^+ may be given. Because of its rarity, AB plasma is not usually available, however, without a patient blood type, but this is not a critical issue because crystalloid may be used for volume expansion.

Red Blood Cells

Red blood cells (RBCs) provide hemoglobin, increase the oxygen-carrying capacity of blood, and, in the setting of severe anemia and thrombocytopenic bleeding, enhance hemostasis (Fig. 8-2). RBCs are indicated for patients with signs and symptoms of anemia such as fatigue, tachycardia, hypotension, mental sluggishness or disorientation, and shortness of breath. Usually these symptoms occur with a hemoglobin level less than 7 g/dL, although in patients with vascular disease in the cerebrovascular or coronary circulation, symptoms may occur with a hemoglobin level of 7 to 9 g/dL. RBC transfusion also are indicated for patients for whom timely improvements in hemoglobin cannot be achieved by erythropoietin, iron therapy, or treatment of the underlying disease.

TABLE 8–1 ABO and Rh(+ or –) Blood Group Compatibility Chart

	RBCs		FFP	
Patient	**Identical**	**Compatible**	**Identical**	**Compatible**
O+	O+	O + or –	O+	O, A, B, AB + or –
A+	A+	O, A + or –	A+	A, AB + or –
B+	B+	O, B + or –	B+	B, AB + or –
AB+	AB+	O, A, B, AB+ or –	AB+	AB + or –
O–	O–	O + or –	O–	O, A, B, AB + or –
A–	A–	O, A + or –	A–	A, AB + or –
B–	B–	O, B + or –	B–	B, AB + or –
AB–	AB–	O, A, B, AB + or –	AB–	AB + or –

FFP, fresh frozen plasma; RBCs, red blood cells.

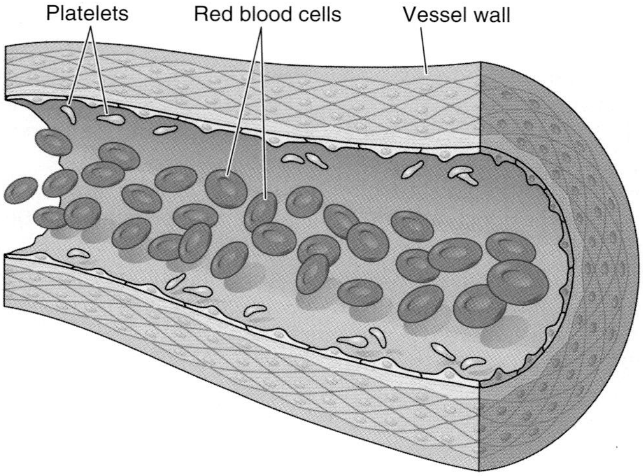

FIGURE 8–2 The hematocrit and platelet function. Red blood cells (RBCs) flow down the middle of this vessel, viewed in a lateral section. The flow of RBCs is layered or laminar, and the coursing red blood cells push the lighter platelets to the outer edges of the flow, enhancing the interaction between platelets and the vessel wall. This interaction is enhanced by higher hematocrits (>25%) and is adversely affected by severe anemia.

The adult dose of RBCs is determined by the clinical situation. The average pediatric dose is 10 mL/kg of patient weight and should not exceed 15 mL/kg. The adult infusion rate is determined by the clinical situation but usually is 1 unit over a period of 1 to 3 hours. The pediatric infusion rate is usually 2 to 5 mL/kg/hr. The expected outcome of RBC transfusion is resolution or prevention of the symptoms of anemia. One unit of RBCs in the nonbleeding medical patient should increase the hemoglobin concentration by 1 g/dL.

It is important to report transfusion reactions to the blood bank. Leukodepleted RBCs and platelets reduce the risk of transmitting cytomegalovirus and minimize the risk of febrile transfusion reactions. Washed RBCs are indicated for patients who experience allergic transfusion reactions such as hives.

Irradiation of RBCs and platelets is indicated to prevent transfusion-related graft-versus-host disease from viable lymphocytes in these components. Neonates, children with congenital immunodeficiency syndromes, organ and stem-cell transplant patients, patients with lymphoid malignancies or in active treatment for cancer, and patients receiving directed donations from blood relatives or human leukocyte antigen–matched platelets, should receive irradiated components. Irradiated components carry no radiation risk to healthcare personnel or the recipient.

Premedication is useful in patients who are transfused frequently. For adults, premedications may include acetaminophen, 650 mg orally or rectally, and hydrocortisone, 50 mg IV. Dosages should be appropriately determined for pediatric patients with the hospital pharmacy.

PEARLS FOR ROUNDS

Fibrinogen levels <100 mg/dL prolong bleeding.

The vitamin K–dependent clotting factors are II, VII, IX, and X.

FFP or vitamin K reverses warfarin (Coumadin). Protamine reverses heparin.

Bleeding patients whose platelets have been impaired by aspirin or nonsteroidal anti-inflammatory drugs may need platelet transfusions, no matter what the platelet count.

Bleeding after cardiopulmonary bypass may be due to inadequate neutralization of heparin. Giving FFP in this setting may worsen the bleeding because FFP provides antithrombin III.

Platelets

Platelets are used in cases where bleeding is due to thrombocytopenia or platelet-function abnormalities. For adults, pooled platelets or single-donor apheresis platelets are usually ordered. These components contain an average of 4×10^{11} platelets per component and can raise the platelet count by 20 to 50×10^9/L in the nonbleeding patient of average size without splenomegaly or platelet alloimmunization. For pediatric patients, the dose is usually one random donor unit per 10 kg of patient weight (or 10 mL of platelets per kg for patients weighing less than 50 kg). Premedication is recommended before the transfusion of platelets.

Plasma

Fresh frozen plasma (FFP) is indicated in the treatment of deficiencies of coagulation proteins for which specific factor concentrates are unavailable or undesirable (factors II, V, VII, and XI); for the treatment of multiple coagulation protein deficiencies in the patient who is bleeding uncontrollably; for reversal of warfarin effect when the patient is actively bleeding or requires emergency surgery and immediate hemostasis is needed before vitamin K can reverse the functional deficiency; in patients who have more than one blood volume transfused within several hours (usually 10 units of packed cells); and prophylactically before invasive procedures such as lumbar punctures in patients with INR more than 1.5.

FFP should be used in patients in whom factor deficiencies and not thrombocytopenia are thought to be the cause of bleeding. Replacement of deficient factors to 25% of the normal level usually results in normalization of the INR and PTT and adequate hemostasis. The dose of FFP is usually 10 to 15 ml/kg, which usually translates into 2 to 4 units per patient.

FFP also may be used in patients with a deficiency of antithrombin III who are undergoing surgery or who require heparin for treatment of thrombosis, if recombinant antithrombin III is not available. FFP also may be used as a replacement in plasmapheresis or transfused alone in patients with thrombotic thrombocytopenic purpura.

FFP should not be used for volume expansion. In adults, FFP may be infused at 200 mL/hr or slower if circulatory overload is a potential problem. In pediatric patients, the rate will depend on the clinical situation but is usually 1 to 2 mL/min.

Cryoprecipitate

Cryoprecipitate is a product derived from plasma that has been frozen and then thawed. It is rich in clotting factors such as factor VIII and fibrinogen. Cryoprecipitate is administered to patients with bleeding due to fibrinogen deficiency, usually with a fibrinogen level less than 100 mg/dL. Cryoprecipitate is not indicated for the treatment of factor VIII deficiency (hemophilia A) or von Willebrand's disease unless highly purified factor preparations are strictly unavailable.

The recommended dose of cryoprecipitate is based on the patient's plasma volume and fibrinogen level. Cryoprecipitate is usually dispensed in pools of 10 units. Each pool of 10 units of cryoprecipitate contains about 2 g (2000 mg) of fibrinogen; therefore a 70-kg person with a hematocrit of 25% and a fibrinogen level of 50 mg/dL has a blood volume of 5000 mL, a plasma volume of 3850 mL (38.5 dL), and needs 100 mg of fibrinogen per deciliter to increase the fibrinogen level to 150 mg/dL. Then 38.5 dL × 100 mg/d/L = 3850 mg or about two 10-unit pools. Cryoprecipitate also can be used to make fibrin glue intraoperatively for patching leaks in dura mater or lacerated areas of the liver.

In adults, platelets or cryoprecipitate should be infused rapidly. The recommended rate is 10 mL/min. In pediatric patients, the infusion rate is determined by the patient's volume tolerance.

Albumin and Hydroxyethyl Starch

Albumin is the chief plasma protein. Salt-poor concentrated albumin may be used to treat shock caused by loss of fluid from circulating blood volume due to burns, surgical procedures, or edema caused by hypoproteinemia, seen in liver and kidney disease. Albumin increases the osmolarity of plasma and draws fluid from tissue into the circulation, increasing the total blood volume. It promotes excretion of Na^+ and maintains normal electrolyte balance. Albumin should be maintained at levels greater than or equal to 2.0 g/dL to achieve these clinical goals. Albumin persists in the intravascular space for more than 24 hours. The dose of albumin needed to increase the serum level can be easily estimated by determining the patient's blood volume in deciliters (conversion factor, 7 dL/10 kg) and multiplying by the difference between the desired and measured albumin levels (g/dL).

PEARLS FOR THE OR

Microvascular bleeding often indicates a platelet defect.

Hypothermia impairs platelet function and can prolong bleeding.

Red blood cells that have been warmed to >40°C before infusion or are infused through lines containing D5W are likely to hemolyze. Blood should never be infused with medications or with any solution other than saline.

Wound drainage contains fibrinolytic substances. Red blood cells from shed blood usually should be washed before use.

Extensive tissue injury may result in significant blood loss without obvious bleeding. A single injury to the thigh may result in 2 to 3 L of blood loss into the large crushed muscle mass.

$$\text{Dose albumin (g)} = \text{Weight in kg} \times [7\ \text{dL}] \div [10\ \text{kg}] \times [\text{desired level} - \text{current level}].$$

Hydroxyethyl starch (HES) is an effective volume expander that may be used for the same indications as albumin. These include volume expansion for patients with hemorrhage, burns, trauma, or sepsis. Plasma volume expansion is very similar to that of albumin, because the HES molecules are similar in size. HES, however, can cause a coagulopathic effect similar to that of dextran; thus it is recommended that no more than 20 mL/kg of HESPAN be used per patient. HES remains in the intravascular space for up to 24 hours. Unlike RBCs, platelets, and plasma, albumin and HES are free from the danger of transmitting transfusion-transmissible diseases. However, a danger of contamination exists during the manufacturing, shipping, and storing processes.

Recombinant Factor VIIa

Recombinant factor VIIa is a recombinant human protein used to treat bleeding in hemophilia patients with inhibitors and to allow major surgery in that population. Administration of recombinant factor VIIa induces hemostasis by directly activating factor X and enhancing the generation of thrombin, bypassing the need for activation of factors VIII or IX. It has been shown to be of significant benefit in clinical trials for hemophiliacs.

Recombinant factor VIIa also has been used successfully in patients with acquired hemophilia or with excessive bleeding due to trauma or thrombocytopenia. An emerging literature exists on its use in those and other situations, including profuse postoperative bleeding due to complications of ulcer or inflammatory bowel disease. Clinical trials are needed, however, to study and justify such practices. In addition, although uncommon, thromboembolic complications, myocardial infarction, and cerebrovascular accidents have been reported in association with its use. Adequate levels of fibrinogen are needed for the thrombin burst triggered by recombinant factor VIIa to work.

Blood Loss

Transfusion component support is critical in the treatment of acute blood loss. In healthy adults, a unit of whole blood (~400 mL) can usually be removed in 15 minutes with trivial hemodynamic effects. When the amount of blood loss rapidly approaches 30% of the blood volume, hypovolemic shock usually occurs. The extent of blood loss may be deduced from the nature of the injury and from the signs of hypovolemia: tachycardia, hypotension, peripheral vasoconstriction, and unappreciable jugular venous pressure. Decreased urine output and evidence of organ ischemia also are signs of hypovolemic shock. Aggressive volume replacement with crystalloid such as Ringer's lactate is critical in the setting of hypovolemic shock because the primary goal is to maintain an adequate oxygen supply to vital organs. Anemia can be tolerated, provided circulating volume is maintained.

The rate of blood transfusion is a function of the hematocrit of the packed cells, the bore of the catheter (larger is faster), and the temperature of the blood (the flow rate doubles as temperature increases from 10°C to 36°C). The injured patient with persistently low blood pressure despite transfusion may still be losing blood or may be septic. After thermal injuries (burns), leakage of fluid and protein occurs from damaged areas. The volume of fluid lost is a function of the size and thickness of the burn. Half of the estimated fluid lost should be infused in the form of crystalloid in the first 24 hours after injury (Ringer's lactate, 4 mL per 1% area burned per kg).

Massive Transfusion

Massive transfusion occurs when a volume equivalent to the patient's blood volume is transfused in a 24-hour period (Fig. 8-3). Acidosis and hypothermia can impair platelet and vessel-wall function and exacerbate blood loss. Intravenous (IV) fluids and transfusions and the patient should be warmed. Dilutional coagulopathy is a major cause of excessive and persistent bleeding in the patient requiring massive transfusion. Transfusion management in such cases requires prompt clinical and laboratory assessment and balanced component therapy. Early and aggressive transfusion is needed for patients with penetrating injuries of the chest, neck, abdomen, and major vessels, and for those with pelvic fractures, severe abdominal injury, and multiple trauma. Aggressive balanced transfusion component therapy can be a life-saving intervention.

Patients can remain hemodynamically stable initially with aggressive crystalloid resuscitation. However, as blood loss approaches and exceeds blood volume—and

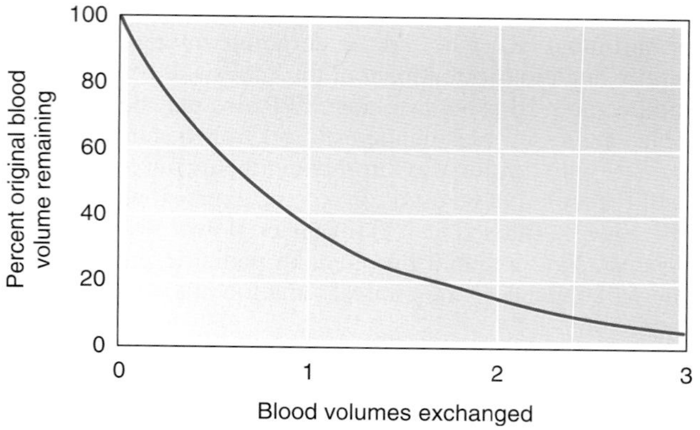

FIGURE 8–3 Dilutional coagulopathy. If a patient with massive bleeding receives only crystalloid resuscitation without early transfusion support, worsening anemia and thrombocytopenia as well as the consumption of clotting factors will lead to a dilutional coagulopathy; hence the need for balanced component support based on clinical status and serial laboratory testing.

particularly as transfusion is delayed—the dilution and consumption of platelets, fibrinogen, and clotting factors can result in a significant bleeding diathesis. Early aggressive transfusion management is indicated.

Serial laboratory tests are a requisite of transfusion management. Complete blood count (CBC), INR/PTT, and fibrinogen should be obtained at regular intervals and the results correlated with the clinical status. As shown in Figure 8-2, the hematocrit affects coagulation because of the influence of RBCs on platelet flow along vessel walls. The hematocrit should be maintained above 25% until blood loss ceases. Subsequently, in young critically ill patients who are not bleeding, lower hematocrits may be adequate to maintain oxygen delivery, and excessive transfusions have been shown to contribute to mortality.

Platelets can be dosed in two pools or apheresis units at a time and should be given at 2- to 4-hour intervals to maintain platelet counts greater than 50,000/mL, or greater than 100,000/mL if optimal hemostasis is desired in the case of bleeding in the lungs, retina, or brain. As noted earlier, FFP replacement of deficient factors to 25% of the normal level usually results in normalization of the INR and PTT. However, when patients are consuming factors due to dilution and trauma, FFP should be given at 2- to 4-hour intervals based on the patient's clinical status and laboratory tests. The recommended dose of cryoprecipitate is based on the patient's plasma volume and fibrinogen level. Fibrinogen levels can be directly and easily measured in the clinical laboratory and should be followed up routinely in these patients.

The existence of preexisting defects of hemostasis should always be investigated, particularly with liver disease, aspirin-containing medications, von Willebrand's disease, or thrombocytopenia. The immediate history of resuscitation contains useful information regarding the duration of hypotension and the extent of resuscitation. If bleeding persists despite aggressive management, sepsis or disseminated intravascular coagulation (DIC) should be considered. A DIC screen should be obtained. Aspects of a patient's clinical course—some reversible—that may be associated with DIC include massive transfusion, blunt trauma, arterial dissection, head injury, acidosis, hypothermia, microthrombi, and multiple organ failure.

Transfusion in Elective Procedures

The preoperative assessment should include a bleeding history, as noted earlier, a review of prescribed and OTC medications, physical examination for stigmata of bleeding problems and liver disease, and, before procedures with moderate to high risk of bleeding, laboratory tests that include a CBC, INR/PTT, and biochemical profile. Patients with a history suggestive of a hemostatic problem, or with abnormalities of platelet number or of coagulation testing, should be further evaluated with hematology consultation.

The question of the appropriate preoperative hemoglobin remains a controversial one. In chronically ill patients with normochromic normocytic anemia, the RBC mass may actually be diminished, and vasodilation associated with anesthesia can lead to severe intraoperative hypotension requiring aggressive fluid resuscitation, a happenstance that may prolong surgery and significantly complicate recovery. At the same time, however, much surgery is performed globally on patients with hemoglobin levels of 8 g/dL or lower, and most survive.

If severe anemia is discovered in a patient en route to elective surgery, it is important to determine the cause. Moreover, if such patients also have cerebrovascular or coronary artery disease, preoperative transfusion may be indicated. Patient informed consent for blood transfusion has become commonplace. It is useful to review the risks of transfusion, which include very unlikely outcomes such as death from incompatible blood (600,000:1) or acquisition of human immunodeficiency virus disease (1,000,000:1), or viral hepatitis (1,000,000:1). The risks also include those of minor reactions including febrile and allergic transfusion reactions. The odds of having such a reaction are 1 in 10.

Limiting blood loss in surgery has become sophisticated and effective. Intraoperative hemodilution is a convenient technique for elective procedures such as orthopedic surgery in young patients. Patients are bled, and their whole blood is saved in the operating room for reinfusion at the end of the procedure. Cardiopulmonary bypass surgery has become much more efficient at limiting blood loss by use of anticoagulated circuits, procoagulant medications, and careful patient-warming techniques. Recently cryopreserved platelets were shown to provide a more effective procoagulant effect than liquid platelets in cardiothoracic surgery, although their use is not routine. Procoagulant medications such as aprotinin are particularly useful in the setting of "re-do" bypass surgery, in which the risk of bleeding is greater. It is important to remember, however, that the most common cause of excessive surgical blood loss remains technical and unrelated to preexisting defects of hemostasis.

Suggested Reading

Blajchman MA, Bordin JO, Bardossy L, et al: The contribution of the haematocrit to thrombocytopenic bleeding in experimental animals. Br J Haematol 86:347–350, 1994.

Hedner U, Erhardtsen E: Potential role of rFVIIa in transfusion medicine. Transfusion 42:114–124, 2002.

Herbert PC, Wells G, Blajchman MA, et al: A multicenter, randomized, controlled clinical trial of transfusion requirements in critical care. N Engl J Med 340:490–416, 1999.

Lynn M, Jeroukhimov I, Klein Y, Martinowitz U: Updates in the management of severe coagulopathy in trauma patients. Intensive Care Med 28:241–247, 2002.

Trunkey DD: Hepatic trauma: Contemporary management. Surg Clin North Am 84:437–450, 2004.

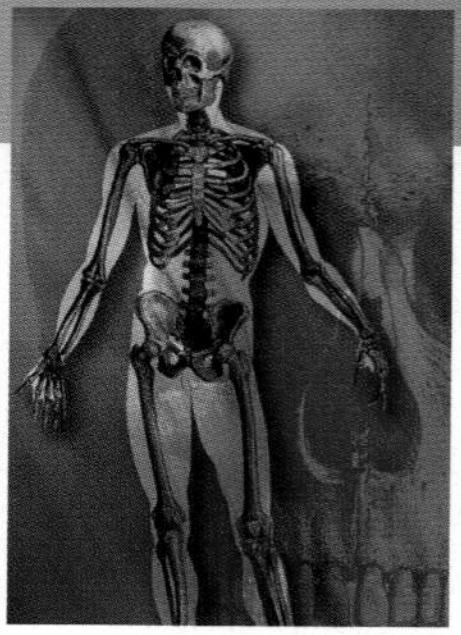

Chapter 9

Wound Healing

THOMAS A. MUSTOE, MD

Wound healing is central to the surgical disciplines, for they inherently involve the controlled creation of a wound. Minimally invasive surgery is based on the premise that smaller incisions reduce morbidity and the potential for complications. An estimated 2000 dressings are on the market and an almost equally large number of approaches to wound management. However, knowledge of a few basic scientific principles provides the student with a rational and straightforward approach. This chapter illuminates the principles of wound healing and their clinical implications.

Basic Wound Healing: Surgical Incisions

A successful surgical outcome requires rapid and strong wound healing initially and subsequent scar modulation to avoid late complications such as stricture, adhesion, and fibrosis.

The tissue response to injury, whether in the skin, intestine, liver, or heart, involves the processes of inflammation, cell proliferation, matrix deposition, wound remodeling, and scar resolution. Each organ has unique characteristics, but the basic principles are fundamentally similar. This chapter focuses on cutaneous and on hollow viscus wounds.

The Three Phases of Wound Healing

Inflammatory Phase

The initial response to injury is hemostasis with a fibrin-platelet clot that entraps red blood cells (Fig. 9-1*A*). The platelets degranulate, releasing platelet-derived growth factor (PDGF), transforming growth factor β (TGF-β), chemokines, and other biologically active proteins. The complement system is activated, and serum-derived fibronectin and fibrin provide a provisional matrix along which cells can migrate.

Within 24 hours, large numbers of circulating polymorphonuclear leukocytes (PMNs) roll and adhere to the capillary endothelium and then transmigrate into the wound through leaky capillaries (Fig. 9-1*B*). These cells are attracted by growth factors, chemokines, and the matrix itself, which enhances cell migration and proliferation via integrins and other cell-surface receptors. The PMNs begin to phagocytose the clot by releasing proteases. They also kill bacteria by releasing free radicals in a process dependent on the local oxygen level. Although PMNs release inflammatory cytokines that can upregulate the inflammatory milieu, they do not release growth factors in quantities sufficient to sustain the wound-healing cascade; now-classic studies have shown that blocking PMN entry into the wound does not decrease wound strength. Mounting evidence indicates that their numbers are tightly regulated and that the presence of too many may actually impair wound healing (see discussion of chronic wounds later).

Within 48 to 72 hours, blood-derived monocytes transmigrate across the capillary beds (Fig. 9-1*C*), differentiate into macrophages, and are activated, releasing a multitude of growth factors including PDGF, TGF-β, keratinocyte growth factor (KGF), fibroblast growth factor (FGF), and vascular endothelial growth factor (VEGF). Macrophages drive the wound-healing cascade through a rapid and enormous amplification, so that the relatively acellular 2- to 3-day-old wound becomes a highly proliferative, intensely cellular wound at 7 days.

PDGF and TGF-β are prototypes for the rich milieu of growth factors in the wound that stimulate cell migration, cell proliferation, and matrix deposition. They also act in an autocrine feedback loop to stimulate additional growth factor production by macrophages and other cells within the wound, such as endothelial cells, perivascular mesenchymal cells, and fibroblasts. VEGF and other growth factors stimulate angiogenesis, an important and necessary component of the wound-healing process.

Along the surface of the wound, exposed collagen matrix stimulates keratinocyte migration from the basal epithelial layer soon after wounding (Fig. 9-1*C*). KGF, produced by macrophages and fibroblasts, is the prototypical growth factor that stimulates keratinocyte proliferation and migration into the wound. If the wound is well approximated, epithelialization is virtually complete at 24 hours. This reestablishes a water barrier. Continued cell proliferation reestablishes a multilayered, keratinized surface within several days. In an open wound, this process can take days to months, depending on the size of the wound, the residual skin appendages, and the condition of the underlying neodermis, or granulation tissue.

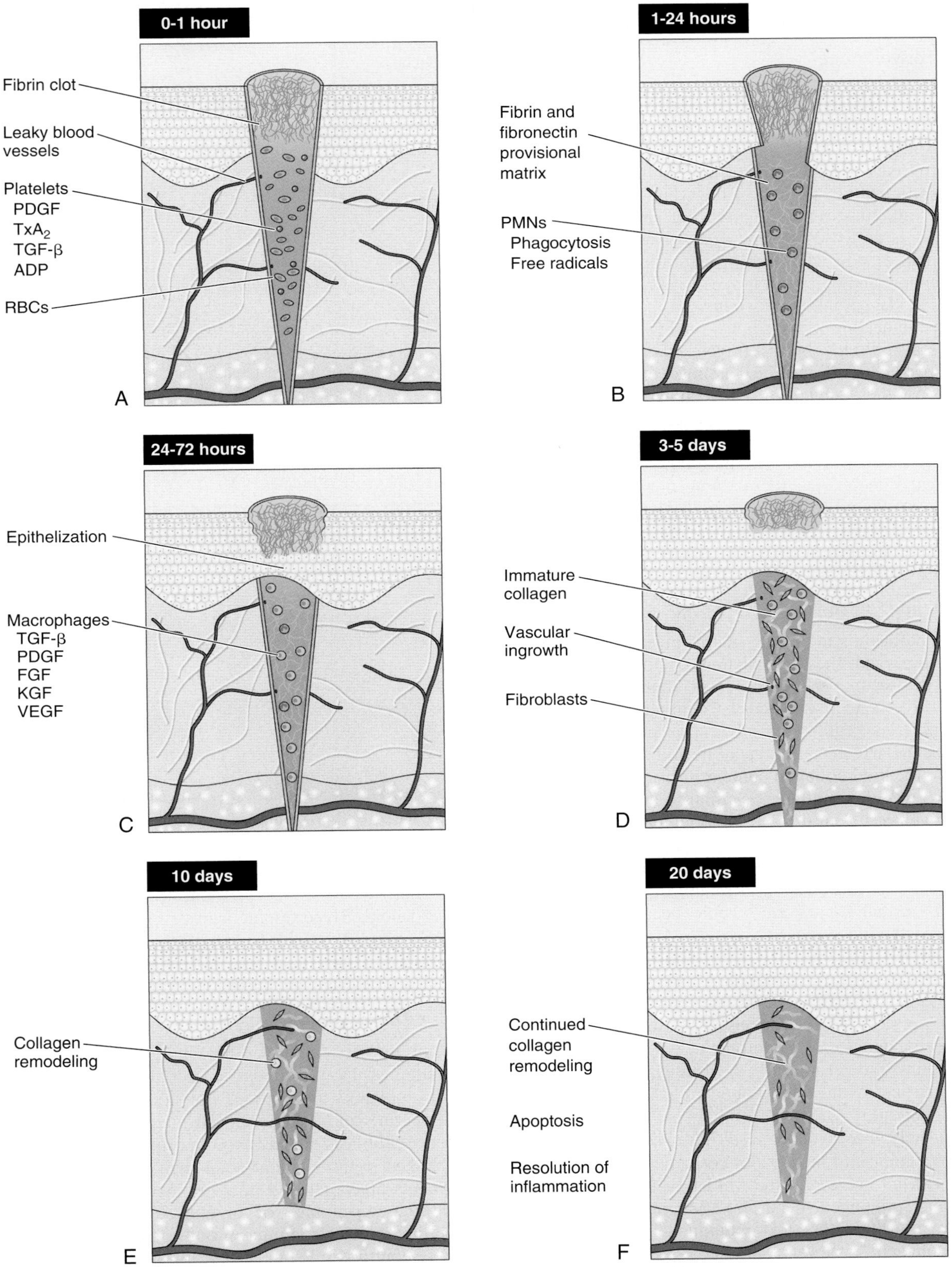

FIGURE 9–1 Schema of the phases of wound healing.

Proliferative Phase

Beginning at about 72 hours after wounding, fibroblasts migrate and proliferate along the provisional matrix, which is made of fibrin and fibronectin (Fig. 9-1*D*). They provide structure to the wound in the form of collagen, the protein responsible for the strength of the wound; proteoglycans; and trace amounts of other matrix molecules.

Although at least 15 types of collagen exist, type I predominates and is the basic structural protein in dermis, bone, tendon, and other soft tissues. It is the most important type of collagen in adult wounds. Type III collagen is produced in healing wounds but exists in greater amounts in fetal tissues. Proteoglycans (glycosaminoglycans), which consist of hyaluronic acid, also are made in large quantities. Because of their long, hydrophilic polysaccharide chains, they hold large amounts of water and are responsible for the high water content in healing wounds and in the dermis. Recent research has demonstrated that proteoglycans and other matrix molecules interact with fibroblasts and other cells in the wound by means of cell-membrane adhesion molecules. As such, changes in the extracellular matrix can lead to alterations in cell motility, protein synthesis, and cell proliferation.

Remodeling Phase

The wound-healing milieu is dynamic in terms of its cellular composition and the organization of matrix molecules. During the second and third weeks after wounding (Fig. 9-1*E* and *F*), the increased density of inflammatory cells and new capillaries begins to resolve. This process occurs by apoptosis, for which many signals are still unknown.

While the total collagen content in the wound increases for 2 to 3 weeks, simultaneous collagen breakdown occurs by collagenases. During this "remodeling" phase, which may last from many months to 2 years, the collagen fibrils become progressively more organized and cross-linked (Fig. 9-2). This increases the strength of the wound up to 70% of normal. Scars are visible because of residual disorganized collagen.

Researchers have observed that in fetuses, wound healing occurs by means of regeneration, in which the dermal architecture after repair is indistinguishable from that of the surrounding skin. Notably, an absence of inflammatory cells and a preponderance of hyaluronic acid is found. Research is attempting to determine whether duplicating some of the characteristics of the fetal wound might lead to reduced scarring in adults.

Fortunately, most wounds result in minimal scars that do not have significant functional or cosmetic consequences. In some cases, however, the inflammatory process is abnormally prolonged. Persistent PMNs and macrophages produce growth factors and inflammatory cytokines that drive collagen synthesis and cell proliferation. This overactivity can lead to hypertrophic scars or, in extreme cases, keloids. Hypertrophic scars develop within the original wound margins. Keloids have a genetic component, are more often seen in pigmented skin, and behave like benign tumors that may spread beyond the original boundaries of the wound.

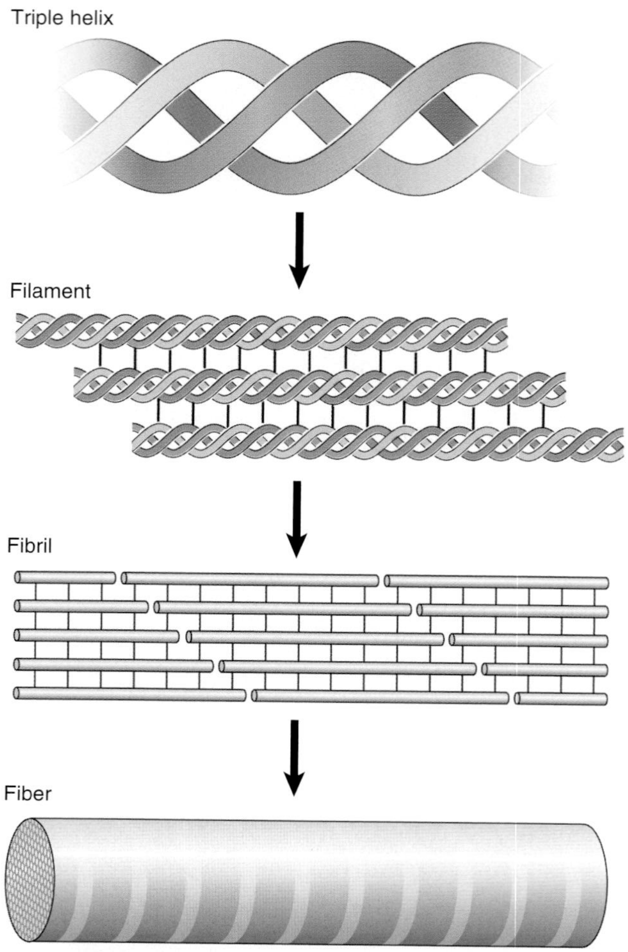

FIGURE 9–2 Type I collagen. Intramolecular cross-linking creates strength.

Wound Contraction

Within the first week of healing and during the early remodeling phase, wounds contract in a process that is still not completely understood. For contraction to occur, a fibronectin- and then collagen-matrix framework must exist. Fibroblasts attach to the matrix via integrins, which are linked to intracellular actin filaments. If enough actin filaments are organized in a strain-type pattern, the cells have the appearance of myofibroblasts. These can be identified on electron microscopy and are characteristic of highly contractile wounds. Fibroblasts act in concert with other fibroblasts to contract the entire framework. They then detach and reattach to the contracted framework to continue the process.

In surgical incisions, this contractile process will shorten or depress scars and is generally undesirable. For circular incisions such as viscus anastomoses, such contracture can result in stenosis. In general, excessive scarring leads to an excessive contraction. Surgical and pharmacologic efforts to control one process must also be directed at the other.

In an open wound, the healing process occurs in part by wound contraction, which pulls mobile skin over the wound to aid in closure. Humans are tight-skinned and have a relative lack of tissue mobility. In an open wound on the lower leg, where the skin is most closely adherent, wound contraction may contribute only 30% to the healing process. In the groin, where the skin is loose and redundant, wound contraction may contribute 90% or more to the process and is much faster because no need exists to create new tissue.

Epithelialization

The processes described earlier involve the dermis and are characteristic of soft-tissue wound repair anywhere in the body. In the skin and the gut, however, epithelial coverage also is critical to successful healing. The keratinized epithelium on the skin forms an important barrier to water, bacteria, and other materials from the environment. In a well-approximated surgical incision, the epithelial cells from the basal layer respond to exposed collagen in the broken basement membrane by mobilizing and rapidly covering the wound within 24 hours.

In a partial-thickness wound (Fig. 9-3) such as a second-degree burn, abrasion, or skin-graft donor site, a minimal loss of dermis occurs, and the wound heals by epithelialization. Under optimal conditions, the new epithelium can traverse an open surface at 1 to 2 mm/day. This speed is limited by epithelial cell motility and by the need for epithelial proliferation. In a partial-thickness wound, epithelial elements are preserved from the dermal appendages such as hair follicles and sweat glands; epithelialization occurs by a confluence of the islands of cells growing out from each dermal appendage. Healing is relatively rapid (7–10 days) for a typical second-degree burn or medium-thickness skin-graft donor site.

For open, full-thickness wounds, the process of epithelialization is prolonged, because the epithelial cells can migrate only from the edges of the wound. For the portion of the wound that does not close by contracture, closure will occur at a maximum rate of 1 to 2 cm/month. In a typical lower-leg ulcer 3 to 4 cm in diameter, in which wound contraction is minimal, the healing process will take 2 to 4 months under optimal circumstances.

The new epithelium interacts with the underlying granulation tissue (fibroblasts, capillaries, inflammatory cells, and matrix). Proteases produced by bacteria or by PMNs degrade the matrix and impair epithelial cell migration. Eschar, necrotic tissue, excess fibrin exudate, or any desiccated material requires enzymatic separation from the underlying collagen framework before epithelial cell migration can occur and thus slow the process significantly. The clinical implications of this are discussed later.

The epithelium has essentially no inherent strength. It is normally attached to the underlying dermis by anchoring fibers. These fibers cross the basement membrane and link to epithelial hemidesmosomes. In the healing wound, the new epithelium takes months to reform completely these hemidesmosome attachments. The new epithelium is

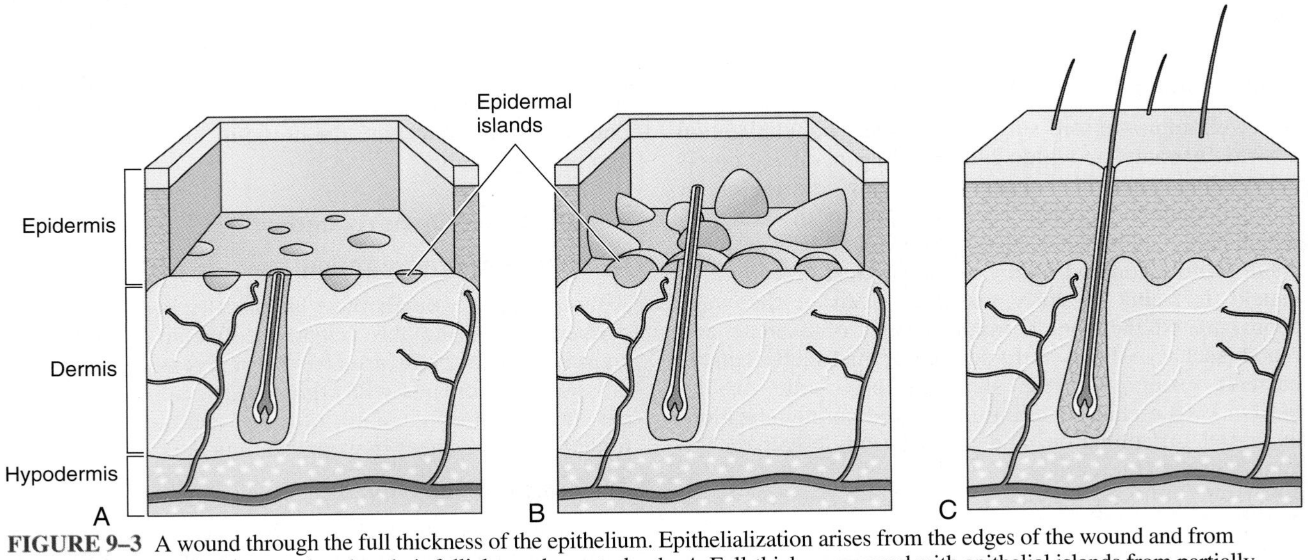

FIGURE 9–3 A wound through the full thickness of the epithelium. Epithelialization arises from the edges of the wound and from epithelial remnants in the wound such as hair follicles and sweat glands. *A*, Full-thickness wound with epithelial islands from partially transected sweat glands and hair follicles. *B*, Epithelialization proceeding from edges, and epithelial islands. *C*, Epithelialization complete.

sensitive to shearing forces and will readily blister or break down in response to trauma. With time, the epithelium will mature, rete ridges will reform, and a full complement of anchoring points will develop. At this point, the epithelium is histologically indistinguishable from normal tissue. The altered appearance and functional differences between mature scar and unwounded skin are due entirely to the altered collagen architecture and to the absence of dermal appendages if they have been destroyed.

Clinical Implications

Surgical Incisions

When to Remove Sutures

If cutaneous sutures are placed, the epithelium will begin to migrate down the suture track immediately. This may cause permanent suture marks. If the suture is closed tightly or if postoperative swelling creates tightness, the suture will begin to cut through the dermis, leaving a visible scar or "railroad tracks." It is therefore desirable to remove cutaneous sutures within 1 week. At this time, however, collagen deposition is not yet complete. Little cross-linking occurs, and it is disorganized. At 1 week, the wound tensile strength is only about 3% of normal; any tension will spread the wound apart. These problems can be avoided by using a subcuticular closure, in which no sutures cross the epithelium that can leave suture tracks. The absorbable sutures commonly used in the dermis (polyglactic acid) maintain their strength for 3 weeks. At that time, the wound strength is about 10% of normal. This is sufficient to prevent wound separation, but not wound spreading. If the tension on the wound is extreme (as in the case of tendon or abdominal fascia), the wounds must be protected from stress for about 6 weeks, at which time wound strength is 35% to 50% of normal.

When to Allow Incisions to Get Wet

In a well-approximated surgical incision, epithelialization is virtually complete within 24 hours. In general, bathing is permissible after that time. Underlying prostheses or foreign materials present an exception to this rule, in which case, any bacteria crossing the wound barrier might result in infection and failure of the surgical procedure. A benefit is found to early washing. Even in the well-approximated incision, a small amount of exudate and blood (eschar) adheres to the surface. If this is left in place, bacteria residing on the skin can proliferate on the nutrient-rich eschar, resulting in delayed epithelialization, increased inflammation, and a deleterious effect on the quality of the scar.

Optimization of Scar Quality

Well-approximated wounds are the keys to good scars. If the wound is closed under tension (such as an incision over the shoulder), the wound must be supported and relieved of tension for several weeks to allow collagen remodeling and cross-linking to occur. Unfortunately, commonly used absorbable polyglactic acid sutures do not prevent scar widening, although they may be sufficient to prevent wound dehiscence. Steristrips and wound immobilization, moreover, are not practical. The easiest way to relieve tension is to use dermal sutures that are nonabsorbable or that will persist for at least 6 weeks.

The most common causes of hypertrophic scars are delayed epithelialization and prolonged inflammation. Applying a semiocclusive dressing to a fresh incision, such as Steristrips or silicone gel sheeting, has been observed to reduce early skin erythema (which presumably indicates inflammation) and to improve scar quality.

Partial-thickness Wounds

Minimizing Discomfort

Although allowing an eschar to form will provide a protective water barrier and is the "natural" way that animals and humans achieve healing of an open wound, the associated desiccation will kill the upper cell layers and extend the depth of the injury slightly. In addition, the eschar is inelastic and will put shear forces on the underlying tissue during motion, causing pain. The use of a semiocclusive dressing such as a polyurethane film will maintain a moist wound environment without eschar formation and allows virtually painless healing. Occluding the wound with a cream will achieve the same effect.

Optimizing Healing

The use of the measures described earlier to achieve painless healing also will optimize epithelialization. Epithelial cell migration and motility are optimized if no eschar is present and the environment is wet. Bacterial growth may occur if the moist environment under an occlusive dressing becomes contaminated. If bacterial contamination is evident, the dressing should be changed and replaced daily.

Full-thickness Open Wounds

Optimizing Epithelialization

Although open wounds have historically been treated by deliberately drying the wounds, epithelial migration is significantly faster in a moist environment. A variety of dressings and creams will achieve this goal. This method has become the standard of care and is one of the fundamental advances in wound care in the last 25 years.

Achieving a Clean Wound

Although this is intuitively beneficial, it is a principle that is often misunderstood and not successfully accomplished. An open wound, which lacks an epithelial barrier, is

PEARLS FOR THE OR

Cutaneous sutures should be removed within 1 week to avoid "railroad tracks."

At 1 week, wounds have 3% of the strength of prewound skin.

At 3 weeks, wounds have 10% of prewounding strength.

At 6 weeks, wounds have 35% to 50% of prewounding strength.

Clean wounds can be achieved by means of dressing changes, water irrigation, mechanical débridement, and detergents.

Hypertrophic scars develop within the original wound margins. Keloids spread beyond the original boundaries of the wound.

In areas where skin is loose, wound contraction may contribute 90% or more to the wound-healing process.

continuously releasing an exudate with a high-protein content because of the leaky capillaries resulting from inflammation. This protein, which consists of albumin, fibrin, and other serum proteins, is adherent and is not easily removed from the wound bed. All open wounds are colonized with bacteria from the surrounding skin surface, and if the protein and cellular debris are not washed off frequently, the bacteria will have a culture medium on which to proliferate. The bacteria will release proteases and will attract PMNs. PMNs will in turn release their own proteases, superoxide radicals, and inflammatory cytokines that will degrade the matrix and create a hostile environment for epithelial cell migration and wound coverage.

Frequent dressing changes, water irrigation, mechanical removal of debris, and detergents can all contribute to a clean wound. Unfortunately, pain or an inability to reach the recesses of an open wound often make achieving a clean wound difficult. Creating a moist wound environment will allow autolysis to occur via endogenous enzymes, making removal of the exudate easier. In general, water irrigation of sufficient duration and intensity is the gentlest and most thorough way to reach the entire surface of a complex wound.

The use of sterile saline, although theoretically ideal, is generally impractical because of its expense. Tap water is cheap, readily available, and far cleaner than a colonized wound. The reduced osmolarity of tap water is a minor issue when compared with the benefits of a truly clean wound.

Wound Débridement:

To achieve a clean wound, débridement may be necessary. If necrotic tissue is within the wound, healing cannot be accomplished until it is removed. Because necrotic tissue is linked via collagen fibrils to surrounding living tissue, simple washing will remove it. Although the body will eventually remove necrotic tissue by means of enzymatic collagenolysis and phagocytosis, increasing bacteria counts in necrotic tissue can result in wound sepsis. The resulting inflammation may prevent healing.

Débridement is accomplished most efficiently with surgery, which usually requires anesthesia and can result in bleeding. An alternative is enzymatic débridement, accomplished through topically applied collagenases and other proteases.

Factors That Impair Healing

Although wound healing usually occurs efficiently, multiple systemic and local factors can impair it. These complicating factors are important in both incisional healing and open wounds. When several such factors are present, problems in healing become common.

Aging

As part of the aging process, cell proliferation, cell motility, and collagen synthesis decrease. The inflammatory response to wounding is dampened, and epithelialization is delayed. Although healing generally progresses without difficulty, if complicating factors are present, open wounds may become chronic, and in the case of surgery, the incidence of complications can increase substantially. Although these issues are progressive with advancing age, they are not generally significant until the seventh and eighth decades. At these ages, sutures should be left in longer, and precautions such as using nonabsorbable sutures for fascia repair should be taken. Skin-graft donor sites may pose difficulties not only in terms of delayed healing, but also because of increased susceptibility to painful blistering due to delayed reestablishment of the hemidesmosomal anchoring of the epithelium.

One benefit to the aging process is an improvement in the cosmetic appearance of scars and a decrease in the deleterious effects of wound healing, such as hypertrophic scars and scar contracture. The improvement in scars with age affords benefit in achieving good results from aesthetic surgery.

Ischemia

The impact of a low-oxygen environment in the wound is multifactorial. Because of the lack of a blood supply at the center of a wound until angiogenesis reestablishes blood flow, normally an oxygen gradient exists in the wound. Short-term changes in oxygen levels are stimuli for angiogenesis, increased cell motility, and increased growth factor production by cells (the "stress" response). If hypoxia is profound, prolonged, or combined with other factors that impair healing, its impact can be severe. Ischemia or ischemic reperfusion injury is central to the etiology of most chronic wounds.

Local wound hypoxia impairs collagen synthesis and may reduce cell proliferation if it is severe or chronic.

PEARLS FOR ROUNDS

The three phases of wound healing are inflammation, proliferation, and remodeling.

PMNs are not necessary for wound healing.

Wounds are fully epithelialized after 24 hours; patients may bathe after this time.

Wounds that are moist epithelialize most quickly. Occlusive dressings best serve this purpose.

Factors that impair healing include aging, tissue ischemia, malnutrition, edema, radiation therapy, steroids, collagen vascular disease, and diabetes

Ninety percent of all leg ulcers are due to venous insufficiency.

In the absence of cellulitis or abscess, pressure sores almost never cause bacteremia and fever.

Wounds in the aged population appear to be particularly susceptible to the negative effects of ischemia. Perhaps the most important negative effect is the impact on the ability of PMNs to kill bacteria. Their chief killing mechanism is the release of superoxides, which are directly dependent on the oxygen levels in the local environment. High bacterial levels, even in the absence of infection, will impair wound healing.

In postoperative patients, the effects of cigarette smoking–induced vasoconstriction, hypovolemia, hypothermia, or excess catecholamines from unrelieved pain can reduce blood flow to the surgical wound, increasing the rate of wound infections and other complications.

Malnutrition or a Catabolic State

Although protein malnourishment and vitamin deficiency are rare in the United States, certain facts are important to keep in mind. Historically, scurvy (vitamin C deficiency) led to open sores because vitamin C is necessary for collagen synthesis. Zinc and copper also are important cofactors for many enzyme systems. Zinc deficiency in particular has been cited as a possible cause of impaired healing. However, it is extremely rare, and measuring zinc levels is typically not cost effective.

Many patients have low albumin levels and are in a catabolic state because of underlying chronic medical conditions. Wound repair requires tremendous net protein synthesis and cellular proliferation. Patients with an albumin level of less than 3.0 mg/dL are at increased risk for surgical wound complications. Because of the long turnover time of serum albumin, transferrin levels may be more informative. However, a paucity of good clinical data fully support the use of either.

From a practical standpoint, if a patient with a chronic wound cannot form healthy granulation tissue in the wound base and no evidence of a decrease in wound size is seen, he or she is at greatly increased risk for failure of a surgical procedure to close the wound.

In burn patients, who are in a high catabolic state with enormous energy loss and protein breakdown, growth hormone has been used successfully to speed healing of skin graft donor sites by putting the patient's metabolism into a more anabolic state.

In general, vitamin and nutritional supplements do not improve wound healing in typical well-nourished patients. Two possible exceptions exist. Patients often rub vitamin E into incisions in an attempt to improve healing and scarring. However, the evidence to support this practice is largely anecdotal. Vitamin A, meanwhile, has been shown to counteract steroid-induced wound impairment in animals and anecdotally appears to be effective in humans taking steroids.

Edema

In normal tissue, each cell is only a few cell diameters removed from a capillary. In systemic conditions such as congestive heart failure, nephrotic syndrome, and venous insufficiency, edema exists. Edema may impair wound healing by several mechanisms: it increases the diffusion distance for nutrients and oxygen; it causes serum extravasation from the capillaries; and it is associated with pericapillary cuffing, which can trap growth factors and provide a diffusion barrier. In many lower extremity ulcers, one of the mainstays of successful therapy is adequate edema control.

Radiation

Radiation leads to progressive fibrosis and the loss of small blood vessels over many years, resulting in local tissue ischemia. In addition, the radiated tissues have a reduced proliferative and synthetic response; radiation ulcers may develop spontaneously years after radiation. Surgical intervention with well-vascularized tissue is frequently the only viable solution.

Steroid Therapy and Chemotherapy

Many patients are taking long-term steroid therapy. Steroids depress collagen synthetic capacity and lead to thinning of the dermis and a decreased response to injury. Immunosuppressive effects are less damaging unless the doses are high enough to depress the bone marrow, as in chemotherapy. Chemotherapy increases susceptibility to infection and depresses the inflammatory phase of wound healing. Clinically, this is rarely a severe problem; many patients can heal wounds while undergoing chemotherapy.

Collagen Vascular Disease

Many patients with collagen vascular diseases take medications such as steroids that impair healing. The autoimmune process itself can cause spontaneous ulcerations and depress healing of chronic wounds. Some such wounds may heal only when the primary process is under control.

Chronic Wounds

In many patients, open wounds heal slowly or not at all. Wounds that have remained open for more than 2 to 3 months are classified as chronic. In aggregate, they are a major national health problem that costs billions of dollars in health care each year. The majority fall into three categories: leg ulcers due to venous insufficiency; diabetic foot ulcers; and pressure sores. Although chronic wounds may occur in all age groups, they are a problem primarily in the elderly. In all three groups, local tissue ischemia or ischemia/reperfusion injury is a contributing factor.

Leg Ulcers

Approximately 90% of all leg ulcers are due to venous insufficiency. However, the differential diagnosis is substantial (Box 9-1).

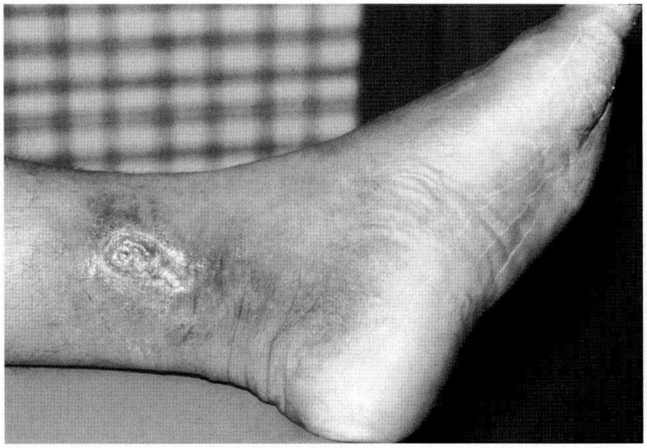

FIGURE 9–4 Venous stasis ulcer.

Evaluation. The initial history and physical examination are important. Venous insufficiency usually follows trauma to the leg, which may have led to an episode of deep venous thrombosis, often undiagnosed. This trauma is typically followed by a history of chronic swelling of the leg when it is dependent. Other etiologies can be ruled in or out by the presence of absence of leg edema, although this is not completely reliable.

On physical examination, venous ulcers are characteristically found on the medial or lateral portion of the leg just above the ankle. They usually are surrounded by hemosiderin deposits and pigmentation as well as subcutaneous fibrosis due to previous injury and red blood cell extravasation through leaky capillaries under increased pressure. This appearance is called *lipodermatosclerosis* (Fig. 9-4). Pulses should be palpable.

A patient with an ulcer in the typical location, the signs of lipodermatosclerosis, good pulses, and a history of dependent swelling without collagen vascular disease can be confidently diagnosed with venous insufficiency.

BOX 9–1 Differential Diagnosis of Leg Ulcers

Venous insufficiency
Arterial insufficiency
Rheumatoid arthritis
Polyarteritis nodosa
Vasculitis
Necrobiosis lipoidica diabeticorum
Sickle cell anemia
Other collagen vascular disease
Squamous cell carcinoma
Münchausen syndrome (self-inflicted)

If atypical aspects of the history or physical are present, further evaluation is necessary. A biopsy can be helpful in diagnosing cancer, collagen vascular disease, vasculitis, or necrobiosis lipoidica diabeticorum (which occurs only in diabetics). Ankle/arm indices and Dopplers are useful for diagnosing arterial insufficiency. Plethysmography, meanwhile, is useful for making a definitive diagnosis of venous insufficiency.

Etiology. Venous ulcers are caused by venous hypertension when the legs are in the dependent position, which is in turn due to incompetent valves and failure of the "calf pump." Increased venous pressure causes a decreased arteriovenous gradient, resulting in decreased tissue perfusion and fibrin cuffing around the small vessels. Although venous hypertension is corrected when the legs are elevated, repeated insults and chronic leg edema lead to ulceration.

Treatment. The principles of moist healing, appropriate débridement, and maintenance of low bacterial levels all are important. However, without addressing the underlying problem of venous hypertension and resultant leg edema, the ulcer will not heal. The importance of edema control has been documented in multiple studies. It can be achieved by means of elastic compression garments, multilayered bandages with outer elastic wraps that achieve stable compression, by sequential pressure pumps, or by simple leg elevation. The most common treatment is a multilayered bandage that achieves compression, absorption of exudate, and moist healing.

For larger ulcers, which may heal slowly, skin grafting can be useful. However, unless the patient can cooperate with long-term edema control, the underlying valvular incompetence will lead to ulcer recurrence.

Diabetic Foot Ulcers

Diabetics are at increased risk for atherosclerosis and ulcers due to arterial insufficiency. They also are more prone to infection and have higher bacterial counts in wounds. Most chronic wounds in diabetics are on pressure points on the feet, such as the heel, metatarsal joint surfaces, and the toes. Patients in whom such ulcers develop are at significant risk for future amputation and have an associated reduction in life expectancy.

Etiology. As diabetics develop neuropathy, their feet are affected first, and they lose the ability to detect excessive pressure from poorly fitting shoes or trauma. As the neuropathy progresses, the intrinsic foot muscles become weak, with a loss of arch support. Charcot joints develop, which allow new pressure points to develop, requiring specially fitting shoes. Twenty to 30 minutes of excessive pressure may cause tissue necrosis to develop over a pressure point.

Evaluation. In the diabetic with neuropathy and a foot ulcer over a pressure point (Fig. 9-5), the diagnosis is straightforward. In the absence of palpable pulses, a low threshold for ruling out large vessel arterial disease with Dopplers and, if necessary, an angiogram is important. Because of the frequent presence of heavily calcified vessels, ankle/arm indices are unreliable.

Treatment. The single most important intervention is adequate protection from excessive pressure. This can be accomplished using offloading shoes, casts, crutch walking, or a wheelchair. The surgeon must débride callus and fibrotic tissue frequently to keep bacterial counts low. Maintaining a moist healing environment also is important.

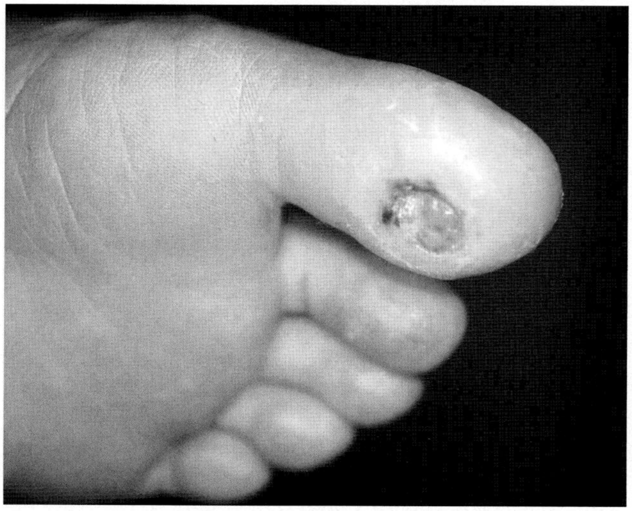

FIGURE 9–5 Diabetic foot ulcer.

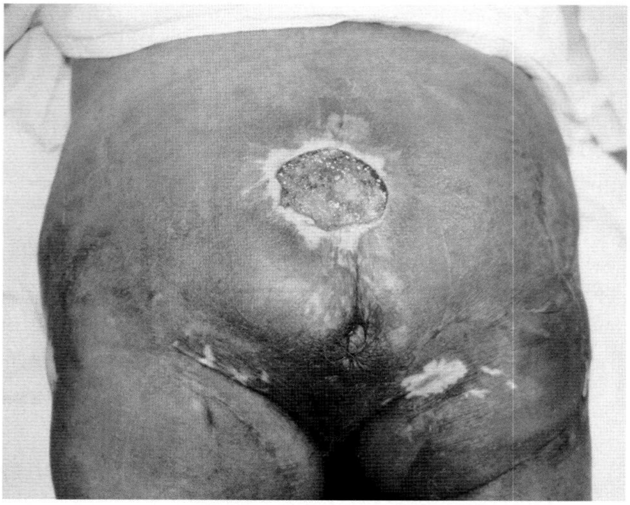

FIGURE 9–6 Sacral pressure ulcer.

Pressure Sores

Pressure sores are perhaps the most common chronic wounds. Advanced age, decreased mental status, incontinence, malnutrition, and other major medical problems increase the risk substantially.

Etiology. Pressure sores are similar to diabetic foot ulcers in that the primary insult is pressure over a bony prominence that exceeds local capillary perfusion pressure (Fig. 9-6). The normal capillary perfusion pressure is about 30 mmHg, whereas the pressure over the trochanter in a recumbent patient reaches 65 mmHg. The resulting lack of perfusion, if constant, may lead to tissue necrosis in as little as 20 to 30 minutes. Shearing forces from turning and skin maceration from incontinence increase the susceptibility to pressure. The patient who is too debilitated to move can develop pressure sores without assisted turning every 2 hours. Paraplegics who lack protective sensation are particularly likely to get pressure sores from sitting in one position for too long.

Evaluation. Diagnosis is straightforward, as the anatomic location is over a pressure point (sacrum, ischium, trochanter, or calcaneus). Osteomyelitis may complicate pressure sores that extend to bone. Probing the wound with a gloved finger is the most cost-effective and accurate diagnostic test. If the wound does not extend to bone, osteomyelitis is unlikely. However, if soft bone is felt, then osteomyelitis probably exists. Simple physical examination in this manner can be 90% accurate. Radiographs are not highly sensitive; unless bony erosion is present, they may appear falsely normal. Bone scans are not helpful either, because they lack specificity; the surrounding inflammation may result in a positive bone scan even without osteomyelitis. The only way to make the diagnosis of bony involvement certain is to perform a bone biopsy. However, this is usually not necessary. A frequent diagnostic issue is whether a pressure sore is the source of fever in a hospital patient with multiple medical problems. An open wound, even if highly exudative, is almost never the cause for significant fever unless surrounding cellulitis is noted. However, if a closed space exists (e.g., under a necrotic eschar), then an abscess can form with resulting high bacteria counts, fever, and even bacteremia.

Treatment. The principles of wound care for open wounds discussed earlier apply here. These wounds are often deep with irregular contours and are frequently contaminated because of their location. Adequate absorption and removal of the exudate to keep the bacteria counts low is very important. Often the amount of necrotic tissue is substantial, and surgical or enzymatic débridement is necessary.

Adequate pressure relief also is crucial, either by frequent turning or weight shifting, or from the use of a suitable pressure-relief bed. Pressure sores can take months to heal, and if bony involvement is present, they may never heal without surgical débridement and flap closure. Unfortunately, the recurrence rates are high if pressure relief on a continual basis is not achieved. Therefore patient education and lifestyle adjustment are important when applicable.

Therapeutic Agents to Optimize Healing

Dressings

Approximately 2000 dressing products are available. It can be confusing to decide which ones are most appropriate, particularly when one is confronted with optimistic marketing claims and the biases of various caregivers. Dressings should accomplish two goals: the wound must be moist, and exudate must be absorbed. Other important goals include infrequent dressing changes (provided that the absorptive power is great enough and the dressing can remain adherent); protection of the surrounding skin from maceration; and minimization of skin injury from adhesive. It must be emphasized that no dressing on the market will accelerate healing over that achieved with a clean wound and moistened gauze.

The traditional moist gauze and tape dressing is inexpensive. However, it requires frequent changes because of its limited absorptive capacity. Tape can irritate the skin, and the gauze can dry out. The traditional "wet to dry" dressings are actually a poor choice, because they allow wound desiccation, which will delay healing. Gauze dressings, when combined with an antibiotic cream, can be useful in aggressively treating a highly exudative wound.

The simplest occlusive dressing is a polyurethane film that facilitates moist healing and has no absorptive capacity. It is particularly useful for superficial wounds that have essentially no exudate, such as skin-graft donor sites. A large number of absorptive dressings fall into the categories of hydrocolloids, foams, hydrogels, alginates, and absorptive powders or pastes (Table 9-1)

Perhaps the most widely used dressings for open wounds are of the hydrocolloid class. They consist of hydrophilic materials combined with a special adhesive. The surface is covered with a polyurethane film that protects the wound and allows moist healing. The adhesive adheres to skin only

TABLE 9–1 Wound Dressings

Classification	Function	Examples
Films	Polyurethane, semiocclusive	Tegaderm
	Some evaporation minimizes maceration	Opsite
	Nonabsorptive, good adhesive	Bioocclusive
Hydrocolloids	Semiocclusive, absorptive, adherent	Duoderm
	Complex hydrophilic polymer	Ultrec
	With a film backing and adhesive	Comfeel
Hydrogels	Synthetic polymers	Vigilon
	Highly absorbent, nonadherent	Intrasite gel
	Used with an external dressing	Geliperm
Alginates	Long-chain hydrophilic polysaccharide	Sorbsan
	Derived from seaweed	Kaltostat
	Absorptive, nonadherent	
	Used with an external dressing	
Foams	Absorptive due to open cell structure	Allevyn
	Nonadherent	Lyofoam
	Used with an external dressing	
Absorptive powders and pastes	Hydrophilic polymers in particulate form	Debrisan
	Absorptive	Duoderm granules
	Used with an external dressing	Bard absorptive
Nonadherent gauze or cellulose combinations	Gauze or cellulose for absorption	Telfa gauze, ointment combination
	Cream or nonadherent porous coating	
	Requires tape or other cover dressing	Adaptic, Xeroform

until the absorptive capacity of the dressing is exhausted. This combination makes these dressings ideal for use on chronic wounds.

Topical Antibiotics

Although topical antibiotics can be useful, they are often inappropriately used as a substitute for many of the principles of good wound care. Reducing the bacterial count in a wound is beneficial, but without effectively removing the exudate, topical antibiotics will merely select resistant organisms without reducing the total bacterial load. Allergic reactions can be a problem with all of the commonly used topical antibiotics. When using topical antibiotics, an ointment or cream base will help to maintain a moist wound environment. Silver sulfadiazene is the most useful first-line topical antibiotic. It has a broad spectrum, does not result in bacterial resistance, sensitizes the skin rarely, and is relatively inexpensive. In addition, complete removal of the white cream from the wound with each dressing change provides an easy end point for the patient to use when cleaning the wound.

Pharmacologic Débriding Agents

Surgical excision of necrotic tissue is the fastest and most effective way to achieve a wound with a healthy wound bed. Enzymatic débriding agents (collaganases and other proteases derived from bacteria) can accomplish the same objective without surgery over a longer period. They should be used only if wound sepsis is not a concern. A semiocclusive dressing left in place for several days can speed up the patient's own autolytic processes, leading to "natural" débridement. This option is relatively inefficient and slow.

Growth Factors

Growth factors are normally present in healing wounds. In animals, the addition of growth factors to impaired wounds has accelerated healing. Multiple clinical trials in humans have produced mixed results, probably because of the complexity and variability of the underlying etiologies and cofactors, the difficulty in conducting clinical trials in chronic wounds, and the presence of proteases that degrade the growth factors.

Nevertheless, after a 7-year process and studies in more than 1000 patients, PDGF (Regranex) was approved in 1997 by the Food and Drug Administration (FDA) for use in diabetic foot ulcers. Studies using PDGF for other indications as well as other growth factors are in current clinical trials.

Artificial Skin Equivalents

Tissue engineering holds promise for treating multiple medical conditions. Perhaps nowhere has more progress toward clinical application been made than in tissue-engineered skin. Several products, which consist of dermis-like matrices with or without synthetic water barrier coverings, have been developed as temporary skin coverage in burn patients.

Tissue-engineered products also have been used in clinical trials on chronic wounds. Apligraf, which consists of a cultured-fibroblast–derived synthetic dermis and a heterologous epithelium, has been successfully used to treat venous ulcers. The FDA approved Apligraf in 1998, for the treatment of refractory ulcers.

Physical Devices for Use in Treating Open Wounds

Whirlpool Treatments. The importance of achieving a clean wound environment without necrotic tissue or protein exudate cannot be overemphasized. Mechanical cleansing or débridement can be quite painful and is potentially injurious to healthy tissue. The gentlest way of achieving a clean wound is by means of water irrigation. Water under pressure from a shower head, dental water pick, or syringe with a catheter tip is effective in removing tenacious protein exudate. Whirlpool treatments were first widely used on burn wounds.

Hyperbaric Oxygen. As discussed previously, many chronic wounds are ischemic. Hyperbaric oxygen (HBO) therapy, during which the patient lies in a hyperbaric chamber set at 2.0 to 2.4 atms and 100% O_2 concentration, can achieve high oxygen levels in the most ischemic wounds for the duration of the treatment. Although oxygen is a necessary component in aerobic metabolism, mounting evidence suggests that it also is a signaling molecule for growth factor production and synthesis of other proteins. A large clinical experience suggests clinical efficacy, but large, prospective, randomized trials have not been conducted. Based on the success of a number of retrospective studies, the use of HBO in recent years has become widespread, particularly for use in diabetic foot ulcers. The length of treatment and other parameters used are still arbitrary.

Electrical Stimulation

Considerable evidence suggests that electrical stimulation stimulates cell proliferation and migration and thus might be useful in wound healing. Several retrospective studies have suggested efficacy in a variety of chronic wounds, but prospective randomized studies are lacking. Nevertheless, the use of electrical stimulation has found widespread acceptance in this country and is usually administered by physical therapists.

Suggested Reading

Mustoe TA: Prevention of excessive scar formation—A surgical perspective. In Téot L, Ziegler UE, Banwell PE (eds): Surgery in Wounds. Berlin, Springer Verlag, 2004, pp 489–495.

Trott AT: Wounds and Lacerations: Emergency Care and Closure, 3rd ed. Philadelphia, Mosby, 2005, pp 1–3.

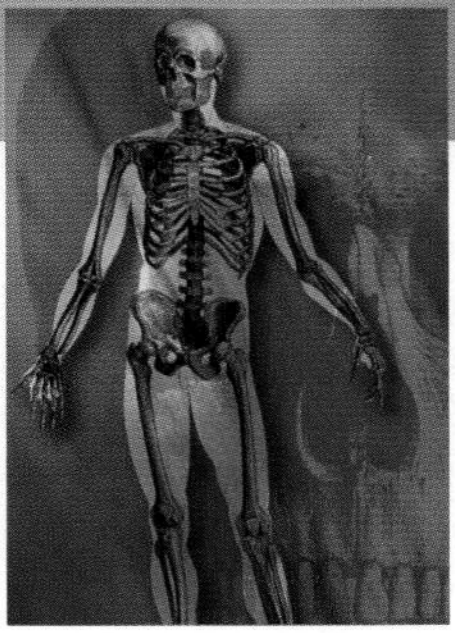

Chapter 10

Prevention and Management of Surgical Infections

RIAD CACHECHO, MD

The body is under constant threat from pathogens, which under optimal conditions can invade the tissues causing infection. Four lines of defense exist: mechanical, chemical, humoral, and cellular; these protect the body against pathogens. Surgical trauma provides multiple opportunities for bacteria to invade the tissues and to cause infection by breaching the host defense barriers.

Host Defense Barrier

The *mechanical* barriers, such as the skin and mucosal membranes, are very effective against microbial invasion. Some of these structures have the ability to secrete *chemical* agents to maintain an acid environment, like the sebaceous glands in the skin and the gastric mucosa, preventing bacterial growth. Any disruption of the barriers by disease, surgery, or trauma will allow the pathogens to invade the involved organ, thus causing an infection.

The *humoral defense* system consists of *immunoglobulins* (Igs) called antibodies and the complement system, both of which work in concert to help lyse the pathogens, attract the polymorphonuclears (PMNs) and the macrophages, and enhance phagocytosis in the area of infection. The five classes of immunoglobulins are IgM, IgG, IgA, IgE, and IgD, each composed of one class-specific heavy protein (H) and two nonspecific light (L) proteins (κ or γ). The amino terminals of the protein chains are responsible for the antibody-antigen binding, whereas the carboxy terminals of the H chains activate the complement cascade and bind to the PMNs and the macrophages, thus presenting the antigen that is already attached to them to the cellular defense system represented by the macrophages, PMNs, and T cells. Each clone of plasmacytes secretes the immunoglobulin (antibody) that targets a specific antigen.

The *complement* system is made of a group of proteins that reside in the serum in a dormant state. Once activated, the complement system releases a number of components that play an important role in the host defense mechanism. The components C3a and C5a increase vascular permeability and attract PMNs and macrophages to the infected area. C3b enhances phagocytosis by opsonization.

Macrophages act as the first line of the *cellular* defense in the body by presenting a "processed" antigen to the T cells, initiating a systemic immune response by way of cytokine secretion. PMNs enter the infected area from the bloodstream by the effect of chemoattractants, such as C5a and the cytokines and inflict direct damage on the pathogens as well as on the host organs. Unfortunately, the damage inflicted by the activated macrophages and PMNs goes beyond pathogen destruction, as secretion of lysosomal enzymes, free radicals, and cytokines delivers an injury to local as well as remote cells in the host.

Cytokines is a term that defines a group of heterogeneous components secreted by the activated macrophages, lymphocytes, and the endothelium. Interferon-γ (IFN-γ) and interleukin-1 (IL-1), secreted by the T cells and macrophages, respectively, are the first cytokines to be secreted during an inflammatory reaction. They are followed by the secretion of the tumor necrosis factor (TNF) and interleukins 6 (IL-6) and 8 (IL-8). In animal and human studies, the symptoms of systemic infection and sepsis were associated with the presence of IL-1 and TNF. In addition, IL-1 promotes the synthesis of acute phase reactants like transferrin and the complement proteins by the liver, further assisting in the defense against infection.

Another important component of the host defense is the *adhesion molecules* that are responsible for neutrophil *margination.* As the activated neutrophil motion slows in the blood vessels, its integrin receptors bind to the endothelial intracellular adhesion molecule (ICAM), an important step that prepares the neutrophils to move across the vascular wall toward the infection or injury site by *diapedesis.*

Resident Microbial Flora

Many microorganisms inhabit the human body and interact positively with the host's defense system, promoting immunity and simultaneously benefiting from its presence within the host. In addition to promoting the development of the immune system in the early stages of life, the microflora prevent pathogens from invading the gut lining by saturating the epithelial receptors used by the pathogens to invade the GI tract (Table 10-1).

TABLE 10–1 Gastrointestinal Microbial Flora

Oropharynx	Staphylococci, streptococcus, lactobacilli, *Bacteroides oralis*
Stomach and upper small bowel	Few gram positives, aerobes, lactobacilli, *Candida* spp.
Lower small bowel	Gram-positive aerobes and anaerobes and some gram-negative colonic flora
Colon	Anaerobes, esp. bacteroides and fusobacterium; aerobes; *Escherichia coli*; *Enterococcus fecaelis*; Enterobacter spp.

Sepsis, Shock and the Systemic Inflammatory Response Syndrome

The immune system reacts in a nonspecific manner to bacterial invasion, to surgical and accidental trauma, and to local inflammatory reactions like pancreatitis. The activation of the complement system, coagulation cascade, macrophages, and PMNs generates a wide range of active mediators, such as lymphokines and adhesion molecules, producing a clinical syndrome that represents the host response to bacterial invasion or to trauma. This syndrome, called the *systemic inflammatory response syndrome* (SIRS), is described by the presence of any two of the following: temperature, more than 38°C or less than 36°C; heart rate, more than 90 beats/min; respiratory rate, more than 20 breaths/min; and white cell count, more than 12,000/mm^3 or less than 4000/mm^3. When SIRS is induced by an infective source, it is called *sepsis*. The term *severe sepsis* is used to identify cases of extreme symptoms and signs of disseminated infection, whereas *septic shock* clearly defines situations of sepsis in which the cardiovascular system is unable to fulfill the metabolic requirements during infection, leading to hypotension, metabolic acidosis, and multisystem organ failure.

The treatment of SIRS, sepsis, and shock must be directed toward drainage of the infected site, debridement of infected or injured soft tissue, and antibiotic therapy, in addition to the support of the failing organs by using mechanical ventilation, renal dialysis, and inotropic agents. The following modalities have been tested over the last decade to break the vicious cycle of inflammatory activation:

1. Monoclonal antibodies to endotoxins, and especially to lipid A, an important activator of the septic response,
2. Monoclonal antibodies to TNF and IL-1, the mediators known to induce the symptoms and signs of sepsis, and
3. Monoclonal antibodies to CD-18, an adhesion molecule that helps in PMN margination.

These mentioned attempts to improve the survival of septic patients have failed because of the multifactorial nature of the disease, the variety of the precipitating factors, and most important, our incomplete understanding of the specific role each mediator plays in SIRS and sepsis. In November 2001, the FDA approved the use of recombinant human activated protein C (Xigris) as a treatment for septic shock. The mechanism by which activated protein C improves survival in patients with septic shock is not understood.

Microbiology

Bacteria are monocellular microorganisms that possess a plasma membrane that envelops the cytoplasm. Their genetic material is segregated in a specific space within the cytoplasm. Gram-positive bacteria have a thick protective cell wall made of peptidoglycan and contain the enzymatic system necessary for the transport of nutrients and electrolytes across the membrane. Gram-negative bacteria have a more elaborate three-layer cellular wall:

1. The outer membrane acts as a physical barrier against antibiotic penetration, allowing certain molecules to penetrate the cell wall and excluding others. It is made of a lipopolysaccharide called *endotoxin*, an important factor for the bacterial virulence. Virulence is thought to be related to the *lipid A* moeity of the endotoxin. Another important role of this layer is its immunogenicity.
2. The cell wall is similar in composition and function to the gram-positive bacterial wall.
3. The lipid inner membrane is separated from the cell wall by a periplasmic space.

Some bacteria have a polysaccharide capsule that protects the microorganism from phagocytosis and shields its surface antigens, thus delaying the formation of antibodies by the host.

The *fungi*, unlike the bacteria, have a nucleus that contains chromosomes. Their cell wall is composed of a polysaccharide known as chitin and may be protected by an external capsule.

The viruses are the most primal infectious pathogens. They are obligate intracellular parasites because they are unable to replicate outside a living cell. Viruses are made of DNA or RNA genetic material called genome. The capsid is the protein cover that surrounds and protects the genome. Some viruses have an external envelope made of a viral protein as well as a layer of lipids and carbohydrates that originates from the host cell, as the viral genome lacks the ability to produce the latter two components. Viral infections start with attachment of the virus to the host cell wall. This step is accomplished by the interaction of the viral envelope or capsid with some specific host cell receptors. This is followed by the penetration of the virus genome into the cell and its release into the cytoplasm. DNA genomes then must travel into the host cell nucleus to induce the transcription of the viral genetic message, whereas the RNA viruses can proliferate in the cellular cytoplasm either directly or by producing a reverse transcriptase, which helps DNA transcription from the viral RNA. This DNA then migrates into the host cellular nucleus and incorporates itself with the host chromosome, leading to the production of more viruses at the expense of the host cell.

Exotoxins

Exotoxins, like hemolysin, coagulase, collagenase, elastase, hyaluronidase, and heparinase, are produced by certain species of bacteria and allow the pathogens to attack the host tissues and inflict injury. Superoxide dismutase and catalase are produced by *Bacillus fragilis* and *Escherichia coli*, respectively. Although not true exotoxins, the two enzymes play an important role in the generation and metabolism of superoxide and hydrogen peroxide, two potent toxic agents. The most potent of all exotoxins are those produced by the *Clostridium* spp. *Clostridium perfringens* produces a cytotoxic exotoxin that causes hemolysis, whereas *C. tetani* produces a neurotoxin.

Antimicrobial Agents

Antimicrobials are chemical agents that help the host fight a microbial invasion by limiting the pathogen's ability to multiply or by inducing physical or biochemical changes in the pathogen that lead to its death. The antimicrobial is called bacteriostatic, if its effect on the pathogen is reversible, and bactericidal, if the effect is irreversible.

Antimicrobials must be considered adjuvant agents to surgery in the management of surgical infections. One must never substitute antibiotic therapy for surgical intervention in the management of life-threatening surgical infections.

Antimicrobial agents affect the pathogens by different mechanisms. For example, penicillins and cephalosporins inhibit cell-wall synthesis, causing death, whereas aminoglycoside bind to the cell ribosomes and interfere with RNA synthesis. Clavulanic acid, sulbactam, and tozbactam are β-lactamase inhibitors combined with some penicillins, such as ticarcillin, amoxicillin, ampicillin, and pipercillin to expand their gram-negative activity while maintaining their effect against gram-positive and anaerobic pathogens.

Antibiotic Resistance

The extensive use of antibiotics led to the increase of strains of pathogens that are resistant to the commonly used antimicrobial. The mechanism by which bacteria develop resistance is variable, depending on the species. It is well established, however, that microorganisms can acquire resistance very quickly after the initiation of the antimicrobial regimen. The author has found a statistically significant increase in bacterial resistance in a group of trauma patients with hollow-viscus injury who were given a 7-day regimen of prophylactic antibiotics compared with a group who received 1 day of prophylaxis (unpublished data). Moreover, the author found that the incidence of vancomycin-resistant enterococci (VRE) at his institution decreased after the use of prophylactic vancomycin was limited to patients who were allergic to penicillin or who were known to be colonized by methicillin-resistant *Staphylococcus aureus*.

Acquired resistance is genetically induced by chromosomal mutation, which is an uncommon event, or with the help of a cytoplasmic material, called the plasmid. The plasmid helps the pathogen build the mechanism necessary to protect it from the effect of antibiotics. The plasmid can be transferred from one microbe to another by different mechanisms.

Empiric Antibiotic Treatment and Prophylaxis

Antibiotics are used to help eradicate ongoing infections. The agents are best chosen based on the culture and antibiotic-sensitivity information. Sometimes the pathogen involved is not readily known, and the choice of antibiotics depends on the surgeon's clinical judgment. This is based on the patient's data as they pertain to the bacteriologic history (i.e., previous urinary tract infection or the source of infection [perforated peptic ulcer vs. perforated diverticulitis]). Empiric antibiotic therapy must be replaced with a more specific regimen as soon as the culture and sensitivity are available, especially when the infection does not respond to the empiric therapy.

The intent of prophylactic antibiotics is to prevent superficial and deep wound infection in the postoperative period. It is accepted that one dose of antibiotic given within 1 hour before incision will decrease the risk of wound infection in clean contaminated and contaminated cases (Table 10-2). Mechanical bowel preparation, in addition to the use of intraluminal and intravenous antibiotic agents, also improves the risk of postoperative wound infection in elective colon surgery. Antibiotics with short half-lives must be

TABLE 10–2 Surgical Wound Classification

Class	Condition	Examples
1	Clean	Breast biopsy, inguinal hernia repair without break in technique
2	Clean contaminated	GI, GU, Gyn organs entered. No gross contamination, minor break in technique
3	Contaminated	Perforated appendectomy, colectomy for diverticulitis, perforated ulcer or bowel, penetrating GI trauma
4	Dirty	Traumatic wounds, burns older than 72 hr, free colon perforation

GI, gastrointestinal; GU, genitourinary.

TABLE 10–3 Prophylactic Regimens for Some General Surgical Procedures

Procedure	Antibiotic Regimen	Bacterial Spectrum
Elective cholecystectomy	First-generation cephalosporin*	Gram +/–
Cholecystectomy for acute cholecystitis	Second- or third-generation cephalosporin*	Gram –
Gastric and proximal small bowel surgery	Second generation cephalosporin*	Gram + and oral anaerobes
Lower small bowel and colon surgery	Ampicillin*/gentamycin/metronidazole or a second-generation cephalosporin*	Gram – and anaerobes
Hernia repair with a prosthesis	First-generation cephalosporin*	Gram + *Staphylococcus aureus*

*Vancomycin for patients allergic to penicillin

repeated in prolonged surgical cases to allow a consistently adequate tissue level. The choice of the antibiotic agent depends on the organ being operated on. It is a standard of care to use prophylaxis for classes 2, 3, and 4 surgical wounds and in class 1 when a prosthesis, synthetic mesh, or a vascular graft is to be used. Although no evidence exists that antibiotics are useful in class 1 wounds, it is accepted that the possible benefit of antibiotics outweighs the risk of a wound infection in the presence of a synthetic prosthesis. Refer to Table 10-3 for recommended prophylactic regimens for common general surgical procedures.

Clinical Presentation of Infections

Infection has systemic symptoms and signs related to the activation of the host inflammatory defense system and local manifestations specific to the involved organ.

The systemic manifestations are fever, chills, malaise, fatigue, tachycardia, tachypnea, and signs and symptoms of hypovolemia, such as dry oral mucosa, hypotension, concentrated urine, oliguria, and anuria in extreme cases. The extent of the symptoms depends on the severity of the infection and the patient's intravascular volume and comorbidities.

The local manifestations of wound or skin infections include erythema, swelling, heat, pain, and tenderness. Fluctuance is found when a purulent collection is present. Loss of function is based on the patient's attempt to immobilize the affected area in a comfortable position, like finger flexion in tenosynovitis and shallow breathing in peritonitis. Leukocytosis (white blood cells [WBCs] >12,000/μL) is commonly seen in acute bacterial infections. Leukopenia may be present in overwhelming infections, and normal WBC count is not uncommon in the elderly and debilitated infected patient.

The Gram stain is an important part of examining the infected patient. Sputum, urine, pus, or exudate must be Gram stained for an immediate identification of the responsible pathogen. Potassium hydroxide, silver, and Giemsa stains are helpful for the identification of fungal hyphae and spores. Mycobacteria can be identified by using the Ziehl-Neelsen stain.

Staining techniques have the ability to direct the clinician to identify a group of pathogens involved in the infection. The specific identification of individual species and their susceptibility to antibiotics is accomplished through the culture of the infected tissue, fluid, or device. The culture media vary. Blood, broth, and agar are the most commonly used media. Quantitative culture is helpful in burn and soft-tissue infections. It is accomplished by providing the laboratory with a known amount of the tissue to be studied, usually a specimen measuring 1 cc. The characterization of the pathogen and antibiotic susceptibility takes 72 hours. The sensitivity to antibiotics is tested by inoculating a medium carrying varying amounts of a specific antibiotic with the bacteria. After 24 hours, the minimal inhibitory concentration (MIC) of an antibiotic is reported as the equivalent of the dilution of the antibiotic that prevents any bacterial growth. MIC is useful when compared with the achievable serum levels of individual antibiotics. As a general rule, antibiotics that can achieve a serum level that is 5 to 8 times the MIC are found to be effective in the treatment of infections.

Wound Infection

The surgical wound classification reflects the risk of postoperative wound infection and dictates the different prophylactic regimens that help in decreasing the risk of infection (Fig. 10-1).

Surgical wound infections have medical and socio-economic implications. Immunocompromised patients are the most vulnerable to infection and its sequelae. The systemic manifestations of chills, fever, loss of appetite, nausea, and vomiting may lead to malnutrition and prolonged hospitalization. The infection of the underlying prosthetic material may be devastating, leading to extremity ischemia in the case of vascular grafts or to a chronically infected wound after hernia repair with a mesh. Bacteremia and distant infections, especially in patients with intravascular catheters and prosthetic devices, could be life-threatening. Abdominal wound infections increase the risk for fascial dehiscence and evisceration or the development of large ventral hernias.

Surgical wound infection is a potentially preventable complication, especially in patients with class 1 and 2

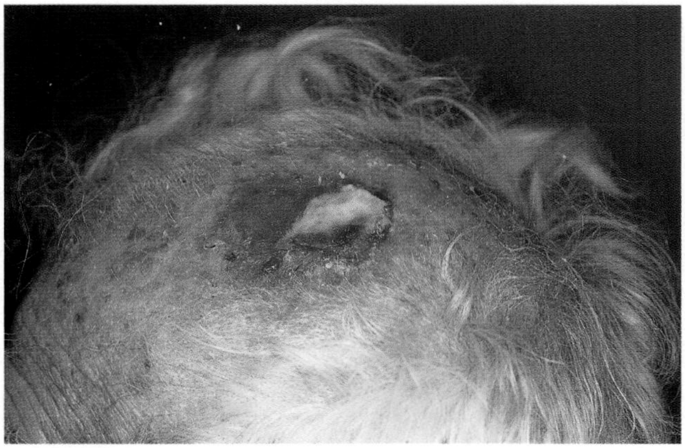

FIGURE 10–1 Wound infection and necrosis at full-thickness skin graft site. (From Stasko T, Clayton AS: Surgical complications and optimizing outcomes. In Bolognia JL, Jorizzo JL, Rapini RP (eds): Dermatology, Vol II. Philadelphia, Mosby, 2003, p 2350.)

PEARLS FOR ROUNDS

Antibiotic prophylaxis:
- No need for prophylactic antibiotics for class I wounds unless a prosthesis is to be implanted. Use a first-generation cephalosporin
- Class II cases:
- Use first-generation cephalosporin for elective cholecystectomy.
- Use first- or second-generation cephalosporin for acute cholecystitis.

Use first- or second-generation cephalosporin for gastric surgery.

Use a mechanical preparation with oral antibiotics (erythromycin base, neomycin) the night before surgery and a second-generation cephalosporin the day of surgery for colon surgery.

Class III cases: trauma, perforated bowel: second-generation cephalosporin or ampicillin/gentamycin/flagyl

Use vancomycin only in penicillin-allergic patients or if methicillin-resistant *Staphylococcus aureus* (MRSA) is documented.

All antibiotics must be given within 1 hour of the incision.

wounds. It can be prevented in part by timing of the skin preparation immediately before incision, because shaving the skin hair of the prospective incision area hours before surgery invites bacteria into the hair roots, thus increasing the risk of wound infection. Applying antiseptic solutions to the patient's skin and the surgical team's hands, by using appropriate surgical techniques that protect the tissues from unwarranted trauma and cleaning the wounds of any foreign material, blood, and debris potentially decreases the risk of infection. As important is the timely use of antibiotics for the clean contaminated cases. Contaminated and dirty wounds pose a difficult problem because their infection rate is high. Débridement of dead tissue and debris and profuse irrigation, in addition to leaving the skin open, could potentially prevent wound infection.

The local signs of wound infection are tenderness, edema, erythema, and sometimes purulent drainage. The diagnosis may be difficult in immunocompromised and obese patients, as the former may not be able to generate an inflammatory reaction typical of the infection, whereas in the latter, the thick subcutaneous tissue may hide the deep-seated infection. In those patients, one must have a high level of suspicion in the presence of systemic symptoms and signs of infection. Computed tomography (CT) scan, fine-needle aspiration, or opening the wound in the involved area may be helpful in confirming the diagnosis of deep infection.

Treatment of infected surgical wounds depends on the severity of the infection. Mild erythema may resolve after the sutures or the staples are removed, whereas a more pronounced local inflammation with or without systemic reaction requires antibiotic therapy. If the infection persists after 48 hours of appropriate antibiotic treatment, abscess formation must be suspected, and the wound must be opened and drained. The choice of antibiotic regimen must be specific for the pathogen if the culture results are available, or empiric based on the surgical wound class and the organ that was operated on; class 1 wounds are usually infected by *Staphylococcus* spp., and less often with *Streptococcus* spp., making a first-generation cephalosporin an appropriate choice. Infections of class 2, 3, or 4 wounds are caused by enteric pathogens and require gentamycin or a third-generation cephalosporin alone for the aerobic gram-negative flora or with metronidazole if anaerobic bacteria are suspected. The treatment must continue for 24 to 48 hours after all the symptoms and signs of the treated infection disappear.

Soft-tissue Infections

Necrotizing fasciitis (Fig. 10-2) is a life-threatening infection that involves the different fascial layers of the body. It is most commonly caused by streptococci, although staphylococci, gram-negative, and anaerobic bacteria may be identified in some cases. Necrotizing fasciitis occurs in contaminated soft-tissue injuries, especially in patients with diabetes or peripheral vascular disease, as well as when the wound is inappropriately closed. Fournier's gangrene is a necrotizing soft-tissue infection that originates in the urethral glands and spreads quickly into the perineal tissue, creating an overwhelming septic condition. Finally, necrotizing

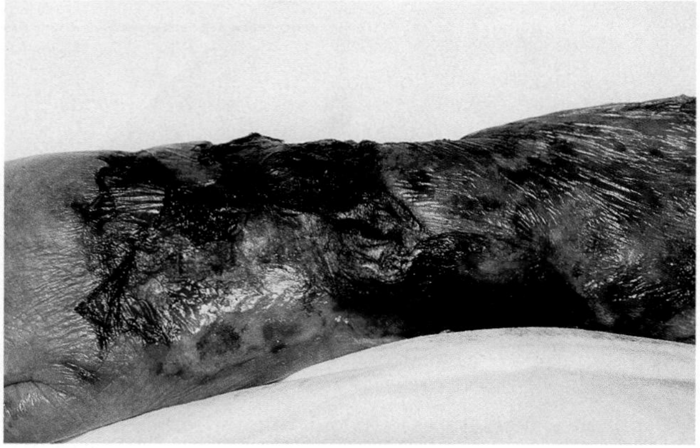

FIGURE 10–2 Necrotizing fasciitis of the upper extremity with erythema and extensive tissue necrosis in an intravenous heroin user. (From Sanchez M: Signs of drug abuse. In Bolognia JL, Jorizzo JL, Rapini RP (eds): Dermatology, Vol II. Philadelphia, Mosby, 2003, p 1415.)

fasciitis is reported after GI surgery most often in immunocompromised and elderly patients.

Whereas a typical wound infection is first seen with low-grade fever, wound erythema, and tenderness 72 hours or later after surgery, the multimicrobial soft-tissue infection manifests itself within the first 48 postoperative hours with a high temperature (103°F), confusion, agitation, and a watery foul-smelling discharge from a discolored, often necrotic wound. Blebs and crepitus could be present if anaerobic bacteria are involved. Typically, a Gram stain of the fluid exhibits a gram-positive or a polymicrobial involvement.

Necrotizing fasciitis (see Fig. 10-2) is a life-threatening infection that requires prompt diagnosis, antibiotic therapy, and aggressive surgical débridement. The antibiotic regimen must cover streptococci as well as gram-negative and anaerobic strains. The surgical management could be challenging to the surgeon and sometimes mutilating to the patient. The limit of débridement should be the limit of tissue necrosis, as any necrotic nidus left behind may lead to further progression of the infection. Débridement must extend to well-perfused tissues, keeping in mind the importance of preserving healthy tissues to allow coverage of vital organs (i.e., vessels, bone, and tendons). If the viability of the surgical margins is questionable, a second look in the operating room or in the intensive care unit is necessary within 24 hours of the initial procedure.

Clostridial infection is the most dangerous of soft-tissue infections. It is most commonly caused by gram-positive rods, *Clostridium* spp. typically; it occurs after a soft-tissue injury in an area contaminated by dirt, such as farm soil. The patient has a simple case of cellulitis with mild systemic symptoms. This is usually caused by *C. tertium* and is responsive to antibiotic therapy. The life-threatening gas gangrene is caused by *C. perfringens*. *Clostridium perfringens* secretes an exotoxin that induces tissue necrosis and putrefaction. This infection spreads to the fascia and muscle groups, thus manifesting itself as an infected, discolored, and foul-smelling wound with crepitus. A simple radiograph will show gas along the muscle and fascial planes. A Gram stain of the wound exudate confirms the presence of gram-positive rods. The treatment of clostridial myonecrosis includes prompt and aggressive surgical débridement along with high doses of penicillin. Hyperbaric oxygen therapy has been helpful in the most severe cases as an adjunct to surgical intervention.

PEARLS FOR THE OR

Did the patient receive prophylactic antibiotic before the incision was made?

In soft-tissue infections, débridement must extend to normal tissues.

Keep the skin open in contaminated cases (classes 3 and 4).

The seven intraperitoneal spaces where abscesses can form:

- Right gutter
- Left gutter
- Right subphrenic space
- Subhepatic space
- Left subphrenic space
- Pouch of Douglas
- Interloop space

Intraabdominal Infections

The most common form of intraabdominal infection is secondary peritonitis originating from a perforated hollow viscus. The bacteriology varies based on the viscus involved. Peritonitis due to perforated peptic ulcer could be sterile early after its onset, because the gastric acid prevents bacterial growth, thus making the inoculum too small to cause an active infection. If untreated, however, oral bacteria (streptococci, staphylococci, lactobacilli, and anaerobes) will induce a bacterial peritonitis. Perforated proximal small bowel (from penetrating trauma, for instance) has the same bacteriology as discussed earlier. The distal small bowel carries a heavier bacterial load of gram-positive and gram-negative aerobes and anaerobes. A colon perforation (i.e., perforated appendicitis, colon cancer, or diverticulitis) inflicts the most severe case of bacterial peritonitis. Anaerobic streptococci, enterococci, *E. coli*, *Klebsiella*, *Enterobacter*, and *Bacteroides fragilis* are usually isolated from colonic peritonitis.

Primary peritonitis, a monobacterial infection, occurs in patients with ascites and patients receiving peritoneal dialysis. The mechanism of this infection is unclear, but typically no visceral perforation is found in these patients. The most common bacteria responsible for this infection are staphylococci, although *E. coli* and other enteric bacteria can be isolated occasionally.

Critically ill patients who have had a secondary peritonitis can acquire what is known as tertiary peritonitis. The infection is facilitated by a weak immune system, poor nutrition, and other poorly understood mechanisms. Extensive clinical evaluation often fails to identify a source of the infection.

Peritonitis presents clinically with both general systemic manifestations and with local abdominal symptoms and signs (i.e., abdominal pain, nausea, vomiting, focal or diffuse tenderness, guarding, and rebound with decreased or absent bowel sounds). The WBC count is usually elevated, with increase in the neutrophils and bands. However, debilitated, immunocompromised, and elderly patients may not have a clear clinical picture. In this situation, radiologic studies, such as CT scan, barium or gastrographin upper GI (UGI) or enema may be necessary for diagnosis.

Primary peritonitis is treated with an antibiotic agent effective against the isolated bacteria. An empiric choice should cover gram-positive and gram-negative microbes until the culture results are available. The peritoneal dialysis catheter may have to be removed if the infection fails to respond to antibiotics. Patients with infected ascites sometimes respond to paracentesis in conjunction with antibiotics. Tertiary peritonitis can be challenging, as the patients affected are often septic and obtunded, difficult to examine, and the radiologic studies may fail to pinpoint a source of infection. Treatment must include a wide-spectrum antibiotic regimen covering gram-positive and gram-negative aerobes and anaerobes, and sometimes antifungal agents. Isolates in this situation may include *Staphylococcus epidermidis, Candida*, and *Pseudomonas aeruginosa*. Nutritional support and persistence in attempting to find a source of the infection are crucial to a good outcome.

The treatment of secondary peritonitis includes empiric or specific antibiotic therapy, abdominal exploration to correct the source of the infection, and sometimes percutaneous drainage, guided by ultrasound or CT scan if the infection is localized. The latter approach is acceptable to control the infection and prepare the patient for a definitive operation to correct the basic pathology, thus making the surgical intervention easier and safer, as is usually the case in patients with appendiceal or diverticular abscesses.

Intravascular Catheters and Devices

Intravascular devices like peripheral intravenous catheters, central lines, pulmonary artery catheters, and arterial lines are commonly used in surgical patients. The catheters are vulnerable to colonization and infection as a result of the skin disruption at the site of insertion, contamination during insertion or during maintenance of the catheter, and bacteremia in patients with remote infections.

Peripheral intravascular catheter infection is easy to diagnose and to treat. Erythema or purulent exudate at the site of insertion is indicative of infection. Removal of the catheter is curative. Empiric antibiotic therapy to cover gram-positive pathogens may be required to treat patients with fever, cellulitis, or lymphangitis.

Patients receiving total parenteral nutrition (TPN) are especially vulnerable to central-line infections, as the high concentration of glucose infused provides an ideal medium for bacterial and fungal growth. Catheter colonization and infection can be prevented by adhering to sterile techniques during insertion, manipulation, and dressing. The central-line culture is done by removing the catheter under sterile conditions and sending the tip for culture or smearing it on a culture medium. The evidence regarding changing the line periodically to prevent line infection remains controversial. *Staphylococcus aureus* is commonly isolated from the line if the contamination occurs during insertion, whereas *S. epidermidis* and yeast are isolated in the immunocompromised patients with long-term central venous access. Gram-negative infections are related to a blood-borne infection. Line colonization is defined as growth of fewer than 10^5 colonies. Line infection is defined as growth of more than 10^5 colonies with no signs of infection and negative blood cultures. Line sepsis is defined as growth of 10^5 or more colonies in a patient with positive blood cultures, with signs of sepsis, or with both.

The diagnosis of central-line infection may be difficult. Erythema or purulent exudate at the site of insertion is evidence of line infection. Sepsis or bacteremia of an unclear origin must be presumed to be related to line infection. In this situation, the line may be either removed or replaced over a wire with a new catheter if the patient is still in need of access. The tip of the suspected catheter must then be sent for culture; if the culture is positive, the central line must be moved to a new site. However, in the critically ill patient with multiple possible sites for sepsis, only an identical bacterial growth from the blood and the tip of the catheter is proof that the line is the source of sepsis. Blood cultures drawn from a central line may be difficult to interpret and must be discouraged. Central-line colonization or infection must be treated with removal of the catheter. If line infection is suspected and the site appears to be clean, the line may be changed over a wire at the same site; the catheter that is removed must then be sent for culture. If the culture is positive, the catheter must be removed from that site. Antibiotic treatment is indicated if the patient has signs of line sepsis or has a positive blood culture. Some authors advocated the treatment of infected lines with antibiotics without removing the catheter in patients with limited access sites.

Vancomycin must be used to cover *Staphylococcus epidermidis* until the culture results are available. The treatment must continue for 7 to 15 days in proven line infections, and for a longer period in immunocompromised or septic patients. The patients who do not respond to therapy within 48 to 72 hours must have the central line removed and cultured and have the antibiotic regimen reviewed. In addition, the diagnosis of suppurative thrombophlebitis must be sought with a duplex ultrasound of the involved vein. Vein excision must be considered in a patient with line infection in the presence of a venous thrombus.

Although it is an uncommon occurrence, arterial line infection must be suspected when the insertion site is erythematous or purulent and when the patient has evidence of infection of an unclear source. The treatment includes removal of the catheter and antibiotic therapy in the bacteremic patient.

Pulmonary artery catheters rarely become infected. Most commonly, the infection is at the insertion site or the tip of the introducer. The diagnosis and treatment are similar to the diagnosis and treatment of central-line infections.

Suppurative Thrombophlebitis

This complication occurs in patients with intravenous catheters. The risk of this infection increases after 72 hours of catheter insertion. It manifests itself as chills, fever, local symptoms and signs of infection, and purulent drainage from the involved vein. If the infected vein is central, the diagnosis may be difficult and should rely on a high degree of suspicion in a patient with gram-positive bacteremia and a duplex study of the vein that is suggestive of vein thrombosis. The treatment includes removal of the catheter, antibiotic therapy to cover gram-positive bacteria, especially *Staphylococcus aureus* and *epidermidis*, and excision of the infected vessel.

Postoperative Pneumonia

Pneumonia is the most common infectious complication in surgical patients. The decrease in the tidal volume due to anesthesia, analgesia, or the pain induced by thoracotomy and laparotomy incisions predisposes the patients to pulmonary atelectasis, disruption of the pulmonary defense mechanisms, and growth of bacteria, leading to pneumonia. Fever (<102°F) in the immediate postoperative period is usually due to atelectasis. Decrease of breath sounds, usually in the base of the lung fields in a patient who is taking shallow breaths, is consistent with atelectasis. A chest radiograph may be helpful in confirming the diagnosis. Encouraging the patient to take a deep breath, cough, and ambulate is effective in the prevention and treatment of this complication. If untreated, atelectasis progresses to pneumonia with high temperature (102°F), confusion, hallucination, hypoxia, and an elevation in the WBC count, in addition to the production of purulent sputum. Empiric antibiotic therapy is appropriate until the sputum culture results are available. *Streptococcus pneumoniae* and *Haemophilus influenzae* are common pathogens in the postoperative patients. Other gram-negative bacteria like *Pseudomonas* must be treated in the patients with a long hospital stay.

Patients on a respirator are at high risk for pneumonia. Immune incompetence induced by the underlying disease and the breach of the pulmonary defense mechanisms by the indwelling endotracheal tube set the stage for bacterial invasion of the pulmonary tissue. The use of aseptic techniques for patient intubation and ventilator management and early patient extubation are important in preventing ventilator-associated pneumonia. The diagnosis of this infection could be difficult, as most of those patients have fever, abnormal chest radiographs, and elevated WBC counts for different reasons. The triad of fever, infiltrate on a chest radiograph, and purulent sputum are accepted as a clinical proof of pneumonia. Some authorities suggest the use of bronchoscopy, protected brush bronchoscopy, and alveolar washing to confirm the diagnosis. The treatment must be aimed against *Pseudomonas* spp., Enterobacteriaceae, and other enteric bacteria.

Aspiration of gastric contents in the elderly and chronically ill patients may lead to a chemical pneumonitis seen as an acute respiratory compromise requiring endotracheal intubation. The diagnosis is based on the witnessed event or on the finding of gastric contents in the airway during intubation. The treatment of this situation is supportive, as the use of antibiotics will not prevent the development of bacterial pneumonia but allows the outgrowth of resistant strains of bacteria that may prove to be difficult to treat once pneumonia occurs. Antibiotics are indicated when the chemical pneumonitis turns into bacterial pneumonia, as proven by the presence of purulent sputum.

Urinary Tract Infection in the Surgical Patient

Indwelling Foley catheters provide bacteria access to the urethra and bladder and cause local inflammation in the urethra, disrupting the local defense mechanisms. The subsequent lack of mucin and IgA secretion and the loss of the cleansing effect of the urinary flow allow the bacteria to invade the urinary tract, causing infection. In the bladder, the catheter causes constant irritation of the mucosa, facilitating the access of bacteria into the bladder wall.

This postoperative complication may be prevented by adhering to aseptic techniques during insertion and by early removal of the catheter. The treatment includes removal of the catheter when clinically appropriate and the use of antibiotics based on the culture results. Empiric antibiotic management must cover *E. coli*, *Klebsiella* spp., and *Pseudomonas* spp., especially in the chronically ill patients.

Suppurative Parotitis

This unusual infection affects the debilitated and dehydrated patients. As parotid secretion declines because of dehydration, the ability of the mucosa in the Wharton duct to secrete mucin and IgA is compromised, allowing bacterial growth and invasion. The most common pathogen is

Staphylococcus aureus. Parotitis occurs with fever and pain, along with erythema and tenderness in the area of the affected gland. The treatment includes hydration, *Staphylococcus* coverage, and sometimes percutaneous drainage of a parotid abscess.

Postsplenectomy Overwhelming Sepsis

The spleen plays an important role in clearing the blood stream from encapsulated bacteria like *Pneumococcus* and *Haemophilus influenzae*. The spleen secretes opsonin and tuftsin, which facilitate bacterial clearance by the spleen and the liver. Postsplenectomy overwhelming sepsis (PSOS) occurs mostly in children who have had a splenectomy for hematologic disease, although it has also been described in the adult trauma population. PSOS occurs as an overwhelming septic crisis that leads to the patient's death in 50% to 70% of the cases. PSOS is best prevented by preserving the spleen when possible. The benefit of spleen autotransplantation remains controversial. The use of life-long antibiotics after splenectomy is not practical and may be ineffective, as only 50% of the PSOS cases are related to *Pneumococcus* and *H. influenzae*, whereas the other 50% are related to a variety of gram-positive and gram-negative bacteria. The polyvalent antipneumococcal and *H. influenzae* vaccines are effective only against the serotypes represented within them. Although they are known to be effective when given before splenectomy in elective situations, it is unclear whether they add any resistance to the trauma patient when given after the splenectomy has been done.

Burn Wound Infection

Refer to Chapter 13.

Acquired Immunodeficiency Syndrome and the Surgeon

Acquired immunodeficiency syndrome (AIDS) is caused by the human retrovirus human immunodeficiency virus 1 (HIV-1) that invades T cells, leading to immunosuppression. Patients with HIV-1 infection may have symptoms and signs that are suggestive of a surgical pathology. These patients are susceptible to the common infections that affect the general population and to specific conditions related to their immunodeficiency. As a general rule, this group of patients must be treated in the same manner in which other patients are treated, especially when potentially life-threatening infections are suspected. These patients are especially susceptible to GI infection with yeast, cytomegalovirus (CMV), and *Mycobacteria avium-intracellulare* (MAI). Abdominal pain could be due to a spectrum of surgical and nonsurgical sources. CMV infection can be seen as colitis, cholecystitis, or as a perforation of the bowel, appendix, or gallbladder. Kaposi sarcoma can affect any part of the GI tract, causing obstruction or perforation. GI lymphoma may be seen with abdominal pain and diarrhea, liver failure, or a perforated viscus. MAI-induced pancreatitis has been described in this patient population. Finally, the anorectal area can be affected by a wide range of bacteria, mycobacteria, fungi, and parasites that manifest themselves as perirectal ulcerations, fissures, and abscesses.

Soft-tissue Infections in the Diabetic Patient

Diabetic patients are vulnerable to skin and soft-tissue infections that could be life threatening (Fig. 10-3). The etiology of the infection is usually mechanical, especially in patients with sensory neuropathy that prevents them from recognizing repetitive trauma or soft-tissue injury, while cutting the nails, for example. Peripheral vascular insufficiency and leukocyte malfunction weaken the patient's ability to contain bacterial invasion and allow the spread of the infection.

The infection manifests itself as a superficial cellulitis, infected ulcer, or an aggressive deep soft-tissue infection involving the muscle and the fascia. The most common pathogens are *Staphylococcus aureus,* followed by *Streptococcus* spp., *Enterococcus* spp., gram-negative bacteria, and anaerobes. Empiric antimicrobial therapy must cover gram-positive, gram-negative, and anaerobic bacteria until more specific characterization of the involved bacteria is available. Although superficial wound culture may give a general idea about the pathogens, intraoperative specimens from the deep tissues better identify the infectious pathogen(s). Immediate débridement of any ischemic tissue is paramount to the control of this infection.

Candida Infection

Yeast infection, especially with *Candida albicans,* has increased, probably as the result of widespread use of

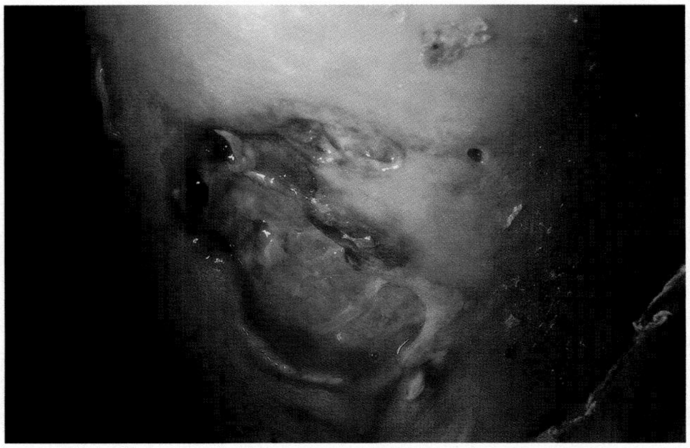

FIGURE 10–3 Infection in upper arm of elderly patient with diabetes. (From Blume JE, Levine EG, Heymann WR: Bacterial diseases. In Bolognia JL, Jorizzo JL, Rapini RP (eds): Dermatology, Vol I. Philadelphia, Mosby, 2003, p 1125.)

antibiotics and because more critically ill and debilitated patients are surviving their original pathology long enough to be afflicted with nosocomial infections. Candidemia has been shown to carry a 45% to 75% mortality. *Candida* species can be cultured from abdominal fluids of patients with perforated viscera. Therapy in this situation is recommended in the immunosuppressed and debilitated patients, as well as in those who are not responding to antibiotic therapy. Fungemia and disseminated *Candida* infection must always be treated. Amphotericin-B and fluconazole are both acceptable for the treatment of *Candida* infection. In patients with candidemic shock, a combination of amphotericin-B and flucytosine may improve the outcome. The systemic toxicity of amphotericin (e.g., renal failure, fluid and electrolytes imbalance) has shifted the interest to fluconazole for the treatment of *Candida albicans*. Amphotericin is still indicated for the treatment of *Candida glabratta* and *kruseii*. The treatment regimen must continue until all signs of infection are resolved.

Viral Hepatitis

Hepatitis A is spread by ingestion of food contaminated with fecal material, whereas the hepatitis B virus spreads through human fluids, such as semen, urine, and saliva. Acute hepatitis is first seen with jaundice, malaise, and sometimes lethargy, with elevation of liver transaminases that persists for 1 to 2 months. Antisurface antibody level increases early in the acute phase, followed by the anti-core antibodies. Chronic active hepatitis affects 15% of patients after the acute viral infection. In rare occasions, the acute hepatitis progresses to fulminant liver failure. Patients receiving hemodialysis, hemophiliacs, and transplant recipients are at high risk for hepatitis B infection. The recombinant hepatitis B vaccine, given in three doses, has been shown to be effective in preventing infection. The vaccine is recommended for healthcare workers who are frequently exposed to human blood products and secretions. Immunity surveillance can be accomplished by measuring anti–hepatitis B antibodies. A booster vaccine dose may be given if the level is low.

Suggested Reading

Anaissie EJ, Bishara AB, Solomkin JS: Fungal infections. In Wilmore DW, Souba WW, Fink MP, et al (eds): ACS Surgery: Principles and Practice. New York, American College of Surgeons, 2005, pp 1484–1502.

Bessey PQ: Metabolic response to critical illness. In Wilmore DW, Souba WW, Fink MP et al (eds): ACS Surgery: Principles and Practice. New York, American College of Surgeons, 2005, pp 1539–1565.

Christou NV: Antibiotics. In Wilmore DW, Souba WW, Fink MP, et al (eds): ACS Surgery: Principles and Practice. New York, American College of Surgeons, 2005, pp 1395–1422.

Dellinger EP: Nosocomial infections. In Wilmore DW, Souba WW, Fink MP et al (eds): ACS Surgery: Principles and Practice. New York, American College of Surgeons, 2005, pp 1423–1440.

Sawyer RG: Intra-abdominal infection. In Wilmore DW, Souba WW, Fink MP, et al (eds): ACS Sugery: Principles and Practice. New York, American College of Surgeons, 2005, pp 1455–1483.

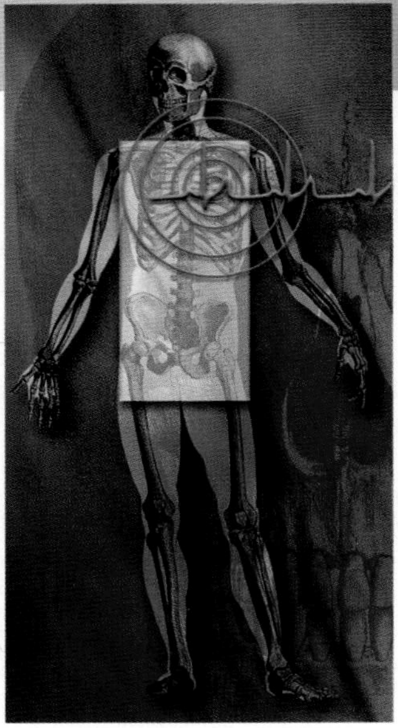

SECTION III

CRITICAL CARE

Chapter 11

Trauma

FREDERICK H. MILLHAM, MD, MBA

The word *trauma* refers to the physical injury of tissues as a result of the transfer of energy. Trauma accounts for around 12% of healthcare expenditures in the United States. More than 36 million Americans per year were injured severely enough to seek hospital care, and more than 150,000 die of injuries annually. The incidence of severe injury is skewed toward the young, as reflected in the admission rates from injury. It is notable that considerably more men die of trauma than do women, although women account for the majority of injuries that occur in the seventh decade and later.

The successful management of patients with complex or multiple injuries requires an organized and efficient approach, using a team of healthcare providers. This approach should be geared toward early recognition and management of life-threatening injuries and shock, as well as the successful identification and eventual treatment of all other injuries.

Approach to the Injured Patient

An organized approach to trauma care is outlined by the Advanced Trauma Life Support course (ATLS). ATLS calls for the injured patient to undergo first a primary survey during which vital signs are measured, the mechanism of injury is ascertained, and an initial examination for life-threatening processes is performed. This examination focuses on the ABCs (**a**irway, **b**reathing, **c**irculation, **d**isability, and **e**xposure). The first priority in all trauma resuscitations is the assessment and management of the patient's **airway**. If a patent and secure airway is not present, then airway control is established before any additional evaluation or treatment occurs. Processes that can interfere with the airway include foreign bodies, direct injury to the airway, and depressed level of consciousness. Maintaining a patent airway may be as simple as performing a jaw-thrust maneuver; however, most trauma patients who require airway management will require more definitive control, such as endotracheal intubation. Airway maneuvers must be performed with the understanding that occult cervical spine injury may be present, and therefore a two-person intubation technique, ensuring that the neck is neither flexed nor extended, is used. For patients with airway injury, such as a massive mandibular fracture, in which the airway is compromised by hematoma and edema or in patients whose anatomic features make laryngoscopic intubation difficult, a surgical airway may be necessary. This is best done by the technique of cricothyroidotomy (Fig. 11-1). A formal tracheostomy should be performed within 24 to 48 hours of performing a cricothyroidotomy.

Once a definitive airway is established, attention is turned to **breathing**, which includes both ventilation and oxygenation. Ventilation, the ability to exchange volumes of air with the environment, can be compromised by direct injury to the musculoskeletal structures responsible for the work of breathing, such as rib fractures. Ventilation also can be compromised by injury to the neurologic structures responsible for the control of breathing. Brain, spinal cord, and phrenic nerve injuries may cause either apnea or compromise of the ability to breathe. Patients who have abdominal injuries may have intraperitoneal bleeding or visceral edema, which pushes up on the diaphragm, limiting the volume available for lung expansion. Finally, patients who are in shock may have very high ventilatory requirements. The amount of air exchange required to remove carbon dioxide may exceed the patient's capabilities. Such patients will accumulate CO_2 and eventually fatigue if not given mechanical ventilatory assistance.

Oxygenation refers to the diffusion of oxygen from inspired air to the blood. Diffusion of oxygen can be impaired by direct injury of the parenchyma of the lung or by aspiration of blood or gastric contents after injury.

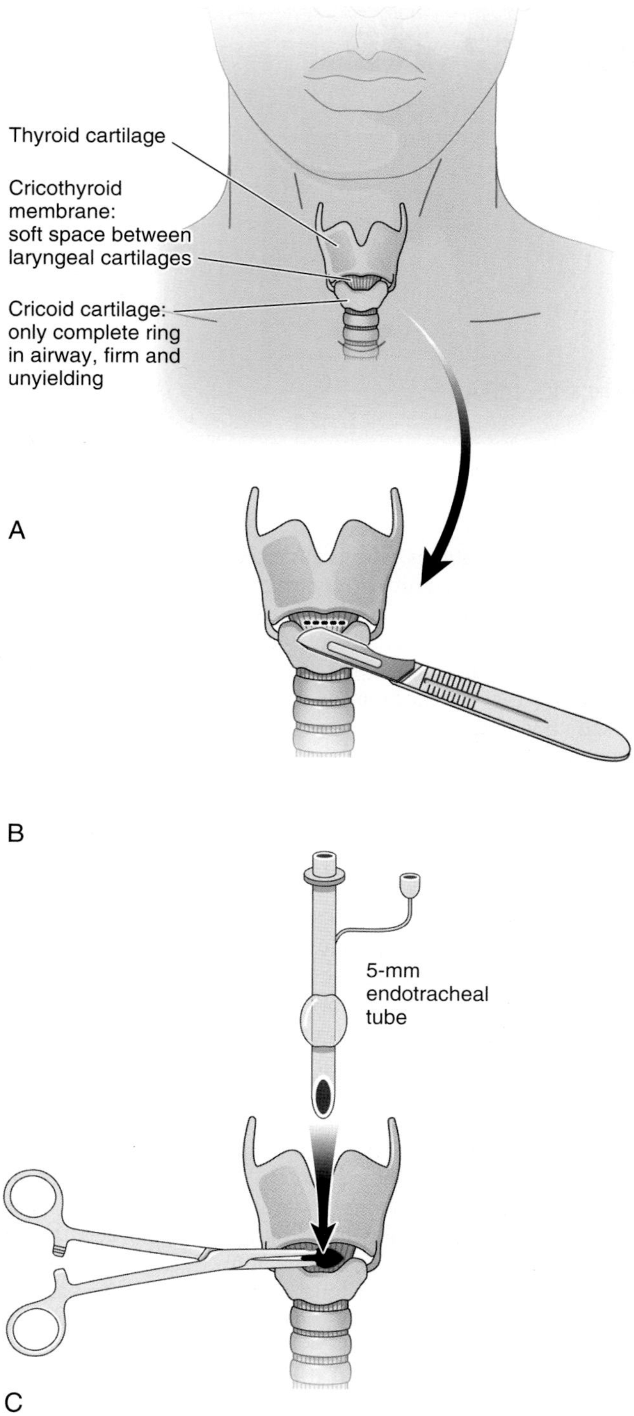

FIGURE 11–1 Emergency cricothyroidotomy. *A*, Anatomy. *B*, Stabilize thyroid cartilage with nondominant hand, and incise membrane transversely. *C*, Open the airway widely with a hemostat. Insert endotracheal tube (ETT) so balloon is 2–3 cm within trachea. Usually a 5-mm ETT is preferred.

Because injured patients may have abnormally low levels of circulating hemoglobin because of blood loss, they are particularly susceptible to hypoxia. Lower oxygen saturation in this setting leads to lower oxygen delivery to tissues and tissue hypoxia. For this reason, all injured patients should be placed initially on high-flow oxygen until it has been determined that they are neither bleeding nor hypoxic. If evidence is noted of problems with either ventilation or oxygenation, patients should be mechanically ventilated.

Circulation is the next area considered in the primary survey. The term *circulation* is used to cover the blood volume and venous access. At the same time that airway and breathing are being evaluated by the team leader, two large-bore intravenous lines are placed by other members of the resuscitation team. If the patient shows any signs of hypovolemia, volume infusion is begun. Any obvious or potential sites of bleeding are identified at this point.

The next step in evaluation is to do a rapid check for neurologic **disability**. This examination usually focuses on level of consciousness, motor strength, sensation and reflexes.

E is for **exposure**, meaning that the patient is completely stripped of all clothing. When patients are unstable, their clothing is usually cut from them with heavy scissors. In most cases, other emergency department personnel remove the patient's clothing while airway and breathing are being addressed by the individual running the resuscitation.

Once the primary survey is completed, and any immediately life-threatening injuries have been addressed, a more detailed physical examination, the secondary survey, is performed. This examination includes careful examination of each area of the body, insertion of nasogastric and urinary catheters when appropriate, and digital rectal examination. If the patient is conscious and able, a medical history, particularly focusing on present medications and allergies, should be obtained. For unstable patients, this may be the last opportunity to obtain such information in the early management phase.

For patients with immediately life-threatening injuries or who are hemodynamically unstable, completion of the secondary survey may be delayed. In cases like this, the secondary survey becomes an ongoing activity, which can continue for several hours or even days. For example, if a patient who has been in a high-speed motor vehicle crash is bleeding from a ruptured spleen, definitive survey of the axial skeleton may be delayed while the bleeding is controlled. Once the patient has stabilized, diagnostic activities can continue. Search for non–life-threatening injuries is staged until the patient is stable enough to undergo whatever radiographic or other procedures are necessary. The secondary survey is thus part of a process of surveillance and dynamic planning that occurs in a milieu of ongoing resuscitation and treatment.

Diagnosis and Management of Shock

Definition and Classification

The modern definition of shock is *a physiological state or syndrome arising from inadequate tissue perfusion.*

Tissues require a constant and uninterrupted supply of oxygen to conduct oxidative metabolism. Hypoperfusion results rapidly in cellular hypoxia. A common finding in all forms of shock is metabolic (lactic) acidosis, reflecting the shift to anaerobic metabolism in tissues that are underperfused. This in turn leads to depletion of intracellular energy stores with resulting breakdown in energy requiring membrane functions and the elaboration of inflammatory mediators and cytokines. These events themselves lead to further cell injury in what can, if untreated, become a remorselessly progressive process.

In 1930, the surgical pioneer Alfred Blalock proposed a classification system defining four categories of shock: hypovolemic, neurogenic, cardiogenic, and vasogenic.* Many modifications have been made to this scheme, but all classification systems follow a common conceptual framework: that deficient perfusion can result from (1) deficient blood volume, (2) deficient cardiac pumping capacity, or (3) dysregulated peripheral vascular tone. In practice, often overlapping physiology is seen; for instance, in severe septic shock, myocardial depression can add a component of cardiogenic shock to the vasoregulatory abnormalities associated with sepsis. We discuss hemorrhagic shock first.

Hypovolemic Shock

Hypovolemic shock was the first state to be described as "shock." It remains the most common form of shock today. As the name indicates, this form of shock is caused by a reduction of circulating blood volume to a point below that necessary to continue adequate tissue perfusion. This can result from the loss of whole blood from hemorrhage or from loss of plasma volume due to processes that cause sequestration of large volumes of fluid outside of the intravascular space, or due to gut losses of fluid as in gastric outlet obstruction or severe diarrhea.

Pathophysiology

In the 1940s, Wiggers performed classic experiments that began to define the physiology of hemorrhagic shock. He bled dogs to sustain a condition of hypotension for from 90 to 120 minutes, after which he reinfused all of the shed blood. The dogs initially returned to a normal blood pressure but slowly deteriorated over the ensuing hours. Most of the dogs died, appearing to be suffering from hypovolemic shock despite having all the shed blood returned. When he repeated this experiment by adding volumes of balanced salt solution, he found that more and more of the dogs survived. Thus it appeared that the state of shock itself produced an obligate fluid requirement beyond the blood loss that produced it. Ultimately he was able to show that dogs required three times the volume of shed blood returned in the form of balanced salt solution (lactated Ringer's). In the 1960s, Shires and others, by using microelectrode studies, were able to demonstrate where the extra volume of resuscitation was going. By monitoring the transmembrane potential of myocytes before, during, and after an experimentally induced hypovolemic shock state, these investigators were able to demonstrate that myocyte depolarization occurred during the shock state. They inferred from this finding that a reversible defect in the functioning of the Na^+/K^+ pump was present.

Thus in severe hemorrhagic shock, fluid moves not only into the intravascular space from the interstitial space, but also into the intracellular space. Therefore in resuscitation of these patients, one must replace not only the lost intravascular volume, but also the volume lost from the interstitial space into the intracellular space.

Workup and Evaluation

A classification system for severity of hypovolemic shock has been established by the American College of Surgeons as part of ATLS. By using observable physical findings, this system describes four classes of hypovolemic shock, each of which is associated with a predictable volume of blood loss (Table 11-1). By estimating the percentage of blood volume lost, one can then predict what volume of crystalloid solution will be necessary for resuscitation. Because the average blood volume for adult males is 7 mL/kg body weight, assuming a 70-kg man, and that fluid requirements will equal three times the blood volume lost, we can arrive at the volumes predicted in the table.

This method is good for a first assessment of blood loss, but resuscitation of seriously injured patients frequently requires a more sophisticated approach. The most reliable laboratory value for assessing depth of shock is a measure of metabolic acidosis. Measuring serum lactate levels is possible; however, this test is not available on an emergency basis at many centers. Base deficit, measured during arterial blood gas determination, is a reliable indicator of both the need for transfusion and the likelihood of multiple organ system failure as a result of shock. If the base deficit is unavailable, pH, corrected for the P_{CO_2} (pHc) by the formula

$$pHc = pH - (.08 \times [40 - P_{CO_2}])$$

is a reasonable indicator of metabolic acidosis and thus depth of shock.

Treatment

Treatment of hemorrhagic shock is determined by the volume of blood lost, the premorbid condition of the patient,

*The scope of this chapter includes only hypovolemic shock, explored as an overarching concept, and neurogenic shock and the obstructive form of cardiogenic shock, discussed with their particular anatomic segments.

TABLE 11–1 Classification of Hemorrhagic Shock*

ATLS Classification	Class I	Class II	Class III	Class IV
Percentage blood volume loss	<15%	15%–30%	30%–40%	>40%
Pulse	Normal	100–120	120–140	>140
Blood pressure	Normal	Elevated diastolic pressure	Systolic hypotension	Marked hypotension
Respiratory rate	14–20	20–30	30–35	>35
Capillary refill	Normal	Slightly delayed	Delayed	Absent
Mental status	Anxious	Agitated	Agitation → Confusion	Confusion, lethargy
Base deficit	–2–2	3–5	6–9	>9
Expected volume of resuscitation	<2000	2000–4500	4500–6000	>6000
Transfusion requirement	No	Occasionally	Usually	Always

*Assuming a 70-kg man.

and whether bleeding has been stopped. Elderly patients or patients with severe coronary artery disease may require transfusion and invasive monitoring for lower absolute levels of blood loss than do younger, fit patients. Class I hemorrhagic shock, as a general rule, requires little or no treatment, provided bleeding has stopped. Patients with class II hemorrhagic shock, who may have a base deficit of 3 to 5, usually require crystalloid infusion and occasionally require transfusion, particularly if bleeding has not been fully controlled. Patients with signs of class III hemorrhagic shock, or who have a base deficit 6 to 9, usually require transfusion. Patients with signs of class IV hemorrhagic shock, or those with a base deficit greater than 9, may die if not given blood urgently. Patients manifesting this degree of shock may require type O negative or type-specific blood as soon as possible.

Resuscitation should continue until acidosis has improved and signs of end-organ underperfusion have stabilized or resolved. Traditionally, it has been believed that earlier fluid resuscitation improves outcome. This assumption has been challenged by authorities who believe that restoration of normal blood pressure with fluid infusion before definitive control of hemorrhage results in excessive bleeding and poorer patient outcomes.

Head Injury

Surgical Anatomy

The head is a frequent target for blows and is prone to strike hard objects such as the ground and automobile dashboards. The encasement of the brain in the rigid bony cranial vault provides some protection for this fragile and complex organ. Supported by the meninges, the brain virtually floats in cerebral spinal fluid (CSF), which can dissipate energy from minor injuries. However, the structure of the skull, a closed space of fixed volume, has important consequences in head injury. The calvarium is incompletely divided by a tough supporting membrane, the tentorium cerebelli, into anterior and posterior compartments. The anterior compartment itself is incompletely divided into a right and left compartment by a similar structure, the falx cerebri. Swelling or expanding masses in the anterior compartment can push, or herniate, brain substance across these incomplete barriers. Most commonly, this occurs transtentorially. In this case, the third cranial nerve, which passes just above the tentorium, is caught between this structure and the swelling brain. Because the area of the brain that usually herniates is known as the uncus, this phenomenon is referred to as uncal herniation and is accompanied by dysfunction of the third cranial nerve, which is manifested by dilatation and lack of constriction response to light of the ipsilateral pupil. Brain substance also can herniate across the falx cerebri. This phenomenon is referred to as subfalcine herniation. No specific physical findings are associated with subfalcine herniation.

The vascular anatomy of the skull and brain also are important in trauma. The middle meningeal artery, which runs laterally up the midportion of the squamous portion of the temporal bone, is prone to injury in temporal bone fracture. The venous drainage of the meninges occurs through small bridging veins that are anchored to the inner table of the skull. These veins also are prone to injury during severe deceleration.

Physiology

Brain function can be assessed easily, by assessing level of consciousness. One of the most common changes in mentation caused by injury is loss of consciousness (LOC). When this occurs, patients are unresponsive to outside stimuli, although vital functions such as respiration continue. Periods of unconsciousness may vary from seconds to hours. Exactly what physiologic insults underlie brief traumatic LOC is unclear. The principal significance of brief LOC is its association with more significant brain injury. Prolonged unconsciousness is referred to as coma. Coma results from major structural brain damage, usually to white-matter areas that serve as vital information pathways within the brain.

Abnormalities of consciousness are graded by using a system known as the Glasgow Coma Scale, or GCS (Table

TABLE 11–2 Glasgow Coma Scale*

Eye opening	**Score**
Spontaneous	4
To voice	3
To pain	2
None	1
Verbal response	**Score**
Oriented	5
Confused	4
Inappropriate words	3
Incomprehensible sounds	2
None	1
Motor response	**Score**
Obeys command	6
Localizes pain	5
Withdraws from pain	4
Flexion	3
Extension	2
None	1

*GCS score, best eye opening + best verbal + best motor response scores.

11-2). The GCS should be measured for all trauma patients as part of the primary survey and repeated frequently in head-injured patients. Worsening conditions within the skull will be reflected by worsening of the level of consciousness and decrease of the GCS. A GCS of eight or less is an indication for insertion of an intracranial pressure (ICP) monitoring device and endotracheal intubation.

Severe injury to the brain also can result in stereotyped postures. The two most common are decorticate and decerebrate posturing. Pressure on the forebrain from mass or swelling reduces the amount of higher cortical control over the thalamus and midbrain. Pain or other stimuli, such as endotracheal suctioning, causes uninhibited reflex responses from the more primitive brain centers. As pressure builds, the first posture to be seen is characterized by arching of the back, flexion of the upper extremities, and extension of the lower. This phenomenon is "decorticate posturing." One can remember decorticate posturing by the "C" made by the upper extremities during this reflex. The word *decorticate* has a hard C sound. As conditions worsen, decerebrate posturing is seen. This posturing consists of flexion and external rotation of the upper extremity and extension of the lower. The upper extremity makes an "S" shape that should remind you of the soft C sound in "decerebrate." If pressure continues to build within the brain, decerebrate posturing will eventually give way to flaccid muscle tone, which precedes brain death.

Because the skull is unyielding, the sum of the volumes of its contents is constant. Brain tissue, CSF, blood, and meninges all occupy the cranial vault. Any process that increases the volume occupied by one of these components must do so at the expense of one of the other components, or must increase the pressure in the cranial cavity, or both. Because blood and CSF are both liquids, and therefore noncompressible, the brain substance itself is compressed and the ICP increases. As mentioned earlier, a mass or swelling in the brain can result in herniation of brain substance through the supporting membranous structures of the cranium. If the ICP increases sufficiently to exceed the perfusion pressure of blood entering the skull (the cerebral perfusion pressure or CPP), cerebral ischemia and eventually brain death will occur. Therefore one of the primary goals of evaluation and management of head injury is to identify patients with the potential for elevated ICP and deliver specific treatment before compromise of cerebral blood flow occurs.

Signs of increased ICP include headache, nausea, vomiting, and somnolence. In cases in which elevated ICP is suspected, systolic blood pressure should be maintained at a level of at least 90 mmHg by any means necessary. Blood from intracranial hematoma should be evacuated as soon as possible. Once ICP is known, the CPP is calculated by the formula

$$CPP = MAP - ICP$$

where MAP is mean arterial pressure. CPP should be maintained at a level of at least 70. CPP is maintained at this level by volume loading with crystalloid or blood transfusion and the use of vasopressors.

When the ICP exceeds 20 to 24, other measures must be taken. The simplest is to elevate the head of the bed to 15 to 30 degrees. This may be done either by placing the head of the bed up, or, if the patient must remain flat, by placing the bed in reverse Trendelenburg position. Patients with high ICP should be kept in darkened rooms, with effort made to keep noise and other stimulation to a minimum. If these measures are ineffective, then more complicated and risky measures must be taken.

The cerebral vasculature is unique in its ability to autoregulate blood flow, and hence the volume of blood, within the cranial vault. One of the most important controlling stimuli of cerebral vasoregulation is the pco_2 of the blood perfusing the brain. As pco_2 decreases, cerebral vasoconstriction occurs. With increasing pco_2, cerebral vasodilatation occurs. It is possible, therefore, to reduce ICP by inducing cerebral vasoconstriction via hyperventilation. This technique is used only when ICP is acutely elevated and unmanageable by other means. Chronic hyperventilation (longer than 48 hours) results in the cerebral vasculature losing its responsiveness to hypocapnia. Thus prolonged hyperventilation should be avoided.

In cases in which extreme brain swelling is noted and ICP is elevated despite these measures, mannitol infusion may be necessary. Mannitol is an osmotic diuretic that increases the serum osmolality and thus may induce some net movement of edema fluid out of the injured brain and into the vascular space. When indicated, mannitol is usually given until the serum osmolarity is between 300 and 310 mOsm/L. Because mannitol is a diuretic, its use will lead to volume depletion, which may worsen CPP. Careful management of blood pressure and CPP must accompany the use of mannitol in head injury.

Cerebral Contusion

Pathophysiology

When the skull is subjected to external forces, the brain, obeying the laws of inertia, will tend to continue moving with respect to the skull and hit the inner table beneath the point of impact. The elasticity of the brain substance may cause a subsequent rebound phenomenon, causing the brain to strike the skull a second time 180 degrees from the point of impact. This is referred to as the coup-contracoup phenomenon.

When the energy delivered to the brain is slight, a small contusion may result. This will appear on computed tomography (CT) scan of the head as a small area of high attenuation because of the small amount of subarachnoid blood, which is present at the area of bruising (Fig. 11-2). As the force of injury increases, hemorrhage may be seen within the substance of the brain. Small contusions usually result in minor changes in mentation, including brief LOC or confusion. Injuries that are more significant can lead to brain swelling, coma, and herniation.

Severe cerebral contusions are associated with the diffuse axonal injury (DAI), in which major damage to the white-matter tracts of the brain results from direct acceleration or deceleration injury. DAI may result in mild to severe neuropsychiatric abnormalities or, in the worst cases, to persistent coma.

Workup and Evaluation

Cerebral contusion should be suspected in any patient who has reported LOC as result of a head injury. Any patient who has a GCS less than 15 also should be suspected of having a cerebral contusion.

Any patient that is suspected of having a cerebral contusion should undergo immediate head CT scanning. Patients who have persistent coma or depressed levels of consciousness several days after injury should undergo magnetic resonance imaging (MRI) scanning to evaluate for DAI.

Treatment

In cases of mild cerebral contusion, observation is sufficient. Many authorities recommend the use of anticonvulsant drugs if subarachnoid blood is seen on head CT. Anticonvulsants may protect against early posttraumatic seizures. No evidence suggests that anticonvulsants will prevent development of long-term posttraumatic seizure disorders.

For patients with GCS of 8 or less, or those who have evidence of brain swelling on CT scan, ICP should be monitored. Outcome from cerebral contusion is variable. Patients with mild contusion frequently return to a normal level of functioning, although many of these patients have persistent neuropsychiatric effects, such as depression and limited attention span, for months or years after injury. Outcome in more severe cerebral contusion is predicted by both GCS on admission and age. Elderly brain-injured patients with low GCS on admission have overall survival rates between 20% and 30%. Patients younger than 30 years, however, have as high as 90% likelihood of good functional outcome, even with low admission GCS.

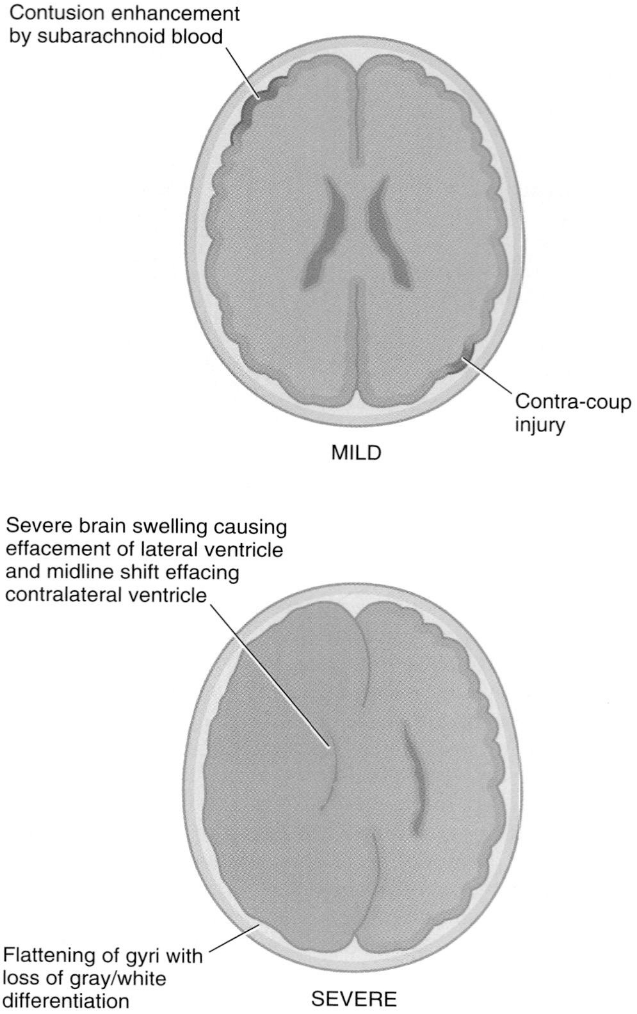

FIGURE 11–2 Computed tomography scan appearance of cerebral contusion.

Subdural Hematoma

Pathophysiology

When the brain is subject to major decelerating forces, the bridging veins, which drain into the dural venous sinuses,

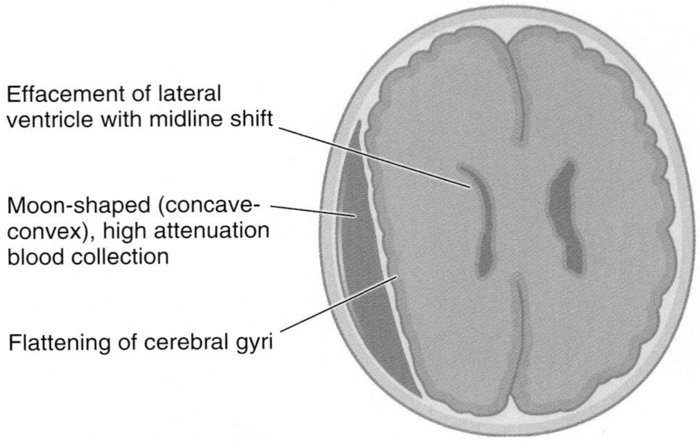

FIGURE 11–3 Computed tomography scan appearance of subdural hematoma.

are prone to tear. Blood leaking from these veins accumulates in the subdural space. Because this space is poorly contained and bordered internally by the relatively soft brain, acute subdural hematomas (SDH) spread widely, forming a "quarter moon"–shaped abnormality visible on CT scan (Fig. 11-3). Because the energy required to cause SDH is high, these patients are usually unconscious at the time of admission because of associated contusion of the brain itself.

Elderly individuals are particularly prone to SDH. Cerebral atrophy elongates the bridging veins, leaving them stretched and more likely to rupture with relatively minor injury. Because the brain is atrophied, more room exists within the calvarium for accumulation of blood before signs of increased ICP occur. Thus elderly patients may appear weeks after a seemingly minor fall with significant SDHs. These are referred to as chronic SDHs.

Workup and Evaluation

Any patient who is suspected of having an SDH should undergo an immediate head CT scan. Because SDH usually occurs in the setting of massive decelerating injury, extracranial injuries are common. All patients with an SDH should be evaluated for potentially life-threatening abdominal and thoracic injuries, as well as cervical spine injury.

Treatment

SDHs smaller than 1 cm in greatest width on CT scan and not associated with a depressed GCS are frequently managed nonoperatively. Otherwise, urgent evacuation, usually with placement of an ICP monitor, is indicated. Because SDH is frequently associated with significant injury to the underlying brain substance, even with early and effective surgical intervention, patients frequently have long-term neurologic impairment.

Epidural Hematoma

Pathophysiology

In contrast to SDH, which is associated with high-energy deceleration injury, epidural hematoma (EDH) may result from relatively low-energy impact on the skull. EDH results from a tear in a dural artery, usually the middle meningeal artery, caused by a depressed skull fracture (Fig. 11-4). Classically, the patient with EDH has received a lateral blow to the temporal bone. Because the blow is relatively low energy, usually no significant parenchymal brain injury is associated with EDH. Thus patients may have brief LOC but usually have a GCS of 15 when initially examined. However, because of the laceration of the middle meningeal artery, blood slowly collects in the epidural space. This process occurs slowly because the dura is tightly adherent to the inner table of the skull. It takes time for blood leaking from the lacerated vessel to dissect the dura from the skull. Eventually the hematoma grows to sufficient size to compress the underlying brain and cause symptoms of increased ICP.

Workup and Evaluation

EDH is characteristically associated with brief LOC after injury, followed by a lucent interval in which the patient has a normal neurologic examination. The lucent interval ends with the patient developing signs of increased ICP, which, if untreated, will result in coma and eventual death.

Because of the association of temporal bone fracture with EDH, any patient with a transverse fracture of the temporal bone should undergo head CT. Similarly, any patient who exhibits worsening headache, nausea, vomiting, or depressed LOC after a blow to the head should undergo head CT.

Treatment

Small EDHs that are smaller than 1 cm in greatest width are occasionally managed nonoperatively. In cases in which

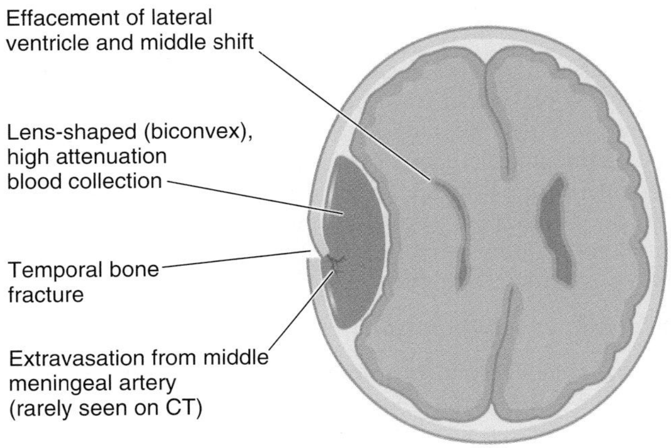

FIGURE 11–4 Computed tomography scan appearance of epidural hematoma.

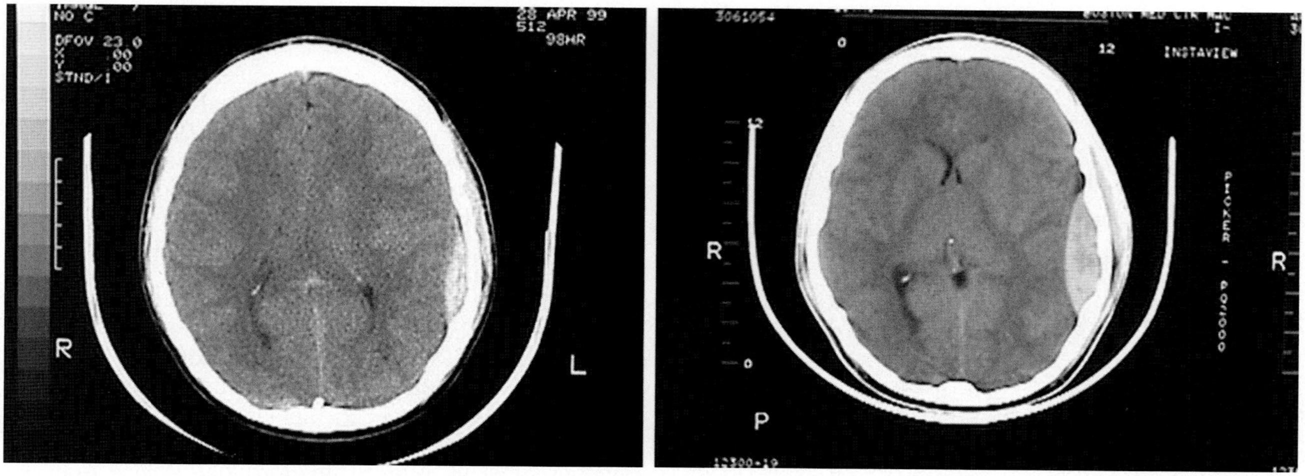

FIGURE 11–5 Evolution of epidural hematoma (EDH). Computed tomography (CT) scans taken 6 hours apart in a 12-year-old after a blow to the side of the head. Glasgow Coma Scale (GCS), 15 on admission. At time of second CT scan, GCS, 13. This study demonstrates significant enlargement of a left temporoparietal EDH.

patients are to be observed with EDH, repeated head CT within 12 hours of admission is advisable to monitor for progression (Fig. 11-5). EDH greater than 1 cm or those associated with neurologic findings should be evacuated as an emergency. Because usually little or no significant injury to the brain is seen in EDH patients who undergo early evacuation, they frequently return to a normal level of neurologic functioning.

Spinal Cord Injury

It is estimated that about 10,000 patients per year in the United States have spinal cord injury. Approximately half of these are due to motor vehicle crashes. Falls, assaults, and athletic injuries account for most of the remainder. Fifty percent of all spine injuries affect the cervical spine; of these, between 35% and 45% result in quadriplegia.

Pathophysiology

The cervical spine is particularly prone to injury due to hyperflexion, hyperextension, rotation, and axial compression. When the integrity of either the bony elements or the ligamentous supports of the spinal column is disrupted, impingement on the spinal canal may occur, with resulting damage to the spinal cord. The spinal cord itself is a delicate structure. Its blood supply is easily disrupted. Once injured, the spinal cord is largely incapable of significant healing.

Workup and Evaluation

All patients who undergo significant deceleration injury or who have significant head or facial trauma should be evaluated for cervical spine injury. When the cervical spine is properly immobilized in an appropriate rigid cervical collar and absolute axial alignment is maintained, any injury to the cervical spine is rendered "stable." Hemodynamically unstable patients should not be diverted from management of shock or other injury for the evaluation of the cervical spine. Such evaluation can be safely delayed until life-threatening issues are resolved. The Eastern Association for the Surgery of Trauma (EAST) has published practice management guidelines reflecting an evidence-based approach to evaluation of the cervical spine. According to the EAST Guidelines, patients who are awake and alert with no mental-status changes and no distracting injuries, are neurologically intact, and have no neck pain, can be considered to have a stable cervical spine. Patients not meeting these criteria should have a cervical spine series containing at least a lateral projection, an anteroposterior view, and an open-mouth odontoid view or a cervical CT scan. Patients who have an altered sensorium and are unable to be evaluated adequately for the presence of either spinal pain or neurologic deficit should have a cervical spine series, as outlined earlier, with the addition of fine-cut axial CT images of C1 and C2.

Treatment

Management of cervical spine fractures may require a rigid collar, external fixation such as halo vest immobilization, or surgical stabilization.

Neurogenic Shock

Pathophysiology

The nerve fibers controlling the sympathetic nervous system exit the spinal cord in the thoracolumbar region. Injury to the spinal cord above this level will cause the loss of all distal sympathetic output. Thus cervical spinal cord injuries are associated with loss of sympathetic vasomotor tone. This results in poor vascular tone in the arterial resistance vessels and pooling of blood. A loss of sympathetic innervation to the heart, bradycardia, and diminished cardiac contractility also may occur. When severe, this phenomenon can result in inadequate tissue perfusion or neurogenic shock. The interruption of sympathetic outflow, and the resulting parasympathetic predominance, results in a constellation of findings that should suggest this diagnosis: bradycardia, hypotension, and (in male patients) priapism.

Evaluation and Workup

Any trauma patient exhibiting either bradycardia or priapism should be assumed to have a cervical spinal cord injury. Under these circumstances, the cervical spine should be immobilized. It should be remembered that patients with spinal cord injuries frequently have other injuries that may be life threatening. It is not uncommon for hypovolemic shock to coexist with neurogenic shock. Therefore a thorough and complete search for additional injuries and sources of shock should be performed.

Treatment

Two physiologic mechanisms exist in neurogenic shock: decreased myocardial contractility and decreased peripheral vascular resistance. In most cases, spinal shock results in relatively mild physiologic derangement, which can be corrected with infusion of modest volumes of balanced salt solution. In some cases, hypotension and malperfusion will persist after volume replacement. In these cases, care should be taken to limit further volume loading, as congestive heart failure may result. Vasopressors with α-adrenergic activity, such as phenylephrine (Neosynephrine), should be added. The end point of resuscitation in neurogenic shock is restoration of tissue perfusion. Parameters such as acid-base balance and urine output may indicate adequate perfusion, even with ongoing hypotension. In cases in which preexisting cardiac disease or hypovolemia makes resuscitation challenging, a low threshold should exist for use of invasive monitoring to guide volume replacement and vasopressor management.

Chest Trauma

Injuries to the thorax cause one of every four trauma deaths in the United States. Because of the concentration of vital structures within the thorax, death from chest trauma can occur from a variety of causes. Exsanguinating hemorrhage may result from injury to the heart or great vessels. Hypoxia or hypercarbia can be caused by injury to pulmonary structures. Tension pneumothorax or pericardial tamponade may lead to fatal obstructive cardiogenic shock. Because of the serious consequences possible, all patients with thoracic trauma should be evaluated in a systematic, thorough, and efficient manner. Both the anterior and posterior surfaces of the chest must be inspected and palpated. The neck should be checked for jugular venous distention (JVD). Both pleural cavities and the heart should be auscultated. A portable chest radiograph should be obtained on all victims of penetrating chest injury and on any patients with possible multisystem blunt injury. Types of chest injuries are presented in Box 11-1.

BOX 11-1 Thoracic Injuries

Life threatening (treat during primary survey)
- Tension pneumothorax
- Pericardial tamponade
- Open pneumothorax
- Massive hemothorax
- Flail chest

Potentially life threatening (treat during the secondary survey)
- Pulmonary contusion
- Myocardial contusion
- Aortic rupture
- Diaphragmatic rupture
- Tracheobronchial injury
- Esophageal injury

Simple Pneumothorax

Pathophysiology

Under normal circumstances, the pleural space is maintained at a pressure less than that of the ambient atmosphere. Any wound that creates a communication between either the external environment or the bronchopulmonary tree and the pleural space will result in the entry of air into the pleural space, or pneumothorax. When air enters the pleural space, an associated collapse of the lung occurs; the lung is no longer distended by the lower pleural pressure.

Workup and Evaluation

Pneumothorax should be suspected in all patients with penetrating injury of the chest or upper abdomen and in all patients with potential multisystem blunt injury. Physical findings for tension pneumothorax include shortness of breath, diminished breath sounds, and hyper-resonance on the injured side. Chest radiograph is diagnostic. Inspiratory/expiratory chest films are useful in cases in which a small pneumothorax is suspected. Occasionally, patients with apparently normal plain films of the chest will have small pneumothoraces seen on either chest or abdominal CT. For patients who are intubated and requiring mechanical ventilation, a sudden increase in the peak inspiratory pressure can signal the presence of a pneumothorax.

Treatment

Very small pneumothoraces in patients with no other injuries, who will not require mechanical ventilation, can be managed with observation alone. A repeated chest radiograph 12 to 24 hours after injury is useful to monitor for progression. Larger pnemothoraces or those occurring in patients who will require positive-pressure ventilation should be treated with a tube thoracostomy. In trauma, pneumothorax may be associated with hemothorax or with elevation of the diaphragm due to hemoperitoneum. Because of these factors, all thoracostomy tubes placed in an injury should be placed in the fourth intercostal space in the midaxillary line. A useful anatomic landmark for location of chest tubes in trauma is just below the tip of the hair-bearing part of the axilla. Because of the possibility of associated hemothorax, all chest tubes placed for trauma should be attached to an underwater suction device.

In cases in which injury to proximal bronchi is present, large amounts of air may be able to pass into the pleural space. In such cases, it is sometimes necessary to place two or more thoracostomy tubes to manage the resulting acute bronchopleural fistula. In extreme cases, surgical repair and or dual lung ventilation is necessary to manage this problem.

Outcomes and Complications

The large majority of simple pneumothoraces will resolve with chest-tube management and require no further treatment. Rarely, empyema or bronchopleural fistula can complicate simple pneumothorax and require prolonged chest-tube drainage or surgical intervention.

Tension Pneumothorax

Pathophysiology

Tension pneumothorax results from an injury to the lung or parietal pleura, resulting in a pleural flap that forms a one-way valve allowing air to leak from the lung or atmosphere into the pleural space but preventing airflow out of the pleural space. Air accumulates in the pleural space, which progressively increases the pressure. Ultimately, the pressure in the pleural space is sufficient to displace the mediastinum toward the opposite hemithorax. The lateral displacement of the mediastinum results in the compression of the vena cavae, thus reducing and ultimately obstructing blood flow into the heart.

This condition of reduced cardiac filling is referred to as extrinsic or obstructive cardiogenic shock. Obstruction of blood flow into the heart can be caused by lateral compression of the mediastinum by a tension pneumothorax, or by extrinsic compression of the right atrium due to pericardial tamponade, which is discussed later. The compensatory mechanisms for both tension pneumothorax and pericardial tamponade are similar. To overcome the extrinsic pressure obstructing cardiac return, a sympathetically mediated adrenergic response causes contraction of venous capacitance vessels, resulting in an increase in central venous pressure (CVP). Thus one of the cardinal signs of extrinsic cardiogenic shock is JVD. Extrinsic cardiogenic shock is the only commonly occurring process to cause JVD in the setting of trauma.

Adrenergic stimulation also causes acceleration of the heart rate. This too is adaptive, as it allows the maintenance of cardiac output in the face of diminished cardiac stroke volume. Extreme tachycardia in chest injury should lead to the suspicion of obstructive cardiogenic shock.

It is important to recognize the importance of these two sympathetic reflexes in the physiologic response to obstructive shock. Until definitive treatment is available, sympatholytic agents (for example, general anesthesia) should be avoided when obstructive shock is suspected.

BOX 11–2 Signs of Tension Pneumothorax

- Respiratory distress
- Tachycardia
- Hypotension
- Tracheal deviation away from affected hemithorax
- Hyper-resonance
- Diminished breath sounds
- Jugular venous distention
- Cyanosis (late finding)
- Escalating peak inspiratory pressure (for patients who are mechanically ventilated)

Workup and Evaluation

Patients with tension pneumothorax are short of breath. Typically, an awake patient will be in obvious respiratory distress. For patients who are obtunded, the diagnosis of tension pneumothorax may be more obscure. Escalating peak inspiratory pressure or decreasing tidal volume may indicate tension pneumothorax (Box 11-2). Chest radiographs are diagnostic (Fig. 11-6); however, if signs of

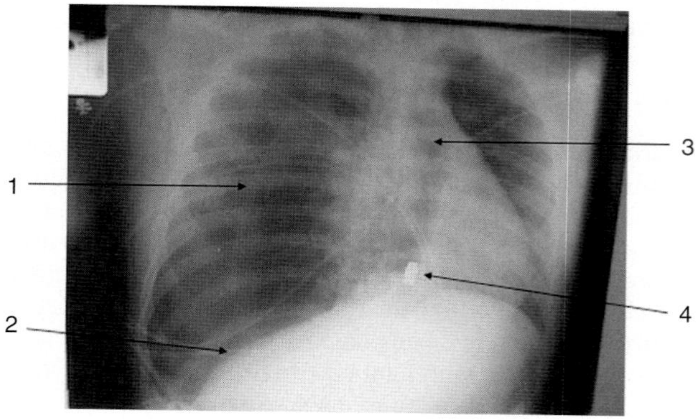

FIGURE 11–6 Tension pneumothorax after a gunshot wound to the chest. 1, Collapsed right lung; 2, depression of the right hemidiaphragm by elevated intrapleural pressure; 3, leftward deviation of trachea; 4, bullet.

tension pneumothorax are present, treatment should be initiated on suspicion of this diagnosis alone. Patients may decompensate while chest radiographs are being obtained.

Treatment

Initial treatment of tension pneumothorax is *immediate* decompression of the affected pleural space by placement of an angiocath in the second intercostal space at the midclavicular line. This maneuver will equilibrate the pressure in the pleural space with the atmosphere, converting the tension pneumothorax to a simple pneumothorax. This will allow the mediastinum to return to the midline and eliminate the compression of the cavae. Definitive management of the now simple pneumothorax by placement of a thoracostomy tube can then be undertaken in an unhurried manner.

Pericardial Tamponade

Pathophysiology

Injury to the heart or the coronary or internal mammary arteries can lead to the accumulation of blood within the pericardial space. Because the pericardium is not acutely distensible, the accumulating fluid within the pericardium allows less space for the heart to fill. Like tension pneumothorax, this process leads to obstructive cardiogenic shock. As intrapericardial pressure increases, the filling of the heart is impeded, and stroke volume decreases. To maintain cardiac output, heart rate increases. The right atrium, having the thinnest wall and lowest intraluminal pressure, is the cardiac structure most easily compressed by the increasing intrapericardial pressure. Eventually, when the pressure outside the atrium (the intrapericardial pressure) exceeds the pressure filling the heart (the CVP), the heart fails to fill, and cardiac output decreases to zero. This decrease can be dramatic and can occur in a matter of seconds (Fig. 11-7). It is therefore necessary to be aggressive in both the suspicion and the treatment of pericardial tamponade.

Workup and Evaluation

Pericardial tamponade is most frequently encountered with penetrating trauma (i.e., gunshot and stab wounds). Although the diagnosis should be suspected in cases of penetrating wounds in proximity to the sternum, patients with stab or gunshot wounds occurring more distally can result in tamponade. Signs of pericardial tamponade are listed in Box 11-3. Patients who demonstrate tachycardia, hypotension, and JVD or elevated CVP in the absence of signs of tension pneumothorax should be considered to have evolving tamponade until proven otherwise. In a hemodynamically stable patient in whom the diagnosis is suspected, emergency echocardiography is diagnostic. When patients are unstable, immediate pericardiocentesis should be performed.

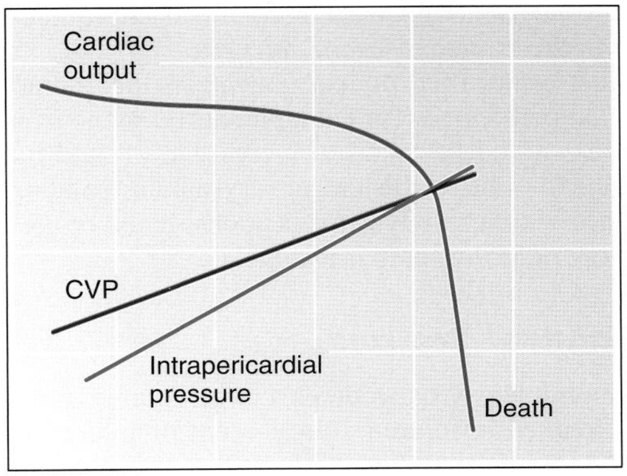

FIGURE 11–7 Physiology of pericardial tamponade. When the intrapericardial pressure exceeds the cardiovascular pressure (CVP), cardiac filling is prevented. Cardiac output decreases, and death occurs. The goal of emergency management of pericardial tamponade is to return to a point on the graph where CVP is greater than intrapericardial pressure.

Treatment

Initial treatment for patients with present and relatively stable vital signs is needle pericardiocentesis. A needle, either an angiocath or a spinal needle, is inserted just to the left of the xyphoid process and angled 45 degrees from horizontal and 45 degrees to the left and advanced. If possible, an electrocardiograph is attached to the needle to monitor for the appearance of a current of injury, indicating that the myocardium has been entered. The needle is aspirated with a large syringe while being advanced. It is not necessary to aspirate all of the intrapericardial fluid, but only to decompress the pericardial space sufficiently to permit the heart to fill. This will usually allow time for the patient to be brought to the operating room for definitive management. Unfortunately, blood that immediately accumulates in the pericardial space will clot. Thus needle pericardiocentesis may not permit sufficient pericardial decompression. In this case, the only alternative is to perform an immediate thoracotomy and operative decompression of the pericardial space. This must be done wherever the patient happens to be

BOX 11–3 Signs of Pericardial Tamponade

- Beck's triad
  - Hypotension
  - Jugular venous distention
  - Muffled heart sounds
- Extreme tachycardia
- Elevated central venous pressure
- Pulsus paradoxus
  - Decrease of systolic pressure by >10 mmHg on inspiration

at the time tamponade is recognized. Frequently this occurs in the trauma resuscitation area.

In the event that pericardiocentesis or thoracotomy cannot be performed (for example, at the scene of injury), measures should be taken to increase CVP and maintain sympathetic tone. Infusion of crystalloid solutions and avoidance of sympatholytic medications should be performed until more definitive care is available.

Abdominal Trauma

The abdominal cavity occupies a large volume of the trunk and is frequently injured. Ten percent of injured patients admitted to our trauma center have documented injuries to abdominal viscera. Because fluid and blood can accumulate in the peritoneal cavity without causing noticeable physical findings, particularly in multiply injured, intoxicated, or neurologically impaired patients, such injuries may be occult to physical examination. The development of CT scanning and ultrasound has greatly improved our ability to diagnose and manage injuries to the abdomen.

Surgical Anatomy

The abdomen is traditionally divided into three areas: the peritoneal cavity, the pelvic cavity, and the retroperitoneum. The upper portion of the peritoneal cavity is relatively protected by the overlying ribs. Injuries occurring between the nipples and midepigastrium may damage structures in either the thorax or abdomen and thus are referred to as thoracoabdominal injuries. Similarly, structures in the pelvis are relatively protected by the surrounding bony pelvic girdle. Structures in the retroperitoneum, such as the duodenum and pancreas, are well protected by surrounding organs and bony structures. When injured, however, their position in the retroperitoneum can make both diagnosis and treatment of injuries to these organs challenging. Because of differences in injury pattern and management, it is useful to consider penetrating injuries and blunt injuries to the abdomen separately.

Penetrating Abdominal Trauma

Injuries caused by piercing weapons, such as knives and spears, and those caused by firearms are referred to as penetrating trauma. Impalement as a result of falls and other nonintentional mechanisms also may result in penetrating injury. Tissue injury is a consequence of energy delivery. Thus it is useful to divide penetrating injury into low-energy and high-energy injuries. Stab wounds deliver low-energy injury to tissues. Gunshot (and shotgun) wounds result in the delivery of much higher energies to tissues. Stab wounds result in laceration and perforation of visceral structures without causing injury to adjacent tissue. Stab wounds do not generally result in tearing or devitalization of the organs injured. Gunshot wounds do cause tearing and devitalization of tissue. The degree of injury from firearms is a direct consequence of the kinetic energy the wounding projectile deposits in tissues. It should be recalled that the formula for kinetic energy is

$$K_e = {}^1\!/_2\, MV^2$$

for projectiles lodging in the body, or

$$K_e = ({}^1\!/_2\, MV^2)_{Entrance} - ({}^1\!/_2\, MV^2)_{Exit}$$

for projectiles traversing the body, where M is mass and V is velocity. Thus injuries from larger projectiles and those with higher velocity will cause more severe injury. Projectiles traveling more than 2000 ft/sec (high velocity) are capable of causing injury well beyond the immediate path of the projectile. In civilian practice, such wounds are, fortunately, rare. Mortality from stab wounds and low-velocity firearms is generally related to injury of a major vascular structure. High-velocity weapons can create wide areas of tissue disruption and necrosis. Such wounds can be lethal without injuring a major vascular structure.

The frequency with which various abdominal organs are injured by penetrating wounds is a function of the surface area and volume occupied. A treatment algorithm for management of penetrating injury is given in Figure 11-8. Management of specific organ system injuries caused by penetrating trauma consists of control and repair of vascular injuries, débridement of dead tissue, and wound management. Most hollow viscous injuries can be managed by primary repair or resection and primary anastomosis.

Blunt Abdominal Injury

Injury to the abdominal viscera is common in cases of high-speed acceleration/deceleration injury and in direct blows to the abdomen. In contrast to injury patterns in penetrating trauma, the organs most commonly injured in blunt trauma are those that are more securely fixed to their surroundings and that, because of their histology, lack structural resilience and elasticity. The spleen, which is tethered to several surrounding structures, and which is notable for a rich blood supply, with a relatively delicate and inelastic structure, is the most commonly injured abdominal organ in blunt trauma.

Before the development of modern diagnostic methods, as many as 17% of patients with major abdominal injury died because of the failure to diagnose intraabdominal hemorrhage in a timely manner. In many patients, the abdominal cavity can accommodate a significant amount of blood before exhibiting significant distention. This factor, combined with the frequent association of blunt abdominal trauma with neurologic injury, significant distracting orthopedic injury, and alcohol or drug intoxication, makes the diagnosis of intraabdominal injury a continuing challenge today. Patients with blunt abdominal injury who exhibit abdominal distention, shock, or peritonitis should undergo immediate celiotomy. In many cases, however, signs of abdominal injury are not evident, and shock may

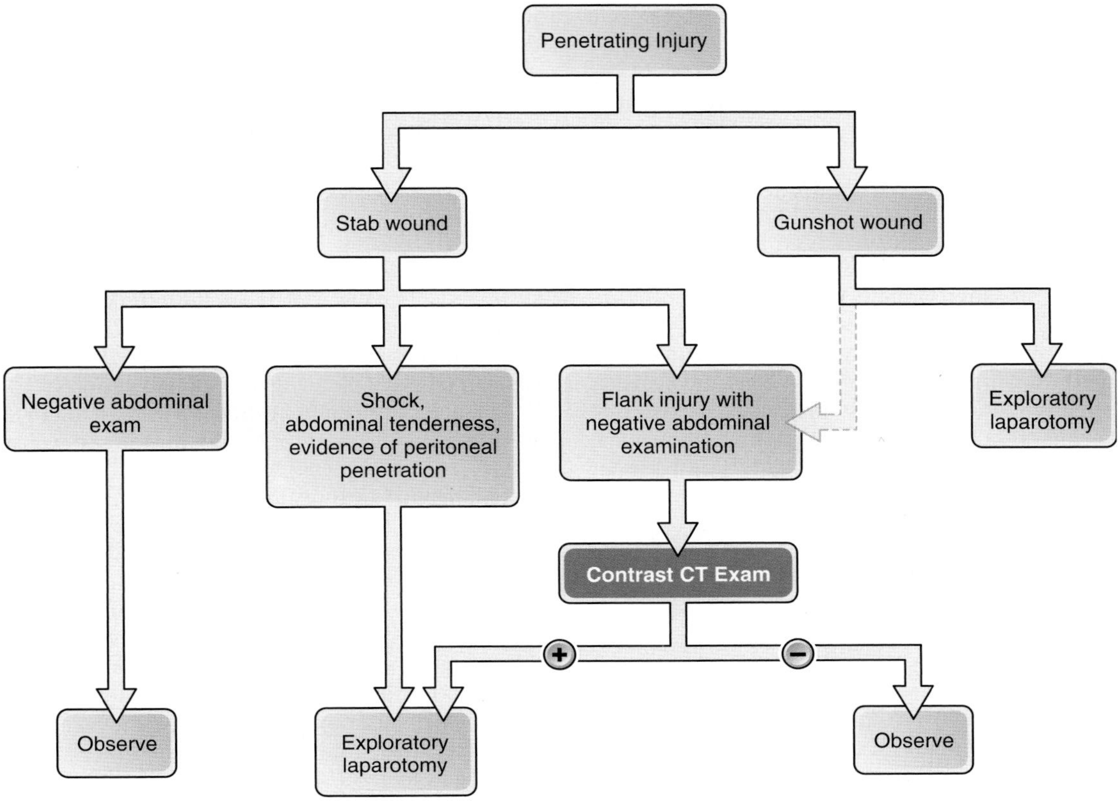

FIGURE 11–8 Management of penetrating injury.

be due to associated extraabdominal injuries. In these cases, additional diagnostic methods must be used. The first major advance in the evaluation of patients with blunt abdominal injury was the development of diagnostic peritoneal lavage (DPL) in the late 1960s. This technique involves placement of a catheter into the abdominal cavity in the emergency department, under local anesthesia. The catheter is aspirated, and if gross blood, bile, stool, or food particles are aspirated, laparotomy is indicated. If nothing is aspirated, 1000 mL of warmed lactated Ringer's solution is instilled into the peritoneal cavity. This fluid is then siphoned off by dropping the infusion bag to the floor. The fluid removed is sent for cell count, amylase, and Gram stain. A positive test is defined as red blood cells (RBCs), more than 100,000 cells/mm^3; white blood cells (WBCs) more than 500 cells/mm^3; amylase, more than 175 U/dL; or Gram stain demonstrating bacteria.

Several disadvantages exist with DPL. It may not be feasible in patients who have undergone prior surgery. The examination itself can cause visceral injury in a small percentage of cases. Most important, bleeding from injuries that do not require surgical management may nonetheless result in a positive result. Currently, ultrasound and CT have largely replaced DPL as the diagnostic methods of choice in abdominal trauma.

Rapid evaluation of the abdomen for the presence of blood is now possible in the resuscitation area with the technique of focused abdominal sonography for trauma (FAST). This method involves the ultrasonic imaging of the pericardium, right upper quadrant, left upper quadrant, and pelvis for the presence of blood. This test has been shown to have a sensitivity of 88%, a specificity of 98%, a positive predictive value of 72%, a negative predictive value of 99%, and an overall accuracy of 97%. In the presence of shock, a positive examination is sufficient to indicate immediate celiotomy.

The availability of high-speed helical CT scanners located near trauma resuscitation areas has made this technology the backbone of the evaluation of blunt abdominal trauma. The ability to identify and grade abdominal injuries accurately by CT has led to the development of nonoperative management schemes for many visceral injuries.

Splenic Injury

The spleen is the most commonly injured organ in blunt abdominal trauma. For the first half of the twentieth century, splenectomy was advocated for most injures of the spleen. However, the realization that the spleen plays an important role of the immunologic response to bacterial infection has resulted in the development of more-conservative methods of splenic injury management.

Surgical Anatomy

The spleen resides in the left upper quadrant posterior and lateral to the stomach. The spleen receives most of its blood supply from the splenic artery, which arises from the celiac axis. The histologic architecture of the spleen serves its function as a filter in the reticuloendothelial system. The arterial elements of the spleen empty segmentally into venous sinusoids, which then drain into a nonsegmental and interconnected venous drainage system. Evidence exists that the parenchyma of the spleen contains more functional smooth muscle in children than in adults. Little fibrous or rigid support of the organ contributes to its propensity for injury. Externally the spleen is supported by as many as eight ligaments, the most important being the gastrosplenic, the splenorenal, and the splenophrenic ligaments.

Pathophysiology

Because of its rich blood supply and delicate structure, the spleen is prone to laceration and hemorrhage. Because the arterial supply of the spleen usually enters the organ in a vertically oriented segmental arrangement, it is thought that transverse fractures of the spleen tend to bleed less than fractures along its long axis. This is because the latter traverse multiple segments, thus injuring multiple segmental arteries. Bleeding from minor injuries to the spleen may be contained within its thin capsule. Rarely, a previously contained subcapsular hematoma may rupture days or weeks after injury, resulting in sudden intraabdominal hemorrhage. Larger injuries are associated with rupture of the capsule and free hemorrhage into the peritoneal cavity. Because the spleen receives 5% of the cardiac output, bleeding from splenic injury can be substantial. In children, the spleen contains smooth muscle elements that may contribute to the arrest of bleeding even in cases of significant injury. Adults, lacking these elements, have a greater tendency to continue to bleed from splenic injuries.

Differential Diagnosis

Splenic injury is frequently associated with fractures of ribs 9 through 12 on the left and should be suspected in any patient with such fractures.

Workup and Evaluation

All patients with blunt abdominal trauma should be suspected of having a splenic rupture. Tenderness in the right upper quadrant or flank should suggest this injury. Irritation of the diaphragm by blood can lead to stimulation of somatic pain fibers that cause the impression of pain in the left shoulder or scapula. It should be stressed, however, that splenic injuries may have no specific physical manifestations on physical examination. A high index of suspicion and low threshold for diagnostic study should be maintained.

Diagnostic studies for the evaluation of splenic injury should be determined by the clinical circumstances. Patients who are hemodynamically unstable with clear-cut abdominal tenderness or distention should undergo immediate celiotomy. In cases in which hemodynamic instability is found but no clear indication of intraperitoneal injury, either FAST or diagnostic peritoneal lavage is indicated. CT of the abdomen is the gold standard for diagnosis of splenic injury in stable patients. All hemodynamically stable patients suspected of splenic injury should undergo abdominal CT as part of their admission workup.

Abdominal CT scanning allows an accurate assessment of the degree of injury to the spleen. A grading system for splenic injuries developed by the American Association for the Surgery of Trauma (AAST) is described in Table 11-3. This scale can be easily used in the grading of splenic injury on CT scan. The likelihood of surgical intervention increases with increasing injury scale. However, the most important single predictor of requirement for surgery is the presence of extravasation of intravenous contrast on a contrast-enhanced abdominal CT scan.

TABLE 11–3 AAST Splenic Injury Scale

Grade	Injury	Description
I	Hematoma	Subcapsular <10% of surface area
	Laceration	Capsular tear <1 cm parenchymal tear
II	Hematoma	Subcapsular 10%–50% of surface area or <5 cm diameter parenchymal hematoma
	Laceration	1–3 cm, not involving a trabecular vessel
III	Hematoma	Subcapsular >50% of surface area, expanding or ruptured. Intraparenchymal hematoma >5 cm diameter or expanding
	Laceration	>3-cm penetration or involving trabecular vessels
IV	Laceration	Laceration of segmental or hilar vessel producing devascularization of >25% of spleen
V	Laceration	Shattered spleen or devascularizing hilar injury

AAST, American Association for the Surgery of Trauma.

PEARLS FOR ROUNDS

Increase in diastolic pressure is the first blood pressure change seen in hypovolemia. When present, it means class II hemorrhagic shock (loss of ~15%–30% of blood volume).

Systolic hypotension is a sign of class III hemorrhagic shock (loss of 30%–40% of blood volume).

Agitation is another sign of shock.

Profound hypotension and apathy are signs of class IV hypovolemic shock (loss of >40% of blood volume).

A normal 70-kg man has approximately 5 L of blood volume (70 mL/kg).

Decorticate posturing includes flexion of the upper extremity (the arm makes a "C" for "deCorticate").

Decerebrate posturing includes extension and external rotation of the upper extremity (the arm makes an "S," like the soft c in "deCerebrate").

The signs of pericardial tamponade include Beck's triad (hypotension, JVD, muffled heart sounds), tachycardia, pulsus paradoxus, and elevated CVP.

Options for managing splenic rupture include observation, embolization, splenorrhaphy, and splenectomy.

Hemodynamic stability and evidence of ongoing bleeding are the most important factors in choosing a treatment strategy for solid-organ injury.

Treatment

Patients who are hypotensive, in shock, or otherwise unstable or are suspected of having intraabdominal bleeding from the spleen, should undergo immediate celiotomy. In patients who have no other significant injuries and the spleen is not shattered or totally devascularized (grade V), splenic salvage can be attempted. A number of techniques exist for preserving splenic tissue under these conditions. The segmental arterial supply of the spleen permits segmental resection of a portion of the spleen. In cases in which more diffuse injury is found, the spleen can be wrapped in prosthetic mesh for control of hemorrhage.

In cases in which shock or complex multisystem injury is present, or in which the spleen has been shattered, splenectomy is the procedure of choice (Fig. 11-9). For cases in which extravasation of contrast from the spleen exists, but the organ itself appears sufficiently intact, angioembolization has been advocated. The addition of angioembolization to the treatment of splenic injury has increased the success rate for nonoperative management to as high as 92% and increased overall splenic salvage to 59%.

Adults who require multiple transfusions to maintain hematocrit after splenic injury are likely to require splenectomy or splenorrhaphy. In children, the ability of the splenic vasculature to constrict in the setting of injury has led some to advocate higher transfusion limits for nonoperative management in this group. A management algorithm for splenic injury is presented in Figure 11-10.

Outcomes and Complications

The proximity of the spleen to the tail of the pancreas makes postoperative pancreatitis a common sequel to splenectomy. Postoperative bleeding, either from inadequate control of the splenic vessels or from failure of splenorrhaphy, occurs in 1% to 2% of patients having splenic conservation procedures. Fewer than 1% of patients undergoing splenic conservation develop splenic abscess as a late complication.

Patients who undergo splenectomy are at risk of developing overwhelming bacterial sepsis. The syndrome of

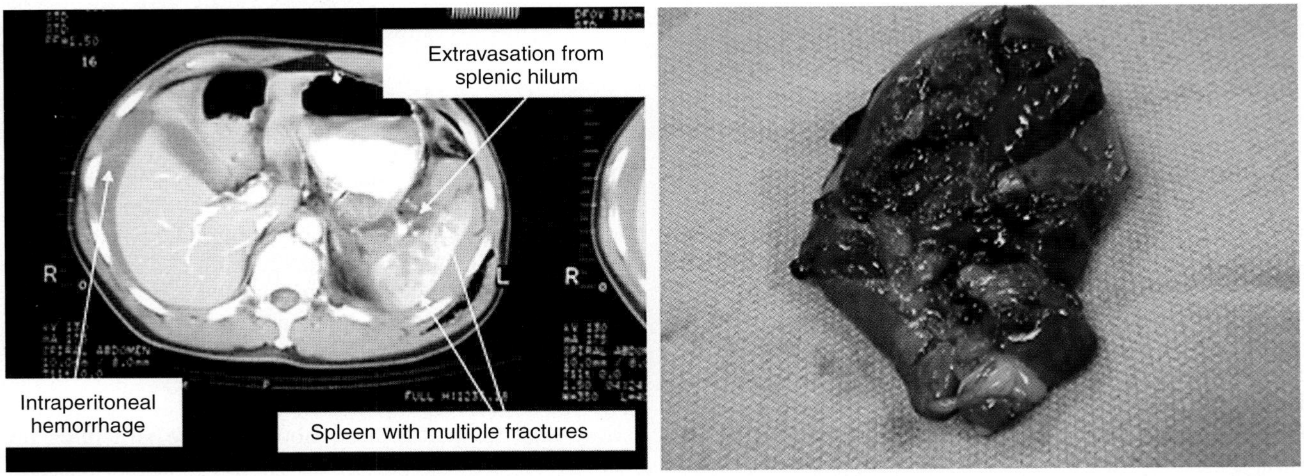

FIGURE 11–9 Grade V (AAST) splenic injury. Computed tomography scan and surgical specimen reveal a shattered spleen. Active bleeding into the peritoneal cavity is demonstrated by extravasation at the splenic hilum and the presence of free intraperitoneal blood.

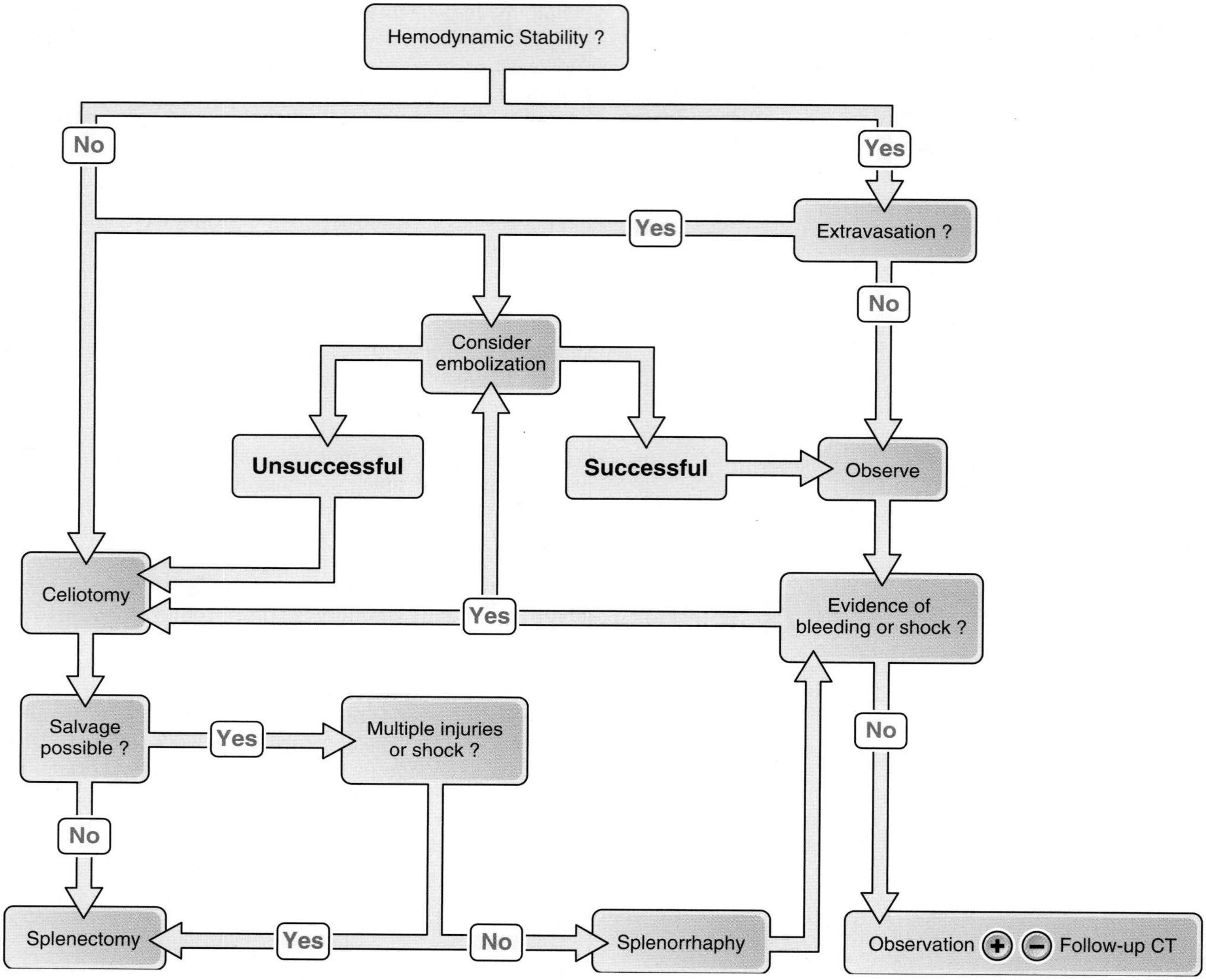

FIGURE 11–10 Management of splenic injury.

overwhelming postsplenectomy sepsis (OPSS) is characterized by abrupt onset of fever, chills, nausea, and vomiting, usually after an upper respiratory tract infection. More than 50% of cases of OPPS occur in the first year after splenectomy, but cases have been reported more than 30 years later. Half of the cases of OPSS are due to infection with *Streptococcus pneumoniae*. Infection with meningococci, *Escherichia coli, Haemophilus influenzae*, staphylococci, and other bacteria have been reported. Mortality rates of 40% to 70% have been reported for OPSS. Long-term follow-up studies indicate that this complication occurs in as many as 1% to 2% of splenectomy patients. To reduce the risk of OPSS, postsplenectomy patients should receive pneumococcal, *H. influenzae*, and meningococcal vaccination.

Liver Injury

The liver is the most commonly injured abdominal organ in penetrating trauma. Most injuries to the liver are minor lacerations and are not life threatening. Overall mortality from liver injury is approximately 10%. As with splenic injury, increasing recognition has developed that liver injuries can, in many cases, be managed nonoperatively.

Surgical Anatomy

The liver receives blood from two sources, the hepatic artery and the portal vein. Both of these structures lie adjacent to each other in the porta hepatis. The liver drains directly into the inferior vena cava by means of three large hepatic veins. Bleeding from liver injuries can originate

PEARLS FOR THE OR

Airway always comes first.

In penetrating trauma, mortality is a function of vascular injury. Address the bleeding first.

In blunt trauma, stop the active bleeding by any means practical, including via angioembolization, packing, or repair, before addressing injuries that are not contributing to blood loss.

When solid-organ bleeding is controllable only by packing, then pack.

Catheters placed during emergencies should be replaced when the emergency has passed.

from any of these structures. The liver secretes bile into the gastrointestinal tract by way of a ductal system draining into the right and left hepatic ducts. The liver is suspended from the diaphragm and retroperitoneum by a series of ligamentous structures and by the hepatic veins themselves. The liver is a relatively inelastic structure and is prone to fracture when subjected to compression or shearing forces. A tendency exists for the liver to fracture along the lobar planes established by the hepatic veins. Thus in severe blunt trauma, the liver characteristically "splits" along the course of the middle, left, or right hepatic veins.

Workup and Evaluation

Any patient who is hemodynamically unstable with obvious signs of intraabdominal injury, such as distended abdomen or peritonitis, should be taken directly to surgery. FAST examination of the abdomen is useful in shock with equivocal abdominal findings. Unstable patients with hemoperitoneum on FAST should undergo immediate exploration. In hemodynamically stable cases, in which injury to the liver is suspected, CT scanning of the abdomen is the mainstay of diagnosis. The AAST liver-injury scale is described in Table 11-4. Examples of CT images of liver fractures are presented in Figure 11-11.

Treatment

In cases in which hemodynamic stability is present, or in which shock is easily resuscitated with 2000 mL or less of crystalloid solution, observation is appropriate. Patients should be monitored carefully for further blood loss. Repeated CT scanning is useful to monitor for further bleeding or expansion of hematoma. Patients who have active extravasation on initial CT scan, but who are reasonably stable hemodynamically, may be managed with angioembolization of the bleeding hepatic artery branch. Patients who are unstable, in deep shock, or who require large volumes of blood for resuscitation should be explored. Several principles should be observed when operating on patients for liver trauma. First, strict attention must be paid to maintaining body temperature during the procedure. Second, red cell and clotting factor replacement must be pursued aggressively. Initial control of the bleeding liver by manual pressure or packing with lap pads is usually possible. When this has been performed, the porta hepatis can be controlled with a vascular tourniquet. If the bleeding is due to injury to either a branch of the portal vein or the hepatic artery, tightening of the tourniquet (Pringle maneuver) will significantly reduce bleeding. If this does not occur, injury to the juxtahepatic vena cava or hepatic veins should be considered. After control of the porta hepatis, the liver should be completely mobilized from the diaphragm and retroperitoneum. This will expose both the suprahepatic and infrahepatic vena cava. If necessary, at this point, vascular control of the cava above and below the liver can be performed. If excessive bleeding or coagulopathy supervenes, the liver should be packed in lap pads and the abdomen closed expeditiously with towel clips or other rapid methods. The patient should be taken then to the

TABLE 11–4 AAST Liver Injury Scale

Grade	Injury	Description
I	Hematoma	Subcapsular <10% of surface area
	Laceration	Capsular tear <1 cm parenchymal tear
II	Hematoma	Subcapsular 10%–50% of surface area or < 10 cm diameter parenchymal hematoma
	Laceration	1–3 cm parenchymal depth, < 10 cm in length
		Intraparenchymal hematoma >10 cm diameter or expanding
III	Hematoma	Subcapsular >50% of surface area, expanding or ruptured
	Laceration	>3 cm parenchymal depth
IV	Laceration	Parenchymal disruption involving 25%–75% of hepatic lobe or 1–3 Counaud segments within a single lobe
V	Laceration	Parenchymal disruption involving >75% of hepatic lobe or >3 Counaud segments within a single lobe
	Vascular	Juxtahepatic venous injuries to either vena cava or hepatic veins
VI	Vascular	Hepatic avulsion

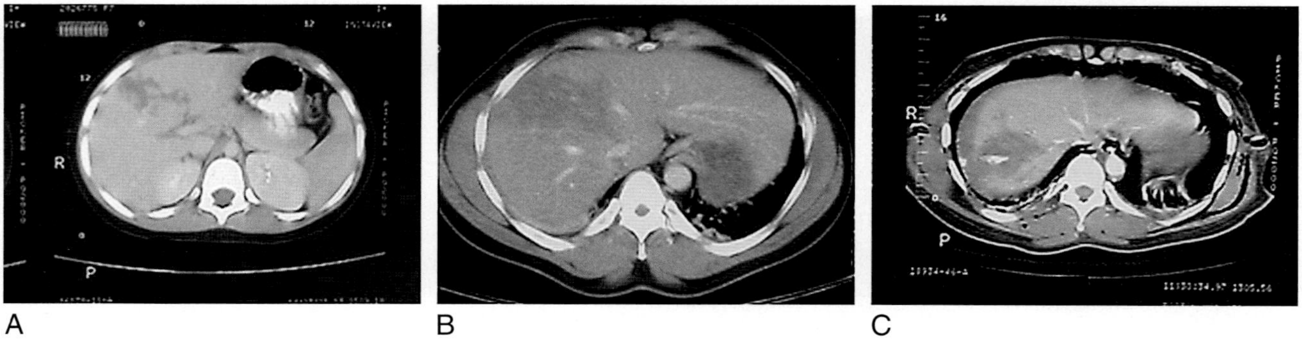

FIGURE 11–11 Computed tomography staging of liver injuries. *A*, Grade III, laceration extending >3 cm into liver substance with no subcapsular hematoma. *B*, Grade IV, laceration involving >24% of right lobe. *C*, Grade V, laceration with parenchymal disruption of >75% of lobe. Note avulsing segments 6 and 7 from the liver with active extravasation.

surgical intensive care unit (ICU) for further resuscitation, with the intention of return to the operating room when stability has been reestablished.

Outcomes and Complications

Appropriate use of damage-control laparotomy techniques and angiography has resulted in a reduction in overall mortality for liver fracture to 10%. Complications resulting from liver injury include bleeding and biliary leak. Bleeding is managed either angiographically or surgically. Biliary leak occurs in as many as 20% of cases but is usually minor, requiring no treatment. In a minority of patients, large amounts of bile may leak into the peritoneal cavity. Surgical management is indicated if bile collections impair respiratory function or cause sepsis or systemic inflammatory response. Bile leakage can be addressed in two ways. Common bile duct pressure can be reduced by endoscopic placement of a stent across the sphincter of Oddi. This will help to establish appropriate prograde drainage in the biliary ductal system and reduce or eliminate bile leakage from liver lacerations. Second, bile collections can be drained externally. Although percutaneous drainage is possible and will work well for small collections, my experience indicates that larger bile collections are better managed with operative placement of large-bore drains.

In a small proportion of patients with liver injury, liver abscesses will develop. This complication can be effectively managed by percutaneous drainage.

The liver, the only visceral organ capable of regeneration, generally heals completely with time, even in cases of extensive laceration. Follow-up CT scans are useful to document liver healing sufficient for resumption of contact sports or active lifestyles.

Renal Injuries

As in other solid abdominal organs, the management of injury to the kidney has undergone considerable evolution over the past 25 years.

Surgical Anatomy

The kidneys enjoy a relatively protected location, partially covered by the ribs and bounded posteriorly by generous musculature. The kidneys are secured within the tough Gerota's fascia, which prevents any movement of the kidneys within the retroperitoneum. Anteriorly, the entire abdominal compartment lies between the kidneys and trouble. The kidneys are susceptible to injury from blunt force applied to the flank and to penetrating injury.

Pathophysiology

The kidneys are highly vascular organs. Injury therefore is usually manifested by hypovolemia. Bleeding into the collecting system may result in hematuria.

Workup and Evaluation

Renal injury should be suspected in patients with blunt or penetrating injury to the flank. The presence of tenderness or hematoma, fracture of ribs 9 through 12, or a flank wound may indicate underlying renal injury. Urinalysis is useful in evaluation of suspected renal injury. Gross or microscopic hematuria is frequently associated with 95% of renal injuries, although absence of hematuria does not exclude renal injury. Vascular injuries to the kidney, in particular, frequently occur without causing hematuria.

For patients who are hemodynamically stable, contrast CT scanning has replaced intravenous pyelography (IVP) in the evaluation of renal trauma. Renal injuries are graded according to degree of parenchymal and vascular injury (Fig. 11-12 and Box 11-4). For patients who require immediate laparotomy, "on-table" IVP is useful not only to demonstrate the extent of renal injury, but also to confirm the presence of a functioning contralateral kidney in case nephrectomy is contemplated.

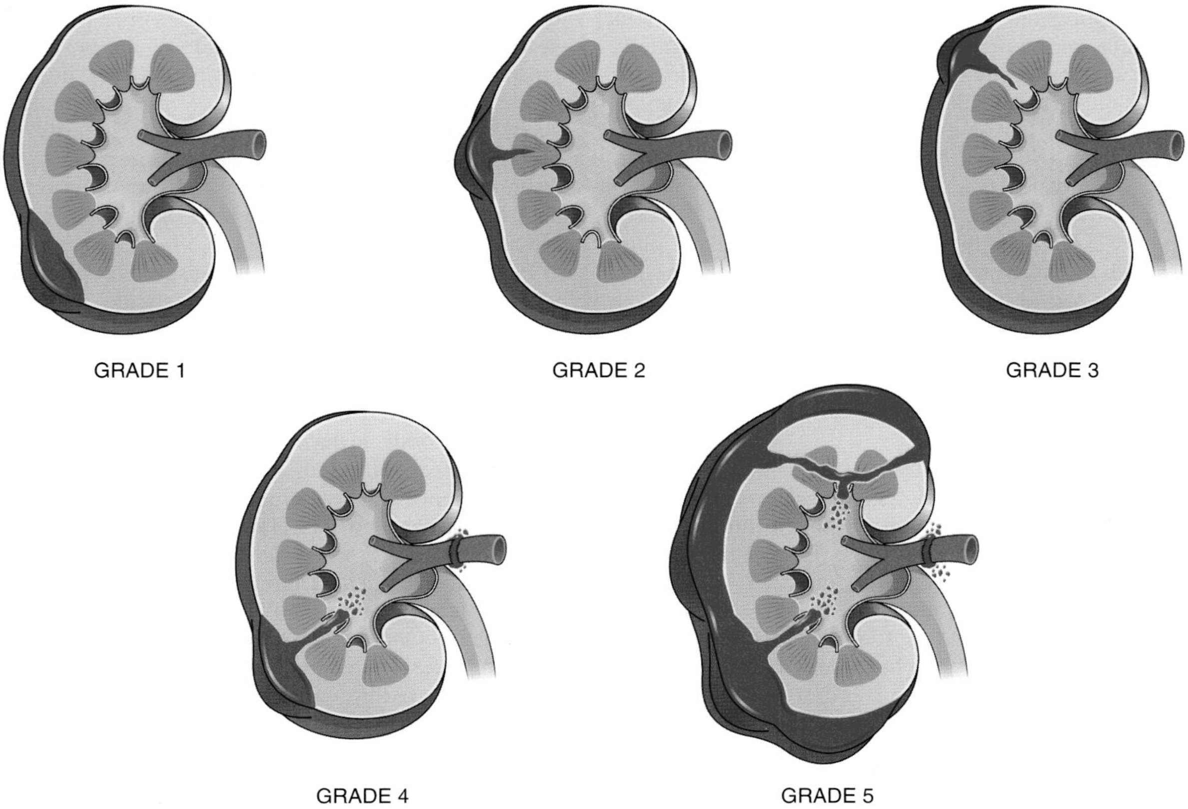

FIGURE 11–12 Renal injury grading (see Box 11-5). (Adapted from Moore EE, Shackford SR, Pachter HL, et al: Organ injury scaling: Spleen, liver, and kidney. J Trauma 29(12):1664–1666, 1989.)

Treatment

Management of renal trauma has become much more conservative over the last 25 years. Indications now for surgical intervention are active bleeding, complete devascularization, and poorly controlled urine leak. Because Gerota's fascia is usually capable of containing bleeding, even "shattered" kidneys can be managed nonoperatively in the setting of hemodynamic stability. Should surgery be required, partial nephrectomy and vascular repair are preferable. This is true especially in penetrating injuries. However, given the present trend to reserve surgery for severe injury, nephrectomy is a frequent outcome in exploration for blunt injury.

When exploration for renal injury is indicated, it is important to obtain control of the renal vessels before opening Gerota's fascia. This tough fascial layer is effective in containing bleeding, which may then recur in large volume when the fascia is opened. Therefore the renal vessels should be controlled close to the vena cava and aorta before exploring the kidney itself.

BOX 11–4 Renal Injury Grading

Grade 1: Contusion
Grade 2: Nonexpanding hematoma, laceration <1 cm without injury to collecting system
Grade 3: Laceration penetrating >1 cm without injury to collecting system
Grade 4: Laceration penetrating through cortex, medulla, and collecting system, or contained injury to renal vessels
Grade 5: Hilar avulsion or shattered kidney

Outcomes and Complications

Bilateral renal injury can result in renal impairment or chronic renal failure. Bilateral injury is rare, however. Common early complications of renal injury are recurrent bleeding and urinoma. Bleeding can be managed with transcatheter embolization or surgery. Urinoma is frequently managed with percutaneous drainage. Provided no obstruction exists to the prograde flow of urine, most urinomas will not require subsequent surgical intervention.

Late complications of renal injury include arteriovenous (AV) fistula and hypertension. AV fistulas are usually managed with transcatheter embolization. Hypertension is usually managed medically, although nephrectomy may be necessary in some cases.

Pelvic Fractures

The pelvis is frequently fractured in high-energy blunt injuries such as falls from heights and motor vehicle crashes. An important part of the secondary survey is to evaluate the pelvis both radiographically and on physical examination. Significant pelvic fractures can be life threatening; thus they frequently have a significant impact on the initial course of treatment.

Surgical Anatomy

The pelvis is a ring of bone, which supports the weight of the trunk and articulates with both the lumbar spine and the lower extremities. Posteriorly, the sacrum articulates with the L5 vertebra and the iliac bones laterally. The sacroiliac joints and the sacral and iliac bones immediately supporting them are frequent sites of fracture. The iliac bones each have three parts: the ilium, the ischium, and the pubis. The ischium and pubic bones are usually referred to together as the superior and inferior pubic rami. These bones are also frequent sites of fracture. The articulation of the pelvis with the lower extremity at the acetabulum is another frequent fracture site.

The bony pelvis is closely associated with soft-tissue structures that are frequently injured as a result of pelvic fracture. A rich plexus of arteries and veins arising from the internal iliac system (also sometimes referred to as the hypogastric system) is closely fixed to the posterior pelvic structures surrounding the sacroiliac joints. Injury to these vessels can cause life-threatening hemorrhage. The rectum, bladder, urethra, and female genital organs also closely associated with the pelvis are prone to injury when it is fractured.

Pathophysiology

The principal physiology associated with severe pelvic fracture is hypovolemia. Injury to vessels of the internal iliac system can result in substantial and catastrophic blood loss. In addition to treatment aimed specifically at arresting pelvic bleeding, aggressive blood replacement may be necessary.

Workup and Evaluation

The pelvis should be directly examined during the secondary survey by palpation and by medial compression of the iliac crests and anterior compression of the pubic symphysis. Shortening of either lower extremity may be associated with acetabular fracture. Careful examination of the perineum for wounds indicating an open pelvic fracture is important. Note should be made of the position of the prostate on digital rectal examination. A "high riding" prostate indicates urethral injury. Rectal examination also should look for evidence of mucosal irregularity or gross blood, indicating associated rectal injury. Most pelvic fractures will be readily identified on the trauma room anteroposterior pelvic radiograph taken as part of the secondary survey.

Patients with an identified or suspected pelvic fracture, who are hemodynamically stable, should undergo rigid sigmoidoscopy and speculum pelvic examination to identify associated injuries. Because urethral injuries are common in males with pelvic fracture, intubation of the bladder should be delayed either until the patient spontaneously voids nonbloody urine, or a retrograde urethrogram has demonstrated urethral integrity.

For patients who are hemodynamically unstable, evaluation for associated visceral injury may require either laparotomy or CT scanning. If other sources of bleeding have been excluded, arteriography is useful to identify arterial bleeding associated with pelvic fracture.

Pelvic fractures are classified based on injury mechanism. The four types are lateral compression (LC), anteroposterior compression (APC), vertical shear (VS), and combined mechanical injury (CM) (Box 11-5 and Fig. 11-13).

BOX 11-5 Young Pelvic Fracture Classification

Lateral Compression (LC)

LC-I Pubic ramus fracture associated with sacral compression on the side of impact

LC-II Pubic ramus fracture associated with Iliac wing fracture

LC-III Pubic ramus fracture associated with contralateral open-book injury

Anteroposterior Compression (APC)

APC-I Symphysis diastasis minimal widening of symphysis and SI joint

APC-II Symphysis diastasis or vertical pubic ramus fracture associated with anterior ligamentous injury to SI joint with widening

APC-III Symphysis diastasis or vertical pubic ramus fracture associated with complete SI joint disruption and hemipelvis separation

Vertical Shear

Symphyseal separation and/or vertical pubic ramus fracture associated with vertical displacement of the hemipelvis

Combined Mechanical Injury

Complex fractures with mixed features. Usually associated with significant extrapelvic injury

SI, sacroiliac.

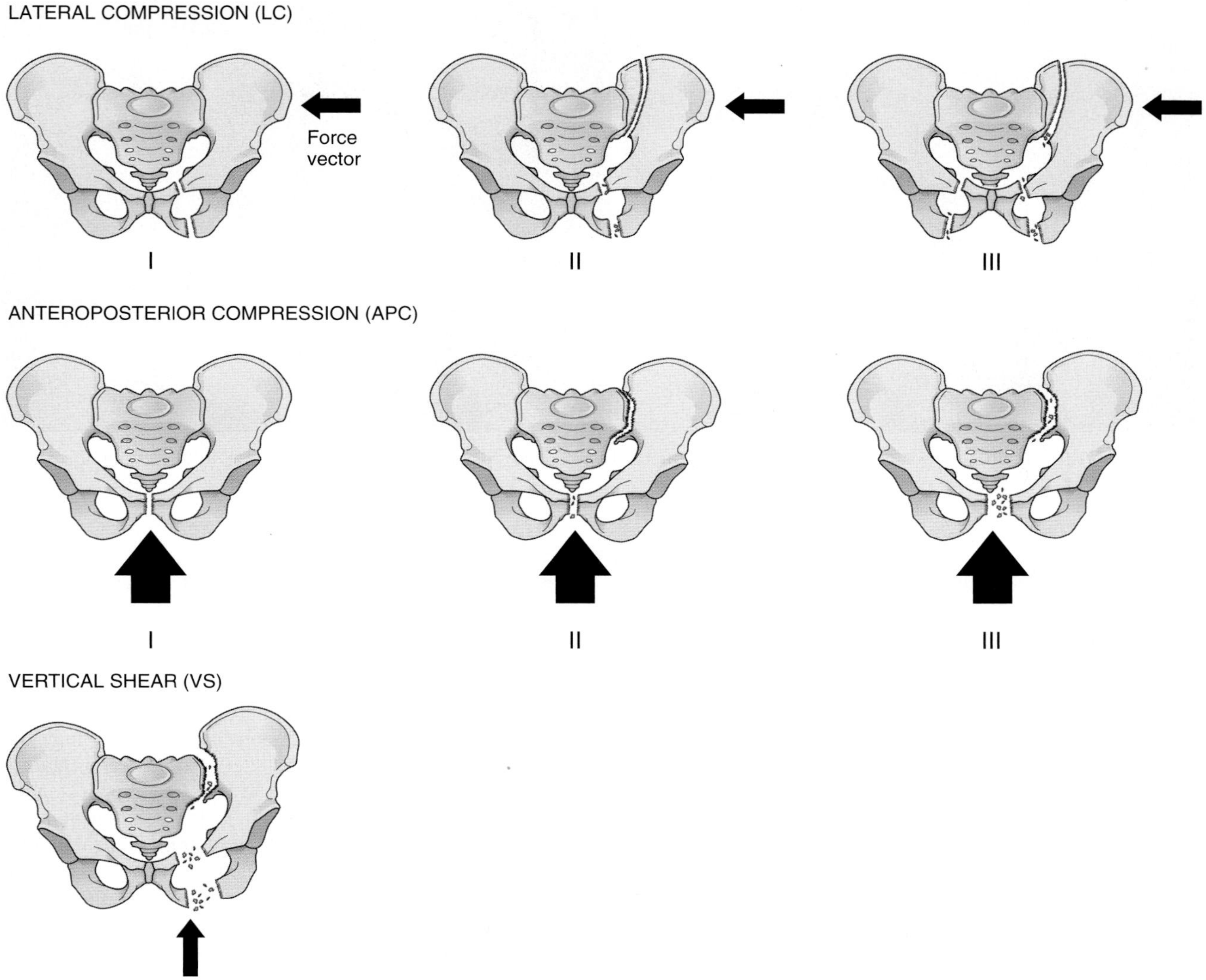

FIGURE 11–13 Young pelvic fracture classification system. Note that combined mechanical injury combines features of LC, APC, and/or VS (see Box 11-4). (Adapted from Eastridge B, Burgess A: Pedestrian pelvic fractures: 5-year experience of a major urban trauma center. J Trauma 42(4):695–700, 1997.)

Treatment

Treatment of pelvic fracture can be divided into three areas of concern. In order of importance, these are management of bleeding, management of associated injuries, and bony fixation.

Management of Bleeding Associated with Pelvic Fractures

Bleeding associated with pelvic fractures can be severe and life threatening. Patients with severe pelvic fractures should be aggressively transfused and appropriately resuscitated with blood products, beginning at the time of identification of the injury. Initial management of pelvic bleeding focuses on stabilizing the fracture and closing the pelvic space into which bleeding is occurring. This is particularly relevant to APC injuries where diastasis of the pubic symphysis and disruption of the sacroiliac region occur. Prehospital measures to control bleeding in this setting include suspension of the pelvis by a posterior sling.

Early hospital management of pelvic hemorrhage includes placement of external fixation devices or C-clamps to restore more normal pelvic geometry in APC-type

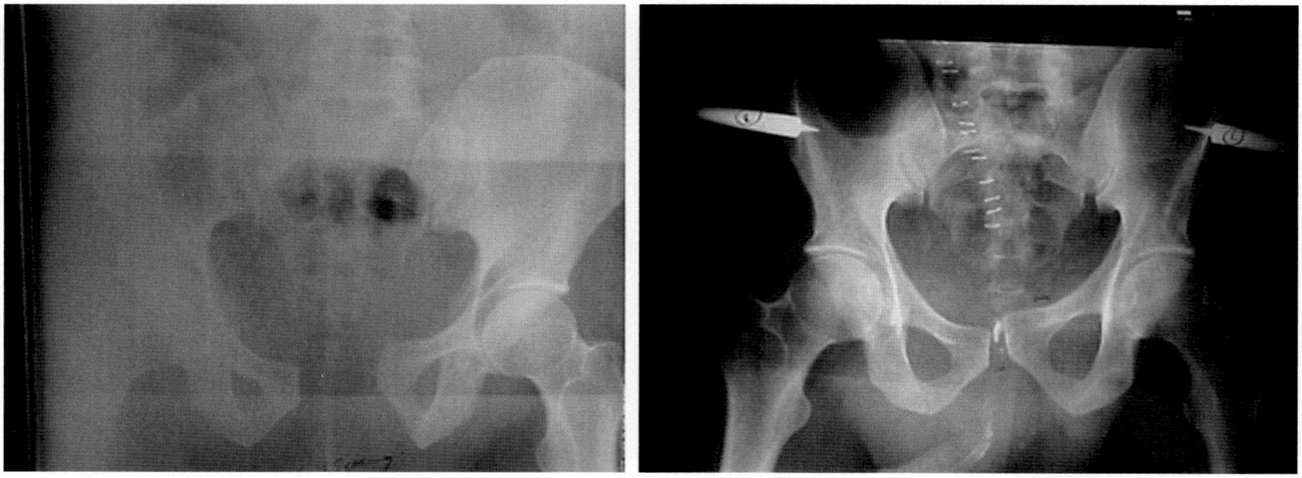

FIGURE 11–14 Anteroposterior compression pelvic fracture, before and after placement of a lateral C-clamp in the setting of severe pelvic bleeding.

fractures (Fig. 11-14). In patients with other life-threatening injuries, external fixation can provide rapid and effective management of pelvic fractures while the other injuries are addressed.

Bleeding patients who have non-APC fractures or those for whom external fixation fails are best managed with arteriographic embolization. Transcatheter embolization is effective in controlling arterial bleeding but does nothing for venous bleeding. Continued transfusion and clotting factor replacement, occasionally to extreme levels, is necessary in cases for whom external fixation and embolization fail. Operative packing of the pelvis is ineffective in controlling arterial bleeding and is not presently recommended for management of pelvic bleeding. If, however, laparotomy is necessary for other reasons, pelvic packing for control of venous bleeding may have some utility.

Management of Associated Injuries

Urethral injuries are most safely managed with placement of a suprapubic cystostomy catheter. Under some circumstances, an experienced surgeon or urologist may be successful in placing a Foley catheter across a urethral injury under fluoroscopic guidance. In this setting, extended catheterization is usually sufficient to facilitate uncomplicated healing. Limited injury to the extraperitoneal portion of the bladder can also be managed, in many cases, with either Foley or suprapubic catheterization. More extensive bladder injuries, or those resulting in free intraperitoneal rupture, usually require operative repair.

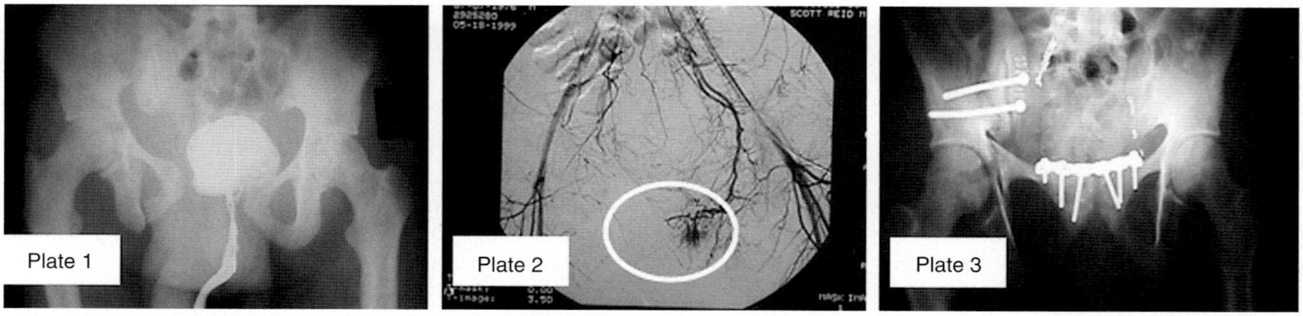

FIGURE 11–15 Sequential studies following the management of an 82-year-old woman with a severe anteroposterior compression III fracture in a motor vehicle accident. A cystogram in the emergency department (Plate 1) demonstrates integrity of the bladder with severe diastasis of the pubic symphysis and posterior sacroiliac disruption. The patient was hemodynamically unstable and was taken directly to arteriography (Plate 2), where bleeding from the left internal iliac system was identified (*circled area*) and successfully embolized. After 12 hours of stabilization in the surgical intensive care unit, definitive fixation was performed (Plate 3). The patient was discharged 2 weeks later.

Anorectal injury associated with pelvic fracture should be managed with fecal diversion, irrigation, and débridement of open wounds. Perineal laceration, particularly when associated with open pelvic fracture, frequently necessitates fecal diversion as well.

Management of Bony Injury

Pelvic fractures that do not involve significant displacement or architectural instability of the pelvis, such as LC I fractures, can be managed nonoperatively. Fractures involving significant distraction of bony elements or structural instability of the pelvis are best managed with internal fixation. In cases in which hemodynamic instability or significant associated injuries preclude internal fixation, external fixation can provide acceptable long term-stabilization and potential for adequate healing. Figure 11-15 demonstrates several steps in the management of a severe APC III pelvic fracture.

Outcomes and Complications

Pelvic fractures have an overall mortality of 8%, though APC III and LC III fractures can result in a mortality rate of 50%. Patients with severe injuries are at high risk for transfusion-related complications, pulmonary embolism, and sepsis.

Suggested Reading

Cantor RM, Leaming JM: Evaluation and management of pediatric major trauma. Emerg Med Clin North Am 16(1):229–256, 1998.

Committee on Trauma of the American College of Surgeons: Advanced Trauma Life Support: Course for Physicians, 6th ed, Chicago, American College of Surgeons, 1997.

Fabian TC, Richardson JD, Croce MA, et al: Prospective study of blunt aortic injury: Multicenter Trial of the American Association for the Surgery of Trauma. J Trauma 42(3):374–380, 1997.

Olshaker JS, Whye DW: Head trauma. Emerg Med Clin North Am 11:165, 1993.

Udekwu PO, Gurkin B, Oller DW: The use of computed tomography in blunt abdominal injuries. Am Surg 62(1):56–59, 1996.

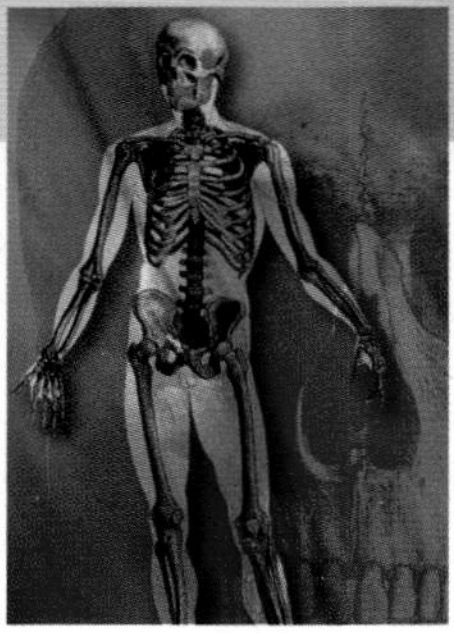

Chapter 12
Critical Care

FREDERICK H. MILLHAM, MD, MBA, LAURA M. PRAGER, MD,
RIE AIHARA, MD, and RICHARD C. DENNIS, MD

The care of the very ill and unstable is one of the most challenging and interesting fields of medicine. The modern surgical intensive care unit (ICU) can be a busy and frightening place. Methods now exist for the mechanical support of nearly every organ system. These technologies are often complex and invasive. In this chapter, we review the common problems treated in surgical ICUs and some of the technologies used in this care. A listing of the specialists commonly required to care for patients in an ICU is presented in Box 12-1. What follows is neither comprehensive nor definitive. We hope that you will find this introduction interesting enough to look more deeply into this fascinating and challenging side of surgical practice.

The Goals of Critical Care

An important goal of critical care is to treat life-threatening disorders. An equally important goal in the care of the critically ill is the prevention and amelioration of the complications of severe illness. Careful attention is given to details such as prophylaxis against deep venous thrombosis, peptic ulceration, and iatrogenic infection. Nutritional support of the critically injured is an important consideration. The final goal of critical care is to preserve the dignity and sanctity of the lives of patients requiring such care. Modern medicine is capable of sustaining the physiologic system long after any rational hope of meaningful recovery is gone. The intensivist must find the boundary between appropriately aggressive treatment to sustain life and futile measures that only prolong suffering. As such, the intensive care specialist must understand not only his or her patient's illness and comorbidities, but also his or her social and cultural milieu. Because ICU patients are frequently unable to express their desires, relationships must be established with family members to help guide the plan of treatment.

Common types of patients found in surgical ICUs include those who are stable but require very close monitoring after complex surgery or trauma who may have a significant incidence of myocardial infarction, dysrhythmias, oliguria, renal failure, electrolyte disturbances, and respiratory failure. Although most of these patients do well, skilled nurses, constant physician supervision, well-trained respiratory therapists, and others are necessary for maximally effective treatment. A second category of patient suitable for admission to surgical ICUs includes postoperative open-heart patients. These patients are often very hemodynamically unstable and frequently require interventions such as vasopressors, antiarrhythmics, inotropes, chronotropes, and mechanical ventilation. A third category of patients commonly admitted to the ICUs includes those with massive trauma, multiple fractures, hypovolemic shock, and pulmonary contusion. These patients require a large number of interventions and an ongoing workup for additional injuries while receiving intensive care.

Respiratory Failure

One of the most common problems encountered in critical care is respiratory failure. The term *respiratory failure* implies a broad variety of pathologic conditions with a common implication: the failure of the lungs to exchange oxygen and/or carbon dioxide adequately between the blood and the alveolar air. We define respiratory failure as a group of conditions resulting in the need for mechanical ventilatory support.

Surgical Anatomy

Anatomical considerations in the management of respiratory failure include the anatomy of the airway and thoracic cavity. Human beings vary widely in the anatomic relations

BOX 12-1 The Critical Care Team

Daily	Special Circumstances
• Intensivist	• Dialysis nurse
• Critical care nurse	• Perfusionist/ECMO specialist
• Respiratory therapist	• Interventional radiologist
• Pharmacist or PharmD	
• Nutritionist	
• Physical therapist	
• Psychiatrist	
• Chaplain	
• Continuing care specialist	

ECMO, extracorporeal membrane oxygenation.

between the structures of the upper airway. In some cases, the larynx is very anterior with respect to the base of the tongue. In these cases, establishing an airway can be challenging. The Mallampati airway classification scheme (Fig. 12-1) is useful in identifying patients with potentially difficult airways. Patients with Mallampati class I airways, where the posterior pharynx and faucial pillars are easily visualized, are usually easily endotracheally intubated. Up to 35% of patients with class II airways, where the faucial pillars and soft palate only are visualized, will have challenging airways, as will nearly all patients with class III airways, in whom none of these structures can be seen.

Pathophysiology

Respiratory failure can develop from pathology of one or more of three areas: the ability to maintain a patent airway, the ability to move air mechanically into and out of the lungs, and the ability to exchange gases within the lung.

Maintaining an adequate airway requires a sufficient level of consciousness to keep secretions and other material from occluding the airway. Respiratory drive is one of the last reflexive activities of the brain to be extinguished and will continue even in profound coma. The ability to cough, sigh, and coordinate the oropharygeal musculature appropriately to sustain adequate airway patency requires a higher level of consciousness. It is generally thought that patients with a Glasgow Coma Scale of eight or less are unable to perform these functions and should have the airway controlled by either endotracheal intubation or surgical airway. The airway also can be threatened by swelling or mass due to trauma, infection, or neoplasm, which also may mandate airway control.

The ability to generate the pressure gradients necessary to fill and empty the lungs can be impaired by conditions affecting the central nervous system, the integrity of the chest wall, or the strength of the muscles of respiration. Narcotic use or abuse, cervical spinal injury, injury to the phrenic nerve, and degenerative neurologic conditions can suppress or block the nervous stimulation of the muscles of respiration, resulting in respiratory failure. Rib fractures, pneumothorax, diaphragmatic rupture, and elevated intra-abdominal pressure can impair the function of the chest-wall musculature. Prolonged severe illness, with extended mechanical ventilation, can result in deconditioning of the muscles of respiration, further prolonging the necessity of mechanical ventilatory support.

Finally, disruption of gas diffusion at the alveolar capillary interface and disturbances of lung perfusion can result in inadequate gas exchange and respiratory failure. Common problems resulting in disordered gas perfusion include pneumonia, congestive heart failure (CHF), and adult respiratory distress syndrome (ARDS). Mismatching of ventilation and perfusion, such as occurs in pulmonary embolus and intrapulmonary shunting, also can result in insufficiency of net gas exchange in the lungs.

ARDS is usually associated with the systemic inflammatory response syndrome (SIRS). The accepted diagnostic criteria for ARDS are listed in Box 12-2. It is characterized

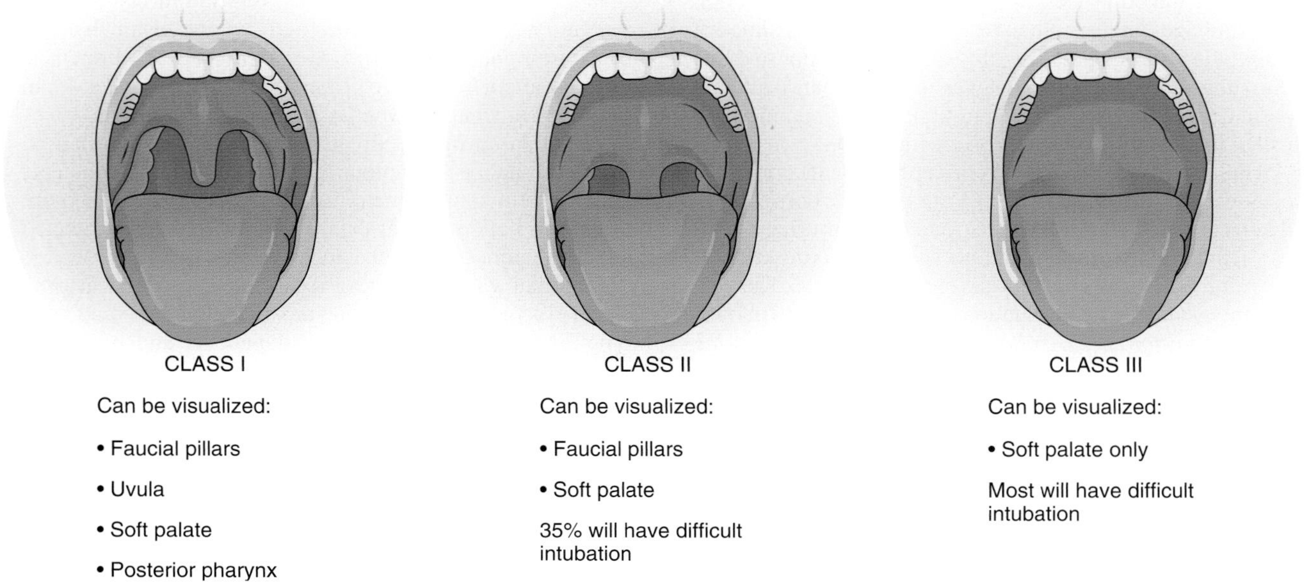

FIGURE 12–1 Mallampati airway classification. (Adapted from Mallampati SR, Gatt SP, Gugino LD, et al: A clinical sign to predict difficult tracheal intubation: A prospective study. Can Anesth Soc J 32(4):429–434, 1985.)

BOX 12-2 Diagnostic Criteria for ARDS

Acute onset
$Po_2/Fio_2 \leq 300$ mmHg
Bilateral interstitial infiltrates
Absence of congestive heart failure

ARDS, adult respiratory distress syndrome.

by damage to the pulmonary capillary membrane, with resultant accumulation of interstitial fluid and alveolar injury. In early or limited ARDS, mild hypoxia develops because of both the filling of the interstitium with protein-rich fluid and the accumulation of fluid within alveoli. As the syndrome worsens, more fluid accumulates in both sites. Type II pneumocytes lining the alveoli are injured, impairing surfactant production. Loss of surfactant causes alveolar collapse and atelectasis to worsen. Worsening ARDS is typified clinically by progressive hypoxia and worsening pulmonary compliance. In severe cases of ARDS, lymphocytes and macrophages invade the pulmonary interstitium. If sufficient numbers of activated immune cells reside in the lung, a self-sustaining process of stimulus and response can become established. In this so-called fibroproliferative ARDS, the lung becomes so inundated with interstitial and intraalveolar fluid that oxygenation and ventilation become impossible. Very few cases of ARDS progress to this stage; in most cases, pulmonary function recovers, although frequently requiring prolonged mechanical ventilation.

Because ARDS is to a large degree driven by immunologically mediated processes, including cytokine activation of macrophages and lymphocytes, several therapies aimed at manipulating or suppressing this immune response have been suggested. Recently it was shown that activated protein C, a naturally occurring anticoagulant, can increase survival in cases of extreme sepsis with ARDS.

ARDS frequently results from septic or inflammatory processes outside of the chest. Patients in whom ARDS suddenly develops should be suspected of harboring occult sites of infection or inflammation, such as leaking anastomoses, infected prostheses, or severe pancreatitis. The rule of thumb in the early evaluation of ARDS is as follows: *Sudden respiratory failure often reflects pathology below the diaphragm.*

Workup and Evaluation

The possibility of respiratory failure constitutes an emergency. Immediate bedside management is required. Physical examination should look carefully for cyanosis, stridor, tachypnea, hypopnea, and paradoxical chest or abdominal movement. Auscultation of the chest to determine the presence and quality of breath sounds is essential. Important adjuncts in the management of respiratory failure are the arterial blood gas measurement and chest radiograph. These studies should be obtained immediately on any patient with suspected pulmonary failure.

The key to managing potential *upper airway* obstruction is careful clinical evaluation. Laboratory tests such as arterial blood gas determination and electrophysiologic monitoring are not useful, as these measurements will become abnormal only after an upper airway crisis has occurred. The sine qua non of upper airway obstruction is inspiratory stridor. Patients who are at risk for upper airway obstruction should be evaluated carefully for early signs of stridor, such as use of accessory muscles and retraction. Auscultation seeking inspiratory wheezing is useful. The best method for evaluating the upper airway is fiberoptic laryngoscopy. This should be performed in any case in which a possibility of upper airway impairment exists. Full-blown clinical stridor is a late finding, often heralding loss of airway patency. When this finding is present, immediate airway control either by endotracheal intubation or tracheostomy is imperative. It is well to remember that one may have only a single chance with endotracheal intubation in a patient with an occluded upper airway. Surgical airway, usually cricothyrotomy, should be performed immediately when endotracheal intubation is impossible in the setting of upper airway obstruction.

The most effective method for following the mechanics of breathing is measurement of spontaneous tidal volume and vital capacity. Patients who have low tidal volume usually manifest a rapid, low-volume breathing pattern. This is best quantified by dividing the respiratory rate by the tidal volume (in liters). If this quotient is greater than 80, mechanical ventilation should be considered. If it is greater than 100, mechanical ventilation is usually mandatory. Vital capacity, the total volume of air that can be inspired and expired in one maximal forced breath, is normally about 70 mL/kg. When vital capacity is less than 10 mL/kg, mechanical ventilation is usually required.

For patients who are already on mechanical ventilation, minute ventilation, the amount of air breathed in 1 minute, is another useful measurement. Generally patients who require minute ventilation greater than 9 L/min will tire if extubated and thus require continued mechanical ventilation.

Abnormal gas exchange is best assessed by measuring arterial oxygen and carbon dioxide pressure and pH. Hypoxia is a common in surgical patients and has many etiologies. In general, hypoxia can be due to hypoventilation, ventilation/perfusion (V/Q) mismatch, or right-to-left shunting. Elevation of Pco_2 indicates hypoventilation. This may be due to obtundation, spinal cord injury, drug overdose, or splinting. V/Q mismatch, such as occurs with pulmonary embolism, is usually associated with hypoxemia, which improves with increasing the inspired oxygen concentration (Fio_2). Right-to-left shunting, such as occurs with patent foramen ovale, will not generally improve significantly with increasing of Fio_2.

Treatment

Mechanical ventilatory support is the foundation of treatment of respiratory failure. Although methods exist for mechanical ventilation without endotracheal intubation, in the surgical patient, intubation is virtually always the most prudent course. Once the patient is intubated, a variety of mechanical ventilatory modes are available. Depending on the clinical circumstance, either volume- or pressure-cycled methods may be used.

For patients with ARDS, worsening pulmonary compliance and hypoxia make mechanical ventilation a nearly uniform requirement. Several mechanical ventilatory treatment modes are available to treat ARDS. The first of these is the addition of positive end-expiratory pressure or PEEP. Loss of surfactant in ARDS leads to alveolar collapse and atelectasis. Increasing the airway pressure at the end of the respiratory cycle can help to keep open alveolar segments that otherwise might close by keeping the alveolar pressure above the critical closing pressure. Increasing the end-expiratory pressure has the effect of increasing the functional residual capacity (FRC) of the lung. Limits exist to the amount of PEEP that can be added in any given case. As PEEP increases, alveolar blood flow can be impaired, which can paradoxically worsen arterial oxygenation. PEEP should be regarded as a drug that has dose-dependent therapeutic responses and toxicities.

In addition to increasing the end-expiratory pressure, the fractional concentration of oxygen (Fio_2) delivered by the ventilator may be increased to compensate for worsening A-a gradient. As with PEEP, excessive Fio_2 can have deleterious effects. Prolonged exposure to alveolar oxygen concentrations greater than 50% can cause pulmonary fibrosis. In the short term, use of 100% oxygen can lead to the absence of sufficient nitrogen in the alveoli to maintain the alveolar pressure above the critical closing pressure once the oxygen in the space has been absorbed by the alveolar capillaries. This phenomenon, known as absorptive atelectasis, or "nitrogen washout," has the unfortunate characteristic of affecting the units with the best ventilation and perfusion. Thus the use of very high oxygen concentrations can, in some cases, actually contribute to worsening hypoxia.

Pulmonary compliance also is significantly affected by ARDS. Compliance represents the relation between pressure and volume in any system. In the case of pulmonary failure, worsening compliance means that delivery of the same tidal volume requires increasing airway pressure. High airway pressure itself can damage the lung and can increase the risk of life-threatening pneumothorax. Therefore one of the aims of ventilator management in ARDS is to manage worsening pulmonary compliance. The net compliance of the pulmonary system reflects the sum of the extra-pulmonary, or chest-wall, compliance and the intra-pulmonary compliance. Efforts by the patient at breathing, coughing, or struggling against the ventilator (commonly called "bucking") can reduce extrapulmonary compliance and thus contribute to poor net pulmonary compliance. The first measure usually taken in the setting of worsening compliance is to establish chemical neuromuscular blockade to remove the impact of extrapulmonary compliance from the system.

When ARDS progresses to the stage at which PEEP and neuromuscular blockade are insufficient, other methods are needed to manage worsening compliance. Intra-pulmonary compliance itself is not a static phenomenon. Rather, any given pulmonary system has a family of compliance curves that depend, in part, on the rate of flow of gas into the lungs. One method for both limiting the peak airway pressure and improving pulmonary compliance is to use pressure-controlled (PC) ventilation. With this method, the ventilator delivers each breath up to a predetermined pressure limit, allowing the clinician to control the peak airway pressure. Pressure-control ventilation has the additional benefit of providing more favorable flow-rate characteristics, specifically a lower dp/dt, meaning that a more favorable compliance value may be exploited. In many cases, acceptable tidal volumes and airway pressures can be attained by changing to pressure-control mode alone. One consequence of this mode, however, is that in severely noncompliant lungs, the peak pressure may be reached at a relatively low tidal volume. In these cases, it is usually preferable to underventilate the patient, accepting the consequent increase in Pco_2, rather than increase the peak pressure, risking further damage to the lung. This approach is called *permissive hypercapnea*.

PEARLS FOR ROUNDS

Sudden onset of adult respiratory distress syndrome (ARDS) may reflect pathology below the diaphragm.

ARDS = (Sudden onset) + (Fio_2/Po_2 <300) + (Diffuse infiltrate) + (No CHF)

Weaning from the ventilator requires
- Adequate mechanical respiratory function
- Adequate ventilation
- Adequate oxygenation

To work up delirium, remember the mnemonic WWHHHIMP: Withdrawal, Wernicke's encephalopathy, Hypoglycemia, Hypoxia, Hypertension, Intracerebral process, Meningitis, and Poisons (drugs).

Catabolic patients require 1.02 g/kg of protein per day.

If the gut works, use it.

Outcomes and Complications

The mechanical ventilator has made survival possible for literally millions of patients with respiratory failure. In some cases, respiratory failure becomes a chronic process requiring prolonged mechanical support. These patients are prone to colonization of the tracheobronchial tree with pathogenic bacteria. Nosocomial pneumonia is thus the principal complication of mechanical ventilation, occurring in a rate directly proportional to duration of mechanical support. The incidence of pneumonia in patients with prolonged mechanical ventilatory support is essentially 100%.

Cardiac Disease

Cardiac disease is another frequent problem requiring critical care. Commonly patients with preexisting cardiac disease who require major surgery are managed by the critical care team to try to reduce the incidence of cardiac-related complications. Other patients with perioperative cardiac complications or with cardiac injury as a result of trauma also are managed by the surgical critical care team.

Pathophysiology

Cardiac diseases are generally divided into ischemic disease, CHF, and rhythm disturbances. All are commonly seen in surgical patients. Ischemic disease, usually due to coronary artery stenosis, is a frequent comorbidity in all patients older than 40 years. Preoperative ischemic disease is an important predictor of perioperative myocardial infarction. Surgery, trauma, and sepsis all increase heart rate and myocardial oxygen demand. If demand is elevated beyond supply, constrained by occlusive coronary artery disease, the underperfused myocardium is prone to infarction.

CHF, due to cardiomyopathy or prior myocardial infarction, also is common. Patients with CHF are prone to volume overload during and after surgical procedures. Patients with severe CHF also may have constrained cardiac output, which limits their ability to respond to the stress of surgery.

Electrical disturbances, chiefly atrial fibrillation, flutter, and conduction disorders, can be exacerbated by surgical interventions, particularly those in the thoracic cage and those associated with large volumes of fluid infusion. This is sometimes related to acute distention of the right atrium due to volume overload or due to postoperative changes in pulmonary blood flow.

Workup and Evaluation

Any patient with a history of myocardial infarction, angina pectoris, CHF, or peripheral vascular disease should be suspected of harboring active myocardial ischemia or congestive failure. Diabetic patients may be particularly prone to cardiac ischemia, yet also are frequently asymptomatic, and thus should be given particular attention. A careful history should be taken, evaluating exercise tolerance, shortness of breath, orthopnea, and paroxysmal nocturnal dyspnea. Physical examination, particularly focusing on the cardiac rhythm, presence of a third heart sound, and rales, should be performed. Patients with signs or symptoms of ischemic heart disease should, if possible, undergo preoperative evaluation including a cardiac stress test. This can be a standard treadmill stress test or an echocardiogram-based evaluation using an inotrope such as dobutamine. Patients with evidence of unstable or reversible ischemic disease should be evaluated for preoperative revascularization, if possible. Patients who have evidence of CHF should have an echocardiogram, looking for evidence of diminished ventricular function, usually reflected in the ejection fraction.

Treatment

It is well established that risk of perioperative myocardial infarction can be reduced by aggressive perioperative β-blockade. Patients with ischemic disease must be managed to avoid periods of excessive myocardial oxygen demand or insufficient supply. Thus blood pressure, pulse, and oxygenation must be maintained within normal limits in these patients.

Perioperative management of CHF first requires assessment of the degree of ventricular impairment. Ongoing assessment of ventricular function before, during, and after surgical procedures can be accomplished by use of a pulmonary artery catheter or transesophageal echocardiography.

The use of pulmonary artery catheters has, in some large series, been associated with poorer outcome. Whether a causal relation exists is unclear. For patients who have compromised ventricular function, the pulmonary artery catheter provides an assessment of intravascular volume, cardiac output, and peripheral perfusion. Figure 12-2 demonstrates the steps in placing a pulmonary artery catheter and the waveforms generated by this device. The ability of the pulmonary artery catheter to estimate intravascular volume status relies on the fact that the pulmonary veins have no valves and therefore provide an uninterrupted fluid column between the pulmonary capillaries and the left atrium. The pulmonary artery catheter has a balloon near its tip which, when wedged against the walls of a branch of the pulmonary artery, blocks the fluid coupling of the catheter tip with the right heart, allowing the catheter tip to "see" only the pressure in the pulmonary capillaries. Because during diastole, the left atrium is itself in direct communication with the left ventricle, through the open mitral valve, the left atrial pressure and hence the pulmonary capillary pressure reflects the left ventricular diastolic pressure. When the left ventricle is overloaded with fluid, the left ventricular diastolic pressure will be high. This will in turn be reflected in elevation of the pulmonary capillary pressure. In this way, this catheter, technically placed in the right heart, allows evaluation of the volume status in the left.

Another useful feature of the pulmonary artery catheter is the ability to measure cardiac output. This is possible

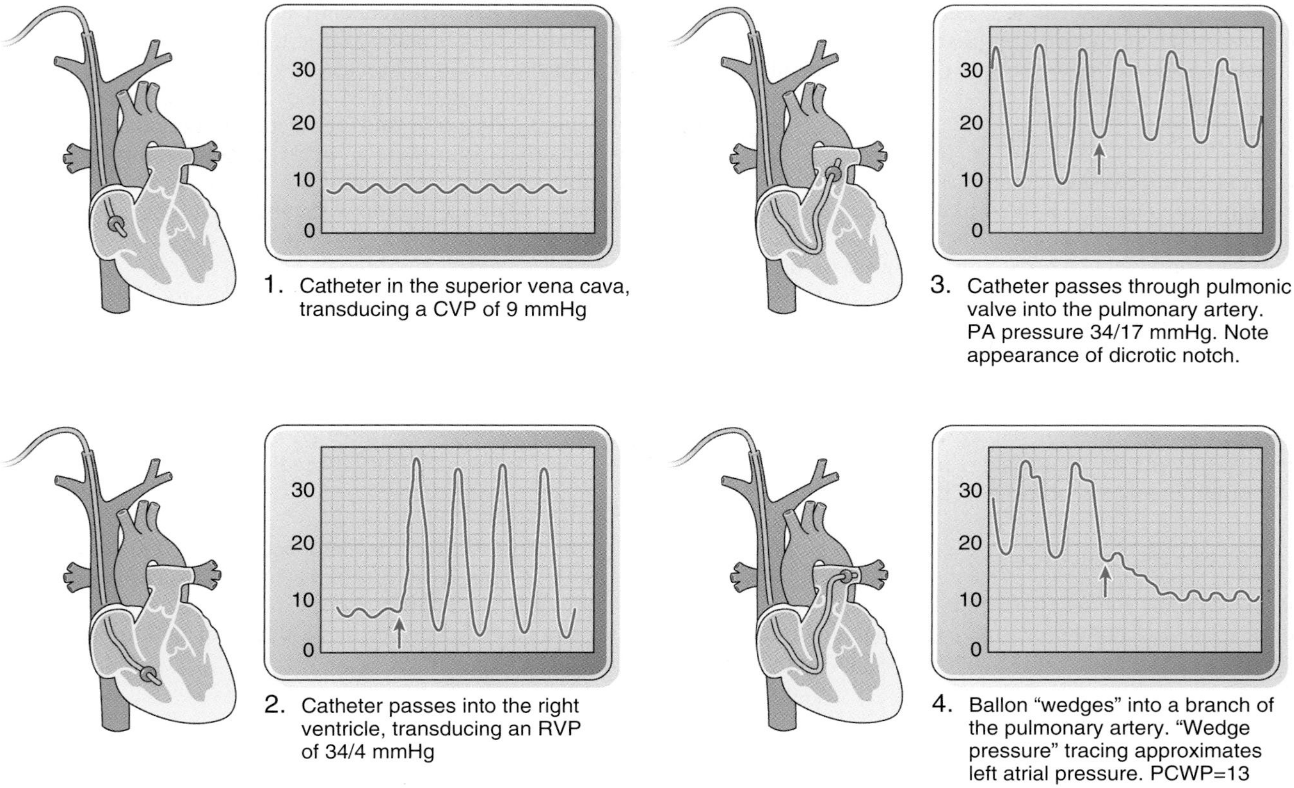
30
20
10
0
1. Catheter in the superior vena cava, transducing a CVP of 9 mmHg
3. Catheter passes through pulmonic valve into the pulmonary artery. PA pressure 34/17 mmHg. Note appearance of dicrotic notch.
2. Catheter passes into the right ventricle, transducing an RVP of 34/4 mmHg
4. Ballon "wedges" into a branch of the pulmonary artery. "Wedge pressure" tracing approximates left atrial pressure. PCWP=13

FIGURE 12–2 Pulmonary artery catheterization. CVP, cardiovascular pressure; PA, pulmonary artery; PCWP, pulmonary capillary wedge pressure; RVP, right ventricular pressure.

because a small rapid-response thermistor placed near the tip of the catheter allows measurement of temperature in the pulmonary artery. When a known volume of cold saline is injected into the right atrium, computer analysis of the temperature washout curve in the pulmonary artery can estimate the cardiac output. It is important to remember that this measurement is dependent on the volume and temperature of the injected fluid being known. A common error is injection of more or less than the customary 10 mL. If less cold saline is injected, the computer will overestimate the cardiac output; if more than the appropriate amount is injected, the computer will underestimate cardiac output.

Finally, by obtaining blood from the pulmonary artery, the "mixed venous" blood gases can be measured. The blood in the pulmonary artery represents the sum of that draining from all capillary beds. Under normal circumstances, the mixed venous blood will have an oxygen saturation of around 75%. If insufficient perfusion is present, tissues will extract more oxygen from the arterial blood than normal. This will in turn reduce the oxygen saturation of the mixed venous blood. This value can then be followed to gauge response to treatments aimed at improving oxygen delivery or perfusion.

When evidence of ventricular failure and volume overload is found, diuresis may indicated. If inadequate perfusion or cardiac output is indicated, a variety of interventions are possible. Inotropes, especially dobutamine, can be useful in augmenting myocardial contractility and improving perfusion (Table 12-1). When chemical support of the heart is

TABLE 12–1 Commonly Used Vasoactive Medications

Agent	Action	Dose
Epinephrine	Nonselective α and β agonist	25–50 μg IV q 5–10 min
Norepinephrine	α and β_1 agonist	2–4 μg/min drip
Dobutamine	Selective β_1 agonist	2.5–25 μg/kg/min
Phenylephrine	Selective α_1 agonist	0.1–0.05 mg IV
Dopamine	Low dose: Dopamine receptor–mediated renal and mesenteric vasodilation	Low dose: 2–5 μg/kg/min
	High dose: $\beta \rightarrow \alpha$ agonism	High dose: 10–50 μg/kg/min

insufficient, mechanical assistance of perfusion may be necessary. This can be accomplished by intraaortic balloon counterpulsation or, in extreme cases, placement of a left ventricular assist device.

Outcomes and Complications

Critical care has substantially reduced the rate of perioperative myocardial infarction and perioperative cardiac death. Aggressive management also has made surgery possible for patients who, in the past, were thought to have prohibitively high mortalities. Nonetheless, the diagnostic and therapeutic maneuvers described earlier are not without their own risks. Pulmonary artery catheters are prone to misinterpretation and can rupture the pulmonary artery or induce right heart block. Transesophageal echocardiography has a low but measurable risk of esophageal rupture. Inotropes can, by increasing myocardial oxygen consumption, induce myocardial ischemia.

Infectious Disease

Bacterial infection is a common finding in the critical care unit. We address two broad topics, iatrogenic infection and septic shock, which are the most important topics in this area for the intensivist.

Iatrogenic Infection

Critical illness is immunosuppressive. Critically ill patients usually require invasive technologies for their care, such as central venous catheters and endotracheal tubes. These two factors make iatrogenic infection a common problem in the ICU. The most common sorts of infection are pneumonia, catheter-related infection, and urinary tract infection. At each of these, a medical device, such as an endotracheal tube, a central line, or a Foley catheter, disrupts the normal defenses against infection. A three-pronged approach is necessary to combat iatrogenic infection: prevention, early identification, and effective treatment.

Prevention

Scrupulous attention to aseptic technique, hand washing, and isolation of patients with resistant organisms is important. Closed catheter suction devices for endotracheal suctioning are useful in reducing iatrogenic pneumonia. All transcutaneous medical devices should be placed under strict sterile technique and changed frequently according to an established policy. Foley catheters should be carefully maintained and be removed or replaced with less invasive devices such as condom catheters at the earliest opportunity.

Early Identification

Looking for sites of iatrogenic infection is part of the daily routine of critical care. All wounds, catheter sites, and draining fluids should be inspected. Careful examination of the chest and review of the pulmonary suction requirements for the past day will frequently allow identification of early pneumonia. Confirmatory chest radiography is useful when new pneumonia is suspected. Examination of the presacral and perineal regions must also be performed to identify decubitus ulceration and perirectal or perineal infection, which may otherwise remain occult. Central venous catheters should be cultured when they are changed, even if their insertions sites appear uninfected.

Effective Treatment

Once an infection is identified, the responsible bacterial pathogen must be isolated, and antibiotic therapy targeted to it. Broad-spectrum antibiotic regimens for monobacterial infections are no more effective than specific antibiotic therapy and encourage the development of antibiotic resistance. If possible, infected medical devices should be removed and if necessary placed at new sites.

Septic Shock

Bacterial sepsis has an incidence of 500,000 to 750,000 cases per year. Mortality rates for sepsis associated with shock range from 30% to 50% and have not changed over the last century despite the addition of antibiotics to the treatment of this process.

Pathophysiology

Great advances in our understanding of the pathophysiology of septic shock have occurred over the last decade. It has been known for some time that bacterial products initiate a cascade of immunologic events that, in the extreme form, can lead to shock. The best described of these bacterial products is lipopolysaccharide (LPS), which is a cell-wall component of gram-negative bacteria. LPS infused alone can cause all the symptoms of bacteremia. LPS probably acts in several ways. The most significant is as a ligand for the CD14 receptor and Toll-like receptor four on macrophages. CD14-TLR4–mediated LPS stimulation causes macrophages to elaborate a number of cytokines and other proinflammatory mediators. Tumor necrosis factor α (TNF-α), interleukin 2 (IL-2), and IL-8 are released. These mediators have several important activities. First, TNF-α and IL-2 are both potent stimulators of additional macrophage-mediator production. This amplifies the original LPS signal severalfold. These inflammatory mediators also stimulate leukocyte release of serine proteases and leukocyte binding to endothelial cells through a P-selectin–mediated process. Inflammatory cytokines also stimulate the release of nitric oxide from endothelial cells and the release of thromboxane and other procoagulant factors from platelets and endothelial cells. TNF-α also is a potent stimulator of fever. This process is referred to as the SIRS.

Clinically, this inflammatory cascade yields the classic constellation of symptoms associated with sepsis: fever, rigors, tachycardia, and hypotension. Relaxation of vascular smooth muscle produces a decrease in peripheral vascular resistance. In the early, compensated stages of sepsis, this decrease in afterload is accompanied by a concomitant increase in cardiac output. Despite this, however, as sepsis worsens, tissue oxygenation is impaired. Through mechanisms as yet poorly understood, oxygen utilization in peripheral tissues is impaired in sepsis. This leads to worsening metabolic acidosis, which, in the terminal phases of the process, is associated with a decline in cardiac output and eventually death.

Workup and Evaluation

Identification of the source of sepsis is of transcending importance in the early workup of septic shock. Often patients are progressively unstable with this process, meaning that the only opportunity for effective treatment is early in the process. In surgical patients, intra-abdominal sepsis is a major concern; if physical examination reveals signs of peritonitis, urgent laparotomy should proceed as soon as the patient has been stabilized. If physical findings are equivocal, cross-sectional imaging of likely sites should be performed. It is essential to identify and ameliorate the source of bacteremia as soon as practical in cases of septic shock.

Blood, urine, and sputum cultures should be obtained on all patients. Central-line sites should be inspected and changed if any suspicion exists of possible catheter-related infection.

Treatment

Supportive treatment of septic shock entails fluid resuscitation and α-adrenergic support of blood pressure, usually with vasopressors such as dopamine or phenylephrine (see Table 12-1). As mentioned earlier, any sites of surgical infection should be appropriately managed. Broad-spectrum antibiotics are administered; agents selected should cover gram-positive, gram-negative, and anaerobic bacteria.

Attempts to modulate the immune response by interrupting LPS, TNF, and IL-2 signaling have failed to improve outcomes in septic shock. Recently, use of activated protein C, a naturally occurring anticoagulant serine protease, showed efficacy in a large randomized clinical trial. Protein C presumably works by interrupting the procoagulant activities of other inflammatory cytokines, improving tissue perfusion, and downregulating the immunologic response to sepsis.

Outcomes and Complications

Sepsis can cause failure of virtually every organ system. Outcomes in septic shock are poor. Mortality rates of 20% to 35% remain, even with the most sophisticated management.

Delirium

Delirium is a reversible altered state of consciousness characterized by cognitive impairment, inability to sustain attention, and perceptual disturbances (i.e., hallucinations). It usually develops rapidly over a short time and fluctuates during the day, often accompanied by reversal of the sleep/wake cycle. Delirious patients can be agitated and belligerent or drowsy and inattentive to the environment. Their cognitive deficits cannot be ascribed to dementia. Delirium is *always* secondary to physiologic change caused by a medical condition. The pathogenesis is poorly understood. Some evidence suggests that an excess of central dopamine, norepinephrine, and glutamate and/or a decrease in cholinergic activity may be causative. Risk factors for the development of delirium include age, premorbid cognitive impairment, and a history of delirium.

The estimated prevalence of delirium in the general medical or surgical patient ranges from 15% to 40%. The presence of delirium is associated with increased morbidity, a poorer overall prognosis, and a longer stay in the hospital. Delirious patients are often agitated and potentially self-injurious; they may attempt to dislodge endotracheal tubes, pacemaker wires, intravenous lines, or indwelling catheters. Therefore it is extremely important to assess a change in mental status, consider the diagnosis of delirium, and, if possible, intervene in a timely fashion.

Differential Diagnosis

Differential diagnosis of delirium includes dementia, depression with psychotic features, schizophrenia, bipolar disorder, and the phenomenon referred to as "ICU psychosis." Delirium is usually distinguishable from these other conditions, but comorbidities can confound diagnosis. Dementia is characterized by a gradual cognitive decline with pronounced memory deficits; late in the course of illness, patients may become aggressive or assaultive. Patients with psychiatric illnesses such as schizophrenia are often delusional and bothered by auditory hallucinations. They are, however, fully awake, alert, oriented, and cognitively intact. The presence of visual hallucinations *always* suggests an underlying organic brain disorder. ICU psychosis is a misleading term used to describe what happens to patients who spend long periods in ICUs. Certainly sensory deprivation, lack of interpersonal contact, prolonged isolation, and immobilization can all *contribute* to a patient's sense of disorientation. However, that experience alone cannot *cause* delirium.

Etiology

Some causes of delirium in critically ill patients are infection, multiorgan system failure, medications used to treat disease, metabolic or electrolyte imbalance, and substance abuse. Other common disease states that can occur with delirium include septicemia, hepatic or renal failure, endocrinologic changes such as hyper- or hypothyroidism, and partial seizures. An easy-to-remember mnemonic is WWHHHIMP. This formula prompts a review of the most common causes of mental status change and/or agitation, particularly those in which prompt intervention is required to prevent permanent damage to the central nervous system (list follows).

Wernicke's encephalopathy is characterized by a rapid onset of a global confusional state, ophthalmoplegia (paralysis of the external recti, nystagmus, and disturbance of conjugate gaze), and ataxia. It is most common in patients who are malnourished and lacking thiamine. Chronic alcoholics are particularly vulnerable. Mental status is marked by disorientation, apathy, inattention, and often lethargy. Treatment is daily thiamine given intramuscularly. The ophthalmoplegia responds to treatment within a few days. The delirium can persist for up to several months.

Withdrawal from many drugs can result in delirium and life-threatening hemodynamic instability. It is often difficult or impossible to obtain a patient's history of prescribed medications or substance use/abuse if the patient has been admitted to the ICU directly from the operating room after a traumatic injury. Common culprits include alcohol, benzodiazepines, narcotics, and barbiturates.

Hypoxia caused by cardiac or respiratory failure or anoxic brain damage in the field or in the operating room can produce delirium. A blood gas should be one of the first things to check when evaluating an agitated, delirious patient.

Hypertensive encephalopathy is a potentially fatal event characterized by an acute elevation in blood pressure, headache, nausea, vomiting, and confusion. It can result in intracerebral hemorrhage. Acute intervention involves administration of a calcium channel blocker or an α_1-adrenergic antagonist.

Hypoglycemia can be associated with agitation, confusion, and ultimately, obtundation. ICU patients are prone to dysregulation of blood sugar due to sepsis, high adrenergic tone, and exogenously administered insulin. Random blood sugar determination should be part of the initial workup of agitation.

Intracerebral events include, for example, traumatic brain injury, subarachnoid hemorrhage, and subdural or epidural hematomas. Frontal contusion in particular is a frequent contributor to agitation in the surgical ICU. Patients with damage to the frontal lobes can exhibit extreme agitation because of the "disinhibition" of lower brain centers.

Meningitis, either bacterial or viral, can cause delirium. This diagnosis is frequently missed in patients who, because of other comorbid factors, cannot complain of headache or neck stiffness. Clinical suspicion of meningitis should remain high, particularly in patients with parameningeal foci of infection. Lumbar puncture is diagnostic.

Poisoning can result from ingestion of prescribed medications or from other exogenous substances. It is advisable to check both serum and urine toxic screens.

Workup and Evaluation

The patient's clinical picture determines the focus of the bedside examination. The goal of the global mental status examination is to assess level of consciousness, orientation, attention, memory, mood, judgment, and behavior. The Confusion Assessment Method for the Intensive Care Unit (CAM-ICU) is the most commonly used standardized tool. This instrument emphasizes the four central features of delirium: (1) presence of acute onset of mental status change with fluctuating course, (2) inattention, (3) disorganized thinking, and (4) depressed level of consciousness. The presence of the first two criteria with either the third or the fourth is sufficient for diagnosis. This scale is being validated and tested in combination with the Glasgow Coma Scale and has shown good interrater reliability, specificity, and sensitivity. Attention should be tested first because, if it is impaired, the remainder of the mental status examination is compromised. Attention can be evaluated by asking the patient to indicate the letters of the alphabet that rhyme with tree. If the patient remains intubated and cannot talk, he or she can be asked to squeeze the examiner's hand as the letters are recited. If attention is preserved, the examiner can use the Folstein Mini Mental Status Exam (Table 12-2) to test orientation, memory, and language function.

Once the diagnosis of delirium is made, a search for etiology begins. One should start with a review of the patient's current and old charts and medication sheets. Has the patient had an episode of delirium before? At what point during admission did the patient's mental status change? Scanning flow sheets will allow determination of hemodynamic instability and of laboratory abnormalities. A

TABLE 12–2 Folstein Mini Mental Status Exam*

Test Exercises	***Score***
Orientation	Maximum
What is the: year season, date, day, month (1 point for each)	5
Where are we: state, country, town, hospital, ward (1 point for each)	5
Registration	
Name three objects	3
Attention	
Serial 7s, 1 point for each up to 5 (alternative: spell "world" backward)	5
Recall	
Ask patient to repeat the three objects listed for Registration, give 1 point for each	3
Language	9
Name: pencil and watch (2 pt)	
Repeat: "no ifs ands or buts" (1 pt)	
Follow a three-stage command (3 pt)	
Read and obey the following:	
Close your eyes (1 pt)	
Write a sentence (1 pt)	
Copy a design (1 pt)	
Total:	**30**

*Assess level of consciousness along the continuum: Alert—Drowsy—Stuporous—Comatose

careful review of the medication sheets is time consuming but invaluable. A list of medications that the patient has received since admission, with timing and dosages noted, could reveal excess dosing or abrupt discontinuation with subsequent intoxication or precipitation of withdrawal. Each patient's clinical presentation is different, and often no identifiable etiology fully explains the mental status change. Most often, the cause of the delirium is multifactorial.

Treatment

Treatment should be directed at the underlying cause of the delirium. If the patient is hypoxic, supplemental oxygen may reverse delirium. If the patient is withdrawing from a narcotic or a benzodiazepine, administering the appropriate medication may alleviate symptoms. If the patient is delirious because he or she is intoxicated from a narcotic or a benzodiazepine, specific antidotes (naloxone and flumazenil, respectively) will reverse the effects. These drugs should be used with caution because too much can precipitate withdrawal. However, in many situations, a patient's symptoms can persist even after appropriate treatment for suspected cause is instituted, as in the case of septic patients who can remain delirious even after initiation of appropriate antibiotics. Sometimes, because of the patient's overall condition, the causative agent (e.g., an immunosuppressive agent) cannot be discontinued.

Neuroleptics remain the mainstay of treatment for the delirious patient. Haloperidol (Haldol) is the drug of choice because it can be given orally or parenterally and because it causes only slight alterations in pulse, blood pressure, and respiration. The intravenous route of administration is preferred because it causes few extrapyramidal side effects. The most significant side effect is the prolongation of the Q-T_c interval, with the potential for causing torsades de pointes ventricular tachycardia. Haloperidol should be give with caution to patients with Q-T_c intervals of longer than 450 μsec and to those who have low potassium or magnesium levels.

In situations in which the delirious patient also is agitated, a benzodiazepine (lorazepam, midazolam, or other sedative-hypnotic [e.g., proprofol]) may be indicated. Neither class of drug provides analgesia, but both are quite sedating. Using these agents can be tricky because even low-dose benzodiazepines can paradoxically contribute to delirium in certain vulnerable patients. However, the sedatives can be extremely effective, particularly when they are used in conjunction with haloperidol. Opiates, the primary analgesics used in critical care settings, should never be used to control agitation or to treat delirium.

Nutritional Support

Nutritional support is a vital component in the care of critically ill patients in the modern ICU setting. The catabolic state of the critically ill renders them susceptible to muscle wasting and protein loss secondary to the catecholamine and cortisol surges that accompany the insult. Initially the body may maintain a fuel supply by the breakdown of fat. With time, however, the body is no longer able to keep up with the demand, and extrinsic sources of energy must be provided to prevent compromise of the immune system, wound healing, and weight loss. This is especially important in patients with underlying malnutrition.

Providing nutritional support in the ICU involves three distinctive steps. The first step is the evaluation of the patients and their individual nutritional requirements. This involves calculation of their basic energy requirements and the amount of protein, carbohydrate, and lipid needed. The second step is to deliver the support by using an appropriate route that can be tolerated by the patient. These include oral supplements, enteral feedings, and parenteral support. The third step is the monitoring of patients for response to treatment and complications. After laboratory data and daily weights, evaluation of nitrogen balance, and making necessary adjustments in the calories provided are all part of providing nutritional support. A number of complications associated with administration of both parenteral and enteral nutrition must be recognized early and treated properly.

Patient Evaluation

Assessing patients for their nutritional status and requirement requires expertise. Detailed medical and nutritional history, clinical evaluation, review of laboratory data, and predicting the effects of the disease state on the patient are all part of a complete evaluation. Patients should be assessed and nutritional support initiated within 48 hours of their admission.

Basal energy expenditure (BEE) is an approximated energy requirement for an individual that is calculated by using the Harris-Benedict equation. This equation takes into the account the difference in weight (W, kilograms), height (H, centimeters), and age (A, years) as well as sex.

$$\text{Men: } 66.5 + (13.8 \times W) + (5 + H) - (6.8 \times A) = \text{kcal/24 hr}$$

$$\text{Women: } 65.5 + (9.6 \times W) + (1.8 \times H) - (4.7 \times A) = \text{kcal/24 hr}$$

To account for the variable physiologic state of patients, the resting energy expenditure (REE) is calculated by multiplying the BEE by 1.1 to 1.4.

Calories are provided in the following three forms: proteins, carbohydrates, and lipids. The protein requirement for a normal individual is 0.6 g/kg/day. However in patients with high protein turnover, 1.02 g/kg/day of protein is required to keep up with the catabolism. In renal insufficiency, some adjustments may be necessary, although many prefer to give the full amount of required protein and consider dialysis rather than compromise nutrition.

Proteins provide 4 kcal of energy for every gram given, whereas carbohydrates and lipids provide 3.4 kcal/g and 9 kcal/g, respectively.

Delivery of Nutritional Support

Nutritional support can now be provided by using either the enteral or parenteral route. The development of total parenteral nutrition (TPN) in the 1960s was a breakthrough in medicine, allowing patients who otherwise could not have been fed to receive nutritional support by solution into a central vein. Enteral feeding formulas were developed in the following decade. It has been shown in various studies that enteral support results in fewer septic complications and improves immune function and wound healing.

The normal mucosal lining of the gastrointestinal (GI) tract provides a barrier against the toxins and bacteria that dwell within the lumen. This function is further supported by peristalsis, immunoglobulins, and mucin that are secreted by the intestinal mucosa. However, when the patients are not fed enterally, the mucosa of the GI tract undergoes atrophy, thereby decreasing this protective function against the bacteria and toxins produced. As a result, bacterial translocation, or the invasion of bacteria across the atrophied mucosal barrier, occurs. Pneumonia, abscess formation, and infection of central lines and prostheses are frequent complications in these patients.

Enteral nutritional therapy requires access into the GI tract. A number of nonoperative and operative methods are used for this. Bedside placement of a nasogastric (NG) tube is the quickest and easiest method in patients who have normal gastric emptying. A lubricated silicone 14F to 16F NG tube or a 5F to 7F weighted feeding tube can be placed through the nostril or mouth and advanced into the stomach. Confirmation of placement is obtained clinically by injecting air into the stomach and auscultating or by obtaining a low chest radiograph. A nasojejunal tube may be placed at the bedside in patients with poor gastric emptying or recurrent aspiration pneumonia. A lubricated, weighted 5F to 7F silicone tube is placed through the nostril or mouth and advanced into the stomach. Passage of the tube through the pylorus can be facilitated by insufflation of the stomach with air, premedication with erythromycin and/or metaclopromide, and positioning the patient in a right decubitus position. After an hour, a kidneys-ureters-bladder (KUB) is obtained to confirm positioning of the tube. If bedside tube placement is unsuccessful, endoscopic or fluoroscopic placement of the tube may be necessary. If long-term tube feedings are anticipated, a surgical or endoscopic-assisted (percutaneous endoscopic gastrostomy; PEG) gastrostomy tube or surgical feeding jejunostomy tube may be placed.

Once placement of the feeding tube is accomplished and confirmed, the selected tube feedings are initiated. The tube-feeding formulations can be divided into polymeric and elemental diets. Most patients with normal GI motility can tolerate the polymeric solutions; however, those patients with conditions such as malabsorption, short-gut syndrome, or severe sepsis may require elemental tube feeds. Polymeric diets provide patients with whole proteins, oils, and complex carbohydrates, whereas elemental diets contain amino acids or short-chain peptides, triglycerides, and oligo- or monosaccharides. The various tube feedings differ in the concentration of calories and the amount of nutrient composition and electrolyte content to suit such conditions as renal and hepatic failure. Some tube feeds contain fish oils and glutamine that are noted to improve the immune function as well as additives to increase the fat, carbohydrate, protein, and bulk content.

Tube feedings are initiated at a low rate of 10 mL/hr and increased by 10 to 20 mL/hr every 8 to 12 hours. It is most important to check for residuals every 4 hours through the NG tube to assess the tolerance. If high residuals (>150–200 mL) or abdominal pain/distention develops, tube feeds should be held and resumed at a lower rate when symptoms subside or the residuals improve.

Patients with prolonged postsurgical ileus, fistulas, pancreatitis, and short-bowel syndrome may require parenteral nutrition to deliver their caloric requirements. Delay in providing calories because of the patient's disease status or inability to tolerate enteral feedings is unwise, only allowing further catabolism and increasing the likelihood of malnutrition.

Parenteral nutrition must be administered through a central venous catheter in the subclavian, internal jugular, or femoral veins. Central lines are required because of the high concentration of the solution, which may sclerose the smaller low-flow veins of the periphery. These catheters must be placed carefully by using the aseptic technique including gowns, masks, cap, and sterile gloves and drapes.

TPN contains a variety of mixture of dextrose, amino acids, and lipids. Lipids can be given mixed in the TPN solution itself (3:1 solution) or hung as a separate infusion. Most institutions have standard formulas that contain 25% dextrose and 4.25% amino acids as well as renal and hepatic formulas with less protein and glucose. However, customized solutions can easily be made. In addition to nutritional elements, various medications may be added to the TPN solutions such as heparin, H2 blockers, and some antibiotics.

Outcomes and Complications

Once the patients are on the stable nutritional support regimen, the efficacy of the therapy must be monitored. This includes assessment of daily weights and regular laboratory tests such as prealbumin, electrolytes, and nitrogen balance. Patients in the ICU are prone to undernutrition because of their high demands as well as their inability to reach goal nutritional therapy because of intolerance of tube feeding or problems with venous access.

A number of infectious and metabolic complications have been recognized with both the enteral and parenteral nutrition. Although enteral feedings are associated with fewer complications, this form of therapy is not without risks. Perforation and obstruction of the GI tract from jejunostomy tubes can occur. NG tubes can be erroneously placed in the tracheal bronchial tree with disastrous consequences. Infectious complications include aspiration pneumonia, sinusitis, and skin breakdown of the tube site.

Serious complications can accompany parenteral nutrition as well. Central-line placement can result in pneumothorax, hemothorax, arterial puncture, arrhythmia, and even cardiac perforation. Displacement of the catheters also can lead to extravasation of the fluid. Catheter infections are common, ranging from a localized cellulitis around the insertion site to profound sepsis septicemia from catheter-related infection.

GI complications from TPN occur from the load of nutrients given to the solution itself or from the lack of GI tract stimulation by tube feeds. Cholestatic jaundice frequently occurs with long-term TPN. Overfeeding carbohydrates can adversely increase the respiratory quotient, complicating weaning and pulmonary management.

Suggested Reading

Bernard GR, Artigas A, Brigham KL, et al: The American-European Consensus Conference on ARDS: Definitions, mechanisms, relevant outcomes, and clinical trial coordination. Am J Respir Crit Care Med 149:818–824, 1994.

Mainous MR, Deitch EA: Nutrition and infection. Surg Clin North Am 74:659–676, 1994.

Marcy TW, Marini JJ: Respiratory distress in the ventilated patient. Clin Chest Med 15:55–73, 1994.

Warren HS, Suffredini AF, Eichacker PQ, Munford RS: Risks and benefits of activated protein C treatment for severe sepsis. N Engl J Med 347:1027–1030, 2002.

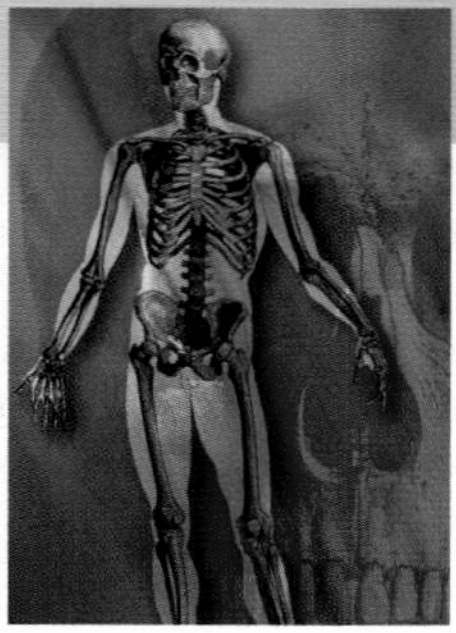

Chapter 13
Burns

JEFFREY R. SAFFLE, MD

In addition to being among the most horrifying and painful of injuries, burns produce a number of severe systemic abnormalities, including shock and fluid sequestration, susceptibility to infection, and metabolic stress, which combine to make major burns a paradigm for the physiologic response to traumatic injury.

Burns are a significant public health problem as well. In the United States, about 1.25 million patients require treatment for burns annually. More than 5500 people die every year of burn-related injuries, primarily from house fires, and about 51,000 patients are hospitalized.

In the last 50 years, improved understanding of the pathophysiology of burn injuries has led to more successful treatment and a corresponding dramatic reduction in the mortality associated with major burns. Physicians use the term "LA_{50}" to describe the burn size (expressed as percentage of total body surface area [%TBSA]), which is lethal to half the patients in a given population. This figure has improved from about 40% TBSA in World War II to more than 80% TBSA today and may be even higher for children and young adults, among whom almost no injury is too severe to preclude the possibility of meaningful survival. Figure 13-1 shows a group of current survival curves for burn patients. Although mortality from burn injury is clearly influenced by patient age as well as burn size, significant improvements in survival have been documented in recent years, even among the oldest patients. Mortality also is affected by the presence of inhalation injury, which approximately doubles mortality for burns of any given size.

Ironically, recent improvements in survival from burns have created new problems that challenge the burn team. As more patients with major injuries survive, they require extensive surgery for skin coverage and reconstruction, prolonged and costly rehabilitation, and psychologically challenging reintegration into society.

Pathophysiology of Burn Injury

The skin serves a number of roles in regulating contact between the organism and the outside world. In this function as a protective barrier, the skin is susceptible to damage from a variety of environmental agents. The term *burn* most accurately refers to injuries caused by excessive heat; however, other types of injuries are often referred to as "burns," including those produced by chemicals, electrical current, ionizing radiation, and friction. These injuries share a common pathophysiologic mechanism, in that they all produce coagulative necrosis of tissues. The amount of necrosis is determined by the intensity of the source of injury (temperature, voltage, pH, etc.), and the duration of contact.

The clinical severity of a burn is a function of the depth and extent of injury. These determine what skin structures are destroyed, the pathologic response to injury, and,

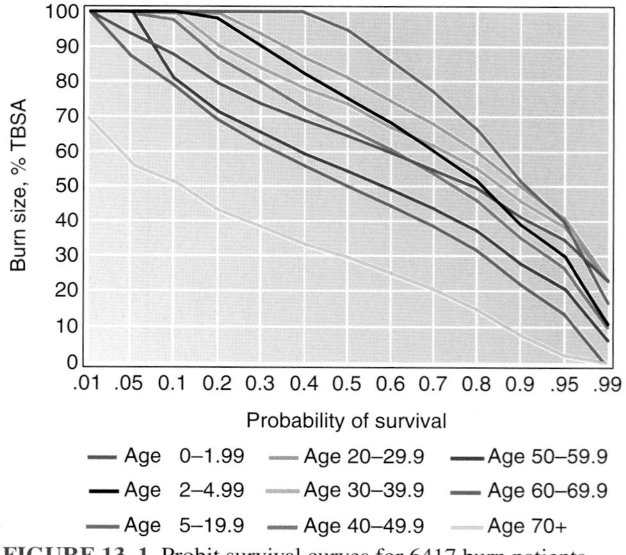

FIGURE 13–1 Probit survival curves for 6417 burn patients treated at 28 burn centers in the United States from 1990 to 1993. For each age group listed, the burn size is expressed on the ordinate, and the probability of survival, on the abscissa. The LA_{50} (burn size that results in a 50% mortality) ranges from 29.5% TBSA (for patients aged 70 and older) to 94.5% TBSA (for patients aged 5 to 20 years). (Adapted from Saffle JR, Davis B, Williams P, et al: Recent outcomes in the treatment of burn injury in the United States: A report from the American Burn Association Patient Registry. J Burn Care Rehabil 16:219–232, 1995.)

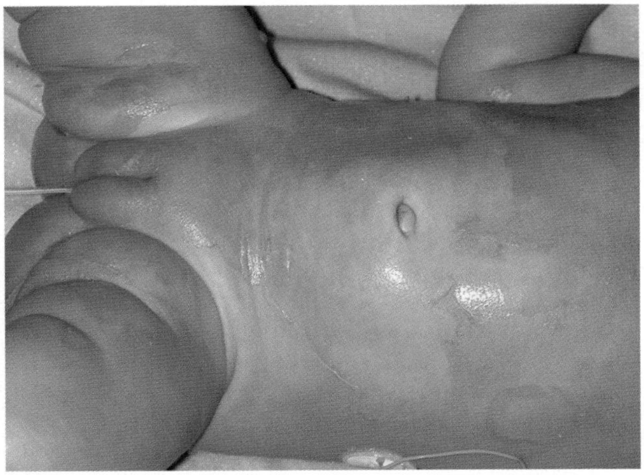

FIGURE 13–2 This child was injured in a bathtub scalding accident and sustained superficial second-degree ("partial-thickness") burns. The wounds display intense erythema. Blisters have been removed in most areas, although residual loose epidermis can be seen at the edges. The wound surface is moist and oozing, whereas the underlying dermis blanches readily with pressure, indicating intact perfusion. The wound is extremely painful, but despite its dramatic appearance, this burn should heal within 7 to 10 days with appropriate treatment.

ultimately, the ability of the wound to heal. Accurate assessment of burn depth also is of great importance in determining appropriate treatment and in predicting outcome. Because the appearance of burn injuries is an essential component of initial evaluation, a number of illustrations are included in the following section.

Skin is composed of a thin outer layer, the epidermis, and a thicker inner layer, the dermis. Epidermis serves as a unique barrier to moisture, bacteria, and chemicals. Epidermis is thin and relatively fragile, with rapid cell proliferation and turnover; accordingly, it is metabolically active and richly vascularized. Epidermis also forms the lining of hair follicles and sweat glands, forming deep "epidermal appendages," which are important for skin regeneration and burn wound healing. Burns limited to the epidermis, called **first-degree burns**, are usually caused by relatively mild trauma such as sun exposure and hot liquids (although both these agents can produce much deeper burns). They are characterized by erythema, mild to moderate pain, and limited physiologic response. Edema formation and evaporative losses are slight. Damaged epidermis does not blister initially, but usually sloughs ("peels") within a few days, as new epidermis rapidly grows to replace it from the basal, germinal layer.

When injury extends into the dermis, a **dermal burn** (also called a **second-degree, or partial-thickness burn**) is produced (Fig. 13-2). Because the dermis is relatively thick, dermal injuries can vary significantly in their appearance, depth, and severity. Such injuries are usually classified as "superficial" or "deep" partial-thickness burns. In **superficial** partial-thickness burns, reactive dilatation of dermal capillaries produces marked erythema, while destruction of the epidermis and increased capillary permeability permit escape of large amounts of fluid into the wound, forming thin-walled blisters and a wet wound surface. Cutaneous nerves, located more deeply in the dermis, are activated but not destroyed; as a result, these superficial burns are usually extremely painful.

In contrast, *deep* partial-thickness burns produce coagulative necrosis of a significant part of the dermis (Figs. 13-3, 13-4, and 13-5). This destroys superficial blood vessels and effectively "seals off" the skin surface from fluid leakage; instead, the fluid that escapes from damaged capillaries collects *beneath* the wound. Such deep burns often have a dry, pale appearance, but can display dark discoloration that does not blanch with direct pressure. These injuries are less painful than more superficial burns.

Healing of burn wounds also depends on the depth of injury. Burn wounds quickly accumulate a coating of opaque, tenacious film called eschar, which comprises dried serum and necrotic dermis. This material will gradually separate from the underlying viable tissue as leukocytes digest it away; the time required for this is a function of burn depth. Simultaneously, epidermis begins to grow upward from viable epidermal appendages, forming tiny islands that enlarge and coalesce, gradually re-covering the wound. Two aspects of this process are important in clinical burn treatment and for long-term results: First, *dermis never regenerates*; it is only replaced by scar tissue. Thus the deeper the dermal burn, the more scar eventually forms. Second, as long as epidermal appendages survive, the wound will eventually "heal" (that is, reepithelialize) on its own. If these appendages are destroyed, the wound can reepithelialize only from the margins, not from the base.

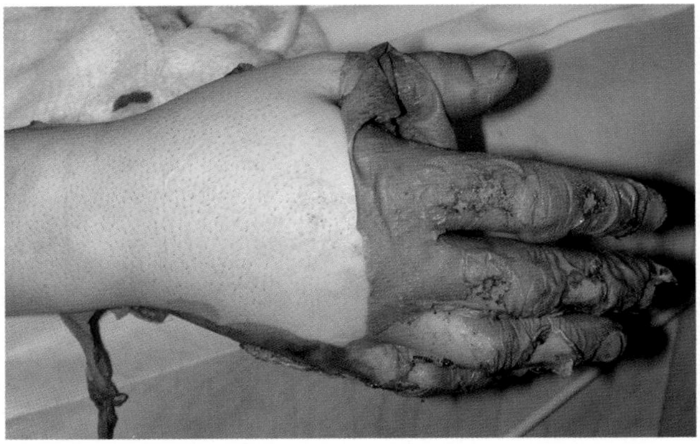

FIGURE 13–3 Deep dermal burns. A man's hand injured while he was priming a carburetor with gasoline. Charred epidermis sloughs readily, revealing pale, dry, relatively painless dermis beneath.

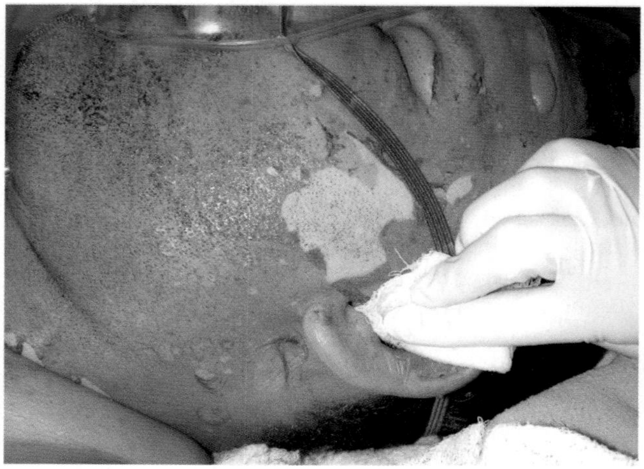

FIGURE 13–4 Deep dermal burn. Facial epidermis is discolored and adherent, but separates with vigorous débridement, revealing the characteristic pale, dry dermis beneath. Note the swelling, particularly of the eyelids.

It is often difficult to determine the exact depth of a burn injury. Wounds of questionable depth can be followed up with conservative treatment, awaiting both the "separation" of eschar and the appearance of epidermal "buds." Most clinicians agree that wounds that display both these features within 14 to 21 days of injury can be allowed to heal spontaneously (Fig. 13-6). Wounds that fail to progress in this period have usually sustained so much dermal damage that scarring will be unacceptable, and a better result will be obtained from skin grafting (see the following).

The most severe burns destroy the entire dermis, producing a **full-thickness** or **third-degree burn.** Such injuries may be a variety of colors, but are invariably dry and relatively insensate (Fig. 13-7). Coagulative necrosis may involve the subcutaneous blood vessels, which is pathognomonic of full-thickness injury. The coagulated dermis is constricted and rigid; as fluid accumulates beneath it, tissue pressure can increase to a dangerous degree, causing vascular compromise. Incision through the burn wound, termed escharotomy, may be required to relieve this compression and restore distal circulation.

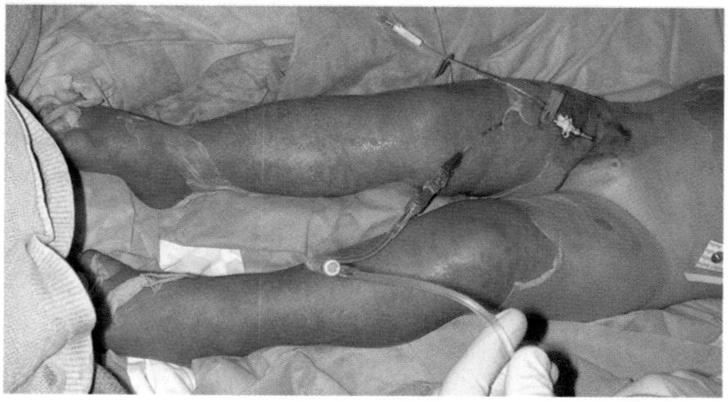

FIGURE 13–5 Deep dermal burn. Another bathtub scald; however, this child's legs are darker red, dry, and do not blanch with pressure. They are deeply injured and eventually required skin grafting.

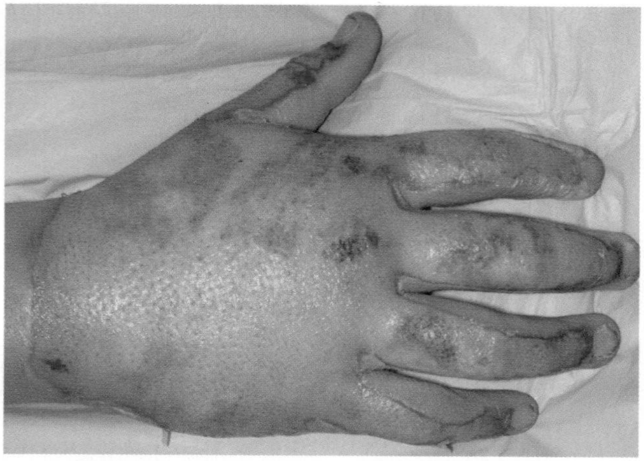

FIGURE 13–6 Healing partial-thickness wound. This hand was burned approximately 10 days earlier. Initially, solid eschar covered the entire hand. It is now "separating" in many areas, revealing translucent pink tissue. Simultaneously, a regular pattern of epidermal "buds" can be seen emerging from the base of the wound. These buds will grow, spread, and coalesce, covering the wound with new epidermis. This wound should heal satisfactorily without surgery.

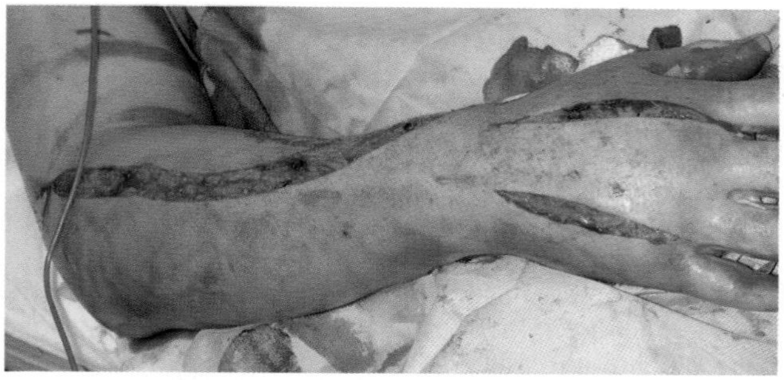

FIGURE 13–7 Full-thickness burn of the hand and forearm. The wound is mottled, dry, and leathery, with little sensation. Escharotomy incisions have been made through some of the burn eschar to relieve compression and improve distal perfusion. Because both epidermal appendages and the entire dermis are destroyed, this wound will require skin grafting for satisfactory healing.

Treatment of the Burn Patient

Victims of burn injury will require a variety of types of care as they progress from acute injury through rehabilitation. Since World War II, specialized burn centers have evolved to provide these treatments, using a coordinated team of physicians, nurses, physical therapists, and others. Although provision of this care is in reality a continuum, with multiple disciplines and treatments involved simultaneously, it is useful to divide burn treatment into four stages: (1) initial evaluation, (2) resuscitation, (3) wound coverage and metabolic support, and (4) rehabilitation. The priority assigned to each of these problems will vary with the magnitude of injury, the patient's response to treatment, and the time after injury. Caregivers must remember that many aspects of care continue throughout these phases, always dictated by the needs of the patient.

Initial Evaluation

Burn patients, just as trauma patients, should be treated according to the principles of trauma management, which are outlined elsewhere in this book. Initial assessment of burn patients requires awareness of problems specific to burn injuries (Fig. 13-8).

Scene Safety: Stop the Burning Process

Although often unstated in trauma algorithms, it is well recognized that accidents can endanger healthcare providers as well as patients. First responders, such as firefighters and emergency medical technicians (EMTs) and those dealing with mass casualties, chemical/biologic agents, and other scenarios, are taught to "secure the scene," protecting against further injury, even before attempting to treat patients. This principle is important for burn patients, as many situations that produce burns can continue to do so after first aid has been rendered. Assure that victims of chemical exposure undergo thorough decontamination before contact with healthcare workers. Extinguish flame burns completely with water, smothering, or rolling patients on the ground *before* applying oxygen, which can reignite smoldering clothing. Cool hot liquids that cannot be removed, such as tar, asphalt, or plastic, with water or moist compresses. Do not approach victims of electrocution until the source of current is shut off. Remember that most people killed by electrical current die of acute arrhythmias; evaluate for cardiopulmonary resuscitation (CPR) immediately.

Primary Survey: The ABCs

As trauma patients, burn victims must undergo a thorough and systematic initial evaluation before attention is focused on the burn wound. Two problems should be evaluated with particular care: airway edema and inhalation injury. Patients with extensive burns of the face and neck can develop airway obstruction from progressive swelling. Like all edema, airway swelling worsens dramatically over the first 24 to 36 hours after injury. Examine patients at risk for this problem carefully and *serially*, and consider early and elective intubation if airway compromise appears likely. Even if patients have no initial problems, complications of

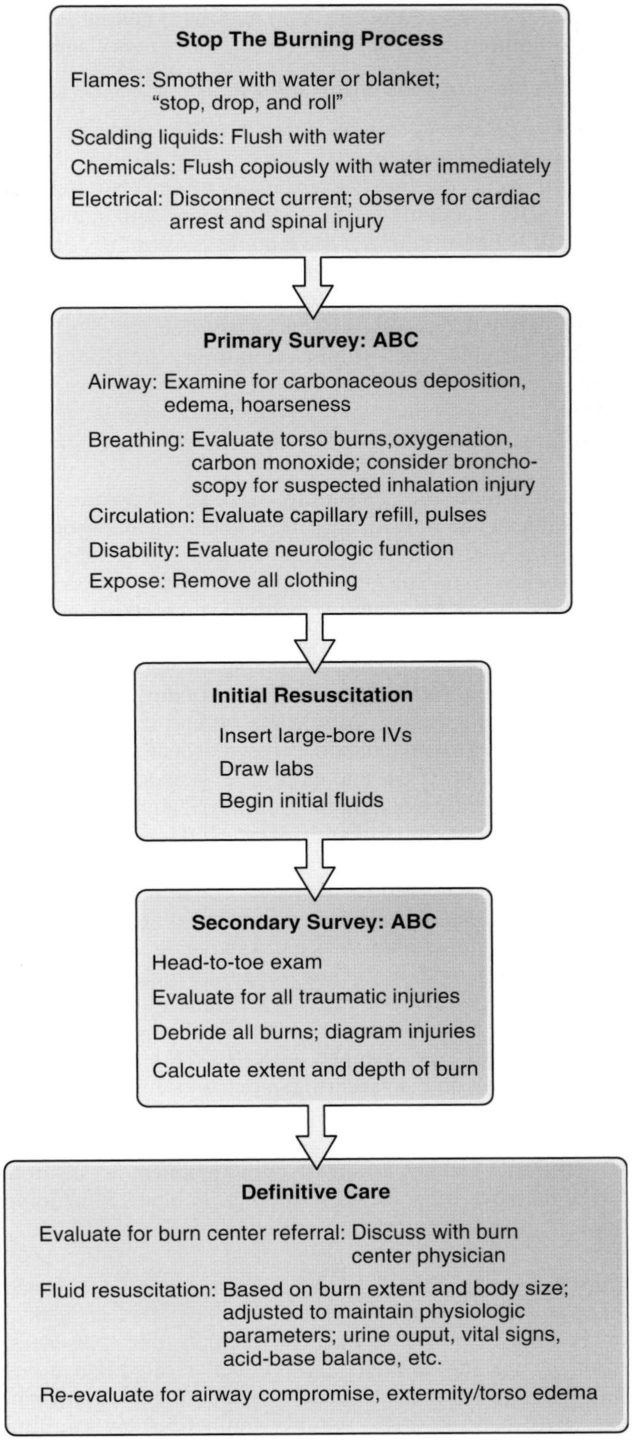
Stop The Burning Process
Flames: Smother with water or blanket; "stop, drop, and roll"
Scalding liquids: Flush with water
Chemicals: Flush copiously with water immediately
Electrical: Disconnect current; observe for cardiac arrest and spinal injury
Primary Survey: ABC
Airway: Examine for carbonaceous deposition, edema, hoarseness
Breathing: Evaluate torso burns,oxygenation, carbon monoxide; consider bronchoscopy for suspected inhalation injury
Circulation: Evaluate capillary refill, pulses
Disability: Evaluate neurologic function
Expose: Remove all clothing
Initial Resuscitation
Insert large-bore IVs
Draw labs
Begin initial fluids
Secondary Survey: ABC
Head-to-toe exam
Evaluate for all traumatic injuries
Debride all burns; diagram injuries
Calculate extent and depth of burn
Definitive Care
Evaluate for burn center referral: Discuss with burn center physician
Fluid resuscitation: Based on burn extent and body size; adjusted to maintain physiologic parameters; urine ouput, vital signs, acid-base balance, etc.
Re-evaluate for airway compromise, extermity/torso edema

FIGURE 13–8 Algorithm for initial evaluation of burn patients.

inhalation injury can occur later, and the potential for this type of injury should be noted during the primary survey.

The Problem of Inhalation Injury

Injury to the airway or lungs from inhaling smoke or steam is termed *inhalation injury*. Although this can occur as an isolated event, the most severe cases of smoke inhalation are usually encountered in combination with cutaneous burns. Inhalation injury is the leading cause of death from house and other building fires, greatly complicates the care of burn patients, and more than doubles the mortality associated with cutaneous burns of any size.

Three distinct types of inhalation injury are recognized; evidence for each should be looked for carefully during the primary and secondary surveys. They are carbon monoxide poisoning, upper airway injury, and lower airway injury.

Carbon Monoxide Poisoning. Carbon monoxide (CO) poisoning can be immediately life threatening and should be strongly suspected in any patient with altered mental status after exposure to smoke. Carbon monoxide, an odorless, colorless gas, is a product of incomplete combustion. Thus fires that smolder are the typical source of CO poisoning. CO binds avidly to hemoglobin, preventing the uptake and transport of oxygen. Symptoms of CO poisoning are primarily neurologic, progressing from headache and confusion with mild exposures to obtundation, coma, and death.

Confirmation of carbon monoxide poisoning requires measurement of carboxyhemoglobin (COHgb) in a blood-gas sample. Remember that, because COHgb is bright red, pulse oximetry gives falsely elevated readings of arterial saturation in this setting. However, treatment should be instituted *immediately* if CO poisoning is suspected and not await results of blood-gas analysis.

Treatment is with high-flow oxygen, which supports the patient, and competes with CO for hemoglobin binding. Unconscious patients should be intubated immediately and ventilated with 100% oxygen until COHgb levels return to normal. Considerable recent interest has been expressed in the use of hyperbaric oxygen (HBO) to treat CO poisoning. Although HBO can reduce the half-life of COHgb, its value is unproven. Do not withhold burn treatment to institute HBO therapy; other life-threatening problems, including burn shock resuscitation, take precedence.

Upper Airway Injury. Patients who inhale superheated gases and smoke can have thermal trauma to the face, palate, or pharynx. Such patients frequently demonstrate hoarseness, stridor, wheezing, and a cough productive of carbonaceous sputum. Initial treatment should be with humidified oxygen, but such patients may require intubation as swelling progresses and should be watched closely.

Lower Respiratory Injury. Lower airway injury (so-called true inhalation injury) is produced not from heat, but from the toxic chemicals contained in smoke. When these chemicals contact the moist lining of the trachea and distal airways, they can produce severe progressive damage, leading to mucosal sloughing, bronchiectasis, plugging, hypoxia, and infection.

It is critical to remember that *even severe inhalation injury may be asymptomatic for up to 72 hours after smoke exposure*. Suspect inhalation injury in any patient exposed to concentrations of smoke, especially in a closed space. Other clues to this diagnosis include burns of the face, neck, or pharynx; carbonaceous sputum, or wheezing. The most accurate test for inhalation injury is fiberoptic bronchoscopy, which usually reveals carbonaceous deposition within the trachea and bronchi, erythema, mucosal sloughing, or a combination of these. A negative bronchoscopy, however, does not preclude the development of respiratory distress. Treat all patients exposed to concentrated smoke with humidified oxygen, and watch closely for evidence of hypoxemia or respiratory distress. Perform endotracheal intubation early if hypoxemia is progressive; patients may require prolonged ventilatory support. Pulmonary infections are frequent, difficult to treat, and can be lethal.

After a rapid primary survey, begin initial fluid therapy. If injuries are extensive, secure IV access and place a Foley catheter to monitor urine output (see later). Begin crystalloids at a generous maintenance rate; formal calculation of fluid requirements can be performed later.

Secondary Survey

Many burn injuries can be associated with other trauma. Multiple trauma can be difficult to diagnose in the presence of a burn, yet be more immediately life threatening than the burn itself. It is therefore critical that *a comprehensive, head-to-toe examination be performed on every burn patient.* This should include initial radiographic studies as needed. Reevaluate these problems during the secondary survey, and plan on serial examinations for patients at high risk.

As an extension of the secondary survey, remove all clothing, and inspect burn wounds. Burns are often treated in the field by application of ice water or cold towels; these should be removed immediately, as they can produce hypothermia and further tissue damage. Keep wounds (and the patient) clean and dry. Débride wounds by thorough washing, remove blistered skin, and shave adjacent hair. At this time, document the extent, depth, and location of burn wounds on a diagram. Because the size of the injury dictates fluid resuscitation, nutrition, and many other aspects of care, calculate the total burn size carefully. Several methods are used for estimating burn size, which is expressed as **percentage of total body surface area** (%TBSA). One widely used method, the "rule of nines," is illustrated in Figure 13-9. Major body parts are assigned multiples of 9% TBSA: 9% each for head and each arm; 18% TBSA for anterior torso, posterior torso, and each leg. Because small children have relatively larger heads and smaller legs than adults, the

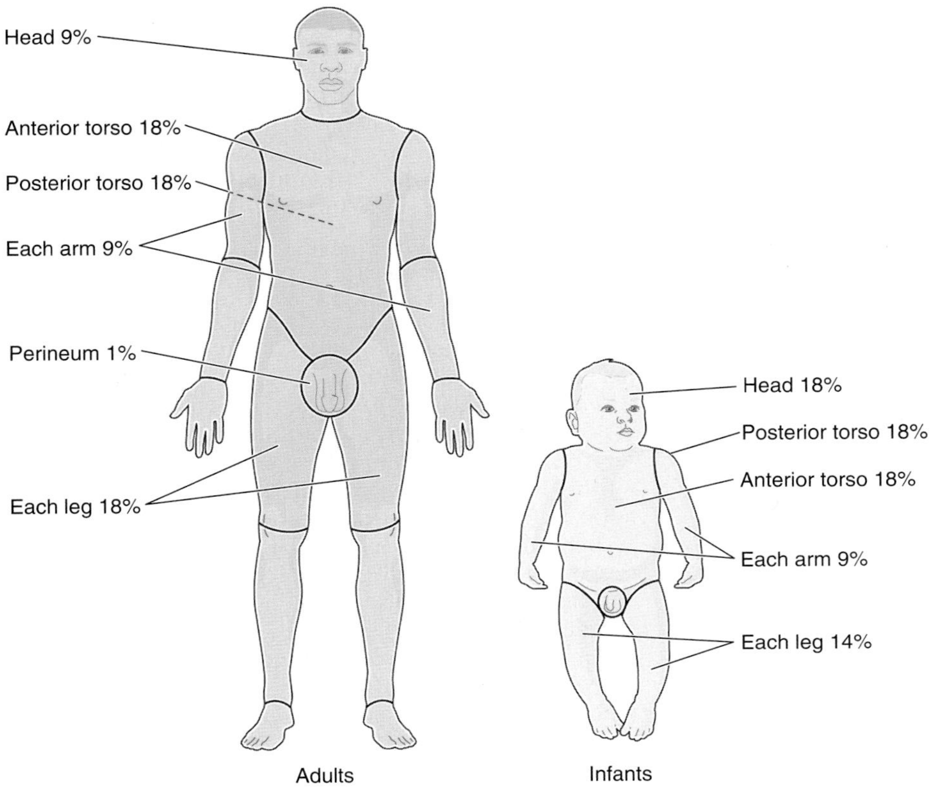

FIGURE 13–9 The "rule of nines" for estimating burn extent. Because infants have significantly larger heads and smaller legs than adults, different rules must be used when evaluating these patients. A simple, practical rule is that the palm of the patient's hand, with fingers, equals 1% of the total body surface area.

algorithm is modified for them, as shown. Another useful, practical rule for evaluating small injuries in patients of any age is that the palm of the *patient's* hand (including fingers) is approximately 1% of his or her BSA. Applying this simple rule can permit fairly accurate and rapid burn assessment.

Do not dress or wrap burn wounds until the secondary survey has been completed and all wounds have been débrided and documented.

Burn Center Referral

Once initial assessment has been completed, the surgeon should consider the optimal setting for care of the burned patient. As mentioned previously, mortality rates from burns have been dramatically improved over the past 50-year period, coincident with development of specialized burn-treatment facilities. In support of this concept, the American College of Surgeons has joined with the American Burn Association to define criteria for referral of patients to burn centers. These include

1. Patients with partial- or full-thickness burns of 10% TBSA or greater.
2. All full-thickness burns.
3. Burns of "specialty" care areas: eyes, ears, face, hands, feet, perineum, major joints.
4. Burns complicated by smoke inhalation or multiple trauma.
5. Burns from high-voltage electrical or chemical injury.
6. Burns in patients with significant comorbid medical problems (e.g., diabetes).
7. Burned children who require specialized pediatric care.

PEARLS FOR THE OR

Tangential excision is the preferred method, removing thin layers of eschar until viable tissue, characterized by punctate capillary bleeding, is encountered.

Methods for covering large wounds include widely meshed skin grafts, temporary coverage with cadaver allografts, synthetic skin substitutes, or cultured epidermal cells.

Infiltration of burn wounds or skin graft donor sites or both with saline solution containing epinephrine can facilitate excision or harvest and markedly reduce bleeding.

Deep partial-thickness burns should be treated with excision and skin grafting to speed healing, reduce the possibility of infection, and improve the ultimate functional and cosmetic result for the patient.

PEARLS FOR ROUNDS

Mortality for major burns is now low. A young adult with burns of 80% to 90% TBSA has a 50% survival.

Smoke inhalation worsens survival because of pneumonia and multiple organ failure. Three types of inhalation injury are carbon monoxide poisoning, upper-airway burns, and lower-airway chemical injury.

Estimate burn extent by using the "rule of nines": Head, arms: 9% TBSA each; anterior torso, posterior torso, each leg: 18% TBSA each. The palm of the patient's hand is 1% TBSA.

Parkland formula for fluid resuscitation: 4 mL lactated Ringer's × body weight (kg) × burn size (%TBSA). This tells you where to start resuscitation, which is subsequently adjusted to patient response. Urine output is the single most important parameter of adequate fluid resuscitation. Remember that edema is progressive throughout fluid resuscitation. The patient should be repeatedly evaluated for compartment syndromes involving the extremities or torso.

Nutritional requirements for burn patients may exceed twice normal. Whenever possible, use enteral nutrition: 30 to 35 nonprotein kcal/kg/day; 1.5 to 2.0 gr protein/kg/day. Fat should not exceed 35% of diet.

Indications for surgery: any burn that does not demonstrate **eschar separation** and **epidermal budding** within 14 days of injury.

8. Patients who will require special social, psychological, or prolonged rehabilitation.

Each category identifies a situation in which treatment by a specialized team will be necessary to achieve the best possible outcome. These criteria have been widely adopted in the trauma-care community. Surgeons treating patients who fulfill one or more of these guidelines should consult the regional burn center. The necessity, method, and timing of transport, as well as the details of initial care, should be determined by the transferring and receiving physician in direct conversation.

Fluid Resuscitation

Once the patient has completed initial evaluation, *the most important goal of initial burn treatment is fluid resuscitation*, and this aspect of care takes priority for 24 to 48 hours. Like any tissue injury, even small burns alter the permeability of blood vessels, resulting in localized leakage of fluid from capillaries and the accumulation of edema. As burns become larger, capillary leakage becomes more pronounced; when burns exceed 15% to 20% TBSA, capillary leakage becomes systemic, leading to significant loss of circulating blood volume, a phenomenon known as **burn shock**. Massive burn injuries (40% TBSA) produce tremendous losses, and many liters of resuscitation fluid may be required to compensate for widespread edema formation.

To help guide successful resuscitation from burn shock, physicians have developed a host of resuscitation regimens. Most call for an initial calculation of fluid requirements based on both burn area and body size, with the majority of the fluid given in the first 8 to 12 hours after the burn, when capillary leakage is most rapid. In perhaps the most widely accepted regimen, the **Parkland formula,** fluid requirements are calculated as follows:

$$\text{Fluid requirements for the first 24 hours} = (4\text{ mL LR}) \times (\text{Kg}) \times (\%\text{TBSA})$$

where LR is lactated Ringer's solution, Kg is patient's weight in kilograms, and %TBSA is burn size as percentage of TBSA.

For example, a man who weights 80 kg, with a 50% TBSA burn, would be calculated to receive (4 mL × 80 kg × 50%TBSA) = 16,000 mL LR, or 16 L of fluid! Half of this would be given over the first 8 hours after injury (1000 mL/hr), and the rest, over the remaining 16 hours.

In beginning fluid resuscitation, remember that patients' responses to resuscitation vary. Fluid requirements can be affected by the depth of the burn, associated injuries (particularly inhalation injury), multiple trauma, and electrical burns, and patient factors such as alcohol abuse, liver disease, diabetes, and others. Children and the elderly frequently require more fluid than is called for by predictive formulas. Resuscitation formulas help the physician decide where to *begin* resuscitation, but subsequent fluid administration must be guided by the response of the patient. The most useful and widely used parameter is the maintenance of adequate urine output (30–50 mL/hr in adults; 1–2 mL/kg/hr in children). Adjust the infusion rate according to urine output, and gradually decrease until a maintenance rate is reached. Monitor vital signs, hematocrit, acid-base balance, and other laboratory tests as well. The use of pulmonary artery catheters and direct measurement of cardiac function is usually reserved for high-risk patients or those who are doing badly with resuscitation. Consultation with a burn center is strongly recommended for physicians inexperienced with resuscitation of major burns.

Edema formation continues throughout resuscitation. In badly burned extremities, accumulation of edema beneath rigid eschar can cause major increases in tissue hydrostatic pressure, leading to impaired capillary perfusion and ischemia, the so-called **compartment syndrome**. Because edema formation is progressive, monitor patients repeatedly by checking peripheral pulses and motor and sensory function. Measurement of intramuscular pressure by using a needle-transducer system can detect extremity compression before ischemia becomes irreversible. When significant circulatory compromise occurs in an extremity, perform **escharotomy** by making an incision longitudinally along the medial or lateral side or both of the supinated limb by using a

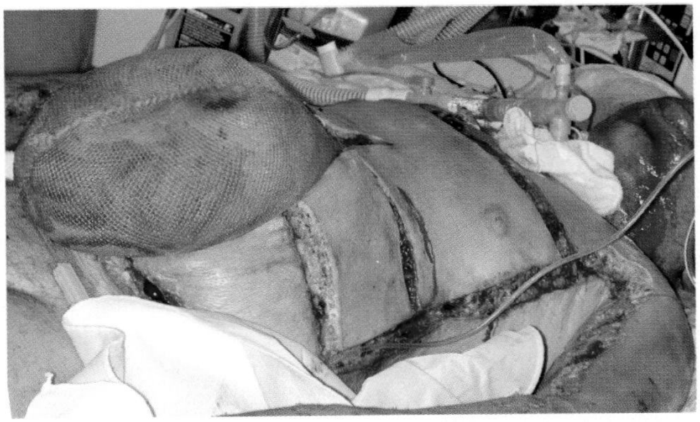

FIGURE 13–10 Massive torso injury. In this man, acute cardiac and respiratory compromise developed because of edema formation of the chest and abdomen. Initially, chest escharotomy incisions were performed to improve respirations. As his condition deteriorated, acute abdominal compartment syndrome developed, manifested by hypotension, oliguria, and respiratory embarrassment. Bladder pressure, measured through the indwelling Foley catheter, exceeded 30 cm water. Decompressive laparotomy led to immediate and dramatic improvement in blood pressure and respiratory mechanics. However, edema prevents the return of his viscera within the abdomen, necessitating creation of a temporary "silo," by using Dexon mesh. Massive edema of his lower face has been treated with tracheostomy.

scalpel or electrocautery (see Fig. 13-7). These incisions can be covered with skin grafts during the subacute phase of burn treatment.

Compression also can occur in the torso, causing respiratory embarrassment; and in the abdomen, causing the **abdominal compartment syndrome**, in which increased intraabdominal pressure leads to venous compression, oliguria, and shock. Patients may require torso escharotomies, or even decompressive laparotomy, to relieve this acute compression (Fig. 13-10).

Wound Coverage and Metabolic Support

This phase of treatment begins immediately after fluid resuscitation and lasts for days to weeks, until the burn wound heals spontaneously or is covered by skin grafts. This is a time of great metabolic and physical stress for the patient, who is in danger of infection and other complications until the burn is successfully closed. Most inpatient care for burn patients occurs during this period.

Care of the burn wound is a labor-intensive process, requiring a team of experts. Wounds must be cleansed and débrided frequently; this removes loose eschar and old topical agents, stimulates blood flow to the wounds, and permits detailed examination of wound healing and potential areas of infection. Simultaneously, physical therapy to improve muscle tone and prevent contractures must be started as soon after injury as possible (see later).

Excision and Skin Grafting

Burn injury causes an intense inflammatory reaction that characterizes the initial phase of wound healing. The continued presence of necrotic eschar on the wound surface also serves as an ideal medium for infection, which in turn stimulates even more pronounced release of inflammatory mediators, causing great metabolic stress and contributing to the generation of multiple organ failure. As recently as 25 years ago, burn eschar was allowed to remain in place until it "separated" spontaneously and developed a bed of granulation tissue that could support skin grafting. This technique subjected patients to prolonged severe pain, hypermetabolism, and risk of infection. In addition, when treated in this manner, even very deep partial-thickness burns were allowed to heal spontaneously, producing thick, unstable scar tissue that was functionally as well as cosmetically unacceptable.

For these reasons, most burn centers now perform **early excision** of burn wounds. In this technique, the eschar of full-thickness and deep partial-thickness burn wounds is cut away until a viable bed is reached. In **fascial excision**, a scalpel or cautery is used to remove the entire skin and subcutaneous fat down to the level of underlying fascia, which will support skin grafting. Although it is rapid and relatively bloodless, fascial excision is disfiguring, and the loss of subcutaneous tissue can result in joint stiffness and poor mobility. In contrast, the technique of **tangential excision**, using dermatomes to remove sequential thin layers of tissue until punctate capillary bleeding is encountered, preserves more viable skin elements, including the deep dermis of some partial-thickness injuries, thereby reducing scarring and disfigurement, while still permitting good skin graft "take." Tangential excisions can be associated with significant bleeding and metabolic stress for the patient, and most experts limit the extent of any single operation to 15% to 20% TBSA. Larger burns are excised by using serial procedures.

Once excised, burn wounds are covered with split-thickness skin grafts obtained from unburned areas of the body. These grafts are harvested by using the same dermatomes that are used for tangential excision, set to a thickness of 0.005 to 0.015 inches. This cuts the skin in the upper to mid-dermis, producing a durable graft, and leaving a bed than can heal spontaneously with little scarring. Infiltration of the subcutaneous tissue beneath the graft (or "donor") site with balanced salt solution is often used to increase skin turgor, which facilitates harvesting; the addition to epinephrine to this fluid reduces bleeding significantly. Skin grafts can be applied as intact sheets (Fig. 13-11) or expanded by cutting numerous small slits in the skin, a technique called "meshing." Meshed grafts are more durable and take readily, although their cosmetic result is inferior to that of sheet grafts.

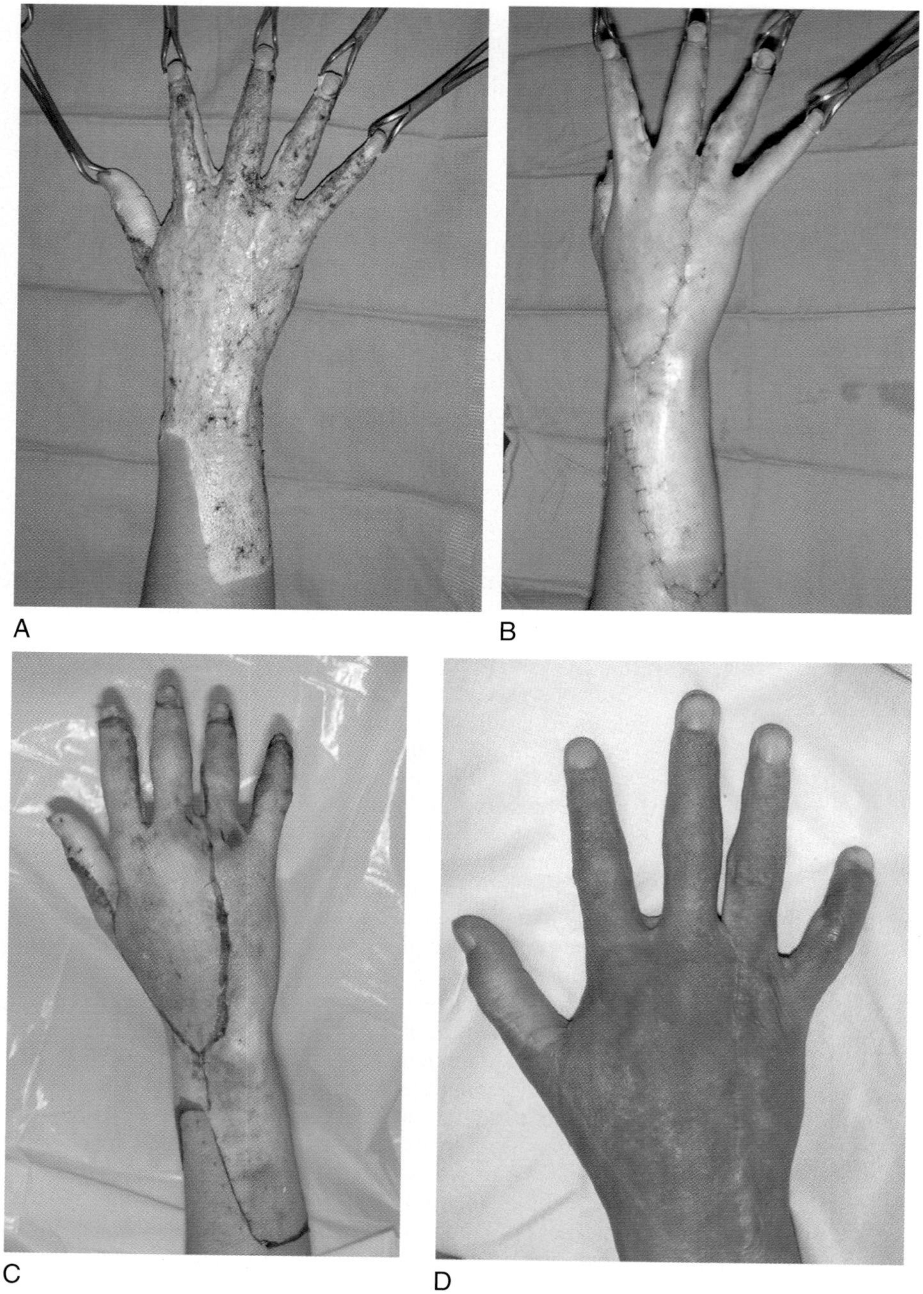

FIGURE 13–11 This man had a deep burn of the hand, similar to that illustrated in Figure 13-7. Escharotomies were necessary to relieve compression. *A*, The hand has undergone tangential excision and is now ready for grafting. You can see the network of capillaries in the subcutaneous tissue. *B*, A "sheet" split-thickness skin graft, harvested from the thigh, has been applied with stables and sutures. *C*, The graft 2 weeks later, showing uniform perfusion and "take." *D*, The result, after 12 months. This patient wore a compressive glove and performed physical therapy throughout this interval.

In treating large injuries, it may be necessary to harvest multiple skin grafts from the same donor sites. This can be done once original donor sites reepithelialize (usually within 14 days of harvest), although reharvested grafts are thinner and more fragile than the original skin. For patients with very large burns, the risk of infection of necrotic eschar increases within a few days of injury, so it is critical to remove eschar quickly. In this situation, a number of techniques can be used to facilitate wound coverage. By increasing the size of "mesh," donor skin can be expanded to several times its original size, permitting coverage of wounds much larger than the donors themselves. Widely meshed grafts produce a "checkered" or "scaled" appearance to the skin; and, because the interstices created by meshing must heal with only

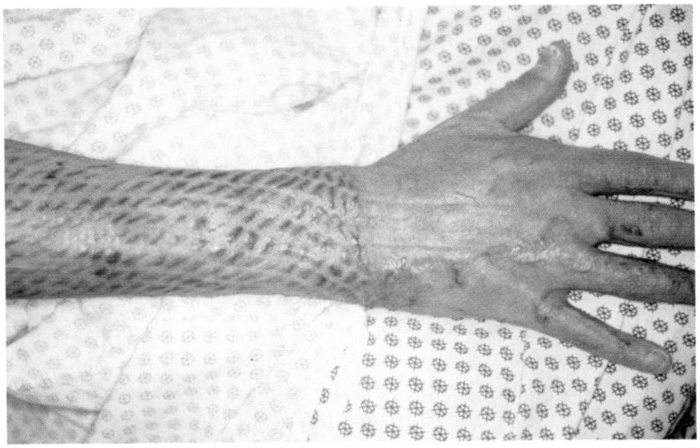

FIGURE 13–12 This man had extensive, deep burns to the forearm and hand. Scarcity of donor sites led to skin grafting with widely meshed skin over the forearm, whereas sheet grafts were used on the hand. The reticular appearance of the widely meshed graft is apparent, although the skin quality is good.

epidermal coverage, they can scar severely (Fig. 13-12). As an alternative, excised burn wounds can be covered with temporary dressings to maintain a clean and viable surface until the patient's donors can be re-harvested. Cadaver allograft skin is excellent for this purpose; it will vascularize just like autograft, although it is eventually rejected. However, cadaver skin can be difficult to acquire, costly, and carries the risk of disease transmission. In recent years, the search for the perfect "artificial skin" has led to development of several biologic dressings that can be used for temporary skin coverage. A number of useful products are available off the shelf. None is ideal, however; most are very expensive and often produce variable results. Finally, it is possible to grow skin in tissue culture. At present, only epidermis can be grown readily, producing an extremely thin, fragile graft. Such grafts can be life saving, but are tremendously costly, and very prone to infection and failure, which can be disastrous. Clearly, the search for an ideal synthetic skin substitute is still under way.

Infection Control

Burns are among the most infection prone of injuries. Although burns initially destroy the bacteria that colonize normal skin, they also remove the epidermal barrier to bacterial invasion and provide nutrient-rich necrotic eschar. As a result, bacteria proliferate rapidly within a few days of injury. When they reach sufficient numbers, they can penetrate viable tissue and invade blood vessels, extending the area of tissue necrosis, and causing **burn wound sepsis**.

Infections have historically been the most frequent cause of death after burns. Fortunately, they are now much less common. Early and aggressive burn wound excision and coverage, improved antibiotics, and critical care share the credit for the greatly improved prognosis for severe burns. It is noteworthy that as physicians have developed techniques for control of bacterial infections, new, more virulent (and resistant) pathogens have evolved that continue to challenge the burn care team, a situation that has been seen in many medical fields. Development of penicillin, topical sulfonamides, and silver nitrate solution in the 1940s reduced mortality from infections caused by *Staphylococcus* and *Streptococcus* species. As use of these agents became more widespread, however, several gram-negative bacteria emerged as major pathogens. In the 1960s, two powerful topical antibiotics were developed and remain in widespread use: mafenide acetate (Sulfamylon), and **silver sulfadiazene** (Silvadene, Thermazene, SSD, etc.). These agents helped control many gram-negative bacteria, which were then replaced by resistant *Pseudomonas* as a dominant pathogen. A number of systemic antibacterials, in addition to topical therapy, have helped control *Pseudomonas* infections. However, this success has been followed by emergence of multiply-resistant bacteria (methicillin-resistant *Staph. aureus, Acinetobacter*, vancomycin-resistant *Enterococcus*, etc.), fungi, and other exotic organisms, as important clinical pathogens in burn victims.

Although infections arising in burn wounds have been largely controlled, other types of infections remain significant problems in the care of burn victims. Foremost among these is pneumonia. As described previously, inhalation injury produces sloughing of tracheobronchial mucosa, mucus plugging of small airways, and bronchiectasis, all of which favor the accumulation of infected secretions. Because pulmonary clearance mechanisms are severely compromised, pneumonia can be exceedingly difficult to eradicate. In addition to posing a serious direct threat to the patient, persistent pneumonia often serves as the source of ongoing inflammation and bacteremia, leading to multiple organ failure and death. This is the major reason that mortality rates are much higher for burn patients with inhalation injury.

A host of other infectious complications can occur in burn victims as well. These include septic thrombophlebitis complicating venous cannulation, and even endocarditis arising from infected central venous lines; osteomyelitis in bone exposed by deep burns; acalculous cholecystitis; and a host of miscellaneous infections in the urinary tract, salivary glands, and elsewhere. Fortunately, most of these infections, like burn wound sepsis, are becoming increasingly rare as more efficient methods of burn treatment have evolved.

Nutritional Support

Burn injuries produce the most severe metabolic response of any form of trauma or illness. The hormonal response to a major burn includes marked elevations of the catabolic hormones epinephrine, cortisol, and glucagon, which increase metabolic rate and stimulate gluconeogenesis to provide substrates for wound healing. In a patient with a major burn, energy utilization more than twice that of a normal person may develop and be maintained for weeks. Much of the increase in energy consumption comes at the expense of muscle catabolism, which can exceed a half-pound of lean body mass per day. Before the use of aggressive nutritional support, burn patients would frequently have progressive nutritional depletion and muscle wasting over the first 3 to 4 weeks of injury and die of pneumonia and other infections, largely as a result of starvation. Now the role of nutrition in recovering from major injury is well understood, but burn victims still pose a number of practical challenges to the treatment team, simply because their nutritional requirements are so great.

Although a variety of techniques for nutritional support exist, enteral nutrition—using the patient's gastrointestinal tract—is clearly superior to intravenous nutrition, which should be reserved for patients with abdominal surgery or other contraindications to enteral feeding. Nutritional support should begin within 2 to 3 days of injury; patients may be encouraged to eat, but many will benefit from immediate placement of enteric feeding tubes for nutritional maintenance. A host of specialized formulas for enteral nutrition exist, but several key components should be provided for burn victims. First, sufficient *nonprotein* calories must meet the needs of the patient and minimize the breakdown of endogenous protein for energy. Patients vary significantly in their caloric requirements, which are affected by such factors as activity, fever, surgery, etc. For that reason, measurement of energy utilization by using indirect calorimetry is preferred by some experts over the estimation of caloric needs by using standardized formulas. The hormonal response to burn injury limits the amount of fat calories that can be used, so fat should not make up more than 25% to 30% of nonprotein calories. Finally, enteral formulas must be high in protein, providing not less than 1.5 to 2.0 grams of protein per kilogram body weight per day, to support wound healing and immune function.

A great deal of recent research has evaluated the role of "customized" formulas for nutrition of patients with trauma, burns, cancer, and other disorders. Specific additives such as Ω-3 fatty acids (which minimize the synthesis of pro-inflammatory prostaglandins), glutamine (which provides direct nutrition to intestinal mucosa), RNA (for protein synthesis), and others have shown some promise in improving outcomes in these disease states, but their use has not yet been universally accepted. Similarly, the use of anabolic hormones such as growth hormone, oxandrolone, and others is an area of active current research, but their use remains largely experimental. At present, the most important aspect of support for burn patients remains the provision of high-calorie, high-protein enteral nutrition sufficient to meet their accelerated metabolic demands.

Rehabilitation

As mentioned previously, recent success in saving the lives of patients with major burn injuries has produced new challenges to the burn team, particularly in the realm of rehabilitation. This phase of care actually starts immediately after the burn (*rehabilitation begins at the time of injury*), becomes increasingly important through the wound-closure period, and becomes the foremost problem in burn care from then on.

Several problems make burn rehabilitation a real challenge. First, healing wounds contain myofibroblasts, which aid the natural closure of open wounds by pulling them together, a process called **contracture**. This process causes progressive restriction in joint motion that can freeze extremities completely and cause major disfigurement. To combat this, patients require time-consuming daily stretching of involved areas, in addition to general therapy to maintain muscle strength and activity. Unless begun soon after injury and maintained rigorously, scar tissue will "set" into significant contractures that may be impossible to relieve without surgical intervention. Because the process of scar maturation lasts for months after injury, therapy must continue for at least that long.

Simultaneously, the accumulation of collagen beneath healed and grafted burn wounds produces unsightly, uncomfortable, and unstable burn scars (Fig. 13-13). Because scars grow and remodel in response to pressure, many experts believe that burn scars can be significantly reduced by having patients wear custom-made tight-fitting garments to combat scar hypertrophy. The use of topical moisturizers and lotions also helps soften scar tissue and reduce the chronic itching that plagues many burn survivors. Although some scars may be amenable to reconstructive surgery, most experts do not attempt such procedures until scars have lost their erythema and rigidity, which can

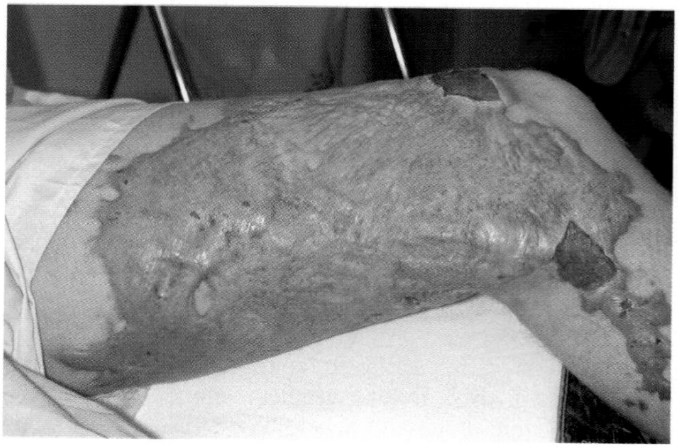

FIGURE 13–13 Severe hypertrophic scarring 18 months after injury. This man has very thick, rigid scar tissue covering his thigh. The ulcerations are typical of hypertrophic scars, which often have unstable epidermal coverage. Although treated with skin grafting, this man did not comply with pressure garments and physical therapy.

take more than a year. In addition, many reconstructive procedures can be obviated by meticulous and successful skin grafting and by diligent attention to physical therapy and the use of burn-scar supports.

Finally, the psychological sequelae of burn injuries have been shown to exceed those of other, less visible wounds. In many burn victims, symptoms of posttraumatic stress disorder may not correlate well with burn wound size and can significantly impede return to a functional lifestyle. Despite these challenges, most patients who survive burn injuries do eventually return to work, school, and home. This success, however, is bought at the price of months of hard work on the part of burn therapists and patients alike.

Suggested Reading

American Burn Association: Practice guidelines for burn care. J Burn Care Rehabil 22:1S–69S, 2001.

Monafo WW. Current concepts: Initial management of burns. N Engl J Med 225:1581–1586, 1996.

Saffle JR (ed): Burns. Prob Gen Surg 20:1–145, 2003.

Sheridan RL: Burns. Crit Care Med 30:S500–S514, 2002.

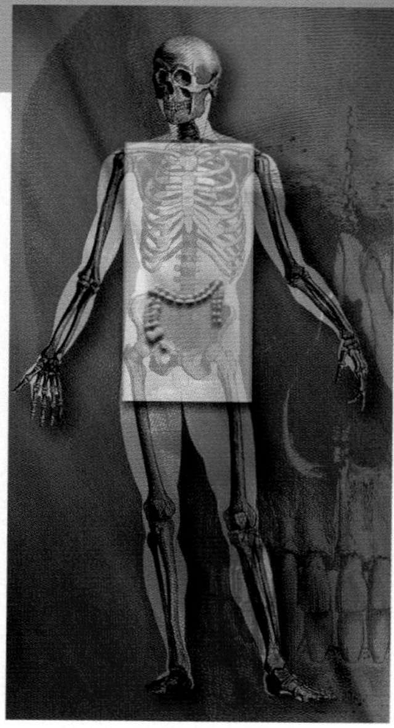

SECTION IV

ABDOMEN

Chapter 14

Acute Abdomen

STEPHEN J. FERZOCO, MD, and JAMES M. BECKER, MD

Acute abdominal pain is one of the most common complaints necessitating a surgical evaluation. It also presents one of the most difficult challenges in clinical medicine. The surgeon must perform a quick, but thorough, assessment and rapidly arrive at an accurate diagnosis in the treatment.

By definition, *acute abdomen* implies severe abdominal pain arising rather suddenly and of less than 24 hours' duration. A careful, thorough evaluation and workup is crucial for appropriate treatment options.

Surgical Anatomy

A detailed knowledge of surgical anatomy is fundamental in caring for these patients. An understanding of the neurophysiology of pain in abdominal organs is important in establishing a diagnosis of the acute abdomen. The embryologic derivation of the structures of the abdomen provides a basis for the location and distribution of pain. Pain arising in structures originating from the foregut, including the stomach, pancreas, duodenum, and biliary tree, localizes to the epigastric region. Pain from the small bowel and right and transverse colon, which are derivatives of the midgut, localize in the periumbilical region, whereas pain from the hindgut derivatives, such as the left colon, sigmoid and rectum, have pain fibers that localize lower in the hypogastric region.

The nerve supply to the parietal peritoneum is derived from the somatic nerves that also supply the adjacent abdominal wall and skin. Sensory pathways for visceral pain are present in the lower thoracic and lumbar splanchnic nerves and in the parasympathetic nerves of the vagus and sacral plexus. In general, two types of abdominal pain occur within an acute abdomen. The first is a steady, well-localized abdominal pain that usually occurs after ischemia, perforation, inflammation, or hemorrhage. The second is intermittent colicky, poorly localized abdominal pain, found with obstruction of the GI tract.

History

The initial evaluation of a patient with abdominal pain is a detailed and thorough history. The time of onset of pain, its location, and change in character and location are all very important.

Timing of the pain can provide surgeons with important information. Determine whether the pain began suddenly or was gradual in onset. A sudden onset of excruciating pain heralds perforation, rupture, or ischemia of a visceral organ. Pain of a gradual onset suggests a subacute process and may include peptic ulcer disease, gastritis, cholecystitis, inflammatory bowel disease, and diverticulitis.

Physical Examination

Once a detailed history has been obtained, the physical examination remains the most important tool that a surgeon can use in determining the cause of the underlying disease process. In a systematic approach, the examiner assesses, inspects, auscultates, palpates, and percusses the patient and attempts to elicit responses that the examiner can use in determining his or her differential diagnosis.

The general assessment of the patient can be determined in the first several minutes. The degree of the patient's discomfort, the restlessness, and position in bed all provide the examiner with clues about the patient's overall state. The patient who lies in bed motionless, unable to answer questions, or appears anxious and in pain is in more distress than the patient who is cooperative, relaxed, and able to answer questions.

The abdomen is then auscultated in all four quadrants for several minutes to be certain of the character of the bowel sounds. The frequency and pitch of bowel sounds are noted, and absence of bowel sounds after several minutes is consistent with an ileus. Bowel sounds that are characterized as high-pitched with splashes, tinkles, and rushes, especially in the presence of abdominal distention, are indicative of a small-bowel obstruction.

The abdomen is then palpated in all four quadrants. It is important that the examiner begin the examination in a nontender quadrant and proceed slowly toward the point of maximal tenderness. During the examination, it is important to correlate physical findings with the patient's own history of the illness. In addition, any evidence of guarding, voluntary or involuntary, as well as spasm, should be noted. The abdomen can then be percussed to determine the degree of abdominal distention. The presence of rebound tenderness suggests peritoneal irritation. This can be elicited by palpation of the abdomen, followed by quick release of the pressure by the hand.

Additional components of the physical examination that can yield important information are the rectal and pelvic examinations, which permit a thorough examination of the lower pelvis. Masses, both firm and fluctuant, as well as areas of tenderness, are noted. The stool should always be inspected and tested for occult blood. The presence of cervical discharge or vaginal bleeding is important, and a bimanual examination can elicit uterine or adnexal tenderness or masses.

Laboratory Tests

In addition to the physical findings, important information leading to a clear understanding of the clinical manifestations is provided by specific laboratory tests. Perhaps the most useful test is the complete blood count (CBC). An elevated leukocyte count and left shift in the differential indicates an active inflammatory process; however, the absence of an elevated white blood cell count does not exclude the possibility of infection. The elderly, diabetics, or the immunosuppressed patient may demonstrate a normal leukocyte count yet have active infection. The hematocrit also can provide clues to the patient's status. An elevated hematocrit can suggest dehydration, whereas anemia can suggest chronic bleeding.

Serum electrolytes can reveal severe hypokalemia seen during severe vomiting or diarrhea. Serum bicarbonate and the anion gap can demonstrate acid-base disturbances and the degree of compensation. Serum electrolyte measurement provides the surgeon an opportunity to correct any electrolyte abnormalities before admission to the hospital or any surgical intervention. Patients with suspected biliary disease should have liver-function tests (LFTs) evaluated. Those with pancreatic involvement also should have serum amylase and lipase tested.

Urinalysis should be performed routinely on all patients. A urinary tract infection can often mimic the signs and symptoms of an acute abdomen. The presence of blood, protein, or glucose offers additional data to the etiology, whereas the urine specific gravity reflects the status of the patient's blood volume. All female patients of childbearing age should have a urine pregnancy test to eliminate that as a source of lower abdominal pain.

Radiographic Imaging

Plain Radiographs

Radiographic imaging can provide much useful information in the diagnosis of an acute abdomen. The standard series of films that should be obtained in a patient with abdominal pain include three views: supine and upright abdominal views as well as a standard chest radiograph. A chest film can reveal a basilar pneumonia, which can cause referred abdominal pain. The presence of free air in the abdomen also can be determined on chest radiograph (Fig. 14-1). Supine and upright abdominal films can reveal intestinal obstruction as well as the presence of air-fluid levels. In addition, fecaliths and kidney stones may be found on the radiographs, aiding in the diagnosis of appendicitis and nephrolithiasis, respectively.

Ultrasound

Ultrasound is another noninvasive radiologic imaging study that provides a safe and painless method of evaluation. This method can visualize and assess a variety of intraabdominal organs such as the liver, biliary tract, pancreas, appendix,

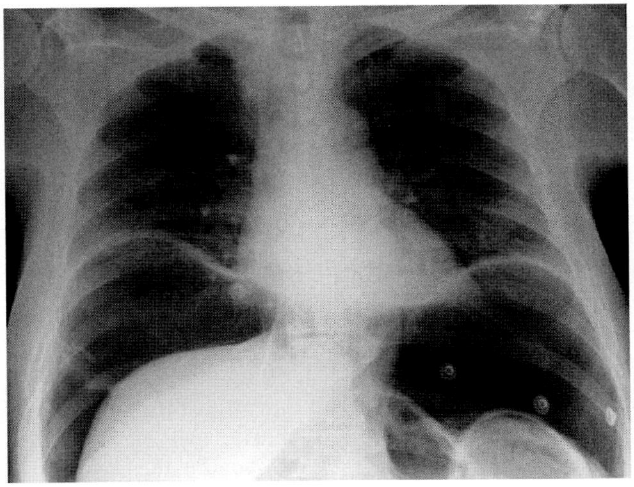

FIGURE 14–1 Upright chest radiograph demonstrating massive intraperitoneal free air. (Photo courtesy of Stephen Ledbetter, MD, Emergency Radiology Division, Brigham and Women's Hospital, Boston, Massachusetts.)

PEARLS FOR ROUNDS

The workup of patients with acute abdominal pain

- Physical examination
A detailed physical examination includes assessment, inspection, auscultation, palpation, percussion, and rectal/pelvic examination.

- Laboratory values
CBC, electrolytes, LFTs, amylase, lipase, and urinalysis can all provide important information in the workup of patients with abdominal pain. A pregnancy test (urine or blood) is mandatory in all women of childbearing age.

- Radiographic tests
Imaging studies such as plain, supine, and upright radiographs, ultrasound, CT, angiography, barium studies, and endoscopy are useful tools for the surgeon in determining a cause of a patient's abdominal pain.

kidneys, spleen, and ovaries. In addition to solid organs, ultrasound can detect free fluid in the abdomen, as well as the degree of ascites. The use of duplex ultrasound also can assess vascular structures such as a ruptured or leaking aortic aneurysm, venous thrombi, and arteriovenous fistulae. Some centers have begun using ultrasound in the workup of abdominal pain in blunt trauma patients. In the right hands, it can provide rapid assessment of the abdomen.

Computed Tomography

Computed tomography (CT) has evolved into another important tool for the surgeon in the diagnosis of an acute abdomen. CT has been proven to be a fast, safe, noninvasive method to provide valuable information for the surgeon. Evaluation of all solid organs, both intraabdominal and retroperitoneal, is provided in great detail. In the diagnosis of hollow organs, such as the small and large intestine, one can evaluate bowel-wall thickness and the presence of air within the bowel wall as well as the mesentery (Fig. 14-2). CT is superior to other radiographic modalities in assessing abnormalities in the kidneys, pancreas, duodenum, and aorta. CT also can detect small amounts of free air in the abdomen, much less than that required in an upright chest radiograph.

Magnetic Resonance Imaging

Magnetic resonance imaging (MRI) continues to provide new uses for today's physicians and surgeons. However, despite its superior assessment of soft-tissue structures and views, MRI is not used in the evaluation of patients with an acute abdomen. The test remains expensive and time consuming and is rarely used in evaluating these patients.

Angiography

Angiography has become a useful therapeutic rather than a diagnostic tool for surgeons when dealing with patients with acute abdominal pain. In patients with bleeding in association with abdominal pain, angiography can be used to confirm the diagnosis, usually after a tagged–red cell scan. Once the bleeding vessel has been identified, therapeutic embolization of the vessel can be instituted.

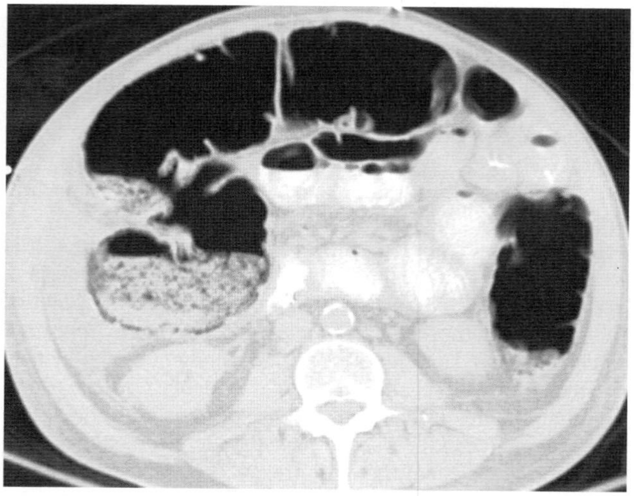

FIGURE 14–2 Computed tomography scan of abdomen, showing pneumatosis of the bowel wall. (Photo courtesy of Stephen Ledbetter, MD, Emergency Radiology Division, Brigham and Women's Hospital, Boston, Massachusetts.)

Barium Studies

With the newer, less-invasive imaging modalities such as ultrasound and CT, the role of barium studies has diminished. They remain useful in aiding in the diagnosis of a carcinoma of the colon, volvulus, as well as determining the extent of mucosal disease in various forms of colitis.

Radionucleotide Scans

Radionucleotide scans came be helpful in localizing the site of bleeding in a patient with presumed GI bleed. Methods include abdominal scintigraphy with [^{99m}Tc]-sulfur colloid and [^{99m}Tc]-labeled red blood cells. Studies have demonstrated the ability to detect bleeding at rates as low as 0.1 mL/min, a rate more sensitive than that of angiography. Whereas angiography can be both diagnostic and therapeutic, radionucleotide scans can be advantageous when bleeding is slow or intermittent.

Endoscopy

The role of endoscopy remains important in the evaluation of the patient with acute abdominal pain. Direct visualization of the GI tract can be both diagnostic and therapeutic. Upper endoscopy can visualize bleeding peptic and duodenal ulcers, as well as outlet obstruction from tumors or strictures. Colonoscopy can reveal inflammation of the colon, neoplasms, intussusception, and volvulus.

Laparoscopy and Laparotomy

Laparoscopy has found an increasing role in the diagnosis and treatment of many patients with abdominal pain. Most commonly, it is used by surgeons when the diagnosis of appendicitis remains unclear, especially in female patients in whom pelvic disease may be included in the differential diagnosis. In addition, patients with acute cholecystitis may undergo laparoscopy as the initial approach in the treatment of their disease. Today, more and more surgeons are using laparoscopy in a variety of their approaches to surgical diseases.

Laparotomy remains the final pathway in many patients with acute abdominal pain. When the patient shows signs of peritonitis or the diagnosis remains unclear with a worsening clinical picture despite a thorough preoperative assessment, abdominal exploration through a midline laparotomy remains the final option.

Presentation of Common Conditions Leading to an Acute Abdomen

Peritonitis (Gastrointestinal Tract Perforation)

Patients with a perforated viscus or peritonitis often have diffuse, severe abdominal tenderness. Their examination is remarkable for guarding and rigidity as well as absence of bowel sounds. These patients also can quickly develop systemic sepsis, and the need for a rapid, accurate diagnosis is paramount. Often an upright kidney-ureter-bladder (KUB) or chest radiograph will reveal the presence of free intraperitoneal air under the diaphragm. If this is discovered, no need exists for further diagnostic studies. The patient must be quickly resuscitated and brought to the operating room for exploratory laparotomy.

Appendicitis

The classic signs and symptoms of appendicitis are mild fever and focal right lower quadrant (McBurney point) pain with rebound tenderness. Anorexia, nausea, and vomiting are common early in the course of the disease. Pain may begin periumbilically and then localize to the right lower quadrant. Patients may report low-grade fever, and a moderate leukocytosis is usually present. A pelvic examination in female patients and a rectal examination in all patients is mandatory. Fecaliths may be found on plain films. Recently, the use of CT has shown promise as a new diagnostic tool for surgeons replacing the more conventional ultrasound (Fig. 14-3).

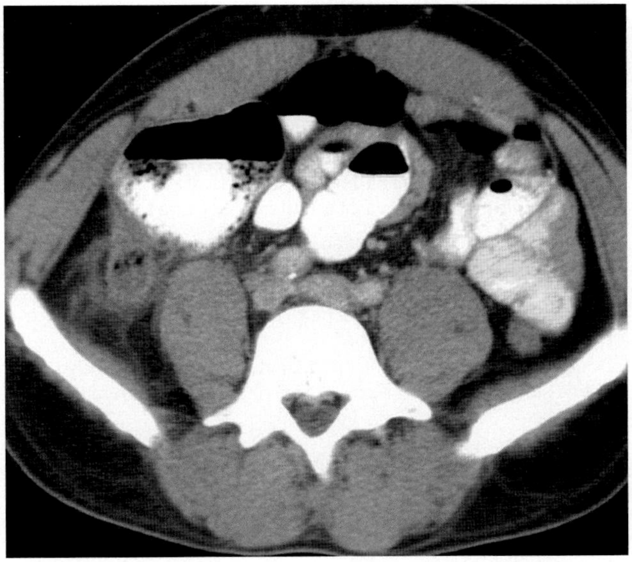

FIGURE 14–3 Computed tomography scan of the abdomen, demonstrating appendicitis. (Photo courtesy of Stephen Ledbetter, MD, Emergency Radiology Division, Brigham and Women's Hospital, Boston, Massachusetts.)

Acute Pancreatitis

Pancreatitis often occurs with a relatively rapid onset of severe epigastric pain, which radiates to the back. Patients also may complain of anorexia, nausea, and vomiting. Tenderness is best elicited in the midepigastric region, and rebound tenderness is not uncommon. Bowel sounds may be hypoactive or absent. Tests that should be ordered include CBC, to determine an elevated white count or a depressed hematocrit due to hemorrhage, as well as a serum amylase and lipase. CT with oral and intravenous contrast is useful to determine the presence of pseudocysts, necrosis, or masses within the gland. Surgery is reserved for patients with an infection or severe pancreatic necrosis.

Cholecystitis

Acute cholecystitis commonly occurs in women between the ages of 40 and 60 years who are overweight and have a previous history of pregnancy. Cholecystitis may be difficult to differentiate from biliary colic, which is often self-limiting. Patients will have right upper quadrant tenderness that is accentuated by inspiration (Murphy's sign) and accompanied by nausea and vomiting. These patients are febrile, and the abdomen may be slightly distended, with guarding. Laboratory tests should include a CBC as well as LFTs, amylase, and lipase. Ultrasound remains the radiographic test of choice to evaluate the gallbladder and biliary tree. Gallstones are often found, frequently accompanied by a thickened-wall gallbladder with pericholecystic fluid. It is important to evaluate the biliary tree to detect dilated ducts or intraductal stones. Hepatobiliary iminodiacetic acid (HIDA) scans can suggest acute cholecystitis if the cystic duct is occluded and the gallbladder fails to take up the radiolabeled bile.

PEARLS FOR THE OR

Laparoscopy versus laparotomy: Laparoscopy is often used for unclear diagnoses in patients with signs of an acute abdomen. Laparoscopic approaches can be quickly converted to a standard laparotomy, if necessary.

Peritonitis/perforation: Patients with signs of peritonitis or found to have perforation of a hollow viscus need surgical intervention.

Appendicitis: Pain that localizes to right lower quadrant accompanied by anorexia, nausea, and vomiting is a classic symptom.

Acute pancreatitis: Patients with acute pancreatitis rarely needs surgical intervention but rather supportive medical care.

Cholecystitis: Laparoscopic approach has been proven safe in both acute and chronic settings.

Diverticulitis: Patients with diverticulitis will require emergency surgery with signs of perforation and significant abscess formation.

Bowel obstruction: Small-bowel obstructions can be initially treated with a nonoperative course including bowel rest and nasogastric suction.

Mesenteric ischemia: Pain out of proportion to physical examination is pathognomonic for mesenteric ischemia.

Ruptured aortic aneurysm: Early detection and intervention are the keys for patient survival.

Gynecologic causes: Ruptured ectopic pregnancy is the most life-threatening gynecologic emergency.

Diverticulitis

Although diverticulosis can occur throughout the colon, diverticulitis most frequently remains limited to the left and sigmoid colon. The incidence of diverticulosis and diverticulitis increases with age. Patients with sigmoid diverticulitis will have left lower quadrant pain that is often accompanied by fever and chills. Examination reveals tenderness in the left lower quadrant and occasionally a palpable mass in the case of a phlegmon. CT with oral contrast is often diagnostic. Interval barium enema or colonoscopy or both provide additional information once the acute inflammatory process has resolved.

Small-Bowel Obstruction

Patients with small-bowel obstruction have nausea, bilious vomiting, and distention. Sharp, colicky abdominal pain is often present as well. In those with advanced stages of the disease, tachycardia, hypotension, and fever may be present. Examination is remarkable for abdominal distention, high-pitched bowel sounds, and a tympanitic abdomen. Laboratory values may reveal hypochloremic, hypokalemic metabolic alkalosis. Supine and upright plain films of the abdomen are very useful for demonstrating dilated loops of small bowel as well as air-fluid levels. CT or an upper GI series can reveal a lead point for the obstruction and may help direct the surgical exploration.

Large-Bowel Obstruction

Patient with large-bowel obstruction have constipation and abdominal distention, and pain is often gradual in onset. The most common causes of large-bowel obstruction include carcinoma of the colon, acute diverticulitis, and volvulus. Physical examination reveals abdominal tenderness and distention. Radiographic tests that aid in the diagnosis include plain films of the abdomen and retrograde contrast studies that help localize the site of obstruction (Fig. 14-4). In the case of volvulus, colonoscopy is both diagnostic and therapeutic.

Mesenteric Ischemia

The presentation of patients with mesenteric ischemia is typically sudden onset of severe abdominal pain. Additional symptoms include nausea, vomiting, diarrhea, and GI bleeding. The classic finding of acute mesenteric ischemia is

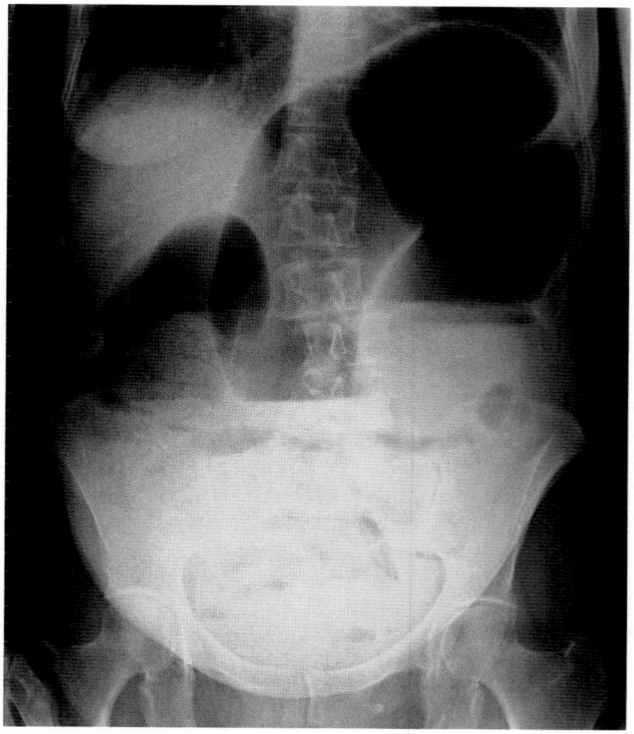

FIGURE 14–4 Plain film of the abdomen, showing large-bowel obstruction with dilated colon. (Photo courtesy of Stephen Ledbetter, MD, Emergency Radiology Division, Brigham and Women's Hospital, Boston, Massachusetts.)

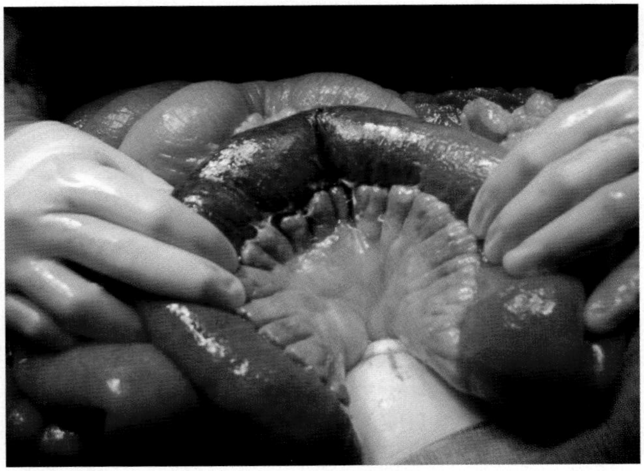

FIGURE 14–5 Intraoperative findings of a patient with ischemic bowel. Note the ischemic segment of small bowel.

pain out of proportion to the amount of tenderness elicited by abdominal palpation. These patients are at risk of suddenly developing signs of overwhelming sepsis with hypotension, tachycardia, and hypovolemia. Plain films are often nondiagnostic. CT can reveal thickened loops of affected bowel with air in the bowel wall (pneumatosis). Once adequately resuscitated, these patients are brought to operation for exploratory laparotomy and removal of diseased bowel (Fig. 14-5).

Ruptured Aortic Abdominal Aneurysm

Patients with ruptured or leaking abdominal aortic aneurysms often have abdominal pain. Their abdominal pain also may be accompanied by back or flank pain. These patients often are first seen in shock and are hypovolemic. On physical examination, a pulsatile supraumbilical mass is present. Patients with known aneurysms who have abdominal pain, shock, and a pulsatile mass are presumed to have ruptured. Although ultrasound, CT, and angiography can confirm the diagnosis, time frequently does not permit obtaining these studies. Surgical intervention with proximal control of the aorta is paramount for their survival.

Gynecologic Causes

Although a variety of gynecologic disorders occur with abdominal pain, the most life-threatening is a ruptured ectopic pregnancy. A detailed gynecologic history should be obtained, and crampy abdominal pain elicited. A pregnancy test should be performed on all women with abdominal pain with the suspicion of a possible pregnancy. Pelvic inflammatory disease is another common cause of acute abdominal pain in female patients between the ages of 15 and 35 years. Patients have crampy lower-quadrant pain and high fever. Most have had a history of pelvic inflammatory disease. Pelvic examination reveals a hyperemic, extremely tender cervix with vaginal discharge. A positive diagnosis can be made with a cervical smear and culture. Ultrasound is useful for the diagnosis of tuboovarian abscess. Other gynecologic causes of acute abdominal pain include ovarian cysts, endometriosis, ovarian torsion, and ruptured uterus.

Nonsurgical Causes

It is important to emphasize that patients with an acute abdomen require surgical intervention. The list of nonsurgical causes is extensive and must be considered before committing a patient to any surgical intervention. Cardiac causes of abdominal pain include acute myocardial infarction and pericarditis. Pulmonary causes include pneumonia of either right or left lower lobes, pleuritis, or pleural effusions. Common GI causes of acute abdominal pain include gastroenteritis, biliary colic, ulcerative colitis, or Crohn's disease. Several urologic conditions can be associated with abdominal pain. These include pyelonephritis, urolithiasis, and renal cysts. Sickle cell anemia is a common hematologic cause of acute abdominal pain. Infectious agents such as *Salmonella* and *Shigella* can produce severe abdominal pain that is usually self-limited. In addition, a patient with acquired immunodeficiency syndrome may have a variety of secondary causes for acute abdominal pain such as cytomegalovirus enterocolitis, lymphoma, Kaposi's sarcoma, and tuberculosis of the GI tract.

Suggested Reading

Eskelinen M, Ikonen J, Liponen P: Contribution of history-taking, physical examination, and computer assistance to diagnose small bowel obstruction: A prospective study of 1333 patients with acute abdominal pain. Scand J Gastroenterol 29:715, 1994.

Memon MA, Fitzgibbons RJ Jr: The role of minimal access surgery in the acute abdomen. Surg Clin North Am 77:1333–1353, 1997.

Silen W: Cope's Early Diagnosis of the Acute Abdomen, 20th ed. New York, Oxford University Press, 2000.

Sucher JF, MacFadyen BV Jr: Imaging modalities for acute abdominal pain. Semin Laparosc Surg 9:3–9, 2002.

Yousaf M, McCallion K, Diamond T: Management of severe acute pancreatitis. Br J Surg. 90:407–420, 2003.

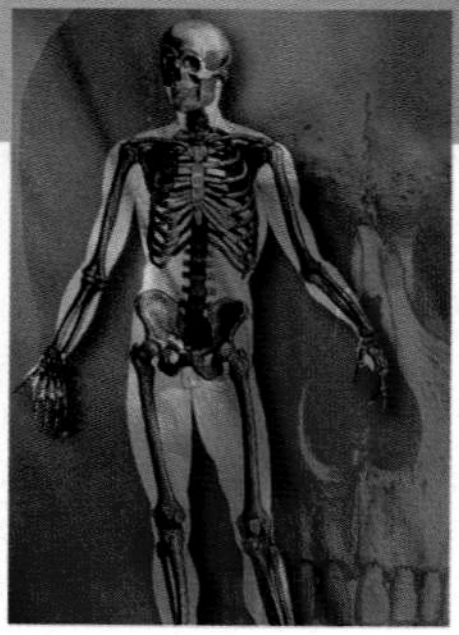

Chapter 15
Appendicitis

MARK E. STOKER, MD

For generations, appendicitis has challenged clinicians. Despite tremendous advances in technology and basic science, this commonplace disease often eludes prompt and accurate diagnosis. This is partly due to the extensive differential diagnosis and varied presentation. A stepwise and logical approach to the diagnosis of acute appendicitis should be possible with a proper understanding of the pathophysiology and with close attention to a detailed history and physical examination and an evidence-based diagnostic evaluation.

The appendix in some lower species plays a role in the digestive process; however, in humans, the appendix has traditionally been thought of as a vestigial organ with little function. More recently it has been thought to have a role in the secretory immune system of the gut. A large number of lymphoid follicles exist, which are part of the gut-associated lymphoid tissue (GALT) producing secretory immunoglobulins. The clinical significance of this is unclear. No clear evidence exists of alteration in immune function after appendectomy.

Surgical Anatomy

The appendix is derived from the caudal portion of the embryonic midgut. During fetal development, it rotates posterior and medial as the cecum enlarges. The base of the appendix begins at the confluence of the three tinea coli and lies about 2.5 cm inferior to the ileocecal valve. The appendix can vary from 2 cm to 22 cm in length. The appendiceal artery arises from the ileocolic artery and travels posterior to the terminal ileum or cecum through the mesoappendix. In the newborn and small child, the appendix has a funnel shape with a wide orifice and comparatively short length. The appendix lengthens, and its orifice narrows with age. This may account for the relative rarity of appendicitis in infants and small children. The base of the appendix is fairly constant in its anatomic position. However, the body and the tip of the appendix may vary considerably in their locations. The appendix may lie in the normal anterior intraperitoneal position. It also may be found in atypical or "hidden" positions such as retrocecal (intraperitoneal or retroperitoneal) or pelvic. The so-called hidden positions may be a cause of atypical presentation and result in an increased risk of perforation because of delayed diagnosis. The position of the appendix also may be altered during pregnancy. With enlargement of the gravid uterus, the appendix will rise above the iliac crest by 5 months of gestation and may lie as high as the right upper quadrant at term.

Incidence, Etiology, and Pathogenesis

It is estimated that in Western populations, the lifetime risk of developing acute appendicitis is approximately 7%. The incidence of appendicitis varies greatly with age. Appendicitis is primarily a disease of adolescents and young adults. It is quite rare in newborns and young children younger than 5 years. The incidence of appendicitis also declines after age 30 years and has an incidence of less than 1% after age 70 years. Acute appendicitis has a slightly higher male predominance in the second and third decades of life. Before puberty and after 30 years, the incidence is roughly equal. Over the past several decades, the true incidence of appendicitis appears to have declined. The cause of this decline is unclear. Some geographic differences appear in the rates of appendicitis, which may be related to dietary factors such as higher levels of dietary fiber and unprocessed foods in less-developed regions. Improvements in reporting can account for only part of this decline.

Obstruction of the appendiceal lumen is seen in approximately 70% of cases of appendicitis. The appendiceal lumen can be obstructed by fecaliths, foreign bodies, tumors, parasites, and lymphoid hyperplasia. The number of lymphoid follicles in the vermiform appendix peaks between ages 10 and 30 years, which coincides with the maximal incidence of appendicitis. Obstruction alone does not account for all cases of obstruction of the lumen of the appendix. Conversely, chronic obstruction by the presence of a long-standing fecalith is often noted in patients who remain asymptomatic. Diverticula and duplications also are seen as rare causes of appendicitis.

In cases of appendiceal obstruction, the pathophysiology is probably similar to that of a closed-loop intestinal obstruction. After obstruction of the appendiceal lumen, mucosal secretions by the lining cells of the appendix continue. Bacterial overgrowth and increasing intraluminal pressure follow. As a result of increasing intraluminal pressure, the surface tension on the wall of the appendix increases. This produces vascular congestion, which ultimately leads to ulceration, necrosis, gangrene, and perforation.

Microbiology

The bacterial flora of the appendix in the healthy state closely mimics that of the colonic environment. Numerous species of both aerobic and anaerobic bacteria have been reported within the normal and diseased appendix. Quantitative cultures obtained at the time of surgery reveal a higher number of aerobic and a higher percentage of anaerobic bacteria in acute appendicitis when compared with those in incidental appendectomy.

Escherichia coli is by far the most commonly found gram-negative organism (67%–75%). *Klebsiella oxytoca*, *Serratia marcescens*, *Enterobacter* spp., and *Acinetobacter* spp. are among other gram-negative aerobes encountered. *Bacteroides fragilis* is the most common anaerobic organism encountered in acute appendicitis. *Pseudomonas* has been reported in 5% to 30% of cases. *Enterococcus* is seen in between 1% and 35% of cases. *Enterococcus* and *Pseudomonas* are more commonly seen in hospitalized patients and those receiving prior antibiotic therapy. It is important to stress that in most cases of appendicitis, the infections are polymicrobial, so the use of intraoperative cultures in acute appendicitis has been shown to be of little benefit. Granulomatous appendicitis also has been reported to be caused by *Yersinia*.

In recent decades, increasing trends toward unusual and opportunistic infections have been seen. The United States and other developed countries have seen an increasing incidence of tuberculosis and human immunodeficiency virus (HIV) infection as well as an increased use of immunosuppressive drugs. As a result, the number of once rare cases of *Mycobacterium*, *Cytomegalovirus*, and other uncommon infectious agents is increasing.

Diagnosis

Over the past several decades, many technical and scientific advances have been made in the treatment of various surgical diseases. Despite these advances, appendicitis still remains a challenge to the clinician. In acute appendicitis, history and physical examination alone should establish a correct diagnosis in the majority of cases. Appendicitis may have a broad range of signs and symptoms. Anatomic variations such as a retrocecal location and pregnancy may render the classic history and physical examination less reliable. At the extremes of age, the diagnosis becomes more difficult because of the relative rarity of the appendicitis. The incidence of perforation in adolescents or young adults is approximately 20%. However, perforation can be seen in as many as 50% of cases in patients younger than 6 years or older than 60 years. One factor that contributes to this diagnostic challenge is the very large differential diagnosis.

History

The evolution of the signs and symptoms of appendicitis closely follow its pathologic progression. Abdominal pain is the most common symptom in acute appendicitis (95%–99%). Early in the disease course, the pain is usually mild to moderate in severity and diffuse in location. The pain may be steady, or it may be intermittent and colicky. These are the hallmarks of visceral pain mediated by the autonomic nervous system and probably reflect obstruction of the appendiceal lumen with increasing intraluminal pressure. After a time, which may vary between 1 and 12 hours, the pain will usually migrate to the right lower quadrant and become more intense. This is somatic pain, mediated by spinal nerves, and will therefore be localized to the site of inflammation. If the inflamed appendix lies in a retrocecal location, the pain may be predominantly in the right flank or back. The appendix may come to lie in the pelvis or left lower quadrant, producing pain in these locations.

Approximately 90% of patients will report anorexia, and most will complain of nausea. Vomiting and diarrhea may be present but are usually not excessive. In small children, frequent diarrhea may be more commonly seen than in an adult population. If vomiting precedes abdominal pain or if anorexia is not present, the diagnosis of appendicitis should be questioned.

With the progression of appendicitis, the pain is often described as being located near **McBurney's point**. McBurney's point is located in the right lower quadrant, two thirds of the distance from the umbilicus to the anterior superior iliac spine. It is important to recognize that approximately 25% of patients with appendicitis have right-lower-quadrant pain as their initial symptom without a prodrome of visceral symptoms. Altogether as many as 50% of patients may have some variation from the classic presentation of appendicitis.

Physical Examination

In acute appendicitis, the physical examination is of the utmost importance and should supersede all else in the diagnosis. Laboratory and radiologic evaluation should serve as supplemental tools to the diagnosis but never replace a properly conducted history and physical examination. Fever should be present in 75% to 85% of all patients with acute appendicitis. A patient's temperature will rarely be higher than 38°C unless the appendix is grossly perforated. Vital signs are usually normal, with the exception of a slight tachycardia, which can be present secondary to pain, fever, or dehydration. In advanced cases of appendicitis with gross peritonitis, in the elderly or mentally infirmed, signs of sepsis and shock, including hypotension, may be present. The later, however, is an exception and should be seen in only a minority of cases.

On initial observation, patients with acute appendicitis prefer to lie motionless as a response to local peritonitis. This is in contrast to patients with colicky-type pain, who may appear restless. The maximal area of tenderness will often be at McBurney's point unless the appendix lies in an atypical location, as mentioned earlier. Patients will often be initially seen with "referred pain," also known as **Rovsing's sign**. This sign is demonstrated by palpation of the left lower quadrant, which produces right-lower-quadrant pain. Voluntary guarding and signs of peritonitis are typical findings in appendicitis. The most classically taught maneuver to diagnose peritonitis is an evaluation for **rebound tenderness**. The rebound examination is performed by deep palpation in the right lower quadrant, followed by a sudden release. This maneuver will produce sudden voluntary guarding because of the irritation of the inflamed peritoneal surfaces. A false-positive rebound examination can be seen because this maneuver will often frighten an already anxious patient. Indirect measures of peritonitis may often be more reliable. Having a patient cough will often elicit right-lower-quadrant guarding. Coughing is a maneuver that most patients do not automatically associate with abdominal pain, and this may more reliably demonstrate true peritonitis. A positive **psoas sign** may indicate an inflamed appendix lying anterior to the psoas muscle. This sign is best demonstrated by extension of the hip or flexion against resistance. Similarly, an **obturator sign** is produced by stretching this muscle with passive internal rotation of the thigh, with the hip in a flexed position. Both the psoas and obturator signs are nonspecific and are present only on occasion.

The finding of a mass in the right lower quadrant often indicates advanced disease with abscess formation. Often a mass effect will be present without an abscess, because of the inflamed omentum and adjacent loops of bowel attempting to wall off the inflammatory process.

A pelvic examination is a critical part of the evaluation of the patient with a suspicion of appendicitis. The pelvic examination is important to rule out gynecologic pathology such as pelvic inflammatory disease. In female patients of reproductive age, the accurate diagnosis of appendicitis can be much more challenging. Negative laparotomy rates in women have been reported as high as 20% to 50%.

A rectal examination also is important in evaluating any patient with abdominal pain. If the appendix is in an intraabdominal or retrocecal position, the rectal examination will be negative. Tenderness on a rectal examination is most commonly seen when the inflamed appendix lies within the pelvis. Gross blood found on fecal examination should be quite rare and lead to the consideration of other diagnoses.

Laboratory Tests

An array of laboratory tests is available to the clinician in the evaluation of the patient with acute abdominal pain. However, when appendicitis is suspected, only a few tests are necessary. The most common laboratory determination is a total white blood cell (WBC) count with a differential count. The majority of patients with appendicitis will have a mild to moderate leukocytosis. A white blood cell count greater than 18,000 to 20,000/cc should raise the concern of perforation. Occasionally, a WBC count within normal range will be seen, but often a left shift will be found, with an increased percentage of polymorphonuclear cells. Approximately 85% to 90% of patients should have an elevation in their WBC count or a left shift. In an otherwise healthy individual, the absence of an elevation in the WBC count should bring into question the accuracy of a diagnosis of appendicitis.

Urinalysis is often helpful to rule out urinary tract infection and renal calculi. A small percentage of patients with appendicitis may have leukocytes, bacteria, and red blood cells in their urine if an inflamed appendix is in proximity to the bladder or ureter. In women of childbearing age, a pregnancy test is important. Ectopic pregnancy is always in the differential diagnosis in this subset of patients. It also is important to identify the woman who has a normal intrauterine pregnancy if she does require more invasive testing or surgical intervention. Appendicitis in pregnancy is discussed later in this chapter.

Most recent developments in laboratory testing for appendicitis have shown little clinical promise. Quantitative levels of interleukin-6 and C-reactive protein have been shown to be elevated in appendicitis. One drawback is their lack of routine availability and slow turnover time in most laboratories.

Radiologic Imaging

History and physical examination should establish or rule out appendicitis in the majority of patients. Radiologic testing becomes more important when the diagnosis is in question. The most common radiographic examination done in the evaluation of abdominal pain is the plain abdominal film or KUB (kidney-ureter-bladder). Radiographs in a supine and upright position are often used in combination. Upright films may demonstrate air/fluid levels associated with a small-bowel obstruction or free air under the diaphragm in the case of a perforated viscus. Findings that may be consistent with appendicitis are a localized ileus, altered right psoas shadow (Fig. 15-1), or a calcified density in the right lower quadrant consistent with fecalith. It must be noted that these findings are nonspecific. In appendicitis, a barium contrast enema may show nonfilling of the appendix; however, this finding will be present in a large number of healthy patients. A barium enema also may show effacement of the cecum by an inflammatory mass. As these findings are

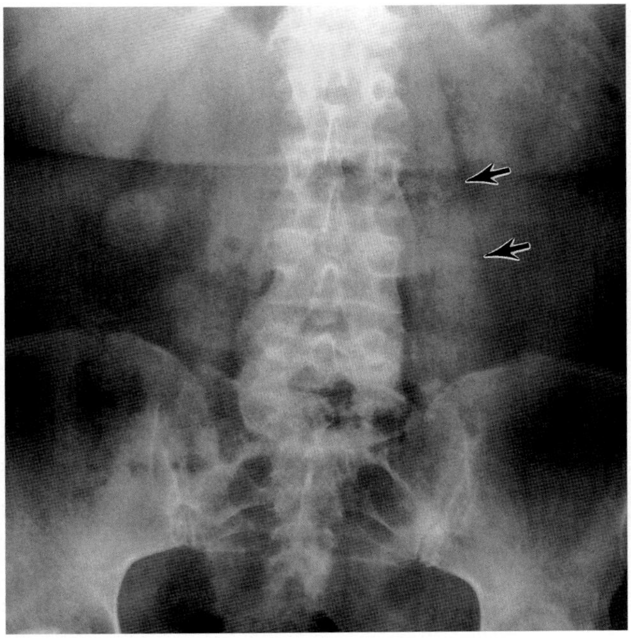

FIGURE 15–1 Kidney-ureter-bladder film demonstrating absence of the right psoas shadow. Note left psoas shadow (*arrows*).

somewhat unreliable, barium enema should be considered only when colon pathology is suspected and should not be part of the routine diagnostic workup for appendicitis.

Nuclear medicine scans have been proposed as a means of localizing an acute and inflammatory process and thereby aiding in the diagnosis of appendicitis. Some clinical trials have shown that technetium 99m hexamethylpropylene amine oxime–tagged leukocyte scan is as high as 95% sensitive and 85% specific. Other trials have failed to demonstrate this level of diagnostic accuracy, and as a result, this type of study has not achieved widespread acceptance.

The use of ultrasound has been widely studied to evaluate patients with right-lower-quadrant and pelvic pain. It is most useful in female patients of childbearing age to rule out pelvic pathology. Its accuracy in appendicitis varies greatly between clinical trials. Ultrasound is very operator dependent. It requires a skilled and dedicated technician to perform the examination adequately. Therefore the results may be less reproducible. In a recent meta-analysis comprising 17 clinical reports of 3358 patients, the overall sensitivity was 84.7%, and the specificity was 92.1%. From this study, it was apparent that the value of ultrasonography was dependent on the likelihood of appendicitis, as determined by history and physical examination. If the clinical impression was highly suggestive of appendicitis, a negative ultrasound could have misled clinicians (negative predictive value, 59%). The opposite was seen if the clinical impression for appendicitis was low, and a high false-positive rate was seen (19%). In this large review, ultrasound was most useful when the probability of appendicitis was indeterminate. Ultrasound also has been widely evaluated in children and in pregnant women. These studies have shown a slightly higher accuracy in these groups. Graded compression ultrasound in pregnant women has produced the best results. With this technique, any large tubular structure seen in the right lower quadrant is compressed with the ultrasound probe. If it is seen to be noncompressible and tender to this evaluation, this is consistent with appendicitis (Fig. 15-2*A* and *B*). Again it must be emphasized that the accuracy of the ultrasound is dependent on the skill and dedication of the ultrasound technician.

Computer tomography (CT) is highly accurate for the diagnosis of appendicitis. Positive and negative predictive values of 95% or greater have been demonstrated. The techniques of the scan can be critical to its results. In standard CT scans of the abdomen, sections of 8 mm to 10 mm are routine. When performing a CT scan for appendicitis, thin sections (2–5 mm) are critical. Oral and rectal contrasts have been shown to increase the diagnostic accuracy of CT, but many authorities consider this unnecessary to diagnose appendicitis. The typical findings of appendicitis are fat streaking in the right lower quadrant consistent with the acute inflammatory response. The appendix itself may be visualized as a thick and inflamed structure (Figs. 15-3, 15-4, and 15-5). Effacement of the cecum or a mass effect in the right lower quadrant may be seen. Some of these findings may be nonspecific, however, when put into the context of the proper clinical picture. CT scanning is the diagnostic modality of choice in many institutions. CT will also disclose other processes such as

PEARLS FOR ROUNDS

The classic history of diffuse periumbilical pain migrating to become more-intense right-lower-quadrant (RLQ) pain is present in only 50% of cases.

Frequency of signs and symptoms: Abdominal pain, 95% to 99%; anorexia, 90%; elevated white blood cell (WBC) count (or simple shift) plus fever, 90%; nausea, vomiting, and/or diarrhea, 85%.

Rebound tenderness is defined as voluntary guarding with sudden release after deep palpation.

Rovsing's sign is defined as referred tenderness and guarding in the RLQ with palpation in the LLQ.

Psoas sign is seen when pain is elicited with flexion of the hip or extension against resistance.

Fever higher than 38°C and WBC more than 20,000 often denotes perforation.

Appendicitis has an extensive differential diagnosis.

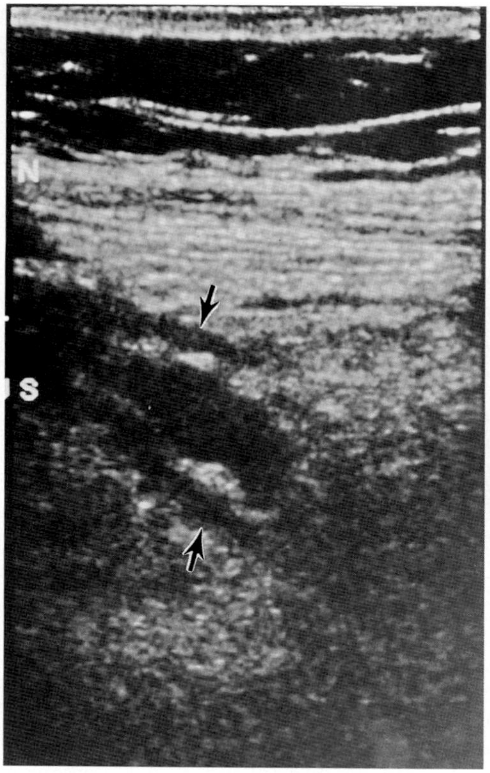

A

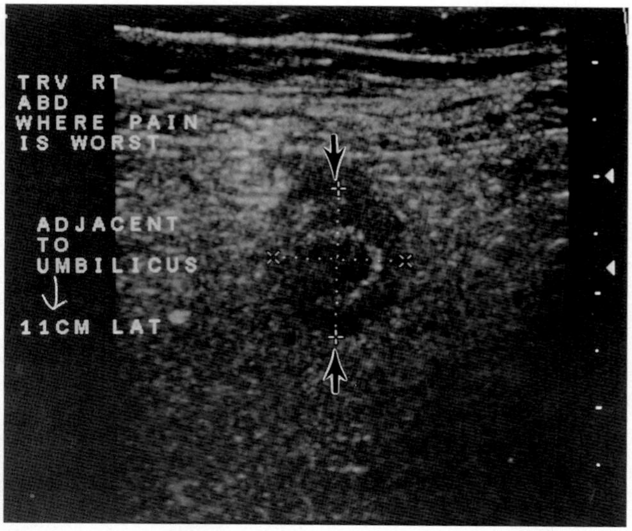

B

FIGURE 15–2 Ultrasound views of inflamed appendix. *A*, Longitudinal view. Hypodense edema surrounding the inflamed appendix (*arrows*). *B*, Transverse view. Inflammatory mass (*arrows*).

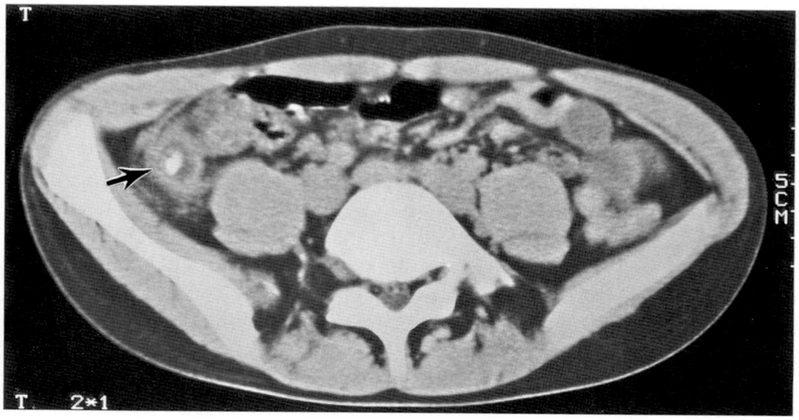

FIGURE 15–3 Computed tomographic appearance of acute appendicitis. Note the calcified fecalith (*arrow*) and the inflammatory fat streaks surrounding the appendix.

periappendiceal abscess, phlegmon, and diverticulitis. The accuracy of a CT scan may be somewhat diminished in very thin adults or small children in whom the fat planes are less prominent, and therefore the CT signs of inflammation may be less pronounced. CT scan has been safely used in pregnancy. However, it may be prudent to avoid this modality during the first trimester, although little hard evidence exists that is detrimental.

Treatment

Antibiotics

Antibiotic use has been most widely studied as an adjunct to surgical appendectomy and is not ordinarily considered a primary treatment. Several small studies have shown success in treating acute appendicitis with antibiotics alone. A high rate of recurrence should be expected if this

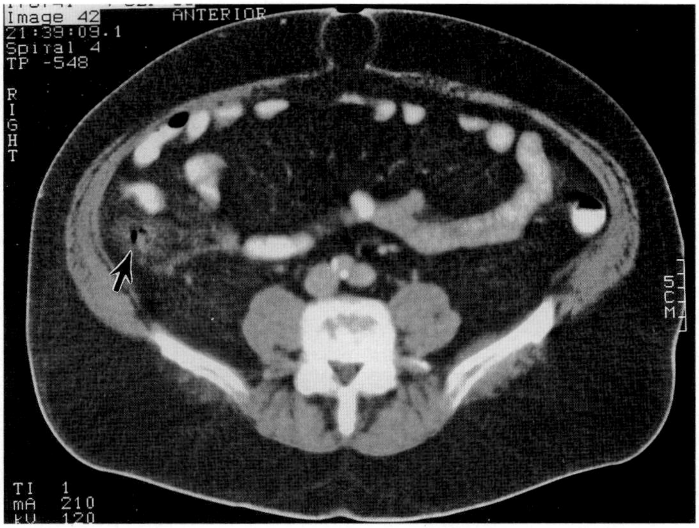

FIGURE 15–4 Computed tomographic appearance documenting "free air" and fat streaking associated with perforated appendicitis.

course of therapy is followed. Surgical removal of the appendix is considered the established standard of care.

Infectious complications due to appendicitis and after appendectomy are the most frequent types of complications seen. These complications can be as simple as minor wound infections or as serious as life-threatening septic shock with multisystem organ failure infection.

The types, indications, and durations of treatment with antibiotic therapy have been the sources of numerous studies and considerable controversy. The most widely accepted use of antibiotics is for wound prophylaxis. Little doubt exists that a single dose of a broad-spectrum antibiotic before surgical intervention will decrease the risk of wound infection substantially. In patients not receiving antibiotic prophylaxis, wound-infection rates have been seen between 9% and 30% in early appendicitis. In late appendicitis, the wound-infection rate approaches 80%. Prophylactic antibiotics administered before appendectomy have been shown to decrease the incidence of wound infection to less than 5% in noncomplicated appendicitis.

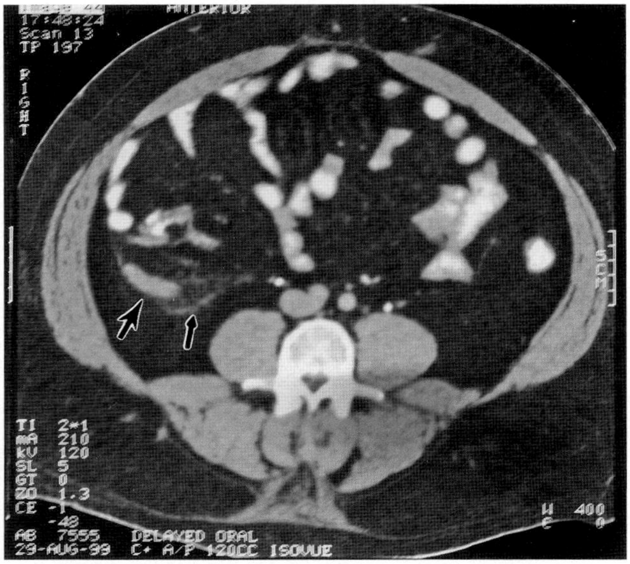

FIGURE 15–5 Computed tomographic appearance of acute appendicitis. *Large arrow* designates the appendix. *Small arrow* marks fat streaking of acute inflammation.

Numerous studies have evaluated the efficacy of different antibiotic agents in the treatment of appendicitis. Aminoglycosides have been used for many decades, have excellent gram-negative coverage, and are inexpensive; however, the cost of monitoring drug levels adds to the total cost of their use. Aminoglycosides carry a risk of ototoxicity of approximately 10% and up to a 25% incidence of nephrotoxicity. Aztreonam has a spectrum of activity similar to that of aminoglycosides against gram-negative aerobic organisms. Ototoxicity, nephrotoxicity, and drug-level monitoring are not a concern with aztreonam. It is therefore considered an excellent choice for combination therapy with either clindamycin or metronidazole (as an agent for the treatment of anaerobic organisms). Cephalosporins have been extensively studied as single-agent broad-spectrum drugs. As single agents, they are less complicated to administer and have, in general, low drug toxicity. Second-generation cephalosporins such as cefotetan and cefoxitin are widely recommended for use in gastrointestinal infections such as appendicitis. Cefamandole and cefoperazone have a lower level of activity against *Bacteroides fragilis* and should not be considered as first-choice drugs for appendicitis. Quinolones such as ciprofloxacin are effective against a wide

PEARLS FOR THE OR

- Administer prophylactic antibiotics before incision.
- Operative approaches include oblique (McBurney) incision, transverse (Rocky-Davis) incision, midline laparotomy, and laparoscopy.
- Location of the appendix may vary between the right lower quadrant (RLQ), pelvic, or retrocecal positions. The tip of the appendix may lie in the RUQ or LLQ.
- The base of the appendix is located at the junction of the three tenia.
- The appendiceal artery lies posterior to the cecum or terminal ileum.
- If appendicitis is not present, a thorough search for other pathology is important (Meckel's, pelvic inflammatory disease, ovarian cyst, etc.)
- In advanced appendicitis or perforation, search for concomitant abscess (pelvic, paracolic gutter, intraloop).
- Consider open packing of the wound for advanced and perforated appendicitis.

variety of aerobic gram-positive and gram-negative bacteria. Quinolones are often used in combination with a second drug such metronidazole, targeting anaerobic organisms. Antibiotics such as imipenem are very effective as single-agent antibiotics. These drugs are often reserved for cases of overwhelming sepsis and hospital-acquired infection and should not be used in routine uncomplicated appendicitis.

The duration of antibiotic therapy has been less well studied. In early appendicitis, a single dose of a prophylactic preoperative antibiotic may suffice as the only therapy. In more complicated appendicitis, postoperative antibiotics may be administered for a very brief course (1 day). In cases of perforated appendicitis, a full 7- to 10-day course of antibiotics is recommended. Often the duration of antibiotic therapy is based on clinical grounds. Antibiotics are often administered until the patient is afebrile for a period of 24 to 48 hours and has made clinical improvement.

Surgical Appendectomy

The gold standard for the treatment of appendicitis is exploratory laparotomy and appendectomy. This has changed little since pioneers such as McBurney made their initial recommendations for prompt diagnosis and surgery in appendicitis. A number of different operative approaches can be taken in appendicitis. Laparotomy can be accomplished through a McBurney incision. This is an oblique incision, which divides the fascia parallel to its fibers, and a muscle-splitting technique is used. A right-lower-quadrant transverse "Rocky-Davis" incision is preferred by many. If the diagnosis were in question, especially in the elderly where other disease processes may be encountered, many surgeons would prefer a lower midline laparotomy incision.

Traditional surgical techniques involve ligation of the appendiceal stump and appendiceal artery and, on occasion, inversion of the appendiceal stump into the cecum with a pursestring-type suture. More recently, surgical staplers have been used to ligate and divide the appendiceal stump. In cases of advanced appendicitis in which the cecum itself has been damaged, a partial cecectomy is occasionally necessary.

A widespread controversy exists over the use of surgical drains in appendicitis. Despite this controversy, some standard recommendations can be made. Intraabdominal drains are usually indicated if a well-formed intraabdominal or pelvic abscess is encountered. Wound drains are to be discouraged. If a case of perforated appendicitis with generalized peritonitis is encountered, the wound should be considered grossly contaminated and packed open for closure by secondary intention or a delayed primary closure.

Periappendiceal Abscess

When the patient with advanced appendicitis is first seen late in the disease course, a well-formed periappendiceal abscess may be present. The optimal treatment of periappendiceal abscess is somewhat controversial. One method of treatment is to perform a CT-guided percutaneous drainage, administer intravenous antibiotic, and perform a delayed "interval appendectomy" when the acute infection has been controlled. This interval appendectomy would usually be performed 4 to 6 weeks after percutaneous drainage. The rationale behind this mode of treatment is to decrease the morbidity of exploration in the presence of an acute septic process. This approach, however, has been demonstrated to increase the length of hospital stay, the cost of treatment, and the duration of illness. With modern supportive care and antibiotic therapy, surgical drainage and appendectomy should be well tolerated by most patients.

Negative Appendectomy

If an exploration for appendicitis has yielded a normal appendix, a thorough search should be made for other pathology including Meckel diverticulum or ovarian cyst (Box 15-1). Consideration should be given to incidental appendectomy with certain exceptions. Incidental appendectomy should not be performed if Crohn's colitis is found to be affecting the cecum, as the incidences of fistulization may be quite high. If other septic processes such as perforated sigmoid diverticulitis are found, they should be treated primarily. The appendix has been used recently in some reconstructive surgeries, and therefore incidental appendectomy has come into question.

Laparoscopy and Laparoscopic Appendectomy

Laparoscopy has been used for many decades to evaluate women with pelvic pathology. In the past decade, with the

BOX 15–1 Differential Diagnosis for Acute Appendicitis

Gastrointestinal
Regional enteritis
Ulcerative colitis
Mesenteric adenitis
Meckel's diverticulitis
Diverticulitis coli
Peptic ulcer
Gastroenteritis
Intussusception
Cholecystitis
Pancreatitis

Gynecologic
Ovarian cyst
Pelvic inflammatory disease
Ectopic pregnancy
Endometriosis
Ovarian torsion

Urologic
Renal stone
Urinary tract infection
Testicular torsion
Epididymitis
Pyelonephritis

Neoplastic
Carcinoid
Colon carcinoma
Lymphoma
Ovarian carcinoma
Pseudomyoma peritonei

Vascular
Aortic and iliac aneurysm
Mesenteric ischemia

Neurogenic
Herpes zoster

Medical
Diabetes
Hepatitis
Sickle cell anemia
Henoch-Schönlein purpura
Sarcoidosis
Porphyria

Other
Spontaneous bacterial peritonitis
Trauma
Lead poisoning
Spider bite

advent of miniature video-chip cameras and refinement in surgical instruments and surgical techniques, surgeons have been performing more advanced laparoscopic abdominal procedures. As a diagnostic procedure, laparoscopy is by far the most accurate, but it also is invasive. In a number of randomized studies to determine the efficacy of laparoscopic appendectomy, many have failed to show a significant advantage of laparoscopic appendectomy over traditional appendectomy. The data from many of these studies show a slightly decreased length of hospital stay but longer operative times and subsequently higher cost. An improvement in postoperative pain control and decreased narcotic use is not found. A slightly faster return to normal physical activity occurs after laparoscopy. With laparoscopic appendectomy, the infection rate seems to be decreased when compared with that of open laparotomy: 4% to 7% versus 8% to 12%. This difference can be partially explained by the preference of many surgeons for laparotomy in cases of perforated appendicitis. The disadvantage of laparoscopy appears to be slightly higher incidences of intraoperative complications. These include trocar injuries, intraoperative hemorrhage, and other technical misadventures. This slightly higher incidence of complications may be attributable to a longer learning curve with laparoscopic appendectomy. With experience, the operative time tends to be very consistent with that of open appendectomy, and the complication rates are low. Many experienced surgeons perform laparoscopic appendectomy for the majority of patients with acute appendicitis. This approach is especially useful in several clinical settings: (1) when the diagnosis is in question, (2) in women of reproductive age, (3) in obese patients in whom laparotomy is more difficult, and (4) in the elderly for whom other disease processes are more common (for example, diverticulitis and malignancy). In young male patients in whom a diagnostic accuracy of 90% is seen, the advantage of laparoscopy is less clear. In small children in whom recovery from appendectomy is so rapid, laparoscopy also has less of an advantage, although it remains useful as a diagnostic procedure.

Postoperative Care

In early appendicitis, postoperative care and hospitalization should be minimized. As previously mentioned, antibiotic therapy in early appendicitis should not be prolonged. Postoperative ileus and recovery from small lower-quadrant incision should be rapid. Many of these patients can be progressed to a diet and discharge within 24 to 48 hours of appendectomy. In more advanced cases of appendicitis, postoperative ileus is not uncommon. When perforation is encountered, a longer course of antibiotics, wound care, and hospitalization is the norm. As with any abdominal surgery, early ambulation, pulmonary toilet, and deep venous thrombosis prophylaxis should be considered.

Complications

Complications after appendectomy are largely related to the health of the patient and progression of the disease at the time of diagnosis and treatment. Technical complications are the exception to this rule and should be uncommon.

Septic complications are by far the most frequently seen problem after appendectomy. The wound-infection rate ranges between 1% and 15% in early nonperforated appendicitis. If perforation has occurred, the wound-infection rate may be as high as 25% to 80%. It is, therefore, common practice to pack these wounds open and to allow the wound to close by secondary intention or to consider a delayed primary closure. Once a wound infection is diagnosed, the primary treatment is to open the wound and to allow drainage of purulent material. If cellulitis is present, administration of antibiotics is indicated. Rapidly spreading abdominal-wall infections such as necrotizing fasciitis, are less common but potentially life threatening. Early recognition, aggressive surgical débridement, and administration of broad-spectrum antibiotics are critical, as these infections carry a high morbidity and mortality rate.

The formation of an intraabdominal abscess after appendectomy is less common than wound infection but has higher morbidity. An abscess is the result of the abdominal host defenses attempting to isolate or "wall-off" an infectious threat. An abscess after appendicitis most commonly forms in the right paracolic gutter, pelvis, or intraloop position in the small bowel. Drainage and antibiotics are the treatments for postoperative abscess. A pelvic abscess can be drained through the rectum, sparing a laparotomy. Other abscesses may require reexploration. The most common treatment for postoperative abscess is CT-guided catheter drainage. This modality is safe and highly effective. On occasion, an intraloop abscess will require surgical drainage, but most should be managed successfully with CT drainage.

Pylephlebitis is the radiographic finding of air in the portal vein. This is a rare presentation of an advanced septic process due to gas-forming organisms. It is most often seen in the elderly, immunocompromised host or in advanced sepsis. This is often a preterminal finding. Septic shock and adult respiratory distress syndrome also are signs of advanced sepsis.

Technical complications of appendectomy should be less common but are nonetheless important. Surgical injury to adjacent structures such as a ureter, bowel, and major vessel may occur. Fistula formation from the appendiceal stump is rare but may be seen if the cecum is grossly involved in the inflammatory process or inadequate technique is used to ligate the stump. Long-term problems such as incisional hernia formation and intestinal obstruction secondary to adhesions may occur. Infertility in young women is a possible sequela of perforation.

Appendicitis in Special Circumstances

Appendicitis and Acquired Immunodeficiency Syndrome

In general, patients with acquired immunodeficiency syndrome (AIDS) from HIV infection pose a unique diagnostic and therapeutic challenge. Patients with HIV infection and a normal lymphocyte count who have relatively intact immune systems can be treated and evaluated as would be any other patient with suspected appendicitis. However, patients with AIDS have a somewhat more complex differential diagnosis. This includes bacterial, parasitic, fungal, and viral infections. Lymphoma and Kaposi's sarcoma also have been reported as being seen with symptoms of appendicitis. Symptoms in the AIDS patient are often more vague and longer in duration than usually seen in otherwise healthy individuals. Immunosuppressed patients often do not have a fever or elevated WBC count. In this subset of patients, laparoscopy can be very helpful in establishing the diagnosis of appendicitis. As in all patients with appendicitis, prompt diagnosis and appendectomy are essential.

Appendicitis in Pregnancy

Appendicitis is seen in approximately 1 in 2000 pregnancies. It is the most common nonobstetric emergency in pregnant women. The diagnosis of appendicitis in pregnancy can be challenging. The normal leukocytosis of pregnancy makes the WBC count unreliable, but a left shift can be seen in pregnant women with appendicitis. Ultrasonography is one of the most common diagnostic modalities, as it is considered safe during pregnancy and also may rule out other pathology. If they are clinically indicated, the clinician should not be deterred from obtaining conventional diagnostic radiographs such as a KUB or even CT scans, as the risk to the fetus is negligible after the first trimester of pregnancy. An important point to consider is that the pregnant patient may have symptoms of appendicitis that do not correlate with the normal location of pain in the nonpregnant female. During pregnancy, the appendix rises out of the right lower quadrant as the uterus enlarges, and at term, it may reside in the right upper quadrant. Prompt diagnosis and early appendectomy are crucial, as perforation increases the risk of fetal death. Laparoscopy has been shown to be safe during pregnancy.

Appendicitis in the Young and Elderly

The diagnosis of appendicitis in patients younger than 6 years and older than 70 years is often delayed. The reason for the delay is diagnosis is usually multifactorial. Appendicitis is often not considered very high on the differential diagnosis in patients in these age groups. The presenting symptoms in these age groups are often more vague and may mislead clinicians. In the extremes of age, perforation is much more common. At the age of peak incidence, approximately 20% of patients will be initially seen with perforation. At the extremes of age, the frequency of perforation has been reported as from 40% to as high as 90%. As a result, the morbidity is correspondingly higher, and mortality rates also are excessive.

Chronic Appendicitis

Many clinicians are skeptical as to the presence of the clinical entity of chronic or recurring appendicitis and will rule out the diagnosis of appendicitis if the patient gives a history of past episodes of similar pain. Others, however, believe that this is a true clinical entity that will be seen in between 1% and 10% of all appendectomies. Several small series of patients with clinical and pathologic evidence of chronic appendicitis have been reported. Many of these initial episodes are followed by recurring right-lower-quadrant pain over a period of weeks to years in duration. At the time of surgical exploration, clinical and pathologic changes of chronic inflammation are identified in the region of the appendix. A majority of these case reports have identified patients relieved of their chronic right-lower-quadrant pain after appendectomy. Rare cases of chronic granulomatous appendicitis have been described. Many of these patients are relieved of their symptoms with appendectomy. However, in a few of these patients, if monitored over long periods, Crohn's disease will develop.

Suggested Reading

Garbutt JM, Soper NJ, Shannon WD, et al: Meta-analysis of randomized controlled trials comparing laparoscopic and open appendectomy. Surg Laparosc Endosc 9:17–26, 1999.

Long KH, Bannon MP, Zietlow S, et al: A prospective randomized comparison of laparoscopic appendectomy with open appendectomy: Clinical and economic analyses. Surgery 129:390–400, 2001.

Ortega AE, Hunter JG, Peters JH, et al: A prospective randomized comparison of laparoscopic appendectomy with open appendectomy. Laparoscopic Appendectomy Study Group. Am J Surg 169:208–213, 1995.

Wagner JM, McKinney WP, Carpenter JL: Does this patient have appendicitis? JAMA 276:1589–1594, 1996.

Wilson EB, Cole C, Nipper ML, et al: Computerized tomography and ultrasound in the diagnosis of appendicitis: When are they indicated? Arch Surg 136:670–675, 2001.

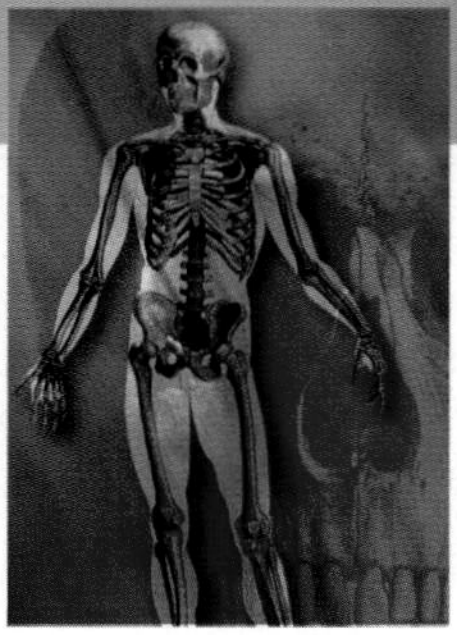

Chapter 16
Hernias

GORDON L. TELFORD, MD

Abdominal wall hernias are very common, occurring in approximately 1.5% of the United States population. Herniorrhaphy is one of the most frequently performed operations. It is therefore important that general surgeons be aware of the physical findings and the management of abdominal wall hernias. A thorough understanding of the detailed anatomy of the structures involved in the repair of abdominal wall hernias and the techniques used to perform these operations is essential.

Inguinal Hernia

Anatomy

The inguinal canal is a cleft in the anterior abdominal wall that is bound anteriorly by the external oblique aponeurosis and posteriorly by the transversalis fascia and to a variable degree by the aponeurosis of the transversus abdominis muscle (Fig. 16-1). Inferiorly it is bound by the inguinal and lacunar ligaments, and superiorly, by the internal oblique and transversus abdominis muscles and their aponeuroses. The spermatic cord in males and the round ligament in females enter the inguinal canal through the transversus abdominis fascia at the internal inguinal ring. The cord then travels the length of the canal and exits through the external oblique aponeurosis at the external inguinal ring.

Pathophysiology

Indirect inguinal hernias come through the internal inguinal ring and enter the inguinal canal. With time, they may extend along the canal and exit through the external ring into the scrotum. They are usually caused by a lack of obliteration of the processus vaginalis during development and are congenital. Direct inguinal hernias come through the posterior wall of the inguinal canal and are a defect in the transversalis fascia. They infrequently extend along the canal and enter the scrotum. The main etiologic factor in direct hernias is any maneuver that increases intraabdominal pressure, such as frequent heavy lifting. Cigarette smoking, advanced age, and chronic illness also are risk factors. Indirect inguinal hernias are the most commonly observed hernias in both sexes and at all ages, even though direct inguinal hernias occur more commonly in older patients, and femoral hernias are more common in women.

Differential Diagnosis

Other masses can occur in the groin and be confused with an inguinal hernia. The bulge from a femoral hernia can be misdiagnosed as being above the inguinal ligament. A lipoma of the spermatic cord can appear as a bulge in the inguinal canal that appears to be accentuated with coughing. Even an experienced examiner can make a misdiagnosis under this circumstance. Inguinal lymphadenopathy, although below the inguinal canal, can be confused with a hernia by an inexperienced examiner. A large hydrocele that extends superiorly to the level of the external ring can usually be distinguished from a hernia by the lack of a bulge in the inguinal canal region and by the palpation of a normal-sized spermatic cord above the hydrocele.

Evaluation

The most important aspect of the evaluation of a patient suspected to have an inguinal hernia is a thorough history and physical examination. Laboratory testing is seldom necessary unless another diagnosis is being considered, such as lymphoma. Most patients are asymptomatic or complain of a bulge in the groin that is more prominent when the patient coughs, stands for a long period, or increases intraabdominal pressure by lifting a heavy object or performing other maneuvers. The bulge can usually be reduced manually or by simply lying down. Pain alone is not indicative of an inguinal hernia.

The examination of a patient for an inguinal hernia is begun with the patient standing. The groin area is inspected for bulges or other pathology. If a bulge is observed, it should be palpated and an attempt made to reduce it. If it is not reducible and is firm or hard, other diagnoses should be considered. Next, the groin should be palpated for a bulge that is accentuated by coughing. The lateral aspect of the scrotal skin is evaginated with the index finger until the external inguinal ring is palpated. If a hernia is present, a bulge is often felt that is also accentuated by coughing. It is important to remember that patients with no hernia can have an impulse with coughing that can be mistaken for a hernia; therefore other evidence for the diagnosis must be

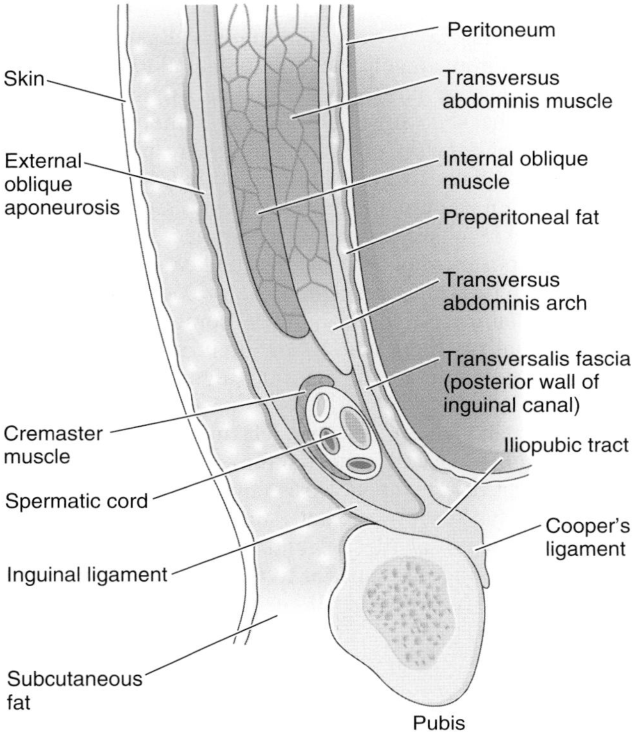

FIGURE 16–1 Sagittal section through the midpoint of the inguinal canal, demonstrating the surgical anatomy. (Adapted from Condon RE, Telford GL: Hernia. In Nora PF (ed): Operative Surgery: Principles and Techniques, 3rd ed. Philadelphia, WB Saunders, 1990, with permission.)

sought. Because coughing accentuates a hernia for only a very brief time, asking the patient to produce a Valsalva maneuver can accentuate the hernia for a much longer period and more reliably demonstrate a bulge. In extremely obese patients, patients who have difficulty standing, and patients in whom the examination is equivocal in the standing position, the examination should be repeated in the supine position by using both coughing and a Valsalva maneuver to attempt to produce a bulge. The differentiation between an indirect and a direct inguinal hernia is of minimal importance because the operative approach is the same. In one approach to distinguishing between an indirect and a direct hernia, thumb pressure is maintained over the anatomic position of the deep inguinal ring, midway between the pubic tubercle and the anterior superior iliac spine, while the patient does a Valsalva maneuver. If the hernia bulge does not appear, the hernia is assumed to be indirect in origin. If a bulge is noted medial to the thumb, it is more likely that a direct or large indirect hernia is present.

Except in patients with an inconclusive examination and patients with unexplained groin pain with no clinical evidence of a hernia, imaging studies are not indicated. Herniography, in which radiopaque dye is injected into the abdominal cavity, has a high rate of diagnostic accuracy in inconclusive cases. CT and ultrasonography also have been recommended in the aforementioned circumstances but have not been studied.

Treatment

Because of the risk of incarceration and strangulation, nonsurgical management of inguinal hernias is not recommended, except in patients for whom any surgical procedure would be of unacceptable risk. Wearing a truss does not guarantee that a groin hernia will remain reduced and not become incarcerated or strangulated.

Many types of repairs of inguinal hernias have been described and can be categorized as follows: (1) anterior or inguinal canal approach, (2) posterior or preperitoneal approach, and (3) posterior laparoscopic technique. Reasons exist to recommend all three.

Anterior (Inguinal Canal) Approach

The skin incision is begun 2 cm above the pubic tubercle. It continues laterally and superiorly to cross the projected position of the internal inguinal ring (at the midpoint between the pubic tubercle and the anterior superior iliac spine). Dissection is carried through the subcutaneous tissue to the external oblique aponeurosis. A small incision is made in the external oblique aponeurosis so that when carried medially, it joins the external inguinal ring at its apex. The underlying muscles and nerves are separated from the external oblique aponeurosis. An incision is made between the fibers of the external oblique aponeurosis in a fashion that connects with the external inguinal ring. Care is taken to identify the iliohypogastric and ilioinguinal nerves. The nerves are mobilized and retracted behind hemostats that catch the edge of the external oblique aponeurosis. The spermatic cord is retracted superiorly, and its attachments to the inguinal ligament are bluntly dissected free.

The cord is then retracted inferiorly, and the internal oblique muscle and its aponeurosis retracted superiorly to expose the plane between these two structures. With blunt and sharp dissection, they are separated. By continuing this dissection inferiorly, the transversalis fascia of the posterior inguinal wall is exposed. It is then possible with anterior retraction of the cord to pass an instrument through the remaining attachments posterior to the cord, and with blunt and sharp dissection, free the cord from all its attachments in the inguinal canal (Fig. 16-2). A Penrose drain is passed beneath the cord for retraction.

If the patient has a direct hernia, no further dissection is necessary. If the patient has an indirect hernia, the cremasteric muscle is divided, and the underlying cord structures bluntly exposed. The hernia sac is identified and opened. A finger is inserted into the sac, and the sac separated from its attachments to the cremasteric muscle and other cord

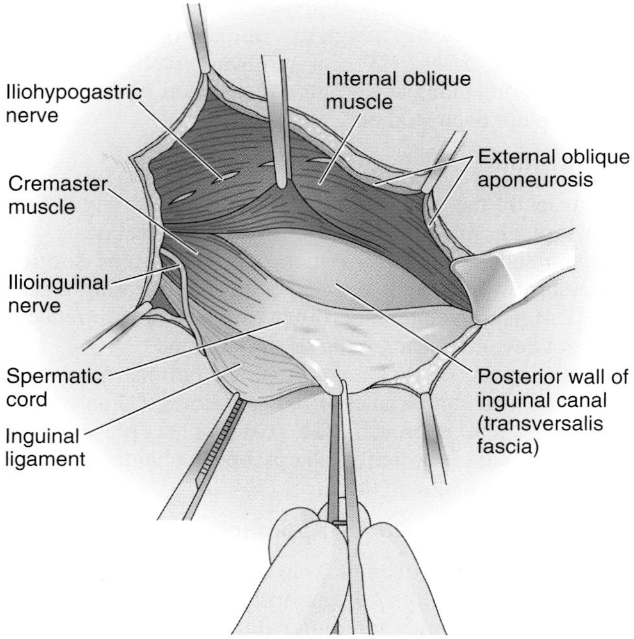

FIGURE 16–2 The spermatic cord has been separated from its attachments in the inguinal canal. (Adapted from Condon RE, Telford GL: Hernia. In Nora PF (ed): Operative Surgery: Principles and Techniques, 3rd ed. Philadelphia, WB Saunders, 1990, with permission.)

structures. If the hernia sac is entirely within the inguinal canal, it should be freed from its attachments to the level of the internal inguinal ring. The sac is examined, and the index finger inserted into the peritoneal cavity to examine for femoral and direct inguinal hernias; appropriate measures are taken to repair the defects if they exist. The sac is twisted, followed by suture ligature at the level of the internal inguinal ring. The redundant sac is excised. If the sac extends into the scrotum, the dissection is carried distally for a reasonable distance, and the sac divided. It is not necessary to excise the entire sac under this circumstance.

A number of options exist for the repair of an inguinal hernia from the anterior approach.

Bassini Repair. The Bassini procedure or one of its modifications is frequently used for indirect and direct inguinal herniorrhaphies. Although the aponeurosis of the transversus abdominis aponeurosis is sufficient for the superior aspect of the repair, the conjoined tendon of the transversus abdominis and internal oblique muscles is more frequently used. These structures are sutured inferiorly to the inguinal ligament, the iliopubic tract, or preferably both. Heavy, braided nonabsorbable sutures are placed every 5 to 7 mm from the pubic tubercle to just medial to the internal inguinal ring (Fig. 16-3). Lateral to the internal inguinal ring, one or two sutures are placed from the transversus abdominis muscle above to the inguinal ligament below. The sutures immediately medial and lateral to the internal inguinal ring are pulled snug, and the tightness of the repair is checked. It should freely admit the tip of a hemostat but not a finger. Based on these results, the repair should be adjusted and the sutures tied (Fig. 16-4). In small indirect inguinal hernias, it is necessary to reconstruct only the internal inguinal ring, and it is not necessary to repair the entire posterior wall of the inguinal canal. The medial sutures can be eliminated from the aforementioned repair. For large indirect inguinal hernias (complete), the entire repair should be performed. For direct inguinal hernias, the sutures lateral to the internal inguinal ring can be eliminated.

If the repair is under tension, a relaxing incision should be performed to reduce the potential for recurrence (Fig. 16-5). The external oblique aponeurosis (superficial lamina of the anterior rectus sheath) is bluntly dissected off the internal oblique aponeurosis (deep lamina of the anterior rectus sheath) beginning just superior to the pubis and continuing superiorly and laterally for 10 cm. The relaxing incision is

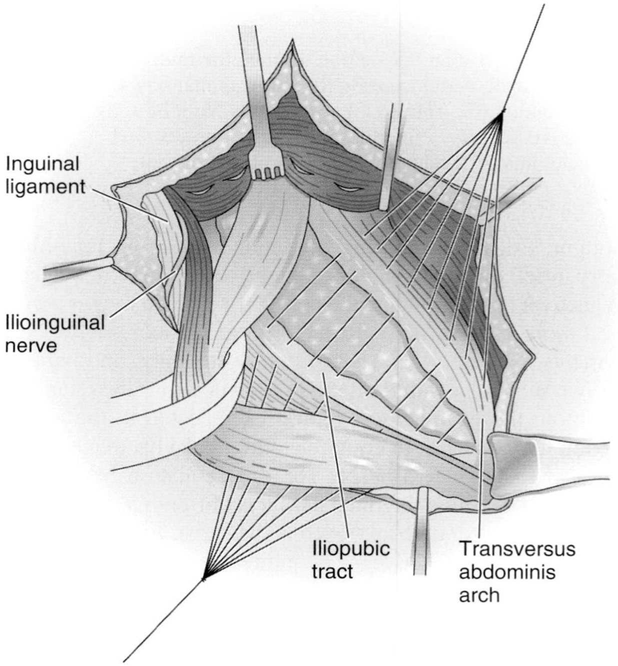

FIGURE 16–3 Placement of medial sutures in iliopubic tract repair of indirect inguinal hernia. Sutures are placed from the pubic tubercle to just medial to the internal inguinal ring. In this illustration, the transversalis fascia has been incised. (Adapted from Condon RE, Telford GL: Hernia. In Nora PF (ed): Operative Surgery: Principles and Techniques, 3rd ed. Philadelphia, WB Saunders, 1990, with permission.)

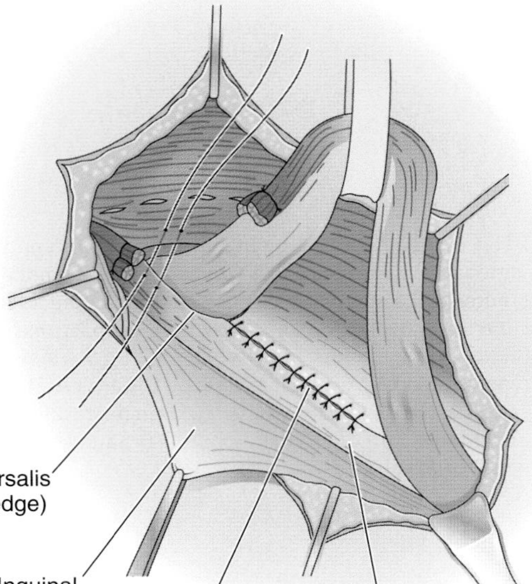

FIGURE 16–4 The sutures medial to the internal inguinal ring have been tied. Sutures used for reconstruction of the lateral aspect of the ring are placed. (Adapted from Condon RE, Telford GL: Hernia. In Nora PF (ed): Operative Surgery: Principles and Techniques, 3rd ed. Philadelphia, WB Saunders, 1990, with permission.)

made in the deep lamina of the anterior rectus sheath, following the line of fusion of the two lamina and exposing the rectus muscle. The incision is begun 2 cm superior to the pubis and is continued superiorly until the tension on the repair is relieved.

The wound is irrigated with warm saline, and meticulous hemostasis is obtained. The external oblique aponeurosis is closed in any acceptable fashion.

Cooper's Ligament (McVay) Repair. The Cooper's ligament repair is thought by some surgeons to be indicated for direct, large indirect, and recurrent inguinal hernias. The anterior approach to the inguinal canal is performed as already outlined. The transversalis fascia of the posterior wall of the inguinal canal is incised from the pubic tubercle to the internal inguinal ring. Cooper's ligament is exposed by using blunt dissection. The repair is performed by suturing the conjoined tendon to Cooper's ligament from the pubic tubercle to the femoral canal by using heavy, braided nonabsorbable suture. The repair continues more anteriorly by suturing the conjoined tendon to the inguinal ligament until an adequate reconstruction of the internal inguinal ring is performed. A relaxing incision is performed.

PEARLS FOR ROUNDS

An acutely incarcerated hernia is a surgical emergency.

The posterior or preperitoneal approach is best for recurrent hernias (open or laparoscopic).

The recurrence rates for inguinal hernias are direct, 5%–10%, and indirect, 1%–5%.

The use of a prosthesis for herniorrhaphies is mandatory only when a suture repair would be under undue tension.

Ventral, incisional hernias frequently occur because of wound infection, obesity, malnutrition, and other factors that lead to poor wound healing.

Prosthetic Repair. When the aforementioned repairs cannot be performed without undue tension, even with a relaxing incision, then a prosthesis must be used to bridge the gap between the margins of the hernia aperture. Either polypropylene or polytetrafluoroethylene (PTFE) mesh is used. The prosthesis is sutured to Cooper's ligament, the iliopubic tract and/or the inguinal ligament inferiorly (Fig. 16-6) and the conjoined tendon or internal oblique aponeurosis superiorly. The lateral edge of the material is slit to allow the spermatic cord to pass through the prosthesis. The lateral aspects of the mesh, once passed around the cord, are then sutured together, incorporating the inguinal ligament and the transversus abdominis muscle (see Fig. 16-6).

Recently various plug techniques have been developed for the repair of groin hernias. They involve the placement of a plug of polypropylene into the hernia defect with or without anchoring sutures. Interestingly, the results of this technique have been very good. The fact that these repairs are performed with minimal or no tension on the repair is probably the main reason for their low recurrence rate. Of course, the absence of tension in the completed repair, no matter which type of repair is performed, is essential to the success of the repair.

Posterior (Preperitoneal) Approach

The preperitoneal approach for the repair of inguinal hernias is ideal for recurrent hernias, incarcerated or strangulated hernias, and complicated hernias. An 8- to 10-cm transverse skin incision is placed 3 cm above the pubic tubercle. A transverse incision is made in the anterior rectus sheath and the aponeurosis of the external oblique muscle. The deeper muscles are separated in the line of their fibers. The transversalis aponeurosis is incised, and the preperitoneal space is entered. The peritoneum is bluntly dissected away from the anterior abdominal wall and the posterior wall of the inguinal canal, and the hernia is exposed. The hernia sac is reduced, and any redundant sac excised and ligated. If the sac cannot be reduced, the

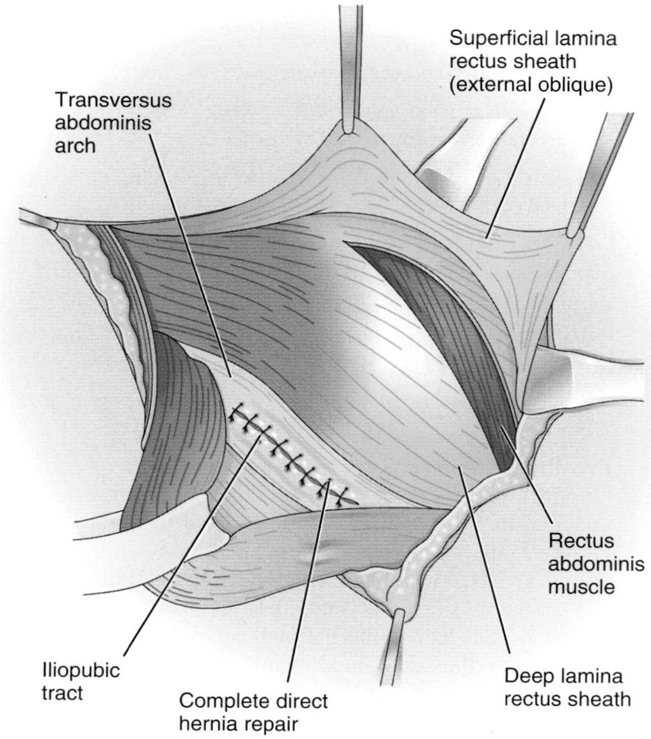

FIGURE 16–5 Relaxing incision in anterior approach to inguinal herniorrhaphy. The incision is made in the deep lamina of the anterior rectus sheath, beginning 2 cm superior to the pubis. This allows the deep lamina of the rectus sheath to relax inferiorly, reducing the tension of the repair. (Adapted from Condon RE, Telford GL: Hernia. In Nora PF (ed): Operative Surgery: Principles and Techniques, 3rd ed. Philadelphia, WB Saunders, 1990, with permission.)

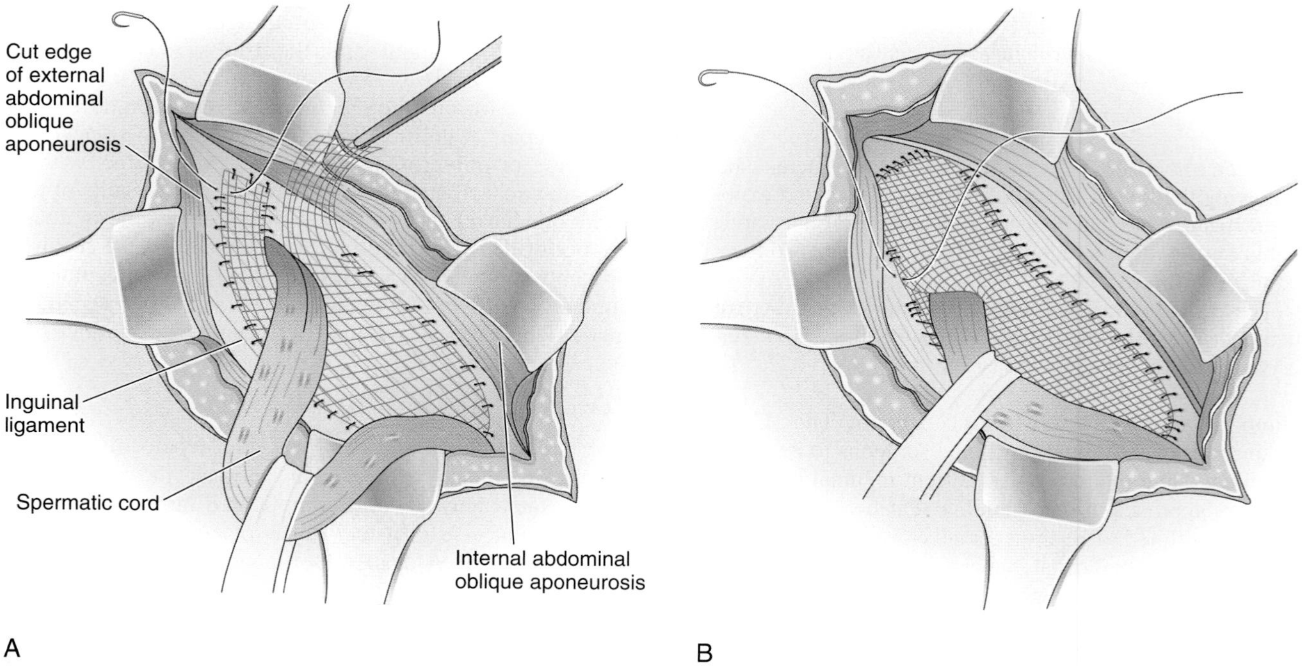

FIGURE 16–6 Use of prosthesis in anterior approach to the repair of an inguinal hernia. *A*, The inferior edge of the prosthesis has been sutured to the inguinal ligament, and the superior edge, to the internal oblique aponeurosis. *B*, The superior aspect of the prosthesis is passed around the spermatic cord and sutured in place. (Adapted from Knol JA, Eckhauser FE: Inguinal anatomy and abdominal wall hernias. In Greenfield LJ (ed): Surgery: Scientific Principles and Practice, 2nd ed. Philadelphia, JB Lippincott, 1997, with permission.)

PEARLS FOR THE OR

The boundaries of the inguinal canal are (1) anterior, the external oblique aponeurosis; (2) posterior, the transversalis fascia and transversus abdominis aponeurosis; (3) inferior, the inguinal and lacunar ligaments; and (4) superior, the internal oblique and transversus abdominis muscle and aponeuroses.

Indirect inguinal hernias come through the internal or deep inguinal ring, whereas direct inguinal hernias come through the posterior wall of the inguinal canal (transversalis fascia).

Two frequently used types of inguinal herniorrhaphies are the Bassini repair, in which the transversus abdominis aponeurosis and the internal oblique aponeurosis (conjoined tendon) superiorly are sutured to the inguinal ligament inferiorly, and the Cooper's ligament (McVay) repair, in which the conjoined tendon superiorly is sutured to Cooper's ligament inferiorly.

The boundaries of femoral canal are (1) anterior, the iliopubic tract and inguinal ligament; (2) posterior, Cooper's ligament; (3) medial, the lacunar ligament; and (4) lateral, the femoral vein.

Hematomas and infections occur in 1%–2% of inguinal herniorrhaphies.

sac is opened, and its contents are reduced. The sac can then usually be reduced. Sutures for the repair are placed from the transversus abdominis arch superiorly to Cooper's ligament and/or the iliopubic tract inferiorly, starting at the pubic tubercle and progressing laterally to the internal inguinal ring (Fig. 16-7). For indirect hernias, one or two additional sutures are placed medial and lateral to the internal ring. The fascial incision is closed in layers.

If the hernia defect is large, it may be necessary to uses a prosthesis. The material is sutured to Cooper's ligament and the iliopubic tract inferiorly and to the full thickness of the abdominal musculature superiorly (Fig. 16-8). Numerous variations on this technique exist, including the Stoppa technique, in which a large piece of material is fixed with only a few sutures.

Laparoscopic Repair

Two main techniques are used for laparoscopic inguinal herniorrhaphy, the transabdominal preperitoneal (TAPP) and the totally extraperitoneal approach (TEPA). In the TAPP technique, the peritoneal cavity is entered, and the repair is performed. In the TEPA technique, the preperitoneal space is entered and, with balloon dissectors, the posterior wall of the inguinal canal is exposed. Prosthetic material is usually used for the repair and is secured to Cooper's ligament inferiorly, the posterior rectus fascia superiorly and medially, and laterally to the transversus abdominis aponeurotic arch. Numerous variations on these techniques have been reported, but the basic concepts of the repairs are the same.

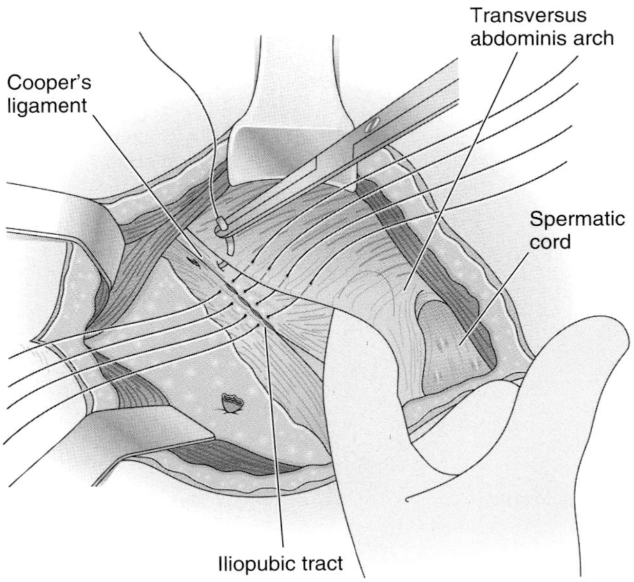

FIGURE 16–7 Placement of sutures in the posterior approach to the repair of direct inguinal hernias. The transversus abdominis arch superiorly is sutured to Cooper's ligament and the iliopubic tract inferiorly. (Adapted from Condon RE, Telford GL: Hernia. In Nora PF (ed): Operative Surgery: Principles and Techniques, 3rd ed. Philadelphia, WB Saunders, 1990, with permission.)

Outcomes

The recurrence rates for direct and indirect inguinal hernias are different. Direct hernias have a recurrence rate of 5% to 10%, whereas indirect hernias recur at a rate of 1% to 5%.

Complications

The risk of wound infection and hematomas is approximately 1%. Symptomatic ilioinguinal and genitofemoral neuromas occur in fewer than 1% of patients.

Femoral Hernia

Anatomy and Pathophysiology

Femoral hernias exit the abdominal cavity through the femoral canal, which is bounded anteriorly by the iliopubic tract and inguinal ligament, posteriorly by Cooper's ligament, medially by the insertion of the iliopubic tract into Cooper's ligament (lacunar ligament), and laterally by the femoral vein (Fig. 16-9). The sac is below the inguinal ligament in the groin or upper thigh area. As stated previously, femoral hernias are more common in women.

Differential Diagnosis

The bulge from a femoral hernia protrudes beneath the inguinal ligament medial to the femoral vessels and is

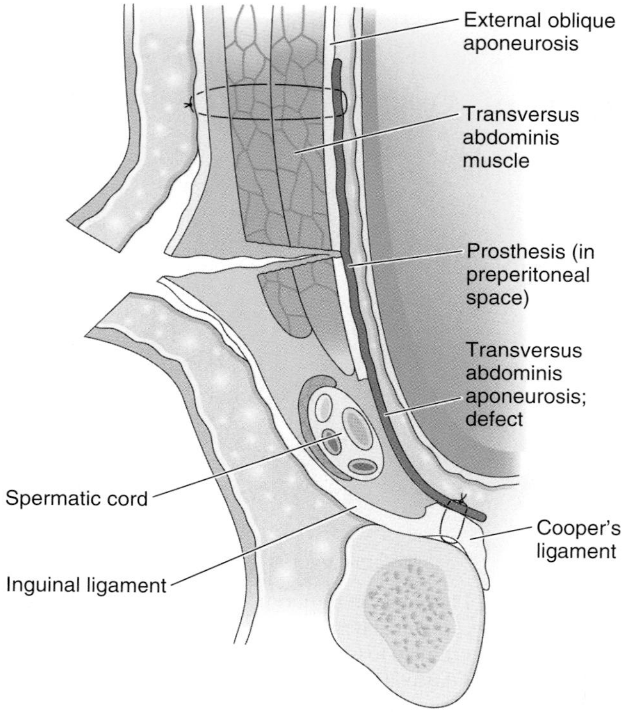

FIGURE 16–8 Placement of the prosthesis in the preperitoneal space in the posterior approach to groin hernia repair. (Adapted from Condon RE, Telford GL: Hernia. In Nora PF (ed): Operative Surgery: Principles and Techniques, 3rd ed. Philadelphia, WB Saunders, 1990, with permission.)

palpable in the thigh just below the groin crease. Because femoral hernias usually have a narrow neck, they can be difficult to reduce. They feel like a small mass and have no impulse on coughing. They therefore can be confused with inguinal lymphadenopathy or a lipoma. They can be misdiagnosed as inguinal hernias and vice versa.

Evaluation

The evaluation is similar to that in patients with a suspected inguinal hernia. The only hint that a patient may have a femoral hernia is groin pain, although no findings may appear on the initial physical examination. Repeated examinations may be necessary to make the diagnosis. As a last resort, herniography, ultrasonography, or CT may be helpful.

Treatment

The only acceptable approach to the treatment of femoral hernias is operative, except for patients in whom any surgical procedure would be of unacceptable risk. The three approaches to femoral hernias are as previously described for inguinal hernias: (1) anterior or inguinal canal approach; (2) open, preperitoneal approach; and (3) posterior laparoscopic approach. In the anterior approach, the hernia is reduced as for inguinal hernias, and a Cooper's ligament repair is used as previously described because of the location of the hernia beneath the inguinal ligament. The open, preperitoneal approach is preferred by many surgeons because of the relative ease with which incarcerated hernias can be reduced. Usually gentle traction and blunt dissection

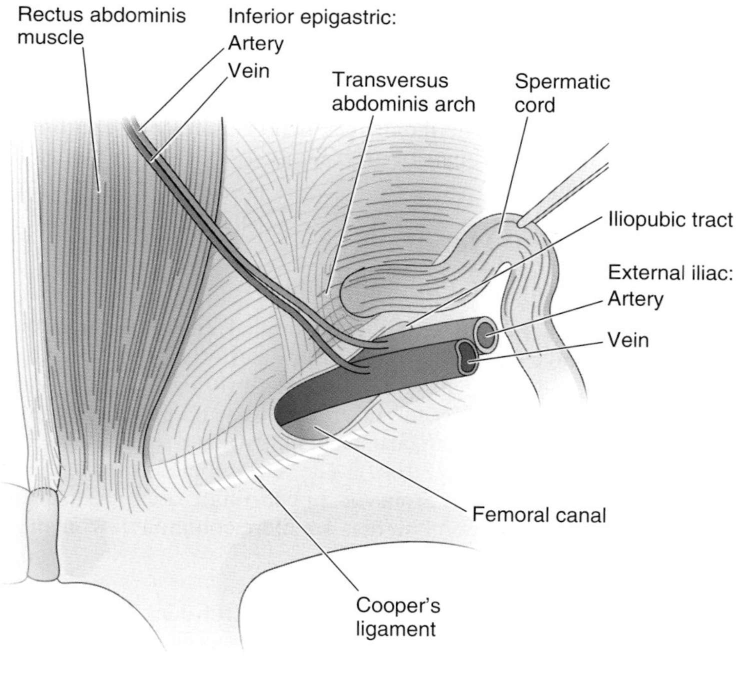

FIGURE 16–9 The anatomy of the femoral canal from the posterior aspect. (Adapted from Condon RE, Telford GL: Hernia. In Nora PF (ed): Operative Surgery: Principles and Techniques, 3rd ed. Philadelphia, WB Saunders, 1990, with permission.)

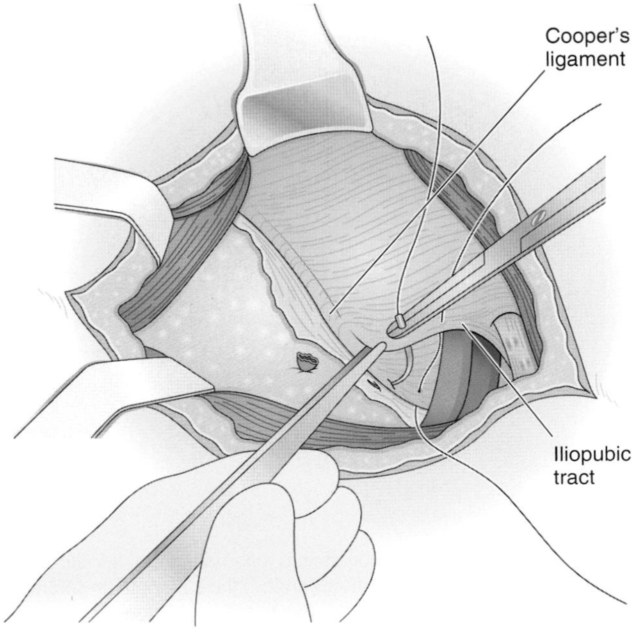

FIGURE 16–10 Posterior approach to repair of femoral hernias. The hernia has been reduced and the sac excised. The repair is accomplished by suturing the iliopubic tract superiorly to the Cooper's ligament inferiorly. (Adapted from Condon RE, Telford GL: Hernia. In Nora PF (ed): Operative Surgery: Principles and Techniques, 3rd ed. Philadelphia, WB Saunders, 1990, with permission.)

are sufficient to reduce the sac from this approach. If the hernia is incarcerated and is not easily reduced, the neck of the sac is released by incising the iliopubic tract medial to the hernia. For the repair, the iliopubic tract is sutured to Cooper's ligament by using heavy, braided nonabsorbable suture (Fig. 16-10). The laparoscopic approach with the use of mesh for the repair, as previously described, is gaining acceptance.

Umbilical Hernia

Umbilical hernias are usually congenital. Those that are acquired frequently occur in patients with increased abdominal pressure from pregnancy, ascites, or morbid obesity. Congenital umbilical hernias usually close spontaneously by age 2 years. Defects that persist beyond age 4 years or defects larger than 2 cm at an earlier age should be repaired.

With a Valsalva maneuver, a bulge is seen at the umbilicus that can be reduced, and the defect palpated. Rarely a lipoma or an epigastric hernia can be confused with an umbilical hernia, but the majority of the time, the diagnosis is correct. Chronically incarcerated hernias can be confused with a lipoma. Unless an indication is found that the diagnosis may be incorrect, no additional testing is necessary before proceeding with surgery.

A supra- or subumbilical incision is made, and the hernia sac is identified. Once the sac is freed from its attachments, it is transected at the fascial level, and its contents are reduced into the abdominal cavity. The defect is closed with simple heavy, braided nonabsorbable sutures. If the defect is large enough that the sutures would be tied under undue tension, a prosthetic repair with an open or laparoscopic technique should be carried out, as is described for ventral, incisional hernias. Recurrence of the hernia is very uncommon, and few complications occur.

Ventral, Incisional Hernia

The vast majority of ventral hernias occur at the site of a previous abdominal incision because of a clinical or subclinical wound infection, inadequate healing of the surgical wound, malnutrition, ascites, pregnancy, chemotherapy, steroids, or other conditions causing strain on the wound. As a result, the fascial edges separate, and a hernia protrudes through the defect. The diagnosis is usually obvious, although small defects can be missed on the initial examination in obese patients. When the patient performs a Valsalva maneuver, a bulge is seen that usually reduces spontaneously when the patient exhales. The edges of the fascial defect are usually palpable. Except in circumstances in which the diagnosis is in question, no further testing is necessary.

Because of the high recurrence rate with the repair of ventral hernias, it is important to alter any conditions that can predispose to recurrence, such as obesity, malnutrition, use of steroids, uncontrolled diabetes, or other conditions, before proceeding with a repair. Otherwise surgical repair of ventral hernias is recommended at the time of diagnosis.

If an open technique is used, the incision used for the original operation is reopened. It is then easier to extend the incision if other defects are identified during exploration of the fascia.

The hernia sac is identified and the dissection continued until normal fascia is identified circumferentially. If the hernia sac is not redundant, it can be held in the reduced position while the repair is completed. If the sac is redundant or a narrow neck to the sac is found and the contents cannot be reduced, the redundant sac should be excised and the contents reduced. Attenuated fascia and scar tissue at the margins of the defect are excised until normal fascia is present at all margins. The remainder of the original wound is explored for additional defects, and the fascial opening is extended if necessary. If the wound can be closed primarily with minimal tension, this is performed with an interrupted technique. If a primary repair can be accomplished without excessive tension, yet the tissues appear weak, an onlay of polypropylene mesh should be performed. The sutures used for the primary repair are

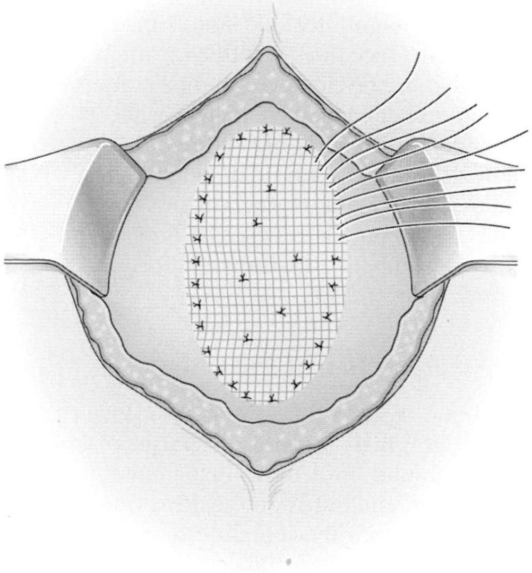

FIGURE 16–11 Completion of the onlay repair of a ventral hernia. The ends of the sutures are passed though the polypropylene mesh and tied. (Adapted from Condon RE, Telford GL: Hernia. In Nora PF (ed): Operative Surgery: Principles and Techniques, 3rd ed. Philadelphia, WB Saunders, 1990, with permission.)

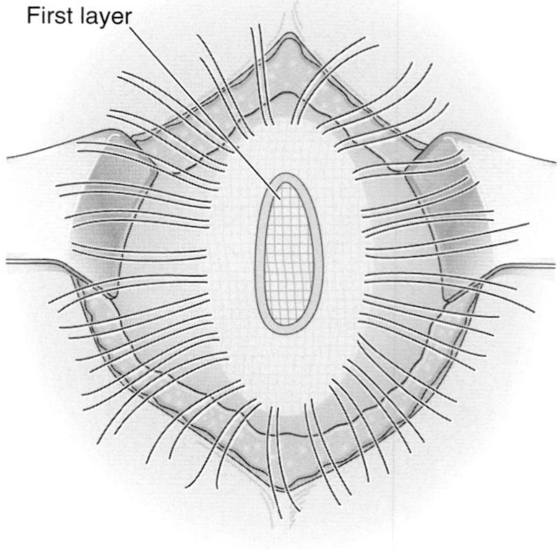

FIGURE 16–12 Two-layer prosthetic repair of ventral hernia. After placement of mattress sutures around the entire circumference of inner layer of the prosthesis, the prosthesis is positioned below the fascia. (Adapted from Condon RE, Telford GL: Hernia. In Nora PF (ed): Operative Surgery: Principles and Techniques, 3rd ed. Philadelphia, WB Saunders, 1990, with permission.)

brought through the mesh. Additional sutures are placed through the full thickness of the abdominal wall fascia 5 cm from the defect and then through the mesh (Fig. 16-11).

If the fascia cannot be approximated without undue tension, a prosthesis or autologous tissue such as fascial lata or a muscle or fascial flap should be used to repair the defect. More recently, laparoscopic techniques have been developed in which a single layer of PTFE is placed intraabdominally by various techniques. PTFE is used because of the tendency of intestines to adhere to polypropylene mesh, resulting in fistulas and infection.

In the open technique, a number of approaches have been described using one layer of material above or below the fascia or two layers of material, one above and one below the fascia. One of the more popular techniques places prosthetic material above and below the fascia with mattress sutures encompassing the full thickness of the abdominal wall fascia and both layers of the prosthesis (Figs. 16-12 and 16-13). PTFE is used for the inner layer of the repair, and polypropylene is used for the outer layer.

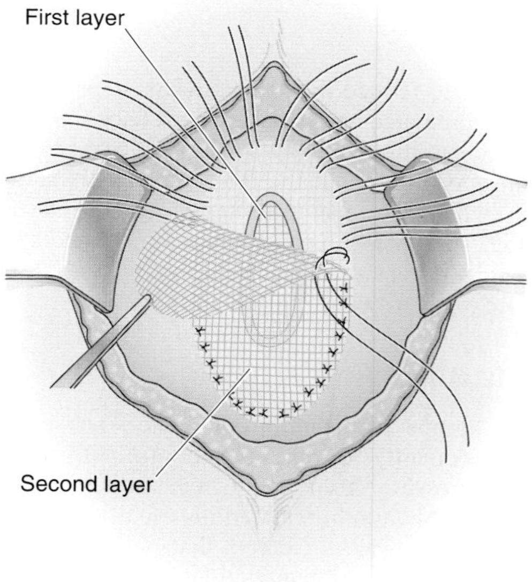

FIGURE 16–13 Two-layer technique of prosthetic repair of ventral hernia. The second layer of prosthetic material is placed superficial to the musculoaponeurotic abdominal wall, and the mattress sutures are passed through the material and tied. (Adapted from Condon RE, Telford GL: Hernia. In Nora PF (ed): Operative Surgery: Principles and Techniques, 3rd ed. Philadelphia, WB Saunders, 1990, with permission.)

Unusual Hernias

Parastomal Hernia

Parastomal hernias occur through the same fascial opening created for an ostomy. They occur more frequently in obese patients. They are distressing to patients because they cause unreliable fitting of ostomy appliances, ostomy retraction, and an unsightly appearance. The preferred treatment is transfer of the ostomy to a new site and primary closure of the hernia defect. If it is not feasible to transfer the ostomy site, primary closure of the hernia defect with prosthetic mesh reinforcement is performed. Primary closure of the hernia alone without mesh reinforcement has a recurrence rate of more than 50%.

Spigelian Hernia

Spigelian hernias occur through the fascia between the lateral edge of the rectus muscle and the semilunar line. These hernias most commonly occur below the semicircular line of Douglas. No posterior rectus fascia exists below the semicircular line, making this area inherently weak. These hernias are frequently interparietal, and the hernia sac is posterior to the external oblique aponeurosis. This makes it difficult to diagnose these hernias, and a CT scan or ultrasonography may be necessary to make the diagnosis, especially in obese patients. Because these hernias often have narrow necks and the risk of incarceration and strangulation is high, these hernias should be repaired when diagnosed.

A transverse incision is made over the hernia, and the external oblique aponeurosis is incised along the direction of its fibers. The sac is identified and dissected from surrounding tissues to its neck. After reducing its contents, the sac is excised. The defects in the transversus abdominis aponeurosis and internal oblique muscles are closed with interrupted, nonabsorbable sutures. The need for the use of prosthetic material is infrequent. Recurrence is rare.

Obturator Hernia

Obturator hernias occur through the obturator canal in the pelvis. The sac exits the pelvis along the obturator vessels and nerve. They are difficult to diagnose preoperatively and occur more frequently in older women. The diagnosis can frequently be made with CT scan. Patients may be seen initially with pain in the distribution of the obturator nerve along the upper medial aspect of the thigh. More often, the patients have signs and symptoms of a complete or intermittent small-bowel obstruction, and the diagnosis is made at the time of exploratory laparotomy.

When the diagnosis is suspected, the abdomen should be entered through a lower midline incision. The sac is reduced, and any compromised intestine is resected. If small, the defect is closed with interrupted sutures; if large, prosthetic mesh should be used.

Lumbar (Dorsal) Hernia

Lumbar or dorsal hernias occur through the posterior abdominal wall in the lumbar region. Grynfeltt's hernia occurs at the superior lumbar triangle, and Petit's hernia occurs at the inferior lumbar triangle. Patients can have a mass in the flank. The differential diagnosis includes soft-tissue tumors, hematomas, abscesses, and renal tumors. A CT scan will usually help in establishing the diagnosis.

Because of the risk of incarceration and strangulation and because these hernias are often large and cosmetically troublesome, they should be repaired. The repair is accomplished transabdominally. The sac and its contents are reduced, and any compromised tissue is resected. Small hernias are repaired by direct repair. Larger hernias are challenging and may require the use of prosthetic material or autologous grafts.

Sciatic Hernia

A sciatic hernia occurs at the greater sciatic foramen. They are extremely rare, and the patients are almost always symptom free until a bowel obstruction develops. The repair is best carried out by a transabdominal approach, although the transgluteal approach is appropriate in reducible hernias. The sac and the defect are handled as described for obturator hernias.

Perineal Hernia

Perineal hernias occur through the muscles and fascia of the pelvic diaphragm. They can be congenital but also occur after perineal procedures, such as abdominal perineal resection of the rectum, prostatectomy, or pelvic exenteration. They are best repaired through a transabdominal approach. After reduction and amputation of the hernia sac, the defect is closed primarily, if small. Large defects require prosthetic material or a myocutaneous flap for the repair.

Suggested Reading

Abrahamson J: Hernias. In Zinner MJ, Schwartz SI, Ellis H (eds): Maingot's Abdominal Operations, 10th ed. Stamford, Conn, Appleton & Lange, 1997, pp 479–580.

Fitzgibbons RJ, Greenburg AG (eds): Nyhus and Condon's Hernia, 5th ed. Philadelphia, JB Lippincott, 2001.

Nyhus LM, Condon RE (eds): Hernia, 4th ed. Philadelphia, JB Lippincott, 1995.

Read RC, Terranova O, Battocchio F, et al: Surgery of hernia. In Nyhus LM, Baker RJ, Fischer JE (eds): Mastery of Surgery, 3rd ed. Boston, Little, Brown, 1997, pp 1795–1881.

Richards AT, Quinn TH, Fitzgibbons RJ: Abdominal wall hernias. In Greenfield LJ, Mulholland MW, Oldham KT, et al. (eds): Surgery: Scientific Principles and Practice, 3rd ed. Philadelphia, Lippincott Williams & Wilkins, 2001, pp 1185–1224.

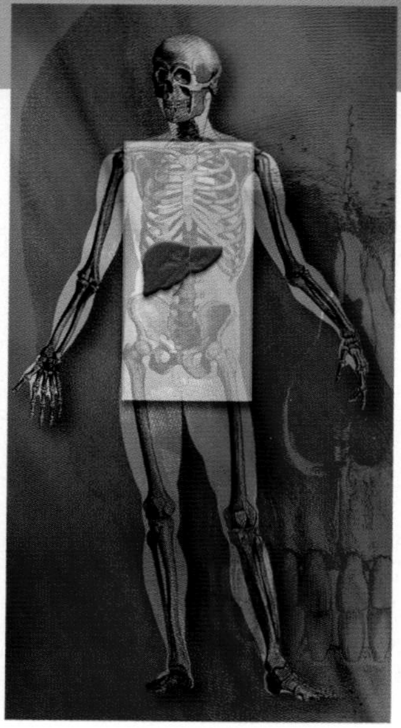

SECTION V

HEPATOBILIARY AND SPLEEN

Chapter 17

Biliary System

TIMOTHY J. BABINEAU, MD, MBA

The biliary system is one of the most variable and complex anatomic areas of the abdomen. As such, it can present a challenge for even the most experienced surgeon operating in the right upper quadrant for either benign or malignant disease. Although the vast majority of the biliary system is within the liver parenchyma, it is the extrahepatic portion of the system that is the site of most biliary operations.

Anatomy

The anatomy of the biliary system is extraordinarily variable, which must be remembered any time surgery is undertaken in the right upper quadrant of the abdomen. This consideration has received recent emphasis with the advent of laparoscopic biliary surgery. In the early 1990s, laparoscopic surgical techniques were adapted to the biliary tree, and laparoscopic cholecystectomy has become the standard treatment for most symptomatic gallstone disease. Unfortunately, early in the evolution of this technique, a number of injuries to the biliary system occurred. These injuries were attributed, in large part, to surgeons' inadequate knowledge of the possible anatomic variations of the biliary tree. A thorough understanding of the normal and variant anatomy is a prerequisite for safe biliary surgery. Normal or classic biliary anatomy is present in only one third of patients, and anatomic variability should always be anticipated (Fig. 17-1).

The biliary system is an organized collection of tubules and ducts that carry bile from the liver parenchyma, where it is produced, into the duodenum and eventually the entire gastrointestinal tract. To understand biliary anatomy adequately, it is useful to consider the intrahepatic system distinct from the extrahepatic system. The intrahepatic system comprises small intrahepatic ducts that coalesce into the right and left hepatic ducts, which drain the right and left lobes of the liver, respectively. The left hepatic duct is longer than the right and will often be the first to dilate from distal obstruction. The right and left ducts subsequently join (usually extrahepatically in the hilum of the liver) to form the common hepatic duct. Once the gallbladder joins the common hepatic duct via the cystic duct, the duct that progresses distally to the second portion of the duodenum is referred to as the common bile duct.

The normal gallbladder is a hollow, pear-shaped viscus with a fluid capacity of approximately 30 mL to 50 mL. The bulbous blind end is termed the *fundus*; the rounded midportion, the *body*; and the narrow distal end, the *neck*. Occasionally, an outpouching of the neck is referred to as the infundibulum or the Hartmann pouch. The cystic duct arises from the neck and varies in length from 3 mm to 3 cm. Its usual insertion into the common hepatic duct is on the lateral aspect, but numerous variations are found. It is particularly this variability in cystic duct/common bile duct junction that, when not recognized, may lead to surgical misadventures and inadvertent injury to the bile duct system (Fig. 17-2).

The common bile duct measures 4 mm to 8 mm in diameter in normal patients. It may become dilated with distal obstruction from a stone or malignancy, in patients who have undergone cholecystectomy, or in patients who are of advanced age. A useful rule of thumb is that patients are often found to have duct diameters (as measured in millimeters by ultrasound [US]) that are equivalent to their age in years divided by 10. For example, an 80-year-old woman may be found to have an 8-mm duct by US. Although its course may be quite variable, the common bile duct typically passes posterior to the duodenum through the head of the pancreas and into the second portion of the duodenum. Before its termination, the common bile duct typically joins with the main pancreatic duct and empties

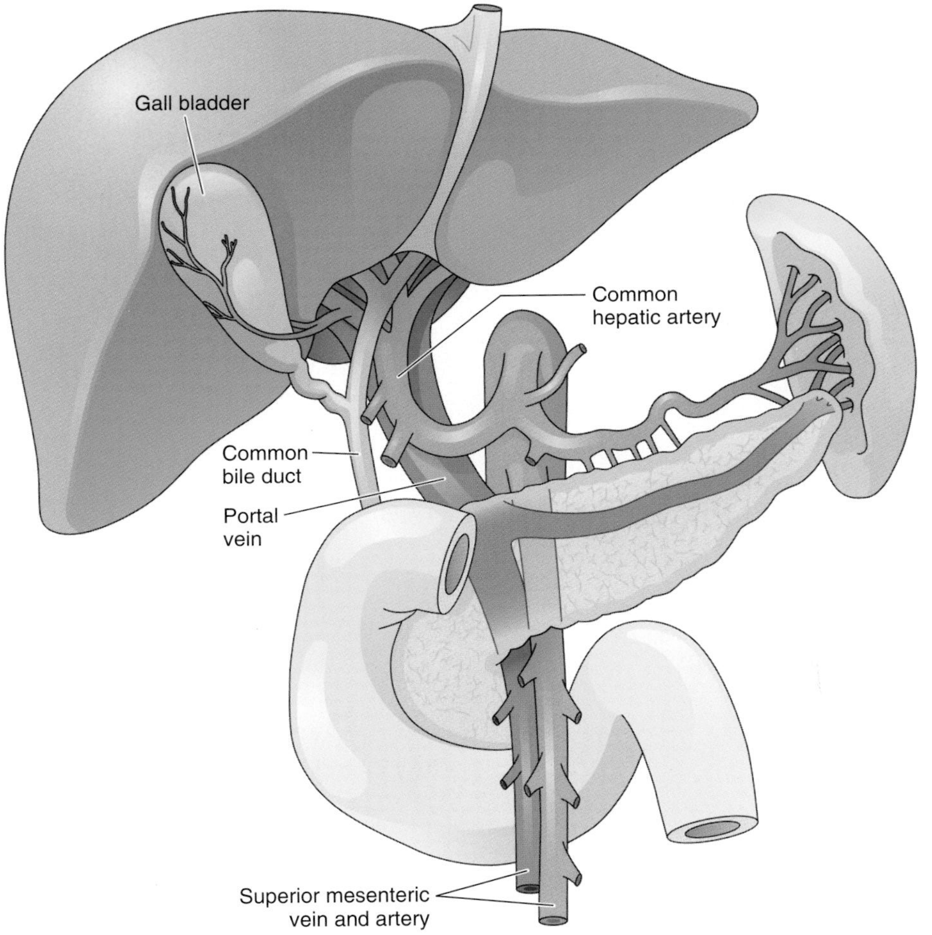

FIGURE 17–1 Normal or classic biliary anatomy.

into the duodenum at the ampulla of Vater. Specialized smooth muscle known as the sphincter of Oddi surrounds both ducts in this area. In response to a variety of stimuli (such as cholecystokinin), the sphincter relaxes (often in conjunction with contraction of the gallbladder) to allow bile flow into the intestinal lumen. Malignant obstruction at this point often gives rise to a typical "double-duct sign" on endoscopic retrograde cholangiopancreatography (Fig. 17-3).

An unusual form of biliary duct cystic disease that affects primarily the intrahepatic biliary system, known as Caroli's disease, deserves special mention. Although classified as a cystic disease of the liver, the process actually involves multiple dilatations of the intrahepatic biliary system, causing the formation of biliary lakes, which appear cystic on imaging studies. It is more accurately classified as a cystic disease of the biliary tree. This syndrome often occurs in conjunction with congenital hepatic fibrosis. Occasionally, intrahepatic calculi develop and, in some patients, carcinoma of the ducts. Patients usually have recurrent attacks of cholangitis and are best managed with surgical debridement and drainage. Endoscopic intervention to drain the biliary tree also may have a therapeutic role in selected cases.

The arterial supply of the biliary system arises from branches of the arterial supply to the liver. Much as in the ductal anatomy, variability is the rule rather than the exception (Fig. 17-4). Modifications of the classic anatomy, in which the liver receives its total inflow from the hepatic branch of the celiac axis, may occur in 25% to 75% of cases. In the typical situation, the celiac artery passes from the aorta anteriorly and trifurcates into the left gastric, splenic, and common hepatic arteries. The common hepatic loops forward and cephalad within the lesser omentum, giving off a caudal gastroduodenal branch supplying the duodenum and pancreas. The proper hepatic artery then continues up toward the hilum of the liver, dividing at a variable point into right and left branches. The blood supply to the gallbladder is via the cystic artery, typically a branch of the right hepatic artery, but also may arise from a "replaced" right (5%), left (10%), or common hepatic arteries (10%). The various anomalous patterns involve a blood supply that originates

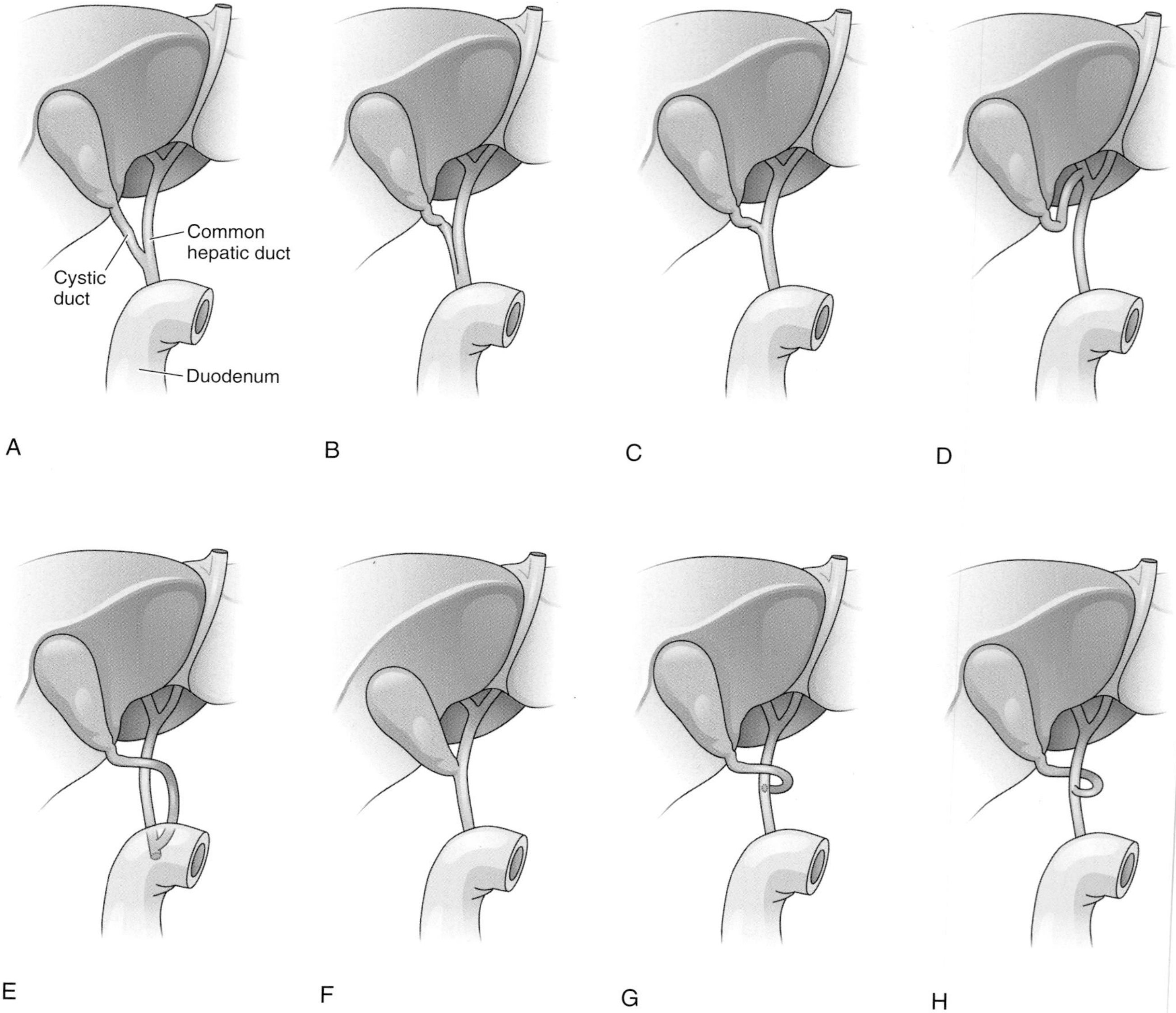

FIGURE 17–2 Variability in cystic duct/bile duct junction. *A*, Normal cystic duct anatomy. *B*, Cystic duct parallel to common bile duct (CBD). *C*, Short cystic duct. *D*, Insertion into right hepatic duct. *E*, Low-insertion cystic duct crossing anterior to CBD. *F*, Absence of cystic duct. *G*, Medial insertion of cystic duct into CBD. *H*, Anterior insertion of cystic duct into CBD.

from the superior mesenteric artery, the left gastric artery, the aorta, and other visceral branches. These variations may be accessory (occurring in addition to the normal arterial supply) or replaced (representing the primary supply to that particular lobe). Occasionally, the right hepatic artery is mistaken (during surgery) for the cystic artery when it runs in parallel with the cystic artery or in the mesentery of the gallbladder (sometimes referred to as a "caterpillar hump"). If mistaken for the cystic artery, it may be inadvertently ligated or injured.

The bile ducts receive their blood supply from small unnamed branches of the hepatic artery. The venous drainage is via the portal venous system. Lymphatics from the gallbladder drain into the cystic duct node (or Calot node), located between the cystic and common hepatic ducts. This node serves as an important potential site of metastatic spread from hepatobiliary malignancies and may help determine the resectability of such lesions.

The triangle of Calot is a critical anatomic area that lies within the porta hepatis and is defined laterally by the cystic

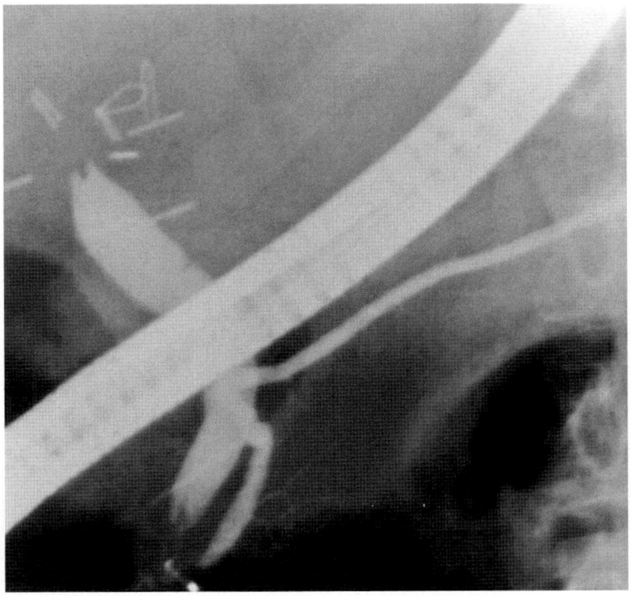

FIGURE 17–3 Endoscopic retrograde endoscopic retrograde cholangiopancreatography with double-duct sign.

duct, medially by the common hepatic duct, and superiorly by the liver parenchyma. This small area contains a number of important structures including the cystic artery, right hepatic artery, cystic node, and a potentially endless combination of arterial and biliary variants. This area must be meticulously dissected during cholecystectomy to avoid inadvertent ductal and arterial injuries. In the setting of acute cholecystitis, this area is often quite inflamed, and dissection can be difficult and hazardous. Nonetheless, a prerequisite for safe cholecystectomy remains the proper identification of the structures within and adjacent to this area.

The hepatoduodenal ligament (also referred to as the porta hepatis) comprises the common bile duct anterolaterally, the proper hepatic artery anteromedially, and the portal vein posteriorly. In addition, the nerves and lymphatics to the liver course through this important structure. Access to the lesser sac is possible posterior to the hepatoduodenal ligament via an opening referred to as the epiploic foramen of Winslow. Vascular control of the liver may be obtained in urgent situations by encircling the hepatodoudenal ligament with the thumb and forefinger and compressing the vascular structures contained within. Such a maneuver is referred to as the *Pringle maneuver* and aids in the control of hemorrhage from the liver parenchyma in traumatic situations or during elective hepatic resections. Compression of the ligament may be undertaken for up to 1 hour in some circumstances, although warm ischemic injury of the liver may result.

Physiology

Bile Production

Healthy patients make and excrete approximately 500 mL to 1000 mL of bile per day. Certain stimuli, such as the release of secretin from the duodenum (in response to hydrochloric acid) and meals rich in fatty foods, increase the production of bile, a green semiviscous fluid, consisting of electrolytes, bile salts, proteins, cholesterol, fats, and bile pigments. The concentration of the electrolytes roughly mirrors that of serum. The pH of bile ranges from 5.7 to 8.6 and tends to be more alkalotic at higher rates of secretion and more acidotic in response to protein stimulation. The major bile salts, cholic, deoxycholic, and chenodeoxycholic acids, are anionic and conjugated with either taurine or glycine. In addition, bile contains unesterified cholesterol, lecithin, and fatty acids. Bile receives its characteristic greenish yellow color from the presence of the pigment bilirubin diglucoronide, a breakdown product of hemoglobin.

The gallbladder functions primarily as a storage organ for bile. Although it also serves the purpose of concentrating bile, humans can (and do) live quite normal lives without their gallbladders. Once bile is produced by the liver, it flows via the common hepatic and cystic ducts to the gallbladder, where electrolytes and some bile pigments are selectively reabsorbed. The exception to this process is bicarbonate, which achieves a concentration twice that of plasma. Mucus also is secreted by the gallbladder (~20 mL/24 hr) and serves as a protective barrier against the lytic action of bile.

After the ingestion of food, the gallbladder contracts and expels its contents into the duodenum via the ductal system. The contraction of the gallbladder occurs simultaneously with the relaxation of the sphincter of Oddi. This process is triggered by the presence of food in the duodenum (particularly fatty foods) and is mediated primarily by cholecystokinin released from the intestinal mucosa.

Gallstone Formation

Gallstones form as a result of solids precipitating out of a solution. Composed primarily of cholesterol, bile pigment, and calcium, gallstones result from the complex interaction of the bile-lecithin micelle and cholesterol. Although cholesterol is insoluble in aqueous solutions, it becomes soluble when incorporated into the bile-lecithin micelle. Lecithin is the predominant phospholipid in bile. Plotting the percentages of lecithin, bile salt, and cholesterol on a triangular area (Fig. 17-5) reveals a narrow area in which the solubility of cholesterol in bile is defined. When this area is exceeded, cholesterol crystals result and often coalesce to form gallstones.

Although most stones contain all three elements (cholesterol, bile pigment, and calcium), the percentages of each element may vary. In Western cultures, the majority of stones are approximately 70% cholesterol and have a characteristic chalky or clay appearance. Bilirubin pigment stones

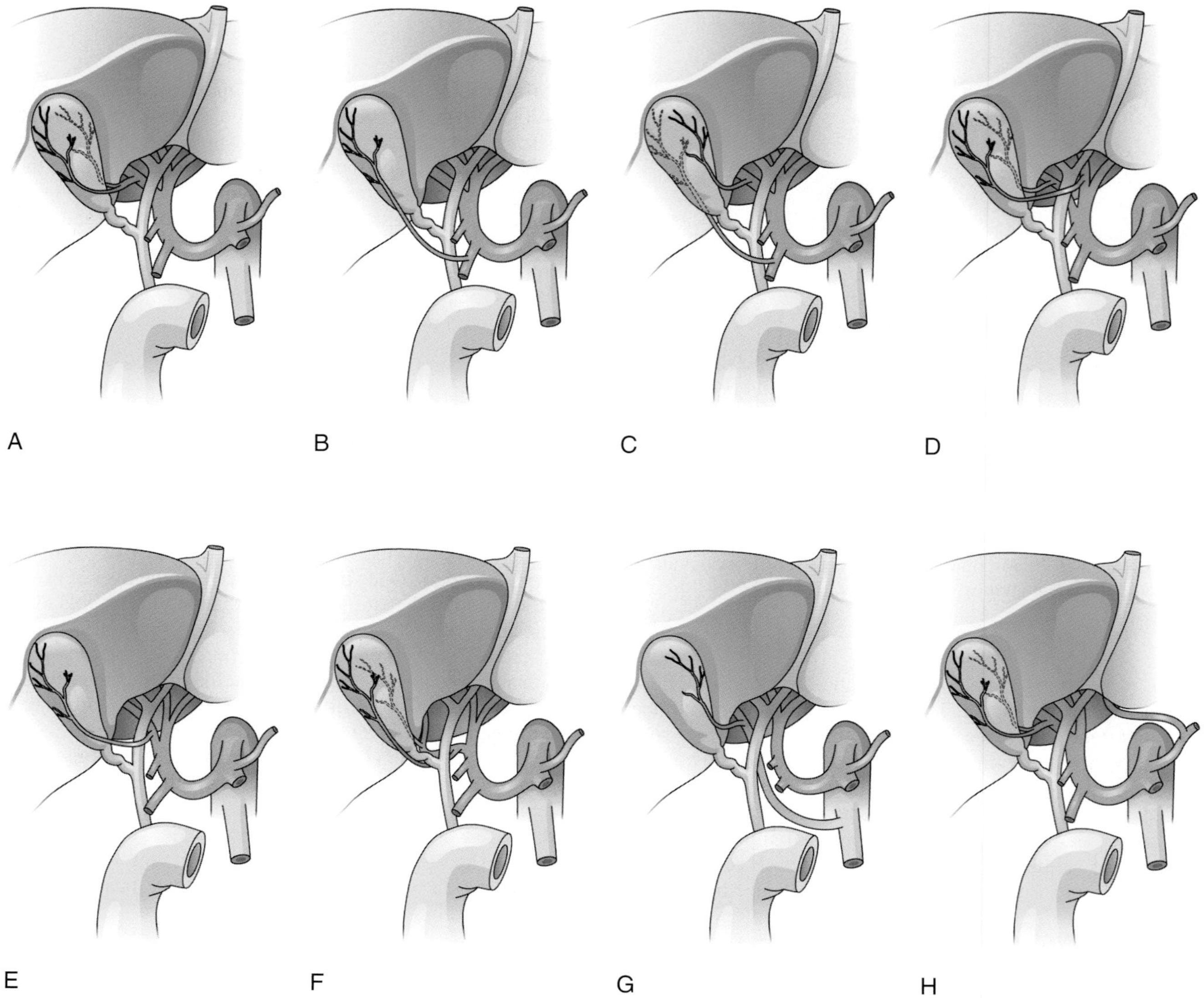

FIGURE 17–4 Anomalies of the arteries to the gallbladder. *A*, Normal cystic artery anatomy. *B–H*, Potential variability in the origin and course of the cystic artery.

are less common in Western cultures and appear smooth and shiny with a green or black surface. Pigmented stones tend to be associated with hemolytic conditions or situations of increased red cell destruction, such as that seen with prosthetic heart valve replacement. Pigmented stones have higher concentrations of calcium and therefore are radio-opaque on routine abdominal radiographs, as opposed to cholesterol stones, which have lower calcium concentrations and are therefore radiolucent.

The question, "Why do some people form gallstones while others do not?" still remains largely unanswered. Although a variety of factors such as ethnicity, bile stasis, bacteria, fungi, hormones, and reflux of intestinal fluid may all play a role, no absolute predictive criteria are known. Pima Indians, for example, have a 70% incidence of gallstones, whereas gallstones are virtually absent among the Masai of Africa. In addition, although *Escherichia coli* and *Streptococcus* spp. have been isolated from gallbladders with stones, infection is frequently absent in many other patients with stones. Reflux of intestinal fluid into the bile also has been inconsistently found in patients with and without gallstones. Finally, stasis of bile flow, probably a major contributor in most cases of gallstone formation, is difficult to quantify accurately and therefore has little predictive value.

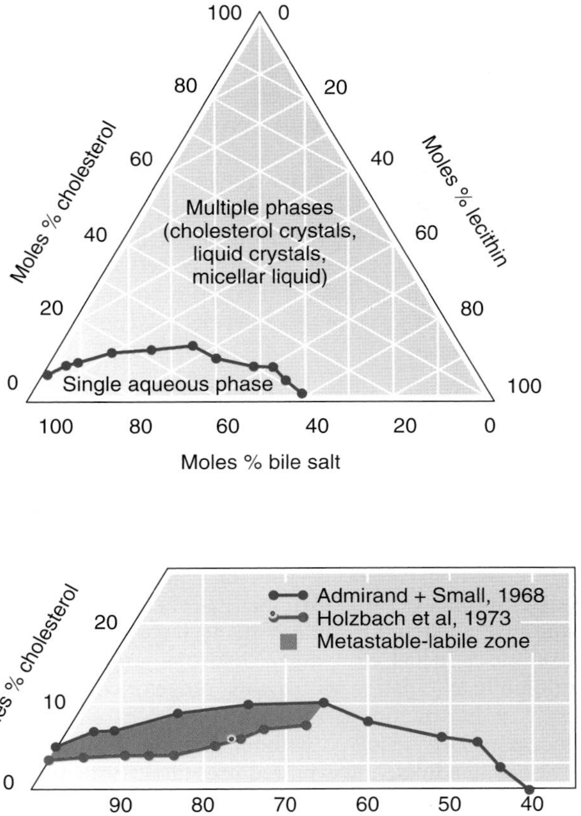

FIGURE 17–5 Triangular diagram in which the amounts of lecithin, bile salt, and cholesterol can be used to express the lithogenicity of bile. Lines are drawn into the triangle perpendicular from the appropriate point on each side of the triangle. If the point at which they intersect is above the blue line, cholesterol is completely soluble; if beneath, the bile is supersaturated. Stone formation can occur in the metastable-labile zone if specific nucleating factors are present. (Adapted from Nahrwold DL: Chronic cholecystitis and cholelithiasis. In Sabiston DC (ed): Sabiston Textbook of Surgery, 14th ed. Philadelphia, WB Saunders, 1991, with permission.)

When bile flow to the intestine is decreased, a corresponding decrease occurs in the liver's output of bile acids and phospholipids and a subsequent decrease in cholesterol solubility. Enterohepatic circulation of bile salts also is decreased when the distal third of the small intestine is resected, which explains the high incidence of gallstone formation in such patients. Prophylactic cholecystectomy should be considered in patients undergoing extensive resection of their distal small intestine because of this increased incidence.

In all likelihood, all of these factors combine in a variety of ways to alter the solubility characteristics of bile. Regimens have been developed in an attempt to alter favorably the solubility characteristics of bile and either prevent gallstone formation or dissolve stones once they form. Such regimens, however, of which chenodeoxycholic acid administration is one example, have met with limited success, as stone dissolution is slow and incomplete. Moreover, stones reform once the medication is discontinued, and significant side effects occur (e.g., nausea, diarrhea, liver dysfunction) from prolonged use of such medications.

Although one cannot predict with certainty who will and who will not develop gallstones during their lifetimes, some characteristics appear more common in patients who eventually develop gallstones. The so-called five Fs have been used to describe a "typical" **f**emale patient who is in her **f**orties, has been pregnant in the past (**f**ertile), is of **f**air complexion, and is a bit overweight (**f**at). Although these characteristics do apply to many patients with gallstone disease, they are by no means all inclusive, and gallstone formation also occurs in a variety of people, including men who are thin and of dark complexion.

Symptomatic versus Asymptomatic Gallstones

It is not known why some people form stones, whereas others do not, or why some stones cause symptoms (i.e., obstruction of bile flow and pain), whereas others do not. It is useful to consider gallstones that are asymptomatic separately from those that cause symptoms.

The exact incidence of asymptomatic gallstones in the American population is not known, but some autopsy reports put the estimate at 20% of women and 10% of men. As more physicians order ultrasonography, increasing numbers of patients who were unaware of the presence of gallstones are found to have them. Asymptomatic gallstones require no specific treatment, and "prophylactic" cholecystectomy to prevent future symptoms is not indicated. Most authorities believe, however, that symptoms will develop in approximately 2% of asymptomatic patients per year. It is simple to infer, therefore, that asymptomatic stones discovered in an elderly patient are much more likely to remain "silent," as opposed to those discovered in a younger person.

Gallstones produce symptoms when they cause obstruction of the flow of bile from the gallbladder or bile ducts into the intestine. Biliary colic (colicky pain referable to the biliary tree) results from the intermittent obstruction of bile flow into the duodenum. The obstruction can occur at any point along the extrahepatic biliary tree, but most typically involves the gallbladder/cystic duct junction. Although it can occur for other reasons, the most common cause of biliary colic (by far) is a gallstone that temporarily blocks the outflow of bile from the gallbladder into the common bile duct. Typically, the attack is triggered by a fatty meal, although attacks may occur with bland diets or at random. The typical symptoms include excruciating pain that is localized to the right upper quadrant or midepigastrium or both. The pain also may radiate through to the back and right shoulder. Patients frequently experience nausea and have the sensation that vomiting will relieve their symptoms. Many patients will induce vomiting to obtain relief. The attacks may last from several minutes to several hours. If the attack is self-limiting, the stone that was blocking the outflow is dislodged, the gallbladder empties, and the pain resolves. Patients with biliary colic alone are usually afebrile with normal white blood cell (WBC) counts and normal liver-function tests. Conversely, if the attack is not self-limiting and the obstruction persists, so too does the pain, and cholecystitis often develops.

It is generally accepted that if patients are good surgical candidates, one episode of biliary colic is sufficient to recommend elective cholecystectomy. This is based on the fact that once a patient has had an attack of colic, he or she is likely to have another. The time interval between attacks can range from days to years. In addition, biliary colic often precedes the development of cholecystitis, a more serious condition and one that often requires urgent surgery. Although an attack of biliary colic that resolves does not represent a surgical emergency, it should not be ignored. Close follow-up with that patient is required, and the risks and benefits of elective cholecystectomy discussed with an experienced surgeon.

Biliary Dyskinesia

Although the precise pathophysiology of biliary dyskinesia is not entirely understood, a small subset of patients has classic symptoms of biliary colic, yet ultrasonography fails to demonstrate the presence of gallstones. Such patients, who may be diagnosed as having biliary dyskinesia, have typical right-upper-quadrant pain, nausea, and vomiting after fatty meals. Although the US of the biliary tree is normal, an underlying functional obstruction may be present from either a "kinked" cystic duct or other aberrant anatomy. Such obstruction often causes the classic symptoms of pain with eating, even in the absence of gallstones. Diagnosis is usually made by a radionucleotide hepatobiliary iminodiacetic acid (HIDA) scan, which reveals less than 35% emptying of the gallbladder after stimulation with cholecystokinin (CCK). Pain that is reproduced with injection of CCK also is supporting evidence for this condition. In all cases of suspected biliary dyskinesia, a thorough search for other causes of abdominal pain must be sought (e.g., peptic ulcer disease, gastroesophageal reflux disease [GERD], pancreatitis) before cholecystectomy is recommended. In four of five patients in whom the diagnosis is confirmed, cholecystectomy provides symptomatic relief.

Gallbladder Polyps

Occasionally, patients are found to have polyps within the gallbladder on US examination. Although rare, gallbladder polyps represent localized overgrowths of the gallbladder epithelial lining, which can manifest as either pedunculated or flat sessile structures. Most authors recommend elective cholecystectomy for lesions larger than 1 cm in diameter. However, smaller polyps located in the neck of the gallbladder have been known to cause outlet obstruction and symptoms of biliary colic. If a polyp is suspected as being the cause of biliary symptoms, then elective cholecystectomy also is warranted.

Hydrops of the Gallbladder

Complete obstruction of the gallbladder outlet, usually by an impacted stone, results in hydrops of the gallbladder. Over time, bile pigments are reabsorbed by the gallbladder, and the organ becomes filled with a clear mucoid material. This condition can occur with or without accompanying cholecystitis. Occasionally, the gallbladder can become quite distended and reach extremely large sizes. Although most cases occur in adults, hydrops may develop in children in association with a wide range of conditions that result in narrowing of the cystic duct. In children, the process usually resolves without treatment. Hydrops that develops in adults, however, requires cholecystectomy.

Diagnosis

Liver-Function Tests

The collection of blood tests used to characterize liver and biliary function has traditionally included the enzymes alkaline phosphatase, serum glutamic-oxaloacetic transaminase (AST/SGOT), serum glutamate pyruvate transaminase (ALT/SGPT), lactic acid dehydrogenase (LDH), and bilirubin. Levels of certain plasma proteins such as albumin and fibrinogen also have been used to assess hepatic synthetic function. The prothrombin time (PT), a measure of coagulability, is the most sensitive test for hepatic synthetic reserve. Patients not receiving anticoagulation medication who are noted to have a prolongation in their PT should be suspected of having underlying severe liver dysfunction.

Alkaline phosphatase is a sensitive measure of biliary obstruction, and its serum level increases with impairment of bile outflow from either benign or malignant causes. Elevated levels (from nonhepatic sources) may be noted with increased osteoblastic activity sometimes seen in the setting of bone metastases from cancer. The source of an elevated alkaline phosphatase can be distinguished by fractionating the isoenzymes based on their heat sensitivity. An elevation in liver enzymes (AST/ALT) is associated with hepatocyte inflammation and is usually seen in the setting of acute cholecystitis, hepatitis, or ischemic injury to the liver. Other conditions also may lead to an elevation in liver enzymes. Finally, elevations in serum bilirubin levels should always raise the suspicion of an underlying obstructive process, although hyperbilirubinemia may be seen in a variety of diseases. Biliary colic is usually associated with a normal serum bilirubin level, whereas acute cholecystitis may produce a slight elevation. Malignant obstruction of the biliary tree produces the most significant increase in serum bilirubin levels.

Ultrasonography

An abdominal US examination is often the first radiologic test ordered with a suspicion of biliary tract disease. It is safe, relatively inexpensive, and noninvasive. Its greatest efficacy lies in identifying gallbladder morphology and contents and in differentiating mechanical from metabolic causes of jaundice. Dilation of the intrahepatic or extrahepatic bile ducts or both is often first diagnosed by US and is highly suggestive of a mechanical cause of jaundice. Conversely, normal-caliber ducts by US would suggest a metabolic or infectious cause for jaundice. In addition, gallbladder-wall thickening and stones often help confirm the clinical suspicion of acute cholecystitis.

Endoscopic Retrograde Cholangiopancreatography in Patients with Biliary Disease

The approach to the diagnosis and management of common bile duct pathology has changed dramatically since the introduction of endoscopic retrograde cholangiopancreatography (ERCP). Developed in the early 1970s, ERCP involves passing a flexible side-viewing endoscope through the mouth into the second portion of the duodenum. A catheter is then inserted (through the endoscope) into the ampulla of Vater, contrast injected into the biliary and pancreatic ducts, and radiologic images obtained. In addition to its diagnostic capabilities, ERCP also has therapeutic capabilities, as sphincterotomy may be performed of the ampulla for extraction of common bile duct stones and relief of obstruction (Fig. 17-6). In acute cholangitis or gallstone pancreatitis with jaundice, ERCP is the initial treatment of choice for common bile duct obstruction. Finally, ERCP is often very useful in establishing a tissue diagnosis when malignancy is suspected.

Before the advent of laparoscopic cholecystectomy, stones within the common bile duct were addressed at the time of operation for gallbladder disease. With the widespread use of laparoscopic surgery to treat symptomatic gallstone disease, however, ERCP has played a prominent role in the management of suspected or confirmed common bile duct stones. Although many centers perform laparoscopic common bile duct explorations (thus obviating the need for ERCP), such a technique can be technically challenging and is not widely available in all hospitals. ERCP remains an invaluable part of the algorithm for diagnosing and managing patients suspected of having common bile duct stones.

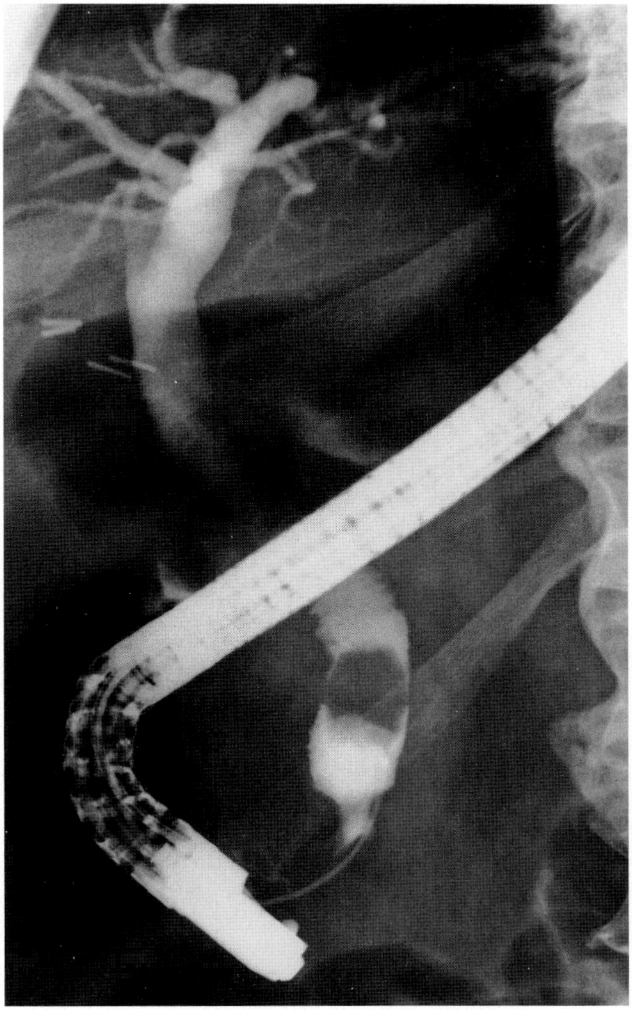

FIGURE 17–6 Common bile duct stone on endoscopic retrograde cholangiopancreatography.

A more controversial issue, however, relates to the timing of ERCP vis-à-vis performing a laparoscopic cholecystectomy. Stated more explicitly, the question is: What are the indications to perform an ERCP before a laparoscopic cholecystectomy? Although much debate continues on this issue, the factors to be considered are (1) the degree of suspicion of common duct stones, (2) the expertise of the ERCP endoscopist, (3) the clinical state of the patient, and (4) the expertise of the surgeon. For patients in whom the suspicion for common duct stones is high (defined as a preoperative bilirubin >2.0 or a dilated common bile duct seen on US or both), a preoperative ERCP is probably warranted. In addition, the likelihood of having to remove the gallbladder via an open approach (during which a formal common duct exploration could be undertaken) should be low. Conversely, for patients in whom the index of suspicion is low (normal bilirubin and normal common bile duct), no indication exists for routine preoperative ERCP. Finally, for patients with a history of gallstone pancreatitis, ERCP is indicated only if jaundice (bilirubin >2) was diagnosed in conjunction with the pancreatitis. For surgeons skilled in laparoscopic common bile duct exploration, however, the role of ERCP has diminished as both a diagnostic and a therapeutic modality.

Recently, magnetic resonance cholangiopancreatography (MRCP) also has found a role in the diagnosis of biliary pathology. In most centers, the sensitivity and specificity appear equal with those of ERCP in diagnosing common bile duct stones. Although it has the advantage of being less invasive than ERCP for diagnosis, it lacks the therapeutic potential of stone extraction seen with ERCP. Its exact role in the diagnostic and treatment algorithm of biliary disease remains to be clearly defined, but its most likely utility will be as a screening tool for suspected common bile duct pathology.

Acute Cholecystitis

Acute cholecystitis, or inflammation of the gallbladder, remains one of the most common conditions encountered by the general surgeon. In the vast majority of cases (>90%), obstruction of the cystic duct by a stone is the initiating event. Typically it is distinguished from an attack of biliary colic by persistent (as opposed to intermittent) right-upper-quadrant pain, fever, elevation in WBCs, and alteration in liver chemistries. After obstruction of the cystic duct, the gallbladder distends, causing subserosal edema, venous and lymphatic obstruction, cellular infiltration, and localized areas of ischemia. Acute cholecystitis is associated with a variety of bacterial pathogens in 50% to 75% of cases. The organisms most frequently cultured from the gallbladder specimen are *Escherichia coli*, *Klebsiella aerogenes*, *Streptococcus fecalis*, *Clostridium* spp., *Enterobacter* spp., and *Proteus* spp. Antibiotic regimens should be tailored to cover these common pathogens. If left untreated, severe, gangrenous cholecystitis (most often seen in diabetic patients) may develop, leading to increased morbidity and mortality from perforation of the gallbladder or overwhelming sepsis. Another potential complication of untreated cholecystitis is perforation of the gallbladder into the wall of adjacent hollow viscera (duodenum, jejunum or colon), causing a cholecystoenteric fistula. If a stone subsequently passes into the hollow viscera, bowel obstruction may result. This condition is referred to as *gallstone ileus*.

Diagnosis

Most patients in whom acute cholecystitis develops will have a history of abdominal symptoms referable to the biliary tree, although some patients have acute cholecystitis as their first manifestation of stone disease. In all cases of acute cholecystitis, persistent right-upper-quadrant pain with peritoneal irritation (rebound tenderness or Murphy's sign) is the most characteristic symptom and sign. Initially the pain is due to the obstruction of the cystic duct with distention of the gallbladder, similar to the pain of biliary colic. However, once inflammation, edema, and ischemia develop, the pain is due to the irritation of adjacent peritoneal surfaces. Like that with biliary colic, the pain is usually located in the right upper quadrant but also may be in the midepigastrium and occasionally radiates to the shoulder and back. However, in contrast to pain from biliary colic, which tends to last only a few hours, pain from acute cholecystitis may last for several days. Similar to biliary colic, however, nausea, vomiting, and anorexia are common in patients with acute cholecystitis.

Physical examination of patients with acute cholecystitis typically reveals an ill-appearing patient with an elevated temperature. Frequently, the inflamed gallbladder can be palpated in the right upper quadrant as a tender, distended mass, although this finding is not uniformly present. Diabetics, in particular, may have severe cholecystitis with minimal findings on physical examination. Murphy's sign refers to the sudden pain from deep palpation in the right upper quadrant during inspiration, as the inflamed gallbladder descends to meet the examining hand. Patients often stop their inspiratory effort during mid-breath. A similar event during US of the right upper quadrant has been termed an *ultrasonic Murphy's sign* as the US probe comes in contact with the gallbladder.

Laboratory findings in patients with acute cholecystitis include an elevated WBC count with an associated bandemia. In addition, liver function tests (particularly AST, ALT, and alkaline phosphatase) are elevated. Total bilirubin is usually moderately elevated (in the 1 to 2 range), although significant elevation (>2) should raise the suspicion of concomitant common bile duct obstruction. Patients first seen very late in their illness may, ironically, have completely normal liver chemistries.

The two most common radiologic studies used for the diagnosis of acute cholecystitis are abdominal US and HIDA scan. Plain radiographs have limited utility because only approximately 15% of gallstones are radio-opaque, and the gallbladder is not visualized on standard roentgenograms. US is usually performed early in the workup of such patients (Fig. 17-7). Questions to be answered by the ultrasound are "Are gallstones present?," "Is the gallbladder distended?," "Is thickening of the gallbladder wall and/or pericholecystic fluid found?," and "Is dilatation of the intrahepatic or extrahepatic bile ducts present?" Radiologists will often use gallbladder-wall thickening as a criterion for the diagnosis of cholecystitis. Significant false positives and false negatives may occur with this finding. For example, patients with low serum albumin and normal gallbladders may have peri-

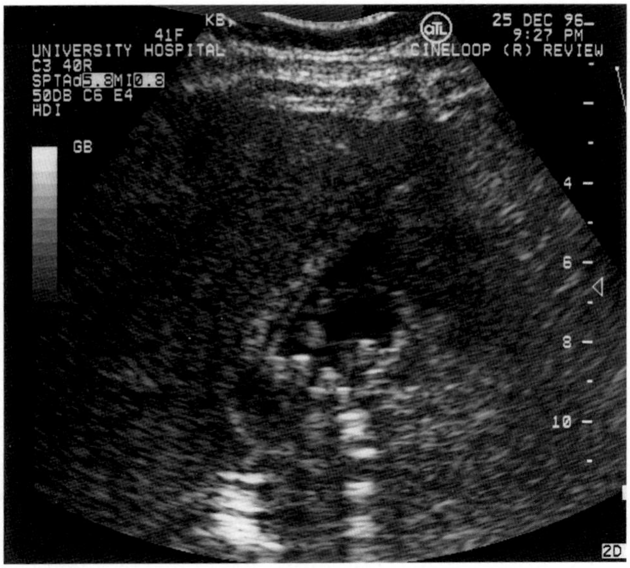

FIGURE 17–7 Ultrasound of the gallbladder with stones and wall thickening.

cholecystic fluid in the absence of inflammation because of generalized anasarca. In addition, patients who have severe cholecystitis may be judged to have normal wall thickness by US. The most reliable US signs are the documentation of stones, a distended gallbladder, and presence or absence of an ultrasonic Murphy's sign. Finally, the diameter of the extrahepatic bile ducts must always be evaluated to exclude the possibility of choledocholithiasis. which may alter the treatment plan.

In patients in whom the diagnosis of acute cholecystitis is questionable, a nuclear medicine HIDA scan may be useful. In patients who do *not* have obstruction of the cystic duct, the scan will outline the extrahepatic biliary system with uptake of dye into the gallbladder, which is referred to as visualization of the gallbladder on HIDA (Fig. 17-8*A*). In patients with cystic duct obstruction, the gallbladder will *not* be visualized (Fig. 17-8*B*). The test is very sensitive in patients who have been eating recently, but has a 10% to 15% false-positive rate in patients who have taken nothing by mouth (NPO) for several days. For this reason, its usefulness in intensive care unit (ICU) patients is somewhat limited. For patients with typical signs and symptoms of acute cholecystitis and a positive US, HIDA scan is usually not necessary to confirm the diagnosis.

Differential Diagnosis

Acute cholecystitis may mimic a number of other acute intraabdominal processes including appendicitis, perforated peptic ulcer, small-bowel obstruction, hepatitis, and acute pancreatitis. In addition, pneumonia, myocardial ischemia, and herpes zoster (shingles) should be included in the differential. A careful history and physical examination, however, can usually distinguish cholecystitis from other causes of right-upper-quadrant pain. An elevation in the serum amylase, occasionally seen in acute cholecystitis, may make the diagnosis of pancreatitis versus cholecystitis difficult. Here, an abdominal computed tomography (CT) scan may be useful to look for the presence of inflammation within the pancreas.

Treatment

Patients suspected of having acute cholecystitis should be admitted to the hospital, made NPO, and started on intravenous fluids. If the diagnosis is confirmed, intravenous antibiotics effective against the common pathogens should be instituted.

Unless contraindications exist (myocardial ischemia, pancreatitis, cholangitis), cholecystectomy should be performed within the first 24 to 36 hours of admission. If patients are first seen later in their illness (e.g., 4 or 5 days), some benefit may accrue to managing the acute illness with antibiotics and deferring definitive treatment (laparoscopic removal) to 6 weeks hence. Because the inflammatory process tends to be the most severe between 72 hours and 1 week of the onset of symptoms, the technical challenge of successful laparoscopic removal is greatest during this period, and the conversion rate to an open procedure may be increased. In all cases, however, an attack of cholecystitis requires eventual removal of the gallbladder, except in very poor-risk patients. Such poor-risk patients may benefit from placement of a percutaneous cholecystostomy tube under US guidance and local anesthesia.

Extracorporeal Shock Wave Lithotripsy

Extracorporeal shock-wave lithotripsy (ESWL) was used in the past to treat selected patients with gallstones. The technique was based on the principle that gallstones fragment when acoustic energy (shock waves) is focused on them. The goal was to fracture the stones into pieces small enough to pass through the cystic duct and sphincter of Oddi, roughly thought to be about 5 mm. Unfortunately, the success rates with this technique were low, and the complication rates, high. This procedure, therefore, has been abandoned.

Gallstone Pancreatitis

It is estimated that approximately 40% of all cases of acute pancreatitis in the United States are due to the passage of gallstones through the common bile duct and temporary obstruction of the pancreatic duct at the ampulla of Vater. How this phenomenon triggers pancreatic inflammation is still not certain, although some evidence suggests that bile reflux into the pancreatic duct through a common channel

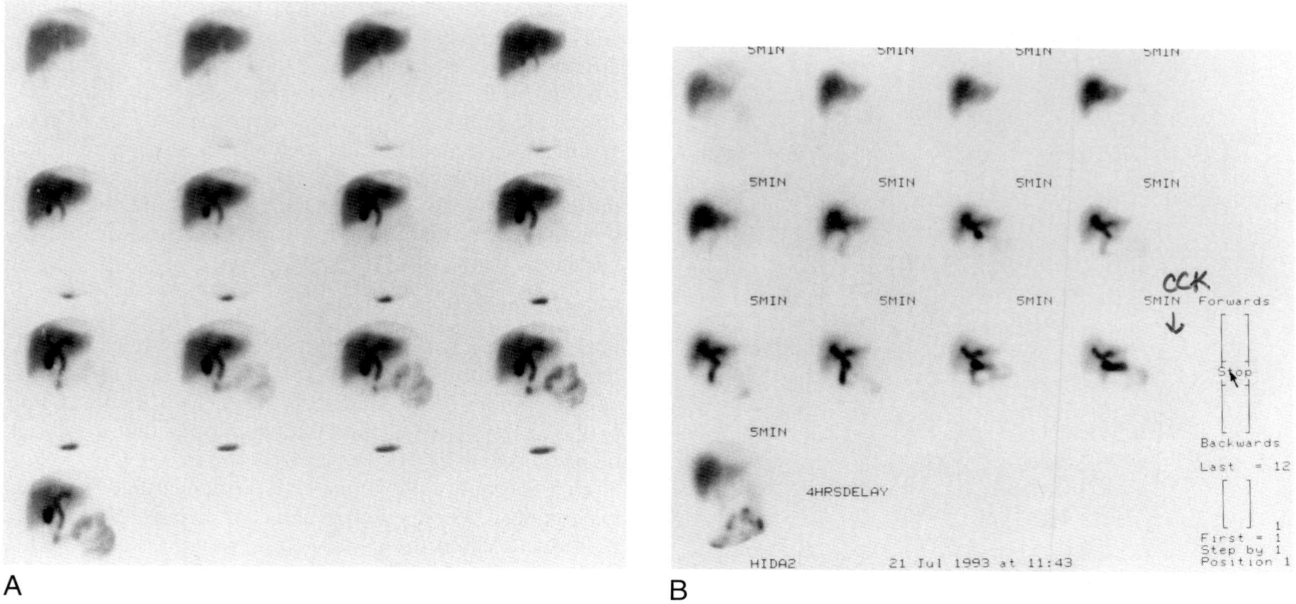

FIGURE 17–8 Hepatobiliary iminodiacetic acid (HIDA) scan with (*A*) and without (*B*) gallbladder visualization.

may damage the duct and increase its permeability to pancreatic enzymes. This mechanism is largely speculative.

Patients with gallstone-induced pancreatitis usually have epigastric pain, often with radiation around through to the back, in association with nausea and vomiting. Elevated serum levels of amylase and lipase are typical early in the course of the disease and, along with clinical findings, often confirm the diagnosis of pancreatitis. In patients with known gallstones and no other of the common causes of pancreatitis, the diagnosis of gallstone pancreatitis can be made with a high degree of reliability, even if gallstones are not seen in the common bile duct by US.

The timing of cholecystectomy in the setting of gallstone pancreatitis depends entirely on the clinical course the pancreatitis follows. In patients with mild to moderate disease, the treatment usually consists of a period of initial observation. If the patient's signs and symptoms improve during the first 48 hours and gallstones are considered the source, then an elective laparoscopic cholecystectomy is usually performed during that hospital admission. If jaundice accompanies the pancreatitis, then a preoperative ERCP is indicated to rule out retained common bile duct stones. In addition, if a patient deteriorates during the first 48 hours, an ERCP also may be indicated to determine whether a stone is impacted at the ampulla of Vater. Careful consideration must be given, however, to the possibility of making the pancreatitis worse with the ERCP. Once the obstruction (if present) is relieved, the pancreatitis becomes the focus of management, and patients are cared for according to the generally accepted principles of pancreatitis management. When the pancreatitis resolves (which may take several weeks), patients are discharged from the hospital and scheduled for an elective cholecystectomy several months later to prevent future attacks.

Laparoscopic Cholecystectomy

In 1992, an NIH Consensus conference concluded, "Laparoscopic cholecystectomy provides a safe and effective treatment for most patients with symptomatic gallstones and indeed, is the treatment of choice for these patients." Although widely accepted today, this recommendation represented a radical shift in the way biliary surgery had been performed for more than a century. What had once been a fairly morbid procedure performed through a lengthy right-upper-quadrant or midline incision and associated with a prolonged recovery was modified to a minimally invasive approach with decreased morbidity and earlier return to normal activities. With the exception of a few relative contraindications (portal hypertension, previous right-upper-quadrant surgery, cirrhosis), most patients are suitable candidates for laparoscopic gallbladder removal. This advent of laparoscopic surgical techniques has made the surgery for biliary tract disease less morbid. Not all patients, however, are amenable to successful laparoscopic surgery, and some patients require conversion during the

PEARLS FOR THE OR

How to perform safe dissection

Gallbladder is retracted superiorly while the redundant infundibulum is retracted laterally to expose the cystic duct—gallbladder junction.

Dissect only the gallbladder—cystic duct junction. Avoid dissecting the common bile duct unless common bile duct exploration is anticipated.

Clearly visualize and confirm all structures before ligating and dividing; always be attentive to the likelihood of biliary and arterial anomalies and variations.

Learn to expect the unexpected: ductal and arterial anatomic variability is the rule rather than the exception.

Calot's triangle is defined by the cystic duct laterally, the common hepatic duct medially, and the liver superiorly.

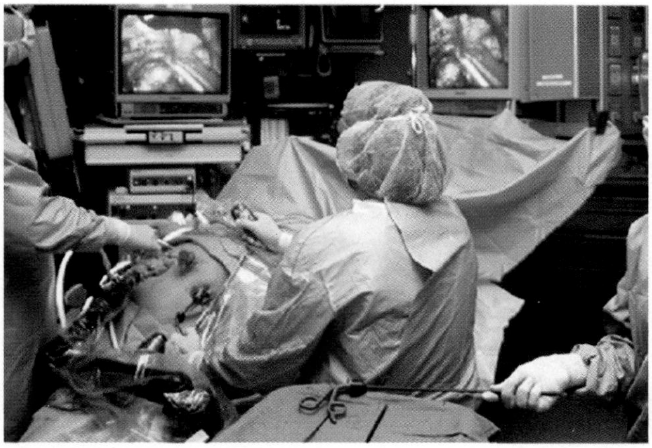

FIGURE 17–9 Typical operating room setup for laparoscopic cholecystectomy.

course of their operation to a traditional open approach. Whereas the conversion rate to an open procedure for elective cholecystectomy is 1% to 2%, the conversion rate for patients with acute cholecystitis ranges from 5% to 10%. This figure is even higher in diabetic patients.

Important Technical Aspects of Laparoscopic Cholecystectomy

Most patients undergoing elective laparoscopic cholecystectomy are managed as day-surgery patients if intraoperative complications do not develop. No special bowel preparation is required for patients undergoing laparoscopic cholecystectomy. After the induction of general anesthesia, patients are positioned supine on the operating table. An orogastric tube should be placed by the anesthesiologist for gastric decompression and removed at the conclusion of the case. Routine decompression of the urinary bladder is not required if the open technique of trocar insertion is used. The abdomen is then prepped and draped in the usual sterile fashion. A small infraumbilical incision is carried down to the fascia. The fascia is then grasped and elevated by using Kocher clamps and incised. A trocar (usually 10 mm) is inserted and secured in place. Carbon dioxide is insufflated under low pressure (15 mmHg), and a series of three trocars is inserted in the right subcostal area. By using instruments developed exclusively for laparoscopic surgery, the operation is begun by retracting the gallbladder superiorly over the edge of the liver, and dissection commences in the triangle of Calot (Figs. 17-9, 17-10, and 17-11). After careful identification, confirmation, and ligation of the cystic duct and cystic artery, the gallbladder is dissected free of the gallbladder fossa and delivered from the abdomen. Hemostasis is meticulously assured, and all trocars are removed under direct vision. The placement of intraabdominal drains is not indicated unless concern exists about the possibility of postoperative bile leak (i.e., from the gallbladder fossa or a tenuously ligated cystic duct). The trocar sites are then closed. Patients are taken to the recovery room where they are allowed to resume a normal diet as soon as they are sufficiently conscious to prevent aspiration. After discharge, most patients can resume normal activities within 5 days after surgery.

The appropriate use of intraoperative cholangiography during laparoscopic cholecystectomy is controversial. Most surgeons use it selectively (cases with suspicion of common duct stones in which ERCP was not performed preoperatively), as opposed to routinely (all cases). Routine use increases operative costs and has not been shown to

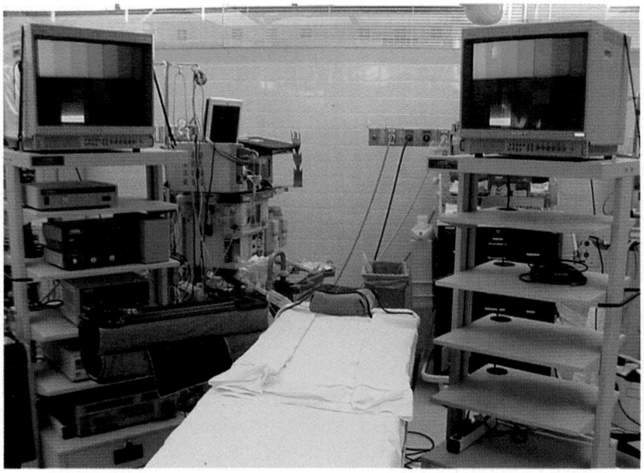

FIGURE 17–10 Typical instrumentation setup for laparoscopic cholecystectomy.

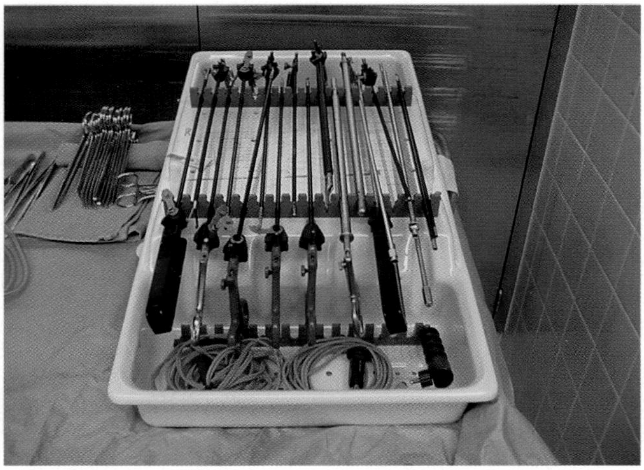

FIGURE 17–11 Typical instruments for laparoscopic cholecystectomy.

prevent biliary injuries. If, however, the anatomy is unclear, cholangiography may be useful in identifying biliary structures. If performed, the cholangiogram must be interpreted correctly by both the surgeon and the radiologist.

The technical aspects of an open cholecystectomy mirror those of a laparoscopic approach in terms of identification of structures and attention to detail. Rather than using laparoscopic instruments and small (trocar) incisions, a right-upper-quadrant or midline incision and traditional surgical instruments are used.

PEARLS FOR ROUNDS

Painless jaundice is an otherwise healthy patient is carcinoma of the biliary system until proven otherwise.

After laparoscopic cholecystectomy, patients should have minimal pain and be able to eat. Nausea, vomiting, and increasing abdominal pain are often early warning signs of a postoperative bile leak or other complication

Ultrasound examinations performed for biliary pathology: Need to know

- presence or absence of stones
- gallbladder wall thickening
- presence or absence of common bile duct dilatation

Patients admitted with acute cholecystitis should ingest nothing by mouth (NPO), given antibiotics, and operated on during that admission

Fractionate the total bilirubin into direct and indirect components to determine obstructive (i.e., surgical) causes of jaundice. High direct suggests obstructive cause for jaundice. High indirect suggests nonobstructive (e.g., hepatic) cause.

Complications of Laparoscopic (and Open) Cholecystectomy

Approximately 5% of patients undergoing cholecystectomy will have minor complications, such as atelectasis or fever or wound infections. In elective cases, the mortality of cholecystectomy is well below 1%. However, in a small percentage of cases, major complications can occur as a result of a technical misadventure. Complications can occur during the initial stages of the operation related to the establishment of the pneumoperitoneum. When the closed technique of insufflation is used, improper placement of the Veress needle may result in insufflation of gas into subcutaneous tissue, omentum, bowel, and vascular structures. For this reason, many surgeons use the Hasson open technique of trocar insertion. Here, the abdomen is entered under direct vision as opposed to blind puncture with the closed Veress technique. In addition, trocar insertion can injure any organ, vessel, or structure in the abdomen and should therefore be accomplished only under direct vision with an adequate cushion of pneumoperitoneum. If perforation of a hollow viscus or vascular structure occurs at any time during the operation, the procedure should be converted to open, and the injury repaired.

Complications related to the cholecystectomy itself include hemorrhage, bile duct injury, biliary leaks, and adjacent organ/vessel injuries. Bleeding may occur from several sources including the cystic artery, the hepatic arteries, the gallbladder fossa, or the abdominal wall site of trocar insertion. The more significant problem is hemorrhage from an uncontrolled vessel, which may result from inadequate ligation or inadvertent injury during dissection. When this occurs, the severity of the bleeding often appears magnified under the amplification of the laparoscope. However, if approached in a calm, methodical manner, most bleeding can be corrected without converting to an open procedure. If bleeding cannot be controlled easily, however, the surgeon should convert to an open procedure immediately. Insertion of additional trocars often aids in the control and exposure of hemorrhage because blind maneuvers and random application of hemoclips pose a threat to vital structures such as the bile duct and hepatic arterial supply.

The most dreaded complication from cholecystectomy, particularly during the evolution of laparoscopic surgery, remains injury to the extrahepatic biliary tree (Fig. 17-12). The most commonly injured bile ducts during laparoscopic cholecystectomy are the right hepatic, common hepatic, and common bile ducts. The lessons learned from injuries inflicted during the days of open cholecystectomy are applicable to laparoscopic surgery. The principle of dividing only what can be positively confirmed is of paramount importance. Meticulous dissection of the area near the infundibulum of the gallbladder to identify the cystic duct/gallbladder junction clearly is a prerequisite safe division of the cystic duct. A similar approach to the cystic artery will

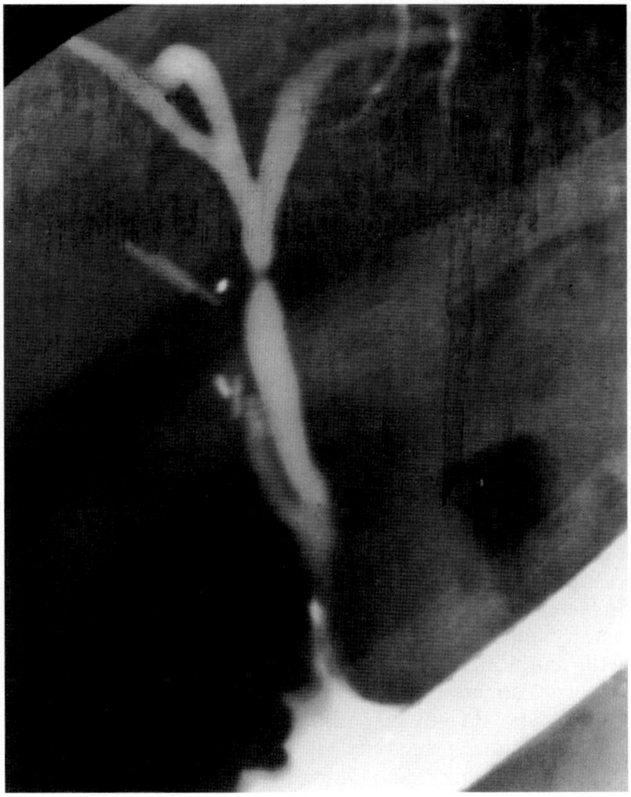

FIGURE 17–12 Bile duct injury from laparoscopic cholecystectomy.

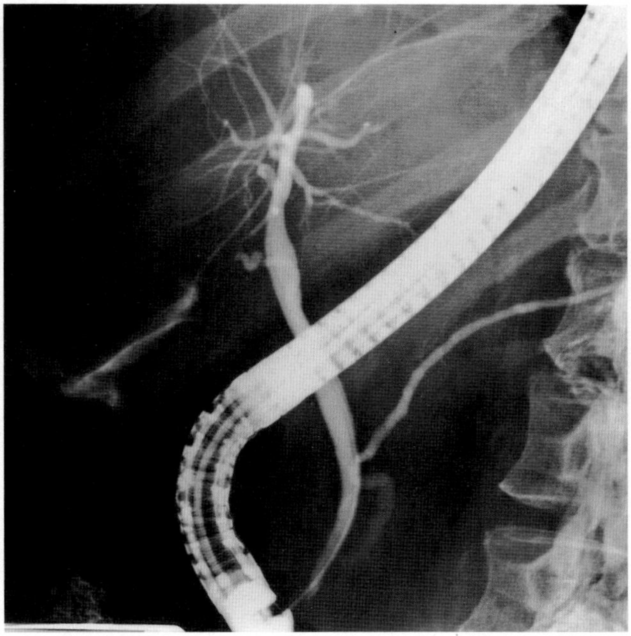

FIGURE 17–13 Bile duct leak after laparoscopic cholecystectomy from cystic duct stump.

decrease the likelihood of injury to the hepatic arterial tree. The morbidity that results from a bile duct injury is directly proportional to the time between the injury and the time it is recognized and definitively repaired. If recognized at the time of the laparoscopic procedure, the injury should be repaired immediately via an open approach and according to the standards previously developed for biliary injuries. If the injury is discovered postoperatively, the patient should be urgently evaluated by a surgeon with expertise in advanced hepatobiliary surgery, and definitive repair should be performed within 48 to 72 hours.

Biliary leaks after laparoscopic cholecystectomy are usually diagnosed when the patient has persistent postoperative pain or unexplained fever (Fig. 17-13). Other early warning signs are pain requiring increasing doses of narcotics or vomiting. If a leak is suspected, imaging studies such as ultrasound or HIDA scan will often confirm the diagnosis. Once it is confirmed, the patient should undergo an ERCP to document the source of the leak and percutaneous drainage of the bile collection. If the source of the leak is the liver bed (most common) or cystic duct, most of these will respond to a nasobiliary stent placed endoscopically in the extrahepatic biliary tree and drainage. If the source of the leak is a major bile duct injury, such as the right hepatic or common bile duct, then immediate operative repair is required.

The gallbladder is occasionally and inadvertently entered during its removal, spilling stones and bile into the abdominal cavity. Recovery of the spilled gallstones is always recommended but not always possible. Most surgeons would not convert an otherwise uncomplicated laparoscopic procedure to an open procedure solely for the purpose of retrieving gallstones. Reports have been made, however, of intraabdominal gallstones leading to delayed complications of bowel obstruction and infection.

Special Considerations

Biliary Disease in Diabetics

Until recently, diabetic patients were thought to be at increased risk for developing gallstones because of the metabolic complications of poor glycemic control. Moreover, diabetic patients with asymptomatic gallstones were recommended to undergo elective cholecystectomy based on a perceived increased morbidity and mortality when acute cholecystitis developed. Recent studies, however, have found no increased risk, and routine prophylactic cholecystectomies in diabetic patients are no longer recommended. It is true, however, that when complications develop in diabetics from their gallstones, they tend to be seen later in their illness, often with a more severe inflammatory response, and may have prolonged hospital stays. In addition, the conversion rate of laparoscopic cholecystectomy to open cholecystectomy has been reported to be higher in diabetic patients, presumably because of the increased inflammatory response and obscured anatomy.

Because it is often described in association with diabetic patients, emphysematous cholecystitis requires special mention. First diagnosed at surgery in 1908 and preoperatively in 1931, emphysematous cholecystitis (or gas gangrene of the gallbladder) results from gas-producing organisms found within the inflamed gallbladder. In one series of 161 cases by Mentzer, approximately one third occurred in diabetic patients. Diagnosis is readily made based on US, history, and physical examination. Treatment in all cases is prompt surgical intervention and appropriate antibiotic coverage.

Finally, diabetes is not a contraindication to laparoscopic surgery. However, the comorbidities associated with diabetic patients (particularly autonomic neuropathy) may lead to a delayed presentation of the biliary illness. These patients often are a unique technical challenge to even the most skilled laparoscopic surgeon, and the conversion rate to an open procedure appears to be slightly higher in this population. Forearmed with this knowledge, the surgeon can anticipate a technically challenging dissection and take extra precautions to identify vital structures.

Hepatic Cirrhosis

Biliary stone disease in patients with hepatic cirrhosis has long been a therapeutic and diagnostic challenge. The incidence of cholelithiasis in patients with cirrhosis has been reported to be as high as 46% compared with approximately 5% to 15% of the general population. Fortunately, most patients remain asymptomatic and do not require surgical intervention. However, if surgery is required, the mortality rate may be quite high. The mortality rate for open cholecystectomy in patients with cirrhosis is reported to be as high as 10% to 30%. Most of these deaths, however, occur in patients with advanced, complicated cirrhosis (Child's class C) who either have excessive blood loss during the operation or develop postoperative hepatic complications and sepsis. Patients with Child's A or B cirrhosis have much less morbidity and mortality, but the rates are still higher than those for the general population. For these reasons, it is generally accepted that patients with cirrhosis and cholelithiasis should be closely monitored and operated on only for significant symptomatic disease.

In the era of laparoscopic surgery, the role of cholecystectomy in patients with hepatic cirrhosis is still being defined. In the late 1980s, surgeons began performing laparoscopic cholecystectomies, but cirrhosis was considered a contraindication. However, recent series have demonstrated that the laparoscopic approach to patients with early cirrhosis (i.e., Child's A) is safe, effective, and does not lead to increased mortality. If severe inflammation is encountered, then a subtotal cholecystectomy (leaving the back wall of the gallbladder attached to the liver) is often the safest approach. Patients with advanced cirrhosis, portal hypertension, and ascites may still be best managed via an open approach if cholecystectomy is absolutely warranted.

Human Immunodeficiency Virus/Acquired Immunodeficiency Syndrome

Abdominal pain and gastrointestinal complications are common in patients with human immunodeficiency virus (HIV) and acquired immunodeficiency syndrome (AIDS), yet few patients require surgery. Diseases involving the biliary tract have been grouped together and classified as AIDS cholangiopathies. This term describes a spectrum of pathologic changes ranging from ampullary papillitis, biliary radical disease, sclerosing cholangitis, infectious cholangiopathies (particularly in patients superinfected with cytomegalovirus), and cholecystitis. In addition, diseases involving the common bile duct appear more commonly in AIDS patients. When cholecystitis develops in patients with AIDS, a higher incidence of the acalculous variety appears, often successfully treated nonoperatively with antibiotics. Cholecystitis from stones, however, also occurs. Patients with AIDS and cholecystitis (from any cause) who do not respond to antibiotic therapy should undergo cholecystectomy. Both laparoscopic and open cholecystectomies are well tolerated in compensated AIDS patients, although the conversion rate is slightly higher than that in the general population at 8.2%. Even patients with very low CD4 cell counts (i.e., <50) have a 50% 2-year survival after cholecystectomy. The presence of AIDS, therefore, should not be considered a contraindication to surgery in those patients that require it.

Critically Ill Patients and Acalculous Cholecystitis

Acute acalculous cholecystitis may develop in critically ill patients who have prolonged stays in the ICU. This phenomenon has become a well-recognized complication of the acute illnesses that often precipitate ICU admission in the first place. In addition, it may result as a complication of the subsequent treatment. Cholecystitis that develops in the ICU differs significantly from cholecystitis that develops in the general population in its etiology, presentation, and treatment. As opposed to the outpatient setting, where more than 90% of cases of acute cholecystitis are due to stone disease, only approximately 10% of cases of cholecystitis in the ICU are due to stone disease, with the remainder classified as *acalculous*.

The precise cause of acalculous cholecystitis is unclear, although biliary stasis and gallbladder ischemia seem to be prerequisites. Bacterial invasion is usually not the cause of acalculous cholecystitis, but rather represents superinfection of an already diseased gallbladder. Diagnosis can be difficult, although pain in the right upper quadrant, fever, and vomiting are signs that should alert the clinician to possibility of acalculous cholecystitis. Unfortunately, these signs also are present in a variety of other ICU conditions not directly referable to the biliary tree. The physical examination is notoriously unreliable, unless a palpable tender mass is present in the right upper quadrant. This is infrequently the case. Routine laboratory investigations are often unhelpful and may be misleading, because most patients will have a leukocytosis and liver-function test abnormalities, findings common in many ICU patients without the disease.

US is the most commonly ordered imaging study when acalculous cholecystitis is suspected. Unfortunately, the sensitivity and specificity of this test vary widely and have been reported to be as low as 50% in some series. Sonographic findings consistent with a diagnosis of acalculous cholecystitis include gallbladder-wall thickening, gallbladder distention, pericholecystic fluid, and sludge within the gallbladder. Gallbladder-wall thickening, thought by some to be the most specific test for acalculous cholecystitis, also is found in a variety of other conditions including hepatitis, hypoalbuminemia, and renal failure. Therefore many clinicians will rely on a radioactive technetium 99m scan (HIDA) to make the diagnosis. If the gallbladder is not visualized within 1 hour (positive HIDA), another scan is performed at 4 hours. Nonvisualization of the gallbladder indicates an obstructed cystic duct in 90% in outpatient settings. However, in the ICU setting, a false-positive rate may approach 50% because of prolonged fasting, decreased cholecystokinin-induced gallbladder contraction, narcotic administration, and total parenteral nutrition (TPN)-induced bile stasis. To overcome these obstacles, some surgeons will administer morphine sulfate in conjunction with the HIDA scan to induce contraction of the sphincter of Oddi. This increases bile duct pressure and diverts bile flow (and contrast) to the gallbladder if the cystic duct is patent. Although this improves the reliability of the test, false negatives and false positives are still common.

When a diagnosis of acalculous cholecystitis is confirmed, the management consists of both medical and surgical therapies. The gallbladder must be removed or percutaneously drained, and broad-spectrum intravenous antibiotics instituted. Because most ICU patients are not surgical candidates, radiologic placement of percutaneous cholecystostomy tubes has become an attractive alternative to surgical removal. However, some patients will have gangrenous acalculous cholecystitis and abscess formation, which may require surgical removal.

Hemobilia

Hemobilia is an unusual manifestation of biliary disease in which gastrointestinal hemorrhage occurs secondary to biliary tract bleeding. It may originate from almost any site along the biliary system, including the liver parenchyma itself or the intra- and extrahepatic bile ducts and gallbladder. Although the blood supply to the liver does not communicate directly with the biliary system, certain conditions, such as trauma, infection, or tumor, may create hemorrhage within the biliary tree. Penetrating or blunt trauma to the liver also may cause hemobilia. Most cases of hemobilia in the United States arise from iatrogenic causes such as liver biopsy, ERCP, and/or bile duct stent placement. Most recently, transjugular intrahepatic portosystemic shunt (TIPS) procedures have been associated with acute hemobilia. Infection, gallstones, and tumors account for the remaining cases.

Clinically, hemobilia may occur early or late in a disease process. The extent of the bleeding may be massive with hematemesis and shock, or minimal with only guaiac-positive stools. Classically, the triad of right-upper-quadrant pain, jaundice, and gastrointestinal bleeding suggests hemobilia as the source of bleeding.

The diagnosis of hemobilia is best made by arteriography. Occasionally, when a distal bile duct source is suspected, ERCP or percutaneous transhepatic cholangiography (PTC) may be useful. However, both procedures may actually cause hemobilia and may obscure the diagnosis. In addition to its diagnostic use, however, arteriography with selective hepatic arterial embolization is the initial treatment of choice for hemobilia. Because most hemobilia originates from an arterial rather than a venous source, selectively placed radiologic catheters can usually identify and embolize the bleeding source. However, if significant bleeding continues after embolization, operative intervention is mandatory.

Carcinoma of the Biliary Tract

Gallbladder Cancer

Carcinoma may occur at any point along the intra- or extrahepatic biliary tree, including the gallbladder. Carcinoma of the gallbladder is the fifth most common cancer of the gastrointestinal tract and the most common biliary tract cancer. Gallbladder cancer is more common in women than in men, occurs in older patients, and is usually quite advanced at the time of diagnosis. Early lesions, such as those discovered incidentally in gallbladders removed for cholelithiasis, are potentially cured with surgery. For most patients, however, the prognosis is dismal, and the usual forms of therapy, such as chemotherapy and radiation, are aimed primarily at palliating symptoms.

Patients with gallbladder cancer often are first seen with signs and symptoms similar to those for benign disease: right-upper-quadrant pain, nausea, vomiting, and jaundice. Occasionally, however, gallbladder carcinoma is completely asymptomatic at the time of diagnosis and is discovered in the course of a workup for painless jaundice. Approximately 90% of patients with gallbladder cancer have concurrent cholelithiasis, often leading to a delay in diagnosis of the cancer. A characteristic sign of gallbladder cancer is calcification of the gallbladder wall, termed *porcelain gallbladder*, and can be seen on either US or plain abdominal radiographs. When discovered, porcelain gallbladder is an absolute indication for cholecystectomy.

If discovered at the time of surgery, gallbladder cancer should be treated by excision of the gallbladder with a rim of surrounding hepatic parenchyma. More radical resections have not been shown to improve survival. Gallbladder carcinomas spread most commonly by direct extension into the liver parenchyma, by direct venous drainage, and through lymphatic channels. Direct extension also may involve adjacent structures such a stomach, duodenum, pancreas, colon, and omentum. If unresectable or widespread metastatic disease is present, efforts should be aimed at palliation of the biliary obstructive component of the disease. A choledochojejunostomy or hepaticojejunostomy can be performed if technically feasible. If tumor involvement prevents this approach, palliative drainage can be achieved postoperatively with PTC or stenting via ERCP.

The 5-year survival for patients with gallbladder cancer is less than 5%, and the median survival is less than 6 months. Long-term survivors are usually those whose gallbladder specimens were found to have in situ carcinoma, discovered during cholecystectomy for benign stone disease. Those patients do not require a second exploration for further liver resection.

Bile Duct Cancer

Adenocarcinomas of the biliary tree, termed *cholangiocarcinomas*, predominate in the extrahepatic biliary tree. As opposed to gallbladder cancer, which is more common in women, bile duct cancers are more common in men. In addition, cholangiocarcinomas tend to be more slow growing than gallbladder cancers, although they share the characteristics of being locally invasive and spreading primarily via lymphatics.

Bile duct cancers are classified primarily based on their location within the biliary tree (Fig. 17-14). Those of the middle and distal thirds (55%) are more easily managed than those of the proximal third (45%). Klatskin tumors refer to those tumors of the proximal third that involve the hilar bifurcation. The Bismuth classification further divides proximal tumors into four types. Type I tumors are those limited to the common hepatic duct; type II lesions involve the right and left hepatic ducts above the hilar bifurcation; and type III and IV are found in the intrahepatic secondary bile duct radicals.

Patients with bile duct cancer classically are initially seen with painless jaundice. If the jaundice has been prolonged and severe, debilitating pruritis is often present. Weight loss, fatigue, and vague abdominal pain also are seen. For distal tumors, the gallbladder may become distended, resulting in a painless, palpable gallbladder termed *Courvoisier's sign*.

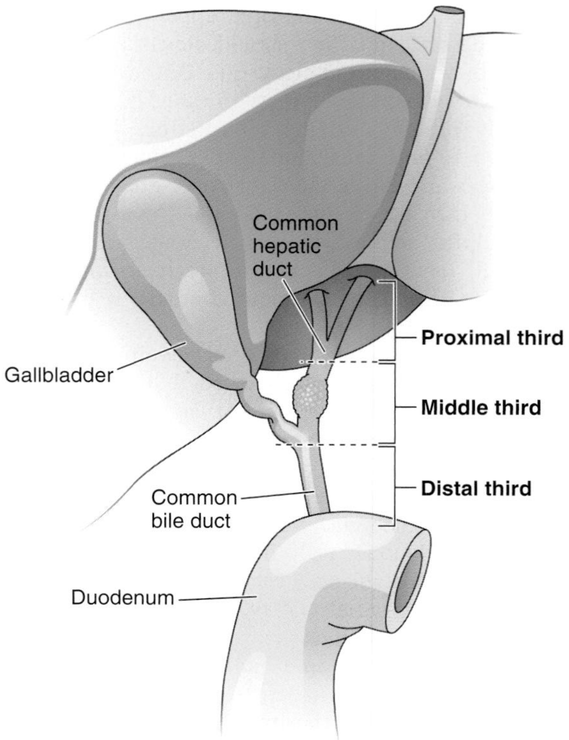

FIGURE 17–14 Bile duct tumors are referenced based on proximal, bifurcation (middle third), and distal bile duct locations.

Serum bilirubin levels greater than 10 mg/dL and elevated alkaline phosphatase levels are common.

US is usually the first imaging study obtained and typically reveals dilated bile ducts. If the lesion is distal, dilated intra- and extrahepatic ducts are seen. With more proximal lesions, however, only intrahepatic ductal dilatation may be seen. The combination of normal extrahepatic bile ducts with dilated intrahepatic bile ducts is highly suggestive of a hilar carcinoma, although it is occasionally seen in cases of severe inflammation of the gallbladder with compression of the cystic duct/common duct junction (Mirizzi's syndrome). Once US has revealed dilated bile ducts, and if a suspicion of malignancy exists, then spiral CT and MRI scans (including MRCP) define the location and extent of the lesion. These modalities are highly accurate at imaging small lesions along the biliary tree and determining their invasion into adjacent portal structures. Once identified, cholangiography via either ERCP or PTC is required to outline the tumor and proximal biliary involvement. In unresectable lesions, these modalities facilitate the placement of external or internal drainage catheters to alleviate the obstructive jaundice.

One of the most challenging aspects of bile duct cancers is determining their resectability both preoperatively and intraoperatively. If no radiologic evidence of unresectability exists, such as vascular invasion or bilateral or multifocal intrahepatic disease, then patients are prepared for surgery. Most surgeons perform a diagnostic laparoscopy as the initial procedure because 20% to 40% of patients will be found unresectable with this technique and thus avoid the morbidity of a laparotomy. If no evidence of unresectability is found by laparoscopy (i.e., no metastatic disease or cirrhosis), then the operation proceeds to formal exploration via an open laparotomy.

The only chance of cure for patients with bile duct cancers is surgical resection with negative margins. The details of the operation are determined by the location of the tumor and extent of spread. Tumors that involve the lower third of the bile duct and ampullary region are resected via a pancreaticoduodenectomy (Whipple procedure). Tumors of the middle third are resected from above the duodenum to the base of the liver, and a biliary enteric anastomosis is performed to the proximal duct. Proximal hilar (Klatskin) tumors are more difficult to deal with because of their proximity to the liver parenchyma. In addition, obtaining negative proximal margins may require including a formal liver resection in conjunction with the bile duct resection. If negative margins can be obtained by performing either a left or right hepatic lobectomy in conjunction with a bile duct resection on the contralateral side, then this aggressive approach is justified. Occasionally, however, margins that are determined to be negative intraoperatively may prove positive on the final pathologic diagnosis. In such cases, the procedure performed is palliative. Liver transplantation has not proven effective in unresectable cases.

The resectability rates for all bile duct cancers is approximately 40%, with lower-third lesions having higher resectability rates and upper-third lesions having lower resectability rates. Overall 5-year survival rates for resected bile duct cancers is approximately 20% with lower-third lesions having higher cure rates (30%) and upper-third lesions having lower cure rates (5%). Distal lesions that can be managed with a pancreaticoduodenectomy tend to have the most favorable prognosis.

Suggested Reading

Babineau TJ, Bothe A: General surgery considerations in the diabetic patient. In Eliopoulos GM (ed): Infectious Disease Clinics of North America. Philadelphia, WB Saunders, 1995, pp 183–195.

Blumgart LH, Benjamin IS: Liver resection for bile duct cancer. In Cady B (ed): Surgical Clinics of North America, Vol. 69. Philadelphia, WB Saunders, 1989, pp 323–339.

Friedman GD: Natural history of asymptomatic and symptomatic gallstones. Am J Surg 165:399–403, 1993.

National Institutes of Health: Consensus statement: Gallstones and laparoscopic cholecystectomy. JAMA 269:1018–1024, 1993.

Warren KW, Jenkins RL, Steele GD (eds): Atlas of Surgery of the Liver, Pancreas and Biliary Tract. Norwalk, Conn, Appleton & Lange, 1991.

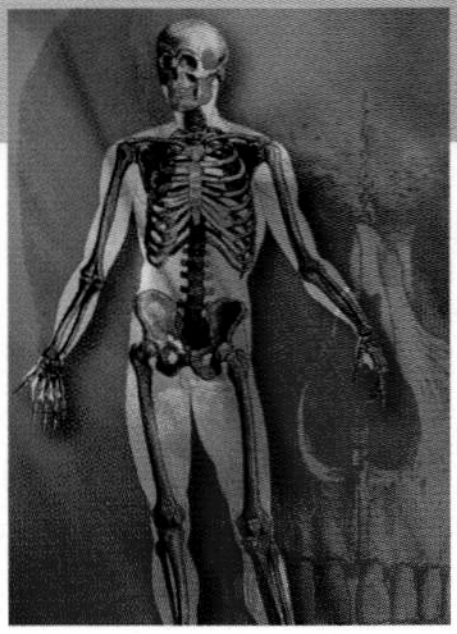

Chapter 18

Liver

TIMOTHY J. BABINEAU, MD, MBA and JAMES J. POMPOSELLI, MD, PhD

Because of the unforgiving nature of the liver and the biliary system, errors in technique or judgment or both can be disastrous for the patient, resulting in lifelong disability or death. For this reason, a high premium exists on performing the correct procedure, without technical misadventure, the first time. Positive outcome requires a balance between sound judgment, technical acumen, and attention to detail. Additionally, the hepatic surgeon of today must be able to integrate surgical options with the broadening array of radiologic and endoscopic treatment options discussed elsewhere in this book.

Surface Anatomy

The liver is shaped like a wedge with its base against the right abdominal wall and its tip pointing toward the spleen. Few intraabdominal organs can be ignored when considering liver surgery. A fibrous capsule of Glisson (or Walaeus) covers the liver. At the porta hepatis, the connective tissue of the capsule is continuous with a fibrous sheath that invests the portal vessels and bile ducts and follows them to their smallest ramifications. The capsular peritoneum reflects onto the diaphragm and forms the right and left triangular ligaments and the falciform ligament. These ligaments hold the liver firmly in place and allow passage of lymphatics, small blood vessels, and nerves.

The falciform ligament connects the liver to the diaphragm and anterior abdominal wall. The lower free edge contains the ligamentum teres, which contains the obliterated umbilical veins and is called the round ligament. In cases of liver disease leading to cirrhosis and portal hypertension, the umbilical veins can recanalize and lead to the development of the "caput medusae," seen as a rich network of superficial veins around the umbilicus. On the surface, the falciform ligament gives the false impression of the division of the liver between the left and right lobes, as mentioned previously. Anatomically, the falciform ligament divides the left lobe of the liver into its medial and lateral segments.

Posteriorly, a large bare area is seen where the liver is attached to the diaphragm and the retroperitoneum. The vena cava lies within the bare area and is held to the liver by a ligament or bridge of liver parenchyma between the caudate and right lobe. During major hepatic resection, division of this ligament is critical in exposing the retrohepatic vena cava to gain access to the hepatic veins.

The hepatoduodenal ligament or porta hepatis connects the liver to the superior part of the duodenum. It is part of the lesser omentum and sheaths the hepatic artery, portal vein, nerves, bile ducts, and lymphatics. Within the hepato-duodenal ligament, the common bile duct lies to the right, proper hepatic artery to the left, with the portal vein posteriorly.

Segmental Anatomy

The division of the anatomic right and left hepatic lobes is a plane that extends from the gallbladder fossa anteroinferiorly to the inferior vena cava superoposteriorly. The right hemiliver contains 50% to 70% of the hepatic volume. This is in contrast to the historical view, which divided the liver into right and left lobes based on the falciform ligament. Each hemiliver contains its own arterial and portal blood supply, bile duct, and venous drainage. This anatomic arrangement allows complete division of the left and right lobes of the liver without total vascular inflow occlusion and permits the relatively new technical surgical innovation of living donor liver transplantation.

The liver can be further divided into eight segments based on blood vessel and bile duct anatomy. Schematically, the liver can be viewed as five cylinders divided into eight segments (Fig. 18-1). The left lobe has medial and lateral segments divided by the falciform ligament and can be viewed as two cylinders lying side by side. The right lobe has anterior and posterior segments and can be viewed as two cylinders lying stacked on top of each other (see Fig. 18-1). The caudate lobe (segment 1) can be viewed as a small cylinder posterior to and between the left and right lobe. The caudate lobe shares its blood supply with each lobe of liver and has its own bile duct drainage. In 1957, Couinaud divided the liver into eight segments based primarily on the vascular supply, as demonstrated by model casts produced from injections of the hepatic artery, portal vein, and bile ducts. Although extraordinarily elegant, these anatomic subdivisions are quite variable because of the extensive arborization of the intrahepatic vasculature.

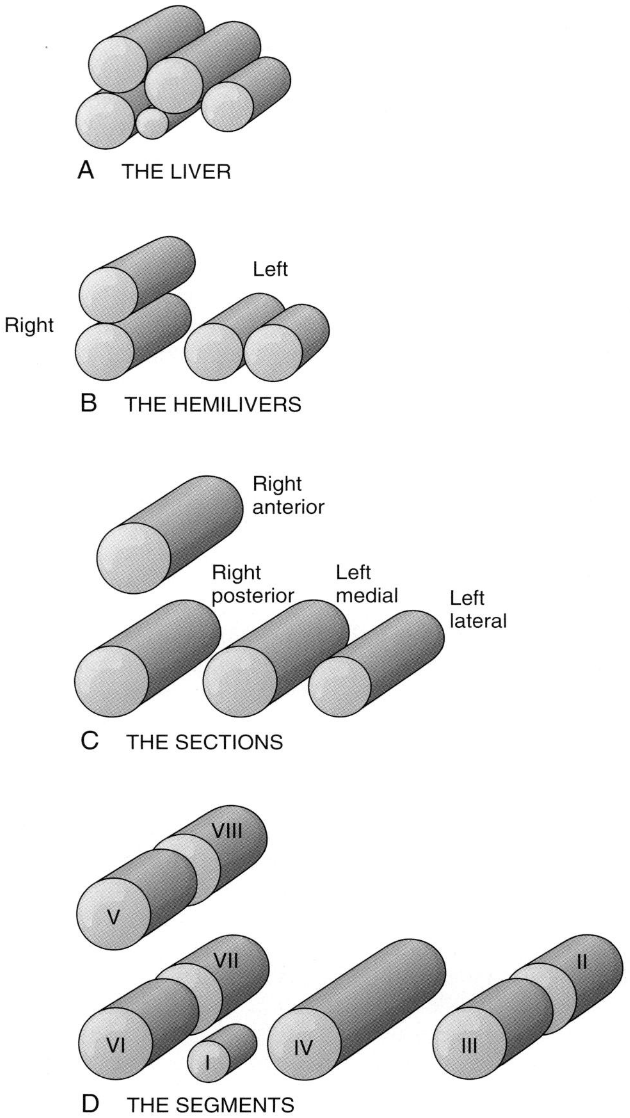

FIGURE 18–1 *A*, The liver can be viewed as five cylinders, arrayed as shown. *B*, *C*, The left lobe is characterized as two cylinders side by side (medial and lateral), whereas the right lobe is shown as two cylinders stacked (anterior and posterior). *D*, The smallest cylinder in between the left and right lobes, and posterior is the caudate lobe. (Adapted from Strasberg SM: Terminology of liver anatomy and liver resections: Coming to grips with hepatic Babel. J Am Coll Surg 184:413–434, 1997.)

However, knowledge of these segments is not just an academic exercise, because planned segmental resection can be carried out in patients with limited hepatic reserve. For resection of large tumors confined to either lobe, anatomic division between lobes can be carried out as well.

Blood Supply

The generous blood supply to the liver accounts, in part, for the respect and caution that surgeons have afforded the liver. Total hepatic blood flow averages approximately 1500 mL/min/m^2. A dual blood supply reaches the liver through the porta hepatis. Oxygenated hepatic arterial blood accounts for approximately 25% of total hepatic blood flow, whereas the nutrient-rich portal blood contributes approximately 75%. The efferent circulatory drainage of the liver is primarily via the three major (right, left, and middle) hepatic veins, which exit the liver directly into the inferior vena cava at the superior posterior margin of the liver. Many smaller branches drain directly into the vena cava from the right lobe and caudate lobe. Approximately 60% of patients have a large accessory right hepatic vein draining the posterior segments, which is frequently omitted in anatomy texts.

The arterial supply of the liver can be quite variable. The common hepatic artery is the largest branch of the celiac artery and, after giving off the right gastric and gastroduodenal branches, continues toward the hilum of the liver as the proper hepatic artery, where it divides into right and left hepatic branches. In 10% to 20% of patients, the right hepatic artery may be "replaced," arising instead from the superior mesenteric artery. Less frequently (~10% of patients), the left hepatic artery also may be replaced, arising from the left gastric artery. Rarely, the common hepatic artery does not arise from the celiac axis but originates from the superior mesenteric artery (completely replaced hepatic artery). The cystic artery is usually an extrahepatic branch of the right hepatic artery but also can have many anatomic variations.

The portal venous system contains no valves and is formed by the confluence of the superior mesenteric, splenic, and inferior mesenteric veins. Within the hepatoduodenal ligament, the portal vein divides into its right and left branches. Some suggestion exists that a preferential "streaming" phenomenon of portal blood flow toward the right lobe may explain the increased incidence of hepatic metastases from bowel cancers found within the right lobe of the liver.

Liver Function and Physiology

The liver performs an extraordinary number of essential metabolic functions that include glucose production and storage, urea formation, synthesis of acute phase and structural proteins, synthesis of clotting factors, and detoxification of drugs and other substances. The liver, either directly or indirectly, influences the substrate formation and utilization of most other organs. In addition to regulating metabolism, the liver has an extensive reticuloendothelial system (RES) that provides a major defense mechanism for the host against infection.

Liver-function Test

The phrase *liver-function tests* is something of a misnomer because these tests often measure liver dysfunction and hepatocellular injury rather than true liver synthetic function. Nonetheless, the collection of tests that has been used to characterize liver function has traditionally included total bilirubin, the enzymes alkaline phosphatase, aspartate aminotransferase (SGOT/AST), alanine aminotransferase (SGPT/ALT), and lactic acid dehydrogenase (LDH). In addition, levels of certain plasma proteins such as albumin, fibrinogen, haptoglobin, and ceruloplasmin have been used to assess hepatic synthetic function. The prothrombin time (PT) is perhaps the most sensitive, commonly available test for hepatic reserve, because it accurately reflects the synthetic ability of the liver. The blood tests for serum albumin, total bilirubin, and PT are used with several clinical parameters such as ascites formation and encephalopathy to assess the severity of liver disease in patients being evaluated for portosystemic shunting or liver transplantation. More recently, the model for end-stage liver disease (MELD) score that uses serum creatinine, PT, and total bilirubin has been used to allocate organs for liver transplantation.

Alkaline phosphatase (ALK) is a sensitive measure of biliary obstruction, and its serum level increases with impairment of bile outflow from either benign or malignant causes. Measured ALK also may be elevated with hepatocellular damage or a space-occupying lesion within the liver. Elevated values (from nonhepatic sources) may be seen with increased osteoblastic activity within bones. Distinguishing the source of an elevation in serum ALK is possible by fractionating the isoenzymes based on their heat sensitivity or obtaining a γ-glutamyl transferase (GGT) level. Serum levels of ALT (also known as SGPT) or AST (also known as SGOT) or both also may be elevated during hepatic disease, drug toxicity, or viral hepatitis. AST also is found in large quantities within heart, muscle, and kidney, as well as liver. However, both AST and ALT reach their highest serum levels when acute hepatocellular damage is present. The etiology of the damage can be from any cause but most commonly stems from infectious etiologies such as hepatitis or "low-flow" phenomena such as shock or ischemic injury.

Defects in the coagulation cascade are multifactorial and commonly seen with both moderate and severe liver dysfunction. A prolongation in a patient's clotting time (as measured by the PT) is usually due to a decrease in vitamin K availability secondary to obstructive jaundice, decreased enterohepatic absorption, or hepatocellular dysfunction with decreased synthesis of prothrombin. In the absence of sepsis or disseminated intravascular coagulopathy (DIC), a prolonged PT that does not respond to the intramuscular injection of 10 mg of vitamin K is an ominous sign of severe liver impairment. Replacement of clotting factors with fresh frozen plasma is often necessary in such patients before invasive procedures that carry a risk of bleeding complications. However, when evaluating a patient for potential liver transplantation, correcting the PT with exogenous fresh frozen plasma eliminates the only true parameter useful in determining the patient's response to therapy.

Physiology

The principal functions of the liver are performed primarily by two cell types, the hepatocytes (or parenchymal cells) and the macrophages (or Kupffer cells). Although intimately related through a series of inter- and intracellular communications, these two cell types perform distinctly different functions. The metabolic functions of the hepatocytes are grouped according to five major activities: (1) provision of energy-fuel substrates, (2) regulation of blood amino acid concentration, (3) synthesis of hepatic secretory and structural proteins, (4) bile acid and bilirubin production, and (5) detoxification of drugs and toxic substances. The hepatic macrophages are specialized endothelial cells located within the sinusoids of the liver that constitute (along with splenic macrophages) approximately 90% of the RES.

Ammonia, which is derived from amino acid metabolism, is detoxified through its conversion into urea within the liver. This energy-requiring process that produces approximately 10 to 20 g of urea nitrogen per day is one of the most teleologically primitive functions of the liver. Along with glucose production, urea production is among the last functions of the liver to fail. An ominous sign in a critically ill patient is profound hypoglycemia in conjunction with a decreasing blood urea nitrogen (BUN). This clinical scenario heralds the end stage of fulminant hepatic failure, and death quickly ensues.

The liver synthesizes 11 proteins that are critical for hemostasis. Vitamin K, which is fat soluble and therefore dependent on bile acid formation, is necessary for the extrinsic clotting pathway and is measured by the PT. Administration of vitamin K often differentiates patients who have malabsorptive-type coagulopathies (seen commonly with obstructive jaundice) from those with impaired synthesis of clotting factors (seen commonly with parenchymal disease). Platelet function also is necessary for clotting and is dependent, in part, on liver function. Although thrombocytopenia is not commonly associated with liver disease, patients with portal hypertension and hypersplenism may have increased platelet sequestration within the spleen that will heighten the potential for bleeding complications.

Diagnostic Imaging of the Liver

Radiologic diagnostic imaging of the liver is performed primarily for the detection and diagnosis of tumors. During the past several decades, the development of computed tomography (CT) scanning, magnetic resonance imaging

(MRI), conventional (external) and intraoperative ultrasonography (US), and most recently, laparoscopy and translaparoscopic US have revolutionized hepatobiliary imaging. Ultrasound is cost effective in locating both benign and malignant lesions of the liver and can determine patency of blood vessels. For further diagnosis, MRI is considered by many to be superior to CT scanning because of its specificity in discriminating hemangiomas and cysts from malignant neoplasms without the need for iodinated contrast material. The development of endoscopic retrograde cholangiopancreatography (ERCP) also has greatly added to the preoperative assessment and treatment of the jaundiced patient. Rapid helical three-dimensional CT scans have been especially helpful for the liver surgeon, because both internal vascular anatomy and volumetric studies can be obtained. During the past several years, laparoscopy and intraoperative US have found a role in the surgical management of hepatic malignancies because of their improved sensitivity in locating small extrahepatic and intrahepatic lesions. These two diagnostic modalities can used together to determine the resectability of either a primary or metastatic hepatic malignancy.

Hepatic Abscesses

Although recognized since the time of Hippocrates, the diagnosis and treatment of liver abscesses remains a challenge to surgeons today. Fortunately, improvements in imaging techniques and antibiotic therapy have helped surgeons in their treatment of these extremely morbid lesions. Two main types of liver abscess are found: pyogenic (or bacterial) and amebic (from amebiasis). Pyogenic abscesses account for nearly 90% of liver abscesses seen in the United States. Although pyogenic and amebic abscess have some common features, the etiology, diagnosis, and treatment are quite different.

The average age of patients with hepatic abscess is between 60 and 70 years. The right lobe is more often involved with solitary pyogenic abscesses, perhaps because of the streaming phenomenon observed within portal blood. Geographic location influences the ratio of pyogenic to amebic abscesses, with a higher percentage of amebic abscesses occurring where amebiasis is endemic. Regardless of the offending organism, the clinical presentations of both types of abscesses are often similar.

Pyogenic Abscesses

Certain conditions predispose patients to the development of a pyogenic abscess. Among the more important clinical processes are biliary tract disease and infections in those areas drained by the portal circulation, such as in diverticulitis, appendicitis, or perforated intestinal neoplasms. Less frequently, bacteremic seeding, trauma, or contiguous suppurative infections may lead to the development of pyogenic abscess. Before antibiotics were routinely used, appendicitis was the most common predisposing factor for the development of pyogenic liver abscess. With current antibiotic use, however, appendicitis is now rarely complicated by liver abscess. Diverticular disease and biliary tract disease (cholangitis, acute cholecystitis) now represent the most common cause of pyogenic liver abscess.

The presenting symptoms and physical findings of hepatic abscess are often varied and nonspecific, and the duration of presentation may range from days to months. The most common presenting complaints are fever (80%–95%), abdominal pain (50%–95%), anorexia and vomiting (20%–60%), fatigue, and weight loss. Physical examination is usually revealing, with abdominal tenderness, hepatomegaly, or a right upper quadrant mass occurring in 20% to 60% of patients. Most patients will have an elevated leukocyte count, with a significant increase in the percentage of immature leukocytes (bands). Liver chemistries vary, with significant elevation of ALK and mild elevation in transaminase levels.

Until the recent advances in hepatic imaging, the radiologic diagnosis of pyogenic hepatic abscess was difficult. Plain abdominal films and chest radiograph findings were subtle, nonspecific, and abnormal only approximately 50% of the time. US and CT scanning, however, have increased the diagnostic accuracy to almost 100%. In addition, these two diagnostic modalities can be used to guide percutaneous abscess drainage and to monitor therapy. Although MRI scanning may give additional information, the US and CT scan remain the diagnostic procedures of choice for suspected hepatic abscess.

In 70% to 100% of cases, cultures from a pyogenic abscess will be positive, whereas blood cultures will be positive in approximately 50% of patients. Enteric gram-negative bacilli, most commonly *Escherichia coli* and *Klebsiella* spp. are the organisms found in these abscesses. Other organisms include *Streptococcus* spp., *Staphylococcus aureus*, *Candida albicans*, *Pseudomonas aeruginosa,* and anaerobic bacteria such as *Bacteroides fragilis* and *Fusobacterium*. Approximately 20% to 50% of abscesses will be polymicrobial, reinforcing the importance of broad-spectrum antibiotic coverage, even when only a single organism has been cultured.

The underlying principle in the treatment of pyogenic liver abscess remains drainage of the abscess. Previously, the gold standard of therapy was open surgical drainage of the abscess with appropriate perioperative antibiotic coverage. Recently, percutaneous drainage under US or CT scan guidance has achieved comparable cure rates with low complication rates. For patients with abscesses that are accessible to percutaneous drainage and for whom surgery is not required to correct the predisposing etiology (i.e., perforated colon carcinoma), percutaneous drainage should be attempted initially. Until recently, the mortality from pyogenic liver abscess exceeded 50%. Recent series have reported an 8% to 22% mortality rate. The complications of liver abscesses are usually related to rupture of the abscess into an adjacent structure or the dissemination of organisms to other organs, resulting in multisystem organ failure.

Amebic Abscesses

The protozoan *Entamoeba histolytica* exists in two forms and causes an intestinal infection through its invasive motile trophozoite. Unlike the cystic form, the motile trophozoite form lives in either the wall or lumen of the colon. Conversely, the cystic form is excreted in stool and can live outside the body (unlike the trophozoite form). Once ingested, the cyst breaks down to release the active trophozoites. The most common extraintestinal complication of infection with *E. histolytica* is an amebic liver abscess, because trophozoites frequently enter the portal circulation, invade the liver, and produce hepatic necrosis with abscess formation.

Patients with this disease in the United States have usually either emigrated from or traveled through regions with endemic amebic disease. Eighty-five percent of patients will have a solitary lesion, and 70% of these will be within the right lobe of the liver. Unlike pyogenic abscesses, amebic liver abscesses do not appear to require any predisposing hepatic dysfunction or underlying parenchymal damage, other than the necrosis created by trophozoite invasion of the liver. Most patients with amebic abscess are men in the 20- to 50-year-old range.

The presentation of patients with amebic abscess is similar to that of those with pyogenic abscess: fever, pain, fatigue, and nausea. Surprisingly, diarrhea is an infrequent presenting complaint, and many patients report no history of amebic dysentery. The vast majority of patients will not have parasites detectable in their stools. Physical examination is often unrevealing, with only a few patients demonstrating a right upper quadrant mass or tenderness. Laboratory tests reveal leukocytosis without eosinophilia, and a nonspecific elevation of liver chemistries. US can make the diagnosis in 90% to 95% of cases, and CT scan may be unnecessary. Finally, serologic tests of an antibody to *E. histolytica* can help confirm the diagnosis. These tests can detect antibody in patients with invasive intestinal amebiasis, as well as in those with extraintestinal amebic infections.

Although percutaneous diagnostic aspiration was performed routinely in the past, a positive US coupled with positive serology has decreased the role for aspiration. However, in cases in which bacterial superinfection is suspected or the abscess cavity is larger than 10 cm and rupture seems imminent, then aspiration and culture may be useful. The fluid obtained from aspiration has various characteristics, but "anchovy paste" is the one most commonly described. Amoebae will be seen on wet-mount examinations in fewer than 50% of aspirates.

The treatment of choice for amebic liver abscess is metronidazole, 750 mg every 8 hours for 10 days. This regimen will be effective in 85% to 100% of patients. Patients who do not respond to this treatment may require surgical drainage or alternative medical therapy (dehydroemetine and chloroquine). Surgery is used as the primary treatment only to treat or prevent abscess rupture, although an attempt at percutaneous drainage is probably warranted initially. In the absence of superinfection or rupture, survival of amebic liver abscess is nearly 100%.

Echinococcosis (Hydatid Disease)

Echinococcal cystic disease of the liver is endemic in much of the world where sheep are raised, although it is relatively uncommon in North America. Infection is caused by *Echinococcus granulosa*, although rarely it may be caused by *Echinococcus multilocularis*. Adult tapeworms of the genus *Echinococcus* are small and generally reside in the canine host without causing disease. Humans are an intermediary host and usually suffer the consequences. Humans become infected by eating canine tapeworm eggs. The eggs then hatch in the duodenum, releasing embryos that cross the mucosal layer and travel into the portal circulation and then other organs of the body. About two thirds of human *Echinococcus granulosa* cysts are found in the liver, with the remainder found in lung, brain, and bones.

The cysts grow extremely slowly and may achieve 5 to 10 cm over the course of years (Fig. 18-2). The wall of the cyst (or hydatid) consists of an outer ectocyst and an inner endocyst. Over the years, the cysts expand because the endocyst secretes a clear fluid that contains the daughter cysts. As the cyst expands, vague abdominal pain is the most common symptom. Once it is suspected, diagnosis is made by indirect hemagglutination and serum immunoelectrophoresis. The Casoni skin test is associated with significant false-positive results.

Surgical therapy should be considered for all patients once the diagnosis is made because anthelmintics such as

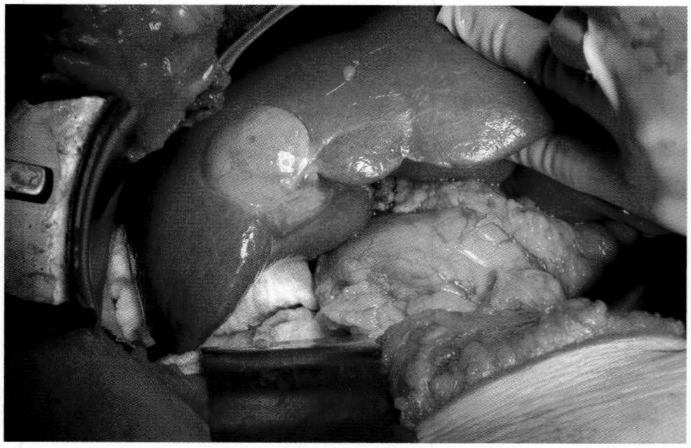

FIGURE 18–2 In situ view of an echinococcal cyst that was diagnosed on routine computed tomography scan after the patient was seen with vague abdominal pain. The lesion was removed with segmental liver resection.

mebendazole have met with limited success. Drug therapy with twice-daily albendazole for approximately 3 months can be curative without surgery in patients who are poor surgical candidates.

The surgical approach varies, depending on the number and location of the cysts. At laparotomy and before attempted excision, the surgeon must first neutralize the daughter cysts, usually by injecting 3% hypertonic saline directly into the largest cyst. After this, the cyst may be unroofed, the contents evacuated, and the cyst removed. Spillage of the contents is avoided because any viable daughter cysts may cause widespread dissemination or anaphylaxis or both.

Hepatic Cysts

Solitary liver cysts are relatively rare, occurring in as few as 1 in 1000 patients. They are benign, slow growing, rarely symptomatic, and usually require no treatment. Occasionally, large cysts are initially seen with dull, vague right-upper-quadrant pain, especially if they occur with hemorrhage or infection of the cyst. If the cyst is large and symptomatic, surgical management offers the best results because aspiration is associated with a high rate of recurrence. If approached surgically, the cyst is excised, and the wall is sent for frozen-section examination to exclude the presence of malignancy. If excision cannot be performed safely (because of the proximity of major vascular structures), then unroofing and free drainage into the abdominal cavity is an acceptable alternative. This can be easily performed laparoscopically for cysts that extend to the surface of the liver.

Unlike simple hepatic cysts, congenital polycystic disease of the liver is defined by the presence of more than one cyst found within the liver (Fig. 18-3). Approximately 50% of patients with adult polycystic liver disease will have renal involvement, whereas in 15% to 75% of patients with polycystic kidney disease, hepatic cystic disease may eventually develop. In hepatic polycystic disease, the cysts are usually located throughout both lobes and can range in size from less than 1 cm to larger than 20 cm in diameter. Like solitary cysts, polycystic disease is frequently asymptomatic and undiagnosed. Symptomatic patients usually complain of epigastric fullness, pain, nausea, and an inability to eat well. Occasionally, progressive kidney failure or a cerebrovascular accident secondary to an associated "berry aneurysm" may be the only presenting symptom. Liver transplantation is indicated for severe symptoms because percutaneous aspiration of multiple cysts is associated with a nearly 100% risk of recurrence, and open surgery is only temporizing for most patients.

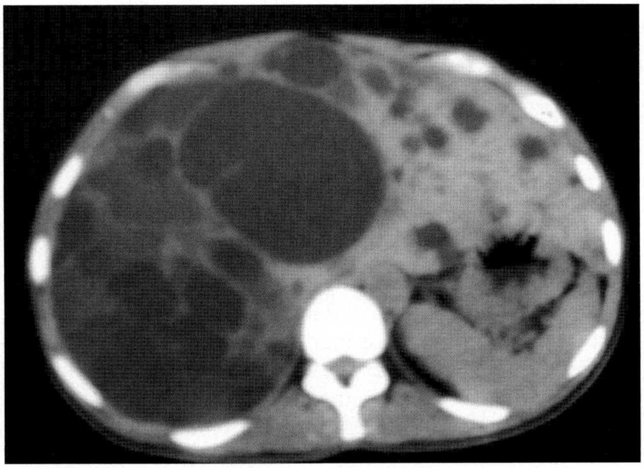

FIGURE 18–3 Computed tomography scan of polycystic liver disease. Cyst fenestration can be performed in this patient, but many with disease this severe will require liver transplantation.

Vascular Diseases

Budd-Chiari Syndrome

Budd-Chiari syndrome comprises a variety of disorders resulting from hepatic venous outflow obstruction. Budd first described the clinical spectrum of abdominal pain, ascites, and hepatomegaly, whereas Chiari was the first to provide the pathological description of the syndrome. Chronic outflow obstruction leads to sinusoidal congestion and centrolobular necrosis.

Patients often have occlusion of the terminal hepatic venules, major hepatic veins, or inferior vena cava. Hypercoagulable states or neoplasms account for most cases of thrombotic occlusion in the West, whereas vena cava webs and membranes are important causes in Asia and South America. The clinical presentation varies greatly from an asymptomatic state to fulminant hepatic failure or end-stage liver disease with cirrhosis.

Screening US can make the diagnosis of Budd-Chiari syndrome most readily. However, patent hepatic outflow does not rule out the disease, and clinical suspicion must remain high. Laboratory tests of blood and ascites are usually not helpful in making the diagnosis but may help characterize the extent of liver injury. Angiography and liver biopsy remain the "gold standard" for the diagnosis and definition of the extent of parenchymal damage. Liver biopsy should be routinely performed on any patient being evaluated for possible surgical correction. As a rule, Budd-Chiari syndrome does not spontaneously resolve, and medical management alone is not sufficient. Treatment options include surgical shunts or liver transplantation. Decompressive shunts must be constructed in such a way to drain blood from the liver while simultaneously draining the splanchnic bed. Therefore simple end-to-side portocaval shunts are not appropriate, because centrolobular congestion is not relieved. Side-to-side portocaval shunts are ideal; however, hypertrophy of the caudate lobe (with its own venous drainage) can make creation of this shunt impossible (Fig. 18-4). The enlarged caudate lobe blocks the surgeon's ability to bring the portal vein down to the vena cava without

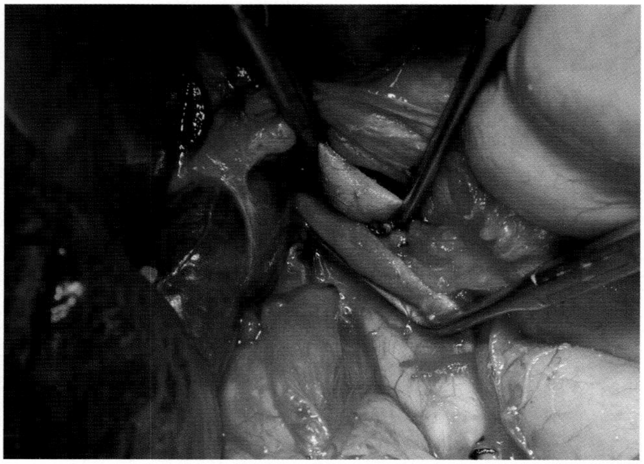

FIGURE 18–4 The surgical setup for side-to-side portocaval shunt. A side-biting clamp is on the anterior aspect of the vena cava, and two straight clamps are on the proximal and distal portal vein. The clamps are maneuvered to bring the portal vein and vena cava into close apposition before anastomosis. This shunt is used for draining portal blood from the liver (hepatofugal flow) and the mesenteric vessels as in cases of Budd-Chiari syndrome.

tension. Alternatively, a mesocaval shunt using prosthetic material made from Dacron or Gore-tex can be used but is less desirable in situations of hypercoagulable states. Therefore we have used the portorenal shunt with the left renal vein as conduit. The renal vein is divided just distal to the gonadal vein, which reverses flow to drain the kidney. The divided renal vein is rotated anteriorly and anastomosed to the posterior aspect of the portal vein. In effect, this creates an autogenous "H" graft and avoids the problems associated with artificial grafts. Transjugular intrahepatic portocaval shunts (TIPS) can be used as a bridge to transplantation in patients with cirrhosis but are prone to fail, with fewer than 40% of TIPS patent at 1 year. Patients with signs of cirrhosis should be rapidly evaluated for liver transplantation before major hepatic decompensation occurs. Liver transplantation has the added benefit of correcting the hypercoagulable state.

Liver Trauma

The liver is the most frequently injured organ in both blunt and penetrating abdominal trauma. In blunt hepatic trauma, most patients can be managed nonoperatively. In penetrating hepatic trauma, surgery is the standard of care. Because of the position in the right upper quadrant, any penetrating or blunt trauma to the lower chest or upper abdomen puts the liver at risk for injury. Approximately 40% of patients who have either operative penetrating or blunt trauma have a simultaneous liver injury.

The management of liver trauma has evolved dramatically over the last decade, from the concept of obligatory surgery for all injuries to one of a selective nonoperative approach with careful observation. In penetrating trauma or when the patient is hemodynamically unstable, immediate surgical exploration should be performed. The operating room should be warmed, and warm intravenous solutions and blood products should be available. The routine use of a cell-saver device can decrease the number of autologous units used, but liberal replacement of coagulation factors with fresh frozen plasma is warranted.

Grade I and II injuries can be controlled with a mixture of direct pressure, electrocautery, and topical hemostatic agents. Argon beam coagulation is especially useful for these injuries if available. Grade III to V injuries require complete mobilization of the liver to assess the injury adequately. In patients with arterial or uncontrolled venous bleeding, the Pringle maneuver using a soft clamp should be performed. The Pringle maneuver involves occluding inflow to the liver by gently clamping across the porta hepatis with either the surgeon's fingers or soft rubber drain used as a noose. Large vascular clamps should be avoided, because trauma caused by the clamp can lead to intimal dissection and hepatic artery thrombosis. In patients who continue to bleed after the Pringle maneuver, total vascular isolation or atrial-caval shunt should be rapidly performed. Vascular isolation can be achieved with clamping the vena cava just above the renal veins and below the diaphragm. Alternatively, a median sternotomy can be performed, and placement of an atrial-caval shunt with an endotracheal tube can be performed. It is controversial whether survival is improved by using atrial-caval shunts after hepatic trauma. The best outcome is obtained when the decision to obtain total vascular isolation is made early.

Complications of Hepatic Trauma

Complications after hepatic trauma can occur early or late after the injury. The acute complications of continued hemorrhage, hypothermia, and coagulopathy are obvious, as discussed previously. Delayed complications can occur days or months after injury and include biloma, biliary fistula formation, abdominal sepsis, hepatic artery pseudoaneurysm, and hemobilia.

Hemobilia

Hemobilia is an unusual manifestation of liver pathology in which gastrointestinal hemorrhage occurs secondary to biliary tract bleeding. It may originate from virtually any site along the biliary system, including the liver parenchyma itself or the intra- and extrahepatic bile ducts including the gallbladder. Although the blood supply to the liver does not communicate directly with the biliary system, certain conditions such as trauma, infection, or tumor may create hemorrhage within the biliary tree. Penetrating or blunt trauma to the liver may cause hemobilia. The majority of cases in this country arise from the iatrogenic trauma of liver biopsy, ERCP, or stent placement. Most recently, TIPS procedures have been associated with a high rate of acute hemobilia. Infection, gallstones, and tumors account for the remaining cases.

Clinically, hemobilia may appear early or quite late in the disease process. The extent of bleeding may be massive, with hematemesis and shock, or minimal, with guaiac-positive stools only. Classically, the triad of right-upper-quadrant pain, jaundice, and gastrointestinal bleeding suggests hemobilia. The diagnosis of hemobilia is best made with arteriography and offers the possibility of treatment with embolization. If bleeding continues after embolization, operative intervention becomes mandatory.

Benign and Malignant Tumors

Solid tumors of the liver are often incidentally discovered in patients without a history of clinical or serologic evidence of liver disease or malignancy. A history of hormone therapy, hepatitis risk factors, and previous neoplasms should be sought in all patients. Routine workup includes CT or MRI imaging as well as hepatitis serologies, liver-function tests, and tumor markers α-fetoprotein (AFP), carcinoembryonic antigen (CEA), and CA19-9. Oral contraceptives may play a role in the development of hemangiomas, focal nodular hyperplasia (FNH), and hepatic adenomas. Therefore oral contraceptive agents should be discontinued in any patient diagnosed with one of these lesions.

In general, patients who are symptomatic and have no contraindication for surgery should undergo surgical resection. Percutaneous biopsy is not necessary before surgery, because this will not alter the treatment plan and can lead to iatrogenic injury or possible dissemination of a malignant lesion. In patients with cirrhosis who will not tolerate liver resection, percutaneous biopsy is helpful because treacherous surgery can be avoided, and malignant lesions can be treated nonoperatively.

Common Benign Hepatic Lesions

Cavernous Hemangioma

Cavernous hemangiomas are the most common benign hepatic tumors with the frequency varying in autopsy series between 0.4% and 20%. The size varies from 1 cm to larger than 20 cm. When larger than 4 cm, hemangiomas are arbitrarily called *giant hemangiomas*. Although they can be found at any age or in any sex group, the majority of hemangiomas are diagnosed in women between the third and fifth decades of life. The precise etiology of cavernous hemangiomas is not clear. Malignant transformation of a cavernous hemangioma has never been reported. Until they reach large size (>10 cm) most cavernous hemangiomas remain asymptomatic. Spontaneous rupture is a very rare presenting complaint, with most patients complaining of vague abdominal discomfort. Surgical treatment, consisting of complete excision by enucleation, is indicated only when significant symptoms (i.e., pain and discomfort) are present. Occasionally, hepatic artery embolization or intraoperative ligation may be used as an emergency measure to control exsanguinating hemorrhage in the extremely rare incident of spontaneous rupture. Once hemorrhage is controlled, subsequent excision of the lesion is recommended.

Imaging with US can establish the diagnosis of hemangioma with confidence in 80% of lesions. Dynamic CT scans show hypodense lesions on the precontrast scans with early peripheral enhancement and progressive centripetal filling on serial scans. MRI scanning is an accurate but expensive technique, with a sensitivity greater than 90%. The lesion is well circumscribed with high signal intensity on T_2 imaging. ^{99m}Technetium pertechnetate–labeled red blood cell pool study shows initial hypoperfusion during the arterial phase, followed by gradual increase of the tracer, peaking 30 to 50 minutes after injection. Sensitivity for lesions larger than 2 cm varies from 70% to 80%, with specificity approaching 100%.

> **PEARLS FOR ROUNDS**
>
> The liver is made up of eight segments, with the anatomic division between the left and right lobe as a line between the gallbladder fossa inferiorly and the vena cava superiorly.
>
> Liver-function tests actually reflect liver dysfunction, with the exception of the prothrombin time (PT).
>
> Administration of fresh frozen plasma to correct liver-induced coagulopathy before bedside procedures is costly and not proven to be effective.
>
> Solitary congenital cyst in the liver means only one. Any patient with the "tell-tale" second cyst has polycystic liver disease by definition.

Focal Nodular Hyperplasia

FNH is the second most common benign solid tumor and also has been referred to as focal cirrhosis, because the center of the lesion often contains bridging fibrosis. Autopsy series have reported an incidence between 0.3% and 0.6%. It is a nonneoplastic lesion seen in patients of all ages and both sexes but more commonly seen in women between ages 20 and 50 years.

The etiologic relation with oral contraceptives is not well established. The incidence of FNH has not increased with the use of oral contraceptives. However, since the introduction of oral contraceptives, the first cases of FNH complicated by hemorrhage were reported. Pregnancy has been shown to induce the growth of tumors, which supports data suggesting that estrogens may affect the growth and hemorrhage of FNH (Fig. 18-5).

US, CT scans, and MRI may see a central scar. US is sensitive to identify a lesion but is usually nondiagnostic. Different from liver metastases, MRI in FNH reveals an

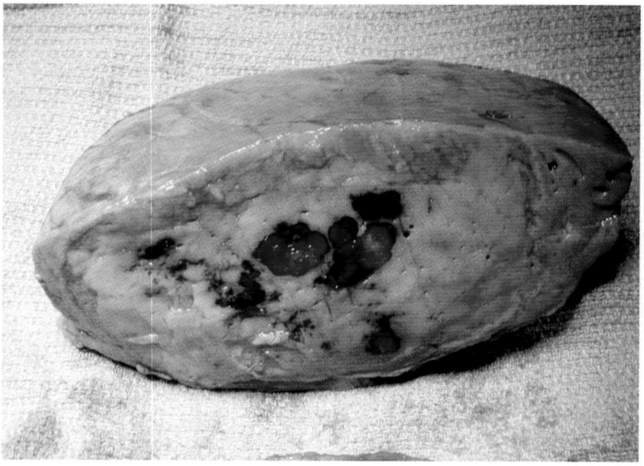

FIGURE 18–5 Resection specimen of focal nodular hyperplasia (FNH) with unusual parenchymal hemorrhage. Usually FNH has cords of scar tissue in a characteristic stellate pattern that can be seen on computed tomography or magnetic resonance imaging scans.

isointense homogeneous central scar on T_1-weighted scans. Angiography is rarely used but can demonstrate a central feeding artery in approximately 60%.

Lesions are generally asymptomatic and are not associated with malignant transformation; therefore the recommended treatment is observation. Surgical resection is recommended for symptomatic lesions or in cases of diagnostic uncertainty.

Hepatic Adenoma

Hepatic adenoma is an uncommon solid liver lesion seen mainly in women of childbearing years. Prior to 1960, only the occasional hepatic adenoma was reported in the literature. After the introduction of oral contraceptive agents, the incidence of hepatic adenoma increased dramatically. The incidence decreased with the reduction of amount of estrogens in oral contraceptives.

Adenomas usually affect young middle-aged women. Ninety-three percent of women affected have a history of oral contraceptive use, many for more than 5 years. The majority of these tumors are symptomatic with the most common complaint of abdominal pain in the midepigastrium and right upper quadrant. Minor trauma can lead to hemorrhage within the adenoma, resulting in significant pain (Fig. 18-6). Volume resuscitation and prompt resection are indicated to prevent further bleeding. Symptoms may include hypotension, shock, and even death if intraperitoneal hemorrhage occurs.

When monitored, adenomas may decrease and even disappear after discontinuation of oral contraceptives. However, tumors may continue to grow. If adenoma is not resected, pregnancy should be avoided because of an

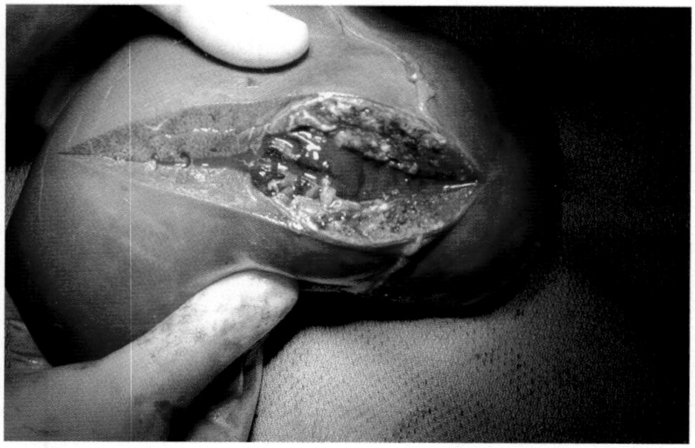

FIGURE 18–6 Young woman with spontaneous hemorrhage of a benign hepatic adenoma. Note the large resection specimen, because these lesions can exhibit malignant transformation and should be treated as cancers. Simple enucleation of these lesions is inappropriate.

increased risk of tumor growth, hemorrhage, and fatal complications. When adenoma is diagnosed, the recommendation is surgical removal because of the risk of malignancy or bleeding complications or both. Because lesions can be viewed as premalignant, formal resection rather than simple enucleation is indicated.

Malignant Neoplasms of the Liver

Primary Lesions

Hepatocellular carcinoma (HCC) is one of the most common malignancies worldwide and is related most often to chronic viral hepatitis, usually in the presence of cirrhosis. Measurement of serum AFP and a US examination may be used to screen for HCC. Survival rates for unresectable lesions are generally dismal, with a 4- to 6-month average life expectancy from the time of diagnosis. Surgical resection and liver transplantation are the treatments that offer the best possibility of long-term survival for patients with HCC. Cholangiocarcinoma (bile duct carcinoma) also occurs in the liver, although less frequently than primary hepatocellular carcinoma. These primary liver tumors arise from different anatomic and cellular locations and are discussed separately.

The epidemiology and etiology of primary HCC is multifactorial and has been related to hepatitis, dietary factors including the ingestion of aflatoxins from contaminated grain supplies, and cirrhosis from any etiology. It has been estimated that cirrhosis secondary to alcohol carries an approximately 10% lifetime risk for the development of HCC, whereas cirrhosis secondary to viral hepatitis carries an approximately 20% risk. Similarly, cirrhosis secondary to hemochromatosis also is associated with an increased risk of HCC.

PEARLS FOR THE OR

Portocaval shunts for Budd-Chiari syndrome must drain the liver and splanchnic circulation to be successful.

Of the benign liver tumors, only hepatic adenoma requires routine resection to prevent bleeding or malignant transformation.

Metastatic colon cancer is biologically privileged, in that cure can be obtained in carefully selected patients with aggressive surgical removal.

HCC may develop within the liver as a diffuse process, a multinodular process, or as a discrete solitary lesion. Although HCC usually arises in a setting of cirrhosis, "fibrolamellar" or well-differentiated HCC that is not associated with cirrhosis can develop and has an improved long-term survival. Frequently, the diagnosis of HCC is obscured by the underlying symptoms of cirrhosis. When HCC is suspected, the diagnostic workup should attempt to differentiate worsening cirrhosis from the onset of cancer through radiologic studies that will define a mass. In addition, the elevation of the serum marker AFP is highly suggestive of hepatocellular malignancy, yet a normal value does not exclude malignancy. Occasionally, angiography may demonstrate the characteristic hypervascular appearance of HCC. Once the diagnosis of HCC is made, patients should be considered for surgical resection if feasible (Fig. 18-7). Extrahepatic metastatic disease, multifocality within the liver (not encompassable with a standard resection), or advanced cirrhosis renders patients unresectable. Although surgeons have operated on patients with cirrhosis in the past, the results have been uniformly dismal, and most surgeons today consider cirrhosis a contraindication to hepatic resection. Patients with small lesions (<5 cm) and cirrhosis should be considered for liver transplantation if no other contraindications to transplant are found. The most suitable candidate for surgical resection is a patient with a solitary lesion arising within a normal liver. Only 30% of patients who are surgically explored will be resectable at laparotomy, and of those resected, only 30% will be "cured" (i.e., have durable disease-free survival). Diagnostic laparoscopy may decrease the number of laparotomies by identifying unsuspected cirrhosis or extrahepatic metastatic spread.

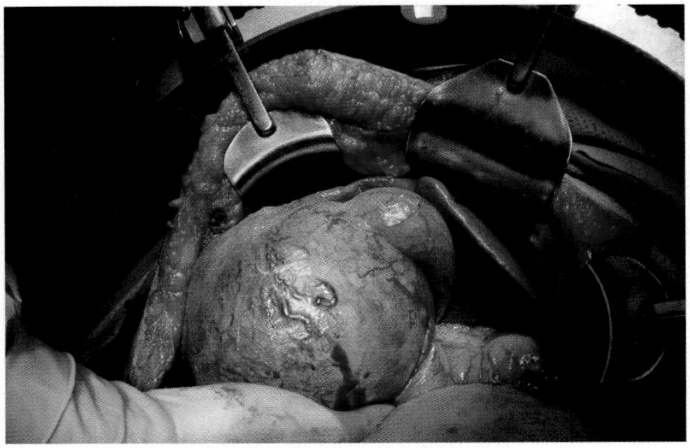

FIGURE 18–7 Large hepatocellular cancer in an elderly man without existing liver disease. The lesion is displacing the gallbladder to the patient's left side. Wide excision with negative margins provides a cure in approximately one third of patients.

Metastatic Lesions

In most countries, malignant tumors metastatic to the liver are much more common than are primary liver tumors. Although virtually any solid tumor has the propensity to metastasize to the liver, it is only carcinoma of the colon and rectum (and some islet cell tumors of the pancreas) that make metastatic lesions amenable to surgical resection. When patients with carcinoma of the large bowel have a "liver-only" pattern of recurrence, which occurs in 3% to 6% of colon resection patients, hepatic resection offers a chance for cure. In patients who undergo curative hepatic resection for colorectal metastases, 5-year survivals of 25% to 35% have been reported. Favorable prognostic signs in these patients are a long disease-free interval (between colonic resection and appearance of hepatic metastasis), few hepatic metastases, a low preoperative CEA level, and a primary colon cancer that was stage II rather than stage III. Of all patients operated on for resection of hepatic metastases from colorectal cancer, only 50% will be found to be resectable at the time of surgery.

The presentation of colorectal cancer metastatic to the liver is variable but usually takes one of three forms, discovered (1) at initial laparotomy for primary cancer resection, (2) as a cause of symptoms, or (3) through an elevated CEA level. If liver metastases are discovered at the time of initial laparotomy for colonic cancer (which occurs in 8% to 25% of patients), the primary tumor should be resected, and the patient should undergo a postoperative evaluation to determine the resectability of the hepatic metastatic disease. An exception to this is the case of a single liver metastasis in which the colonic operation has gone smoothly and the hepatic resection represents a relatively minor additional procedure (i.e., "wedge" resection).

Other primary cancers that rarely give rise to liver metastases amenable to surgical resection include islet cell cancers of the pancreas, carcinoid tumors, and leiomyosarcomas. Rarely, palliative resections of metastatic carcinoid tumors of the liver may be indicated, even in the presence of extrahepatic spread.

Hepatic Resection

Hepatic resection remains the treatment of choice for a wide array of malignant and benign conditions. Up to 70%

of the healthy adult liver can be electively removed with full recovery in most cases. Liver resection that removes more than 70% of the original liver volume is associated with severe cholestasis, progressive liver failure, sepsis, and death. The unique ability of the liver to regenerate restores the functional liver volume to 85% to 100% of the original volume within several months. During periods of metabolic stress such as with a technical or postoperative complication, liver regeneration can be interrupted. Therefore meticulous intraoperative and postoperative care is essential for favorable outcome.

Advances in liver imaging using volumetric CT scanning have revolutionized preoperative planning for liver surgery (Fig. 18-8). Accurate three-dimensional depictions of arterial and venous anatomy as well as segmental volume measurement can predict the amount of liver tissue lost during resection. Dramatic improvement in surgical outcome over the last several decades has provided the impetus in performing living donor liver transplantation (LDLT) using either right or left lobe grafts obtained from healthy donors (Fig. 18-9).

With improvements in surgical technique, pre- and postoperative care, and advanced anesthetic techniques, hepatic resection can now be performed with low mortality in many centers. For hepatic surgery to be successful, the liver surgeon must adequately assess and prepare the patient preoperatively, pay meticulous attention to detail intraoperatively, and be capable of managing the potential complications postoperatively. Because of the unforgiving nature of the liver, surgeons who have not been trained in all aspects of hepatic surgery and care of the postoperative liver patient should not attempt major hepatic resection. A complete understanding of the anatomy and variations of the

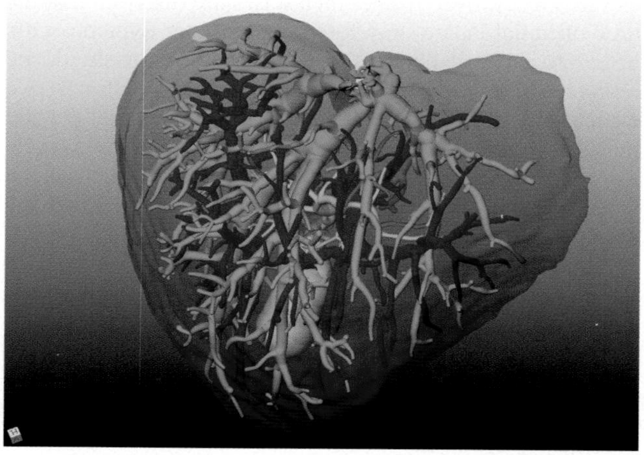

FIGURE 18–8 Advances in imaging software provide three-dimensional views of the liver with internal anatomy and accurate volume assessment.

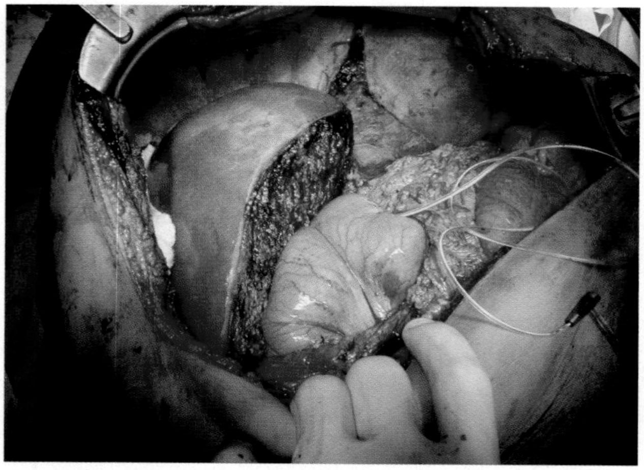

FIGURE 18–9 Completed live-donor liver transplant using a right lobe graft resected from a healthy donor. Outcome is similar to that with traditional cadaveric transplantation but puts a healthy donor at significant risk for postoperative complication. The biliary tree has been reconstructed by using a Roux-en-Y hepaticojejunostomy.

liver is a critical prerequisite for performing new techniques such as cryosurgical or radiofrequency ablation.

Preoperative testing should include a complete history and physical examination, complete blood count, liver-function tests, chest radiograph, electrocardiogram, and coagulation studies. A coagulation defect should be corrected preoperatively with either vitamin K or fresh frozen plasma or both. Particular attention should be focused on the nutritional status of the patient, because preoperative nutritional support may decrease postoperative complications in severely malnourished patients. Postoperatively, patients may have massive “third space” requirements with major extracellular fluid sequestration. Metabolic alkalosis is a common problem when large amounts of blood products are given and can be corrected (if significant) with the central venous administration of 0.1N hydrochloric acid. Usually a transient increase in the serum bilirubin and other liver-function tests occurs postoperatively, but these should return to baseline within 7 to 10 days. A persistently elevated bilirubin suggests biliary obstruction and warrants a diagnostic evaluation. Persistent elevations in hepatocellular enzymes suggest an infectious complication or vascular injury. Serum albumin levels also transiently decrease, but no beneficial effect of supplemental albumin administration is known.

The hepatic surgeon of today must use a multidisciplinary approach in the care of the patient with liver disease. A concerted effort between the surgeon and the diagnostic and invasive radiologist, hepatologist, anesthesiologist, and critical care teams affords the best opportunity for favorable outcome.

Suggested Reading

McDermott WV, Cady B, Steele G, Khettry U: Primary cancer of the liver: Evaluation, treatment and prognosis. Arch Surg 124:552–555, 1989.

Meyers WC: The liver. In Sabiston DC, Lyerly HK (eds.): Textbook of Surgery: The Biological Basis of Modern Surgical Practice, 15th ed. Philadelphia, WB Saunders, 1997.

Steele G, Ravikumar TS: Resection of hepatic metastases from colorectal cancer. Ann Surg 210:127–138, 1989.

Strasberg SM: Terminology of liver anatomy and liver resections: Coming to grips with hepatic Babel. J Am Coll Surg 184:413–434, 1997.

Warren KW, Jenkins RL, Steele GD (eds.): Atlas of Surgery of the Liver, Pancreas, and Biliary Tract. Norwalk, Conn, Appleton & Lange, 1991.

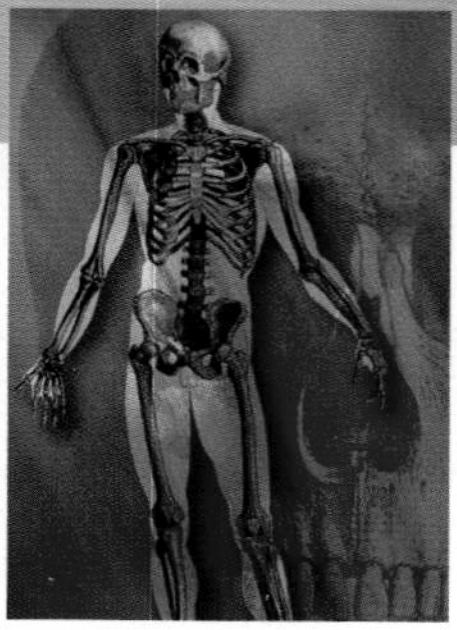

Chapter 19

Portal Hypertension

ALEXANDER S. ROSEMURGY, II, MD, FRANCESCO M, SERAFINI, MD, and MATTHEW J. D'ALESSIO, MD

Anatomy of the Portal Circulation

The mesenteric and portal venous systems receive most of the venous blood of the gastrointestinal tract and account for about 70% of hepatic blood flow. Portal blood is postcapillary and therefore somewhat deoxygenated, but because of copious flow (about 1 L/min), it can adequately supply the hepatic parenchyma with oxygen and substances absorbed from the gut.

The confluence of the splenic vein and the superior mesenteric vein forms the portal vein dorsal to the neck of the pancreas and ventral to the body of the second lumbar vertebra (Fig. 19-1). The splenic vein receives blood from the spleen, lower esophagus, stomach, pancreas, and, via the inferior mesenteric vein, blood from the left colon and upper rectum. The superior mesenteric vein receives blood from the pancreas, small intestine, appendix, right colon, and transverse colon. Just superior to the head of the pancreas, the portal vein receives two small branches: the pyloric vein and the left gastric (coronary) vein, which drain venous blood from the stomach. These latter two branches are important in portal hypertension because they can act as low-resistance collaterals out of the portal vein.

The extrahepatic portion of the main trunk of the portal vein is 4 to 5 cm long. Its cephalad portion is located in the hepatoduodenal ligament, which also contains the common bile duct and the hepatic arteries. The portal vein is located posterior and medial to the common bile duct.

The portal vein bifurcates at the inferior edge of the liver into the right and the left branches of the portal vein. The right branch of the portal vein has a shorter extrahepatic course and, just after entering the hepatic parenchyma, divides into several smaller branches. The left branch of the portal vein is 2.0 to 3.5 cm long, tracks transversely across the base of the liver, and enters the liver parenchyma anterior to the caudate lobe.

Under normal conditions, venous collaterals between the portal and the systemic venous circulation are of small caliber and little consequence. In patients with portal hypertension, these collaterals, acting as outflow conduits from the high-pressure portal system, become larger and are referred to as varicose veins or varices. Varices can carry a formidable amount of blood, and consequently, rupture of these veins can result in fatal hemorrhage.

Physiology of the Portal Circulation and Pathophysiology of Portal Hypertension

Normal portal pressures are 5 to10 mmHg. Portal hypertension is defined as a sustained pressure in the portal vein more than 12 mmHg. Portal hypertension results from increased resistance to blood flow at some point along the portal venous circulation. Depending on the site of the disease process causing increased resistance to portal flow, portal hypertension can be defined as prehepatic, intrahepatic, and posthepatic (Box 19-1).

Intrahepatic portal hypertension is subdivided into presinusoidal and postsinusoidal, depending on where increased resistance to flow occurs. Intrahepatic postsinusoidal portal hypertension is the most common form of portal hypertension in the United States, most frequently caused by cirrhosis due to excessive alcohol consumption or hepatitis C virus. Notably, portal hypertension caused by cirrhosis is associated with liver dysfunction, whereas other causes of portal hypertension generally are not associated with hepatic insufficiency.

Total hepatic blood flow, normally approximately 1.5 L/min, is a combination of portal venous flow and hepatic arterial flow. In the normal individual, about two thirds of the total hepatic blood flow is derived from the portal vein, and about one third is derived from the relatively oxygen-rich arterial system. Total hepatic blood flow generally is regulated such that a decrease in portal blood flow results in an increase in arterial flow and vice versa. Several substances are able to affect total blood flow to the liver (Table 19-1).

In cirrhosis, as a consequence of the disarray of the hepatic architecture and increased sinusoidal resistance, portal blood flow to the liver decreases. Therefore to meet the metabolic demand of the hepatocytes, hepatic arterial inflow increases. This is called *arterialization of the liver*. With cirrhosis, the hepatic artery can account for 40% or more of total liver blood flow. This increase in hepatic arterial blood flow may not completely offset the reduction

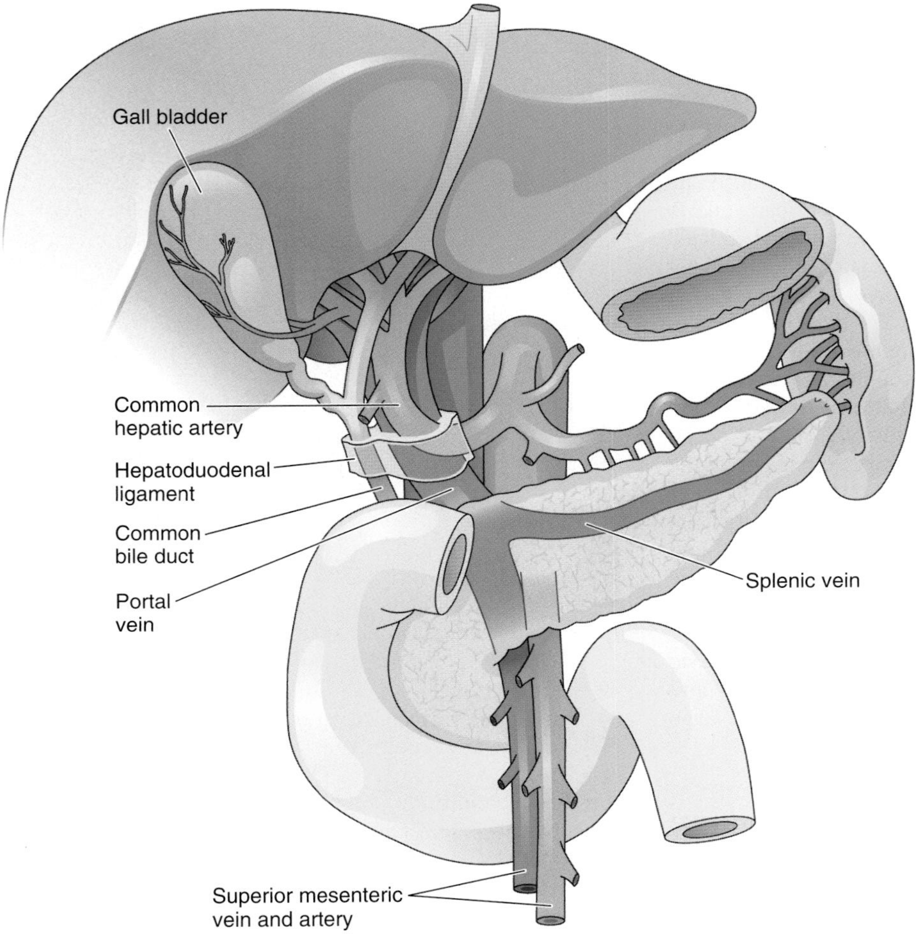

FIGURE 19–1 The portal vein originates from the junction of the superior mesenteric vein and the splenic vein. The portal vein is the most posterior structure of the hepatoduodenal ligament.

BOX 19–1 Classification of Portal Hypertension

Prehepatic portal hypertension	Portal vein thrombosis Increased splenic vein flow Splenic vein thrombosis (left-sided portal hypertension)
Intrahepatic portal hypertension	
Presinusoidal	Schistosomiasis Reticulosis Sarcoidosis Congenital portal fibrosis Idiopathic portal hypertension
Postsinusoidal	Cirrhosis
Posthepatic portal hypertension	Hepatic vein thrombosis (Budd-Chiari) IVC thrombosis/compression Congestive heart failure

IVC, inferior vena cava.

TABLE 19–1 Endogenous Effectors of Hepatic Blood Flow

Decrease Hepatic Blood Flow	Increase Hepatic Blood Flow
Hypocarbia	Glucagon
Sympathetic nerve stimulation	Prostaglandins
Angiotensin	Prostacyclin
Vasopressin	Nitric oxide
Somatostatin	Gastrin
Serotonin	Secretin
Halothane	VIP
Enfluorane	Cholecystokinin

VIP, vasoactive intestinal peptide.

in portal blood flow; nonetheless, arterial flow will sometimes be the only blood flow to the liver. For example, in patients with thrombosis of the portal vein or with cirrhosis and reversal of portal flow (hepatofugal flow), the liver parenchyma depends entirely on hepatic arterial inflow.

Important systemic hemodynamic characteristics of portal hypertension include low peripheral vascular resistance and increased cardiac output. Both of these are, in part, due to intrahepatic and extrahepatic shunting; the former is related mostly to fibrosis of the liver parenchyma, and the later resulting mostly from progressive growth of a network of extrahepatic portasystemic collaterals. The most notable sites of extrahepatic portasystemic shunting are the following:

- From the portal system through a network of esophagogastric varices to the azygos vein and superior vena cava. In this pathway from the portal vein to the azygos vein, the coronary vein is one of the most important collaterals (Fig. 19-2).
- From the left branch of the portal vein through the umbilical vein to the subcutaneous periumbilical and epigastric veins, resulting in a remarkably impressive network of dilated cutaneous veins of the abdominal wall called *caput medusae*.
- From the portal vein through the inferior mesenteric vein to the mesocolic veins of the distal colon and rectum to the hemorrhoidal veins, resulting in large anorectal varices prone to bleeding. Clinically these varices are recognized to be hemorrhoids (see Fig. 19-2).
- From multiple small portal collaterals through countless retroperitoneal veins to the inferior vena cava (IVC), named Retzius's circulation. This large network of veins, along with the other portasystemic shunting, results in the reduction of systemic venous resistance and increased cardiac output (see Fig. 19-2).

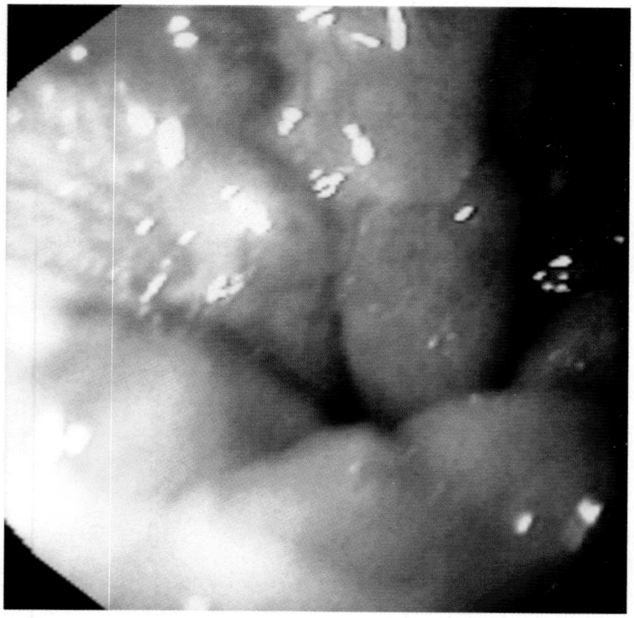
FIGURE 19–3 Endoscopic view of large esophageal varices.

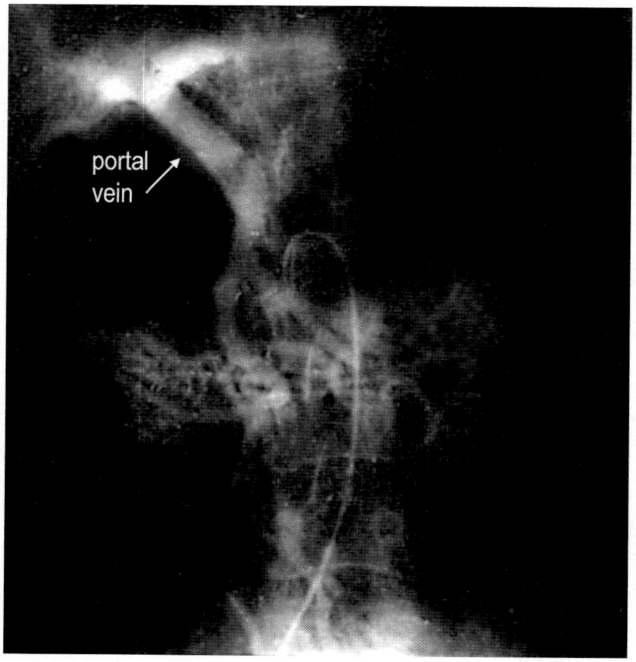

FIGURE 19–2 Contrast study of the portal vein showing the extensive collateral circulation in a patient with portal hypertension. These portasystemic collaterals are known as varices.

Esophagogastric collaterals have received considerable attention because of their relevance in clinical practice. These collaterals are the varices noted during upper endoscopy in patients with portal hypertension (Fig. 19-3). The amount of blood flowing through the esophagogastric varices toward the azygos vein can be as high as 300 mL/min and can be a source of fatal bleeding.

Etiology of Portal Hypertension

Prehepatic portal hypertension can be due to extrinsic compression or thrombosis of the portal vein. Portal vein occlusion and the resultant prehepatic portal hypertension are most commonly caused by mass effect from pancreatic or biliary tumors, pancreatitis, or hematologic disorders.

Intrahepatic presinusoidal causes of portal hypertension are common around the world, but uncommon in the United States. Schistosomiasis causes intrahepatic presinusoidal portal hypertension and is the most frequent cause of portal hypertension in the world. This disease is generally caused by the parasite *Schistosoma mansoni*, which is endemic in the Caribbean as well as the Near and Far East. This organism, absorbed through the gut mucosa, travels through the portal vein and lodges in the intrahepatic branches of the portal vein. The parasite causes an intense inflammatory response, because of egg deposition, and subsequent formation of granulomas within the portal spaces. The characteristic histologic appearance is a "pipe-stem fibrosis" in the presinusoidal spaces, which causes increased resistance to blood flow in the portal vein and presinusoidal portal hypertension.

Intrahepatic postsinusoidal causes of portal hypertension are most common in the United States. In Western countries, alcohol, hepatitis C virus, and chronic biliary obstruction are the most frequent causes of portal hypertension. Damage to hepatocytes and subsequent healing results in fibrosis with altered architecture of liver parenchyma (i.e., cirrhosis). Cirrhosis leads to increased resistance to portal blood flow and portal hypertension. Unlike other forms of portal hypertension, postsinusoidal causes of portal hypertension are usually associated with impaired hepatic reserve. Progression of cirrhosis can be halted if the agent causing hepatic injury is eliminated. Patients with cirrhosis, depending on the stage of the disease, may have hepatic reserve adequate for normal life.

From autopsy studies, it is estimated that 3% to 5% of the North American population have cirrhosis. This potentially represents a monumental problem; however, only a small percentage of people with cirrhosis eventually require treatment for portal hypertension and its complications.

Portal hypertension also can be caused by obstruction of venous outflow from the liver. This can result from hepatic vein obstruction, within or outside the liver parenchyma, and suprahepatic vena caval obstruction. Budd-Chiari syndrome, or thrombosis of the venous outflow from the liver, is a well-recognized cause of posthepatic portal hypertension. Although the etiology of Budd-Chiari syndrome often remains unknown, polycythemia vera is a frequently identified cause, as well as paroxysmal nocturnal hemoglobinuria, oral contraceptive use, and hereditary or acquired hypercoagulable states.

Chronic congestive heart failure also may result in a posthepatic type of portal hypertension, but it rarely causes the formation of gastroesophageal varices because the portal vein–to–systemic venous pressure gradient is not increased. Notably, congestive heart failure can significantly exacerbate preexisting portal hypertension and lead to exsanguinating variceal hemorrhage by increasing pressure in preexisting varices.

Liver Function

As noted, the amount of underlying liver function is usually related to the cause of portal hypertension. Postsinusoidal causes of portal hypertension, so common in Western countries, are generally associated with notable impairment of hepatic function. In the United States, portal hypertension is generally due to cirrhosis and therefore is frequently associated with significant impairment of liver function. Accordingly, this chapter focuses on portal hypertension due to cirrhosis, because it is the most frequent cause of portal hypertension encountered in the United States.

When treating patients with cirrhosis, the physician must consider the severity of portal hypertension together with liver function. Knowledge of hepatic reserve is important because it will predict how people will tolerate various therapeutic measures directed at treating complicated portal hypertension. Hepatic reserve will thereby ultimately influence the type of therapy offered to a particular patient. Unfortunately, hepatic reserve is often difficult to determine. Commonly used indicators of hepatic reserve are routine clinical laboratory tests, the Child's classification, the Child-Pugh score, and the Model for End-Stage Liver Disease (MELD) score.

Routine clinical laboratory tests generally include the group of serum chemistries called *liver-function tests*. These tests include measurements of albumin, bilirubin, alkaline phosphatase, transaminases serum glutamic oxaloacetic transaminase (SGOT) and serum glutamate pyruvate transaminase (SGPT), and cholesterol. Most of these parameters do not reflect liver function; rather, alkaline phosphatase, SGOT, and SGPT are better measures of biliary obstruction or ongoing hepatic parenchymal injury. Serum cholesterol, albumin, and bilirubin, as well as prothrombin time (PT), are more reflective of liver function, as they indicate synthetic and detoxifying activities of the liver. However, these tests do not detect subtle loss of liver function. Abnormalities in these tests may not occur until more than 80% of normal liver function is lost. Furthermore, these tests can be significantly altered by occasional events such as binge drinking, blood transfusions, stress, and trauma, and may not accurately reflect hepatic reserve.

Child's classification (Table 19-2) was defined more than 40 years ago to assess hepatic reserve and to predict mortality with portosystemic shunting. The classification is based on assessment of five routine clinical parameters: ascites, encephalopathy, nutritional status, albumin, and

TABLE 19–2 Child-Turcotte Classification (1964)

	Class A	Class B	Class C
Albumin (g/dL)	>3.5	3.5–3.0	<3.0
Bilirubin (g/dL)	<2	2–3	>3
Encephalopathy	None	Minimal*	Advanced†
Nutritional health	Excellent	Good	Wasting
Ascites	None	Moderate*	Refractory†

*Controlled with medications.
†Not controlled with medications, requiring hospitalization and more aggressive intervention.

TABLE 19–3 Child-Pugh Score (1973)

Points	Albumin (g/dL)	PT*	Bilirubin (g/dL)	Ascites	Encephalopathy†
1	>3.5	<4	<2	Mild	0
2	3.0–3.5	4–6	2–3	Moderate	I–II
3	<3.0	>6	>3	Severe	III–IV

Score A = 5–6 points; Score B = 7–9 points; Score C = 10–15 points.
*Seconds beyond normal.
†Grade of encephalopathy.

serum bilirubin. Each parameter is assigned a qualitative value of A (best), B, or C (worst). Class assignment is determined by the poorest grade given any one of the five parameters. For example, if a patient is noted to have a grade of A for four parameters and a grade of C for one parameter, the patient belongs to class C.

Although simple and applicable, excessive subjectivity and sometimes poor specificity are the most important limitations of Child's classification. The assessment of the volume of ascites is difficult, even with ultrasound or computed tomography (CT) scans. The definition of encephalopathy is most arbitrary, lacking any well-accepted objective scoring system. Nutritional status also is difficult to determine. Patients with cirrhosis are generally malnourished. However, assessment of their nutritional status using routine physical examination or other indices of malnutrition can be quite imprecise. Low serum albumin levels, which indicate chronic malnutrition, can be related to poor liver synthetic function, renal disease, stress, or acute illness, and may not specifically reflect the nutritional health of the patient. Similarly, hepatic dysfunction, biliary stasis, or excessive bilirubin load (seen with multiple blood transfusions) can affect the serum bilirubin level.

To improve its ability to quantify hepatic reserve, the original Child's classification was revised to the Child-Pugh score (Table 19-3). The Child-Pugh score uses three laboratory parameters (serum albumin, serum bilirubin, and PT) and two clinical indices (ascites and encephalopathy). A numeric score is assigned, depending on the value of each parameter, and ultimately, the class (A, B, or C) is assigned based on the resultant numeric score. The severity of encephalopathy is determined in a scale of four grades, in which grade 1 defines a patient with mild transient euphoria, and grade 4 indicates a comatose patient not responding to painful stimuli. Even though the Child-Pugh score would seem to be an improvement, it has not had a significant clinical impact beyond the original Child's classification. Like Child's classification, the Child-Pugh score is affected by many factors. For example, acute alcohol ingestion can make liver function appear much worse by altering mental status, worsening ascites, by causing hepatocyte inflammation (alcoholic hepatitis), or a combination of these. In this way, a patient with alcoholic cirrhosis could belong to two different Child's classes or have two different Child-Pugh scores, one before and one after an alcohol binge, even within a 24-hour interval.

The MELD is a recently developed formula for predicting short-term (<2 years) survival after transjugular intrahepatic portasystemic shunts (TIPS). Its application has been broadened and is thought to be an accurate measure of hepatic reserve and to predict survival for patients with cirrhosis. Three laboratory parameters, the serum bilirubin, the serum creatinine, and the international normalized ratio (INR), are used. The MELD score is calculated as

$$\text{MELD score} = (0.957 \times \log_e[\text{creatinine mg/dL}] + 0.378 \times \log_e[\text{bilirubin mg/dL}] + 1.120 \times \log_e(\text{INR}) + 0.643) \times 10$$

Convenient MELD score calculators can be found on the internet. A MELD score of 18 carries a median survival of 3 months; a score of 15 carries a median survival of 6 months; and a score of 13 has a median survival of 1 year.

Despite its shortcomings, Child's classification, owing to its easy applicability and clinical utility, is used worldwide to quantify severity of cirrhosis and to predict outcome after surgical intervention. It correlates closely with operative mortality and survival after portacaval shunting. MELD scores are becoming increasingly relied on and more widely applied.

More accurate quantitative determinations of hepatocyte function can be undertaken with more sophisticated tests (Table 19-4), which are unfortunately not widely available. These tests are used primarily in centers specializing in the treatment of hepatic disorders.

TABLE 19–4 Tests of Liver Function

Name of the Test	Function Measured
Aminopyrine breath test	Microsomal function
Caffeine clearance test	Microsomal function
Galactose elimination capacity	Metabolic capacity
Low-dose galactose clearance test	Hepatic perfusion
Indocyanine green clearance test	Hepatic perfusion
Albumin synthesis test	Synthetic function

A well-studied test of hepatic metabolic capacity is the galactose elimination capacity. This is determined by measuring the clearance from the serum of a large intravenous bolus dose of galactose, which depends on the ability of hepatocytes to phosphorylate galactose and convert it to glucose. The galactose elimination capacity accurately predicts prognosis in the care of patients with cirrhosis and portal hypertension, including those undergoing portacaval shunting. Unfortunately, the lack of availability of an easy assay for galactose has limited the applicability. Antipyrine clearance, the aminopyrine breath test, the lidocaine clearance test, and the caffeine clearance test are other measures of liver function. They specifically measure the microsomal activity of hepatocytes. The variability of results obtained with these tests has prevented the acceptance of each as the gold standard in determining liver function.

Unfortunately, no ideal or universally accepted measure exists of hepatic reserve in patients with cirrhosis and portal hypertension. Because the implications of accurately predicting hepatic reserve in cirrhotic patients undergoing treatment for complicated portal hypertension are so profound, the development of a simple, reliable, reproducible, and universally accepted measure of liver function would be a major advancement in the care of patients with cirrhosis and portal hypertension. Today, Child's classification and the Child-Pugh score are being replaced by the MELD score as the standard assessment of hepatocellular reserve and outcome in cirrhosis, denoting the first significant clinical progress in this field in the last 30 years.

Portal Hypertension and Variceal Bleeding: Early Evalution and Treatment

Patient Presentation

The collaterals between the portal and systemic venous systems are thin-walled veins. With elevation of portal pressures, these veins become distended and are called *varices*. The presentation of patients with portal hypertension and variceal bleeding will vary, depending on the amount and acuity of ongoing blood loss. Patients with low levels of continuous (occult) blood loss will be seen initially with weakness, anemia, and iron deficiency. Given the chronic nature of this process, patients with occult blood loss may be in profound ill health. On physical examination, they will appear tired, pale, and, given the lack of acute hemorrhage, normal blood pressure. More commonly, the presentation of patients with variceal bleeding is dramatic, manifesting with hematemesis, melena, or hematochezia, indicating massive gastrointestinal blood loss.

Patients with portal hypertension can bleed from virtually anywhere in the gastrointestinal tract. Most commonly, however, massive blood loss occurs from esophageal or gastric varices or both. Blood loss from other sites due to portal hypertension should lead to similar resuscitation, evaluation, and prompt treatment.

In patients with cirrhosis, one cannot assume gastrointestinal hemorrhage to be caused by variceal hemorrhage. Patients with significant liver disease and cirrhosis are more prone than is the general population to peptic ulcers and other gastrointestinal tract pathology. Because of their poor general health and often self-destructive lifestyle, they frequently bleed from peptic ulcers. Additionally, vomiting can result in a Mallory-Weiss tear and bleeding from the lower esophagus. Severe esophagitis or gastritis can result in notable, although more often chronic, blood loss. For a patient with known cirrhosis and esophagogastric varices with signs of massive gastrointestinal hemorrhage, extravariceal bleeding should always be considered while prompt initiation of resuscitation and diagnostic measures is undertaken.

Patient Examination

First and foremost in the evaluation of patients with suspected bleeding varices is a comprehensive clinical evaluation. Evidence of ascites, encephalopathy, and extremity wasting is sought. The presence of any of these would denote advanced cirrhosis and poor hepatic reserve. Palmar erythema and cutaneous spider angiomata often are seen, evidence of increased cardiac output and low peripheral vascular resistance, and represent further signs of advanced cirrhosis.

A general assessment should quickly define the acuity of patient illness. Gross hematemesis and melena, with signs of hemorrhagic shock, should denote severe hemorrhage and indicate the necessity for expedient treatment. Vital signs, mental status, and the rate of clinically apparent ongoing blood loss will dictate early care through the ABCs (airway, bleeding, circulation) of resuscitation. Airway protection and prevention of aspiration of blood into the tracheobronchial tree are critical, particularly in the presence of encephalopathy due to underlying liver disease. Patients with marginal respiratory reserve or an inability to protect their airway should be intubated before any intervention because of the high risk of aspiration. Once the airway has been secured and mechanical ventilation initiated, intravascular volume should be reestablished, and bleeding should be stopped as soon as possible.

Patients with portal hypertension and bleeding varices often have notable hematologic abnormalities. Anemia can be a consequence of both acute and chronic blood losses. With the latter, iron-deficiency anemia may occur. Coagulation defects may be the result of ongoing blood loss, impaired synthetic ability of the liver, or hypersplenism. In patients with bleeding, whatever the site, it is imperative to correct coagulation abnormalities with fresh frozen plasma and parenteral vitamin K. Thrombocytopenia in patients with portal hypertension is often a consequence of platelet sequestration in the spleen. It is futile to transfuse platelets to correct thrombocytopenia, because administered platelets are quickly sequestered.

Numerous abnormalities may be noted on laboratory testing. Electrolyte abnormalities may occur as a consequence of diuretic therapy, excessive alcohol consumption, fluid shifts, acute blood loss, or resuscitation. Serum levels of albumin, bilirubin, and cholesterol, as well as the PT, should be determined to gain an assessment of liver function and to serve as a guide to replacement of clotting factors.

Evaluation of patients with cirrhosis and bleeding varices should involve screening for hepatitis and human immunodeficiency virus (HIV) infection. Hepatitis screening may define the cause of cirrhosis as well as provide information that could direct therapy. Patients with notable viremia may be treated differently from patients with long-standing, end-stage hepatitis and cirrhosis without viremia. Evidence of HIV infection should be sought. Choice of therapy for portal hypertension may be altered, depending on expectations of survival with HIV infection and acquired immunodeficiency syndrome (AIDS).

Liver biopsy can lead to the definitive diagnosis, the possible etiology, and the histologic classification of cirrhosis. The degree of active hepatitis, potentially confusing the clinical picture of hepatic reserve, may be defined by biopsy. Generally, biopsy is not undertaken in the emergency setting because of risk and time of processing the sample.

At the completion of the physical examination and with the return of laboratory values, each patient should be assigned a Child's class or Child-Pugh score and a MELD score. Accepting the limitations of these scoring systems, they remain the best method to predict prognosis and are helpful in determining definitive treatment.

Early Resuscitation

In caring for patients with portal hypertension and gastrointestinal hemorrhage, after securing the airway, consideration must be directed toward replenishing intravascular volume. In planning resuscitation, it is important to estimate the magnitude and acuity of blood loss. Small gastrointestinal hemorrhages can be handled with isotonic crystalloid, such as Ringer's lactate solution. In the presence of significant hemorrhage, transfusions of packed red blood cells should be used early. An adequate hemoglobin level should be maintained. Fresh frozen plasma should be administered to improve underlying coagulopathy associated with and contributing to major hemorrhage.

Because large volumes are often required for resuscitation, it is appropriate to establish central venous access and to monitor either central venous or pulmonary artery pressures to guide resuscitation. Usually the internal jugular vein is the best site of access because hematomas at this site are more controllable than are those complicating subclavian venipuncture. It is important not to over-resuscitate patients in this setting. If infused volumes excessively increase central venous pressure (e.g., to 20 mmHg) portal venous pressures will increase dramatically (e.g., to 40 mmHg), leading to massive distention of varices and promotion of ongoing bleeding. *Over-resuscitation will perpetuate variceal bleeding*. Goals of resuscitation should be normalization of blood pressure and volume status, with reestablishment of adequate urinary output.

Early after patient arrival to the hospital, therapy for bleeding varices should be initiated promptly. During early evaluation and resuscitation, initial therapy can be begun before a definitive diagnosis has been established. Therapy before diagnosis is not optimal, but variceal bleeding can be so morbid that treatment should be initiated based solely on clinical suspicion.

Pharmacotherapy

The initial therapy beyond resuscitation given to patients with cirrhosis and bleeding varices is pharmacologic. It is often initiated before endoscopic diagnosis and therapy because it is readily available, relatively nontoxic, and generally efficacious. These interventions usually will not exacerbate a gastrointestinal bleeding disorder unrelated to portal hypertension and may be helpful.

Vasopressin and octreotide are the staples of pharmacologic intervention. Vasopressin has been the mainstay of therapy for patients with portal hypertensive bleeding for several decades. Intravenous vasopressin should be initiated at a dose of up to 1.0 units/min (not to exceed 20 units over a 20-min period), and gradually decreased to 0.4 units/min. Vasopressin is relatively contraindicated in patients with known coronary artery disease, as it decreases myocardial blood flow by producing coronary vasospasm. If used in elderly patients or in patients with known coronary artery disease, vasopressin therapy should be combined with intravenous nitroglycerin infusion. Furthermore, vasopressin promotes fluid retention and accumulation of ascites; therefore infusion ideally should not exceed 72 hours.

Octreotide is increasingly used relative to vasopressin because of less toxicity. Octreotide (a synthetic somatostatin analogue) does not have adverse effects on coronary blood flow and does not promote fluid retention and ascites. Randomized trials comparing octreotide to vasopressin have documented equivalency in controlling bleeding and 30-day mortality. Octreotide is administered as an IV bolus of 50 to 100 units followed by an infusion of 50 to 100 U/hr. Treatment with these drugs is usually continued for 2 to 4 days, while more definitive therapy is planned and undertaken.

Endoscopic Sclerotherapy and Banding

Early endoscopy is of paramount importance in the evaluation and treatment of patients with cirrhosis and suspected variceal hemorrhage. Endoscopic evaluation of the upper gastrointestinal tract must be initiated early in the management of these patients. Colonoscopy also may be necessary, as bleeding may be located lower in the gastrointestinal tract. Generally, endoscopy in this setting has three major functions:

The first function is to define the cause and the site of bleeding. This may be straightforward, or it may be nearly impossible, as the esophagus, stomach, and duodenum can be full of clot, or in the case of colonoscopy, the colon may be full of stool and clot. It is important to make a distinction between bleeding due to portal hypertension and bleeding from other causes, such as peptic ulcer disease, Mallory-Weiss tear, esophagitis, or cancer.

The second function of early endoscopy is to determine the size and location of varices and to plan adequate treatment. For example, if bleeding is due to small varices localized to the esophagus without evidence of gastric varices, the chances of success with endoscopic treatment are higher than 90%.

The third function and ultimate goal of early endoscopy is therapy. Direct control of variceal hemorrhage by using endoscopy is possible. Esophageal varices, much like hemorrhoids, may be banded endoscopically or may be injected with a sclerosing solution, without deleterious influence on liver function. Larger varices are harder to treat endoscopically and are more likely to rebleed. Varices that are extremely large are very difficult to band, as the band may include only the anterior wall of the varix. Banding only the anterior wall will not obliterate the varix and may potentially exacerbate bleeding due to anterior-wall necrosis. These patients are often better served by sclerotherapy. In the United States, the most commonly used sclerosants are sodium tetradecyl sulfate and sodium morrhuate. The sclerosant is usually injected directly into the varix, although some endoscopists prefer to inject the substance along the sides of the varices (paravariceal injection). Several studies have failed to document an advantage of one technique over the other. In general, gastric varices are not amenable to endoscopic treatment and more often require portal decompression. Gastric varices are not amenable to sclerotherapy or banding because the stomach wall is thin, and perforation is more likely to occur.

Potential complications of endoscopic sclerotherapy and banding are many, although actual major complications are infrequent. Major variceal rehemorrhage, occurring specifically from a sclerotherapy site or from an inappropriately applied band, is considered a complication of treatment. Conversely, rehemorrhage from a site not previously treated is generally a failure of rather than a complication from endoscopic management. Rehemorrhage from a varix, whether because previous therapy failed or because it was missed, may be treated by repeated endoscopic sclerotherapy or banding.

Esophageal perforation is an uncommon, though devastating, complication of sclerotherapy. Ulceration of the esophageal mucosa at the site of sclerotherapy or banding is seen more often. Ulcers may appear up to 1 week after treatment and can be a source of considerable rebleeding. Healing of significant ulcerations can result in late stricture formation.

The mortality directly attributed to endoscopic treatment of bleeding varices is small (1%–2%). Banding seems to have fewer complications, with lower rates of stricture and ulcer formation, and to be more effective at controlling bleeding than is sclerotherapy in the treatment of esophageal varices. In some circumstances, repeated endoscopic therapy can be considered definitive treatment for patients who have bled from esophageal varices. To be definitive, treatment will require several sessions over a prolonged period with the goal of obliteration of the varices. However, chronic endoscopic therapy may not be always applicable. Some patients may not be able to commit to a treatment based on scheduled periodic appointments. Other patients may live in rural areas, distant from medical facilities. Patients with gastric or intestinal varices or both are not candidates for long-term endoscopic therapy.

Balloon Tamponade

For patients with ongoing bleeding not controlled by pharmacologic measures and not amenable to treatment by endoscopic intervention (or for whom the treatment failed), balloon tamponade by using the Sengstaken-Blakemore (S-B) tube should be the next consideration, while preparation for portal decompression or other definitive treatment is being undertaken.

The S-B (Fig. 19-4) double-balloon catheter is inserted per *os* into the stomach. To prevent aspiration, suction is attached to the balloon catheter proximal to the esophageal balloon so that secretions or blood will be suctioned, preventing aspiration into the tracheobronchial tree. After insertion, the location of the tip is confirmed by radiograph to lie in the stomach. Then the gastric balloon is inflated with 250 to 300 cc of air, and the location of the tip is checked again by radiograph. After ensuring adequate positioning, 0.5 to 1.0 kg of traction is applied to the tube. This secures the balloon up into the gastroesophageal junction and compresses fundal and cardial varices. If bleeding continues, the esophageal balloon is inflated, generally to 30 mmHg pressure. After the S-B tube has been correctly placed, the nasoesophageal tube and the gastric port of the S-B tube are both connected to intermittent suction to evacuate secretions from the esophagus and stomach. Attention must be given to the lips of the patient to ensure that pressure necrosis does not occur.

The S-B tube should not be left in place with balloons inflated for more than 48 hours. By 48 hours, patient stabi-

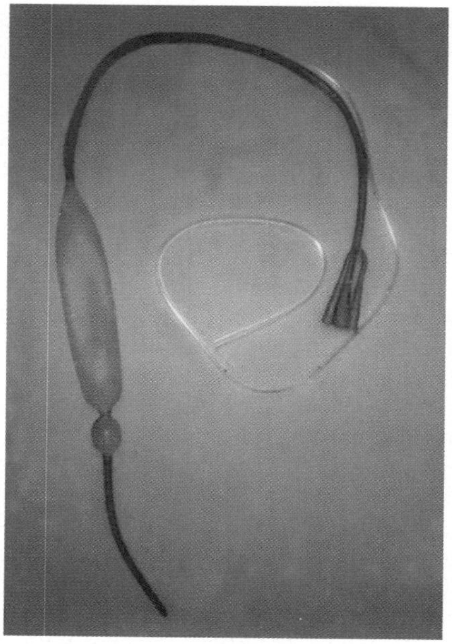

FIGURE 19–4 The Sengstaken-Blakemore tube. A nasogastric tube is attached to the Sengstaken-Blakemore tube to evacuate oropharyngeal secretions that would otherwise accumulate proximal to the esophageal balloon.

PEARLS FOR THE OR

When treating portal hypertension, hope for the best, but be prepared for the worst. Any operation undertaken on patients with cirrhosis and portal hypertension can lead to substantial blood loss.

The dissection of the inferior venal cava and portal vein is greatly facilitated through the use of a blunt, smooth instrument (e.g., Yankauer suction tip). Often numerous varices are seen within the retroperitoneum and porta hepatis; these can bleed quite substantially. Liberal use of ligatures or electrocautery or both is a must.

When undertaking the small-diameter H-graft portacaval shunt, the first anastomosis to be constructed is that between the graft and the vena cava. It is important to remove a wedge of the vena cava wall when making the venotomy to assure adequate outflow from the graft. Care must be used to avoid injury to the bile duct, gallbladder, and hepatic artery.

Check intraoperative pressures before and after shunting. After the shunt is completed, seek a decrease in portal vein pressure of at least 10 mmHg and a portal vein–to–vena cava gradient of less than 10 mmHg. The presence of a thrill in the vena cava cephalad to the shunt will confirm shunt patency.

lization should have occurred, and coagulopathy, corrected. Beyond 48 hours, the risk of ulceration and pressure necrosis due to the balloon becomes excessive.

Definitive Treatment for Patients with Bleeding Varices from Cirrhosis and Portal Hypertension

General Considerations

Patients not amenable to nonoperative management or for whom it has failed, including endoscopic sclerotherapy or banding, require more definitive treatment of their bleeding and underlying portal hypertension. Ideally, operative intervention is best undertaken under elective circumstances. Emergency or urgent operations offer a higher degree of risk. In addition, most surgeons would prefer the opportunity to optimize the coagulation profile, purge the gastrointestinal tract, obtain true informed consent, and assess liver function to plan the best immediate and long-term care.

Considerations of Child's class, MELD score, age, cause of cirrhosis, general health, and patient reliability are important issues in assigning therapy. Patient compliance, reliability, and the availability for follow-up are particularly important factors when choosing therapies requiring multiple applications with significant failure rates, such as prolonged pharmacologic therapy with repeated endoscopic sclerotherapy and banding. Specifically, long-term propranolol and nitrate therapy requires patient diligence and can reduce patient performance status, undoubtedly affecting compliance. For long-term sclerotherapy or banding to be effective, multiple sessions over an extended time are required, presupposing commitment by the physician and patient.

Before assignment of definitive therapy, several questions must be asked:

1. Is active liver disease present?
2. What is the patient's hepatic reserve?
3. Is nonoperative nondecompressive therapy an option?
4. Will this patient be served best by portal decompression, selective devascularization, or transplantation?
5. Is this the right time for operative intervention?

Answering these questions will help the surgeon assign the best therapy for each individual patient. Options for definitive treatment are hepatic transplantation, portal decompression by either a surgical shunt or TIPS, or a devascularization procedure.

Hepatic Transplantation in the Management of Variceal Hemorrhage due to Cirrhosis and Portal Hypertension

Once the acute hemorrhage has been controlled, considerations for definitive management are made. The definitive management for patients with cirrhosis and portal hypertension is liver transplantation; however, it also is the approach that requires the most resources and patient compliance. Because of the magnitude of this approach, as well as limited availability of organs for transplantation, it *should not* be considered to be the first-line therapy for all patients with variceal hemorrhage.

In 1967, Dr. Thomas Starzl first reported a patient with cirrhosis who lived for 13 months after liver transplantation. Advances in immunosuppression, organ procurement, surgical techniques, and anesthesia have helped to reduce perioperative mortality and improve long-term survival after transplantation. Liver transplantation is currently undertaken in approximately 70 centers in the United States. Although transplantation is the definitive therapy, several considerations must be addressed about the applicability of this therapy for a given individual:

- The ultimate need for transplantation should be determined by measures of hepatic reserve. Patients with cirrhosis and portal hypertensive bleeding with marginal or inadequate hepatic reserve should be considered for transplantation. Hepatic reserve has been historically difficult to assess accurately. Today, the MELD score is used most frequently. A MELD score of 18 or more indicates the need for imminent transplantation, and a score of more than 13 implies the need for transplantation at some point.
- Some patients who will benefit from liver transplantation are precluded because of lack of availability in their immediate area. Although medical transportation has reduced this problem, it remains an issue.
- Transplantation and subsequent immunosuppressive medications are expensive and may not be available to patients without adequate funding.
- Active alcoholics, patients with excessive viral load, and patients with HIV are not considered good transplant candidates. Given the epidemiology of cirrhosis in the United States, a substantial percentage of patients with portal hypertension are precluded from having transplantation.
- A severe shortage exists of livers available for transplantation.
- Transplantation is best not done as an emergency because an adequate transplant evaluation and the associated psychosocial tests and interventions cannot be completed.
- Patients with acute variceal hemorrhage will often be too ill to survive a liver transplant operation.
- Hepatic transplantation carries no guarantee of success. Even after excluding alcoholic patients, patients with excessive viral loads, as well as those who are profoundly ill and in extremis, transplantation still carries a notable perioperative mortality and 1-year failure rate. Nevertheless, if a patient lives to 1 year after hepatic transplantation, long-term survival rates with a functioning graft are high.

It is important to stress that the definitive indication for liver transplantation is based on functional hepatic reserve. If life expectancy is short because of end-stage liver disease, transplantation should be strongly considered, given adequate psychosocial support and financial resources. If hepatic reserve is adequate for long-term survival after recovery from the acute hemorrhage and control of alcohol consumption or viral load, transplantation is best deferred.

Operative Portal Decompression in the Management of Variceal Hemorrhage due to Cirrhosis and Portal Hypertension

Patients with adequate hepatic reserve for whom nonoperative treatment for variceal bleeding fails, or who are at significant risk for rebleeding, should be considered for portal decompression. Portal decompression can be undertaken operatively or achieved through radiologically guided techniques, such as the TIPS. Surgical portacaval shunts are classified as selective and nonselective, depending on the focus of the shunt. Selective shunts focus on decompression of the esophagogastric variceal complex without specific intent to decrease overall portal pressures. Nonselective shunts decompress the esophagogastric variceal complex by directly reducing mesenteric and portal venous pressures. Nonselective shunts are further classified as total and partial shunts, depending on the degree of decompression achieved. Nonselective total shunts completely decompress the portal system, with a residual portal vein–to–IVC pressure gradient near zero. Examples of this type of shunt are the end-to-side, side-to-side, and large-diameter (≥16 mm) H-graft portacaval shunts; the large-diameter mesocaval shunt; and the proximal splenorenal shunt. These shunts are no longer applied and have only historical interest. Nonselective partial shunts preserve a degree of the portal vein–to–IVC pressure gradient in an attempt to restore a normal portacaval gradient. Examples of partial shunts are the small-diameter (8 mm and 10 mm) H-graft portacaval shunt, the narrow-diameter (10 mm) side-to-side portacaval shunt, and the small-diameter mesocaval shunt.

Selective shunts do not directly reduce the pressure gradient between the portal vein and the IVC. Rather, they selectively decompress the esophagogastric variceal complex. The most prominent selective shunt is the distal splenorenal shunt, often referred as the Warren shunt.

More recently, TIPS has been received with enthusiasm by many. TIPS is discussed in more detail later in this chapter. In short, it allows direct portal decompression without an abdominal operation. The shunt consists of a stent, deployed across the substance of the liver, connecting the portal vein to the hepatic vein, introduced via a transjugular approach. The amount of portal decompression attained is determined by the diameter of the stent used.

PEARLS FOR ROUNDS

Altered mental status in patients with cirrhosis and portal hypertension (encephalopathy) is a warning sign of poor hepatic reserve and would generally contraindicate shunting until resolved.

Doppler ultrasound of the portal vein is useful in determining portal vein patency. Computed tomography angiography and visceral angiography also are used. A portal vein with good flow and caliber is required for shunting.

Patients with portal hypertension with an acute upper gastrointestinal hemorrhage should be admitted to the intensive care unit. The patient's airway is secured, and the patient is appropriately resuscitated with crystalloid, packed red blood cells, and fresh frozen plasma. Invasive monitoring (e.g., Swan-Ganz catheter) may be helpful in guiding resuscitation. An octreotide infusion should be initiated early. Expedite upper endoscopy, and a Sengstaken-Blakemore (S-B) tube should be readily available. Review S-B tube management so that its use will be appropriate, safe, and effective.

Thrombocytopenia is common in patients with portal hypertension. The inclination to transfuse platelets should be resisted, as platelet transfusions will have little effect because of portal hypertension and splenic sequestration.

TIPS has rapidly achieved a widely accepted role in the management of patients with acute variceal hemorrhage, although probably functioning best as a bridge to imminent transplantation.

Nonselective Shunts

Total Portacaval Shunts. The techniques of total portal decompression have remained essentially unchanged for the last 50 years. Total portal decompression can be attained through the end-to-side portacaval shunt, the large-bore side-to-side portacaval shunt, the large-bore prosthetic H-graft portacaval (and mesocaval) shunts, and the proximal splenorenal shunt (Fig. 19-5). Even though these shunts are anatomically different, they all share a fundamental characteristic: they achieve equalization of pressures between the portal vein and the vena cava by completely diverting portal blood into the IVC.

The end-to-side portacaval shunt is the prototypical nonselective total shunt. The construction of this shunt requires division of the portal vein near to its bifurcation and an end-to-side anastomosis between the portal vein and the IVC. It eliminates portal blood flow to the liver. The large-bore side-to-side portacaval shunt involves constructing an anastomosis between the side of the portal vein and the side of the IVC. This shunt diverts nearly all of the antegrade portal blood flow into the caval system and, furthermore, may siphon blood out of the liver with retrograde (hepatofugal) flow through the portal vein into the IVC. In this way, the large-bore side-to-side shunt may rob the liver of more than portal blood flow.

Proximal splenorenal shunts belong to the group of nonselective shunts providing total portal decompression. Splenectomy is an integrated part of this operation. The splenic vein is divided near the splenic hilum, mobilized from the pancreas, and sewn to the renal vein in an end-to-side fashion. Functionally, this shunt is a large-bore side-to-side portacaval shunt. In spite of early enthusiasm for the proximal splenorenal shunt, longer follow-up indicated that this shunt offered no real advantage when compared with end-to-side or the side-to-side portacaval shunts. Splenic vein thrombosis, and thereby shunt occlusion, has been associated with this shunt.

Large-diameter H-graft portacaval shunts are another way to attain total portal decompression. They are constructed by using a polytetrafluoroethylene (PTFE) or polyester prosthetic vascular graft, 16 to 20 mm in diameter, sewn end-to-side to the portal vein at one end of the graft, and end-to-side to the vena cava at the other end. They have similar hemodynamics and share similar outcomes with large-bore side-to-side shunts. They can be easier to construct than a native side-to-side portacaval shunt but are more prone to thrombosis than the direct anastomosis.

Nonselective total shunts offer good control of variceal hemorrhage, as they totally decompress the portal venous system. However, totally decompressing portacaval shunts are seldom applied now, as total diversion of portal blood flow is associated with a significant incidence of encephalopathy and progressive liver deterioration, which may be as high as 50%.

Partial Portal Decompression. Increased awareness of the deleterious effects of total portacaval shunts, including high rates of postoperative encephalopathy, led surgeons to seek alternative ways to decompress the portal system. Based on observations that varices rarely bleed if the portal vein–to–IVC pressure gradient is less than 12 mmHg, the concept of partial portal decompression was devised. Partial shunts attempt to create a physiologic replacement for the numerous thin-walled portasystemic collaterals with a single low-resistance shunt. By reducing the portasystemic gradient below a critical level, but not ablating it altogether, variceal hemorrhage is prevented, yet prograde portal blood flow (hepatopedal flow) is maintained, reducing postshunt liver dysfunction and encephalopathy.

Early partial shunts were developed by constructing a small-diameter direct side-to-side portacaval anastomosis. Unfortunately, results were not promising, as dilation of the shunt occurred, with loss of partial decompression noted at short-term follow-up. True partial portal decompression was not achieved until the development of the small-diameter prosthetic H-graft portacaval shunt. This shunt is constructed by using an 8-mm PTFE ring-reinforced graft, which is sewn in an end-to-side fashion to the vena cava and then to the

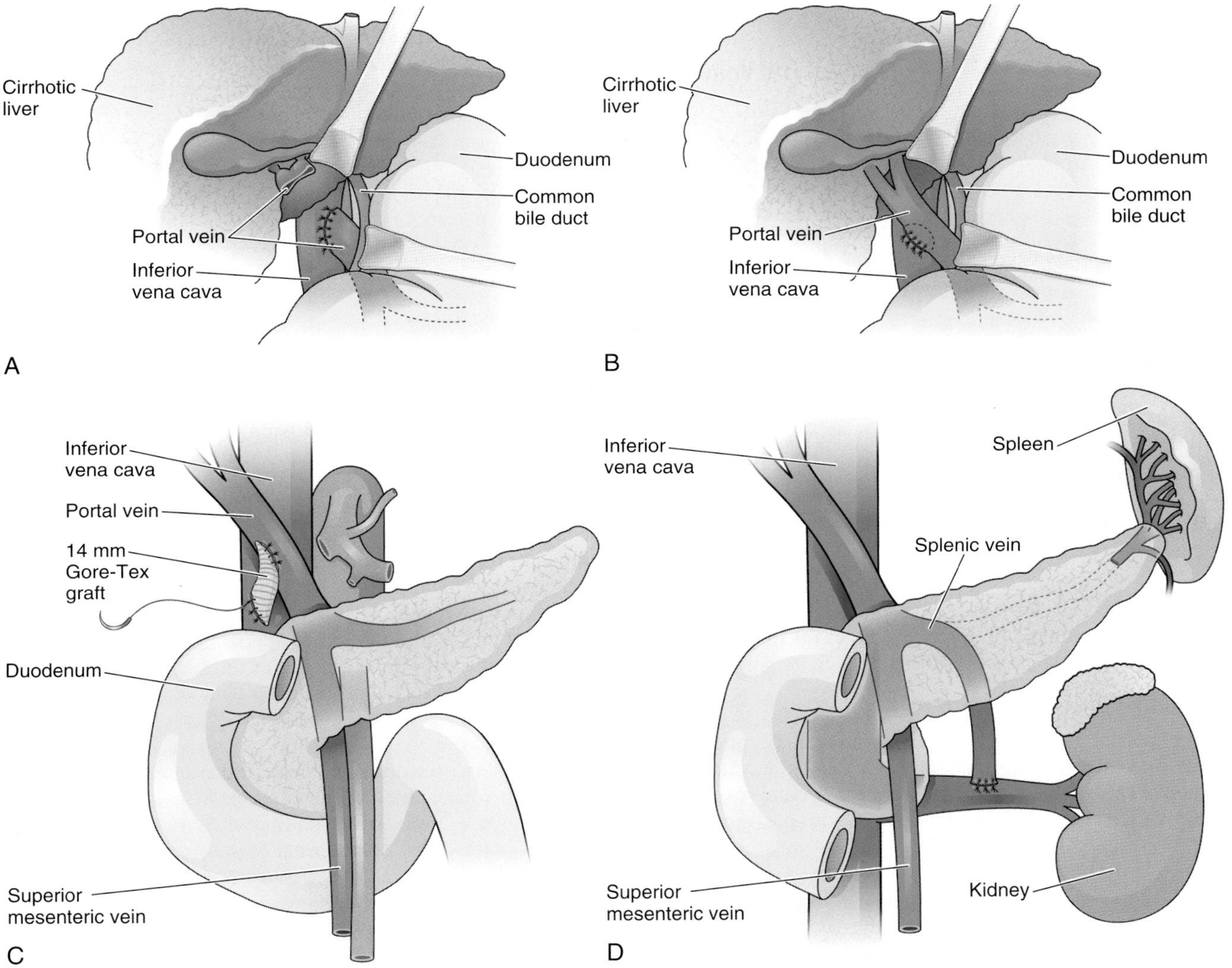

FIGURE 19–5 Nonselective total portasystemic shunts. *A*, End-to-side portacaval shunt. *B*, Side-to-side portacaval shunt. *C*, Large-diameter prosthetic H-graft mesocaval shunt. *D*, Proximal splenorenal shunt.

portal vein by using nonabsorbable monofilament sutures (Fig. 19-6). After shunting, portal pressures should be noted to decrease by more than 10 mmHg, and the gradient between the portal vein and the IVC should be less than 10 mmHg but should not approach zero. A postoperative transfemoral cannulation of the shunt and the portal vein is shown in Figure 19-7. Partial portal decompression attained through this technique maintains a portal vein–to-IVC pressure gradient (Table 19-5) and preserves hepatoportal blood flow in 90% of shunted patients. Not surprisingly, partial shunts are associated with significantly lower rates of postoperative encephalopathy than is seen with total shunts.

The results seen after small-diameter H-graft portacaval shunting have been favorable. The indication for shunting in most patients is bleeding from esophageal varices previously treated with sclerotherapy or banding and/or bleeding gastric varices. Both esophageal and gastric varices are noted in nearly half of patients. Postoperative mortality rate is less than 10% with most postoperative deaths occurring as a result of liver failure in patients of Child's class C. Shunt occlusions, both early and late, are infrequent. Early shunt thrombosis can be treated with catheter-directed thrombolysis, resulting in reestablishment of flow in nearly all cases. Long-term shunt patency and freedom from variceal rebleeding exceeds 90% at 7 years. Ascites resolves in nearly two thirds of patients after shunting and is otherwise considerably improved. Long-term survival is directly related to pre-shunt Child's class (Table 19-6). The

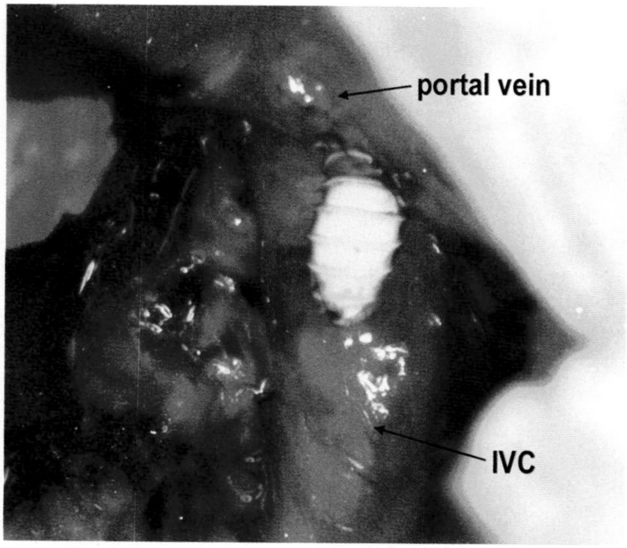

FIGURE 19–6 Small-diameter H-graft portacaval shunt.

majority of long-term survivors belong to Child's class A or B, reinforcing the notion that portacaval shunting is best tolerated by those patients with adequate hepatic reserve.

Selective Variceal Decompression

Like partial shunting, selective variceal decompression was introduced as an alternative to totally decompressing shunts. The intent of selective variceal decompression is to stop variceal bleeding by providing a low-pressure decompressive pathway from the gastroesophageal variceal complex while leaving the portal circulation undisturbed, thereby preventing postshunt liver dysfunction. The distal splenorenal (Warren) shunt is the prototypical selective shunt. This shunt involves division of the splenic vein at its junction with the portal vein and sewing the cut end of the splenic vein to the left renal vein. This shunt provides a low-pressure outflow conduit for the gastroesophageal variceal complex which drains into the renal vein (Fig. 19-8). To prevent recollateralization through the substance of the pancreas, it is important to ligate the numerous venous branches between the splenic vein and the pancreas. A further caveat of this operation is devascularization, separation of the gastroesophageal variceal complex from the portal venous circulation, and includes ligature of numerous veins, most important the left gastric (coronary) vein and the gastroepiploic vein.

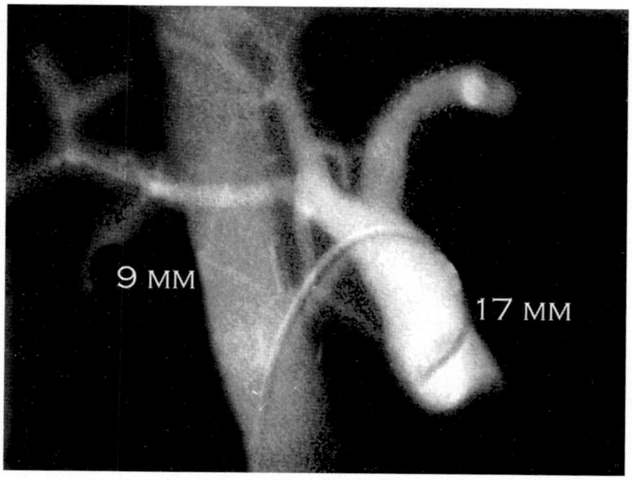

FIGURE 19–7 Postoperative transfemoral cannulation of the small-diameter prosthetic H-graft portacaval shunt. The shunt is patent with a portal vein–to–inferior vena cava gradient of 8 mmHg.

TABLE 19–5 Preshunt and Postshunt Portal Vein and Systemic Venous Pressures after Small-diameter H-graft Portacaval Shunt (mean ± SD)

Hemodynamics	Preshunt	Postshunt
Portal vein (mmHg)	30 ± 5.3	20 ± 5.5
Inferior vena cava (mmHg)	12 ± 5.2	14 ± 5.0
Portal vein–vena cava gradient (mmHg)	18 ± 4.7	6 ± 3.5

Results with the distal splenorenal shunt are acceptable, as postshunt variceal bleeding is infrequent and encephalopathy is largely avoided. Trials comparing endoscopic sclerotherapy with distal splenorenal shunting have noted that the distal splenorenal shunt is associated with low periprocedural mortality, less variceal rehemorrhage, and comparatively low postshunt encephalopathy. However, significant drawbacks are associated with the distal splenorenal shunt. It is a technically difficult operation, with highly variable success rates reported in the literature. Because portal pressures are not directly addressed, in many patients, particularly those with severe cirrhosis, ascites tends to develop postoperatively. Patients with hepatofugal (retrograde) flow and ascites are not good candidates for this type of shunt. Furthermore, portal vein and splenic vein (shunt) thrombosis occur at a significant rate. Nonetheless,

TABLE 19–6 Survival Stratified by Child's Class after Small-diameter H-graft Portacaval Shunt

Child's Class	30 Days	1 Year	3 Years	5 Years
A	94%	88%	57%	75%
B	92%	79%	60%	43%
C	80%	62%	40%	30%

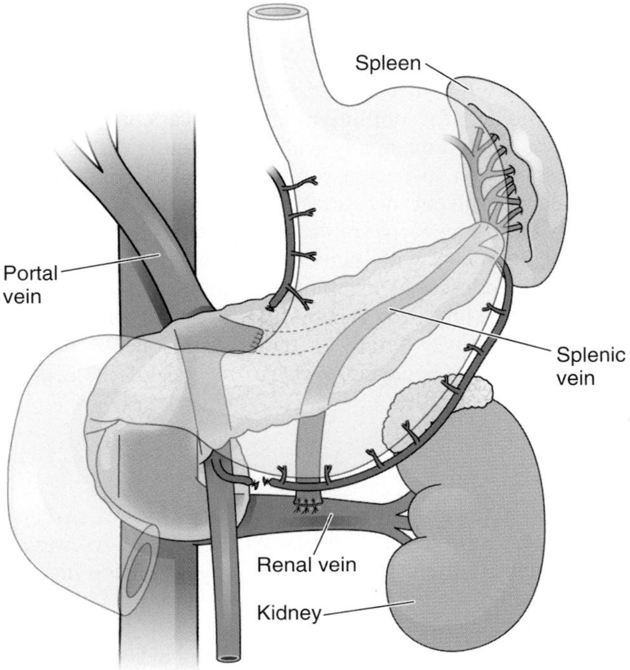

FIGURE 19–8 Distal splenorenal shunt.

the distal splenorenal shunt continues to be a widely accepted method in achieving variceal decompression because of good long-term results.

Transjugular Intrahepatic Portasystemic Shunt for Nonoperative Portal Decompression in Patients with Cirrhosis and Variceal Hemorrhage

TIPS shunts are radiologically placed portacaval shunts. This shunt, originally conceptualized in the 1960s, involves accessing the superior vena cava through the internal jugular vein. A guide wire is passed down through the IVC into the right hepatic vein and then across the liver substance and into the right portal vein. The tract between the portal vein and the hepatic vein is then dilated, allowing communication between the portal and systemic venous systems. Shunt patency was dismal until the addition of endovascular stents in the early 1990s. These stents are deployed across the tract through the hepatic parenchyma, leading to far more acceptable shunt patency rates (Fig. 19-9). Initial short-term success with TIPS, its relative ease of performance, as well as the perceived benefits of avoidance of an abdominal operation led to the rapid acceptance of TIPS as a first-line therapy in the treatment of complex portal hypertension.

Although TIPS can achieve nonoperative portal decompression, it remains fraught with significant periprocedural morbidity and relatively poor long-term patency. Stenosis and occlusion remain common problems, requiring close shunt surveillance, and frequent reinterventions are often required to maintain shunt patency (Fig. 19-10). Shunt occlusions are particularly problematic, as they are frequently associated with rehemorrhage.

TIPS has been compared with small-diameter prosthetic H-graft portacaval shunts in a prospective randomized clinical trial comparing 132 randomized patients of similar age, gender, causes of cirrhosis, and Child-Pugh scores. Early and late shunt occlusions were a greater problem after TIPS. Thirty-day mortality was similar (12%) after each shunt, but by 1 year, mortality after TIPS was 25%, and after the surgical shunt, it was 15% ($P = .07$). Overall 3-year survival was significantly higher for those receiving the small-diameter H-graft portacaval shunt compared with TIPS. Because of the high rate of reinterventions required by those receiving TIPS, overall cost of care was significantly higher for those patients undergoing portal decompression by TIPS.

Both the small-diameter prosthetic H-graft portacaval shunt and TIPS will achieve partial portal decompression. TIPS has higher rates of rebleeding, mortality, occlusion, and revision. TIPS is most optimally applied in patients with variceal bleeding and poor hepatic reserve (MELD score, ≥18) needing a bridge to imminent transplantation, or for those whose medical comorbidities would preclude an abdominal operation. Given its superior results and durability, the small-diameter H-graft portacaval shunt

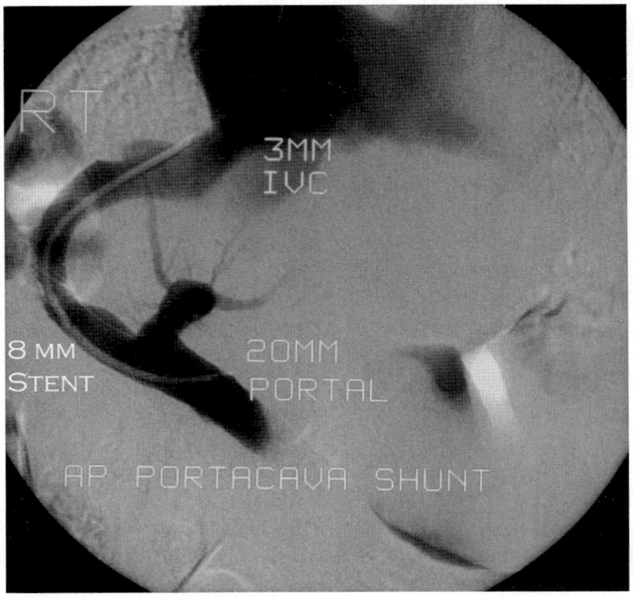

FIGURE 19–9 Contrast study of a transjugular intrahepatic portasystemic shunt (TIPS).

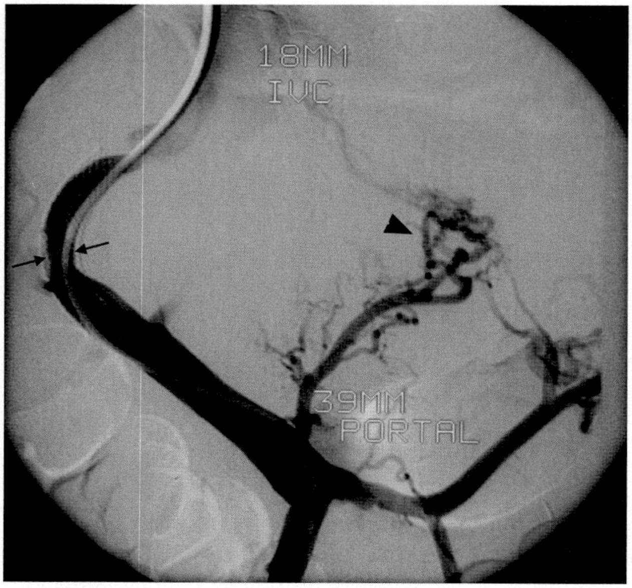

FIGURE 19–10 Transjugular cannulation of a transjugular intrahepatic portasystemic shunt showing stenosis (arrows), foreshortening of the stent, and recurrent varices (arrowhead). Revision of this shunt required placement of an additional stent.

should be considered preferentially to TIPS for portal hypertensive patients with variceal hemorrhage and adequate hepatic reserve.

Devascularization Procedures in the Management of Variceal Hemorrhage due to Cirrhosis and Portal Hypertension

Devascularization refers to the interruption of venous collaterals between the portal vein and the bleeding variceal complex. Generally, these procedures interrupt collaterals from the portal vein to the gastroesophageal varices, disconnecting the portal vein from venous collaterals of the stomach and esophagus. This requires ligation of the coronary, pyloric, gastroepiploic, and short gastric veins, as well as numerous unnamed venous collaterals posterior to the stomach. The operation generally includes splenectomy and, infrequently, esophageal transection.

Lack of widespread acceptance of devascularization procedures has largely been a consequence of poor long-term outcomes and high periprocedural morbidity. The operations generally increase portal pressures, leading to postoperative accumulation of ascites, reduced functional capacity, prolonged recovery, and late rebleeding. In Western countries, devascularization procedures are used mainly as salvage therapy for variceal hemorrhage, when shunts are contraindicated because of portal vein or splenic vein thrombosis.

Long-Term Therapy to Prevent Rebleeding

For patients with cirrhosis and portal hypertension who are not candidates for definitive therapy, variceal bleeding should be treated medically with propranolol, as this agent has been shown to decrease portal pressures. Endoscopic surveillance with chronic variceal sclerotherapy and banding reduces the frequency of rebleeding episodes and improves survival, compared with medications alone. Patients require scheduled endoscopic examinations and repeated sclerotherapy or banding. As a general rule, no matter what type of nondecompressive therapy is undertaken, once a patient has bled from esophageal varices, the risk of rebleeding can be as high as 70%.

Ascites

Free fluid in the abdominal cavity is called ascites. Ascites can arise because of different causes (Box 19-2). Ascites as a consequence of cirrhosis and portal hypertension has the characteristics of an exudate, rich in protein with poor opsonizing capacity.

Management consists of a diet restricted in sodium (≤2 g of sodium/24 hr) and limited in fluid intake (1500 mL/24 hr). Diuretics, like aldactone (≤400 mg/day) and furosemide (≤160 mg/day) are useful in controlling ascites and are considered integral parts of therapy. Ascites is called "refractory" when it is not controlled with maximal medical therapy. Patients with refractory ascites are of Child's class C, have limited hepatic reserve, limited life expectancy, and are at high risk for complications with any intervention. Goals of intervention are largely to provide symptomatic relief and must be carefully weighed against the periprocedural morbidity:

BOX 19–2 Causes of Ascites

Liver disease	Cirrhosis
	Fulminant hepatic failure
	Budd-Chiari syndrome
Malignancy	
Cardiac failure	
Infectious diseases	Schistosomiasis
	Tuberculosis
	Chlamydia
Renal disease	Peritoneal dialysis
	Nephrotic syndrome
Pancreatitis	Pancreatic fistula
Chylous ascites	Trauma
	Iatrogenic
	Congenital
Miscellaneous	Mesenteric venous thrombosis
	Idiopathic

- High-volume paracentesis. This is undertaken at the bedside by using local anesthesia. Protein loss, ascitic leak, and infections are complications of this treatment. Relief of ascites is only short-term, as ascites reaccumulates, and repeated paracentesis is required.
- Peritoneovenous shunt. The Leveen and the Denver shunts are two unidirectional shunts that evacuate ascites from the peritoneal cavity and infuse it into the central venous system. Complications of peritoneovenous shunts include occlusion (50% within 3 months), disseminated intravascular coagulation, and infection. Patency at 6 months is uncommon, requiring shunt revision.
- Portal decompression (usually attained through TIPS) provides good control of ascites. TIPS has been shown to be superior to peritoneovenous shunts in a randomized trial comparing the two methods for control of ascites. The risks of encephalopathy and liver deterioration associated with portal decompression must be balanced against the benefits of relieving ascites. TIPS is often used as a bridge to transplantation.

Suggested Reading

Bosch J, Abraldes JG, Groszmann R: Current management of portal hypertension. J Hepatol 38:S54–S68, 2003.

Knechtle SJ: Portal hypertension: from Eck's fistula to TIPS. Ann Surg 238:S49–S55, 2003.

Rosemurgy AS, Zervos EE: Management of variceal hemorrhage. Curr Probl Surg 40:263–343, 2003.

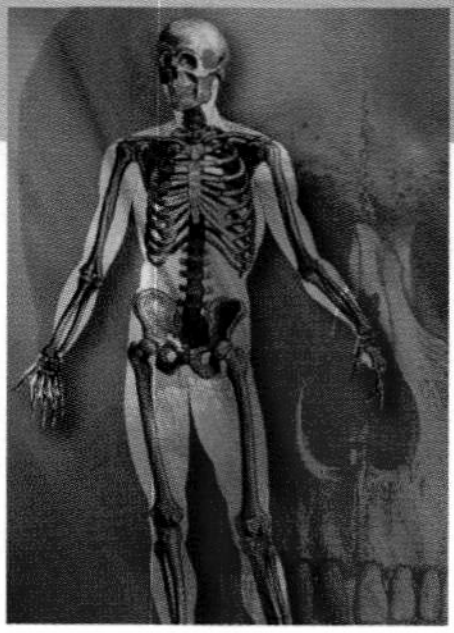

Chapter 20

Spleen and Hematologic Disorders

DAVID McANENY, MD

Anatomy

The spleen is of mesenchymal origin and develops as nodular folds of cells within the layers of the left dorsal mesogastrium, the primordial blood supply of the upper gastrointestinal tract. This portion of the mesogastrium eventually becomes the vasa brevia, the short gastric vessels, and the spleen rotates to the left upper quadrant of the abdominal cavity. The average size of the spleen is about 150 g, the size of a fist. However, an adult's spleen can range in weight from 50 g to as large as 5 kg in certain hematologic conditions.

The spleen is a vascular intraperitoneal solid organ. Its hilum abuts the tail of the pancreas, and the organ is suspended from the adjacent structures by "ligaments" that define their attachments: splenophrenic, splenorenal (or lienorenal), splenocolic, and gastrosplenic (Fig. 20-1). The proper splenic artery perfuses the spleen, with a contribution from an inferior polar artery within the splenocolic ligament. (The short gastric arteries infrequently perfuse some of the spleen, although the blood in these vessels usually flows from the spleen to the stomach.) The splenic artery is a major branch of the celiac axis that runs a transversely oriented, serpentine course in the retroperitoneum. The venous drainage of the spleen complements the arteries. Short gastric veins are located within the gastrosplenic portion of the greater omentum. However, the majority of blood flow from the spleen is via the splenic vein. This vein is immediately inferior to the splenic artery, and it is adherent to the posterior aspect of the body and tail of the pancreas. The confluence of the splenic and superior mesenteric veins, and occasionally of the inferior mesenteric vein as well, creates the portal vein. The lymphatic ducts develop in the white pulp near the trabeculae, coalesce at the splenic hilum, and enter hilar nodes.

A dense capsule invests the organ, and thick trabeculae extend into the parenchyma. This connective tissue contains myofibroblasts that are responsible for the modest ability of the human spleen to contract and expel pooled blood. Spleens of other mammals, particularly dogs, have a more impressive contractile ability.

The microanatomy of the spleen is unique (Fig. 20-2). The vascular branches are segmental, with no significant collateral circulation. Arteries divide into trabecular branches that pierce the parenchyma and are buttressed by a reticular lattice of lymphocytes. These lymphocytes constitute the white pulp that is evident on cross section of the spleen as 1-mm to 2-mm nodules. (The designation of pulp by color refers to the gross appearance.) A relatively straight central artery traverses the white pulp within a cylinder of predominantly T lymphocytes, the periarterial lymphatic sheath (PALS). Nodules of B lymphocytes develop from local expansions of the PALS and contain germinal centers. In concordance with other nodal tissue, the germinal centers evolve with antigen exposure, and enlarged nodules are known as Malpighi's corpuscles. The marginal zone is defined by less dense aggregates of lymphocytes that abut the PALS.

The central artery divides into branches to the white pulp and into penicillar arterioles that enter the red pulp. The red pulp is composed of a maze of sinuses that are supported by splenic cords (of Billroth). These cords are composed of a scaffold of reticular cells and fibers, supporting erythrocytes, macrophages, lymphocytes, plasma cells, and granulocytes. The endothelial cells of the sinuses are elongated and in line with the axis of the sinus. In addition, these cells have sparse interdigitations, permitting blood cells to enter and exit the sinuses. Macrophages from the cords extend dendritic processes through the interstices between endothelial cells and directly into the sinuses, where they can detect foreign antigens.

Two models are proposed for the passage of blood within the microcirculation of the spleen. The open-circulation model purports a communication of the penicillar arterioles with the cords of Billroth and not directly into the splenic sinuses. In this way, blood percolates along the processes of the cordal macrophages before entering a sinus from the extravascular space. In the closed-circulation model, the splenic arterioles are believed to communicate directly with the sinuses. Blood cells would have to exit and then reenter the sinuses to be exposed to the macrophages of the cords. It may be that both mechanisms actually exist. Regardless, this microcirculation is special in that no enclosed circuit exists between arteries and veins. The sinuses eventually coalesce into trabecular veins, complementing the trabecular arteries, before the blood leaves the spleen in segmental splenic vein branches.

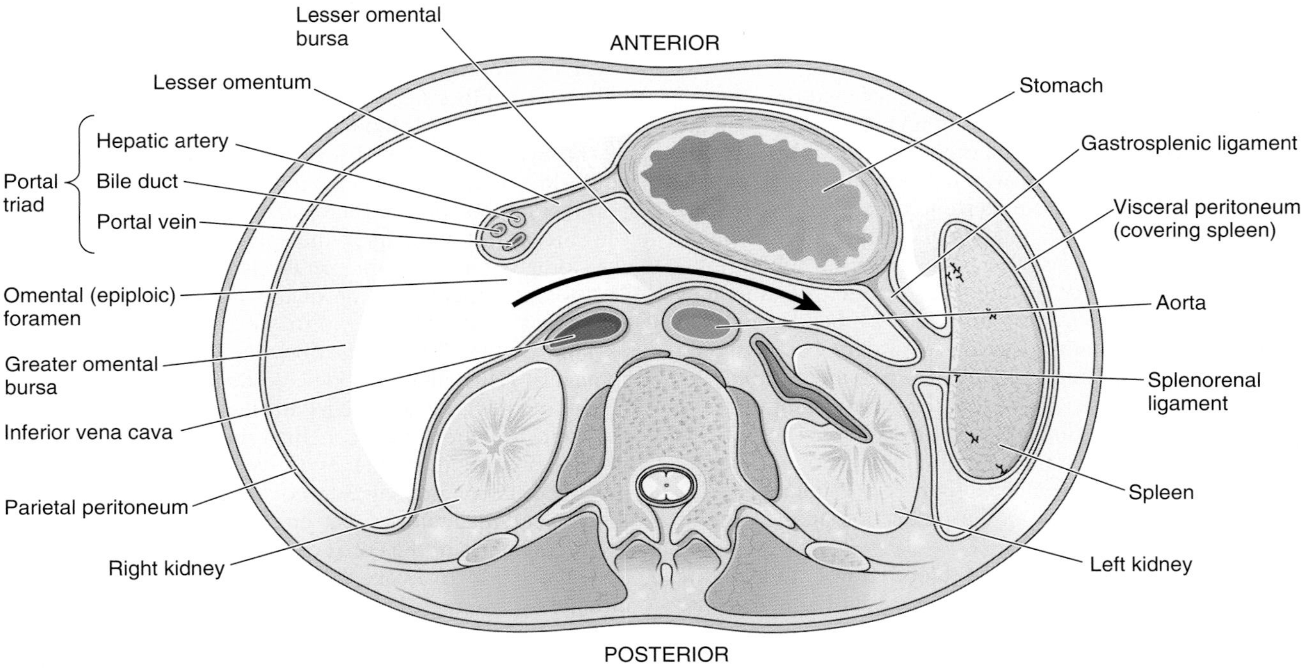

FIGURE 20–1 The short gastric vessels reside in the gastrosplenic ligament. The proper splenic vessels course through the retroperitoneum.

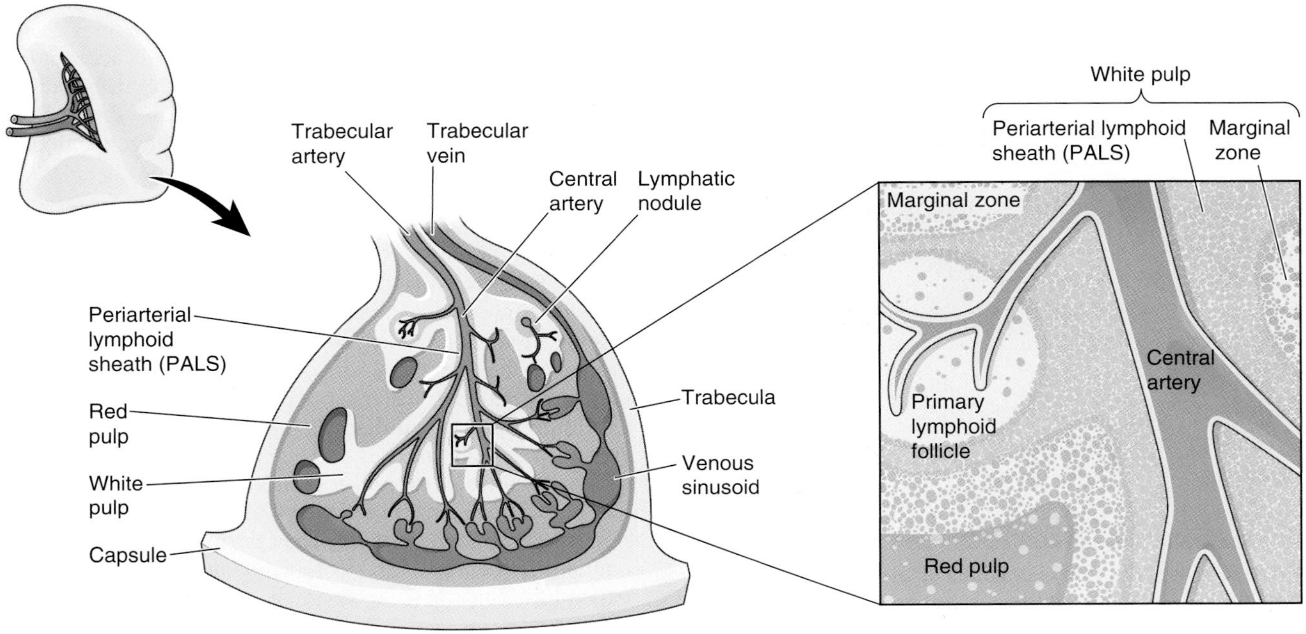

FIGURE 20–2 Microanatomy of the spleen.

Physiology

Galen called the spleen *misterii plenum organum*, the Organ Full of Mystery. Hippocrates attributed the removal of excess water to the spleen. Plato maintained that the spleen served as the cleansing organ of black bile. Aristotle contended that the spleen was not only a filtering organ, but also a "bastard," or counterfeit, liver. He proposed the spleen as an organ of hematopoiesis, although this blood certainly could not be as pure as that from the nobler right-sided organ, the liver. In the 12th century, Maimonides asserted the blood-purifying properties of the spleen. Even in the early 18th century, nervous disorders were assigned to the spleen, including hypochondria and melancholia.

Physicians now recognize that the microanatomy of the spleen is inexorably linked to its physiology. The primary functions of the spleen include filtration of blood, "pitting" of erythrocytes, and specific and nonspecific immunity. The spleen plays a lesser role in the production and storage of blood cells.

Each minute, about 2 L of blood flows through the spleen, where foreign bodies and senescent blood cells are removed from circulation. Most of the filtration process is performed in the marginal zone of the white pulp and by the macrophages of the cords of Billroth. Defective erythrocytes lose cell membrane plasticity and consequently their ability to maneuver through the cords of Billroth and into the sinuses (Fig. 20-3). This pertains to both senescent cells and diseased cells (e.g., hereditary spherocytosis). Stagnant blood in the pulp cords creates a viscous, acidotic, and hypoxic milieu that is particularly hostile to defective erythrocytes. Fragile red blood cells (RBCs) are less capable of oxidative phosphorylation in this glucose-poor environment and are thus vulnerable to phagocytosis by cordal macrophages. This process is known as *culling*. The spleen also culls other defective cells and particles, such as bacteria, from the blood. Erythroclasis is a method of erythrocyte destruction that involves the fragmentation of cells. In contrast to culling, the fragments return to the peripheral blood but are removed on later passages through the spleen. In this manner, the spleen also plays a role in the storage of iron and the metabolism of hemoglobin.

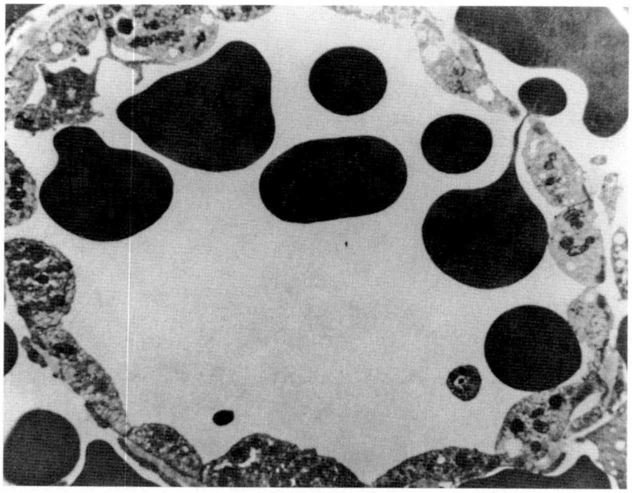

FIGURE 20–3 Electron micrograph of an erythrocyte passing from the cord of Billroth into a splenic sinus lumen. (From Neiman RS, Orazi A: Disorders of the Spleen, 2nd ed. Philadelphia, WB Saunders, 1999.)

Another critical function of the spleen is the ability to maintain the integrity of erythrocytes. This process, known as *pitting* (Fig. 20-4), describes the removal of nuclear remnants (Howell-Jolly bodies), denatured hemoglobin (Heinz bodies), intracellular parasites (e.g., malaria), and siderotic granules (Pappenheimer bodies). An inclusion detains a portion of the erythrocyte outside the sinus, where cordal macrophages remove the inclusion bodies so that the cell may return to the circulation.

Macrophages of the cords of Billroth act in concert with the white pulp to evoke a specific immune response to circulating antigens, but the macrophages also are capable of a nonspecific phagocytosis of unopsonized particles. It is important to note that whereas the spleen contains more than 15% of the body's B and T cells at any moment, primarily in the white pulp, these cells do circulate and are not assigned exclusively to the spleen. The marginal zone may be the initial site where antigens are detained and processed by macrophages. The antigens next penetrate the germinal center, where the B-cell response is coordinated by T-helper cells. The B lymphocytes of the germinal centers express predominantly immunoglobulin M (IgM) and IgG. Perhaps the concentration of antigens in the marginal zone and their relatively slow transit through this area account for the efficiency of the spleen's extraordinary response to previously unrecognized antigens. In contrast, the liver is more effective than the spleen in clearing antigen-antibody complexes once high levels of a specific antibody are already established. Studies of splenectomized patients provide further insight into the spleen's role in immunity. Some have suggested a diminished elaboration of antigen-specific IgM in these patients, whereas others have implicated an impaired IgG response to antigens as the cause of inefficient opsonization of particulate antigens. Finally, the spleen likely produces the opsonins tuftsin and properdin, immunoregulatory peptides that enhance phagocytosis.

Although extramedullary hematopoiesis is found in the spleen in certain diseases, the organ is not normally a site of hematopoiesis, even in fetal life. Another function that has been attributed to the spleen is that of a reservoir for pooled peripheral blood. The normal human spleen contains less than 40 mL of blood and does not appreciably expand or contract, in contrast to the canine spleen. Nonetheless, an adult's spleen can store up to one third of circulating platelets.

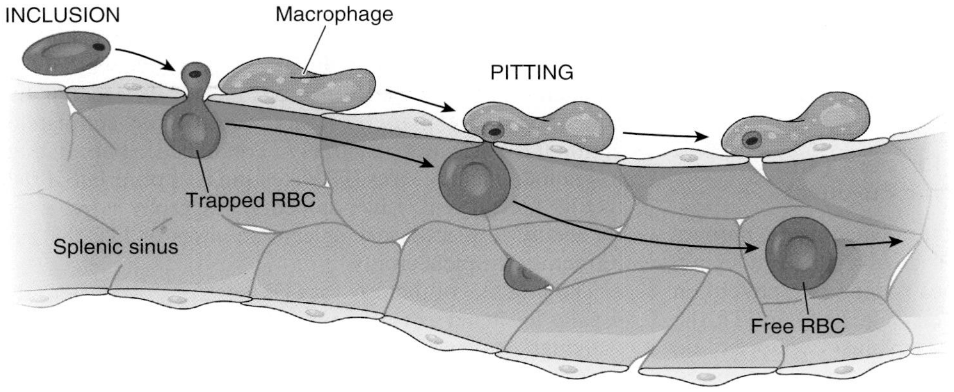

FIGURE 20–4 A Howell-Jolly body is removed from an erythrocyte through the process of "pitting." The inclusion precludes the complete passage of a red blood cell into the sinus. A cord-related macrophage extracts the Howell-Jolly body, releasing the erythrocyte into the sinus. (Adapted from Weintraub LR: Splenectomy: Who, when, and why? Hosp Pract 29(6):27, 1994, with permission.)

Pathology of the Spleen

Autoimmune Hemolytic Anemia

Autoimmune hemolytic anemia (AIHA) was one of the first autoimmune diseases to be described; it is characterized by the antibody-mediated destruction of RBCs. The temperature at which an antibody is most active classifies autoimmune hemolysis. Warm antibodies (IgG) are active at 37°C, whereas cold antibodies (IgM) are usually active at less than 32°C. Intravascular hemolysis occurs when complement proteins C5 through C9 attach to circulating RBCs. In extravascular hemolysis, macrophages phagocytize RBCs that are coated with antibodies, complement molecules, or both.

Warm AIHA occurs in 1 of 50,000 to 80,000 people and accounts for two thirds of cases of immune hemolysis. Most patients with warm-antibody AIHA have an idiopathic form. The others have an associated disease such as a solid tumor, a lymphoproliferative disorder (e.g., leukemia, lymphoma, or multiple myeloma), or another autoimmune disorder (e.g., systemic lupus erythematosus, rheumatoid arthritis, or scleroderma).

In warm AIHA, erythrocytes are coated with either IgG alone or IgG and complement molecules; the antibody attaches to the Rh locus or to one of the minor Rh determinants on the cell membrane. The RBCs are destroyed primarily by splenic macrophages that express specific receptors for the Fc fragment of the IgG molecule. Because of the high concentration of IgG in the white pulp, the majority of hemolysis in warm AIHA occurs in the spleen. Conversely, IgM-coated cells are generally destroyed in the liver; splenic macrophages do not have receptors specific to IgM.

The presentation of AIHA is a function of the acuity of the anemia and the extent of any associated systemic disease. Most signs and symptoms are related to the depressed hemoglobin level: fatigue, lightheadedness, dyspnea on exertion, and pallor. About half of the patients will experience enlargement of the spleen and liver, and one third will have fever, adenopathy, or jaundice. Congenital hemolytic anemias, drug-induced hemolysis, alloimmune hemolysis (e.g., hemolytic disease of the newborn or transfusion reaction), RBC enzyme deficiency disorders, and the hemolytic-uremic syndrome must be considered in the differential diagnosis. The diagnosis of AIHA is established in anemic patients by a positive direct antiglobulin (Coombs) test. A complete blood cell count, peripheral blood smear, reticulocyte count, and liver chemistries are evaluated, and a bone marrow biopsy is occasionally performed to exclude a lymphoproliferative disease.

Immunosuppression with corticosteroids is usually the first line of treatment for warm antibody AIHA, as steroids probably downregulate the membrane Fc-receptor site on the macrophage. The great majority of patients respond to steroids within 10 to 14 days. However, fewer than one third of patients have a sustained remission. About half require long-term steroids, and 10% to 20% do not respond at all to steroids. Other medical treatments include γ-globulin, cyclophosphamide, azathioprine, danazol, plasma exchange, and even splenic irradiation. The occupation of the Fc receptors by free IgG likely explains the efficacy of high-dose intravenous γ-globulin.

Because IgG-coated RBCs are destroyed in the spleen, the surgical removal of the organ is an important treatment for those who fail to respond to steroids. In a collected series of 316 patients with warm antibody AIHA, splenectomy resulted in a 60% response rate. The author's experience suggests that practically all patients with idiopathic AIHA successfully respond to splenectomy, with more than 80% achieving a complete response (a normal hemoglobin and reticulocyte count without subsequent medical therapy or transfusions). In contrast, among patients who have AIHA associated with a systemic illness, the likelihood of a complete response is only 20%, whereas an additional one third will have a partial response. Therefore splenectomy is certainly indicated for idiopathic AIHA. Even in AIHA due to systemic disease, a splenectomy may be worthwhile to ameliorate the need for transfusions and the degree of chronic immunosuppression. It is important to understand that a splenectomy is not indicated for cold agglutinin AIHA. In this IgM-mediated syndrome, hemolysis is intravascular rather than in the spleen.

Immune Thrombocytopenic Purpura (and Thrombotic Thrombocytopenic Purpura)

Immune (formerly "idiopathic") thrombocytopenic purpura (ITP) is similar to AIHA in that it involves the production of IgG autoantibodies that specifically bind to a protein on the surface of a peripheral blood cell (Fig. 20-5). In ITP, the antibody is directed primarily against epitopes on glycoprotein IIb/IIIa of the platelet membrane. The spleen is one of the sites of production of the antiplatelet IgG antibody. Furthermore, the reticuloendothelial system is responsible for the destruction of IgG-coated platelets, and the spleen is the primary site of this sequestration.

About 15,000 new cases of ITP occur in the United States each year. Its diagnosis is one of exclusion, in that no single confirmatory test exists. A low platelet count, a normal bone marrow, and the lack of other sources of thrombocytopenia define the condition. The differential diagnosis includes drug-related (e.g., heparin) thrombocytopenia, myelodysplastic syndromes, congenital thrombocytopenia (in children), lymphoproliferative diseases, and other autoimmune diseases. Although ITP is usually idiopathic, it also may be associated with a systemic disease such as lupus.

The natural history of ITP is difficult to define, but it seems to convey a mortality rate of 4% when untreated. The deaths generally involve older patients with profoundly depressed platelet counts. Adult ITP typically has an indolent, chronic course, and this constitutes most of the discussion that follows. Conversely, ITP among children is classically acute and severe, but it resolves spontaneously with a permanent remission in most cases. In pediatric cases, the sexes are equally affected, whereas about 70% of adults with ITP are women.

The severity of the thrombocytopenia dictates the presentation, and ultimately the management, of ITP. Patients with platelet counts more than 50,000/mm^3 are usually asymptomatic and do not require therapy. Those in whom the platelet counts are between 30,000/mm^3 and 50,000/mm^3 bruise easily with mild trauma, whereas spontaneous bruising (e.g., purpura) or prolonged bleeding with injury occurs when the counts are 10,000/mm^3 to 30,000/mm^3. Spontaneous mucosal bleeding (e.g., epistaxis or gastrointestinal bleeding) can occur with platelet counts less than 10,000/ mm^3, and these patients also are at risk for central nervous system hemorrhages. However, even the most severe thrombocytopenias usually do not result in a major bleeding episode.

The evaluation of thrombocytopenia includes an examination of a peripheral blood smear; a bone marrow biopsy reveals a normal or increased number of megakaryocytes. The bone marrow should probably be aspirated to confirm the diagnosis if a splenectomy is planned, or to exclude a myelodysplastic disorder if the patient is older than 60 years. Assays for antiplatelet antibodies are not routinely conducted, but human immunodeficiency virus (HIV) testing is appropriate if risk factors are present. Liver-spleen scintigraphy is reserved for identifying accessory spleens in cases of ITP that are refractory to splenectomy.

The first line of therapy for ITP includes corticosteroids, usually instituted as prednisone at a dosage of 1 mg/kg/day. Although patients who experience a complete remission with a course of steroids will have done so within 4 weeks, perhaps only 20% of adults will have a sustained response. Active, severe bleeding is managed with combinations of steroids, intravenous immune globulin, and anti-RhD immune globulin. Platelet transfusions are reserved for severe hemorrhage, but the antiplatelet antibodies limit their efficacy.

When patients fail to respond sufficiently to steroids or do not tolerate them, splenectomy is generally the next line of therapy, and it can result in complete responses of ITP in 70% to 80% of patients. ITP is probably the most common hematologic condition for which splenectomy is performed. The surgeon should conduct a thorough search for accessory spleens, and the spleen is gently handled to avoid leaving remnants of viable tissue (splenosis). Steroids and intravenous immune globulin can be used to boost the platelet count before surgery; some investigators believe the responses to these measures correlate with the likelihood of success after splenectomy. However, others relate younger ages and higher preoperative platelet counts to better responses to splenectomy.

The persistence or recurrence of thrombocytopenia after splenectomy is a vexing problem. This situation can imply the presence of residual splenic tissue (e.g., accessory spleen[s] or splenosis), persistent antiplatelet antibodies with destruction of the platelets elsewhere in the reticuloendothelial system, or an initially errant diagnosis. If functioning splenic tissue is present, Howell-Jolly bodies will typically be absent on an examination of the peripheral blood smear. Liver-spleen scintigraphy (with indium 111–labeled platelets or technetium 99m pertechnetate–labeled RBCs), including intraoperative scanning, is valuable in identifying accessory spleens that may account for 10% to 40% of cases of recurrent ITP. The removal of accessory spleens controls recurrent ITP in about two thirds of patients. In the absence of potentially removable splenic tissue, the usual treatments for recurrent ITP include corticosteroids, anti-RhD immune globulin, and intravenous γ-globulin, although the last is particularly expensive and has recently been in short supply. Other medical options include azathioprine, cyclophosphamide, colchicine, vincristine, vinblastine, danazol, and plasmapheresis, but sustained

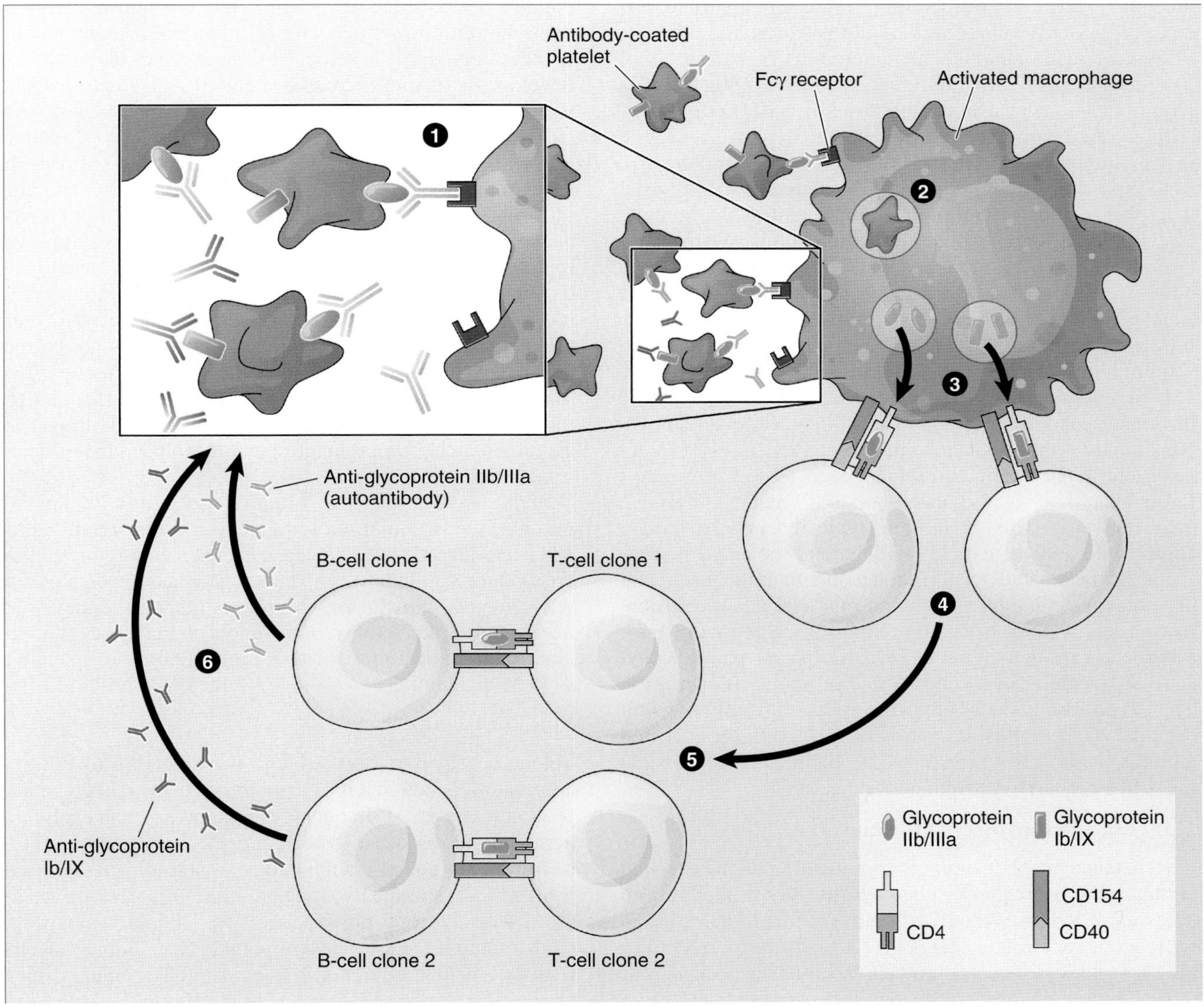

FIGURE 20–5 Pathogenesis of epitope spread in immune thrombocytopenic purpura. The factors that initiate autoantibody production are unknown. Most patients have antibodies against several platelet-surface glycoproteins at the time the disease becomes clinically evident. Inset: Glycoprotein IIb/IIIa (*blue ovals*) is recognized by autoantibody (*orange*), whereas antibodies that recognize the glycoprotein Ib/IX complex have not been generated at this stage (1). Antibody-coated platelets bind to antigen-presenting cells (macrophages or dendritic cells) through Fcγ receptors and are then internalized and degraded (2). Antigen-presenting cells not only degrade glycoprotein IIb/IIIa (*blue ovals*), thereby amplifying the initial immune response, but also may generate cryptic epitopes from other platelet glycoproteins (*blue cylinders*) (3). Activated antigen-presenting cells (4) express these novel peptides on the cell surface along with co-stimulatory help (represented in part by the interaction between CD154 and CD40) and the relevant cytokines that facilitate the proliferation of the initiating CD4-positive T-cell clones (T-cell clone 1) and those with additional specificities (T-cell clone 2) (5). B-cell immunoglobulin receptors that recognize additional platelet antigens (B-cell clone 2) are thereby also induced to proliferate and synthesize antiglycoprotein Ib/IX antibodies (*green*) in addition to amplifying the production of antiglycoprotein IIb/IIIa antibodies (*orange*) by B-cell clone 1 (6). (Adapted from Cines DB, Blanchette VS: Immune thrombocytopenic purpura. N Engl J Med 346(13):995–1008, 2002, with permission.)

responses to these medical measures are uncommon. When the platelet count is greater than 30,000/ mm^3 and no bleeding develops, observation alone may suffice. Of course, alternative diagnoses should be entertained.

Thrombocytopenia is encountered in 5% to 15% of patients with HIV, including a variant of ITP that occurs with an incidence of about 65 cases per 10,000 patients. Although the pathophysiology seems to be consistent with that of standard ITP, our experience suggests that the size of the spleen is often greater in HIV-related ITP. The initial therapy includes antiretroviral agents, anti-RhD immune globulin, and intravenous immunoglobulin. When these efforts fail, splenectomy is indicated and has been tolerated quite well. The response rate is comparable to that of standard ITP, and the absence of a spleen does not seem to influence long-term survival or the rapidity of progression to acquired immunodeficiency syndrome (AIDS).

Five features define the rare syndrome of thrombotic thrombocytopenic purpura (TTP): hemolytic anemia, a consumptive thrombocytopenia, central nervous system disorders, renal dysfunction, and fever. However, perhaps fewer than half of patients with TTP manifest all five characteristics. This syndrome typically occurs among adults, with a slight female predilection. The cause of TTP seems to be related to a vascular endothelium insult that promotes platelet aggregation and microvascular occlusion. Although splenectomy had been historically invoked for TTP, standard therapy now involves plasmapheresis and steroids, resulting in a survival rate of about 70% to 80%. The benefits of splenectomy for TTP are currently not well established, and this operation is reserved for selected patients who fail to respond to the standard medical measures or who have frequent relapses.

Congenital Hemolytic Anemias

Certain congenital hematologic conditions result in abnormal erythrocytes. Hereditary spherocytosis, transmitted as an autosomal dominant trait, is due to a defect in spectrin, an RBC membrane protein. This defect prevents spectrin from binding with cytoskeletal proteins, resulting in a change of the cell morphology from a biconvex disk to a sphere. A rare and milder variant of spherocytosis is elliptocytosis, which involves an alteration of spectrin from its normal tetrameric protein to a dimeric configuration, forming an elliptical cell. In both conditions, the abnormal cell shape imparts rigidity to the membrane, impeding the passage of the cell from the splenic cords into the sinuses and promoting sequestration of erythrocytes.

The destruction of abnormal RBCs results in anemia, jaundice, splenomegaly, and cholelithiasis, and the diagnosis is readily established by an examination of the peripheral blood smear. Hereditary spherocytosis is the most common congenital anemia that requires a splenectomy. Conversely, elliptocytosis warrants a splenectomy only when an overwhelming percentage of erythrocytes are affected. As these are congenital conditions that may be first seen in childhood, the timing of splenectomy calls for a thoughtful balance between the degree of hemolysis and the risks of overwhelming postsplenectomy infection. A concomitant cholecystectomy also may be necessary if gallstones develop from the increased hemoglobin load that the hemolysis engenders.

Thalassemia is typically found in people of Mediterranean heritage and is transmitted as a dominant trait. In thalassemia major, a decreased number of β-globin chains of hemoglobin are produced in comparison to α chains, causing the latter to precipitate along the erythrocyte membrane. Therefore the resultant anemia is due to the diminished rate of hemoglobin synthesis rather than to red blood cell destruction. The peripheral blood smear reveals target cells, nucleated RBCs. Splenectomy does not correct the underlying disease, but it may affect the frequency of transfusions. The operation is not ordinarily performed for thalassemia, but it can be indicated for patients with painful splenic infarcts, symptomatic splenomegaly, and significant transfusion requirements.

Sickle cell anemia is often associated with splenic infarcts, the eventual consequence of which is an "autosplenectomized" state. However, acute splenic-sequestration crises can result in abrupt splenomegaly and hypersplenism, with major transfusion requirements, and they can necessitate splenectomy. Pain and splenic abscesses are additional indications for the removal of the spleen in sickle cell anemia.

Splenomegaly

Splenomegaly is discovered in fewer than 1% of hospital admissions, although it is probably more evident in outpatient practice. The most frequent causes of splenomegaly are hematologic diseases, liver disorders, and infections; it is uncommonly due to primary spleen pathology. Congestive heart failure, storage diseases, and inflammatory disorders are relatively rare predisposing conditions. Among the hematologic sources are lymphoma, leukemias, myelofibrosis, hemolytic anemias, and hemoglobinopathies. Chronic liver disease is responsible for portal hypertension, which in turn produces splenomegaly and hypersplenism. Infectious causes include endocarditis (e.g., with intravenous drug use), mononucleosis, malaria, tuberculosis, and a host of other agents. AIDS also can result in splenomegaly, as a primary disease or in association with disseminated organisms. Massive splenomegaly is generally due to non-Hodgkin's lymphoma, chronic lymphocytic leukemia, hairy cell leukemia, or myelofibrosis, and it is reviewed later in the chapter.

Inexplicable splenomegaly warrants an investigation. Beyond a thorough history and physical examination, a review of the peripheral blood smear, a complete blood cell count, and various imaging studies, the evaluation is tailored to the clinical scenario. For example, lymphadenopathy, progressive splenic enlargement, and massive splenomegaly are typically associated with hematologic diseases. A lymph node biopsy or a bone marrow aspiration may establish a diagnosis. Abnormal liver chemistries or evidence of portal hypertension imply liver disease and might provoke a liver biopsy. Fevers strongly suggest an infectious disease, the diagnosis of which may be determined by cultures or a peripheral node biopsy.

Viral and other benign conditions certainly cause splenomegaly, so an enlarged spleen in an asymptomatic patient may be observed for a few months. A splenectomy will eventually be necessary to establish a diagnosis in about 10% of cases of splenomegaly. However, most splenectomies for splenomegaly are performed to treat a hematologic disorder, to palliate pain or early satiety, or to ameliorate the hypersplenism associated with a hematologic disease.

Red-pulp hypertrophy leads to hypersplenism, with exuberant blood cell destruction. This occurs in myeloproliferative disorders, lipid-storage diseases, and portal hypertension, although early red-pulp infiltration also is encountered in certain lymphoproliferative disorders (e.g., hairy cell leukemia). The hypersplenism is particularly pronounced with myelofibrosis and myeloid metaplasia, whereas the pancytopenia associated with portal hypertension is relatively mild and rarely warrants a splenectomy or portosystemic decompression. Conversely, splenectomy is indicated for significant, transfusion-dependent cytopenias, and it is efficacious in more than 75% of patients with non-Hodgkin's lymphoma, Hodgkin's disease, and chronic lymphocytic leukemia.

Neoplasms of the Spleen

Hemangiomas are the most common lesion of the spleen. They are generally asymptomatic and are usually discovered serendipitously with imaging studies. A splenectomy is not necessary for a hemangioma, unless it is symptomatic or quite large, or if the diagnosis is in doubt. Benign lesions of the spleen also include hamartomas, littoral cell angiomas, and other rare tumors. These neoplasms usually require a splenectomy to establish a diagnosis and to remove potentially malignant tumors (Fig. 20-6).

About three fourths of splenic cysts are nonepithelialized pseudocysts that form after a remote trauma. In the United States, true splenic cysts are rarely parasitic, although this type predominates in parts of the world where *Echinococcus* is endemic. Nonparasitic true cysts comprise the congenital and neoplastic types. The latter include epidermoid (the most common) and dermoid cysts, as well as lymphangiomas and cavernous angiomas. Splenic cysts are often discovered fortuitously, or they might initially be seen with a dull abdominal pain, referred pain to the left shoulder, or a vague left-upper-quadrant fullness. A history of previous trauma raises the likelihood of a pseudocyst. Although computed tomography (CT) scanning and ultrasonography demonstrate the presence of a cyst, they usually cannot distinguish between true and false types. Furthermore, significant cysts might be at risk of rupture or hemorrhage. Therefore it usually is best to remove the cyst, with either a splenectomy or a spleen-preserving resection. When the clinical situation suggests the possibility of a pseudocyst due to trauma, a laparoscopic resection of the exposed portion of the pseudocyst wall can be performed, although the pathologist must confirm that the cyst wall does not have an epithelialized lining. Omentum is placed into the resultant cavity to obliterate the space. As for true cysts, a splenectomy may be necessary; a partial splenectomy is an attractive option, especially for children.

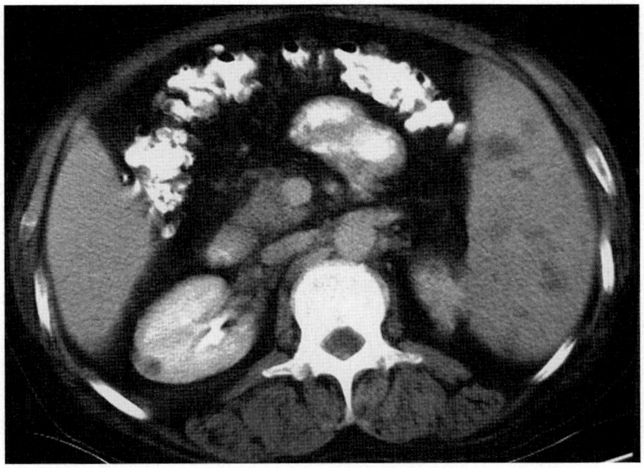

FIGURE 20–6 Computed tomography scan demonstrating multiple hypodense lesions throughout the spleen. A splenectomy was performed both for diagnostic purposes and because of hypersplenism (that proved to be due to cirrhosis). The final pathology of the spleen revealed littoral cell angiomas.

Although the involvement of the spleen by non-Hodgkin's lymphoma usually implies systemic disease, the spleen also can harbor a primary focus of lymphoma. This may manifest as splenomegaly of unknown etiology, with a broad differential diagnosis, as reviewed earlier. The development of symptoms (e.g., pain, satiety) or significant cytopenias, or the persistence of splenomegaly without a diagnosis, warrants a splenectomy. In certain situations (e.g., when aggressive chemotherapy or bone marrow transplantation or both are contemplated for non-Hodgkin's lymphoma), a splenectomy may be performed to reduce the bulk of disease. Nevertheless, most cases of non-Hodgkin's lymphoma do not require a splenectomy, and staging laparotomies are rarely performed for this disease.

Staging laparotomies were formerly conducted frequently for Hodgkin's disease. However, because of refinements in chemotherapy and radiation therapy, and considering the hazards of overwhelming postsplenectomy infection in children, this operation is no longer commonly practiced. Alternatives such as partial splenectomy or hand-assisted

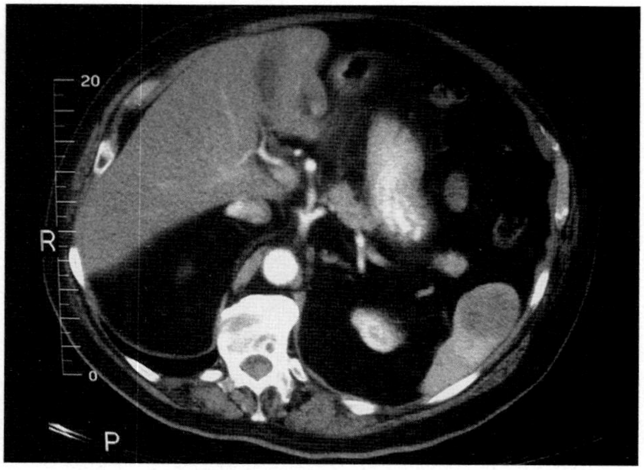

FIGURE 20–7 This patient underwent a splenectomy for an isolated melanoma metastasis.

laparoscopic techniques could revive some role for surgery in Hodgkin's disease.

Despite the vascularity of the spleen, it is rarely a site of metastases. Secondary tumors in the spleen have been seen with melanoma (Fig. 20-7), and with ovarian, colorectal, lung, and breast primary cancers, among others. It is probably reasonable to remove the spleen in selected cases when the metastatic spread is isolated and no tumor progression manifests over an interval of time.

Splenic Abscess

Splenic abscesses are rather rare. However, the frequency of these abscesses seems to be increasing, probably as a result of immunosuppression from chemotherapy, transplantation, HIV, and intravenous drug abuse. Recent series describe immunosuppressed conditions in one third of patients with splenic abscesses. More than half of the abscesses are caused by hematogenous dissemination (e.g., endocarditis). Other etiologies include superinfection of infarcted tissue, contiguous spread from an adjacent abscess, and direct trauma with contamination (including iatrogenic). In about 10% of patients, the inciting septic focus is not identified.

The vast majority of patients with splenic abscesses have fevers, whereas fewer than half experience abdominal pain, splenomegaly, or a pleural effusion. Approximately two thirds of patients have a leukocytosis, but the white blood cell count is usually not dramatically elevated, possibly because of previous antibiotics. Thrombocytosis is a nonspecific finding that affects a minority of patients and may imply an underlying hematologic disorder. Blood cultures are positive about half the time. However, only half of these cultures coincide with the bacteriology of the abscess. *Staphylococcus*, *Streptococcus*, *Salmonella*, and enteric bacteria account for most of the isolated organisms, whereas no bacteria grow in about 10% of cases. Mycobacteria and fungi are being encountered more frequently, reflecting the growing number of immunosuppressed patients.

Scintigraphy and ultrasonography can be valuable diagnostic modalities, but CT scanning is currently the most sensitive imaging study (Fig. 20-8). Reports describe solitary, unilocular abscesses in two thirds of patients, with multiple abscesses in one fourth. Our experience has been that, even when the abscess cavity seems to be unilocular and well defined on CT scan, it often permeates the splenic tissue in an infiltrative pattern.

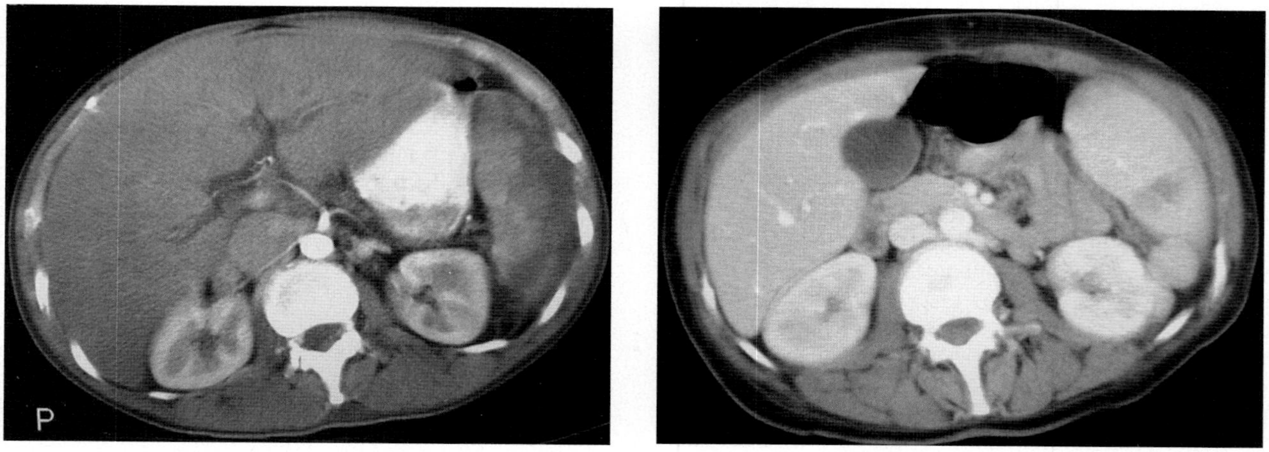

A B

FIGURE 20–8 *A*, This patient's splenic abscess permeated the parenchyma, resulting in heterogeneous changes by computed tomography scan. *B*, This patient had a radiographically focal splenic abscess. Although the abscess might have been amenable to a percutaneous drainage, her clinical condition warranted an urgent operation. Both patients recovered well after splenectomies.

PEARLS FOR THE OR

Splenic ligaments include the splenophrenic, splenorenal (lienorenal), splenocolic, and gastrosplenic.

Accessory spleens are present in 10% to 40% of patients.

The most common indications for splenectomy in United States are immune thrombocytopenic purpura, trauma, and iatrogenic injury.

The primary functions of the spleen are blood filtration, "pitting" of erythrocytes, and immunity.

Splenectomy is the most definitive management of a splenic abscess. A role exists for radiologic-guided percutaneous aspiration or drainage in critically ill patients and perhaps in children, in whom splenic preservation is desirable. These techniques are successful in two thirds of properly selected patients who have unilocular abscesses that contain thin pus. However, a salvage splenectomy is necessary in about one third of these patients when a prompt eradication of sepsis does not occur. Antibiotics alone have been successful in a few cases, but are not ordinarily considered the standard of care. Notable exceptions to this rule include mycobacterial and fungal abscesses. These represent systemic infections and are treated as such, even though a splenectomy will be necessary in some instances for cure or diagnosis. Splenic abscesses are associated with a 12% overall mortality, but death rates increase to 25% among immunosuppressed patients.

Rupture of the Spleen

Traumatic

The management of splenic injuries has dramatically changed during recent years, as concerns about overwhelming postsplenectomy infection have fostered a philosophy of splenic preservation. This is especially apparent with blunt abdominal trauma in adults, to whom surgeons have applied the lessons gleaned from the nonoperative management of pediatric spleen injuries. A CT scan is performed to evaluate significant blunt trauma to the abdomen in the hemodynamically stable patient. Injuries to the spleen are scored, with grade I being a modest laceration or subcapsular hematoma and grade V describing a major hilar vascular disruption (Table 20-1). When splenic injuries are identified, finer CT images are obtained to define the injury precisely and to demonstrate extravasation of contrast.

Nonoperative management of splenic injuries may be practiced when the patient is hemodynamically stable, the CT scan does not define other abdominal injuries that warrant a laparotomy, the hilar vessels are not completely severed, and spleen-related transfusion requirements are minimal (e.g., ≤2 units). This philosophy can even be applied to spleens with underlying pathology, such as in mononucleosis and HIV. Nonoperative protocols include bed rest, observation in a monitored setting with serial abdominal examinations, and frequent hematocrit levels. When the CT scan suggests active extravasation of intravenous contrast from the spleen or a "blush" of contrast (representing a pseudoaneurysm) within the parenchyma, percutaneous angiographic embolization is an option for the stable patient. However, brisk, uncontained extravasation should probably prompt a laparotomy, unless resources are available for an immediate embolization. Another CT scan is obtained in the subsequent days to evaluate a change in clinical status or to reassess a more severe (e.g., grades III or IV) injury. If this approach succeeds, another CT scan in 6 to 8 weeks is helpful to gauge healing, to recognize pseudocyst formation, and to dictate a safe return to contact sports or strenuous activity. (Laboratory data suggest a normalized wound-breaking strength of splenic lacerations in 6 weeks.)

In several recent series of blunt trauma to the spleen, preservation of the organ has been effected in about 70% of cases. Moreover, among patients selected for nonoperative management, success rates of 90% to 98% have been reported, often regardless of age or neurologic impairment. Nonoperative management is applicable to grade III and IV injuries, although these wounds are more likely to require an embolization or a laparotomy. Pachter's experience reflects a consistent rate of splenectomies during the past two decades, although nonoperative management of adults with spleen injuries increased over time, from 13% to 54% of the group,

TABLE 20–1 Spleen Injury Scale (1994 revision)

	Grade*	Injury Description
I	Hematoma	Subcapsular, <10% surface area
	Laceration	Capsular tear, <1cm parenchymal depth
II	Hematoma	Subcapsular, 10–50% surface area; intraparenchymal, <5 cm in diameter
	Laceration	1 to 3-cm parenchymal depth that does not involve a trabecular vessel
III	Hematoma	Subcapsular, >50% surface area or expanding; ruptured subcapsular or parenchymal hematoma Intraparenchymal hematoma >5 cm or expanding
	Laceration	>3 cm parenchymal depth or involving trabecular vessels
IV	Laceration	Laceration involving segmental or hilar vessels producing major devascularization (>25% of spleen)
V	Laceration	Completely shattered spleen
	Vascular	Hilar vascular injury that devascularizes spleen

*Advance one grade for multiple injuries, up to grade III.
Data from the Organ Injury Scaling Committee of the American Association for the Surgery of Trauma.

with a commensurate decline in splenorrhaphies. Interestingly, in that same series, 15 of the 16 infections that occurred were among splenectomized patients, who composed only one quarter of the cohort.

When hemodynamic instability is attributed to abdominal blunt trauma, an expeditious laparotomy is necessary. A splenorrhaphy may be accomplished by a variety of techniques. These include the use of topical hemostatic agents, direct compression, electrocoagulation, argon beam coagulation, sutures, fibrin glue, creation of a buttress with omentum or a bioprosthesis (e.g., Polyglactin knitted mesh), and partial resection of the spleen (possibly using radiofrequency technology). The most critical maneuver of a splenorrhaphy is the complete mobilization of the spleen so that it is fully exposed. It must be noted that the presence of multiple injuries, hemodynamic instability, or a shattered, devascularized spleen still warrants a splenectomy.

Patients with penetrating abdominal trauma undergo laparotomies as clinically indicated and in accordance with the trauma center's practice. This generally implies empiric surgery for gunshot wounds and selective exploration for stab wounds. The same principles apply to splenorrhaphy and to splenectomy for penetrating injuries as for blunt trauma. If a laparotomy is not clinically indicated for a stab, but the wound suggests a potential hazard to the spleen, a CT scan may be performed, and splenic injuries can be managed as described earlier.

It seems that the incidence of overwhelming post-splenectomy infection is lower for traumatically ruptured spleens than in the setting of hematologic diseases. Some investigators ascribe this phenomenon to splenosis: the autotransplantation of splenic fragments onto peritoneal surfaces. Therefore when ruptured spleens are removed, the surgeon might wrap morcellated pieces of spleen tissue within the omentum. Scintigraphy has confirmed the viability of these fragments over time, and they seem to be capable of pitting and culling. However, the preservation of the spleen's native immune function has not been confirmed.

Iatrogenic

In 1882, Trendelenburg reported an incidental splenectomy in conjunction with the resection of a retroperitoneal tumor. Iatrogenic injuries to the spleen occur in fewer than 1% of laparotomies, although an incidence of 1% to 3% is associated with operations involving the left colon, the stomach, and the esophagus. Moreover, these injuries account for one third of splenectomies in many medical centers.

Incidental splenectomies during gastrointestinal operations have resulted in an increased chance of sepsis, wound infections, pulmonary complications, and mortality. The septic complications include subphrenic abscesses, with an incidence of 3% to 9%. Splenectomies performed in conjunction with resections of gastric cancers seem to impart an increased likelihood of infections, complications in general, and perhaps diminished long-term survival. One report related decreased long-term survival for Dukes' stage C colorectal cancer when a simultaneous splenectomy was performed. As with traumatically injured spleens, splenorrhaphy is an attractive option for preserving the spleen that is incidentally injured during an abdominal operation. The surgeon must weigh the risks of asplenia versus the amount of blood already shed, the degree of the injury, the likelihood of repair, and the extent of surgery that remains.

PEARLS FOR ROUNDS

Warm-antibody autoimmune hemolytic anemia (AIHA): Immunoglobulin G (IgG)–coated red blood cells are destroyed in the spleen. The spleen is removed when patients fail to respond to steroids, with a 60% success rate. Splenectomy is not indicated for cold-agglutinin (IgM-mediated) AIHA.

Immune thrombocytopenic purpura: The spleen produces antiplatelet antibodies and destroys IgG-coated platelets. Steroids form the first line of therapy; splenectomy is the second line, with a 70% to 80% response rate. Steroids, intravenous immunoglobulin, or anti-RhD may be given preoperatively to increase the platelet count.

Nonoperative management of spleen injuries requires hemodynamic stability, no other injuries warranting laparotomy, intact hilar vessels, and minimal transfusion requirements.

Overwhelming postsplenectomy infection (OPSI): fulminant, flulike symptoms progress to septic shock in 24 hours; half die. Lifetime incidence is about 3% to 5%, typically in children or in adults with hematologic diseases, and within 2 years of splenectomy. *Streptococcus pneumoniae, Haemophilus influenzae*, and *Neisseria meningitides* are the most common bacteria in OPSI.

Splenomegaly is usually due to hematologic diseases, liver disorders, and infection. Massive (>1500 g) splenomegaly is most commonly due to myelofibrosis, non-Hodgkin's lymphoma, chronic lymphocytic leukemia (CLL), and hairy cell leukemia.

Spontaneous

Spontaneous ruptures of the spleen generally occur in the presence of underlying infections, hematologic diseases, neoplasms, or connective tissue disorders. Anticoagulation or thrombolytic therapy also may contribute to these ruptures. The most common cause of spontaneously ruptured spleens worldwide is malaria, whereas the most common cause in the United States is mononucleosis. Infiltrative diseases such as amyloidosis also can be responsible for spontaneous ruptures.

Splenomegaly develops in about 50% of cases of mononucleosis and in practically all cases of acute malaria infection. Small infarcts, tears, and subcapsular hematomas may occur when the splenic parenchyma expands. As a result, relatively minor insults such as coughing or vomiting might incur a rupture. Patients are first seen with abdominal pain, anemia, tachycardia, hypovolemia, and left-upper-quadrant tenderness and guarding. Pain referred to the left shoulder is known as Kehr's sign.

The management of the spontaneously ruptured spleen is similar to that for blunt trauma. When the patient is hemodynamically stable and the rupture is contained, nonoperative therapy with bed rest and volume resuscitation is reasonable. However, hemodynamic compromise or CT scan evidence of an uncontained hematoma warrants a laparotomy with either splenorrhaphy or splenectomy.

Sinistral Portal Hypertension

Sinistral (left-sided) portal hypertension results from a thrombosis or occlusion of the splenic vein. Venous drainage from the spleen consequently returns to the portal circulation via the short gastric veins, and varices develop when the capacity of these veins is overwhelmed. This condition exists in up to 40% of patients with chronic pancreatitis, and it also can occur with pancreas tumors. More than two thirds of cases are due to primary pancreas pathology.

Gastroesophageal varices, splenomegaly, and normal liver function characterize sinistral portal hypertension. In contrast to the esophageal varices that are classically seen in portal hypertension, gastric varices are encountered predominantly in sinistral portal hypertension. Variceal bleeding is confirmed by endoscopy, whereas CT scanning and magnetic resonance imaging are valuable for the assessment of the pancreas and the portal system. Splenectomy is advised for active gastric variceal hemorrhage or for significant episodes of recurrent bleeding. However, considering the low likelihood of recurrent hemorrhage and the general condition of these patients, the role of prophylactic splenectomy is questionable.

Splenectomy

Indications

Splenectomies are performed for the situations outlined earlier in this chapter. These include autoimmune disorders, congenital anemias, inexplicable splenomegaly, hypersplenism, splenic lesions, and injury. The most common indications for splenectomy in the United States are ITP, trauma (mostly blunt), and iatrogenic injury during abdominal surgery. The operation can be performed with a formal laparotomy or with laparoscopic techniques.

Preoperative Preparation

As always, a thorough history and a physical examination are in order to assure that the patient is medically fit for the operation, possibly including the physiologic effects of a pneumoperitoneum. A complete blood cell count is necessary, especially in hypersplenism cases, along with coagulation studies when indicated. Corticosteroids, intravenous immunoglobulin, and anti-RhD immune globulin may be administered in cases of ITP to augment the platelet count before the operation. Platelet or RBC transfusions also can be given, although circulating antibodies could promptly destroy these blood products in ITP or AIHA, respectively. Therefore when transfusions are required, they are often reserved until the splenic vascular pedicle has been secured. Vaccinations are given to minimize the chances of overwhelming postsplenectomy infection, as described later in the chapter. Preoperative splenic artery embolization (via percutaneous techniques) can be performed to diminish the vascularity and size of the spleen, but it is controversial and not a standard practice. It is discussed later with respect to massive splenomegaly.

Although a splenectomy is classified as a "clean" case, it is reasonable to administer a first-generation cephalosporin as prophylaxis against wound infection. This is particularly true for patients who have hematologic diseases or associated injuries, or perhaps for laparoscopic surgery that involves multiple wounds and a longer operative time.

Open Splenectomy

An open splenectomy is performed through a left subcostal, a midline, or, uncommonly, a left paramedian incision. Our group favors a subcostal incision, especially for massively enlarged spleens, although a midline incision could be more appropriate if other procedures are to be performed.

Once proper exposure of the left upper quadrant is established, a meticulous search is performed for accessory spleens, which are found in perhaps 10% to 40% of patients. These lymph node–sized remnants of spleen tissue are usually located in the splenic hilum, along the pancreas tail, within the ligaments of the spleen, or in the greater omentum, but they also can be found in the lesser omentum or the pelvis. When it is necessary to remove an accessory spleen, it is probably best done early in the operation. (A hematoma in the omentum can later be mistaken for an accessory spleen, or the original discovery may have been forgotten.) A liver biopsy may be useful for staging some patients.

The surgeon is careful to avoid distracting viscera away from the spleen so that an incidental laceration of the fragile capsule is not incurred. Instead, the spleen is manually retracted anteriorly and medially, and the splenophrenic and lienorenal ligaments are incised to mobilize the organ fully. The surgeon divides the portions of the greater omentum that contain the short gastric vessels and the splenocolic attachments. This can be done with a combination of clamps, ligatures, electrocoagulation, and the harmonic scalpel. Finally, the splenic hilar vessels are carefully secured with clamps and ligatures or with a vascular stapler. When bulky adenopathy or perisplenitis is present, the tail of the pancreas can be drawn into the splenic hilum and injured during the hilar dissection. The ligation of the splenic artery immediately before the division of the vein permits an autotransfusion of some blood from the spleen. Our group has not found the early ligation of the splenic artery (via the lesser sac) to be beneficial, as reviewed later with respect to massive splenomegaly. It is essential to assure hemostasis before wound closure; topical hemostatic agents are valuable when oozing is evident along the cut edges of tissues. Drains should not be placed for ongoing blood loss, although they are indicated for splenic abscesses or when an injury to the pancreas is entertained.

Subtotal splenectomy has been advocated in selected situations in an attempt to obviate the hazards of overwhelming postsplenectomy infection. These cases have included massive splenomegaly (e.g., Gaucher's disease, myeloid metaplasia), pediatric hematologic diseases (e.g., hereditary spherocytosis, HIV-related ITP), traumatic ruptures of the spleen, pancreas resections, and operations for portal hypertension. More than 75% of the spleen is removed, but the superior pole of the organ is left in situ, and it remains perfused by the most proximal short gastric vessels. The spleen must be fully mobilized to conduct this resection safely.

Laparoscopic Splenectomy

The popularity of laparoscopic surgery for the gallbladder and other organs has led to the application of minimally invasive techniques to splenectomy. Several series have demonstrated that experienced surgeons can safely perform this demanding operation for many diagnoses. Some surgeons have demonstrated that laparoscopic splenectomy is superior to the open technique for ITP and for other diseases that involve small spleens. Contraindications to a laparoscopic splenectomy may include a debilitated medical status with intolerance of a lengthy procedure or of a pneumoperitoneum, extensive intraperitoneal adhesions, a significant bleeding diathesis, pregnancy, massive splenomegaly, and significant perisplenitis or a splenic abscess.

Surgeons have reported a variety of laparoscopic splenectomy techniques; this chapter also expresses the author's current preferences. The patient is placed in the supine position on a "beanbag," whereupon a nasogastric tube and a Foley catheter are inserted. Rolled blankets are placed beneath the patient's left side to support a 45-degree lateral decubitus position. The standard laparoscopic splenectomy uses four trochars (10 mm–12 mm): one at the umbilicus, one in the midline of the epigastrium, and two along the left umbilical line. A diagnostic laparoscopy (with a 30-degree or 45-degree laparoscope) is performed initially to identify synchronous pathology, to search for accessory spleens, and to determine if the spleen is of a size suitable for laparoscopic removal. The patient is tilted into the reversed Trendelenburg position and rolled as necessary to facilitate exposure and appropriate tension on the tissues being dissected. The splenic attachments are divided in an inferior to superior sequence, often leaving the superior splenophrenic ligament intact until the end of the operation to prevent too much mobility of the spleen. A combination of clips and the harmonic scalpel is used for hemostasis, although clips should be avoided near the hilum, where a stapler may be applied. The major splenic vessels are either secured with ligatures or transected with a vascular staple; the author favors the latter method.

The most confounding portion of the operation has been the removal of the spleen from the peritoneal cavity. Some surgeons place the organ in a sterile specimen bag and extend the length of a trochar wound to permit a safe extraction. Others pulverize the spleen within the specimen bag to allow the removal through a smaller wound. However, the package inserts of some bags specifically state that the Food and Drug Administration has not confirmed the strength of the bag to withstand morcellation. The potential danger is that if the integrity of the bag becomes compromised, spleen fragments could be deposited in the peritoneal cavity, resulting in splenosis and the recurrence of diseases such as ITP or AIHA.

The author's version of laparoscopic splenectomy has evolved over a few years, and it now includes a hand-assisted technique. Two 12-mm trochars are inserted along the left umbilical line and a limited periumbilical midline incision is created to a length (in centimeters) that is commensurate with the surgeon's hand width (by glove size). Various commercially available devices maintain a pneumoperitoneum and permit the surgeon's nondominant hand to manipulate the spleen while the dominant hand performs the dissection with laparoscopic instruments. This method has decreased operative time, improved the ease of hemostasis, reduced the need for some disposable items (e.g., trochars, retractors, and specimen bag), and eliminated problems with extraction. The size of the periumbilical incision is not much larger than would be an extension of a trochar wound for organ retrieval. The hand-assisted technique also may expand the ability to remove large spleens safely or to conduct a staging laparotomy expeditiously. Parenthetically, the benefits conferred by laparoscopic splenectomy do not seem to be lost with hand assistance.

Many series suggest that, in comparison with open splenectomy, the laparoscopic operation results in less pain, a more rapid advance of diet, and a shorter hospital stay. For example, patients remain hospitalized 4 to 6 days after an open splenectomy, in contrast to 1 to 3 days for the laparoscopic counterpart. Furthermore, operative morbidity may be reduced as a dividend of smaller incisions and less respiratory discomfort. Conversely, the costs of the longer operating room time and of disposable equipment often make this more expensive than an open splenectomy. Some studies contend that the diminished hospital stay and perhaps fewer complications will offset the greater operating room costs. Of course, it is easily conceivable that technologic advances and the economies of scale of capital equipment will eventually make laparoscopic splenectomy both more efficient and less expensive. In addition, operative time should decline as the surgeon's experience increases.

Postoperative Complications

Open or laparoscopic, a splenectomy is a major operation, especially considering the types of underlying conditions that require the removal of the spleen. In most series, the incidence of operative mortality is about 1% to 2%, ranging from none to 10% and depending on the age and debility of the patient. In addition, in up to one third of patients, some complication develops. Beyond the general morbidity of any major operation, splenectomy confers specific risks. Pulmonary problems, such as atelectasis, a left pleural effusion, and pneumonia, have been classically associated with this operation. A disruption of the pancreas may result in acute pancreatitis, a pseudocyst, or a fistula, but these are fortunately rare.

Postoperative hemorrhage develops in perhaps 5% of splenectomies, primarily for massive splenomegaly and myeloproliferative disorders with a significant thrombocytopenia. The bleeding is typically due to oozing from cut surfaces rather than from an actually bleeding vessel. If transfusion requirements persist, a reexploration is necessary to assure the absence of correctable, "surgical" hemorrhage and to evacuate a substantial hematoma that could serve as a nidus for infection.

The incidence of subphrenic abscess formation after the removal of a massive spleen is about 2% to 4%. A multivariate analysis correlates the development of a postsplenectomy intraabdominal abscess with a synchronous gastrointestinal or biliary operation, corticosteroid use, the diagnosis of leukemia, and blood loss. However, the size of the spleen is not a factor. Overwhelming postsplenectomy infection is separately considered later.

Patients with myeloproliferative diseases and hematologic malignancies have an increased propensity for thromboembolic complications. Portal vein thrombosis is a particularly feared complication, and it may even occur spontaneously without a splenectomy. The propagation of clot from an enlarged splenic vein stump is probably an initiating event of portal vein thrombosis. Hypercoagulability and portal hypertension are other critical factors. Harbingers of postsplenectomy portal vein thrombosis include any combination of inexplicable fever or sepsis, nausea, diarrhea, ileus, elevated liver chemistries, ascites, nonspecific abdominal pain, or peritonitis (due to mesenteric ischemia from venous thrombosis). In the absence of peritonitis, the diagnosis is established by color-Doppler ultrasonography or by CT scanning with intravenous contrast. Anticoagulation and empiric antibiotics are probably necessary for a significant portal vein thrombosis; furthermore, thrombolytic therapy is cautiously administered in selected cases. Of course, a laparotomy and bowel resection is indicated if peritonitis develops because of infarcted gut. A thrombectomy also may be performed to preserve viable bowel.

Certain complications are particular to laparoscopy. These include the adverse hemodynamic effects of a pneumoperitoneum; the development of a pneumothorax, pneumomediastinum, or subcutaneous emphysema; and thermal injury to adjacent viscera (e.g., from electrocoagulation or a harmonic scalpel).

Overwhelming Postsplenectomy Infection

Laboratory confirmation of the link between asplenia and infection in animals was presented in 1919. King and Shumaker were the first investigators (in 1952) to formally propose this association in humans. Overwhelming postsplenectomy infection (OPSI) describes a fulminant infection that classically develops in an asplenic patient. This condition typically begins with flulike symptoms, but rapidly escalates to profound septic shock in less than 24 hours, resulting in death in approximately half of its victims. Although OPSI can develop in any patient who has undergone a splenectomy, it occurs most frequently among children or in adults with underlying hematologic disorders, usually within 2 years of the operation. The incidence of OPSI is difficult to determine, but recent figures estimate a lifetime risk as high as 3% to 5%. Interestingly, the removal of the spleen for HIV-related ITP does not seem to confer an increased risk of infection.

The majority of OPSI cases are caused by polysaccharide-encapsulated bacteria strains such as *Streptococcus pneumoniae*, *Haemophilus influenzae,* and *Neisseria meningitidis.* The absence of the spleen's phagocytosis capability and of its opsonizing antibodies makes these patients susceptible to infection by bacteria with the antiphagocytic coat. The spleen can promptly elaborate a type-specific IgM against these bacteria. Furthermore, once the organisms are coated with antibodies, the spleen is the most efficient phagocytic organ. Conversely, the liver can handle organisms against which high antibody levels are already present, but it cannot produce opsonins or effectively clear circulating antigens that have not been previously encountered. That youngsters and infants have not yet developed specific opsonizing antibodies against these bacteria explains their higher risk of OPSI in comparison to that of adults.

An expeditious diagnosis of OPSI is critical and relies on a high level of suspicion. The peripheral blood smear should be examined for organisms, and cultures of blood, urine, and sputum are obtained. (In addition to these encapsulated bacteria, protozoa such as malaria and babesiosis can cause OPSI.) A lumbar puncture may be necessary, especially in children. An evaluation of the clotting parameters is essential to identify disseminated intravascular coagulation. Blood-volume resuscitation and broad-spectrum antibiotics (e.g., vancomycin, ceftriaxone, and clindamycin) should be instituted immediately, allowing for antibiotic resistance patterns.

The most effective therapy for OPSI is prevention, through vaccinations, empiric antibiotics, and education of the patient about this phenomenon (Box 20-1). The polyvalent pneumococcal polysaccharide vaccine (e.g., Pneumovax, Merck & Co., Inc.) covers most of the serotypes responsible for pneumococcal infections in the United States. Although the timing of vaccination has not really been studied, it stands to reason that the vaccine is most effective in eliciting a sound immune response if administered before the splenectomy. Vaccination is still recommended after emergency splenectomy, but it may be best to delay for several days until the postoperative immunosuppression subsides. Repeated vaccinations against *Streptococcus pneumoniae* may be necessary every 5 to 6 years to sustain a proper antibody level. Vaccines for *Haemophilus influenzae* and *Neisseria meningitidis* are most suitable for children and for selected adults. An annual influenza virus vaccine may be indicated as well. Medical records should acknowledge the patient's asplenic state, and a medical-alert bracelet may be prudent as well.

Prophylactic oral antibiotics are probably warranted for youngsters and perhaps for HIV-infected adults who have undergone splenectomy. Choices of therapy include penicillin, amoxicillin, and trimethoprim/sulfamethoxazole. For adults, the author provides a standing prescription for an antibiotic that is to be taken at the onset of flulike symptoms. The patient also is counseled to call the primary care physician, hematologist, or surgeon immediately if this scenario occurs. The asplenic patient should avoid exposure to ticks and mosquitoes, and special plans should be devised for patients who travel to lands in which malaria or babesia is endemic. Of course, the best prevention of OPSI is the preservation of the spleen, such as by avoiding or delaying splenectomies in particularly young children and by the judicious practice of splenic salvage for trauma cases, including iatrogenic injury.

Both the gravity and the rarity of OPSI must be emphasized to the patient. Striking a wise balance between terror and complacency, the clinician should assure that the patient appreciates the nature of this entity and complies with these measures.

BOX 20-1 Overwhelming Postsplenectomy Infection Instructions for the Patient

If flulike symptoms develop (e.g., muscle aches, fevers), especially during the next 2 years, you should immediately contact your hematologist and/or primary care physician. (Contact your surgeon if you cannot locate the other physicians.) In addition, you should start taking an antibiotic, as prescribed. (You will receive a prescription for penicillin VK, Bactrim, or erythromycin on discharge from the hospital.)

Flulike symptoms can be related to a rare, but aggressive, infection that may develop when the spleen is absent. If these symptoms occur, they are possibly due to an ordinary episode of the flu, but the above measures should be taken for your safety in the event of the rare, aggressive infection.

You received vaccinations before (or occasionally after) the operation. Contact your physician or hematologist to schedule repeated Pheumococcus vaccinations every 5–6 years. In addition, you should have an annual influenza vaccine.

We suggest that you wear a medical alert bracelet to indicate that you have had your spleen removed (e.g., http://www.medicalert.org).

Avoid exposure to ticks and mosquitoes. Contact your primary care physician or hematologist before traveling to regions where malaria or babesia is endemic.

Massive Splenomegaly

Massive splenomegaly refers to spleens that weigh 1500 g or more. Most cases of massively enlarged spleens are due to myelofibrosis, non-Hodgkin's lymphoma, chronic lymphocytic leukemia, or hairy cell leukemia. These spleens are generally removed because of hypersplenism, symptoms such as altered gut function (e.g., early satiety) and pain, or to establish a diagnosis. (Hypersplenism develops with the malignant infiltration of red pulp that is typical of myelofibrosis and hairy cell leukemia.) It has long been thought that the removal of massive spleens is associated with an increased risk of complications and perhaps of deaths. Although that may be true, the author's group recently used logistic regression models and meta-analysis to demonstrate that the patient's age and the nature of the underlying illness actually dictate the operative morbidity and mortality. After one adjusts for these factors, the size of the spleen is not a determinant of risk.

Various technical maneuvers have been proposed for the safe removal of the massive spleen. Some surgeons have advocated the injection of epinephrine directly into the splenic artery, whereas others ligate the splenic artery via the lesser sac early in the operation, in hopes of reducing blood loss. Our experience indicates that early splenic artery ligation does not reduce blood loss, transfusion requirements, or the incidence of complications or deaths; but it does significantly prolong the duration of surgery. A minimally invasive method of reducing the perfusion and size of the spleen involves the percutaneous infusion of embolizing particles into the splenic artery within 24 hours of splenectomy. However, we contend that, when major blood loss occurs during the removal of massive spleens, it is generally from the venous circulation and would not be affected by disrupting arterial flow. Because splenic artery embolization carries some morbidity (e.g., splenic abscess, pancreatitis, pancreas necrosis, and splenic vein thrombosis) and can be quite painful, we believe it should be applied only in carefully selected cases. In certain circumstances, radiation therapy or chemotherapy has been used to shrink the spleen.

We favor a generous left subcostal incision for the removal of the massive spleen. This provides excellent exposure for the early division of the splenic attachments so that the organ is mobilized out of the subphrenic space and into the wound. The hilar vessels can be safely dissected once they are exposed on both the anterior and posterior aspects. Massive splenomegaly is often associated with bulky hilar adenopathy and perisplenitis that can confound the identification of the tail of the pancreas. If the pancreas is disrupted, a drain should be left in the subphrenic space. However, drains are not routinely warranted, especially for the evacuation of blood.

Suggested Reading

Cines DB, Blanchette VS: Immune thrombocytopenic purpura. N Engl J Med 346:995–1008, 2002.

Katkhouda N, Mavor E: Laparoscopic splenectomy. Surg Clin North Am 80:1285–1297, 2000.

Lynch AM, Kapila R: Overwhelming postsplenectomy infection. Infect Dis Clin North Am 10:693–707, 1996.

Ooi LL, Leong SS: Splenic abscesses from 1987 to 1995. Am J Surg 174:87–93, 1997.

Uranus S, Pfeifer J: Nonoperative treatment of blunt splenic injury. World J Surg 25:1405–1407, 2001.

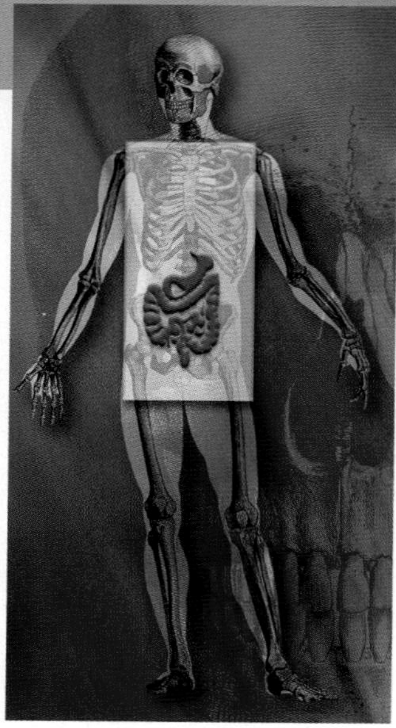

SECTION VI

GASTROINTESTINAL

Chapter 21

Colon and Anorectum

DAVID C. LONGCOPE, MD, and JOHN H. PEMBERTON, MD

Surgical Anatomy

Colon

The colon is approximately 150 cm long. The inner layers of the wall are similar to those of the small bowel: mucosa, submucosa, and circular muscle (muscularis propria). The outer longitudinal layer is slightly different, however, consisting of three bands (teniae coli) that extend from the base of the cecum to the rectosigmoid junction, where they coalesce and form an even layer enveloping the rectum. The cecum is the most proximal part of the colon and also is the most capacious. The appendix is found at its base, where the teniae coli converge. The ileocecal valve is interposed between the large and small bowel. The valve is usually competent, meaning that air and stool in the cecum cannot reflux into the small bowel. This is especially important when the large bowel is obstructed; as air continues to enter the cecum, it becomes distended and, as per Laplace's law (wall tension equals the radius times the change in pressure), it is the most likely spot to perforate. If the ileocecal valve is not competent, air escapes back into the small bowel, and perforation is less likely. The right and left colon, and usually the cecum, are retroperitoneal structures. They develop in the peritoneal cavity and then become fused to the retroperitoneum before birth and so, by definition, are actually secondarily retroperitoneal. This fusion allows easy mobilization back into the peritoneal cavity for resection. The transverse colon and sigmoid colon are intraperitoneal and can be rather redundant. The greater omentum is fused to the transverse colon and, with careful dissection, can be separated from it without injury to either structure. The two flexures, hepatic and splenic, refer to the two angulations in the colon at the liver and spleen, respectively. The splenic flexure is usually more superior and lateral, and thus more difficult to mobilize during surgery. Because of its close proximity to the spleen and frequent colosplenic attachments, if care is not taken during surgery on this part of the colon, splenic injury results. The duodenum lies just posterior to the hepatic flexure and should be identified and avoided during mobilization of this structure. The right and left ureters lie posterior to the right and sigmoid colon, respectively, and also should be identified during surgery on these parts of the colon.

The blood supply to the colon comes from the superior and inferior mesenteric arteries (Fig. 21-1). The superior mesenteric artery (SMA) supplies the colon up to the splenic flexure via the ileocolonic, right colic, and middle colic arteries. The left colic and sigmoidal branches via the inferior mesenteric artery (IMA) supply colon distal to the splenic flexure. The colic arteries branch and form the marginal artery, or marginal artery of Drummond, which usually runs the entire length of the colon. The venous drainage of the colon is into the portal system via the superior and inferior mesenteric vein. The lymphatic drainage parallels the arterial system with many lymph nodes from pericolic to periaortic, so that a proper cancer resection, encompassing lymphatic drainage to the involved part of the colon, requires proximal ligation of the artery that supplies that area of the colon.

Rectum

The rectum has a wider diameter than most of the rest of the colon, except for the cecum. It is 12 to 16 cm long, starts at about the level of the sacral promontory, and ends at the dentate line of the anal canal. The anterior aspect of the upper 4 to 6 cm of the rectum has a serosal surface and is within the peritoneal cavity. The rest of the rectum lies within the extraperitoneal tissue of the pelvis and has no serosal lining. The teniae coli spread out at the

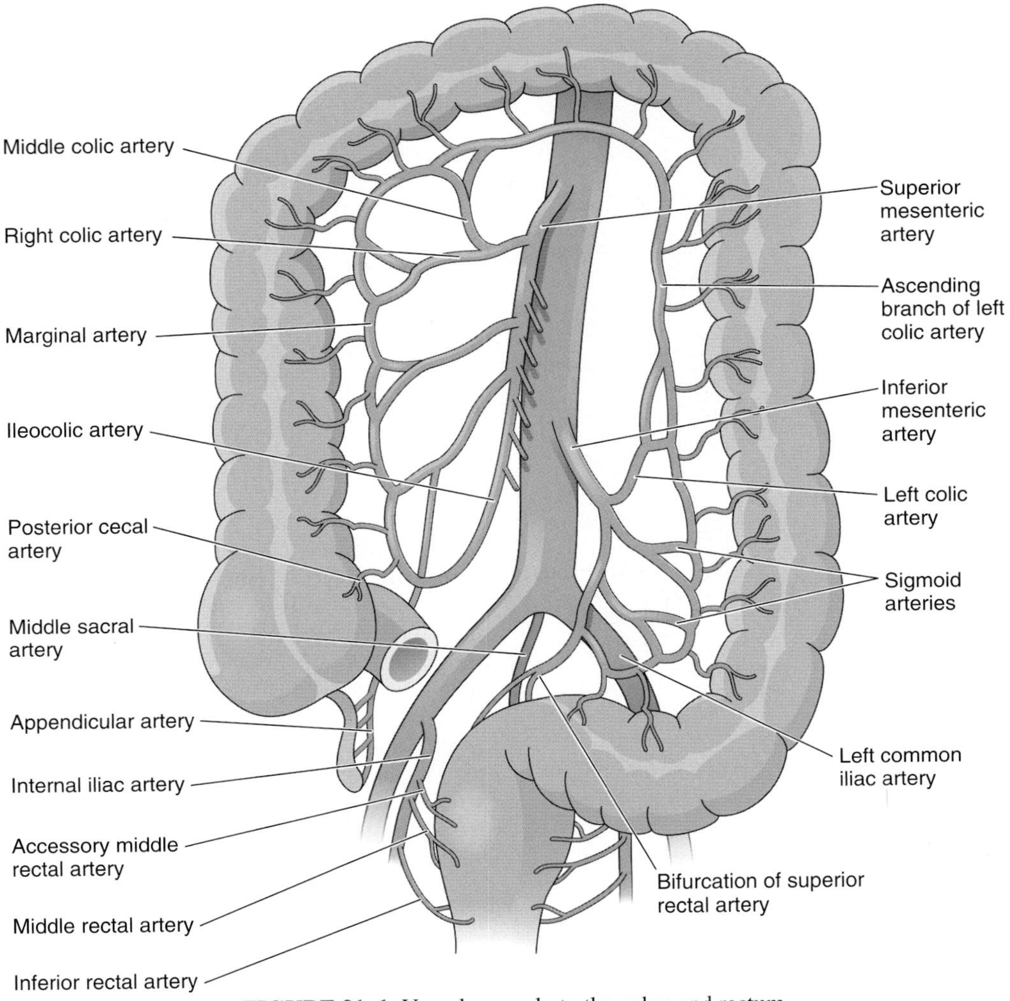

FIGURE 21–1 Vascular supply to the colon and rectum.

rectosigmoid junction to form one uniform, longitudinal muscle layer around the rectum. In women, the vagina lies anterior to the lower rectum, forming the thin and rectovaginal septum. In men, the prostate and seminal vesicles lie anteriorly and are usually identified during distal dissection of the rectum (Fig. 21-2). The anal canal is 3 to 5 cm long and extends from the termination of the levator ani muscles to the anal verge. The internal and external sphincter muscles, dentate line, anal glands, and hemorrhoidal veins all lie within the anal canal. The external sphincter is composed of skeletal muscle and is therefore under voluntary control. The internal sphincter is an anatomic continuation of the circular muscle of the rectum and is thus composed of smooth muscle and is under anatomic neural control. The dentate line is the point of transition of the columnar epithelium of the mucosa and the squamous epithelium of the anoderm. The anal glands start at the dentate line and usually terminate in the space between the internal and external sphincters.

The superior hemorrhoidal artery provides blood supply to the upper rectum. The middle and inferior hemorrhoidal arteries arise from the internal iliac and supply the middle and lower rectum. This difference in origin becomes significant with colonic ischemia due to disease or emboli in the mesenteric arteries. The rectum is usually spared because of its arterial supply from the iliacs (Fig. 21–3*A*). Venous drainage of the rectum and hemorrhoid plexi to the dentate line is into the portal system. The external hemorrhoid plexi, which lie beneath the anoderm, drain systemically. The lymphatic drainage of the rectum also parallels the arterial system (Fig. 21-3*B*). The upper rectum drains along the superior mesorectal artery into the periaortic nodes, whereas the middle and lower rectum drains to the iliacs. The anal canal drains into the inguinal

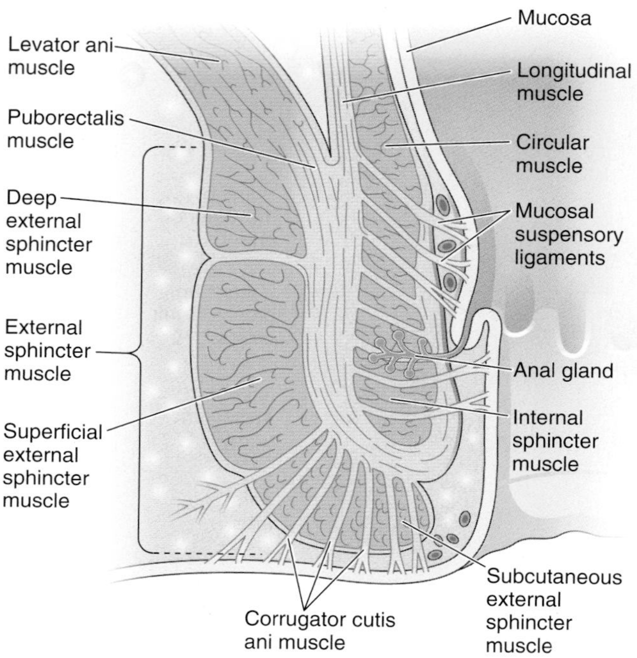

FIGURE 21–2 The anal canal.

nodes, where lymph node metastases from anal tumors can often be palpated.

Nerves: Colon

Innervation of the Colon

The sympathetic and parasympathetic nerves innervate the colon and run with the arterial supply. Colonic contraction and aborad propagation are inhibited by the sympathetic nerves and stimulated by parasympathetic ones. The colon also harbors an internal or enteric nervous system, a description of which is beyond the scope of the chapter.

Innervation of the Rectum and Anus

Sympathetic innervation is via the aortic plexus (prevertebral) and superior hypogastric plexus. This plexus forms into the hypogastric nerves, which travel to the lateral pelvic plexus. Along the course from the superior hypogastric plexus and the pelvic plexus, the parasympathetic nerves (nervi erogentes) join the hypogastric nerves. The nervi erogentes arise from sacral nerves 2, 3, and 4. The pelvic plexus provides visceral branches to the periprostatic plexus, bladder, ureters, prostate, rectum, etc. Parasympathetic innervation mediates erection, whereas sympathetic stimulation causes ejaculation. Finally, the pudendal nerves, arising from the sacral plexuses S_2 to S_4, innervate the external anal and urethral sphincters. The puborectal muscle is *separately* innervated by a branch of S_3 and S_4 lying on top of the pelvic floor.

Physiology

The colon has two main functions: to absorb water and store content. Neither is mandatory for survival. Approximately 1500 mL of ileal effluent is received by the cecum over a 24-hour period, and all but 200 mL is absorbed, most by the right colon. Through a combination of contractions (retrograde, segmental, and mass), content makes its way to the sigmoid colon and rectum, where it is stored before elimination. Normal elimination occurs every 8 to 72 hours. Resection of part of the colon can lead to a decrease in water absorption and a more liquid stool consistency. Resection of the rectum (with preservation of the anal canal) usually results in an increase in frequency of bowel movements due to loss of storage capacity. Intestinal gas is made up of nitrogen, oxygen, carbon dioxide, hydrogen, and methane. It comes from one of three sources: swallowing, breakdown products of intestinal bacteria, and diffusion from the bloodstream. The vast majority of intestinal gas comes from swallowing, and thus the passage of flatus usually signifies a patent intestinal tract. The colon also contains a large concentration of aerobic and anaerobic bacteria, including *Bacteroides fragilis* and *Escherichia coli*. These are of little consequence during normal health but are quick to cause illness when they escape the confines of the intestinal tract (i.e., perforation). Preoperative mechanical (oral cathartic) and antibacterial preparation of the colon effectively reduces the incidence of infection from enteric bacteria during elective bowel surgery.

The internal and external sphincters make up the high-pressure zone (HPZ) of the anal canal. The HPZ maintains fecal continence because pressures in the anal canal are always higher than those in the rectum. Unlike the voluntary external sphincter, the internal sphincter is in an almost constant state of contraction. It relaxes only in an involuntary, reflexive response to straining and distention of the rectum. Absence of a relaxation response to rectal distention is diagnostic for Hirschsprung's disease. The puborectalis muscle also plays an important role in fecal continence. This muscle creates an angle of about 90 degrees between the rectum and the anal canal. During defecation, the muscle relaxes, thus facilitating opening of the anorectal anal sphincter, in turn facilitating defecation.

Normal transit time through the colon is 30 to 40 hours; it is rarely more than 70 hours. Transit is determined by oral ingestion of radio-opaque markers, which are then followed by periodic radiographs to evaluate their rate of progress or by scintigraphic techniques. Abnormalities of defecation are observed on defecography, which evaluates function of the pelvic floor during evacuation. A complete workup of constipation should encompass both of these

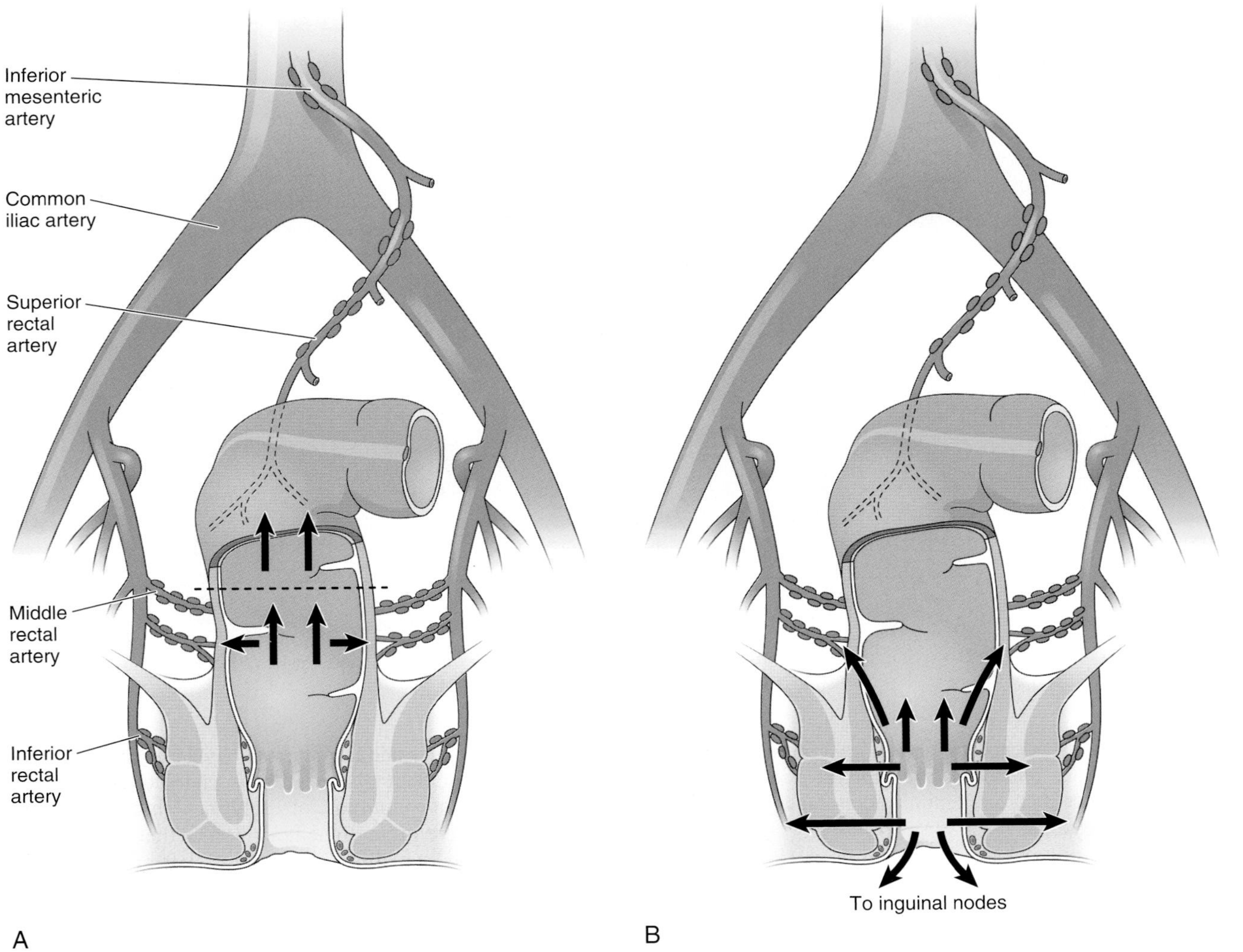

FIGURE 21–3 *A*, Arterial and lymphatic drainage of the rectum. *B*, Lymphatic draining of the anal canal. (From Gordon PH, Nivatvongs S (eds): Principles and Practice of Surgery for the Colon, Rectum, and Anus, 2nd ed. St. Louis, Quality Medical Publishers, 1999, with permission.)

studies, as well as colonoscopy or barium enema, to rule out any obstructive causes. Anal sphincter function can be evaluated with anorectal manometry.

Colon Polyps

The several types of colon polyps are divided into one of three categories: nonmalignant, premalignant, and malignant. Polyps are generally described as being either sessile (flat) or pedunculated (on a stalk). They can occur at any age with a variety of different symptoms or no symptoms at all.

Pathophysiology

Hyperplastic polyps are a common form of nonmalignant polyps. They are asymptomatic, and although they are often found in the presence of other polyps, are thought not to put the patient at increased risk for an adenoma or cancer. Therefore their presence alone requires no increase in surveillance. Rarely more than a few millimeters in size, a biopsy can confirm the histology, or they may be coagulated.

Juvenile polyps are usually found in patients younger than 10 years and are nonmalignant hamartomas. They often occur with rectal bleeding, and more than one can be present. Endoscopic excision is all that is necessary, and no further follow-up is needed.

Adenomas, benign by definition, are premalignant polyps, and their peak incidence occurs around age 50 years. Histologically they can be tubular, villous, or mixed. Tubular adenomas are more likely to be pedunculated,

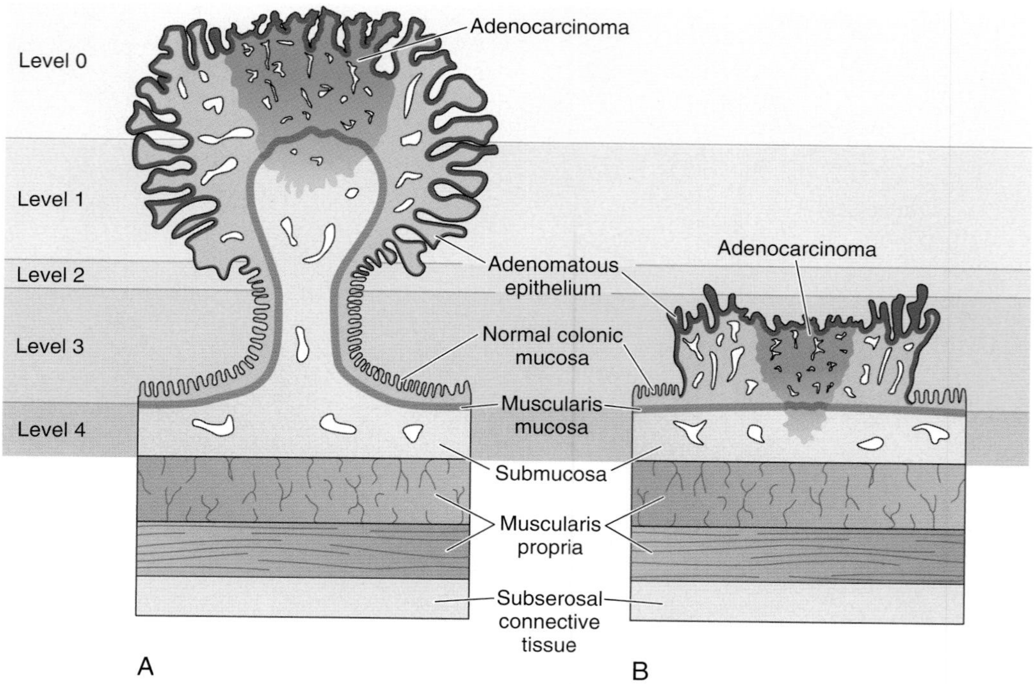

FIGURE 21–4 Staging system of Haggitt for carcinomas of pedunculated *(A)* and sessile *(B)* polyps.

whereas villous adenomas are more commonly sessile. Although villous adenomas are more at risk to contain a focus of cancer than are tubular adenomas, the treatment for both is the same.

Malignant polyps are the same as a cancer and are treated with formal bowel resection, the exception being either polyps completely removed transanally, or pedunculated polyps with cancer in the tip and no presence of lymphovascular invasion or invasion into the stalk. These patients can be followed up with endoscopic surveillance.

The most reliable staging system for polyps complicated by a cancer is Haggitt's. Figure 21-4 illustrates this staging system for pedunculated and sessile polyps.

Level 0 Intramucosal carcinoma, not invasive
Level 1 Invasive into submucosa *in the head*
Level 2 Invasive to the neck
Level 3 Invasive into stalk
Level 4 Invasive into submucosa of the *bowel wall*

Only level 4 invasion is associated with lymph node involvement, and this occurs in about 10% of patients. Kikuchi and colleagues defined the classification of *sessile* polyps by dividing invasion into Sm1, Sm2, and Sm3. Sm1 is invasive into the upper one third of submucosa; Sm2, to the middle one third; and Sm3, to the lowermost one third. Only Sm3 invasion is associated with a significant risk of lymph node invasion (>20%).

Familial adenomatous polyposis (FAP) is an inherited, autosomal dominant disease that is characterized by the development of hundreds of polyps within the colon. These polyps are premalignant adenomas that appear at an early age, and two thirds of patients that are diagnosed when symptomatic will already have a carcinoma. Families susceptible to this disorder should be screened with endoscopy at an early age so that cancer can be avoided by early surgical treatment. Without treatment, cancer will develop in essentially 100% of patients with FAP at an average age of 40 years. Colonoscopic screening for patients at risk for FAP should start before age 20 years. These patients also are at risk for small bowel adenomas, so upper endoscopy is used to aid in their diagnosis and treatment. A genetic variant of FAP is Gardner's syndrome, which, in addition to colonic polyps, includes desmoid tumors, supernumerary teeth and lipomas, and other soft-tissue lesions.

Symptoms

Patients with symptomatic polyps most commonly are first seen with rectal bleeding. They also can have obstruction, prolapse through the anus, change in bowel habit, or increased mucus production. Although rare, some villous adenomas cause dehydration and hypokalemia because of a high rate of secretion. Most polyps, however, are asymptomatic and found on routine endoscopy.

Differential Diagnosis

On barium enema, retained stool can sometimes appear as a polyp. The best way to evaluate this is with colonoscopy. Different types of polyps can be differentiated by endoscopic excisional biopsy, or by partial tissue biopsy if they are too large to be removed. *Pseudopolyps* are seen most often in ulcerative colitis. They are not true polyps but are actually islands of viable mucosa surrounded by denuded areas.

Workup and Evaluation

History and Physical

The history should elicit symptoms, if any, and any family history of polyps or cancer. Often no results are found on physical examination in a patient with polyps. If the polyp is palpable on digital rectal examination, the size, consistency, location, and presence of fixation to surrounding tissue should be documented.

Laboratory and Imaging Tests

A complete blood count (CBC) is all that is necessary with a history of bleeding. Electrolytes can be obtained if concern is present for a secretory polyp, and coagulation studies, for a history of a bleeding disorder.

An anorectal ultrasound can be helpful to look for malignant invasion in a large rectal polyp. Otherwise, no imaging is necessary for colon polyps.

Treatment Alternatives

Expectant

Adenomas are considered premalignant, and these should always be removed. A small hyperplastic polyp can be left alone without incident, but one must be certain that it is not an adenoma, and this is not always possible without polypectomy.

Medical

No acceptable medical treatment exists for colon polyps. Some studies suggest regression of polyps in FAP patients treated with nonsteroidal medications; however, this is experimental.

Surgical Techniques

Most polyps can be removed via the colonoscope, by using either a snare or biopsy forceps. Retrieval of the polyp is important to evaluate the histology and look for the presence of cancer. Polyps too large to remove with the colonoscope require formal surgical excision. Polyps with evidence of invasive cancer (Haggitt level 4, Sm3) also need formal surgical excision, unless they are pedunculated and no evidence of lymphovascular invasion or invasion into the stalk is found.

Laparoscopic colon resection is an excellent option for polyps too large to be removed colonoscopically. Laparoscopic resection, when compared with open resection, generally takes longer, but patients recover more quickly and have less pain. Identification of the polyp laparoscopically can sometimes be difficult; therefore preoperative tattooing or intraoperative colonoscopy may be necessary. The least traumatic operation is to mobilize the part of the colon with the polyp and make a small incision in the colon (colotomy). The polyp is then removed, and the colotomy is closed. However, colotomy with polypectomy should not be performed if the polyp has the potential to be malignant, as this can worsen a patient's prognosis. In this case, formal bowel resection should be performed (see later).

Patients with FAP and Gardner's syndrome will require proctocolectomy eventually because of the inevitable development of cancer. In the past, these patients initially underwent a subtotal colectomy with anastomosis of the ileum to the rectum to avoid a permanent ileostomy for as long as possible. The rectum was removed if polyps became unmanageable by endoscopic excision. However, with the advent of ileal pouch–anal anastomosis, these patients are more commonly undergoing this operation initially and avoiding the ongoing risk of cancer and the subsequent need for a second resection (see later).

Outcomes

Hyperplastic polyps and hamartomas require no further follow-up. A single adenoma can be followed up with a repeated colonoscopy in 3 to 5 years. Large or multiple adenomas should be followed up in 1 to 2 years. If concern is present about incomplete resection of a polyp, follow-up should be sooner.

Complications

Colonoscopy carries roughly a 0.05% to 0.5% risk of perforation. Although this can sometimes be treated with nasogastric decompression and IV antibiotics if diagnosed immediately, surgery is usually required. Bleeding from the polypectomy site can usually be arrested by colonoscopic cauterization. Laparoscopic and open resection for benign polyps carries the risk of bleeding, infection, anastomotic leakage, and injury to the ureter, small bowel, or spleen.

Colorectal Cancer

The incidence and mortality rate of colon cancer has been declining in the United States during recent years. It is estimated that yearly, 130,000 to 140,000 Americans are diagnosed with colon cancer, with about 55,000 deaths. Colorectal cancer (CRC) is evenly distributed among men and women and, although seen as early as age 20 years, the peak incidence is in the seventh decade of life. Five percent of people diagnosed with colon cancer are younger than 40 years.

Pathophysiology

The cause of colon cancer is thought to be a combination of environmental and genetic factors. Having a first-degree relative with colon cancer increases one's risk 2 to 4 times the average. Specific inherited genes such as oncogenes (K-*ras*), tumor-suppressor genes (*APC*, *p53*), and mismatch-repair genes also have been implicated. Colon cancers that develop in the young are more often found in the presence of one of these inherited genes, as opposed to cancers that develop in the elderly. However, despite this evidence, most patients that are diagnosed with colon cancer have no known genetic predisposition.

Of all the environmental factors, diet is believed to play the largest role. It is believed to be the reason that the incidence is higher in the United States than in undeveloped countries. Diet also is thought to be part of the reason that Americans have a higher incidence than do Japanese living in Japan, but not higher than Japanese living in the United States. Although the exact mechanism is still debated, most agree that a diet high in fat and low in fiber is the prime culprit. Alcohol and smoking also increase the risk of developing colon cancer, but not as strongly as diet. Last, obesity, increased bile acids, and sedentary lifestyle have long been suspected to increase one's risk, but the data are less conclusive.

Adenocarcinoma accounts for the vast majority of CRCs. It can be found throughout the colon and rectum, from cecum to anal canal; it has a preponderance to develop distally. Although more than half of all cancers develop distal to the splenic flexure, a slow increase has been noted in the ratio of right-sided to left-sided cancers. The cause is unknown, but it has led to a more aggressive use of colonoscopy in symptomatic patients. Although the exact time frame is unknown, it is generally accepted that it takes 10 years for a polyp to become malignant. This is concluded from the finding that the peak incidence of polyps in the general population is at age 50 years, whereas the peak incidence of cancer is at 60 years of age.

Adenocarcinoma is seen pathologically in four forms: ulcerative, polypoid, annular, or diffusely infiltrating. Ulcerative, the most common, has a central depression, surrounded by raised edges. Polypoid cancers are large polyp-shaped cancers. An annular carcinoma is a circumferential lesion, most notable for its "apple core" appearance on barium enema. A diffusely infiltrating carcinoma appears as a thickening of the bowel wall and is often flat and can be difficult to diagnose. It is by far the least common.

Dukes originally described staging for rectal cancer in 1932. This has been extended to include colon cancer, and several changes have since been made, the best received and useful being that by Astler and Coller. Dukes' A refers to a tumor that invades into but not through the submucosa. Dukes' B1 is tumor invasion into but not through the muscularis propria, and B2 is invasion through it. Neither stage A nor stage B has lymph node involvement. Dukes' C1 and C2 are the same as B1 and B2, but with positive nodes. Dukes' D refers to any tumor with evidence of distant spread. More recently, a shift toward using the tumor-node-metastasis (TNM) classification (Box 21-1) and the subsequent staging system (Box 21-2) has occurred.

BOX 21-1 TNM Classification for Colorectal Cancer

Primary Tumor

T0 No evidence of primary tumor
Tis Carcinoma in situ
T1 Invasion into submucosa
T2 Invasion into muscularis propria
T3 Invasions through muscularis propria and into subserosal or pericolic fat
T4 Invasions through serosa and/or into adjacent organs or structures

Regional Lymph Nodes

N0 No nodal metastasis
N1 1–3 positive lymph nodes
N2 ≥4 positive lymph nodes

Distant Metastasis

M0 No distant metastasis
M1 Distant metastasis

BOX 21-2 Staging System for the TNM Classification

Stage 0		Tis	N0	M0
Stage I	A	T1	N0	M0
	B_1	T2	N0	M0
Stage II	B_2	T3	N0	M0
	B_3	T4	N0	M0
Stage III		Any T	N1	M0
		Any T	N2	M0
Stage IV		Any T	Any N	M1

Symptoms

Colon cancer is first seen with a variety of symptoms including rectal bleeding (occult or gross), anemia, weight loss, obstruction, perforation, abdominal pain, general malaise, or a change in bowel habits or stool caliber. It is sometimes found on routine colonoscopy done for a history of polyps or a family history of colon cancer. Fecal occult blood test (FOBT), although not an ideal test because of its poor sensitivity and specificity for detecting colon cancer, remains in widespread use because of its low cost, ease of use, and noninvasiveness. Its poor specificity is due to the fact that of all patients with a positive FOBT, 5% to 10% will have a colon cancer, and 20% to 30% will have colon polyps. One half of all colon cancers will test positive for FOBT, thus lending to its poor sensitivity. Recently, however, FOBT has been found to decrease overall mortality from colon cancer, thus solidifying its place in colon cancer screening for the near future.

Differential Diagnosis

Although the most common cause of rectal bleeding is hemorrhoids, the most common presenting symptom of colon cancer is rectal bleeding. Thus anyone middle-aged or older, or with a family history of colon cancer, complaining of rectal bleeding, should have a full colon evaluation. Other causes of rectal bleeding are diverticulosis, arteriovenous malformations, ischemia, inflammatory bowel disease (IBD), anal fissure, infectious colitis, peptic ulcer disease, noncolonic gastrointestinal (GI) malignancy, or Meckel's diverticulum. Anyone with a positive FOBT and a normal colon evaluation should undergo upper GI endoscopy. Colonic obstruction, either partial or complete, is the presenting symptom in colon cancer 10% to 20% of the time. Obstruction also can be due to ischemia, diverticulosis, volvulus, or fecal impaction. Perforation from colon cancer is unusual and is the presenting symptom 3% to 6% of the time. Usually it is a small, localized perforation, often found as an inflammatory mass on computed tomography (CT) scan. This can often be confused with diverticulitis, which is often treated nonoperatively. If surgical resection is not planned, colonoscopy should be performed as soon as the inflammation subsides to rule out the presence of carcinoma. Anemia can be due to blood loss (i.e., bleeding malignancy, peptic ulcer disease), hemolysis (i.e., spherocytosis), or decreased red blood cell production (i.e., iron or vitamin B_{12} deficiency). Weight loss, general malaise, and abdominal pain are very nonspecific symptoms and can be due to a variety of diseases, surgical or nonsurgical, malignant or benign, and abdominal or systemic.

Workup and Evaluation

History and Physical Examination

A complete history should include duration of symptoms, last colon evaluation (if any), history of polyps or cancer, or family history of polyps or cancer. More ominous symptoms include abdominal pain, weight loss, or partial obstruction. Symptoms of metastatic disease like jaundice or hemoptysis are rare. Physical examination should be thorough and include abdominal examination, full lymph node examination, and rectal examination. On abdominal examination, one should try to palpate the tumor if possible and evaluate for hepatomegaly. One also should look for evidence of obstruction by way of distention, tympanic percussion, or high-pitched bowel sounds on auscultation. If tumors are palpable on digital examination, one should note the location (anterior, posterior, left, right), whether it is fixed to surrounding structures, and approximate distance from the anal verge.

Laboratory Tests and Imaging

A complete blood count to evaluate for anemia along with standard electrolytes should be routine. LFTs (liver-function tests) and a CEA (carcinoembryonic antigen) level are standard to check for possible signs of metastatic disease. However, normal levels by no means rule out distant spread.

A chest radiograph should be checked for pulmonary metastasis. A CT scan of the abdomen/pelvis is generally not necessary for colon cancer, because the liver will be examined at the time of surgery when biopsies can be obtained of suggestive lesions. However, a scan is beneficial if metastatic disease will preclude or change the operation planned. A CT scan is helpful for rectal cancer to check for local involvement. An ultrasound or CT scan should be done if a laparoscopic resection is planned because one is unable to palpate the liver effectively. An anorectal ultrasound is helpful for rectal tumors to evaluate bowel-wall involvement if one is considering transanal excision. Recently, the flexible intrarectal ultrasound technique has improved the sensitivity and specificity for ultrasound for depth of tumor invasion (>95%), but lymph node imaging is unrelated (<75%). A colonoscopy should always be performed, if not already done, to evaluate the entire colon for synchronous polyps and cancers.

Treatment Alternatives

Expectant

Nonoperative treatment, even in the face of distant spread, will often result in obstructive symptoms necessitating surgery long before the patient dies of the disease. Thus surgical intervention, even if just intestinal diversion, is recommended unless underlying medical conditions would preclude the patient surviving long enough for this devastating condition to result.

Medical

Preoperative treatment with radiation, and more recently chemotherapy, is useful in rectal cancer, especially when invasion into local organs, such as the bladder or prostate, is present. Although reports exist of obliteration of the tumor with adjuvant therapy alone, this is still not an acceptable form of treatment.

Surgical

Complete surgical excision remains the only accepted way to cure a patient with colon cancer. The type of excision performed is very much dependent on the location of the tumor as well as on the presence of any other suggestive lesions (Fig. 21-5). The proximity of the lesion to the anal sphincter is what defines whether the patient will need a permanent colostomy. Tumor involvement of the sphincter

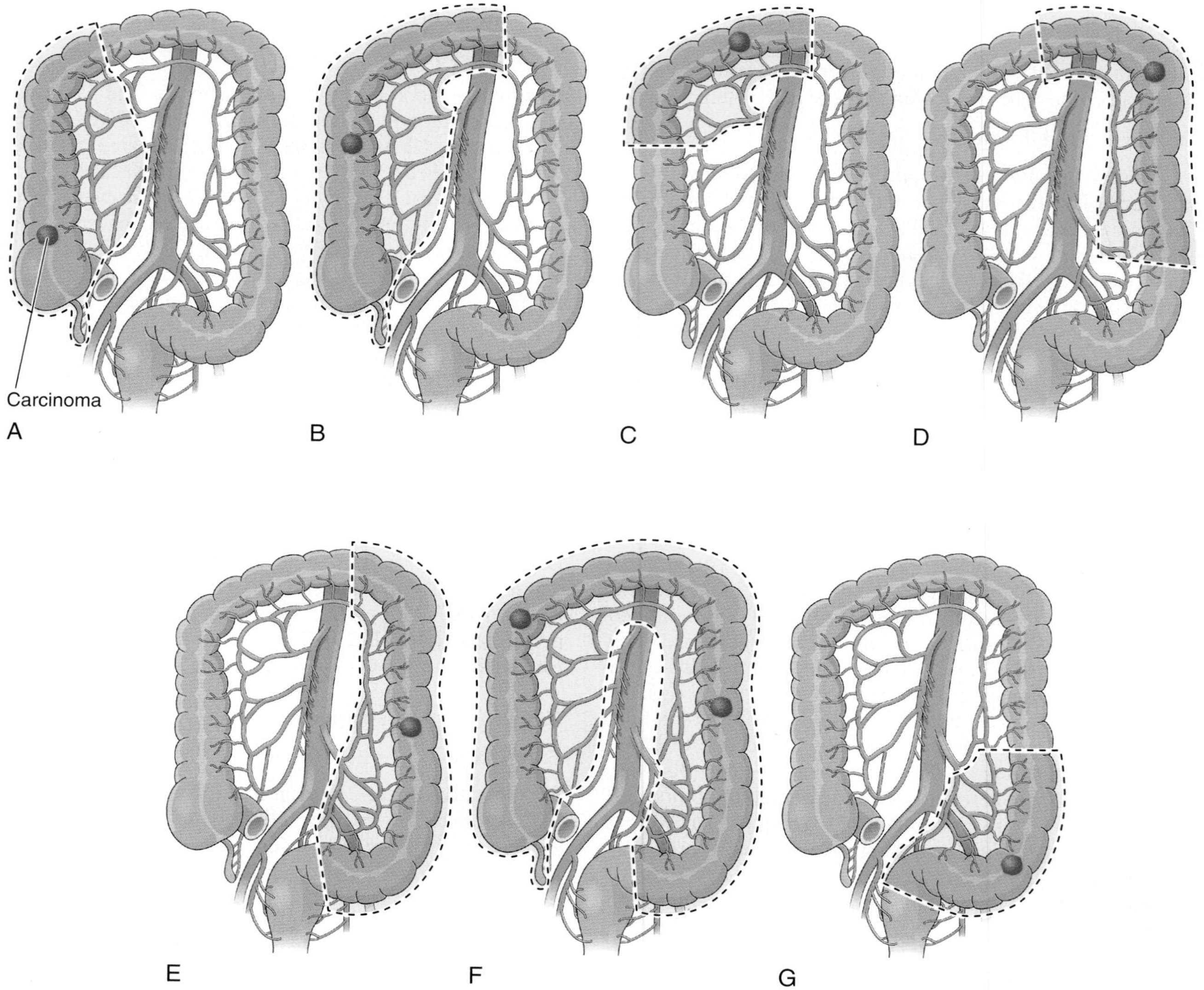

FIGURE 21–5 Extent of colonic resection depends on location of the tumor. *A*, Right hemicolectomy. *B*, Extended right hemicolectomy. *C*, Segmental resection of the transverse colon. *D*, Left hemicolectomy. *E*, Extended left hemicolectomy. *F*, Abdominal colectomy for synchronous colon cancer. *G*, Sigmoid resection.

complex, or involvement within 2 cm of it, usually necessitates a colostomy, as a 2-cm margin is considered the safe, minimum margin of resection. Depending on the size of the tumor and the size of the patient's pelvis, most other tumors can be resected and still allow a safe anastomosis of the colon.

The night before surgery, the patient should take a mechanical bowel prep (i.e., Go-Lytely, Fleet's Phospho-soda) along with an oral antibiotic prep to minimize the risk of operative infection. Patients that may need a colostomy should have the site marked preoperatively (by a stomal therapist, if available) at a place that is comfortable and is easily reachable.

Techniques

Exploration of the abdomen for evidence of metastatic disease should include palpation of the liver and of the ovaries, if present. Location of the colonic lesion should be confirmed by gentle palpation before mobilization of the colon for resection. All lymphatic drainage of the lesion should be included with the resection. Because this involves at least one named vascular trunk, the colon

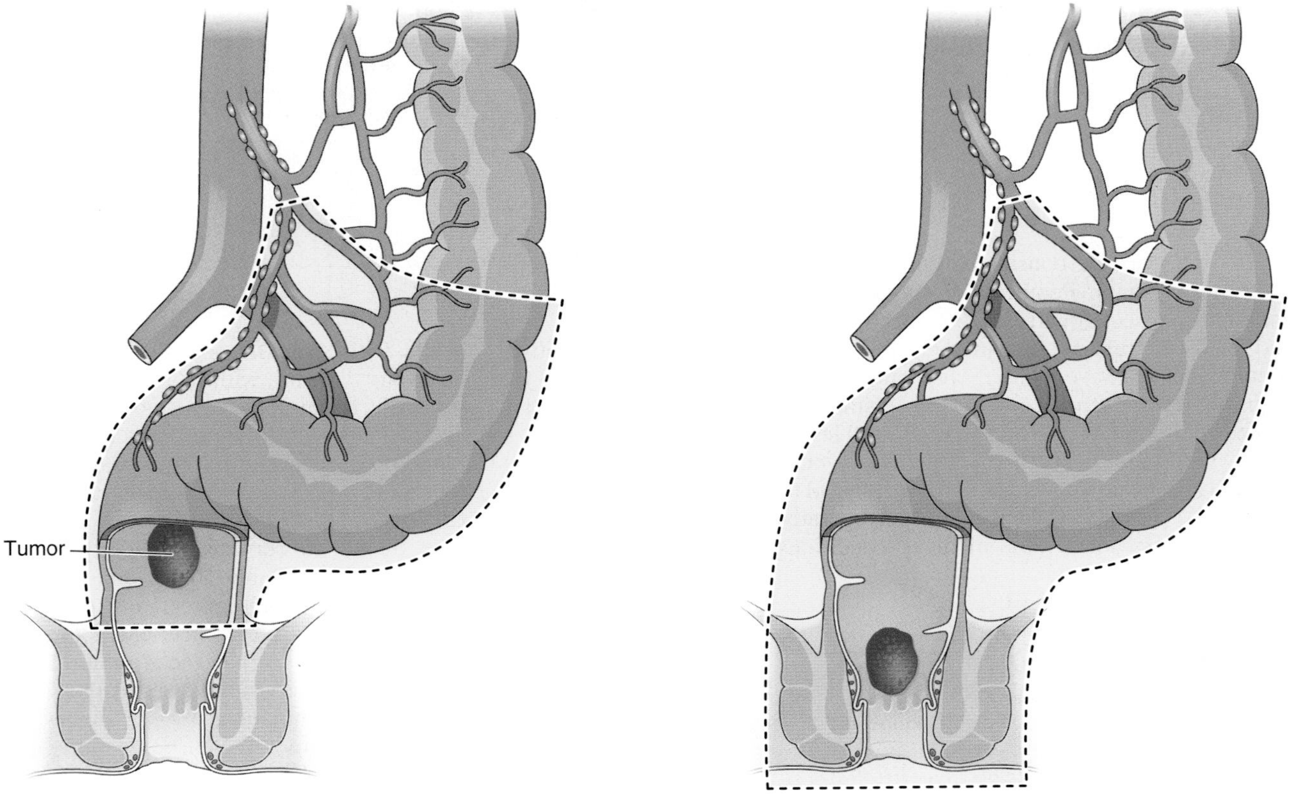

FIGURE 21–6 Extent of rectal resection. *A*, Low anterior resection. Tumor location is above the pelvic floor. *B*, Abdominal perineal resection. Tumor is close to anus and coloanal anastomosis is not indicated.

supplied by this vessel is taken as well. Thus getting at least 2-cm margins around the tumor is usually not a problem. Right-sided colon lesions are resected with a right hemicolectomy, and left-sided lesions are usually amenable to a left hemicolectomy. Extended right or left hemicolectomy, or a transverse colon resection, can be used for lesions in the transverse colon. Lesions in the mid to lower rectum are more difficult because of the physical constraints of the pelvis, and sometimes a 2-cm distal margin is all that can be achieved. Resection of the distal sigmoid or rectum, where an anastomosis is possible, is referred to as a low anterior resection. Excision of lesions in the mid to lower rectum should include the total mesorectum to decrease local recurrence rates (Fig. 21-6). An anastomosis can consist of a single layer of sutures, a double layer of sutures, or staples, but as the anastomosis is lower in the pelvis, the utility of the stapler can be more appreciated.

An abdominoperineal resection is reserved for rectal cancers that are close to the anal sphincter and require their excision for an attempted cure. This resection results in a permanent colostomy, usually in the left lower quadrant. The rectum is mobilized as low as possible from the abdomen, and then the resection is completed from the perineum, where a generous incision includes the anal canal and tumor. The levator muscles and skin are then completely closed to reconstruct the pelvic floor.

A transanal excision is an acceptable way to excise early, low-lying rectal tumors with low morbidity. However, no lymph nodes are obtained for evaluation. Thus it is an accepted treatment in patients with T1 lesions, but more controversial for T2 lesions. It is an ideal procedure in elderly patients with comorbidities, who cannot tolerate a full resection. Healthy patients who undergo transanal excision for lesions deeper that T2 (usually due to underdiagnosing from preoperative ultrasound) should have a full resection.

Laparoscopic resection for colon cancer has recently been shown in a large multicenter trial to be as oncologically safe as traditional open surgery. The benefits are quicker postoperative recovery and decreased pain.

Outcomes

Colon cancer is a potentially curable disease, and the overall prognosis depends on the stage (Box 21-3). Recurrence more than 7 years after surgical resection is

BOX 21–3 5-Year Survival by Dukes' Staging Classification for Curative Resection of Colon Cancer

Dukes A	75%–90%
Dukes B	60%–75%
Dukes C	30%–55%

rare, so patients are considered cured if they are disease free after 7 years. People with stage I tumors that are completely resected carry a 70% to 80% 5-year survival and require no further adjuvant therapy. Patients with stage II colon cancers have a 60% 5-year survival and generally require no further treatment. However, studies are looking at the benefit of chemotherapy for T3-4N0 lesions, and it is being used more often in otherwise young, healthy individuals. Stage III cancers (those with spread to the lymph nodes) are usually treated with postoperative chemotherapy unless coexisting medical conditions make it prohibitive. Patients with stage III colon cancer have a 45% 5-year survival. Patients with stage IV disease (distant spread) have a mean survival of about 2 years. However, selected patients with limited spread to the liver or lung can be cured. Reports exist of 30% 5-year survival for patients undergoing curative resection of metastatic colon cancer to the liver.

PEARLS FOR THE OR

Watershed areas of the colon (poor blood supply): splenic flexure (Griffith's point), rectosigmoid junction (Sudeck's point)

The strongest layer of the bowel wall: submucosa

Requirements of a good bowel anastomosis: Good blood supply, tension free, air tight (for rectal anastomosis tested with a proctoscope)

Two structures to be identified and avoided during right hemicolectomy: duodenum, right ureter

Distal point of resection of sigmoid for diverticular disease: coalescence of teniae coli

Always perform a thorough, bimanual examination of the liver when operating for colorectal cancer.

A good oncologic resection of a colon cancer involves proximal ligation of the named vessel(s) supplying the length of bowel being removed.

A good oncologic resection of a rectal cancer involves total mesorectal excision (for mid and distal rectal tumors) and a proximal ligation of the inferior mesenteric vessels, just distal to the left colic.

Three most common locations for internal hemorrhoids: right anterior, right posterior, left lateral

Successful treatment of a fistula-in-ano requires identification of the internal opening.

Proper treatment of a thrombosed external hemorrhoid involves excision of the hemorrhoid, not incision, and expression of the clot.

TABLE 21–1 Comparative 5-Year Survival by the TNM Classification after Curative Resection for Colon Cancer vs. Rectal Cancer

	Colon Cancer	Rectal Cancer
Stage I	70%	70%
Stage II	60%	55%
Stage III	45%	40%
Stage IV	5%	5%

Stage for stage, rectal cancer has a slightly worse prognosis than colon cancer (Table 21-1), and for this reason, adjuvant treatment is more aggressive. Because it has a higher incidence of local recurrence, chemotherapy and radiation therapy are used for any rectal tumor T3 or worse. Preoperative radiation is usually used if the rectal tumor is fixed on digital examination, or with suggestion of invasion to surrounding structures on preoperative CT scan or anorectal ultrasound. T2 rectal tumors resected via transanal excision should have external-beam radiation if no further excision is planned. Occasionally, a transanal excision is performed on a rectal lesion thought to be a T1 or T2, if it is subsequently found to be a T3 on final pathology. Because of a high rate of local recurrence, these patients should undergo a low anterior resection (LAR) or abdominoperineal resection (APR) unless their medical condition prohibits such an operation. Factors that worsen prognosis, independent of stage, are poorly differentiated tumors and tumors that cause obstruction or perforation.

Complications

Colon resection for cancer carries the same risks as colon resection for any other disease. The risks are bleeding, abdominal abscess, anastomotic leak, splenic injury, ureteral injury, small-bowel injury, wound infection, incisional hernia, deep vein thrombosis (DVT), myocardial infarction, stroke, and death. Surgery in the pelvis carries an increased risk of DVT, as well as a risk of sexual dysfunction in men.

Diverticular Disease

A diverticulum is a saclike protrusion off of the bowel. A true, or congenital, diverticulum is made up of the entire bowel wall, whereas a false, or acquired, diverticulum consists of just mucosa and submucosa protruding through the muscle wall of the bowel. The diverticula in the colon are acquired, and their presence is referred to as *diverticulosis*. They are commonly an incidental finding at endoscopy or on barium enema, whether few or many.

Pathophysiology

In the United States, diverticulosis is present in 5% to 10% of people age 45 years, 50% to 60% at age 60 years, and almost 80% at age 80 years. Although they can be found anywhere in the colon, 85% to 90% reside in the sigmoid. A diverticulum is usually found next to the tenia coli at the site of penetration of a nutrient artery, where the bowel wall is weakest (Fig. 21-7). It is much less prevalent in nonindustrialized societies, being found in less than 1% of the population in North Africa. It is thought to arise from increased intraluminal pressure in the colon due to slow fecal transit. Diets high in fat and low in fiber are thought to be the main culprit.

Although usually asymptomatic, a diverticulum that becomes inflamed or perforates or both will result in diverticulitis. This occurs in 5% to 10% of patients with diverticulosis over a 5-year period, increasing to 35% over a 20-year period. However, only about one fourth of these patients will require surgery. Diverticulitis is 3 times more likely in men than in women, and 20% are younger than 50 years.

Symptoms

Diverticulitis usually occurs with fever and left-lower-quadrant pain. Constipation is more common than diarrhea, but either may be seen, as well as nausea or vomiting. Diffuse abdominal pain can be a sign of free perforation into the abdomen. A redundant sigmoid can produce symptoms in any quadrant of the abdomen. Rectal bleeding is rare with diverticulitis, and its presence should cause one to look for an alternative diagnosis. Recurrent episodes of diverticulitis can lead to a colonic stricture from the healing process. Occasionally, a patient may be seen solely with obstructive symptoms: nausea, vomiting, abdominal distention, and/or absence of flatus. Pneumaturia is a sign of a colovesical fistula, a complication of diverticulitis.

Bleeding from the nutrient artery into the diverticulum can lead to hematochezia. Commonly, these patients have no other symptoms except acute onset of profuse rectal bleeding. This usually stops on its own, although the loss of blood can lead to dizziness or syncope.

Differential Diagnosis

Left-lower-quadrant pain is a presenting complaint in patients with many other entities including abdominal aortic aneurysm, IBD, ovarian cyst or abscess, gastroenteritis, hernia, or kidney stone. A perforated colon cancer can occur in a similar fashion, and a colonoscopy should be obtained when the symptoms abate to rule this

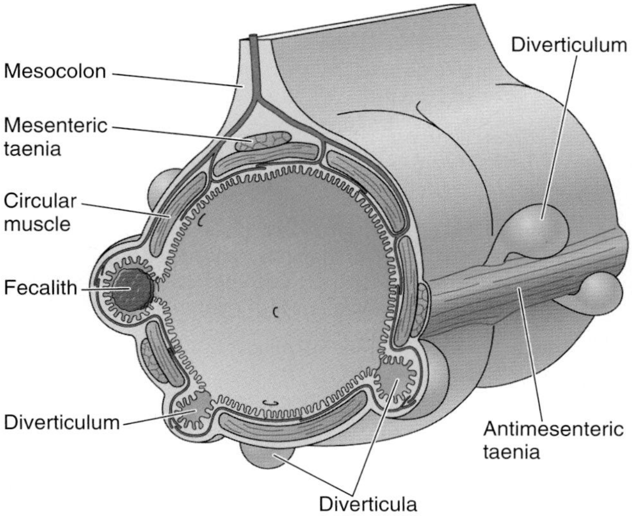

FIGURE 21–7 Diverticula form at relative weak spots in the muscular wall of the colon where vessels enter.

out. Profuse rectal bleeding, as seen with diverticulosis, is uncommon with other diseases, except for arteriovenous malformations and Meckel's diverticulum (these latter patients usually are younger.) However, colon cancer, IBD, ischemic colitis, and hemorrhoids should be considered. A colonic stricture can be caused by cancer most commonly, as well as IBD or ischemia.

Workup and Evaluation

History and Physical Examination

Diverticulosis must be present for diverticulitis to develop, so one should attempt to obtain a history of this from a previous barium enema or colonoscopy. Diverticulitis usually occurs with pain localized to the left lower quadrant, gradual in onset. A patient with a mild case may have symptoms for many days before being seen, whereas more severe cases may appear within 24 hours. A previous episode is significant if it was treated with antibiotics or hospitalization. Cessation of flatus and bowel movements can be a sign of obstruction, and a diet should be withheld. Presence of pneumaturia, fecaluria, or recurrent urinary tract infections is evidence of a colovesical fistula. On examination, a mass in the left lower quadrant is sometimes appreciated from the surrounding inflammation. Any evidence of peritonitis warrants immediate surgery. A malignancy is more likely if bleeding or a mass is found on rectal examination.

With diverticular bleeding, a history of previous episodes is very important. If previous bleeds have occurred, the severity (i.e., transfusions) and type of workup done should be noted. Physical examination is usually unremarkable, but bleeding hemorrhoids should be ruled out. Again,

PEARLS FOR ROUNDS

Causes of colonic obstruction (in order): cancer, diverticular disease, volvulus
Cecal volvulus (in general): younger patient, radiograph shows "coffee-bean" pointing to left upper quadrant (LUQ), treatment is surgical
Sigmoid volvulus (in general): elderly patient, radiograph shows "bent inner tube" pointing to right upper quadrant (RUQ), treatment is endoscopic decompression followed by elective surgery (if patient is not high risk)
The recurrence of a sigmoid volvulus is as high as 60% after endoscopic decompression.
Chemotherapy recommended for colon cancer stages: Tany, N1or2, M0; or Tany, Nany, M1
Chemotherapy and radiation therapy recommended for rectal cancers: T3or4, N0, M0; or Tany, N1or2, M0
Most common cause of rectal bleeding: hemorrhoids
Most common presenting symptom of colorectal cancer: blood per rectum
From 5% to 10% of patients with a positive fecal occult blood test will have colon cancer.
50% of patients with colon cancer will have a positive FOBT.
Incidence of rectal bleeding in patients with diverticulitis: less than 5%
A diverticular abscess can be treated successfully with percutaneous drainage about 75% of the time.
An attack of diverticulitis should be documented by CT scan or elevated WBC and treated and allowed to defervesce before elective surgery is considered.
Virtually all colon cancers start as an adenomatous polyp.
Colorectal cancers most commonly metastasize to the liver and the lung.
Three most common causes of rectal pain: fissure, abscess, thrombosed external hemorrhoid
One third of drained perirectal abscesses will subsequently form a fistula-in-ano.

rectal examination is important to rule out rectal malignancy. If hypotension is present, the patient should be urgently resuscitated with intravenous fluids. Two large-bore IVs should be placed, and blood should be sent for type and cross-match.

Laboratory Tests and Imaging

A CBC is important to evaluate for leukocytosis and anemia. When abdominal pain is present, amylase and lipase can help evaluate for pancreatitis. Electrolytes also are helpful, and a urinalysis should be sent if any urinary symptoms are noted. When a diagnosis of mild diverticulitis is certain, no imaging is necessary immediately, but a colonoscopy or barium enema should be performed when symptoms abate. For more severe cases, a CT scan of the abdomen and pelvis will not only show the presence of inflammation, mesenteric stranding, abscess, perforation, or colovesical fistula, but it also sometimes shows a mass, raising suspicion of a cancer.

For a diverticular bleed, a tagged RBC scan can be helpful to show ongoing bleeding, as most patients are no longer bleeding by the time they see a physician. With active bleeding, a mesenteric angiogram will localize the site within the colon. Surgery should rarely be directed by a tagged RBC scan alone. Alternatively, a colonoscopy can identify the site if active bleeding is seen, although this can be difficult if much blood is present in the lumen.

Treatment Alternatives

Expectant

Diverticulitis will rarely improve without some form of intervention. A diverticular bleed, conversely, usually stops before anything can be done. Episodes can be single or multiple, but if the site cannot be identified, little can and should be done except transfusion, unless it is life threatening.

Medical

Mild patients with diverticulitis can be treated as outpatients with oral antibiotics (ciprofloxacin and metronidazole) for 7 to 10 days. More severe cases require admission and treatment with IV antibiotics. Clear liquids can be given until symptoms improve. If an abscess is present on CT, this can usually be drained percutaneously by an interventional radiologist, with a success rate of 75%, but should still be followed by surgery. Percutaneous drainage allows resolution of the inflammation and avoidance of a colostomy. Worsening of symptoms with medical treatment at any time necessitates surgery.

Diverticular bleeding has been treated successfully with either embolization or IV pitressin by using interventional techniques, but bowel wall ischemia or necrosis or both have been reported.

Surgical Techniques

When peritonitis is present, emergency operation is indicated. Otherwise, surgery is reserved for complications of the disease (stricture, fistula, or abscess), failure of medical treatment, recurrent episodes (usually three or more), and episodes in immunosuppressed patients and those younger than 40 years. Only about 25% of patients with diverticulitis will require surgery. It is important to document the presence of diverticulitis, not just diverticulosis, before operating. This is done with either an elevated white blood cell (WBC) count with left lower quarter (LLQ) pain or positive CT scan findings. The mere presence of LLQ pain and diverticulosis is not reason enough to operate.

Surgery for sigmoid diverticulitis requires resection of the entire sigmoid to prevent recurrence. The distal margin is the point of coalescence of the teniae coli, the anatomic starting point of the rectum. Mobilization of the splenic flexure is usually required to create a tension-free anastomosis. Surgery is ideally done in an elective setting with resection and primary anastomosis, thus avoiding a colostomy. Emergency surgery in the presence of an abscess or unprepped bowel necessitates a resection and colostomy. In unstable patients, sometimes all that can be done safely is a proximal-loop colostomy and drainage of the abscess. In these last two scenarios, colostomy closure or sigmoid resection or both are done at a later date (usually 3 to 6 months).

Laparoscopic surgery is an option for patients undergoing elective sigmoid resection. A circular stapler is used for the low colorectal anastomosis. Some evidence suggests that these patients recover more quickly and with less pain than do those undergoing resection via open laparotomy.

Sigmoid resection with anastomosis is the operation performed for bleeding diverticulosis once the site is identified. Even in an emergency setting, primary anastomosis can often be performed, as the blood acts as a natural cathartic. Again, resection at the upper border of the rectum is important. Sigmoid resection without identifying the actual site of bleeding is a risky proposition, as the true cause, such as a right-sided diverticulum or arteriovenous malformation (AVM), can remain and continue to bleed. Persistent, life-threatening lower GI bleed of unknown etiology requires a subtotal colectomy, which carries a high morbidity and mortality rate. This is rare.

Outcomes

Patients undergoing elective resection for diverticular complications do very well; however, the recurrence rate of diverticulitis has been reported to be as high as 10% after surgical resection. This can be due to inadequate distal sigmoid resection as well as recurrence of symptoms that were initially due to other causes (i.e., irritable bowel syndrome). The latter reason stresses the importance of documenting leukocytosis or sigmoid inflammation or both on CT scan before resection. Recurrent diverticulitis requiring surgery is very rare.

Complications

Elective sigmoid resection with primary anastomosis carries a leak rate of 5%. This usually requires surgical reexploration, temporary colostomy, and drainage of the pelvis. Other immediate complications are abscess, bleeding, ureteral injury, and splenic injury. Injury to the pelvic nerves is less common than with a rectal resection. Long-term complications include incisional hernia, small-bowel obstruction from abdominal adhesions, and anastomotic stricture.

Colonic Volvulus

Pathophysiology

A volvulus is a twisting of the bowel on itself, creating a loop and causing an obstruction at both the beginning and the end of the loop. This causes a "blind loop," meaning that nothing within that part of the bowel can escape orally *or* aborally. In the colon, this can occur in the sigmoid or the cecum, being up to 3 times more common in the former. It is an uncommon cause of colon obstruction in the United States, behind cancer and diverticular disease. In underdeveloped countries, it is the leading cause of colonic obstruction. The majority of patients are older than 65 years, and it is commonly associated with institutionalized and psychiatric patients. The exact etiology is unclear, but it is thought that sedentary lifestyle and constipation play a role. When involved, the cecum and ascending colon are typically intraperitoneal, never having developed their retroperitoneal attachments. However, this is merely considered a risk factor, as up to 10% of the population will have this incidental finding, and in very few of those will a cecal volvulus develop. When the sigmoid is involved, it is typically large and redundant. It is hypothesized that a high-residue diet, present in areas where this condition is most common, causes stretching of the sigmoid over time, thus putting one at increased risk for a volvulus.

Symptoms

Patients most commonly are initially seen with abdominal distention, often quite marked. Pain is often present and typically crampy. Cessation of flatus and bowel movements is usually due to the obstructive component of this condition. Nausea and vomiting may be present and are more common with cecal volvulus. In a few instances, patients may give a history of similar, less acute episodes that resolved spontaneously. These may be due to spontaneous detorsion of the volvulus.

Differential Diagnosis

As mentioned previously, cancer is the most common cause of colonic obstruction and should be considered in the presence of rectal bleeding or radiographs atypical for volvulus. Diverticular disease also can cause colonic obstruction, but bleeding should not be present, and a previous history of diverticulitis may or may not be elicited. A cecal bascule is a redundant cecum that folds over on itself and causes an obstruction and/or blind loop. Differentiating this from a cecal volvulus is difficult and purely academic, as they are both treated similarly. Colonic pseudo-obstruction (Ogilvie's) can appear in a similar fashion and in a similar patient population. Water-soluble contrast enema can help differentiate between the two conditions.

Workup and Evaluation

History and Physical Examination

Because of the high incidence of institutionalized patients with this condition, obtaining a good history can often prove challenging. Symptoms of poor appetite, abdominal distention, and absence of bowel movements have typically occurred within a few days of presentation. A history of bleeding, weight loss, or diverticulitis should lead one to consider an alternative diagnosis. On examination, the abdomen is distended, tympanitic to percussion with positive bowel sounds, and may have mild tenderness. Severe or rebound tenderness or rigidity is a sign of perforation or ischemia, and emergency surgery is mandatory. The rectal vault is typically empty with a sigmoid volvulus.

Laboratory Tests and Imaging

A CBC is usually normal, with an elevated WBC being a possible sign of bowel compromise. Electrolytes may show dehydration if oral intake has been poor.

Plain abdominal radiographs can often make the diagnosis. The classic finding for cecal volvulus is an air-filled colon in the shape of a coffee bean, pointing to the left upper quadrant. A sigmoid volvulus is commonly described as a "bent inner tube" pointing to the right upper quadrant. When the diagnosis is unclear, a water-soluble contrast enema can often make the diagnosis. This shows termination of the contrast at the volvulus, forming the shape of a "bird's beak." If the contrast flows freely to the cecum, a volvulus is not present.

Treatment Alternatives

Expectant

A volvulus will occasionally reduce spontaneously, but this is rare. Typically some form of intervention is required and should be attempted.

Medical

A sigmoid volvulus can be reduced with a proctoscope or flexible sigmoidoscope from 80% to 85% of the time. This should always be attempted first if the patient is hemodynamically stable and without signs of peritonitis. Successful reduction usually results in a profound release of air and stool. Placement of a rectal tube into the sigmoid helps prevent immediate recurrence while the edema resolves. Endoscopy should be halted and surgery pursued if severe ischemia or necrosis is seen. Recurrence rates can be as high as 60%, making most advocate elective surgery if the patient's medical condition permits. Often this is done during the same hospitalization, with a rectal tube in place to help prevent recurrence while the colon is being prepped for surgery.

Endoscopic reduction of a cecal volvulus is more controversial. The failure rate is much higher, and the risk of complication from unsuccessful attempts causes many to shun this approach. If endoscopic reduction is successful, surgery is still recommended because of high recurrence rates.

Surgical Techniques

Several surgical approaches exist for cecal volvulus. If the cecum is viable, cecopexy or tube cecostomy is commonly used. If the bowel is nonviable, right colon resection with either an anastomosis or ileostomy should be performed. When the bowel is perforated, an ileostomy is necessary. For a sigmoid volvulus, a resection with primary anastomosis is the best option in the elective setting. The one caveat is that if the patient is fecally incontinent, a permanent colostomy is a good option. In the unprepped colon, a colostomy should be performed after sigmoid resection, with closure at a later date being dependent on the patient's medical condition.

Outcomes

Cecopexy has the benefit of avoiding an enterotomy, but carries with it a recurrence rate as high as 25%. Tube cecostomy is much more effective, but can be difficult for the patient to deal with. The site usually closes spontaneously when the tube is removed. Resection with anastomosis carries essentially no recurrence, but it is a bigger operation with a higher morbidity.

Complications

The biggest risk to life is the patient's underlying medical problems. Mortality rates range from 20% to 30%, when emergency surgery is required, to as high as 50% when gangrenous bowel is present. An elective operation is more optimal, but an anastomosis still carries a 5% to 10% risk of leakage. This is weighed against the risk of recurrence from a lesser operation, or no surgery at all.

Anorectal Disorders

Hemorrhoids

Hemorrhoids are actually vascular cushions within the anal canal, thought to aid in maintaining fecal continence. Internal hemorrhoids are found above the dentate line where little to no sensation is present, and are covered with mucosa. The blood inside the hemorrhoids is arterial. External hemorrhoids are found below the dentate line and are covered with anoderm.

Pathophysiology

Internal hemorrhoids usually enlarge from constipation and straining. This does not completely explain the etiology, however, as some patients with large hemorrhoids deny the presence of either symptom. Pregnancy predisposes women to hemorrhoids, but these usually resolve after delivery. Internal hemorrhoids are typically described in four degrees (Box 21-4). Thrombosis and necrosis occur if the hemorrhoids are not reduced. Anatomically, internal hemorrhoids are most often present in the left lateral, right posterior, and right anterior positions of the anal canal.

BOX 21-4 Classification of Internal Hemorrhoids

First degree	Bleeding without prolapse
Second degree	Prolapse outside the anal canal with spontaneous reduction
Third degree	Prolapse outside the anal canal requiring manual reduction
Fourth degree	Prolapse that will not reduce (incarcerated) outside the anal canal

Symptoms

Internal hemorrhoids are first seen with rectal bleeding, prolapse, or both. It is important to realize internal hemorrhoids are *not* painful unless a thrombosed external hemorrhoid component is present. The bleeding is often mild, either on the tissue paper or a few drops in the toilet. Occasionally, though, it can be profuse (patients describe squirting blood while straining), filling the toilet bowl. Typically patients bleed only during bowel movements. External hemorrhoids, conversely, are quite painful. Bleeding is uncommon unless the clot has eroded through the skin from pressure necrosis. The pain is typically worse in the first 48 to 72 hours, and then subsides over the next several days.

Differential Diagnosis

Although hemorrhoids are the most common cause of rectal bleeding, carcinoma is the most serious and should always be considered until proven otherwise. Other causes of rectal bleeding include diverticulosis, arteriovenous malformations, IBD, and ischemia. Anal fissures cause rectal bleeding as well, but this bleeding is usually mild. In the presence of portal hypertension, varices may form in the anal canal and rectum because of portosystemic shunting. These are not hemorrhoids and are not treated as such. Rectal prolapse is sometimes mistaken for hemorrhoids. This is usually a circumferential protrusion of rectal mucosa (or wall) reproducible with straining, and actual hemorrhoids are typically absent on examination. Rectal pain, as seen with thrombosed external hemorrhoids, also can be seen with anal fissures and perirectal abscesses. Anal skin tags and hypertrophied anal papillae are often confused for hemorrhoids.

Workup and Evaluation

History and Physical Examination

A history for hemorrhoids should include the initial onset of symptoms, the number of remissions and relapses, worsening symptoms, and any previous treatment. The presence of prolapse and the need for reduction is important for deciding on a treatment. A history of constipation and straining also is important, as this will have to be addressed in the final management plan. Recent weight loss, change in stools, or a family history of colon cancer should heighten one's concerns about a possible malignancy. As always, it is important to know of any recent endoscopic or barium enema evaluation of the colon. If pain is present, the type and duration will help differentiate it from other causes. Whereas the pain from a thrombosed hemorrhoid is usually recent in onset and constant, a fissure is often more chronic, hurting mostly during and after defecation.

On examination, a thrombosed external hemorrhoid can be diagnosed merely from external inspection. If the diagnosis is clear, a digital examination is not only extremely painful but also unnecessary as long as some form of follow-up is prescribed. Internal hemorrhoids, if not prolapsed, are best diagnosed by anoscopy. One should note which columns are inflamed by their anatomic position. Even with a history of profuse hemorrhoidal bleeding, examination rarely shows active bleeding.

Laboratory Tests and Imaging

Laboratory tests are generally not helpful for this condition, unless a history of profuse bleeding causes concern that the patient may be anemic.

No imaging study for hemorrhoids has proven as beneficial as a thorough examination. Occasionally and embarrassingly, however, angiography is performed for GI bleeding, and a bleeding hemorrhoid is identified.

Treatment Alternatives

Expectant

External hemorrhoids will almost always resolve on their own if one can ignore the pain. It is the discomfort that usually causes a patient to seek some form of management. Recurrence is unpredictable, regardless of the form of treatment. If left untreated, internal hemorrhoid symptoms will wax and wane, with an overall direction toward worse. Rarely will they resolve completely, except after pregnancy. Most patients will seek treatment for concern over the bleeding and prolapse.

Medical

Thrombosed external hemorrhoids should be treated with warm soaks, stool softeners, and pain medicine if the symptoms are abating. This typically occurs more than 48 hours after onset when the clot is beginning to be reabsorbed. At this time, attempts to excise the clot can be less fruitful, and pain from the procedure can be as bad as that from the resolving thrombosis. In general, if patients are seen within 4 days of onset, excision is indicated. If patients are seen later than 4 days, sitz baths and reassurance are the treatments of choice. Internal hemorrhoids can often improve by avoiding constipation and straining. A high-fiber diet, increased liquid intake, bulking agents, and stool softeners are very effective.

Surgical Techniques

Painful thrombosed external hemorrhoids that are not improving or are worsening should be excised. This can almost always be done in the office and consists of excising the clot, vein, and part of the overlying skin in an elliptical fashion under local anesthesia. Removing just the clot is incomplete and can lead to persistent bleeding or rethrombosis.

Internal hemorrhoids that are advanced, bleeding, and that *do not* prolapse (first degree) or fail medical management can be treated in one of two ways. The simplest is by banding, which can be done in the office (Fig. 21-8). The hemorrhoid is pulled into the bander by either a clamp or suction, and a small rubber band is applied at the base. This is done with the aid of an anoscope, and it is important to place the band on the mucosa above the dentate line where no sensation exists. The banded tissue sloughs in 4-8 days, sometimes with a small amount of bleeding. Up to two bands can be placed at one time, and repeated bandings may be necessary for large hemorrhoids. Surgical excision of internal hemorrhoids is best for large or prolapsed hemorrhoids or for those that fail banding. This is performed in the operating room under local with IV sedation, spinal, or general. The patient is placed in the prone, jackknife position, and the buttocks are separated with adhesive tape to aid exposure. An anal retractor is used to expose each hemorrhoidal column to be excised. Injecting the anal canal with local anesthetics and 1:200,000 epinephrine before excision can aid in hemostasis. The column is then excised in a longitudinal ellipse, extending from the most proximal aspect within the rectum, out onto the anoderm (Fig. 21-9). The entire column is removed down to the internal sphincter, which should be identified by its white fibers and left uninjured. Bleeding can be stopped with either cautery or suture ligation at the base of the incision. The edges of the mucosa are then undermined slightly to allow tension-free closure with a running, absorbable stitch. Typically, all three columns are removed to prevent recurrence, unless they are completely uninvolved, or concern exists about anal stenosis from excessive tissue loss. The most important aspects of this procedure are hemostasis, complete excision of the hemorrhoidal tissue without injury to the sphincter, and avoidance of excessive tissue excision, which can lead to anal stenosis.

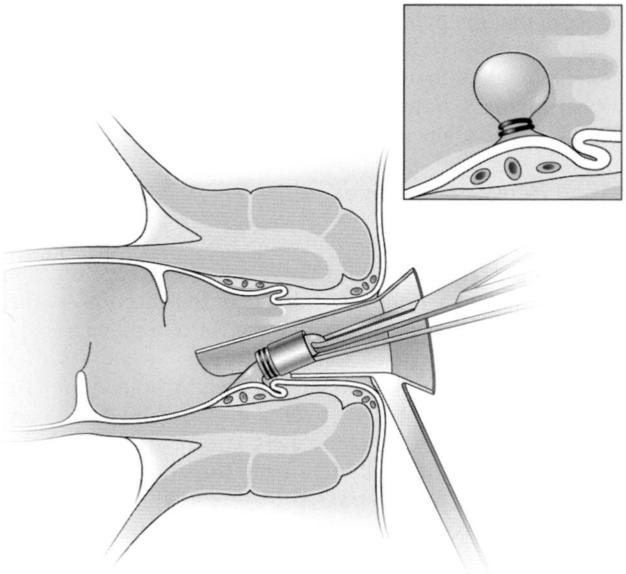

FIGURE 21–8 Rubber-band ligation of a first-degree internal hemorrhoid.

Outcomes

Excellent results follow surgical excision of thrombosed external hemorrhoids when the vein is included. Successful banding of internal hemorrhoids depends on the number of bands placed. As many as 80% of patients state that their condition is much improved after a single ligation, but barely half are completely asymptomatic. Results are better with multiple bands. Surgical excision of internal hemorrhoids gives the best results when all three vascular cushions are excised.

Complications

Although uncommon, complications of excising thrombosed external hemorrhoids are limited to bleeding, infection, or recurrence. With banding of internal hemorrhoids, the biggest risk, although rare, is overwhelmingly sepsis, and several deaths have been reported. Bleeding, severe pain, thrombosis, and urinary retention make up the majority of the 5% to 6% complication rate. Surgical excision carries the same risks as banding, in addition to incontinence and anal stenosis. The latter is secondary to removing too much anoderm. Postoperative bleeding from the suture line can sometimes require a return to the operating room. Reinspecting all suture lines at the completion of the case and oversewing those that are oozing can help to prevent this problem.

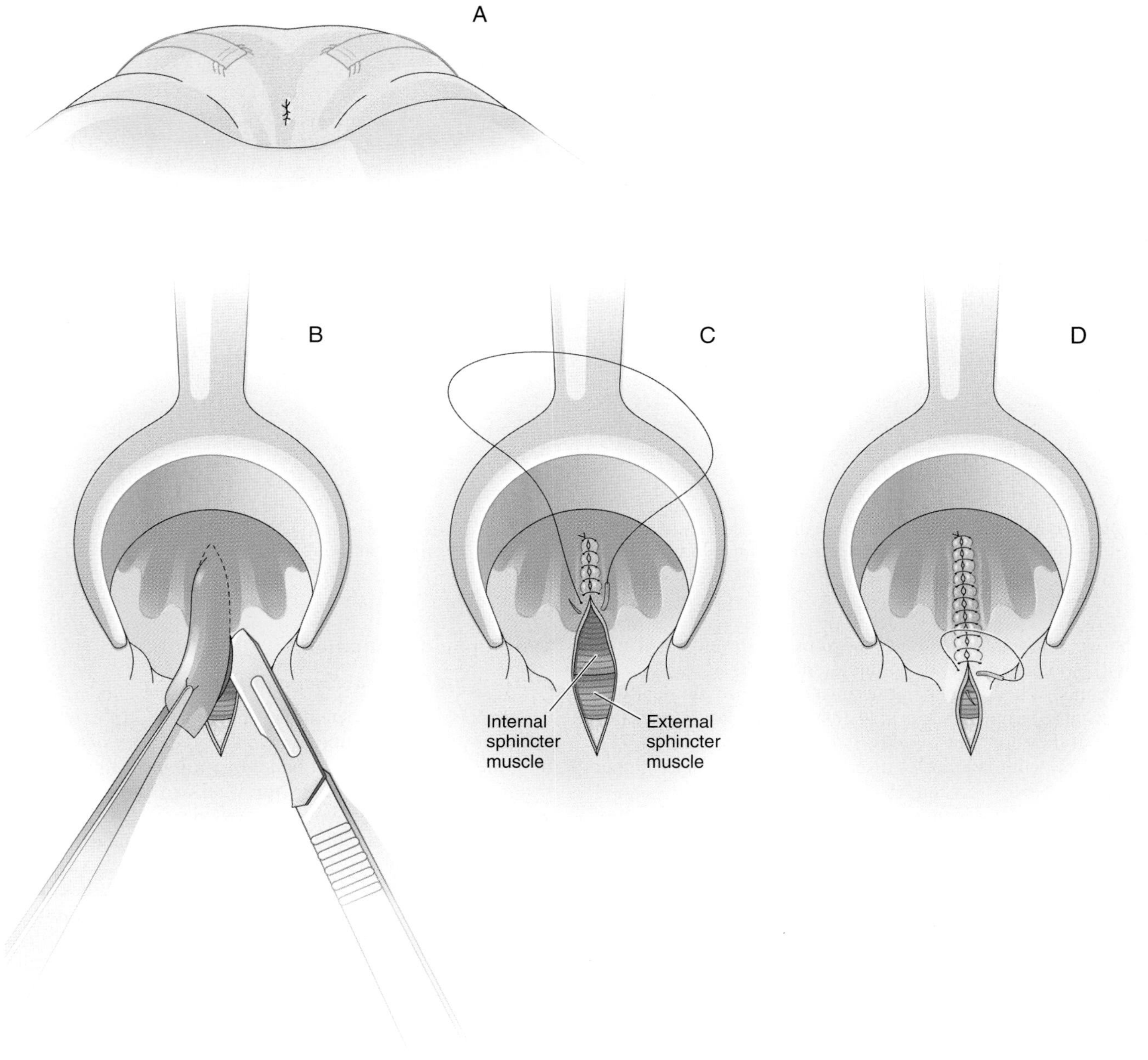

FIGURE 21–9 Classic "closed" hemorrhoidectomy. *A*, Prone jackknife position. *B*, Excise column. *C*, Identify sphincter muscle. *D*, Close edges using absorbable sutures.

Anorectal Abscess/Fistula-in-Ano

Pathophysiology

Most anorectal abscesses are believed to be cryptoglandular in origin (Fig. 21-10). An abscess starts from an infected anal gland, which begins at the dentate line and terminates within the intersphincteric space. The infection can remain within this space or extend by fistulizing into the ischiorectal, supralevator, or perianal space. Most commonly, it extends into the ischiorectal space, and the patient has a swollen, red, tender area on the buttock. Drainage of this abscess then creates a fistulous connection

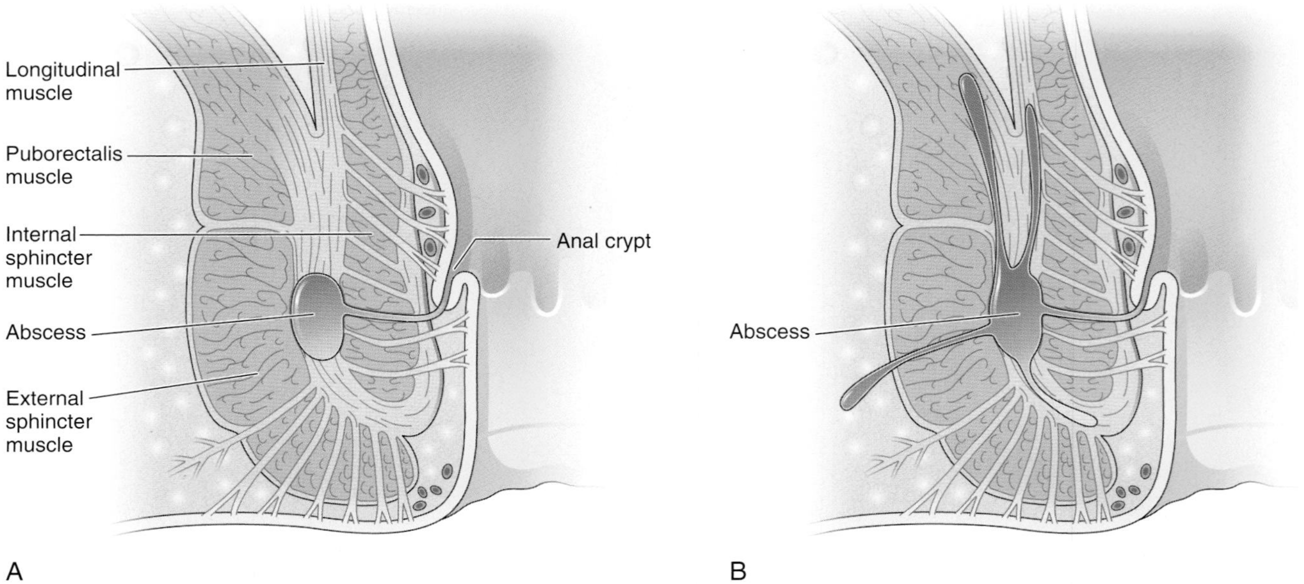

FIGURE 21–10 Cryptoglandular origin of anal abscess. *A*, Note the infection starting in the anal crypt and extending intrasphincterically to form an abscess. *B*, Extensions from the intramuscular abscess occur in several directions.

between the anal canal and the skin. However, this fistula will spontaneously be obliterated in 50% to 70% of patients. When it does not, it must be opened surgically to prevent recurrent infections. Fistula tracks follow Goodsall's rule, if they are not caused by Crohn's disease (Fig. 21-11). Patients with Crohn's disease have a much higher incidence of anorectal abscesses than does the general population. They can sometimes be the initial presenting symptom of the disease. Patients with recurrent or multiple abscesses should be evaluated for Crohn's.

Symptoms

Most anorectal abscesses are first seen with a painful, red, swollen area on the perianal skin. The symptoms usually develop over 1 or many days. Occasionally, the abscess will drain spontaneously, and the patient will have a fistula. The fistula will produce persistent tenderness with a mucus discharge. A small opening near the anus is usually seen. Recurrent abscesses are almost always due to the presence of a fistula. An intersphincteric abscess will often cause rectal pain, but no abnormalities will be seen. A digital examination will be extremely painful, but a mass will not always be palpable, because they can be small.

Differential Diagnosis

Anorectal pain is usually due to an abscess, fistula, or thrombosed hemorrhoid. Physical examination should easily differentiate these three conditions.

Workup and Evaluation

History and Physical Examination

A patient with diabetes can have a more extensive infection than the symptoms would predict. A history of multiple abscesses should make one think of a persistent fistula and/or Crohn's. Pain for weeks to months or the presence of bleeding would make one think more of a thrombosed hemorrhoid or anal fissure. External examination of the anal area usually provides a diagnosis. A digital examination can sometimes show an internal abscess but should be abandoned if the patient is in severe pain and the diagnosis is obvious. The extension of swelling and erythema onto the scrotum or crepitus is a sign of perineal necrotizing fasciitis (Fournier's gangrene), which requires immediate surgical debridement and which is life threatening.

Laboratory Tests and Imaging

A WBC may be helpful if the diagnosis is in question, but usually this is unnecessary. Rarely needed, a CT scan is helpful for a supralevator abscess.

Treatment Alternatives

Expectant

An abscess will often erupt through the perianal skin if a patient seeks no treatment. On presentation to a physician, an undrained abscess should be opened.

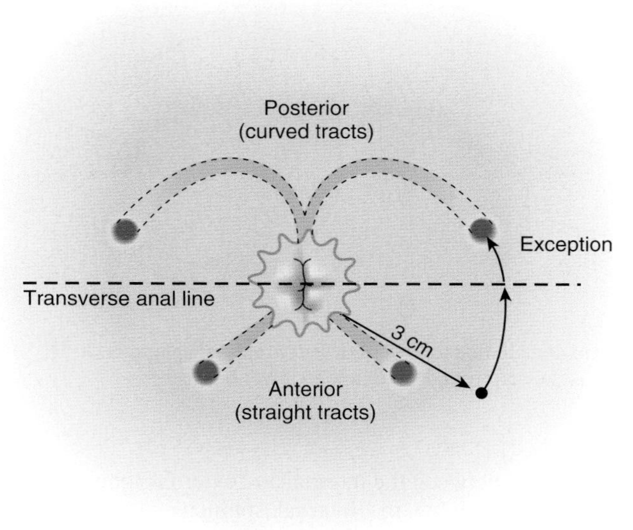

FIGURE 21–11 Goodsall's rule.

Medical

Antibiotics alone have no role in the treatment of an anorectal abscess. If an abscess has adequately drained on its own, antibiotics may help the induration subside. Perianal cellulitis will sometimes develop in neutropenic patients, but they are unable to form pus. Because no abscess is present to drain, antibiotics will usually resolve this condition.

Surgical Techniques

Anorectal abscesses often can be drained in the office or in the emergency department under local anesthesia. Spinal or general anesthesia is needed for complex abscesses (i.e., Crohn's), large abscesses, and in those patients who cannot tolerate any pain. A cruciate incision is made over the most fluctuant area. A packing is placed initially to provide hemostasis and should be removed within 12 to 24 hours, and then warm soaks for 20 minutes, 3 times a day are begun to aid healing. Repacking is painful and unnecessary. The patient should be seen within 10 days to make sure a fistula is not present. Antibiotics are generally not necessary unless the patient is diabetic or impressive induration or cellulitis is present.

A fistula-in-ano requires probing under spinal or general anesthesia. This can be done in one stage, if superficial, or two stages if it encircles the sphincter muscle. A probe is used to identify the tract, and if no external anal sphincter muscle is incorporated, the tissue is divided down to the probe, and the tract curetted. If muscle *is* involved, a "cutting" seton is placed to allow fibrosis of the tract, so that division at a second stage will decrease the chance of incontinence.

Outcomes

Most patients do very well with outpatient drainage. Recurrences are usually due to inadequate drainage, a persistent fistula, or the presence of Crohn's disease.

Complications

Fistula formation after an abscess is not a complication but is the nature of the disease. A fistulotomy carries a risk of incontinence if the sphincter is partially divided. If this is a concern, it should be carried out in multiple stages.

Anal Fissure

Pathophysiology

Anal fissures are small tears in the anoderm typically in the posterior midline, although sometimes seen anteriorly. Any fissure off the midline should raise suspicion for Crohn's disease. They are most commonly caused by the passage of a large or hard stool; however, diarrhea can sometimes be the culprit. Often healing on their own, they sometimes require medical or surgical management. Failure to heal has been ascribed to persistent trauma from hard stools, poor blood supply, spasm of the internal sphincter, or a combination of these. Chronic fissures (>3 weeks) often have a sentinel skin tag at the distal aspect caused by inflammation.

Symptoms

The small size of a fissure belies the great amount of pain it can cause. This pain is usually initiated with each bowel movement and can last several hours. The expectant pain with defecation can compound the problem by causing increasing constipation and harder stools. Blood also can be seen and is usually on the tissue.

Differential Diagnosis

Patients with anal pain usually have a fissure, an abscess, or a thrombosed *external* hemorrhoid. Physical examination easily differentiates these conditions. Rectal bleeding, as discussed earlier, requires at least an endoscopic examination of the rectosigmoid, if not a full colon evaluation.

Workup and Evaluation

History and Physical Examination

Commonly, the onset of symptoms can be pinpointed to a day, and often to the passage of a hard stool. Pain often subsides between bowel movements, and sometimes for longer, until recurring under the same conditions. Bleeding should not be profuse. Examination generally shows a small, radial tear in the anoderm, with or without a sentinel skin tag, and internal sphincter muscle fibers can sometimes be identified at the base of the tear. Identification can

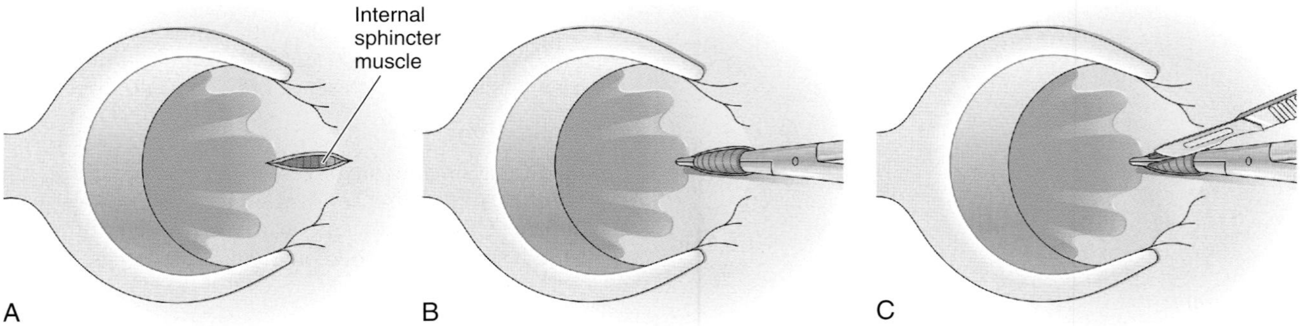

FIGURE 21–12 Lateral internal sphincterotomy. *A*, Incision is made from dentate line to lower border of internal sphincter. *B*, Internal sphincter is dissected off external sphincter. *C*, Internal sphincter is incised from dentate line to lower border.

be difficult in patients who are large, have a long anal canal, or cannot relax because of severe pain.

Laboratory Tests and Imaging

Laboratory tests are unnecessary. Imaging studies are not helpful.

Treatment Alternatives

Expectant

Fissures will sometimes heal on their own but will often recur unless the diet is adjusted. Symptoms that bring a patient to the physician's office require some form of treatment.

Medical

The best form of initial treatment is correcting the constipation with a high-fiber diet, increased liquid intake, and the addition of a bulking agent and a stool softener. Sitz baths and lidocaine jelly applied to the fissure can sometimes decrease the pain until the fissure is healed. This approach in acute anal fissures will lead to healing in the majority of patients (85%). Chronic (>3 weeks) and recurrent fissures do not respond as well. Recently, nitroglycerin paste has been used placed on these chronic fissures; the hypothesis being that the nitroglycerin will improve blood supply to the area and aid in the healing process. This is applied in a 0.2% paste to the anal opening twice a day. Results in Europe have been far better than those in the United States. Severe headache, a reported side effect, mandates discontinuation of the medication.

Surgical Techniques

Fissures that fail conservative management are best treated with surgery. The most widely used approach is a lateral internal sphincterotomy (Fig. 21-12). This can be performed under local, spinal, or general anesthesia. With the sphincter mechanism on slight stretch, one can easily feel the groove between the internal and external sphincter. The anoderm overlying the internal sphincter is then incised (most commonly over the left lateral wall of the anal canal), and the muscle is then divided up to the dentate line. The incision is then sutured closed. The fissure can either be excised or left alone.

Outcomes

Medical management is effective about 50% of the time. About 33% of medically treated patients will ultimately fail. Most recurrences, however, will continue to respond to conservative treatment. Surgical treatment is extremely effective, with symptoms resolving 95% to 98% of the time.

Complications

The biggest risk of sphincterotomy is incontinence. Incontinence to gas or liquid is reported to be as high as 30% after surgical treatment. This almost always is temporary, resolving within a few weeks. Infection and bleeding are rare occurrences.

Suggested Reading

Bell AM, Pemberton JH, Hanson RB, Zinsmeister AR: Variations in muscle tone of the human rectum: Recordings with an electromechanical barostat. Am J Physiol 260:917, 1991.

Drossman DA, Degnon Associates: Rome II: The Functional Gastrointestinal Disorders, 2nd ed. McLean, VA, 2000, p 382.

Fazio VW, Fletcher J, Montague D: Prospective study of the effect of resection of the rectum on male sexual function. World J Surg 4:149, 1980.

Ferrara A, Pemberton JH, Hansen ESR: Relationships between anal canal tone and rectal motor activity. Dis Colon Rectum 34:4–5, 1993.

Ferrara A, Pemberton JH, Hanson RB: Preservation of continence after ileoanal anastomosis by the coordination of the ileal pouch and anal canal motor activity. Am J Surg 163:83–89, 1992.

Goldberg SM, Gordon PH, Nivatvongs S: Essentials of Anorectal Surgery. Philadelphia, JB Lippincott, 1980.

Goligher JC: Surgery of the Anus, Rectum, and Colon, 5th ed. London, Bailliere Tindall, 1984.

Heald RJ, Moran BJ: Embryology and anatomy of the rectum. Semin Surg Oncol 15:66–71, 1998.

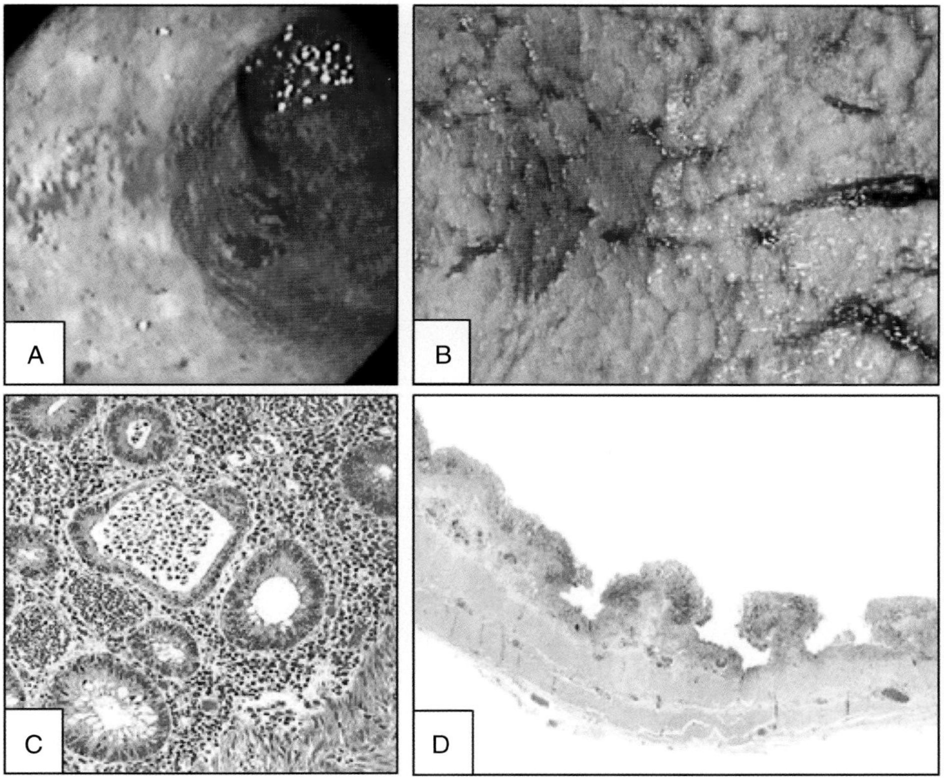

FIGURE 22–1 Ulcerative colitis. *A*, Endoscopic view of the sigmoid colon. *B*, Resected rectosigmoid mucosa showing swollen, congested, and ulcerated mucosa. *C*, Hematoxylin-eosin (H&E)-stained histologic section of mucosa showing crypt abscess and basal plasmacytosis. *D*, H&E-stained whole-mount section showing broad-based, undermined ulcers confined to the mucosa. Note the absence of fibrosis with no evidence of transmural inflammation.

hallmark of UC, tenesmus, fecal urgency, mucoid rectal discharge, crampy abdominal pain, and fever can accompany the advanced condition. Extraintestinal manifestations of UC can be observed in a number of organ systems, including articular disorders, lesions of the skin and oral cavity, liver and biliary tract disorders, thromboembolic disease, and vasculitis.

In addition to the clinical sequelae, endoscopic and histologic evaluations greatly facilitate the diagnosis. Endoscopically, the mucosa of affected areas of the colon can appear granular and friable (Fig. 22-1*A*). After resection, mucosa of affected areas typically appear swollen, congested, and ulcerated (see Fig. 22-1*B*). As the disease worsens, these affected areas can contain superficial ulceration accompanied by a mucopurulent exudate. The diagnosis is further confirmed histologically by a marked abundance of inflammatory cells such as neutrophils, lymphocytes, plasma cells, and macrophages within the lamina propria as well as crypt abscesses and basal plasmacytosis (see Fig. 22-1*C*). Microabscesses accompanied by neutrophils and mucin-depleted goblet cells also are evident within the colonic crypts. As the disease progresses, the inflammatory infiltrate becomes more marked and is accompanied by the production of cytokines, chemokines, and other proinflammatory mediators that can perpetuate and exacerbate inflammation. A typical whole-mount section (see Fig. 22-1*D*) shows broad-based undermined ulcers confined to the mucosa with no evidence of fibrosis or transmural inflammation.

Crohn's Disease

In sharp contrast to UC, in which the disease is confined to the colorectal mucosa, CD is characterized by a segmental inflammation that can affect any portion of the alimentary tract. Ileocolitis or inflammation of the large and small intestine occurs in approximately 40% of CD patients and is the most common presentation. Inflammation isolated to either the small or large intestine are the second and third most common distributions of CD, respectively, whereas involvement in other portions of the alimentary tract is considerably less frequent. Depending on the location and severity, endoscopy can reveal severe disease with stricturing typically associated with CD (Fig. 22-2*A*). After resection, affected areas can show fissuring ulcerations (Fig. 22-2*B*) as well as fistulae, sinus tracts, and abscesses that, when present, can facilitate a differential diagnosis. The clinical manifestations associated with CD tend to be more varied than those with UC because, in part, of the heterogeneity of inflammation along the alimentary tract. Because the predominant distribution appears to be in the

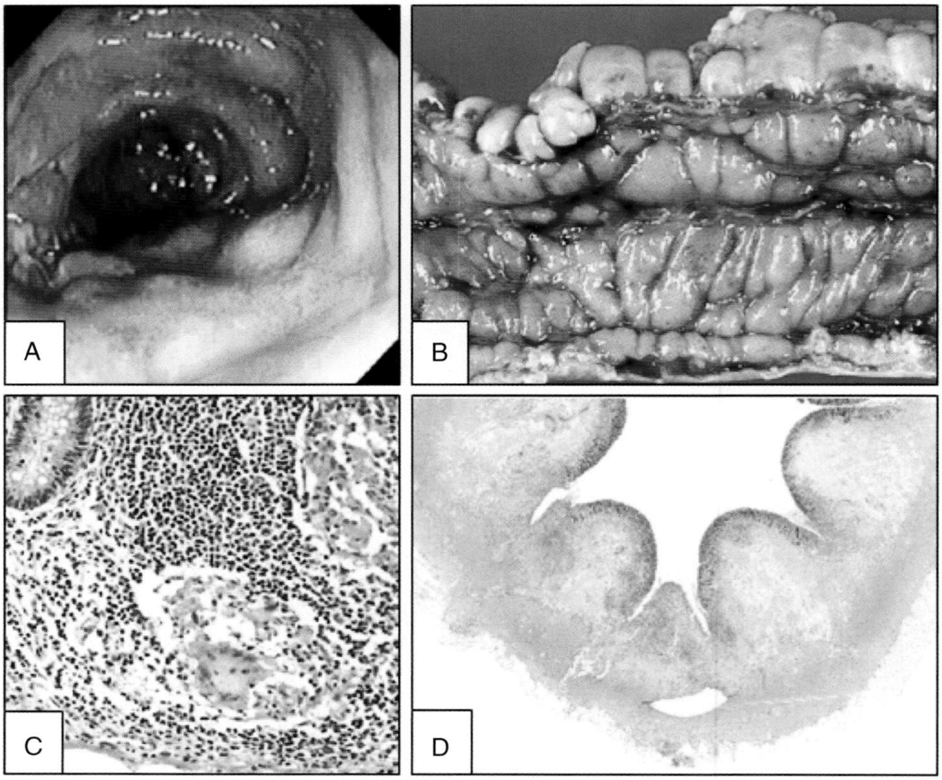

FIGURE 22–2 Crohn's disease. *A*, Endoscopic view of the sigmoid colon with severe disease and strictures. *B*, Resected rectosigmoid showing fissuring ulcerations. *C*, H&E-stained histologic section of deep mucosa showing lymphoid aggregate and giant cell granulomas. *D*, H&E-stained whole-mount section showing ulcers lined by inflamed granulation tissue with submucosal and subserosal fibrosis. Pale blue nodules in submucosa and subserosa correspond to lymphoid aggregates and granulomas.

ileum and ascending or right colon, right lower quadrant pain is frequently noted. Diarrhea also is common, as are weight loss and fever.

The lesions associated with CD typically extend transmurally beyond the mucosa and submucosa, reflecting perhaps a more complex inflammatory process. Inflamed tissues are often characterized by marked infiltrates of macrophages and lymphocytes that can extend deep into the intestinal wall. Deep mucosal areas can often contain lymphoid aggregates and giant cell granulomas (Fig. 22-2*C*), which can lead to the formation of noncaseating granulomata in 50% of the CD patients. Deep, fissuring, or serpiginous ulcers can be present in more advanced cases and can lead to fistula formation. Intramural collagen deposition leading to submucosal and subserosal fibrosis can be remarkable (Fig. 22-2*D*), and in concert with edema and inflammation, can contribute to bowel wall thickening and stricture formation.

Medical Therapy

A number of common therapeutic doctrines guide the treatment of UC and CD, and these principles of medical therapy can be similar for either disease. Although the primary therapy for uncomplicated UC and CD is medical, surgery is often used for specific complications that are discussed later. The goal of any therapeutic regimen is to control the acute and chronic inflammatory processes, but other factors that might play a role in therapy, such as the patient's nutritional status, should be considered. Important differences exist between the treatment of UC and CD, such as the response to drug therapy, type and severity of drug-related complications, as well as their continued use after surgical therapy, which must be carefully considered when monitoring these patients.

Ulcerative Colitis

Once the diagnosis of UC has been clearly established, the decision regarding the implementation of medical therapy depends on the severity of symptoms and on the extent and severity of disease, as indicated by the patient's clinical history, endoscopic or radiographic studies, and histologic evaluations. Drugs commonly used in the treatment of various stages of UC include sulfasalazine and its acetylsalicylic acid (ASA) analogues, corticosteroids, immunomodulators, suppressive antimetabolites, and certain antibiotics (Box 22-1). Symptomatic antidiarrheals and antispasmodic agents also can be used in combination therapy.

Sulfasalazine has been a mainstay in the management of the chronic UC since the early 1950s. Sulfasalazine consists

BOX 22-1 Drugs Commonly Used in the Medical Management of Ulcerative Colitis

Active Disease

Mild–Moderate Disease
- **Distal colon**
  - Sulfasalazine or 5-ASA (oral or topical)
  - Topical corticosteroid
  - **Extensive colitis**
  - Sulfasalazine or oral 5-ASA

Moderate–Severe Disease
- **Distal colon**
  - Topical or oral 5-ASA
  - Topical corticosteroid
  - Prednisone
  - Infliximab
- **Extensive colitis**
  - Prednisone

Severe–Fulminant Disease
- **Distal or extensive colitis**
  - Intravenous corticosteroids
  - Intravenous cyclosporine

Maintenance Therapy
- **Distal colitis**
  - Sulfasalazine or 5-ASA (oral or topical)
  - Azathioprine or 6-MP
- **Extensive colitis**
- Sulfasalazine or oral 5-ASA
- Azathioprine or 6-MP

5-ASA, 5-animosalicylic acid; 6-MP, 6-mercaptopurine.

of an antibacterial sulfapyridine moiety chemically linked to 5-aminosalicylate (5-ASA), a potent anti-inflammatory. Bacterial cleavage in the colon liberates the ASA moiety that is believed to be the active component, exerting its pharmacologic action through the inhibition of the mucosal prostaglandin synthesis. Most of the drug's relatively common side effects are attributable to the sulfapyridine moiety. Sulfasalazine has been found to be effective in treating 75% to 80% of patients with mild to moderate disease but does little for patients with severe disease.

In an effort to eliminate the side effects associated with sulfapyridine, newer ASA derivatives of sulfasalazine, such as 5-ASA and 4-ASA, have become the primary therapy of mild to moderate UC. To facilitate the drug in reaching the target site of active mucosal inflammation, tablets are coated and dissolve only at an alkaline pH typical of the terminal ileum or colon. In studies to date, these compounds have been shown to be as efficacious as sulfasalazine in treating mild to moderate acute UC, as well as in maintenance therapy. Other common therapeutic modalities for treatment of mild to moderate distal UC are topical corticosteroids such as steroid enemas, foams, and suppositories.

Patients with moderate to severe UC may require systemic therapy. These patients initially can be managed with topical steroid therapy and oral sulfasalazine or ASA. If they do not respond to this regimen, oral corticosteroids are introduced and have become the mainstay of therapy during acute attacks. A single daily dose of prednisone between 40 and 60 mg is effective in inducing remission. If clinical symptoms and sigmoidoscopic findings improve, the steroid dosage can be tapered after several weeks. Although steroids may be useful in controlling symptoms in patients with continuing activity, maintenance therapy with low-dose corticosteroids for patients with inactive disease has not been demonstrated to prevent relapse. Patients must be monitored carefully for the long-term adverse sequelae of corticosteroid use, including hypertension, hyperglycemia, cataracts, osteoporosis, and osteomalacia.

A number of immunosuppressive agents have been used for the management of UC, including azathioprine and its metabolite, 6-mercaptopurine. Because immunosuppressive agents do not produce a clinical response for several months, they have no role in treatment of acute flares of UC. Cyclosporine, which has a more rapid onset of action, has been advocated for the treatment of severe, steroid-refractory UC; however, significant risk of irreversible cyclosporine-associated nephropathy and infectious complications also may occur.

Approximately 10% to 20% of patients with severe UC have a clinical course that ultimately requires hospitalization. These patients generally need nutritional support, with either intravenous hyperalimentation or total parenteral nutrition (TPN) and correction of anemia. Patients with more active disease or toxicity require parenteral steroids such as hydrocortisone. TPN plays no primary role in ameliorating the inflammatory response in UC but allows nutritional maintenance and repletion during the treatment phase. During an acute episode of severe colitis, narcotic pain medications and antidiarrheals should be avoided to prevent provocation of toxic megacolon. Once the patient has responded clinically, oral foods can be started, and the patient can begin receiving oral steroids as parenteral steroids are tapered.

Although some evidence supports a microbial factor in the etiology of UC, the therapeutic role of antibiotics remains controversial. Antibiotics such as metronidazole and ciprofloxacin are still widely prescribed for UC; however, clinical trials in patients with acute UC have shown limited efficacy.

Crohn's Disease

As in UC, the primary goal of the medical treatment for CD is to induce and maintain remission. Standard therapy for active CD depends largely on the location, extent, and severity of the disease and consists mainly of the same drugs used in the treatment of UC, such as

BOX 22-2 Drugs Commonly Used in the Medical Management of Crohn's Disease

Active Disease

Mild–Moderate Disease
- Sulfasalazine or oral 5-ASA
- Metronidazole
- Prednisone
- Azathioprine or 6-MP
- Infliximab

Severe Disease
- Prednisone
- Intravenous corticosteroids
- TPN or elemental diet
- Infliximab
- Intravenous cyclosporine

Perianal or Fistulizing Disease
- Metronidazole or alternative antibiotic
- Azathioprine or 6-MP
- Infliximab
- Intravenous cyclosporine

Maintenance Therapy
- Sulfasalazine or oral 5-ASA
- Metronidazole
- Azathioprine or 6-MP

5-ASA, 5-animosalicylic acid; 6-MP, 6-mercaptopurine; TPN, total parenteral nutrition.

PEARLS FOR ROUNDS

In sharp contrast to ulcerative colitis (UC), in which the disease is confined to the colorectal mucosa, Crohn's disease (CD) is characterized by a segmental inflammation that can affect any portion of the alimentary tract. The lesions associated with CD typically extend transmurally beyond the mucosa and submucosa, reflecting perhaps a more complex inflammatory process.

Ulcerative colitis usually is first seen with bloody diarrhea, abdominal pain, and fever.

Extraintestinal manifestations of UC are observed in a number of organ systems, including articular disorders, lesions of the skin and oral cavity, inflammatory disorders of the eye, liver and biliary tract disorders, thromboembolic disease, and vasculitis.

The principal categories of drug treatment for UC include symptomatic antidiarrheal and antispasmodic agents, sulfasalazine and its analogues, corticosteroids, immunosuppressive antimetabolites, and certain antibiotics.

Standard medical therapy for active CD depends largely on the location, extent, and severity of the disease, and consists mainly of the same drugs used in the treatment of UC, such as corticosteroids, anti-inflammatory agents, and immunomodulators.

corticosteroids, anti-inflammatory agents, and immunomodulators (Box 22-2). In addition, a new class of highly efficacious biologic response modifiers aimed at neutralizing the deleterious effects of the proinflammatory cytokine TNF-α are gaining widespread use in the treatment of CD and more recently UC. Unlike those with UC, the management of fistula and abscess formation associated with CD can often become treatment goals unto themselves. These conditions can frequently be complicated by intra-abdominal sepsis that can significantly complicate and, in some cases, preclude medical therapy.

The indolent nature of CD often attenuates the response to therapy compared with that for UC, and the disease tends to advance despite apparent clinical inactivity or even remission. Hence, it may be more difficult to achieve total clinical remission and to discontinue medical therapy completely. Medical therapy for the management of colonic CD can be quite similar to that for UC. Patients with active colonic CD respond well to sulfasalazine at doses similar to those used for UC, whereas patients with small-bowel involvement show significant improvement with prednisone. Despite a satisfactory response to treatment of Crohn's colitis, manifestations such as steady weight loss, diarrhea, and a decline of general health seem to persist in many patients. Recurrent problems of Crohn's colitis include perianal disease, perineal fistula formation, and perirectal abscesses associated predominantly with left-sided colonic disease. The use of immunomodulatory agents has become efficacious and reasonably safe for selected patients with CD. Indications for treatment with azathioprine and 6-mercaptopurine include managing moderate to severe disease activity as well as fistulizing, refractory, and steroid-dependent CD. Although the addition of these immunosuppressive agents can facilitate and maintain remission, the initial response may require several months.

The management of CD of the small intestine is often similar to that for colonic CD, but treatment can be complicated in patients having disease manifestations in both the small intestine and colon. Acute inflammatory episodes with stricturing and intestinal obstruction are a common presentation in patients with ileal involvement. Although flare-ups generally respond to corticosteroids, as these episodes recur and fibrosis develops, steroid therapy becomes less effective, and surgical decompression may be required. Progressive fibrotic involvement of the small intestine, perhaps compounded by one or more surgical resections, can result in a significant loss of absorptive surface. Because CD is generally catabolic, subsequent nutritional deficiencies due to lack of absorption can significantly impair the patient's overall health. Significant improvements in TPN formulations have led to its increasing role in managing these patients. TPN has been used with increasing frequency in severely ill patients as a means of resting the bowel and preparing poorly nourished patients for surgery. TPN also can be efficacious in treating children with extensive small-bowel CD or short-bowel syndrome who are exhibiting severe growth failure associated with CD.

As mentioned earlier, a number of new therapeutic modalities are revolutionizing the treatment of patients with moderate to severe refractory CD. Perhaps at the forefront of the newer agents are the biologic therapies such as infliximab, a monoclonal antibody that blocks the action of TNF-α, an important cause of the inflammation in CD. Infliximab is effective in inducing remission, but usually an immunosuppressive is required to keep patients in remission. Studies are in progress to determine the long-term effects of this medication since serious life-threatening and fatal side effects have occurred. Infliximab is beneficial in the treatment of fistulous CD as well. Other treatments that reduce TNF-α production, such as thalidomide, are efficacious in treating patients with chronically active, steroid-dependent CD. Other newer treatments for CD include the use of probiotics such as lactobacilli and bifidobacteria, especially in maintaining remission.

Surgical Therapy

Ulcerative Colitis

Approximately 20% to 30% of patients with chronic UC will undergo proctocolectomy within a decade after diagnosis, not only because of the chronic, debilitating nature of the disease and the high incidence of relapse, but also because of the significant risk of malignant degeneration. Numerous indications for surgery are seen in these patients, each with unique implications with respect to both timing and surgical options. Surgical intervention is indicated for any of the following conditions: unremitting hemorrhage, fulminating UC that is unresponsive to therapy, obstruction from stricture, high-grade dysplasia or frank colonic cancer, overwhelming systemic complications, toxic megacolon, and intractability. With the advent over the last two decades of sphincter-sparing operations for patients with any of the aforementioned complications associated with UC, it has become critically important to avoid standard proctectomy and to diagnostically distinguish patients with UC from those with CD.

Numerous surgical options exist for patients with UC because the disease is essentially cured after the removal of the colon and rectum. Elective operations for UC include total proctocolectomy with either a Brooke or continent ileostomy (Kock pouch), subtotal colectomy with either ileostomy or ileorectal anastomosis, or colectomy with mucosal proctectomy and ileal pouch–anal anastomosis (IPAA). When single-stage total proctocolectomy with ileostomy was the only alternative, patients frequently delayed surgery to the point at which their health and lifestyle were significantly compromised. Although this surgical procedure eliminated all disease-bearing tissue, the significant physical, psychological, and social implications of a permanent abdominal ileostomy, or Brooke ileostomy, remain poorly accepted by most patients, particularly the young and physically active. Hence, surgeons began to seek alternatives to total proctocolectomy with ileostomy. With the advent of newer surgical alternatives such as IPAA, patients and physicians are electing surgery much earlier in the course of disease.

Subtotal colectomy with either the construction of a Brooke end ileostomy (Fig. 22-3), and Hartmann closure of the rectum or an ileorectal anastomosis (Fig. 22-4) has been used in the surgical treatment of UC for decades. If an ileorectal anastomosis is performed, the abdominal stoma can be eliminated, and with the preservation of the pelvic autonomic nerves, impotence and bladder dysfunction are rare. In any of the surgical emergencies described earlier, subtotal colectomy with ileostomy is the preferred surgical procedure, and although full continence is usually preserved, it does not eliminate all disease-bearing tissue contained within the retained rectum. The procedure is associated with a number of postoperative complications, including small-bowel obstruction and leakage of the anastomosis between the ileum and the disease-bearing rectum. The operation is clearly contraindicated in patients with sphincter dysfunction, severe rectal disease, rectal dysplasia, or frank cancer.

In an effort to overcome the inherent problems associated with a Brooke ileostomy described earlier, Kock developed the continent ileostomy. Constructed entirely of ileum, the intestinal pouch serves as a reservoir for stool, with an ileal conduit connecting the pouch to a cutaneous stoma (Fig. 22-5). The operation was later modified by the addition of an intestinal nipple valve between the pouch and the stoma to facilitate evacuation with a soft plastic tube passed through the valve via the stoma. Although the operation eliminates all disease-bearing tissue and has advantages over the Brooke ileostomy such as offering the patient both continence and the freedom of an external appliance, the continent ileostomy has been associated with a high number of complications. These include a high rate of mechanical, functional, and metabolic complications that have limited its clinical usefulness. Although few Kock pouches are being constructed now, the continent ileostomy may be useful in patients who have already undergone total proctocolectomy and ileostomy and desire to undertake a continence-restoring procedure.

These early operations were curative, but patients continued to have significant long-term psychosocial and medical complications, compelling surgeons to seek alternatives to total proctocolectomy with ileostomy. Because UC is a mucosal disease confined to the colon and rectum, no need mandates ablation of the entire rectum,

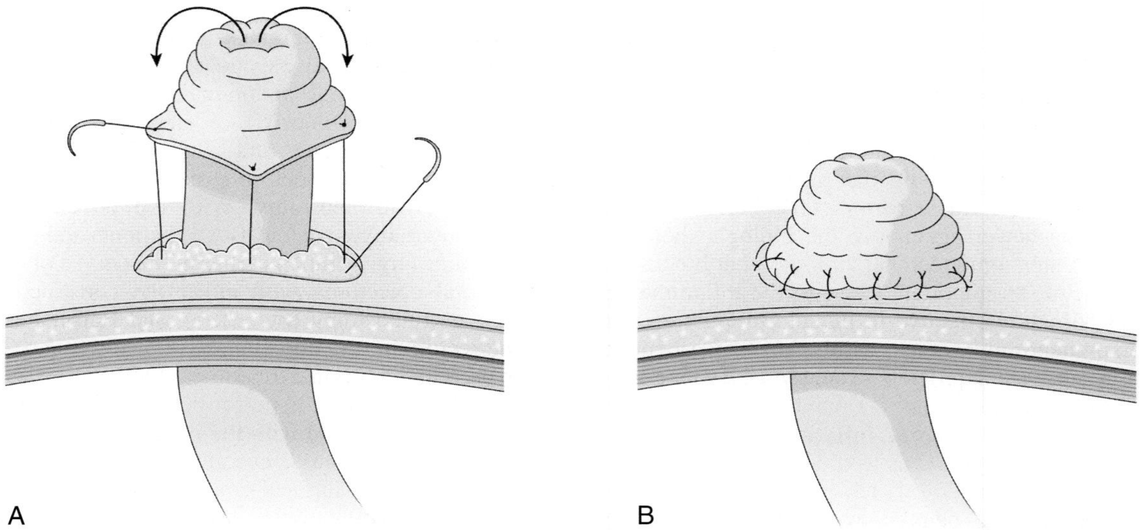

FIGURE 22–3 Construction of an end ileostomy. *A*, The terminal ileum is brought 5 cm through an abdominal wall defect, everted. *B*, It is sutured to the more proximal ileal seromuscularis and the dermis to mature the ileostomy.

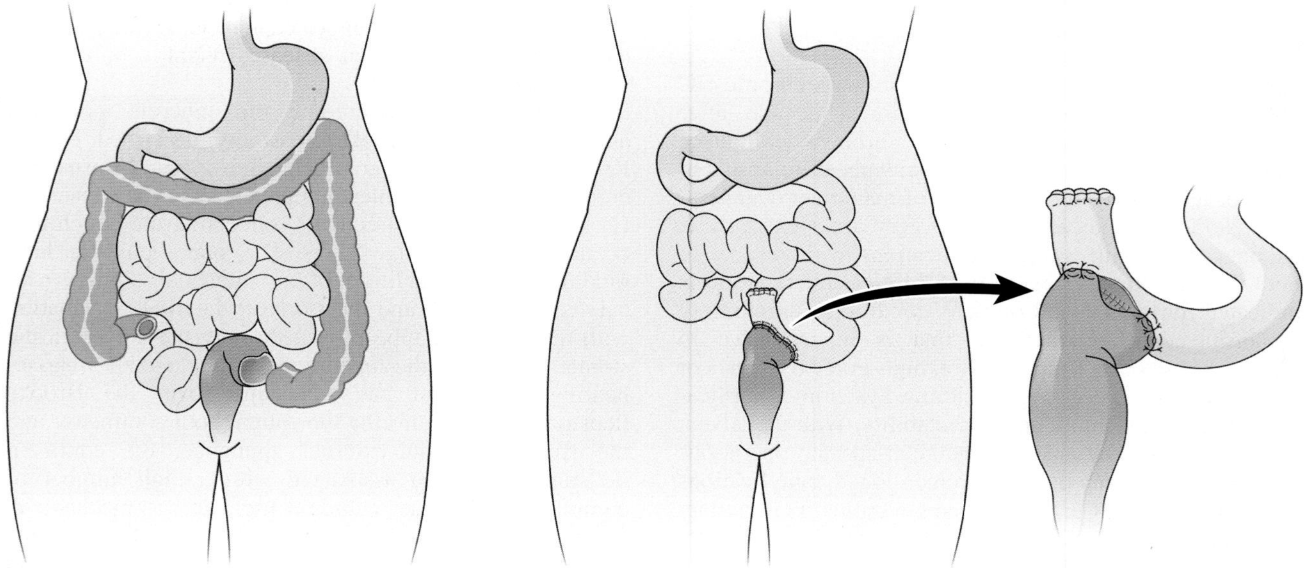

FIGURE 22–4 Ileorectal anastomosis after abdominal colectomy. This represents a nondefinitive operation for selected patients with chronic ulcerative colitis.

anus, and anal sphincter. Instead, the rectal mucosa can be selectively dissected out and removed down to the dentate line of the anus. By carefully preserving the rectal muscular cuff and anal sphincter, we can reestablish continuity of the intestinal tract by extending the ileum into the pelvis endorectally, and circumferentially suturing it to the anus in an end-to-end fashion (Fig. 22-6). This approach offered the advantages of a total proctocolectomy by removing all diseased tissue, and because the pelvic dissection is confined to the endorectal plane,

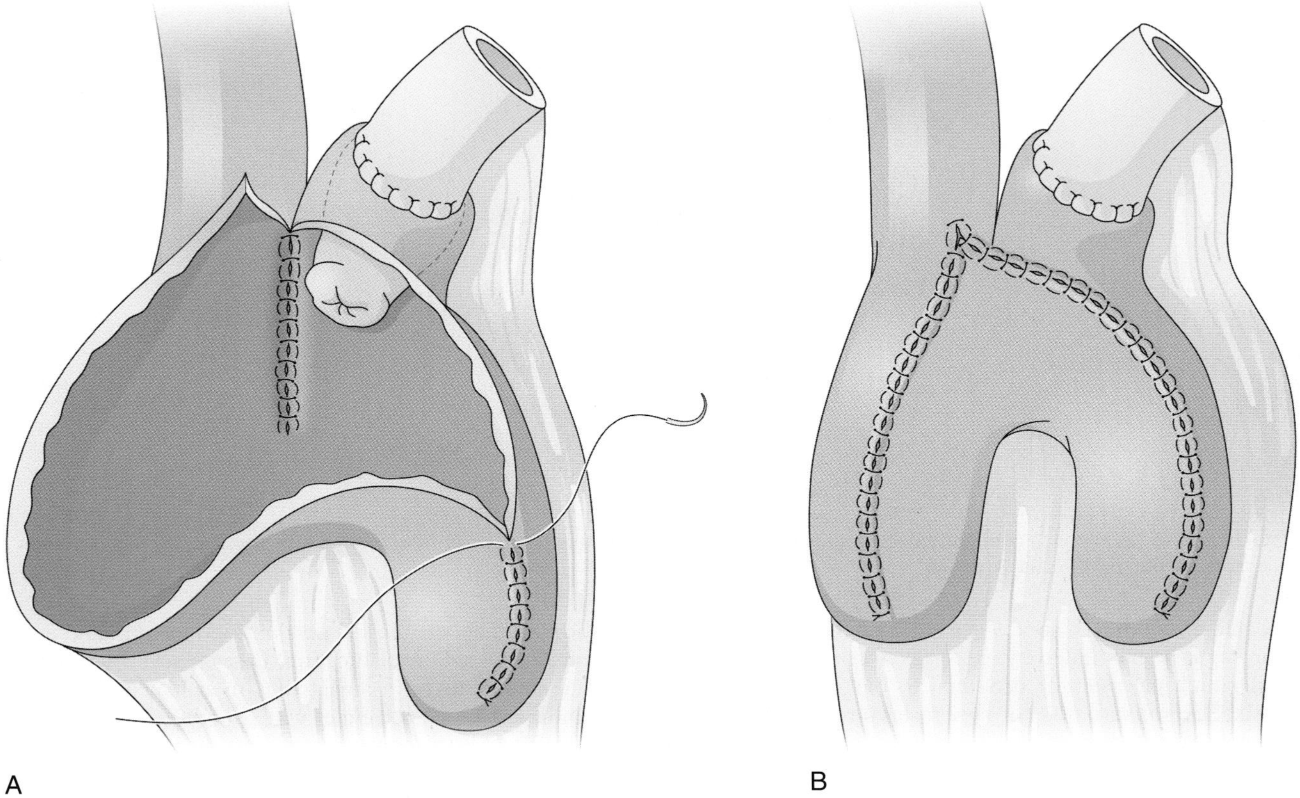

FIGURE 22–5 The continent ileostomy or Kock pouch consists of an ileal reservoir and nipple valve constructed by intussuscepting the efferent limb and (*A*) fixing it in place with sutures or staples. This provides a continent internal intestinal reservoir (*B*) that the patient can drain by intubating the pouch through the flush cutaneous stoma several times throughout the day.

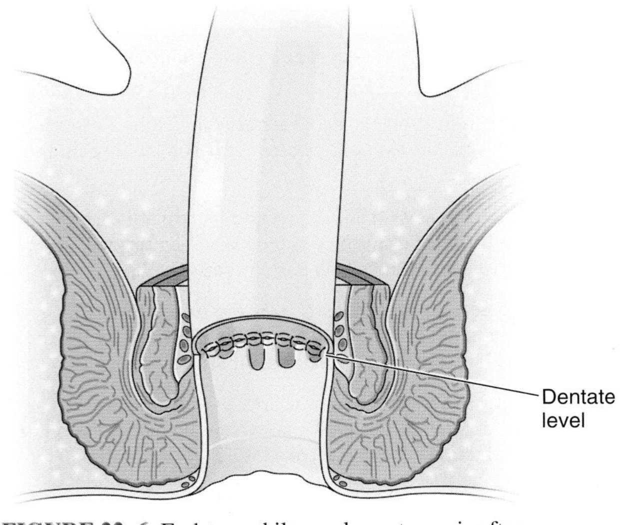

FIGURE 22–6 End-to-end ileoanal anastomosis after colectomy, mucosal proctectomy, and endorectal ileoanal pull-through.

parasympathetic innervation to the bladder and genitalia are preserved. This procedure is sometimes still used in very young children but infrequently in adults.

The success of early sphincter-sparing operations prompted the increasing clinical application of the IPAA procedure in the early 1980s. The long-term results of the Kock pouch were not as promising as initially anticipated, and significant surgical advances had been made in the IPAA technique. By the mid 1980s, various reports demonstrated that acceptable morbidity could be achieved with the IPAA procedure. Despite variable and unpredictable functional results, subsequent studies identified criteria for selecting patients that were associated with significant functional improvement. Perhaps of most importance, patients require adequate preoperative anal sphincter tone and function to achieve and maintain acceptable postoperative continence. This requirement prompted the development of anal manometric techniques to quantitate sphincter function and identify potentially ideal surgical candidates.

Ileal compliance was shown to be inversely correlated with stool frequency in patients after the end-to-end

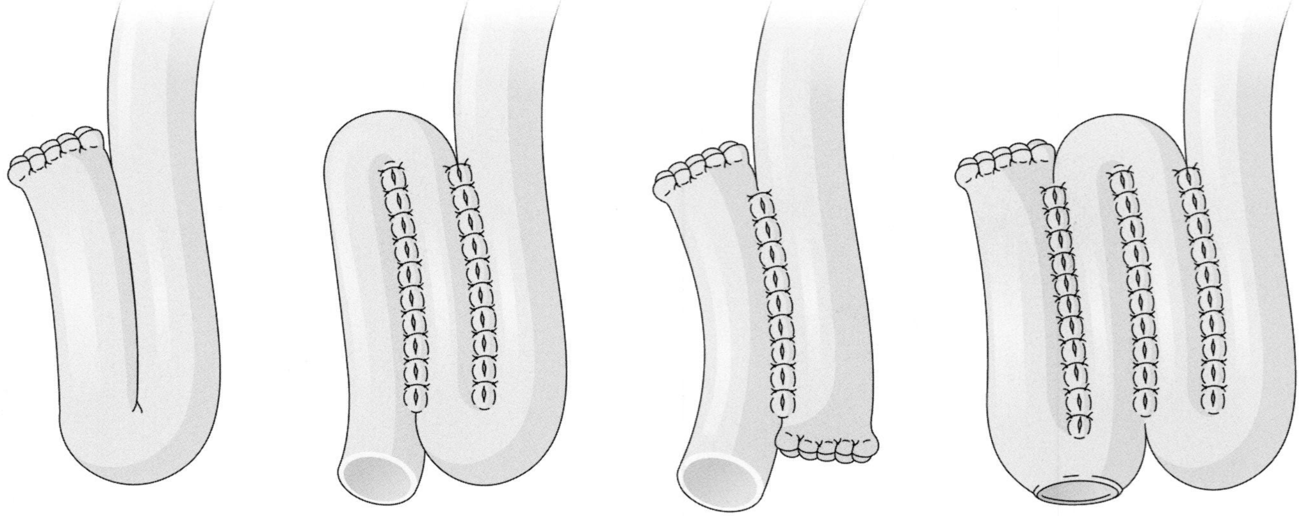

FIGURE 22–7 Ileal pouch configurations in patients undergoing ileal pouch–anal anastomosis. From left: J-pouch, S-pouch, side-to-side isoperistaltic pouch, and W-pouch.

ileoanal anastomosis, so it was suggested that ileal adaptation might be facilitated by the surgical construction of an ileal pouch or reservoir proximal to the ileoanal anastomosis. Several variations of ileal reservoirs were proposed and constructed, including the J-pouch, S-pouch, W-pouch, and lateral side-to-side isoperistaltic pouch (Fig. 22-7). Studies comparing the functional results after ileoanal anastomosis with and without an ileal reservoir have demonstrated that stool frequency was significantly reduced in adult patients in whom an ileal pouch was constructed. By using a temporary diverting loop ileostomy, which allows fecal diversion during the early weeks after surgery to allow ileal pouch and ileoanal anastomotic healing, the incidence of postoperative complications such as pelvic sepsis and anastomotic dehiscence can be significantly reduced.

The operation is performed in two stages for the majority of patients. The first stage consists of abdominal colectomy, mucosal proctectomy, endorectal IPAA, and diverting loop ileostomy. During the second stage, performed at least 8 to 12 weeks after the initial operation, the loop ileostomy is closed, and the fecal stream is resumed. As discussed previously, when an emergency colectomy is required, the operation is further staged. The first stage consists of abdominal colectomy, ileostomy, and Hartmann closure of the rectum. During the second stage, the rectal mucosa is dissected free, and then the IPAA is performed with loop ileostomy. The loop ileostomy is closed in approximately 8 to 12 weeks.

It was thought initially that only patients who were young and had relatively quiescent disease were candidates for IPAA; however, many surgeons are now comfortable in offering the procedure to patients in their sixth or seventh decade if they are in relatively good health and have adequate anal sphincter function. Disease severity has been found neither to be associated with enhanced operative morbidity nor to correlate with subsequent functional results. The most important criterion for electing IPAA is

PEARLS FOR THE OR

Indications for surgical intervention for ulcerative colitis (UC) include unrelenting hemorrhage, fulminating acute UC that is unresponsive to therapy, obstruction from stricture, suspicion or demonstration of colonic cancer, toxic megacolon, somatic and sexual growth in children, and intractability.

The primary indication for initial surgery in Crohn's disease (CD) of the small intestine is obstruction due to fibrosis and stricture.

Subtotal colectomy with ileostomy and Hartmann closure of the rectum is the operation of choice when an urgent situation arises in a critically ill patient with Crohn's colitis.

Subtotal colectomy with ileostomy is the procedure of choice in the emergency setting, or if the diagnosis of UC, as opposed to CD, cannot be clearly established.

Colectomy, mucosal proctectomy, and endorectal ileal pouch–anal anastomosis (IPAA) has become the operation of choice for patients with refractory UC.

Although the major early operative morbidity after IPAA is bowel obstruction, the most frequent late complication in patients undergoing IPAA is ileal pouch dysfunction or pouchitis, which has been reported to occur in up to 50% of patients undergoing this procedure for UC.

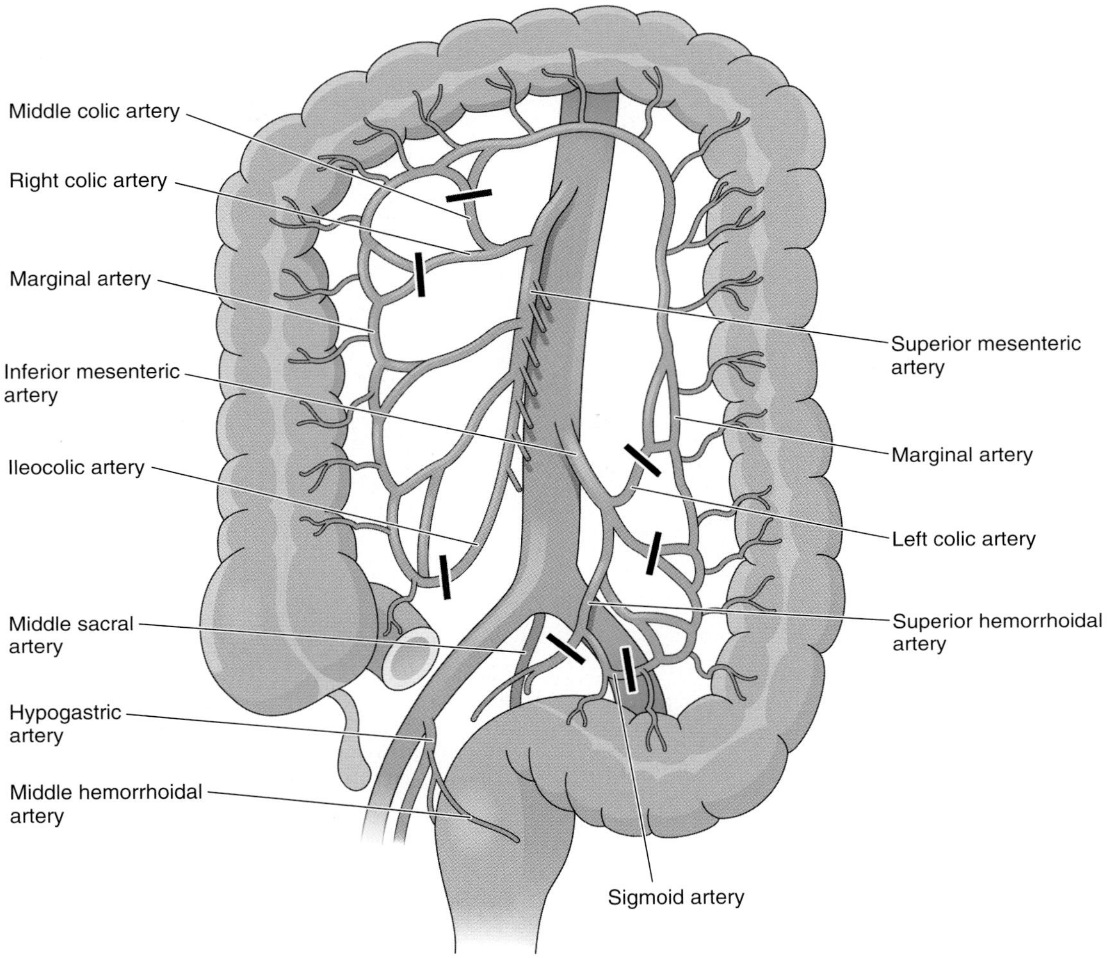

FIGURE 22–8 Arterial blood supply to the colon showing mesenteric divisions before total colectomy.

that the patient fully understands the physiology and technique of the operation and has realistic expectations about the outcome. Optimally, potential candidates for IPAA should be seen several weeks before surgery for flexible sigmoidoscopy and anorectal manometry.

Ileal Pouch–Anal Anastomosis

Colectomy with mucosal proctectomy and ileoanal anastomosis is performed as a two-team operation with the patient placed on the operating table in a modified lithotomy position. One team carries out a standard colectomy through a midline abdominal incision. The mesentery of the colon is divided at a convenient distance from the bowel wall (Fig. 22-8). The proximal rectum is mobilized and transected above the levator ani sling. Simultaneously, the transperineal rectal mucosal dissection is accomplished by the rectal team. Exposure is facilitated by a Lone Star retractor and hooks. A circumferential incision is made at the dentate line with a needle-tip electrocautery, and the rectal mucosa is carefully dissected away from the anal sphincter and then the rectal muscularis (Fig. 22-9). With the mucosal dissection completed, a 15-cm ileal J-pouch is constructed by using two firings of a mechanical stapler applied sequentially through an enterotomy in the apex of the pouch. The ileal pouch is extended into the pelvis endorectally, and its apex is opened and sutured circumferentially to the dentate line (Fig. 22-10). The loop ileostomy is then constructed 40 cm proximal to the pouch (Fig. 22-11). Approximately 4 weeks after the initial operation, standardized radiographic studies are performed to assess the integrity of the ileal pouch and ileoanal anastomosis, as well as continence. Eight weeks after the first stage, anal manometry is repeated and ileal pouch capacity is measured. The loop ileostomy is then closed by

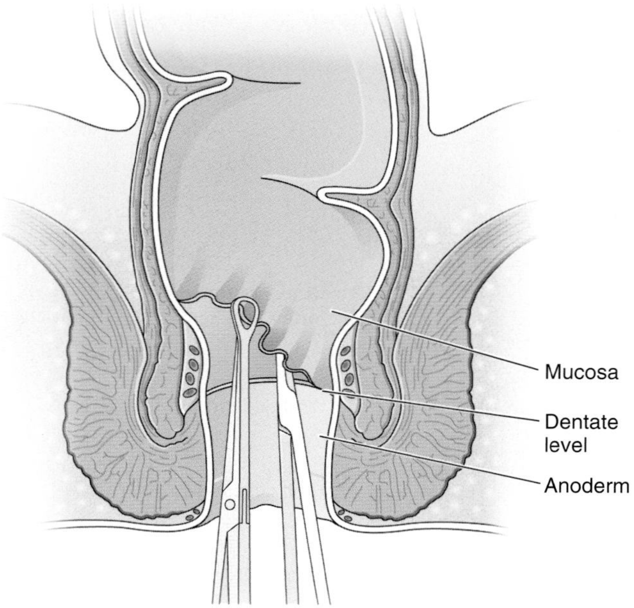

FIGURE 22–9 Transanal mucosal proctectomy. A circumferential incision is made at the dentate line, and the rectal mucosa is carefully dissected away from the anal sphincter and the rectal muscularis.

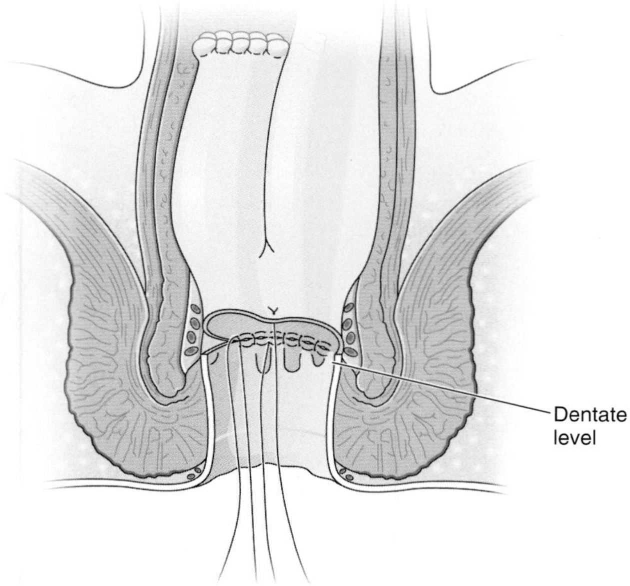

FIGURE 22–10 Creating the ileal J-pouch–anal anastomosis. The ileal J-pouch is secured to the sphincter in each quadrant with a suture. The purse-string stitch closing the enterotomy is cut to allow the apex of the pouch to open. An anastomosis is then created between the apex of the pouch and the anoderm with interrupted absorbable sutures.

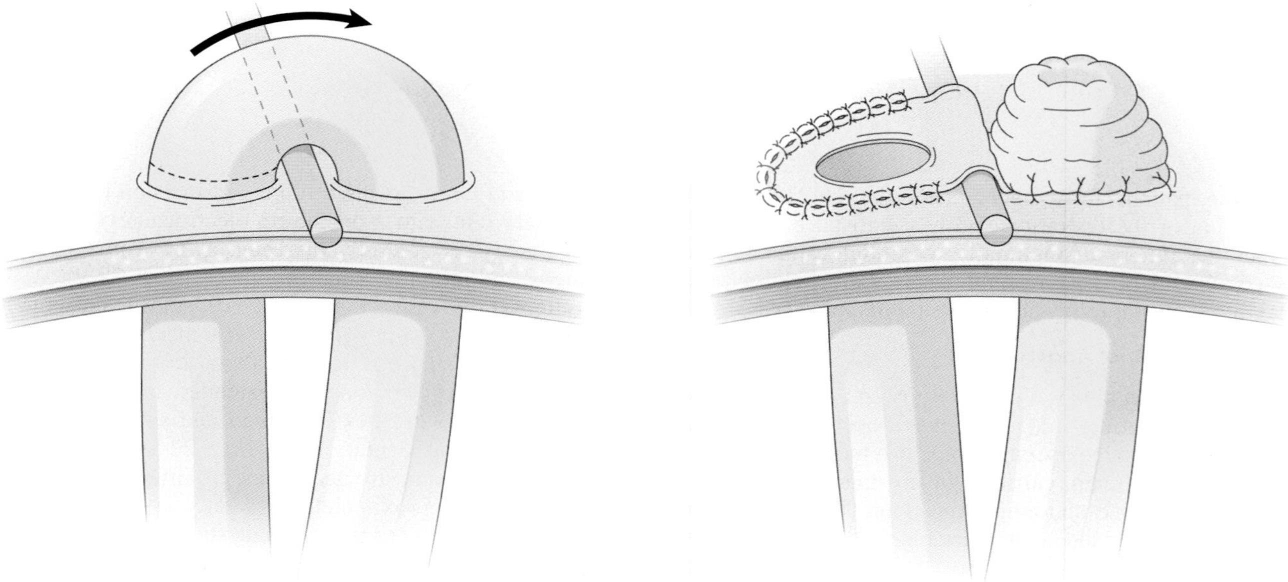

FIGURE 22–11 A loop ileostomy is constructed 40 cm proximal to the ileal pouch and matured over a rod.

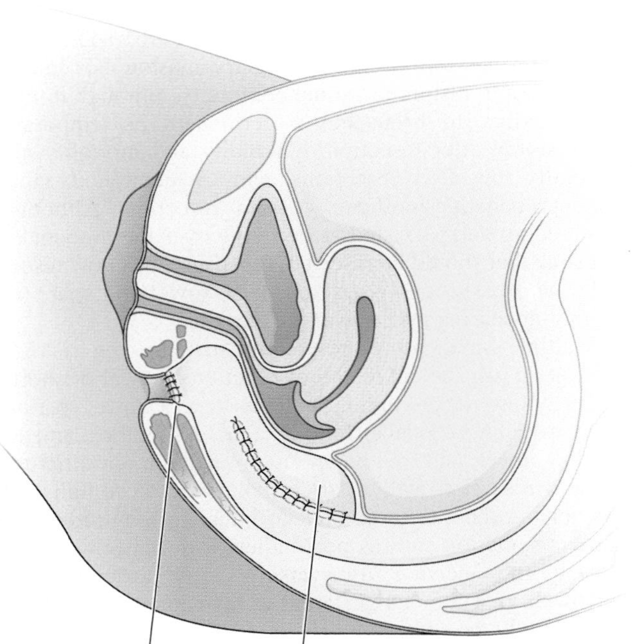

FIGURE 22–12 A sagittal view of the ileal pouch showing the anastomosis to the anus at the dentate line after mucosectomy.

using a stapling technique, which has greatly simplified this operation line (Fig. 22-12).

Among the most common postoperative complaints after IPAA are poor stool consistency, increased stool frequency, and nocturnal leakage. In an effort to control stool output, patients have been given loperamide hydrochloride, a synthetic opioid antidiarrheal agent, and supplementary fiber. In addition, patients are placed on a high-fiber diet.

One author's (J.M.B.) experience with more than 700 patients, of whom 86% were operated on for UC and 14% for familial adenomatous polyposis coli (FAP), supports the absence of mortality and the low morbidity that can be achieved with this operation. Experience and careful adherence to a standardized operative technique have played a major role in the success of this operation. No operative deaths occurred in both series, and the overall operative morbidity after IPAA was about 10%, primarily due to adhesion-related bowel obstruction. Although a 1% to 5% failure rate necessitated conversion to permanent ileostomy, satisfactory results have been reported in several large clinical series that showed a significant improvement in bowel function and quality of life after IPAA in patients with chronic UC. Other series again stress the point that that increased experience decreases the risk of postoperative and pouch-related complications and improves long-term outcome.

Although results with mucosal proctectomy and IPAA have been excellent, divergent points of view exist regarding intraoperative technique and its effect on anal physiology and functional outcome. Alternative approaches that eliminate distal mucosal proctectomy have been proposed in which the distal rectum is divided near the pelvic floor, leaving the anal canal largely intact, and then the ileal pouch is stapled to the top of the anal canal. The rationale for this approach is based on the premise that retaining the mucosa of the anal transition zone will preserve the anatomic integrity of the anal canal and improve fecal incontinence. Although several studies suggested that patients have improved sensation and better functional outcomes after preservation of the anal transition zone, this has not been documented by prospective study.

Nonspecific, idiopathic inflammation of the ileal pouch or pouchitis is the most common late postoperative complication after restorative proctocolectomy for UC. A recent review of the literature through 2004 reported that the incidence of pouchitis in patients after IPAA was as high as 50%. Although pouchitis can occur at any time after ileal pouch construction, most patients experience the initial episode within the first 2 years of the ileostomy closure. Pouchitis has been reported to occur primarily in patients undergoing the procedure for UC, and rarely occurs in patients who have had the procedure for familial polyposis. Pouchitis can have any number of symptoms including increased stool frequency, watery diarrhea, fecal urgency, incontinence, rectal bleeding, abdominal cramping, fever, and malaise. A similar syndrome has been reported in patients with Kock continent ileostomy pouches. In some patients, pouchitis can be accompanied by extra-intestinal manifestations such as primary sclerosing cholangitis, arthritis, skin lesions, and eye problems. Patients with preoperative extraintestinal manifestations associated with UC experience a higher incidence of pouchitis. Although the etiology of pouchitis is unknown, purported causes include early undetected Crohn's disease, bacterial overgrowth or bacterial dysbiosis, either primary or secondary malabsorption, stasis, ischemia, or nutritional or immune deficiencies.

Pouchitis remains a clinically defined syndrome, in part because no clear diagnostic criteria exist. Fortunately, a short course of ciprofloxacin and metronidazole is successful in treating about two thirds of patients with pouchitis. The remaining patients have recurrent pouchitis, which responds to repeated ciprofloxacin and metronidazole therapy, or a chronic, unresponsive form.

Crohn's Disease of the Small Intestine

Unlike that of UC, the surgical management of CD still remains particularly challenging for surgeons primarily because of concerns over multiple surgeries, the limitations imposed by the potential for a shortened small bowel, and the transmural, fistulizing, and skip-lesion nature of the disease. Most CD patients will require at least one operative procedure within their lifetime. The initial sites of involvement within the gastrointestinal tract as well as the length of time the patient has had the disease are both determinants for surgery. Whereas patients with early involvement in the terminal ileum and cecum are most likely to require surgery, those with disease confined to the colon or rectum appear to require less surgical intervention. Despite anatomic differences in disease manifestation, more than 75% of patients with CD require surgery by 20 years, and 90% by 30 years. The significant frequency of surgery is not only related to the chronic nature of the disease, but also to the high incidence of postoperative recurrence. Additional surgery may be required to deter fulminant complications associated with CD such as hemorrhage, perforation, obstruction, abscess formation, or toxic dilation of the colon.

The primary indication for initial surgery in CD of the small intestine is obstruction due to fibrosis and stricture. These patients generally have a long history of stenotic complications, and although surgery is usually elective, emergencies can arise. Most patients benefit from resection or strictureplasty and report an improved quality of life and remission of disease, but recurrence is common, and 33% to 82% of patients will require a second operation, and 22% to 33% will require more than two resections. Acute bowel obstructions can often be managed conservatively with IV fluids and decompression of the stomach, which generally allows time to localize the stricture by radiographic techniques or endoscopy. If conservative management fails, surgical intervention becomes necessary.

Once the patient with CD either has a medically unresolvable obstruction of the small intestine or becomes refractory to conventional therapy, a surgical decision must be made in the best interest of the patient. Surgeons are guided in these decisions by the principle that CD is a recurring disease that can involve the entire gastrointestinal tract. Thus the intended surgery must have a specific and limited objective, with as little bowel as possible either manipulated or resected. Because surgery for CD is not curative, only palliative, a bigger resection is not necessarily beneficial. Surgical alternatives that have been used to treat obstructions associated with CD include intestinal bypass or diversion, resection, and strictureplasty.

Although diversion of the intestinal stream around the diseased bowel segment while leaving that segment intact was once the procedure of choice in the management of CD of the terminal ileum or ileocolic region, studies have now shown that intestinal bypass should be avoided except in certain circumstances. Bypassed segments are prone to bacterial overgrowth and persistent inflammation, with the potential for abscess, bleeding, perforation, or malignant degeneration. Thus intestinal bypass is seldom used, except in CD of the duodenum.

Surgical resection of the diseased intestinal segment is the operation most frequently performed for CD of the small intestine. In most cases, primary anastomosis can be undertaken to restore intestinal continuity, although it may be necessary to bring out a permanent or temporary enterostomy after resection. Morbidity and mortality are generally low after resections, and as mentioned, most patients benefit significantly from resection. Although some controversy existed at one time over the amount of intestine that should be resected, most surgeons now resect only the grossly involved segment of bowel and spare all normal-appearing intestine at the margins.

Multiple small-bowel resections increase the risk of leaving an insufficient length of functional bowel or short-bowel syndrome, prompting surgeons to seek bowel-sparing alternatives. A surgical technique of increasing the diameter of the bowel and relieving an obstruction or stricture without resection, called strictureplasty, is accomplished by incising the strictured area of intestine longitudinally, applying traction sutures perpendicular to the bowel, and closing the incision transversely, thus widening the narrowed area. For longer areas of narrowing, the bowel immediately proximal and distal to the stricture can be sutured from side to side. Multiple strictureplasties can be performed during a single operation or can be combined with resection and anastomosis, if necessary. Although this procedure involves placing sutures directly into diseased bowel, complications associated with the strictureplasty are low. With more that two decades of experience in performing strictureplasty for treatment of symptomatic intestinal strictures secondary to CD, most surgeons agree that it is a safe, effective means of providing long-term surgical palliation to selected patients with CD. Recent advances include minimally invasive, laparoscopic ileocecal resections, as well as the effective use of strictureplasty in patients with duodenal CD. Additional efforts are being made to manage strictures nonoperatively by using hydrostatic balloon dilatation. This technique involves inserting a balloon into the strictured area through an endoscope, followed by inflation to dilate the stricture. This procedure appears to be relatively painless and safe, but it is uncertain how long the benefit lasts. Strictureplasty is contraindicated in the presence of acute inflammation, perforation, or abscess around the intestine. The unanswered question regarding strictureplasty is whether preservation of the diseased bowel involves a long-term risk of malignancy.

Crohn's Disease of the Colon and Rectum

The indications for surgery in Crohn's colitis are different from those in ileocolonic CD. A greater number of patients have intractability, fulminant disease, or anorectal disease and require emergency surgery. Although a simple loop ileostomy can relieve toxic dilation, some surgeons prefer to perform a total proctocolectomy and ileostomy. The total proctocolectomy alleviates the acute inflammatory process, but it is associated with a high morbidity rate in acute disease and may be overly aggressive in eliminating any option for restoration of continence. Therefore most surgeons believe that the most satisfactory operation in an emergency is subtotal colectomy with ileostomy and Hartmann closure of the rectum. This procedure allows removal of most of the disease-bearing tissue and the establishment of a firm histologic diagnosis, but it does not preclude the opportunity for a subsequent sphincter-sparing ileorectal anastomosis.

For patients undergoing elective operative intervention for treatment of colorectal CD, several alternatives are available, ranging from the use of a temporary defunctioning ileostomy to resection of segments of diseased colon or even the entire colon and rectum. Although it was originally thought that the temporary defunctioning ileostomy procedure might provide temporary improvement of systemic, colonic, or anorectal symptoms, several studies have shown that only 15% had intestinal continuity restored. Others have advocated the use of an ileostomy as a staged procedure in preparation for later resection; however, currently available perioperative care now precludes this approach.

The surgical management of patients with segmental involvement of the colon or rectum with CD remains controversial. Segmental resection with primary anastomosis, potentially applicable in 6% to 20% of patients, does adhere to the conservative principles of the surgical management of CD and avoids either a permanent ileostomy or the potential for a poor function after total abdominal colectomy with ileorectal anastomosis. However, not only is the morbidity and mortality rate high, but segmental resection is associated with a high recurrence rate of between 30% and 50% within 5 years and a reoperative rate of 45% within 5 years and 60% within 10 years. Hence, some surgeons advocate total abdominal colectomy. However, most surgeons would agree that despite the higher recurrence rate after segmental resection, it might delay the need for permanent ileostomy for several years and should be considered.

In most cases of Crohn's colitis, the disease affects much of the colon including the rectum. However, sufficient rectum is spared to consider rectal preservation after abdominal colectomy and subsequent ileorectal anastomosis in about one fourth of patients. Ileorectal anastomosis is associated with 3% mortality and 5% to 10% incidence of anastomotic leakage, and a clinical recurrence approaching 50% to 70% at 5 to 10 years, with nearly two thirds of patients requiring subsequent operations. Although some surgeons attempt primary ileorectal anastomosis even in the case of mild Crohn's proctitis, this has, for the most part, been associated with a high complication rate and a poor functional result. Most surgeons instead perform ileorectal anastomosis at the time of abdominal colectomy only if the rectum is completely and unequivocally spared, or if, after a staged subtotal colectomy with ileostomy and Hartmann closure of the rectum, it manifests sustained absence of disease.

As suggested earlier, subtotal colectomy with ileostomy and Hartmann closure of the rectum may be the operation of choice when an urgent situation arises in a critically ill patient with Crohn's colitis. This operation also may be an acceptable elective alternative, particularly in patients in whom uncertainty exists about the inflammatory status of the rectum, in those in whom perianal abscess precludes proctectomy, and finally in those in whom uncertainty exists about the diagnosis of CD versus UC. The mortality and morbidity of elective subtotal colectomy is low. After subtotal colectomy, three potential outcomes include staged proctectomy in patients with severe Crohn's proctitis, ileorectal anastomosis if the rectum remains spared, or maintenance of the status quo. In this latter group of patients, one must consider the risk of the development of rectal carcinoma.

The most aggressive approach for the management of diffuse Crohn's proctocolitis is total proctocolectomy and Brooke ileostomy. This approach may be necessary in up to 55% to 60% of all patients. When performed electively, this operation is associated with a low mortality and a 20% clinical recurrence rate after 10 years. Despite this operation's apparent success, significant complications include chronic perineal wound problems and a higher incidence of ileostomy complications such as fluid and electrolyte problems, vitamin B_{12} malabsorption, and bile acid malabsorption.

Ileal pouch–anal anastomosis, the operation of choice for UC, is contraindicated in the primary surgical therapy for Crohn's colitis; however, the procedure has been proposed for selected patients with no evidence history of small-bowel or anal involvement for whom rectal resection is mandatory, as an alternative to coloproctectomy with definitive end ileostomy. Others have suggested the staged conversion of a Brooke ileostomy to a continent ileostomy in selected patients who, after several recurrence-free years, desire restoration of continence. When not performed on carefully selected patients, these operations are associated with a high incidence of failure, requiring resection of the pouch and conversion to Brooke ileostomy with a subsequently shortened ileum.

Although they are controversial, it appears that similar conservative principles should be applied to the surgical management of Crohn's colitis. Segmental colectomy may be indicated for isolated areas of colonic involvement. Proctocolectomy is indicated for patients with extensive, diffuse colorectal disease. Subtotal colectomy with ileostomy is indicated in the emergency setting, and ileorectal anastomosis may be carried out if the rectum is spared. Pouch operation should be avoided in patients with frank CD but may be applicable to selected patients and those with indeterminate colitis.

If recurrence after surgery for CD anywhere in the gastrointestinal tract is defined as a return of symptoms, including pain, fever, diarrhea, and weight loss, about 20% of patients have recurrence by 2 years, 30% by 3 years, and approximately 50% by 5 years. Most surgical recurrence also appears to be predictable, based on the site of initial involvement. Thus patients with ileocolonic CD have a 53% recurrence rate, those with small intestinal CD have a 46% recurrence rate, and those with colorectal CD have a 40% recurrence rate. In comparing strictureplasty with resection, it is important to focus on the specific site of surgery. The data suggest that the site-specific recurrence rate, approximately 2%, is comparable for both strictureplasty and resection. Overall, when followed up for 5 years, approximately one fourth of patients with either resection or strictureplasty require reoperation for recurrent disease at the site of previous resection or strictureplasty.

Suggested Reading

Becker JM, Stucchi AF: Ulcerative colitis. In Greenfield LJ, Mulholland MW, Oldham KT, et al (eds): Surgery: Scientific Principles and Practice, 3rd ed. Philadelphia, Lippincott Williams & Wilkins, 2001, pp 1070–1089.

Becker JM, Stucchi AF: How I do it: Proctocolectomy with ileoanal anastomosis. J Gastrointest Surg 8(4):376–386, 2004.

Egan LJ, Sandborn WJ: Advances in the treatment of Crohn's disease. Gastroenterology 126:1574–1581, 2004.

Fiocchi C: Inflammatory bowel disease: etiology and pathogenesis. Gastroenterology 115(1):182–205, 1998.

Hanauer SB: Medical therapy for ulcerative colitis 2004. Gastroenterology 126:1582–1592, 2004.

Larson DW, Pemberton JH: Current concepts and controversies in surgery for IBD. Gastroenterology 126:1611–1619, 2004.

Sartor RB, Sandborn WJ (eds): Kirsner's Inflammatory Bowel Diseases, 6th ed. New York, WB Saunders, 2004.

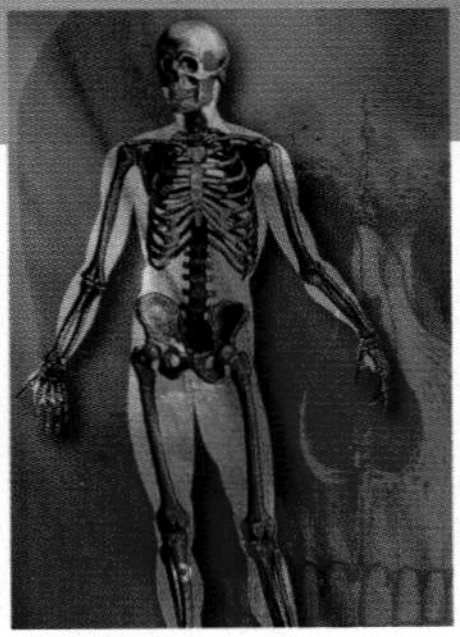

Chapter 23
Motility Disorders

ERICA A. BROTSCHI, MD

The well-being of patients and successful outcome of surgery depend on effective function of the gastrointestinal (GI) tract. Surgical practice includes evaluating patients with altered bowel function, and managing patients with "ileus," or temporary paralysis of the GI tract after surgery, anesthesia, or trauma. Therefore surgeons should understand the physiology of the GI tract and how surgery and medications affect intestinal motility.

Anatomy of the Intestine

The primary role of the GI tract is to absorb water, electrolytes, and nutrients. Most of this absorptive function occurs in the small intestine. The small intestine is divided into three named sections: the duodenum, extending from the stomach to the ligament of Treitz, the jejunum, and the ileum. The jejunum refers to the proximal two fifths of the intraperitoneal small bowel, whereas the ileum refers to the distal three fifths. The total length of the small intestine is approximately 2.5 to 3 m. The colon is about 1 to 1.5 m in length. Absorption occurs as food and secretions are propelled through the GI tract by contractions of the smooth muscle making up the intestinal wall. Three muscular layers are found in the intestine. An inner layer of muscle called the muscularis mucosa runs throughout the submucosa of the GI tract. The outer muscle of the intestine consists of two smooth muscle layers, an inner circular layer and an outer longitudinal layer (Fig. 23-1). In the small intestine, these two layers are continuous, but in the colon, the longitudinal muscle fibers are gathered into three bundles called taenia. The longitudinal muscle bundles come together to form a continuous layer in the rectal wall.

The enteric nervous system is a complex network of nerves located in the intestinal wall and mesentery. It consists of two neural plexuses: the submucosal (Meissner's) plexus between the muscularis mucosa and the circular muscular layer, and the myenteric (Auerbach's) plexus between the circular and longitudinal muscle layers. The enteric nervous system receives input from local receptors and nerves and also exchanges signals with the central nervous system (CNS) through autonomic nerves.

Control of Intestinal Motility

Three mechanisms control smooth muscle contraction: (1) a myogenic mechanism producing rhythmic contraction within the muscle itself, (2) the enteric nervous system, and (3) numerous peptide gastrointestinal hormones.

Myogenic control of GI smooth muscle arises from rhythmic electrical activity within the specialized muscle cells (Cajal cells), similar to the intrinsic pacemaker activity within heart muscle. Myogenic control allows large numbers of cells to contract in an organized pattern. GI smooth muscle shows an intrinsic rhythmic fluctuation of membrane potential at rest, called *slow waves* or BER (basic electrical rhythm).

This provides a pacemaker function to organize contraction along a segment of smooth muscle (Fig. 23-2). The slow-wave frequency of the intestinal muscle cells varies along the intestine, with higher frequencies in the proximal intestine. The gradient of slow-wave frequency allows contraction to be propagated from one muscle cell to

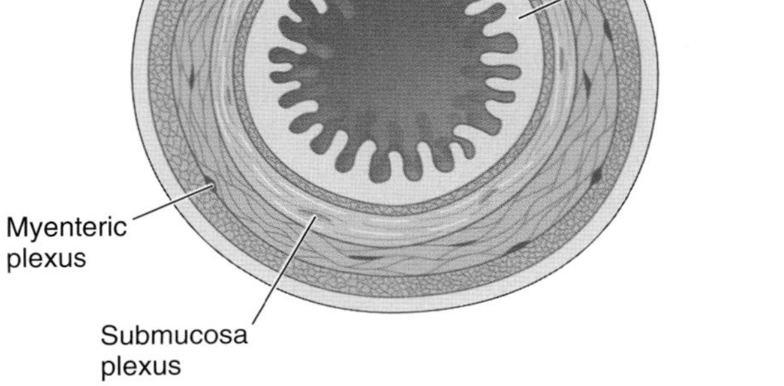

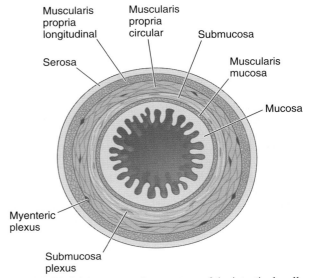

FIGURE 23–1 Neuromuscular anatomy of the intestinal wall. The circular and longitudinal muscle layers together make up the muscularis propria.

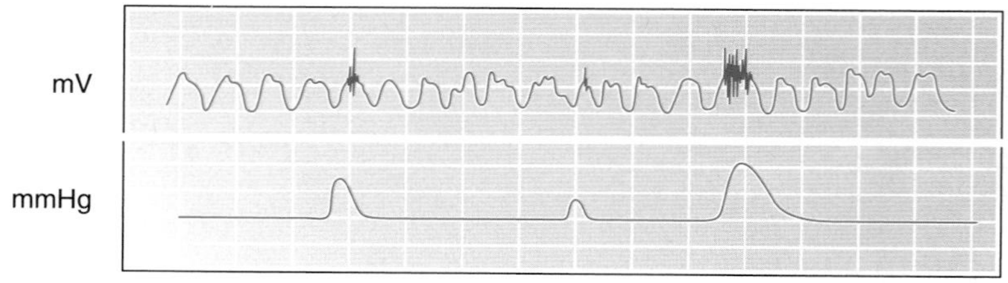

FIGURE 23–2 *Upper tracing*, Myoelectric slow waves recorded from smooth muscle, with superimposed spike potentials. *Lower tracing*, Muscle tension is shown, with the association between spike potentials and muscle contraction.

another in an aborad (proximal to distal) direction in the intestine.

The *enteric nervous system* stimulates contraction of the intestinal muscle. Muscle contraction results when a neurotransmitter such as acetylcholine interacts with receptors on muscle cells to depolarize the muscle membrane. Calcium enters the muscle cells to cause muscle contraction. This results in measurable changes in the electrical potential of the membrane, called spike potentials or action potentials. The enteric nervous system releases multiple contractile and relaxatory neurotransmitters to regulate intestinal contraction. The enteric nervous system includes the parasympathetic (cholinergic) and sympathetic (adrenergic) nerves that have traditionally been called the autonomic nervous system.

The major effect of *parasympathetic nerves* is to stimulate GI function and motility. The major parasympathetic neurotransmitter is acetylcholine. Acetylcholine causes GI smooth muscle to contract by stimulating muscarinic (atropine-sensitive) receptors. Many GI hormones that cause intestinal contraction act by releasing acetylcholine from intrinsic nerves in the intestinal muscle. In contrast, the effect of *sympathetic nerves* on GI function is mainly inhibitory. Sympathetic nerves are called *adrenergic*, because they release epinephrine or norepinephrine, neurotransmitters that also are synthesized in the adrenal medulla.

In addition to these autonomic neurotransmitters, dozens of other neurotransmitters are found in the enteric nervous system. These include many of the well-known CNS neurotransmitters such as serotonin, dopamine, and adenosine triphosphate. Nitric oxide (NO) is an important GI neurotransmitter causing smooth muscle relaxation. The enteric nervous system also includes several dozen peptide GI hormones.

The *GI hormones* are neurotransmitter peptides synthesized in nerves or in specialized neuroendocrine cells in the GI mucosa and pancreas. Some of these peptides such as cholecystokinin also are found in large amounts in the brain. Among the most widely studied of the GI hormones are cholecystokinin, gastrin, vasoactive intestinal peptide, substance P, and somatostatin. These peptides interact with specific receptors on nerves, smooth muscle, or other organs.

Many peptide hormones are neurotransmitters that are released from enteric nerves to coordinate intestinal function and peristalsis. Some peptides also function as endocrine hormones that are released into the blood to control organ function at distant sites. For example, cholecystokinin is released from cells lining the duodenum and jejunum to cause gallbladder contraction and stimulate pancreatic enzyme secretion.

Normal Patterns of Motility

Intestinal contraction is regulated to maximize the absorption of nutrients while food is passing through the GI tract. Effective absorption requires propulsion, mixing, and reservoir capacity in the GI tract. A pattern of tonic and segmenting contractions in the intestine allows this to occur (Fig. 23-3). During fasting, the small intestine exhibits a sweeping contraction wave called the *migrating myoelectric complex* (MMC). In the colon, strong sweeping contractions occur occasionally, about six per 24-hour period. These contractions originate in the ascending colon and move distally, propelling the fecal content. Colon contractile activity increases with feeding and with waking from sleep.

Defecation is a process involving both reflex and voluntary activity. Normally two sphincters close the anal canal. The internal anal sphincter is a thickened area of the circular smooth muscle that makes up one layer of the rectal wall and is continuous with the circular muscle layer throughout the intestine. The external anal sphincter is continuous with the striated muscle of the pelvic floor and is under voluntary control. When a colon contraction

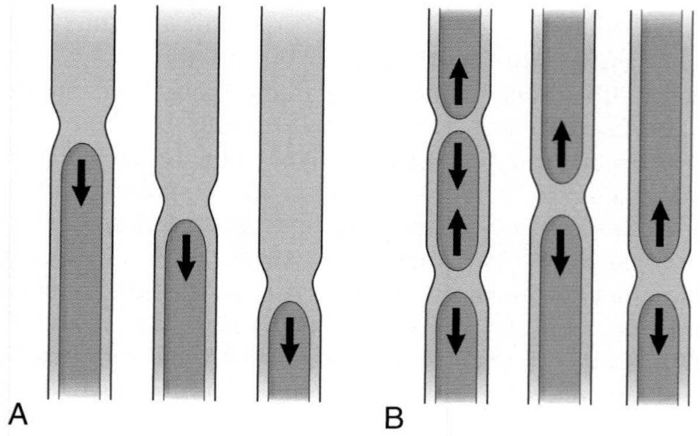

FIGURE 23–3 *A*, Aborad movement of an intestinal peristaltic contraction. *B*, Segmental contraction of the bowel.

distends the rectum with feces, the internal sphincter relaxes (rectal inhibitory reflex), and the external sphincter contracts, producing the urge to defecate. Defecation is controlled by nerve pathways in the sacral cord, regulated by the CNS. Defecation occurs when the internal sphincter relaxes reflexively and the external sphincter is relaxed voluntarily. Muscles of the pelvic floor relax, which helps to straighten the anorectal canal, and contraction of the abdominal muscles increases intraabdominal pressure.

Clinical Measurement of Intestinal Motility

Various tests can be used to measure intestinal motility in patients.

Abdominal plain radiographs, in both flat and upright projections (often referred to as kidneys-ureters-bladder [KUB] and upright) are part of the initial workup for obstruction or abnormal bowel motility. Important findings include the distribution of gas between the small bowel and colon, the amount of bowel distention, and the presence of air/fluid levels. Plain radiographs may show the site of obstruction and whether obstruction is complete or incomplete. Gas distending the entire small bowel and colon suggests paralytic ileus instead of mechanical obstruction.

Abdominal CT scanning with luminal contrast is the most useful test to evaluate for obstruction. In addition to showing what areas of the bowel are distended, the passage of oral contrast can demonstrate whether obstruction is partial or complete. CT is particularly useful in postoperative patients who may have prolonged ileus or obstruction. CT scanning also is reasonably accurate for diagnosing intestinal obstruction due to tumors or other masses and for diagnosing bowel ischemia or infarction.

Endoscopy can be a valuable test for diagnosing obstruction, particularly in the esophagus, stomach, and colon. Endoscopy gives specific information about the cause of obstruction, and biopsies can be obtained. Colonoscopy also can be used to decompress a dangerously distended colon caused by volvulus or pseudo-obstruction. Care must be taken during endoscopy not to insufflate air that increases distention beyond an obstruction.

Contrast fluoroscopy of the upper and lower GI tract (*UGI series with small-bowel follow-through* and barium enema) can be used to identify specific sites of obstruction in the upper and lower GI tract. Placing barium above a high-grade intestinal obstruction can lead to complications, so these studies are most useful with partial obstructions.

Measurement of colonic transit time is a test used in otherwise healthy people with severe chronic constipation. The patient is fed a collection of small radio-opaque marker pellets, and abdominal radiographs are obtained daily until the markers have passed.

Anal manometry can diagnose abnormalities in anal-sphincter function and defecation. This test includes measuring patients' ability to sense distention of a balloon in the rectum, and measurement of relaxation and contraction pressure in the internal and external anal sphincters. Radiographs of the lateral pelvis during evacuation of rectal contrast material (cinedefecography) also may show abnormalities in rectal and anal sphincter contraction and relaxation responses.

Disorders of Intestinal Peristalsis

Intestinal Obstruction

Mechanical obstruction of the large or small intestine is a common cause of abnormal intestinal motility. Patients with obstruction report a change in bowel pattern, with complete obstruction leading to cessation of flatus and stools. Complete obstruction of either the small or large intestine can rapidly evolve into a surgical emergency involving intestinal ischemia and necrosis, so accurate diagnosis is mandatory.

Small-bowel obstruction (SBO) is most commonly caused by intraperitoneal adhesions, usually scarring from prior abdominal surgery. This can result in twisting of intestine around an adhesive band or narrowing of the intestine by layers of scar tissue. The second most common cause of SBO is incarceration or trapping of small intestine in a hernia. Incarceration can occur with any abdominal-wall or pelvic hernia, including inguinal, femoral, and umbilical hernias, as well as less-common hernia types. Bowel also can become trapped and obstructed in incisional hernias of the abdominal wall, especially those with narrow fascial openings. Within the abdomen, bowel can herniate through developmental or surgical defects in the omentum or mesenteries. The third common cause of SBO is blockage by metastatic tumor, arising from cancers such as colon, ovary, or lung cancer.

Obstruction at the level of the ileocecal valve resembles SBO and may be due to colon cancer or cecal volvulus. Other less common causes of SBO include Crohn's disease of the ileum, strictures due to radiation or surgery, foreign bodies, gallstones that erode into the intestine (gallstone ileus), intussusception, and primary small-bowel neoplasms. Congenital abnormalities of the intestine such as duplication, stenosis, or Meckel's diverticulum may cause SBO in infancy or childhood.

Obstruction leads to distention of the intestine above the blockage, with gas and fluid accumulation within the obstructed lumen. Peristaltic patterns become abnormal, progressing to loss of peristalsis if obstruction is complete. In SBO, the patient often experiences severe midabdominal pains, usually of a "crampy" intermittent nature, due to strong peristaltic waves proximal to the obstruction. Anorexia and nausea are present, and vomiting is common. Vomiting is more likely with more proximal obstruction, and vomitus may be foul-smelling or "feculent" because of bacterial overgrowth. Patients often are severely dehydrated because of fluid and electrolyte losses into the bowel lumen and from vomiting.

The evaluation for possible SBO includes a careful history and physical examination to determine the etiology of the obstruction and to assess the patient's general medical state. The history of hernias, abdominal surgery, or cancer must be determined. Physical examination should include checking vital signs and skin turgor for signs of dehydration. An abdominal examination should check for scars and assess the degree of abdominal tenderness. Peritoneal signs such as percussion tenderness or cough tenderness suggest ischemic or gangrenous bowel. A rectal examination with stool test for occult blood is essential. The finding of blood suggests a luminal malignancy or ischemic bowel. Measurement of hematocrit, white blood cell count, electrolytes, blood urea nitrogen (BUN), and creatinine will show how much dehydration and metabolic derangement exists. Flat and upright abdominal films should be obtained to determine the level of obstruction, and abdominal CT scan should be considered, particularly if bowel ischemia or tumor is suspected (Fig. 23-4).

Initial treatment includes nothing by mouth, nasogastric (NG) suction, and IV fluids. Most patients need a Foley catheter and hourly urine measurement to assess hydration. Patients are assumed to have incomplete obstruction if they continue to pass flatus or stool and have gas distal to the presumed obstruction on abdominal radiograph. Patients with incomplete obstruction may be treated with continued bowel rest and suction for several days while a definite diagnosis is made. Approximately half of incomplete SBOs resolve with NG suction. Patients with evidence of complete obstruction (no flatus, no stool, and little gas below the obstruction on radiograph) may require emergency laparotomy as soon as their medical condition permits. In approximately one third of complete SBOs, the obstruction results from a loop of bowel twisting within a hernia sac or under an adhesive band. The twist creates a *closed-loop obstruction* with occlusion of the mesenteric blood supply. Closed-loop obstructions proceed to gangrene and intestinal perforation. Concern over the risk of perforation gave rise to the surgical dictum, "The sun should not rise or set on a small bowel obstruction." Operative management of SBO includes careful inspection of the entire small bowel at laparotomy, repair of hernias, lysis of adhesions, and resection of any intestine that does not appear viable. The prognosis after surgery depends on the etiology of the obstruction and whether dead bowel was found at exploration.

Large-bowel obstruction is most commonly due to cancer of the colon or rectum. Other causes include inflammation or chronic stricture from diverticulitis or colitis. The colon also can be obstructed because of volvulus, or twisting of redundant colon. The common causes for SBO (adhesions, hernia, and metastatic tumor) seldom produce large-bowel

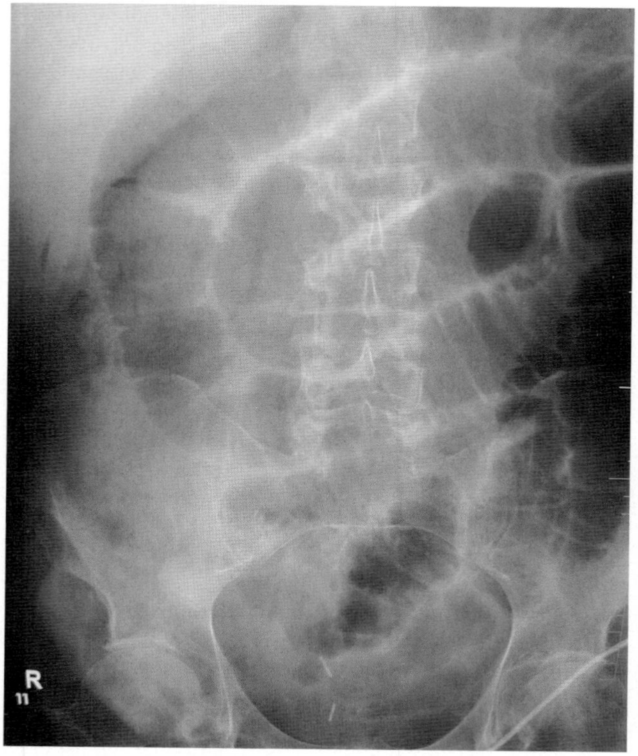

FIGURE 23–4 Abdominal radiograph of a patient with postoperative small-bowel obstruction. Note the multiple dilated loops of small bowel, the absence of gas in the colon, and the surgical clips in the pelvis.

obstruction. The symptoms of large-bowel obstruction differ from those of SBO. In large-bowel obstruction, vomiting and anorexia are usually absent. Pain, although common, tends to be mild and diffuse in the lower abdomen. Patients often have constipation (decreased frequency of bowel movements) or obstipation (cessation of bowel movements) and abdominal distention as their main complaints.

Obstruction of the large intestine may lead to gangrene and perforation of the cecum due to elevated cecal pressure. Patients with a cecal diameter greater than about 9 cm on abdominal radiograph are at high risk of perforation and should have urgent diagnosis and surgical management.

Diagnosis depends on a history of altered bowel habits and physical findings of abdominal distention. Marked abdominal tenderness or peritoneal tenderness suggests ischemia of the distended bowel. Rectal examination and testing for occult blood should always be done, particularly because palpable rectal tumors may cause complete obstruction. Flat and upright radiographs of the abdomen will usually identify the level of obstruction, and a low-pressure contrast enema will confirm the obstruction. The urgency of surgical intervention depends on the degree of colon dilatation, more than on the etiology of the obstruction. If the colon is severely dilated above the obstruction, a risk of cecal gangrene exists, and rapid surgical intervention is required. Treatment should be started with NG suction and hydration. Operative management involves resection of the obstructed segment of colon, if possible, and formation of a colostomy in most cases. If the patient is too ill to undergo colon resection, decompression of the colon proximal to the obstruction can be achieved with a colostomy or cecostomy, and the obstruction can be resected at a later operation. The outcome of surgery depends mainly on whether colon perforation and peritoneal contamination occurred before surgical intervention.

Postoperative Ileus

Paralytic ileus refers to temporary paralysis of intestinal function due to surgery, medical illness, or trauma. Surgery of the abdomen or retroperitoneum is particularly likely to stop normal motility. In surgical patients, dissection into the peritoneal cavity and manipulation of the colon appear to be important factors in inducing ileus. Different portions of the GI tract recover from postoperative ileus at different rates. The small intestine usually resumes peristalsis within 5 to 10 hours of surgery if obstruction is not present. The stomach often recovers function within 24 to 48 hours, and the colon is the last segment of the GI tract to resume normal contraction. Therefore patients who have had major abdominal surgery are usually not fed until colon peristalsis has resumed, as shown by the passage of gas or stool. This may not occur until 3 to 5 days after surgery.

Specific factors in postoperative patients can result in prolonged failure of the intestine to resume function. Common causes of prolonged ileus include excessive use of narcotic pain medicine, intestinal obstruction with a history of bowel distention, low serum albumin, and electrolyte abnormalities (low potassium, magnesium, calcium, sodium, or phosphorus).

Certain surgical procedures may result in disturbances to GI motility. Vagotomy, or division of vagus nerves to the stomach, is performed as therapy for peptic ulcer and also may be part of surgery to the esophagus or gastroesophageal junction. Vagotomy paralyzes gastric motor function and may result in prolonged failure of the stomach to empty, especially after repeated operations on the stomach. Another surgical procedure that can directly affect intestinal peristalsis is duodenal transection and anastomosis, such as occurs in the pylorus-preserving pancreaticoduodenectomy (Whipple procedure). Duodenal transection can result in prolonged failure of motility due to loss of duodenal pacemaker function. In contrast, resection of the distal small intestine and colon appears to have only a brief effect on bowel peristaltic patterns.

Clinically, ileus is characterized by the absence of flatus and stools and accumulation of gas and fluid within the bowel lumen. Patients often feel nauseated or vomit if they are not treated with NG suction. Physical examination reveals a distended, tympanitic abdomen; and bowel sounds are decreased until gastric function resumes. Prolonged postoperative ileus can be confused with early postoperative bowel obstruction due to edema, adhesions, or kinking of bowel loops. Ileus can often be distinguished from mechanical bowel obstruction by the presence of gas throughout the paralyzed small and large intestine on radiograph (Fig. 23-5). Abdominal CT scan with contrast, or radiographs with luminal contrast, may be useful to determine whether mechanical obstruction is present.

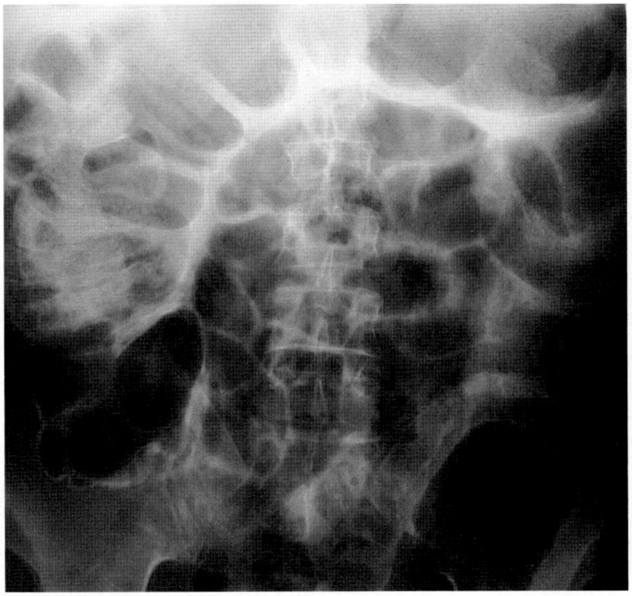

FIGURE 23–5 Abdominal radiograph of a patient with large-bowel obstruction due to sigmoid tumor. Note the dilated loops of colon and small bowel. This resembles the appearance of severe ileus, except that no gas is seen in the rectum

The treatment of postoperative ileus includes nothing by mouth, with NG suction if bowel dilatation or nausea is present. If ileus persists beyond the expected time, the patient's medications should be reviewed, and electrolytes and albumin checked. Workup for intraperitoneal abscess should be considered, and IV nutrition begun. Various attempts to treat intestinal ileus with hormones and drugs have been unsuccessful, but time leads to resolution of the ileus if nutrition is maintained and no obstruction or untreated infection is present.

Medical Causes for Abnormal Intestinal Motility

Chronic systemic diseases that interfere with the function of visceral nerves or muscle may cause abnormal motility

PEARLS FOR THE OR

Complete small-bowel obstruction usually requires urgent laparotomy because of the risk of closed-loop obstruction and intestinal gangrene.

Partial small-bowel obstructions can usually be treated nonoperatively initially with nasogastric (NG) suction and hydration.

Cecal dilatation of 9 cm or greater requires urgent colonoscopic decompression or surgical management, whether it is due to obstruction or to pseudo-obstruction.

Factors that increase the duration of postoperative ileus include preoperative bowel distention, intraperitoneal dissection, and surgery on the colon or rectum.

The two anal sphincters are the internal sphincter, a thickening of the smooth muscle layer of the rectal wall, and the external sphincter, striated muscle arising from the levator muscles. Only the external sphincter is under voluntary control.

in the intestine. The most common systemic disease affecting GI motility in developed countries is diabetes mellitus. The neuropathy associated with poorly controlled diabetes can interfere with normal contractile patterns throughout the GI tract. Infectious diseases causing visceral neuropathy include trypanosomiasis (Chagas' disease) and Cytomegalovirus infection. Other systemic diseases that often affect intestinal function include scleroderma, amyloidosis, and hypothyroidism.

Chronic intestinal pseudo-obstruction (CIP) refers to a heterogeneous group of rare genetic diseases of intestinal nerve and muscle. These patients have failure of intestinal peristalsis due to degeneration of neurons or muscle cells. Patients are first seen with abdominal pain and distention and may have either constipation or diarrhea. Hyperalimentation may be required for nutrition in severe cases.

Acquired intestinal pseudo-obstruction (megacolon and Ogilvie's syndrome) are relatively common conditions, in contrast to true genetic pseudo-obstruction. The colon loses normal peristaltic activity as a result of bed rest, gaseous distention, and medications. Chronic colon dilatation usually occurs in long-term hospitalized patients, particularly in patients receiving anticholinergic or antidopaminergic medication. The colon becomes long and dilated (*megacolon*), and patients may have severe constipation. This abnormality has been called "institutional colon." The long and distended colon is at high risk for volvulus, particularly sigmoid volvulus, causing acute obstruction.

Acute colon dilatation (Ogilvie's syndrome) occurs in patients hospitalized for medical illness or surgery who had previously normal colon function. This condition of *acute pseudo-obstruction* involves a localized ileus with dilatation and loss of peristalsis in the right and transverse colon, and was described by Ogilvie in 1948.

Marked colon distention due to either acute or chronic pseudo-obstruction can result in ischemic perforation of the cecum. Cecal distention can cause perforation without obstruction being present. The cecum is the segment of the colon most likely to perforate, because its large diameter results in increased wall tension during distention (Laplace's law: Tension = Radius × Pressure/2.) Because of the risk of perforation, colon dilatation is considered a surgical emergency when the cecal diameter on abdominal radiograph is greater than 9 cm, whether or not an obstruction is present.

Patients with acquired pseudo-obstruction of the colon are initially seen with abdominal distention and inability to pass flatus. Generalized abdominal pain is common. Abdominal radiographs demonstrate marked dilatation of the colon. Initial treatment includes NG suction, hydration, and treatment of electrolyte disturbances. Colonoscopy should be performed to decompress the colon if possible, and more than one colonoscopy may be necessary. If the cecum cannot be decompressed by colonoscopy, surgery is required to inspect and decompress the right colon, often with a cecostomy or ileostomy. Right colectomy is necessary if cecal distention has progressed to gangrene.

Disorders of Defecation

Anorectal dysfunction occurs in a subgroup of patients with severe constipation who are unable to expel stool from the rectum. Some of these patients have an internal sphincter that does not relax in response to rectal distention (adult Hirschsprung's disease). Other patients are unable to relax the voluntary external sphincter or the puborectalis sling muscle to permit defecation. The surgical treatment of Hirschsprung's disease in adults may include surgical weakening of the sphincter (posterior myectomy) or endorectal pull-through operations (Soave or Duhamel operations), which remove the abnormal segment of smooth muscle. Patients with abnormal function of the voluntary external sphincter may respond to biofeedback therapy.

Severe idiopathic constipation occurs in occasional healthy patients, usually female, who have persistent constipation despite standard treatment with fiber and laxatives. These patients may have stool frequency of less than one per week despite laxatives. Some of these patients have *idiopathic colon dysmotility* with extremely long transit time in the colon. Evaluation includes anal manometry to rule out adult Hirschsprung's disease, or cinedefecography to rule out other abnormalities of anorectal function. Severely affected patients may benefit from subtotal colectomy with ileorectal anastomosis.

Fecal incontinence is a common problem, particularly in patients with neurologic impairments. Fecal incontinence may be due to loss of cerebral control over defecation (e.g.,

PEARLS FOR ROUNDS

In the normal recovery from postoperative ileus, the small intestine resumes peristalsis first, followed by the stomach. The colon recovers last and may take 3 to 5 days to resume function.

In a postoperative patient with prolonged ileus and possible bowel obstruction, abdominal computed tomography scan with luminal contrast is the most useful test.

In a patient with prolonged postoperative ileus, remember to check the medication list for narcotics and other drugs that inhibit transit; also check the electrolytes and the serum albumin.

The first test to rule out intestinal obstruction is usually a flat and upright radiograph of the abdomen. The most reliable radiographic sign of small-bowel obstruction is decreased gas in the colon.

Truncal vagotomy or resection of the ileum will cause postprandial (bile salt) diarrhea in many patients. Resins that bind bile salts (e.g., cholestyramine) are effective treatments.

in dementia or spinal cord injury). It also may be due to loss of adequate contraction of the internal or external sphincters. Weakness of the internal sphincter leads to leakage of liquid stool and may be due to anal trauma or prior anal surgery. The most common site of internal sphincter weakness is the posterior midline, leading to a "keynole anus" deformity. Bulk-forming agents such as soluble fiber (Metamucil) help control this form of incontinence by preventing liquid stool. Weakness of the external sphincter allows incontinence for solid stool and is often due to major neurologic impairment. In a cooperative patient, this form of incontinence can be managed by establishing a bowel regimen with scheduled enemas or defecation.

Chronic constipation is common, particularly among elderly patients taking multiple medications.

When a patient has complaints of constipation, it is important to obtain a description of bowel habit and review medications to look for possible causes. The physician should perform a rectal examination, including examination of the stool for occult blood. If evidence of GI blood loss, a family history of colon cancer, or a recent change in bowel habit is found, a colonoscopy should be recommended.

Other Colon Motility Disorders

Irritable bowel syndrome (IBS) is a functional disorder of colon motility, in which no obvious anatomic abnormality is present. Patients complain of abdominal pain and distention, often with alternating diarrhea and constipation. Manometric studies of the colon show that patients with IBS have increased pain with colon distention. The symptoms of IBS may resemble those of colitis, so colonoscopy to rule out colitis is appropriate before diagnosing IBS in a patient with intermittent diarrhea.

Diverticulosis is a common anatomic abnormality of the colon, in which mucosa and submucosa herniate through the muscular wall of the colon, forming multiple outpouchings. Diverticuli develop at sites where blood vessels pass through the colon wall. Diverticulosis may result from high luminal pressures in the colon, and manometric studies indicate higher luminal pressures in the colons of patients with diverticulosis. Epidemiologic studies suggest that low fecal volume due to a refined Western diet is an important factor in the pathogenesis of diverticulosis, so increasing dietary fiber may be helpful. Complications of diverticulosis that require surgical management include free perforation of a diverticulum with peritonitis, large-volume lower GI bleeding from a diverticular blood vessel, or diverticulitis, an acute inflammation of the colon due to confined perforation of a diverticulum.

Bile-salt diarrhea may follow resection of the ileum, where bile salts are normally absorbed, or may occur after vagotomy. Division of the main vagal trunks increases gastric emptying and may increase intestinal motility, and diarrhea can occur after all techniques of vagotomy. The common effect of vagotomy in humans is postprandial diarrhea, due to rapid transit of bile acids into the colon. This can usually be treated effectively with resins such as cholestyramine, which bind bile acids.

Effect of Medication on Intestinal Function

Many common medications alter the contractility of the intestine and may cause constipation or diarrhea in people without underlying intestinal abnormalities. Many patient complaints about bowel function are related to medication. Drugs alter GI motility by several mechanisms:

1. Interaction with receptors in the brain or spinal cord
2. Interaction with receptors on intestinal muscle cells or intrinsic nerves
3. Changes in the contractility of smooth muscle cells due to altered calcium influx
4. Changes in fluid secretion or resorption in the intestinal lumen, leading to changes in stool consistency and volume

Drugs That Decrease Intestinal Motility

Opiates inhibit intestinal propulsion by effects on receptors in the CNS as well as receptors in the intestine. Opiates decrease propulsive contractions in the intestine, while increasing muscle tone. This leads to slow intestinal transit, increased water absorption, and constipation. Opiates are used clinically to control diarrhea, but prolonged use produces physiologic dependence.

Anticholinergic drugs are used to block excessive motor activity or spasticity in the GI tract and urinary tract. The prototype for this group of drugs is atropine, a competitive inhibitor of the muscarinic receptor for acetylcholine. Acetylcholine is the major neurotransmitter stimulating motor activity in the GI tract, and many other hormones work by releasing acetylcholine from intrinsic nerves. Atropine and related drugs, including belladonna derivatives and oxybutynin, cause decreased peristalsis and constipation. Certain antipsychotic drugs, including the phenolthiazine drug chlorpromazine, have considerable anticholinergic activity. Long-term effects of these drugs may include chronic constipation and megacolon.

Somatostatin analogues, including the drug octreotide, mimic the effects of the peptide hormone somatostatin. Like somatostatin, these agents act on smooth muscle cells and nerves to block the stimulatory effect of GI peptide hormones. Octreotide is clinically useful in treating GI fistulas because it inhibits GI secretion.

Calcium-channel antagonists are drugs used widely to treat hypertension and ischemic heart disease. Calcium-channel antagonists decrease smooth muscle tone by decreasing calcium influx into smooth muscle cells. The decrease in vascular smooth muscle tone reduces blood pressure. In the GI tract, these drugs commonly cause constipation by decreasing tone and contractility in intestinal smooth muscle.

Drugs That Increase Intestinal Motility

Laxatives cause increased defecation by adding bulk, altering fluid and electrolyte secretion into the bowel lumen, or increasing contractility. Many common laxatives contain salts or osmotic agents that are poorly absorbed. This causes fluid accumulation in the intestinal lumen. Solutions containing magnesium salts, phosphates, or sulfate act by this mechanism. Other osmotic laxatives include polyethylene-glycol solutions (e.g., Colyte) that are used for bowel preparation for procedures, as well as lactulose and sorbitol. The common laxatives biscodyl and castor oil act both to increase luminal fluid absorption and to stimulate colon motility.

Many laxatives cause decreased colon contractility with prolonged use, leading to laxative dependence. The treatment of constipation should include adequate dietary fiber and oral liquid, with a bulk-forming agent such as psyllium powder when necessary.

Cholinergic drugs stimulate secretion and motility throughout the GI tract by interacting with acetylcholine receptors. Drugs in this class, such as bethanechol, may be used in surgical patients to treat urinary retention. Cholinergic drugs have been tried in postoperative patients to shorten postoperative ileus but have not led to significant improvement.

Anti-dopaminergic drugs may increase gastric emptying and are useful to treat gastroesphageal reflux and to control nausea and vomiting. Some of these drugs also increase intestinal motility. Metoclopramide acts in the stomach as a dopamine antagonist and also by releasing acetylcholine. Metoclopramide promotes gastric emptying by increasing antral contractility and accelerates small intestinal transit time. Domperidone is another dopamine antagonist that is used as an antiemetic. Cisapride is a benzamide drug that stimulates GI motility, probably by releasing acetylcholine from enteric nerves. Cisapride increases motility of the esophagus, small intestine, and colon. It was used to treat gastroesophageal reflux as well as gastroparesis and severe constipation but is no longer on the market because of serious cardiac side effects. Erythromycin, an antibiotic, increases gastric emptying and may increase small bowel transit through its interaction with receptors for the peptide hormone motilin.

Prostaglandins are a group of biologically active lipids derived from arachidonic acid. The prostaglandin E analogue misoprostol is used clinically to decrease gastric acidity. Most prostaglandins cause diarrhea by stimulating adenylate cyclase activity in mucosal cells. The resulting elevation of mucosal levels of cyclic adenosine monophosphate causes increased fluid secretion into the intestine.

Suggested Reading

Bassotti G, Iantorno G, Fiorella S, et al: Colonic motility in man: Features in normal subjects and in patients with chronic idiopathic constipation. Am J Gastroenterol 94(7):1760–1770, 1999.

Davis L, Lowman RM: An evaluation of cecal size in impending perforation of the cecum. Surg Gynecol Obstet 103(6):711–718, 1956.

Ogilvie WH: Large-intestine colic due to sympathetic deprivation. A new clinical syndrome. Dis Colon Rectum 30(12):984–987, 1987 (Reprinted from British Medical Journal 2:671–673, 1948).

Pfeifer J, Agachan F, Wexner SD: Surgery for constipation: a review. Dis Colon Rectum 39(4):444–460, 1996.

Tack J, Vanden Berghe P: Neuropeptides and colonic motility: It's all in the little brain. Gastroenterology 119(1):257–260, 2000.

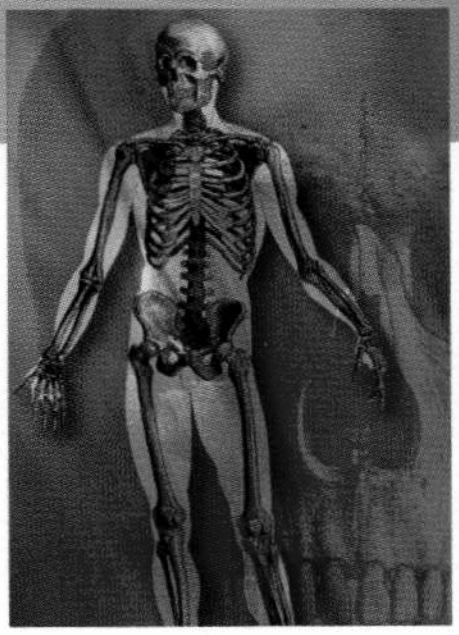

Chapter 24
Pancreas

JAMES A. MADURA, II, MD, HARRY M. RICHTER, III, MD, and
RICHARD A. PRINZ, MD

Anatomy

The pancreas originates from two separate embryologic outpouchings of the primordial foregut. The dorsal pancreatic bud and its duct arise from the duodenum, whereas the ventral pancreatic bud and its duct arise from the bile duct. Around week 6 of gestation, the ventral pancreatic bud, which is attached to the bile duct, rotates posteriorly around the duodenum to fuse with the dorsal bud and form a single organ. The duct systems of the two pancreatic buds fuse as well. The primordial ventral duct becomes the main pancreatic duct, known as the duct of Wirsung. The dorsal pancreatic duct remains as a small accessory duct, called the duct of Santorini, and enters the duodenum separately. The main pancreatic duct joins the common bile duct just above its junction with the duodenum. The head and uncinate process of the pancreas lie within the sweep of the duodenum, to the right of the superior mesenteric artery and superior mesenteric and portal veins. The neck is that portion anterior to the superior mesenteric vessels, whereas the body and tail lie to the left of the superior mesenteric vessels, anterior to the splenic vein (Fig. 24-1). The head, neck, and uncinate process of the pancreas receive blood supply via the pancreaticoduodenal branches of the gastroduodenal and the superior mesenteric arteries. The body and tail are nourished by branches of the splenic artery. The pancreas receives parasympathetic innervation from the celiac division of the vagus nerve and sympathetic innervation from the splanchnic nerves, chiefly through the celiac ganglion. The pancreas also is served by the gastrointestinal intrinsic nervous system.

The pancreas is a mixed exocrine (80% by mass) and endocrine gland (20% by mass). Insulin, glucagon, and somatostatin are secreted respectively by the beta, alpha, and delta cells located within the numerous islets of Langerhans distributed throughout the pancreas. The exocrine pancreas consists of discrete subunits called *acini* (Box 24-1). These aggregates of secretory cells synthesize and release digestive enzymes. The exocrine secretion from each acinus is collected into a small ductule, which merges with other ductules ultimately to form the pancreatic duct. The cells that line the pancreatic ductules secrete an aqueous electrolyte solution rich in bicarbonate.

The pancreatic acini consist of 20 to 50 acinar cells distributed spherically around a pancreatic ductule (Fig. 24-2). Each acinar cell is a truncated pyramid, with its narrow apex oriented in contact with the ductal lumen. These cells produce digestive enzymes in great quantity. After synthesis, these enzymes are stored in zymogen granules within the intracellular compartment. The proteolytic enzymes and phospholipases are synthesized and stored intracellularly as inactive proenzymes, whereas lipase, amylase, and nucleases are synthesized in active form. This minimizes the risk of accidental enzymatic autodestruction of the acinar cell. Further intrinsic protection is provided by the inclusion within zymogen granules of small amounts of trypsin inhibitor. Finally, a cofactor molecule necessary for the activity of the enzyme lipase, known as colipase, is synthesized as an inactive procolipase. The contents of the zymogen granules are released through the apical cell membrane into the pancreatic ductule by the process of exocytosis.

In contrast with the pancreatic acinar cells, the pancreatic ductule and duct cells secrete an aqueous electrolyte solution. The cationic component of the ductal secretion consists of sodium and potassium ions in a concentration similar to that in plasma. The anions are chloride and bicarbonate, whose relative concentrations depend on the secretory state of the gland. Under basal conditions, total duct-secretion volume is small, and chloride is the predominant anion. When stimulated, ductal secretion increases dramatically, and bicarbonate replaces chloride as the predominant anion. Thus during physiologic stimulation such as ingestion of a meal, pancreatic juice is an alkaline, bicarbonate-rich fluid.

The volume of pancreatic juice secreted by a healthy human is estimated to be about 1 L/day. Basal or fasting pancreatic exocrine fluid output is relatively small and fluctuates with the phases of the interdigestive motility pattern known as the *migrating motor complex* (MMC). After ingestion of a meal, neurohumoral mechanisms profoundly stimulate the pancreas to secrete juice rich in both digestive enzymes and bicarbonate. Pancreatic duct secretion of water and bicarbonate is stimulated chiefly by the hormone secretin. This polypeptide is released from the duodenum and upper jejunum mainly in response to the presence of hydrochloric acid (HCl) within the upper

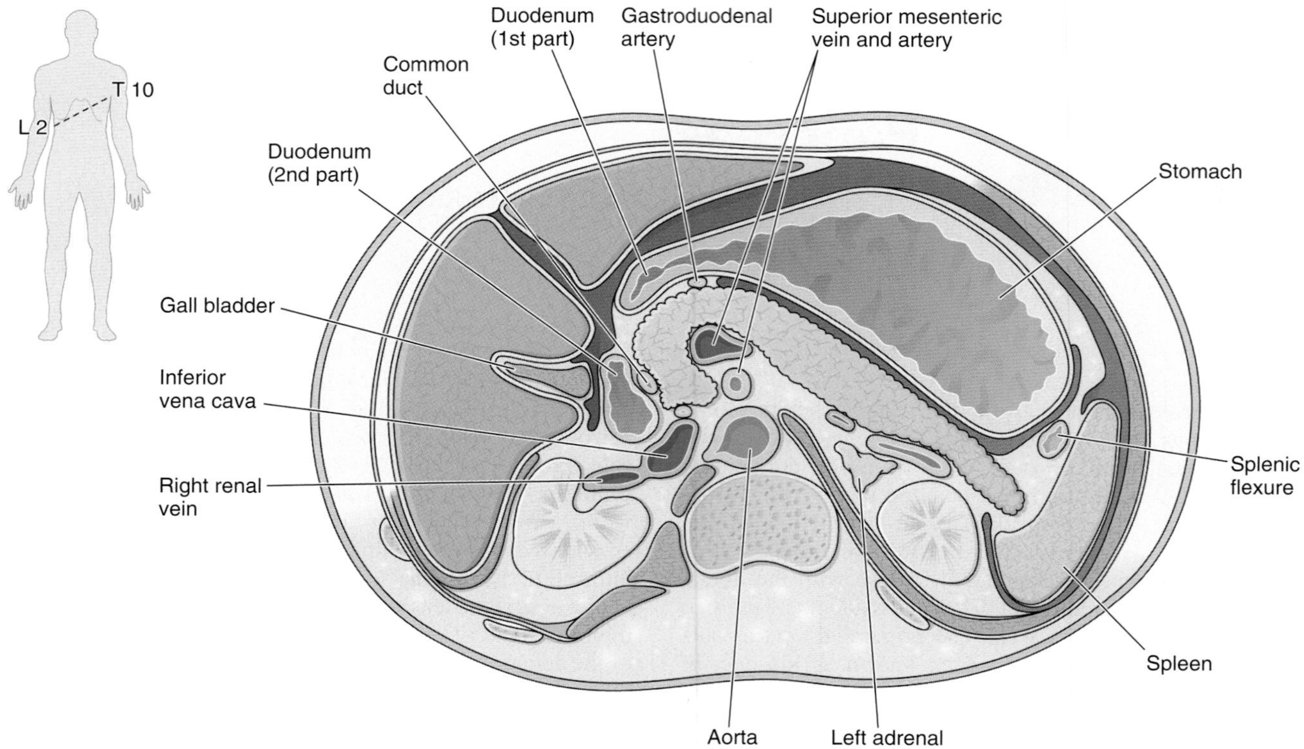

FIGURE 24–1 Anatomic relations of the pancreas, as demonstrated by oblique transverse section through the upper abdomen.

small bowel. The resulting outpouring of alkaline pancreatic juice helps neutralize acid in the duodenal lumen, thus acting as a classic physiologic negative-feedback loop. The control of pancreatic enzyme secretion is somewhat more complex. The hormone cholecystokinin (CCK) is released from the duodenum and upper jejunum in response to nutrients, in particular, fatty acids, amino acids, and oligopeptides. This hormone directly stimulates pancreatic acinar cell secretion. Direct hormonal stimulation by CCK stimulation is not the only initiator of acinar secretion. Enteropancreatic neural activation of cholinergic reflexes, including vagovagal reflexes, probably stimulates the majority of acinar enzyme-rich secretion. CCK appears to facilitate and augment this enteropancreatic neural response.

When pancreatic juice enters the lumen of the duodenum, the proteolytic enzymes arrive as inactive proenzymes. The duodenal brush-border enzyme enteropeptidase (enterokinase) cleaves a peptide fragment from trypsinogen to form activated trypsin. Trypsin then further autoactivates additional trypsinogen molecules, as well as the other proenzymes and procolipase within the duodenal lumen. Pancreatic enzymes function optimally at neutral pH; lipase especially is irreversibly denatured at low pH. The alkaline pancreatic juice, together with duodenal bicarbonate secretion and bile, balances the HCl secreted by the stomach to provide a neutral environment within the upper small intestine. The normal healthy pancreas enzyme secretion is about 10-fold the amount necessary to achieve complete intraluminal digestion. Thus malabsorption due to pancreatic insufficiency usually represents at least a 90% loss of exocrine function.

BOX 24–1 Digestive Enzymes Secreted by the Pancreas

Proteases*	Lipases
Trypsin	Nucleases
Chymotrypsin	RNase
Elastase	DNase
Carboxypeptidase A and B	Amylase
Phospholipases*	
Phospholipase A and B	

*Secreted as inactive proenzyme

Acute Pancreatitis

Acute pancreatitis is a common, potentially lethal disease causing a variable spectrum of pancreatic inflammation. In

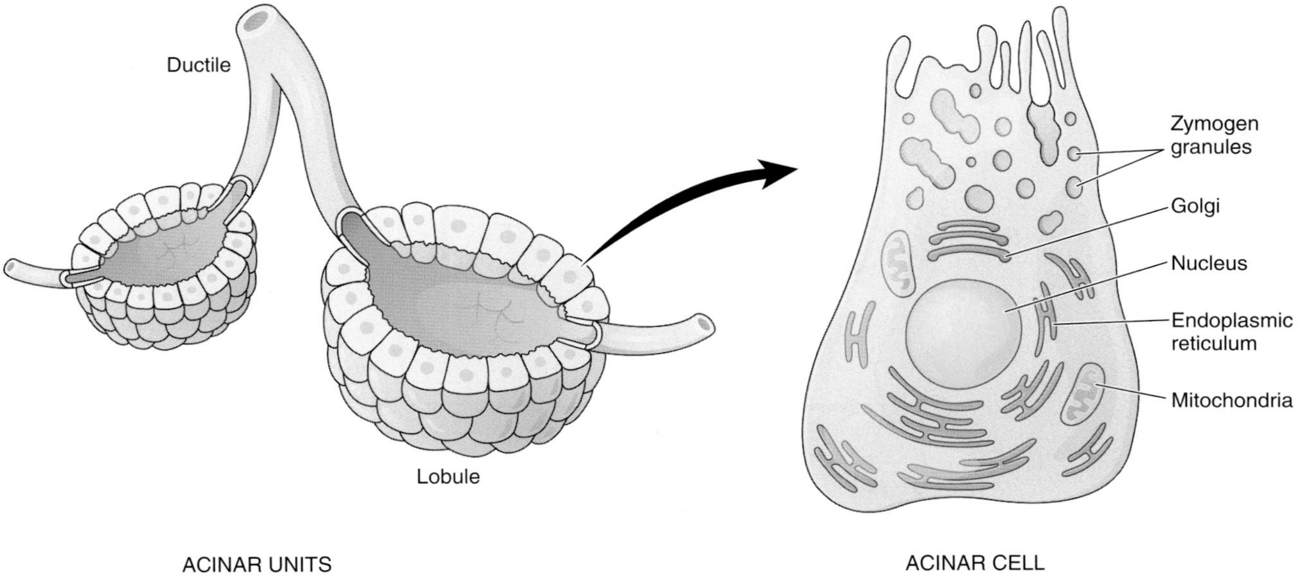

FIGURE 24–2 *Left*, Arrangement of pancreatic acini, the subunit of pancreatic exocrine function. *Right*, Pancreatic acinar cell, which synthesizes and secretes digestive enzymes.

its worst form, pancreatic necrosis, regional tissue destruction, and systemic compromise occur. The severity of an attack appears to be determined almost at its inception, and many of the mechanisms involved remain obscure.

Etiology

Throughout the world, alcoholism and gallstones account for about 80% of acute pancreatitis. Acute alcoholic pancreatitis occurs, almost always, after a minimum 5 to 7 years of regular, heavy ethanol ingestion. In only a small minority of alcoholics will acute pancreatitis ever develop, implying multifactorial causation. A gallstone in the common bile duct (choledocholithiasis) may incite acute pancreatitis as it passes through the sphincter of Oddi en route to the duodenum. It does so, at least in principle, by transiently obstructing pancreatic duct flow, and perhaps also by promoting reflux of bile into the pancreatic duct. As with alcoholic acute pancreatitis, the exact mechanisms remain uncertain. Perhaps 10% of attacks remain idiopathic, in spite of thorough investigation. The remainder are due to drugs that are toxic to the pancreas, viral infections (e.g., mumps), hyperlipidemia, hyperparathyroidism, trauma, anatomic anomaly, pancreatic duct obstruction due to tumor or pancreatic stone, or an autoimmune process.

Pathogenesis

Although the known causes of acute pancreatitis are many, the resulting cellular events involved are probably similar and may be portrayed as a unified scheme. The pancreatic acinar cells segregate inactive proteases and other inactive and active digestive enzymes within the zymogen granules. These are maintained separate from lysosomes, which contain substances capable of activating trypsin. Soon after a generic event that triggers acute pancreatitis, the extracellular release of enzymes (exocytosis) is blocked, and trypsin becomes activated within the cell. The latter occurs because the segregation of zymogen granules and lysosomes is lost; the contents of these two components become "colocalized." Lysosomal molecules, probably cathepsin-B, cause activation of trypsinogen. Active trypsin will then catalyze the activation of other intracellular digestive proenzymes. Activated enzymes damage the acinar cell and its membrane, leading to their release into the retroperitoneum, the peritoneal cavity, and the systemic circulation.

Local pancreatic injury is followed by influx of leukocytes and macrophages, which, together with the pancreas itself, elaborate numerous mediators of inflammation and the systemic inflammatory response (Fig. 24-3). Vasoconstrictors may cause pancreatic ischemia, a hallmark of severe pancreatitis and a contributor to pancreatic necrosis. Among many mediators, current interest is focused on tumor necrosis factor (TNF), interleukin-1 (IL-1), and platelet-activating factor (PAF). Timely inhibition of mediators such as these could in theory moderate pancreatic and peripancreatic destruction and ameliorate the systemic effects of pancreatitis, such as hypotension, respiratory failure, and renal failure, or a combination of these.

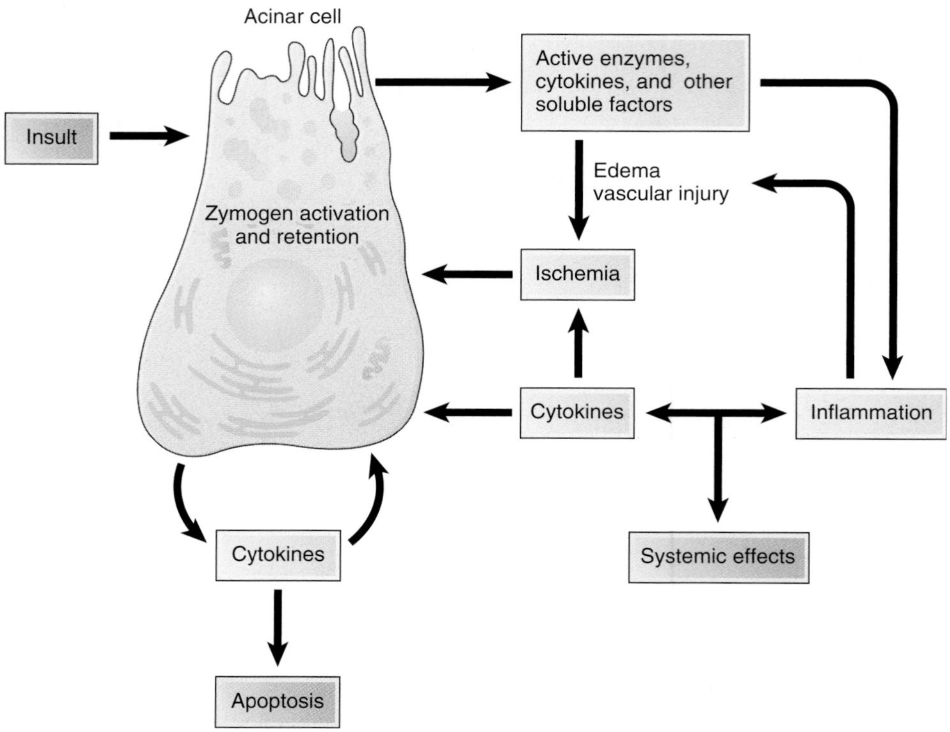

FIGURE 24–3 Pathophysiology of acute pancreatitis: generalized scheme. (Adapted from Karne S, Gorelick FS: Etiopathogenesis of acute pancreatitis. Surg Clin North Am 79(4):699–710, 1999.)

Clinical Presentation

The predominant symptom of acute pancreatitis is severe, constant epigastric pain. The onset is rapid, although not so sudden as that of perforated duodenal ulcer. The pain frequently radiates through to the back and may be partially diminished by sitting and leaning forward or lying curled in a fetal position. Nausea and vomiting are nearly universal. The symptoms cause most patients to seek medical attention within 6 to 12 hours of the onset of pancreatitis, although delay is often seen among inebriated patients. The patient appears acutely ill and is usually tachycardic. Hypotension denotes a severe attack. The abdomen is quiet, tender, and full to palpation in the epigastrium.

Diagnostic Tests

The simplest laboratory test that suggests the diagnosis of acute pancreatitis is an elevated serum amylase level. Acute acinar cell injury causes a rapid increase in serum amylase. Normal kidneys efficiently clear amylase, so that typically serum amylase may have returned toward normal by the third or fourth day of the attack. A number of acute abdominal surgical emergencies, such as perforated duodenal ulcer, cause hyperamylasemia, but rarely to the level of elevation seen in acute pancreatitis. The severity of pancreatitis does not correlate with the degree of amylase elevation. Patients with acute biliary pancreatitis tend to have very high amylase levels, even during a mild attack, presumably because the pancreas was completely normal at the outset. A lesser elevation of serum amylase is usually observed in acute alcoholic pancreatitis, especially during a second or subsequent attack. Serum lipase is as sensitive as serum amylase measurement and somewhat more specific as a marker of acute pancreatitis than is elevated amylase, and the elevated serum level persists for a day or two longer than does the amylase. Thus patients first seen 2 or 3 days into an attack of acute pancreatitis may still demonstrate elevated lipase levels.

Plain abdominal radiographs are useful mainly to exclude other conditions, such as perforated peptic ulcer or mechanical small-bowel obstruction. Ultrasound of the abdomen may disclose edema of the pancreatic substance if it is seen, but often it is obscured by overlying bowel gas, which acts as an acoustic barrier. Ultrasound is most useful to diagnose gallbladder stones and also can accurately calibrate the common bile duct diameter, suggesting choledocholithiasis if distended. A contrast-enhanced abdominal computed tomography (CT) scan (although often unnecessary) dependably diagnoses acute pancreatitis. The severity of the attack and its outcome can be graded and correlated to the CT appearance of the pancreas and parapancreatic tissues. Finally, regions of necrosis within the pancreatic substance can be precisely identified by CT scan after rapid bolus infusion of intravenous contrast (Fig.

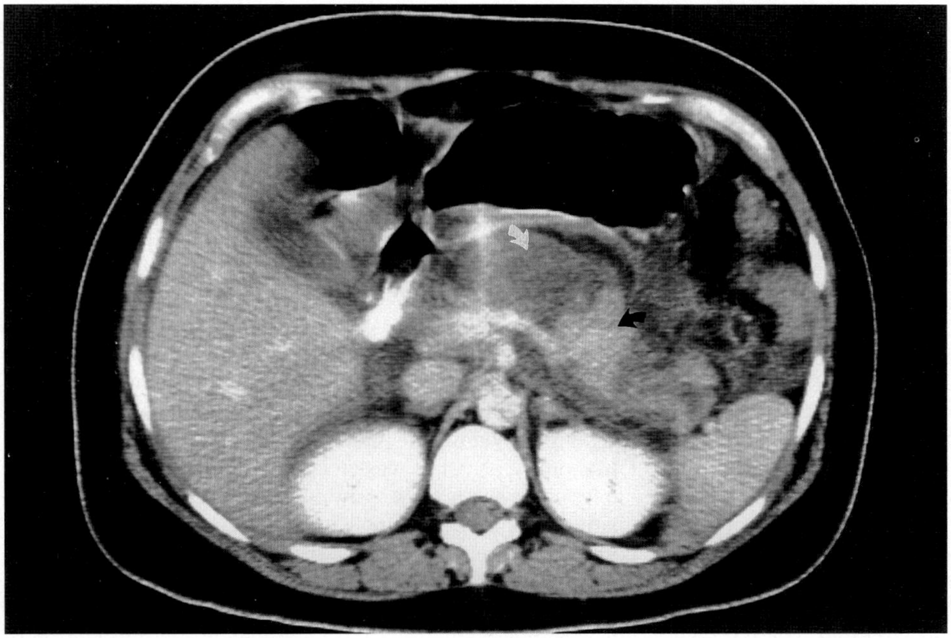

FIGURE 24–4 Computed tomography scan of pancreas body and tail after bolus infusion of intravenous contrast. Severe acute pancreatitis with necrosis. Regions of viable pancreas demonstrate contrast enhancement (*black arrow*), whereas regions of necrotic pancreas do not (*white arrow*).

24-4). Viable pancreatic tissue will enhance, whereas necrotic pancreatic tissue will not, allowing estimation of the fraction of pancreas that is necrotic.

Prediction of Severity

Between 70% and 80% of all attacks of acute pancreatitis are mild, resulting in little short- or long-term morbidity and virtually no mortality. The remainder are severe attacks, involving a variable fraction of pancreatic necrosis, and are associated with extensive short- and long-term morbidity and a mortality rate between 10% and 30%. Predicting severe pancreatitis soon after hospital admission allows early triage to intensive care for supportive treatment. To this end, several systems of severity measurement have been developed and correlated with outcome. Of these systems, the best known is the scoring system devised by Ranson and associates (Table 24-1). They identified 11 "criteria," five of which were determined on admission and six others at 48 hours after admission, which correlated with ultimate risk of morbidity and mortality. Patients exhibiting two or fewer of the prognostic criteria are likely to survive a relatively mild attack; those with three to six criteria have progressively more severe disease and a greater probability of death, whereas those with seven or more criteria will almost certainly not survive. The Ranson prognostic score has the advantages of strong clinical correlation and a simple, universally available data set; its disadvantage is that the ultimate prognostic calculation requires 48 hours of hospitalization. The condition of the pancreas and parapancreatic tissue on CT scan of the abdomen also can be correlated with clinical outcome. The appearance of pancreatic edema alone portends uncomplicated recovery, whereas severity and infectious complications correlate with the quantity of parapancreatic fluid collections seen (Table 24-2). In the future, serum or urinary markers of necrosis may predict the severity of pancreatitis.

Management of Mild Pancreatitis

When mild acute pancreatitis is diagnosed by clinical criteria and serum amylase and/or lipase levels, a confirmatory CT scan is unnecessary. Although recovery without specific treatment is the rule, all patients are watched closely in a hospital setting, because rapid deterioration is not always

TABLE 24–1 Ranson's Criteria for Severity of Acute Pancreatitis*

On Admission	At 48 Hr
Age >55 yr	Hematocrit decrease >10 percentage points†
WBC >16,000 cells/mm^3	Serum calcium <8 mg/dL
Serum glucose >200 mg/dL	Base deficit >4 mEg/L
Serum LDH >350 units/L	BUN increase >5 mg/dL†
AST >250 U/dL	Arterial pO_2 <60 mmHg
	Fluid sequestration >6 L‡

*Criteria are modified slightly for gallstone pancreatitis.
†Compared with admission values.
‡Fluid volume infused minus urine and nasogastric tube output.
WBC, white blood cell; LDH, lactate dehydrogluase; AST, aspartate aminotransferase; BUN, blood urea nitrogen.

TABLE 24–2 Grading of Acute Pancreatitis by CT Criteria

Grade	CT Characteristics
A	Normal
B	Focal or diffuse pancreas enlargement
C	Abnormal pancreas and peripancreatic inflammation
D	Single pancreatic fluid collection
E	2 or more pancreatic fluid collections and/or presence of gas

CT, computed tomography.

predictable. Management consists of nothing by mouth, hydration with intravenous crystalloid solution, and analgesia as needed. Prophylaxis against deep venous thrombosis with low-dose subcutaneous heparin or sequential calf compression or both should be routine. Alcoholic patients must be assessed for risk of alcohol withdrawal syndromes. Laboratory tests on admission should include either an arterial blood gas measurement or oxygen saturation measured by pulse oximetry. Oral intake of liquids is resumed when the abdomen is soft and nontender, which usually correlates with a normalized serum amylase level. If the liquids do not exacerbate the attack, the diet can then be advanced as tolerated. A right upper quadrant ultrasound is performed in all patients, even alcoholic patients, because they too may harbor gallstones. Nasogastric suction and gastric antisecretory agents are rarely indicated.

Management of Severe Pancreatitis

Severe acute pancreatitis is usually evident on initial clinical assessment; if not, the grave situation declares itself within the subsequent 24 to 48 hours. Early mortality from severe acute pancreatitis results from cardiovascular or respiratory failure or both. Thus patients are managed in an intensive care unit, with urinary, central venous pressure, and arterial catheters; cardiac and pulse oximetry monitoring; and close observation. Profound and ongoing intravascular volume loss results from fluid sequestration within the retroperitoneum as well as a diffuse capillary leak that causes generalized edema. Intravascular volume is maintained by crystalloid infusion, titrated to maintain adequate tissue perfusion. Inotropic cardiac support is used as needed once intravascular volume repletion is achieved. Packed red blood cells are transfused as needed to maintain adequate oxygen-carrying capacity. Respiratory function frequently worsens precipitously in the first 24 hours, requiring endotracheal intubation and ventilatory support. Analgesia and sedation are liberally administered, as is stress ulcer prophylaxis.

No pharmacologic therapy now dependably ameliorates the severity of the pancreatitis or decreases the risk of systemic complications. Neither octreotide, a somatostatin analogue that inhibits pancreatic exocrine secretion, nor various protease inhibitors have improved mortality. Newer therapies targeting mediators of the pancreatic and systemic inflammatory response could in theory improve outcome, especially if administered very early in the attack. One such agent, a PAF antagonist called lexipafant, showed promise in initial laboratory investigations, but so far has not proved beneficial in clinical trails. Because retroperitoneal and peritoneal exudate contains activated digestive enzymes and a host of other vasoactive and inflammatory mediators, peritoneal dialysis might logically improve the condition of patients with severe acute pancreatitis. Several trials report amelioration of the cardiovascular collapse associated with a severe attack, although overall hospital mortality due mainly to late infectious sequelae was not altered. Although peritoneal dialysis is not now widely practiced, it still has a role in patients who are progressing toward death in spite of all other measures. Finally, operation has almost no role early in the course of severe acute pancreatitis, except to rule out another suspected cause of the acute abdomen or to resect gangrenous bowel that has developed as a complication of the severe pancreatitis.

Necrosis and Infection

Severe acute or necrotizing pancreatitis is synonymous with some necrosis of the pancreatic parenchyma or the surrounding retroperitoneal tissue or both. The presence of pancreatic necrosis can be detected by dynamic CT scanning or by serum markers, if available. The probability of complications and of death correlates with the amount of necrotic pancreas. When 20% or less of the gland undergoes necrosis, secondary pancreatic infection is rare, and survival is expected. If 50% or more of the gland is necrotic, secondary infection becomes probable, and mortality reaches as high as 50%. Secondary infection of necrotic pancreatic and parapancreatic tissues is relatively common and is the principal cause of mortality from severe acute pancreatitis. Infecting organisms are usually enteric gram-negative bacilli, but infection with gram-positive organisms and fungi is now recognized as well. Most likely, the gram-negative organisms translocate from the colon or small bowel and travel via the peritoneum, lymphatics, or mesenteric veins to the pancreatic bed. A trend toward reduced pancreatic infection (as well as other systemic infection) has been shown after the prolonged use of newer antibiotics, which effectively penetrate pancreatic tissue. However, infections that develop in patients treated with prophylactic antibiotics tend to involve resistant organisms. One standard prophylactic antibiotic regimen gaining acceptance uses imipenim-cilistatin begun soon after admission and continued for at least 2 weeks. Other methods to prevent translocation, such as early enteral feeding, when possible, have been shown to decrease secondary pancreatic infection. These patients have many intravenous and invasive monitoring catheters. These are potential portals for entry of gram-positive organisms that can secondarily infect the pancreas. Rigid adherence to appropriate infection-control measures is required to minimize this risk.

Infected pancreatic necrosis, when it occurs, is the most dreaded and lethal complication of severe acute pancreatitis. The condition becomes apparent most frequently during the third or fourth week of hospitalization and is marked by fever, increasing pain, tenderness, and fullness in the upper abdomen. The patient usually appears septic. CT scan may reveal extraluminal retroperitoneal gas, which is a radiographic hallmark of infected necrosis (Fig. 24-5). Percutaneous image-guided fine-needle aspiration of the pancreas, with immediate Gram stain and culture of the aspirate, can reveal the presence of organisms that are diagnostic of infected necrosis. Infected pancreatic necrosis is almost always fatal without aggressive débridement and drainage of the retroperitoneum. The standard for wide débridement is an open laparotomy, although laparoscopic and endoscopic techniques are being described and developed. Surgical strategy ranges from débridement with closed suction and irrigation of the retroperitoneum to multiple planned operative débridements every 2 to 3 days until all necrotic material is removed. All approaches are time and labor intensive but offer the only chance for survival of the majority of patients.

Sterile pancreatic necrosis is associated with severe acute pancreatitis, but unlike infected pancreatic necrosis, it is usually managed without the need for urgent operation. Acute peripancreatic fluid collections frequently arise. These may include reactive serous effusions but likely represent secondary or even main pancreatic ductal disruption, with resultant leak of pancreatic juice into the lesser peritoneal sac or other anatomic spaces surrounding the pancreas. These acute collections will often resorb spontaneously, requiring no specific treatment. If infection of the fluid is suspected, or if pain and tenderness are increasing, the collections may be percutaneously aspirated or even drained. In some centers, endoscopically placed transpapillary drains are inserted into the pancreatic duct, occasionally through the disruption into the fluid collection, to accomplish drainage. Finally, if such collections do not spontaneously disappear and do not require early drainage, they may evolve into a pancreatic pseudocyst.

A few patients with sterile pancreatic necrosis fail to improve in spite of optimal, protracted conservative care. These patients deserve operative exploration and pancreatic debridement on the grounds of failed nonoperative treatment, coupled perhaps with the suspicion that a smoldering, occult infection has eluded discovery. The operation is delayed as long as is practical, to allow areas undergoing necrosis to demarcate and liquefy. This makes the débridement technically easier. The pancreas and adjacent tissues are débrided and drained, provision for enteric feeding is established, and the abdomen is closed with the expectation that the need for reoperation will be unlikely.

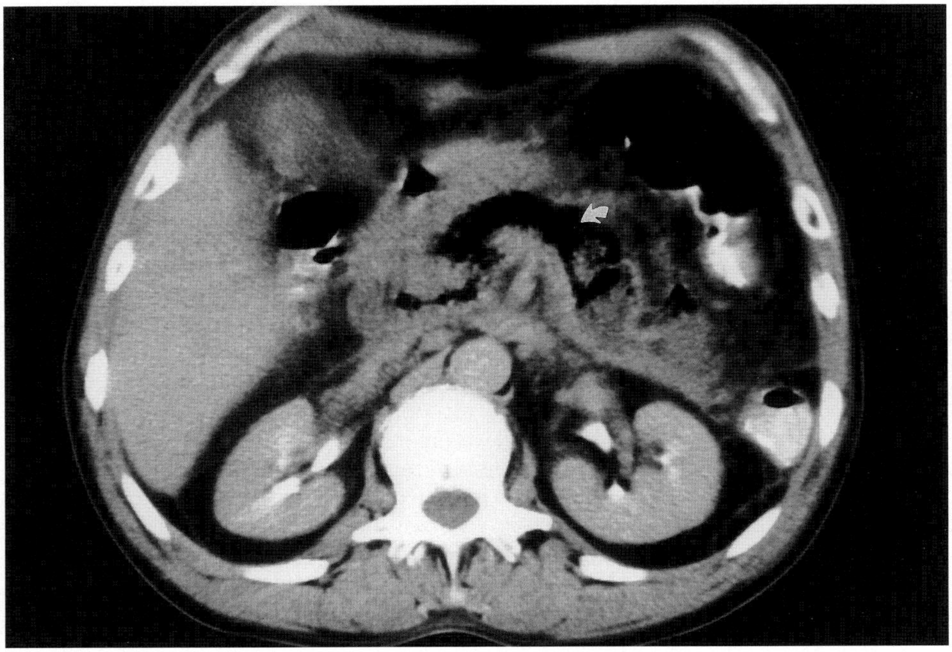

FIGURE 24–5 Computed tomography scan of pancreas. Infected pancreatic necrosis. Pancreas is greatly enlarged and extraluminal retroperitoneal gas is apparent (*arrow*).

Biliary (Gallstone) Pancreatitis

Gallstones are the most common cause of acute pancreatitis in most series around the world. The relation between acute pancreatitis and the passage of a gallstone through the common bile duct and into the intestinal tract was proven by the demonstration of gallstones in the filtered feces of patients with acute nonalcoholic pancreatitis. Anatomically, the common bile and the pancreatic ducts join to form a common channel shortly before entering the duodenum. A gallstone that even transiently blocks the common channel can give rise to the reflux of bile into the pancreatic duct, at a pressure greater than normal pancreatic duct pressure (Fig. 24-6). Perhaps this transient situation triggers a sequence of events resulting in acute pancreatitis. Clearly the offending gallstone need not be large; "biliary sludge" and even biliary "microlithiasis" appear to be capable of provoking acute pancreatitis, although perhaps by a different mechanism. As a rule, gallstone pancreatitis patients have multiple small gallstones within the gallbladder, a comparatively wide cystic duct (promoting passage into the common bile duct), and a distinct common channel of the bile and pancreatic ducts. A number of patients thought to have recurrent idiopathic pancreatitis have been cured by surgical removal of an apparently normal gallbladder, suggesting the gallbladder to be the source of unnoticed tiny stones or microlithiasis.

Diagnosis

Nonalcoholic patients with acute pancreatitis are very likely to have biliary lithiasis as the underlying cause. The presence of gallstones within the gallbladder virtually secures the diagnosis. A distended common bile duct seen by ultrasound further suggests the recent passage of a stone. Serum bilirubin or alkaline phosphatase or both may be mildly elevated, but often both are normal. If the ultrasound fails to reveal gallbladder stones or sludge, and other rare causes are excluded, the next diagnostic step includes endoscopic retrograde cholangiopancreatography (ERCP). A sample of bile may be obtained to examine for microscopic crystals (this can be achieved by duodenal drainage as well), and small stones or anatomic anomalies may be identified.

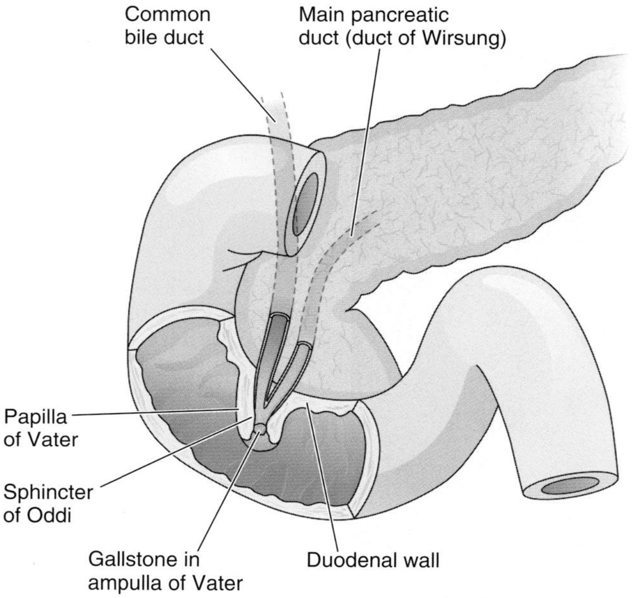

FIGURE 24–6 Mechanism of acute gallstone (biliary) pancreatitis. Stone transiently obstructs common channel of the pancreatic and common bile ducts.

Management

Gallstone pancreatitis is usually mild, resolving clinically within 2 to 4 days. Serum bilirubin and alkaline phosphatase are typically normal or return to normal within this period, suggesting a low probability of persistent stone(s) within the common bile duct. Cholecystectomy eliminates the source of further stones and thus prevents recurrent pancreatitis. An intraoperative cholangiogram is performed (unless it has been undertaken preoperatively). If pancreatitis resolves but liver-function tests suggest persistent stone in the bile duct, then preoperative ERCP with papillotomy and stone extraction is appropriate, followed by prompt cholecystectomy.

Severe gallstone pancreatitis is managed like severe pancreatitis of any cause. Usually, the inciting stone has passed, leaving the bile and pancreatic ducts unobstructed. Routine, early ERCP is therefore not warranted. However, if a stone is persistently obstructing the ampulla of Vater, then endoscopic stone extraction is attractive. Not only does the decompression benefit the pancreatitis, but obstructive jaundice and the risk of cholangitis are minimized as well.

Chronic Pancreatitis

Chronic pancreatitis is an irreversible, progressive inflammatory disease of the pancreas characterized by pain, fibrosis, and progressive loss of exocrine or endocrine function or both. The early course of this disease may often be manifest by repeated attacks of acute pancreatitis. It occurs in men more frequently than in women, and excessive alcohol consumption is usually the cause in developed countries. Average age at diagnosis of alcoholic pancreatitis is 35 to 45 years, with an 11- to 18-year history of 150 to 175 g of daily alcohol ingestion.

Worldwide estimates of the incidence of chronic pancreatitis range between 2 and 10 per 100,000 population per year, with a prevalence of 30 per 100,000 persons. The incidence is generally thought to be increasing. Regional differences are not completely explained by differences in alcohol consumption. According to estimates of the Commission on Professional and Hospital Activities, chronic pancreatitis ranks as the 27th most common

BOX 24-2 Indications for Surgery in Chronic Pancreatitis

- Pain refractory to medical management
- Inability to exclude pancreatic malignancy
- Complications
  - Pseudocyst
  - Biliary obstruction
  - Duodenal obstruction
  - Splenic vein thrombosis
  - Pancreatic fistula
  - Colonic obstruction
  - Pancreatic ascites

BOX 24-3 Causes of Chronic Pancreatitis

- Alcohol
- Obstruction
  - Pancreas divisum
  - Congenital strictures
  - Acquired strictures
    - Acute pancreatitis
    - Trauma
    - ERCP
  - Neoplasm
    - Pancreatic
    - Periampullary
- Toxic substances
  - Tropical pancreatitis
  - Hypercalcemia
  - Hyperlipidemia
- Autoimmune
- Idiopathic

ERCP, endoscopic retrograde cholangiopancreatography.

digestive disease in the United States, with a three-fold higher prevalence in the black male population.

The majority of care for chronic pancreatitis is directed toward ameliorating pain, but a substantial amount of resources also is spent on treating complications. In more than one half of chronic pancreatitis patients, pancreatic diabetes will develop; one third of these patients will be insulin dependent, and nearly 50% will eventually require surgical intervention for pain or other complications. As many as one half of all patients will die within 20 years of their diagnosis of chronic pancreatitis, a rate much higher than that of their age-matched population.

Optimal care of the patient with chronic pancreatitis relies on supportive medical management of endocrine and exocrine insufficiency and pain. Surgical intervention is generally reserved for intractable pain and specific complications such as pseudocyst or biliary or intestinal obstruction (Box 24-2).

Etiology

Chronic pancreatitis appears to be a multifactorial process involving both a genetic predisposition and environmental factors (Box 24-3). Alcohol use is by far the number one cause of chronic pancreatitis in the Western world, accounting for an estimated 70% of the cases in the United States and Europe. In about 10% of chronic alcoholics, chronic pancreatitis will develop, roughly the same percentage of alcoholics in whom hepatic cirrhosis develops. Ingested alcohol results in direct damage to the acinar cell with increased concentration of protein secretion, decreased production of bicarbonate, and decreased fluid volume, as demonstrated in experimental models and in patients with alcoholic pancreatitis. This combination appears to result in protein and calcium precipitation within the pancreatic duct system, subsequent ductal obstruction, activation of pancreatic enzymes, and autodigestion of the gland. Over time, a fibrotic response results in permanent ductal abnormalities, calcification, and stone formation.

Dietary factors, high fat and high protein, and trace mineral insufficiency, may have an epidemiologic association with chronic pancreatitis. Another theory suggests that the presence of an acinar cell product, lithostatin or pancreatic stone protein, prevents calcium precipitation. Decreased concentrations of lithostatin and decreased levels of lithostatin messenger RNA have been found in the pancreatic juice and acini of patients with chronic calcific pancreatitis, suggesting a genetic component of risk for developing the disease. Alcohol-induced derangement of lipid metabolism also has been postulated to induce the periacinar fibrosis and changes associated with alcoholic pancreatitis. The range of experimentally identified abnormalities supports the multifactorial nature of the disease.

Another form of chronic pancreatitis, tropical pancreatitis, may be caused by protein malnutrition and cyanogens found in cassava root. The clinical and histologic features of tropical pancreatitis are nearly identical to those of alcoholic chronic pancreatitis. Obstructive pancreatitis results from both congenital and acquired ductal obstruction, as in pancreas divisum, congenital and acquired strictures, and neoplasia. Unlike alcoholic pancreatitis, the obstructed pancreas shows uniform inflammatory changes with preserved ductal epithelium and rare protein plugs. The hypothesis that high intraductal pressure results in pancreatitis has been proposed, based partly on the demonstration of high intraductal pressures in these patients.

Additional causes of chronic pancreatitis include hypercalcemia, hyperlipidemia, autoimmune diseases, and hereditary pancreatitis. The mechanism by which pancreatitis develops in these situations is unclear, as it is in the 20% of patients with idiopathic chronic pancreatitis.

Diagnosis

Patients with chronic pancreatitis typically are first seen with persistent midepigastric pain, often with a thoracolumbar component. The pain may be exacerbated by eating and by alcohol consumption. Nausea, vomiting, and hemodynamic instability are less frequent than with acute pancreatitis. Examination often reveals upper abdominal fullness and tenderness with frequent associated signs of malnutrition

BOX 24–4 Proposed Factors Producing Pain in Chronic Pancreatitis

Ductal hypertension
Autodigestion
Parenchymal ischemia
Perineural inflammation

and occasionally jaundice. Pancreatic calcification, diabetes mellitus, and steatorrhea, the classic triad of chronic pancreatitis, occur in fewer than 25% of cases, although two thirds of patients will have an abnormal glucose tolerance test at the time of presentation. Radiologic evidence of pancreatic calcification is pathognomonic and is present in 30% to 50% of patients.

Pain is present in 75% of patients. Initially the pain is characterized by recurrent attacks but tends to become persistent, with variable periods of remission. Occasionally it will "burn out" over time. The etiology of pain is uncertain. Box 24-4 lists some of the proposed factors. The most recent theory suggests hypoxia and damage to local sensory nerves with exposure to inflammatory irritants such as histamine, prostaglandins, and pancreatic enzymes.

Laboratory values are limited in evaluation of chronic pancreatitis. Pancreatic enzyme levels (amylase, lipase) may be elevated in acute exacerbations but are not a good measure of chronic disease, pancreatic function, or pancreatic reserve, nor do they correlate with symptoms. Functional studies are cumbersome and are rarely required to diagnose chronic pancreatitis. However, stimulated pancreatic secretions collected from the duodenum (amylase, lipase, trypsin, chymotrypsin, and bicarbonate), urine (NBT-PABA test, and pancreolauryl test), or serum (P-isoamylase, and trypsin), provide reliable estimates of pancreatic functional reserve and can be useful in evaluating treatment strategies. Serum liver enzymes and leukocyte counts may identify important information regarding complications of the disease.

Imaging

Plain abdominal radiographs reveal pancreatic calcification in fewer than 50% of patients and are otherwise nonspecific in chronic pancreatitis. Transabdominal ultrasound can determine important information regarding the size and consistency of the gland, characteristics of the biliary tree, and the presence of complications. A skilled ultrasonographer may achieve 70% sensitivity in diagnosing the disease.

CT approaches 90% sensitivity and 100% specificity in diagnosing chronic pancreatitis and should be considered in all suspected patients to classify their disease and determine the presence of complications and surgically correctable lesions (Fig. 24-7). CT may be the only imaging study necessary in most cases. ERCP may provide important information regarding ductal anatomy. The small but finite incidence of serious complications related

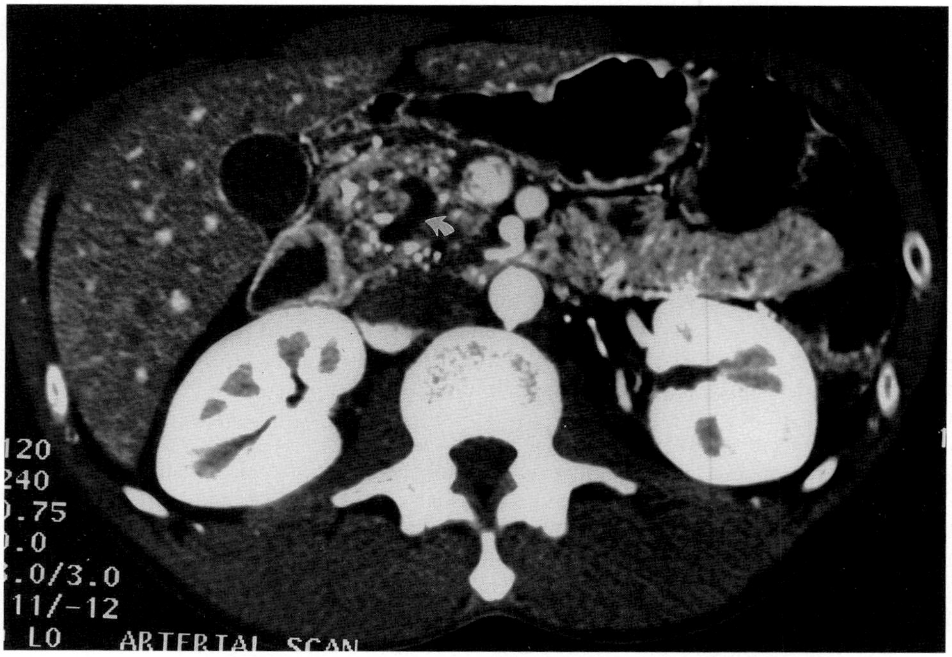

FIGURE 24–7 Computed tomography scan of chronic pancreatitis demonstrating calcification of gland and dilated pancreatic duct in the head of the gland (*arrow*).

to ERCP should limit its use to those patients that require anatomic definition not provided by other imaging studies and in patients suspected of ampullary or ductal obstruction amenable to ERCP treatment.

Magnetic resonance imaging (MRI) and MRI cholangiopancreatography (MRCP) are rapidly evolving and may eventually replace both CT and diagnostic ERCP. This technology provides definition of soft tissues and ductal anatomy. Likewise, endoscopic ultrasound is becoming more available and may play a role in the evaluation of patients with chronic pancreatitis.

Medical Treatment

Medical treatment of chronic pancreatitis consists primarily of supportive care. Pain relief, metabolic and nutritional support, as well as pancreatic endocrine and exocrine support are the mainstays of medical therapy.

Pain control is difficult, often requiring opiate analgesics. Abstinence from alcohol must be the initial goal, as alcohol consumption predicts recurrent pain, even after surgical intervention. Oral pancreatic enzyme supplementation and octreotide may provide modest pain relief, probably because of reduced pancreatic secretion. Because opiate addiction increases in proportion to duration of disease, nonsteroidal anti-inflammatory drugs should be prescribed early and over the long term, with opiates reserved for exacerbations and intractable pain. Some authorities recommend surgical intervention before the prolonged administration of opiates.

Malnutrition is common because of fear of pain after eating, as well as poor dietary habits and nutritional problems in the alcoholic population. Attention should be directed at providing a low-fat diet with adequate protein and calories and vitamin supplementation. Parenteral or jejunal feedings may be required in certain situations such as preoperative preparation and episodes of acute exacerbation.

Pancreatic exocrine insufficiency necessary to produce protein malabsorption does not occur until a loss of 90% of acinar mass has occurred. However, steatorrhea, or fat malabsorption, is a common and often troublesome problem in patents with chronic pancreatitis. In addition to requiring lipase from the pancreas, complete digestion of lipids depends on salivary and gastric hydrolysis, alkalinization in the duodenum, and adequate bile acid concentrations; all of which may be diminished in alcoholics. Pancreatic exocrine enzyme replacement is indicated to help ameliorate steatorrhea. Present enzyme preparations include enteric-coated and encapsulated forms to aid delivery of active enzymes and decrease the volume of administration. Gastric acid suppression also may be necessary to provide an adequate pH environment for enzyme activity.

Endocrine insufficiency in chronic pancreatitis is manifested primarily as pancreatic diabetes. Its treatment is similar to that for other forms of diabetes, in that it may be controlled by diet, oral hypoglycemic agents, or insulin.

TABLE 24–3 Selection of Operation for Chronic Pancreatitis

Anatomic Consideration	Procedure
Disease limited to tail of gland	Distal pancreatectomy
Obstruction in head of gland	
Dilated pancreatic duct	LR-LPJ
Nondilated pancreatic duct	Whipple, DPPHR
No obstruction in head of gland	
Dilated pancreatic duct	LPJ
Nondilated pancreatic duct	Distal resection (40%–95%), total pancreatectomy
Unable to tolerate major operation	Neurolysis?
Failure of primary drainage/resection	Additional resection, neurolysis
Inability to rule out malignancy	Resection

LPJ, lateral pancreaticojejunostomy; LR, local resection; DPPHR, duodenum-preserving pancreatic head resection.

Surgical Treatment

Surgical intervention for chronic pancreatitis is most commonly performed for chronic intractable pain. Additional indications for surgical intervention are listed in Box 24-2. The choice of operation depends on the anatomic considerations in each patient (Table 24-3). Pancreatic and biliary ductular anatomy should be carefully evaluated preoperatively. Improvement in perioperative preparation and care has allowed routine performance of surgical procedures on the pancreas with very low mortality and morbidity. Contemporary series of operations for chronic pancreatitis demonstrate mortality rates less than 3% and complication rates less than 20%, comparable to other major intraabdominal operations.

In a minority of patients, stenosis or stricture of the ampulla of Vater may be treated with simple sphincterotomy or sphincteroplasty. Initial results with this technique revealed improvement in pain but were short-lived and correlated with alcohol abstinence. Although these procedures have been successful in limiting recurrent acute bouts of pancreatitis in pancreas divisum, no benefit has been realized in chronic pancreatitis. This experience suggests that sphincterotomy and pancreatic duct stenting will have little effect on the long-term management of chronic pancreatitis from other etiologies.

The pancreatic duct in chronic pancreatitis is usually either dilated diffusely or in a beaded ("chain-of-lakes") pattern. A dilated pancreatic duct is best treated with internal drainage of the pancreatic duct into a Roux-en-Y limb of jejunum. Historically, 8 mm was considered the lower limit of dilation considered amenable to internal drainage, but the procedure has proved tenable and successful in relieving pain in patients with duct dilation of

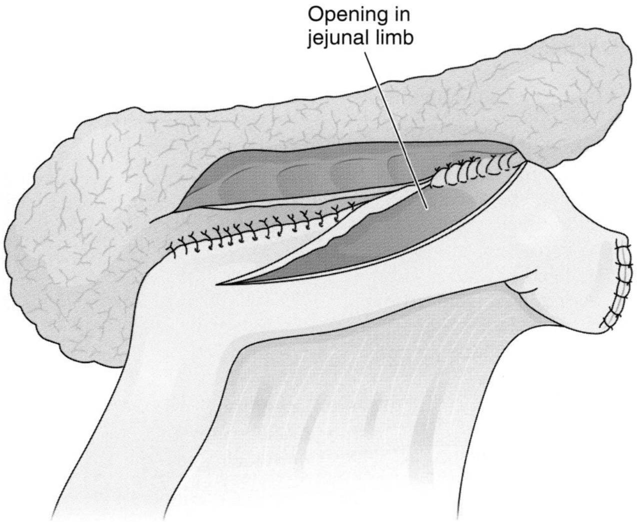

FIGURE 24–8 Lateral pancreaticojejunostomy. Dilated pancreatic duct is opened and sutured to an opening made in a Roux-en-Y limb of jejunum.

greater than 5 mm. The Partington-Rochelle modification of the Puestow operation (lateral pancreaticojejunostomy, LPJ) (Fig. 24-8) has resulted in good to excellent relief of pain in 70% to 80% of patients. Concomitant procedures to address complications such as pseudocyst and biliary obstruction can be incorporated into the jejunal limb. No evidence exists that surgery improves pancreatic function, as was hoped by the pioneers of ductal drainage procedures.

The Frey procedure is based on the concept that the head of the pancreas and uncinate process may not be completely drained by longitudinal pancreaticojejunostomy. This procedure entails a "coring out" or local resection of the head of the gland combined with LPJ (LR-LPJ). Results have been promising, with only 13% of patients reporting no pain relief. Another proposed mechanism for the success of this operation is the reversal of ischemia or ductal hypertension that has been irritating sensory nerves in the head of the gland.

When the pancreatic duct is not dilated, decompressing procedures are not feasible. However, patients may obtain relief of pain with pancreatic resection. Debate continues on the merits and complications of partial (40% to 80%) distal pancreatectomy, subtotal (95%) distal pancreatectomy (Child's procedure), pancreaticoduodenectomy (Whipple's procedure), and total pancreatectomy. Duodenum-preserving pancreatic head resection (Beger's procedure) has shown excellent pain relief that is comparable to that with a Whipple procedure, when performed in the 10% to 30% of chronic pancreatitis patients with an inflammatory mass in the head of the gland (Fig. 24-9). Pancreatic

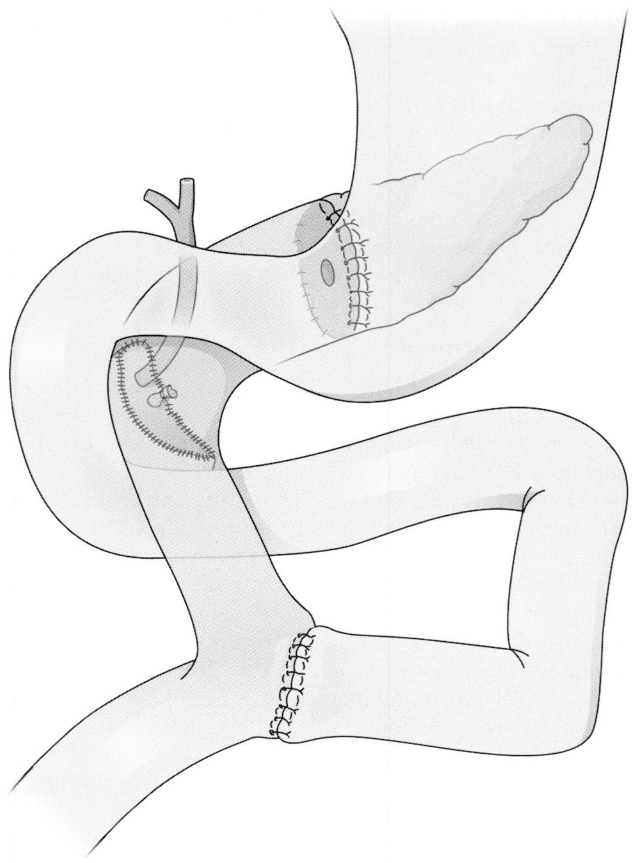

FIGURE 24–9 Beger procedure. The head of the pancreas has been resected, leaving the duodenum intact, and the area has been internally drained into a Roux-en-Y limb of jejunum.

insufficiency resulting from resection procedures is generally proportional to the extent of resection, with severe exocrine insufficiency and a particularly brittle and difficult-to-control form of pancreatic diabetes at the extreme. Attempts at autologous pancreatic islet cell transplantation at the time of pancreas resection were initially promising, but enthusiasm for the technique has waned because of less than satisfactory long-term results.

Several approaches to nerve ablation have been proposed, based on the theory that the pain of chronic pancreatitis is related to inflammatory involvement of the splanchnic nerves. Extraperitoneal, intraperitoneal, thoracic, and thoracoscopic splanchnicectomy as well as complete denervation procedures have been attempted to treat the pain of chronic pancreatitis. Results have been unpredictable, often unconfirmed, and with limited follow-up. Neurotomy may be considered in patients who have not obtained relief of pain after surgical drainage or resection procedures.

Pancreatic Pseudocyst

Pancreatic pseudocysts are walled-off collections of fluid and debris resulting from disruption of the pancreatic duct and are most commonly associated with acute and chronic pancreatitis. Pseudocysts will develop in up to 10% of patients after an episode of acute alcoholic pancreatitis. They also may occur after trauma or in association with a neoplasm. The wall is vascularized inflammatory tissue without an epithelial lining and may contain pancreatic parenchyma. Pseudocysts may occur in any region of the gland and are multiple in 10% to 15% of patients. Fluid collections occurring within 3 weeks of an acute episode of pancreatitis are considered acute fluid collections, and 30% to 40% of these collections will resolve spontaneously.

The most common presentation is abdominal pain, present in 90% of patients. Physical examination will often reveal a tender abdominal fullness or mass. Nonspecific complaints of nausea, vomiting, early satiety, and weight loss are common. More dramatic presentations may result from free intraperitoneal rupture, intracyst hemorrhage or infection, gastric variceal bleeding resulting from splenic or portal vein thrombosis, or intraperitoneal hemorrhage from adjacent pseudoaneurysm rupture. Laboratory findings are nonspecific, although amylase elevation is common. Imaging with CT is preferable, but ultrasound is nearly as sensitive and can be recommended for follow-up to determine interval changes in size (Fig. 24-10).

Sampling of a postpancreatitis fluid collection is rarely indicated. However, if a preceding episode of pancreatitis has not occurred, fluid cytology and chemistry can help differentiate a pseudocyst from a more likely mucinous or serous cystic neoplasm.

The natural history of asymptomatic pseudocysts reveals that nearly half remain stable, decrease in size, or completely resolve at 1 year of follow-up, irrespective of size. However, pseudocysts larger than 6 cm are more likely to require operation during follow-up. Pseudocysts present for more than 12 weeks almost never resolve spontaneously and have a high rate of complications. Therefore current management of pancreatic pseudocysts takes into account the presence or absence of symptoms, the age and size of the pseudocyst, and the presence or absence of complications. Postpancreatitis fluid collections that are asymptomatic in a stable patient can be followed up with monthly imaging to evaluate resolution, stability, or enlargement. Failure to resolve or evidence of enlargement is an indication for intervention. If, conversely, the pseudocyst is symptomatic, early intervention should be considered. Generally, a period of 6 weeks is desired before surgical intervention to assure adequate maturation of the cyst wall.

The preferred operative management of a pseudocyst is internal drainage into the gastrointestinal tract. This may be accomplished by anastomosis of the opened cyst wall to the stomach (cystogastrostomy; Fig. 24-11), duodenum (cystoduodenostomy), or a Roux-en-Y limb of jejunum (cystojejunostomy), depending on the location of the pseudocyst (Fig. 24-12). Multiple pseudocysts can be addressed simultaneously by connecting the pseudocysts and draining as one, or separately draining each cyst into a Roux-

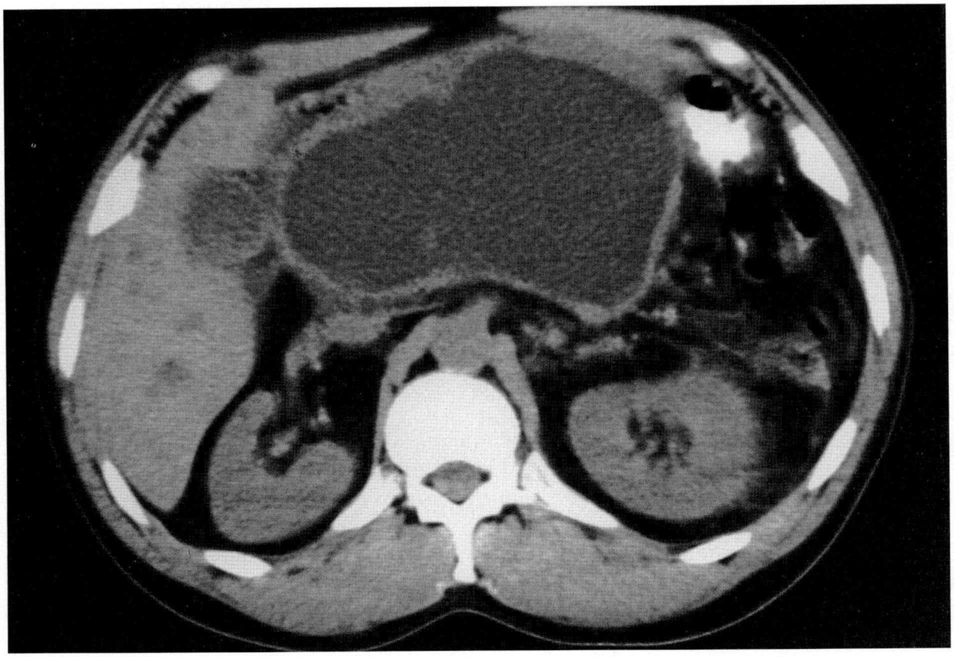

FIGURE 24–10 Computed tomography scan of a large postpancreatitis pseudocyst.

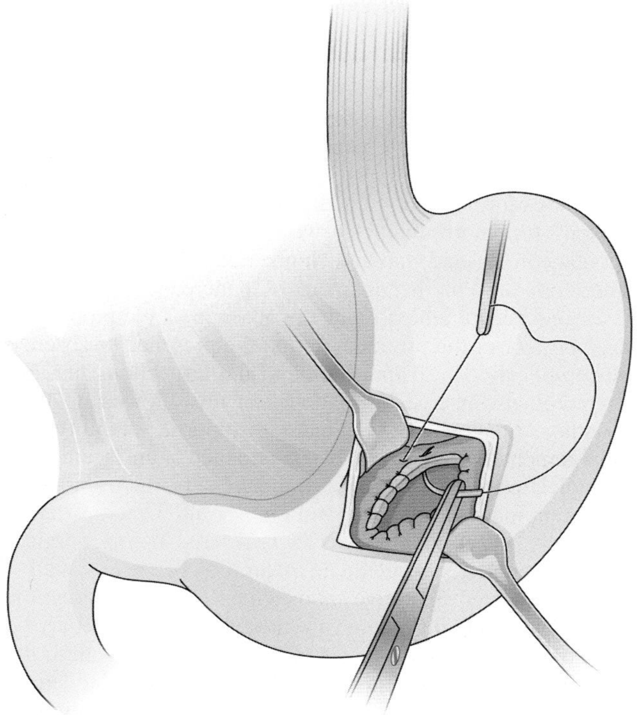

FIGURE 24–11 Cystgastrostomy. Anterior wall of stomach has been opened, and the posterior wall is opened into the pseudocyst. The posterior stomach wall is then sutured to the cyst wall with a hemostatic locking suture.

en-Y jejunal limb or a combination of these internal drainage procedures. A lateral pancreaticojejunostomy also should be added when the pancreatic duct is dilated. A biopsy of the cyst wall should be obtained on all occasions, as cystic neoplasms of the pancreas can mimic a pseudocyst. Infected pseudocysts are generally treated as pancreatic abscesses.

Simple aspiration of pseudocysts will fail to resolve the fluid collection in as many as 80% of patients. Prolonged catheter drainage has demonstrated better resolution rates but may take months of drain maintenance. New endoscopic techniques that place an endoprosthesis through the intestinal lumen into the pseudocyst and that bridge the pancreatic duct disruption with a pancreatic duct stent are currently being analyzed.

Adenocarcinoma of the Pancreas

The incidence of pancreatic cancer has steadily increased over the past 50 to 60 years to a present annual incidence of about 10 new cases per 100,000 people in the United States. It accounts for over 24,000 deaths annually in the United States, making it the fifth leading cause of cancer death behind malignancies of the lung, large intestine,

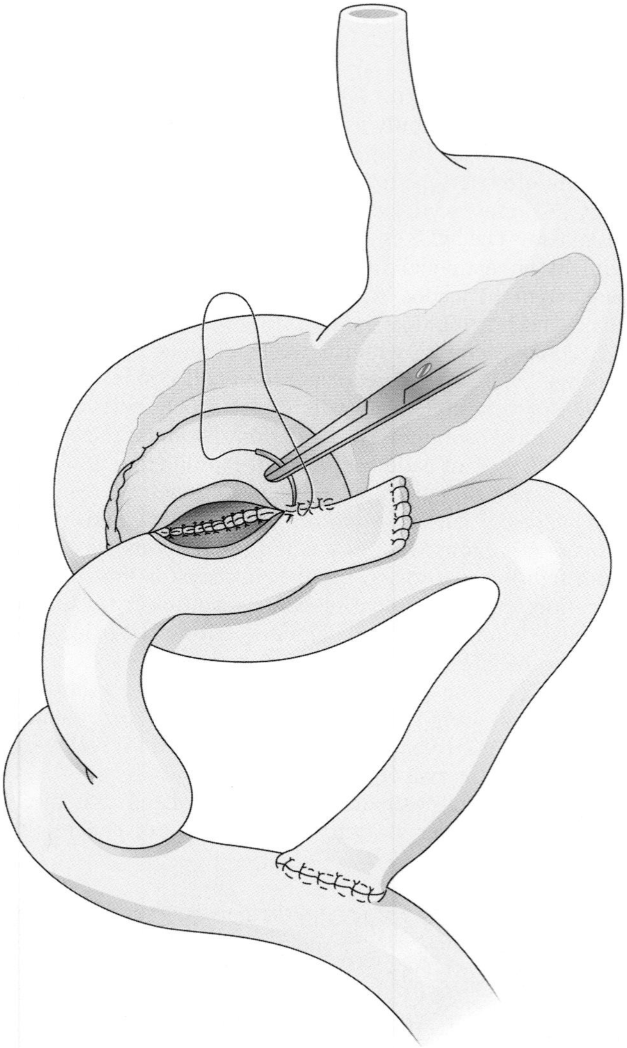

FIGURE 24–12 Cystojejunostomy. Pseudocyst is opened and sutured to the opening in a Roux-en-Y limb of jejunum.

breast, and prostate. Ductal adenocarcinoma accounts for 90% of cases, with 80% of pancreatic cancer occurring in the 60- to 80-year-old population.

The etiology is largely unknown, but genetic and environmental factors have been implicated. A number of reports document familial occurrences of pancreatic cancer in addition to being one of the malignancies in the *Cancer Family Syndromes* described by Lynch. More recent evidence has shown frequent chromosome gains, losses, and mutations, especially with tumor-suppressor genes *p53*, *DPC4*, and *MTS1,* and point mutations in the oncogene k-*ras*. A strong association exists with cigarette smoking and exposure to some chemical carcinogens, and less convincing associations with diets high in fat and red meat, coffee consumption, diabetes, cholelithiasis, and after partial gastrectomy.

Prognosis of pancreatic cancer remains poor because of its aggressive nature and frequent regional and distant metastasis at the time of presentation. At most, only 20% of patients will have a resectable tumor. Fewer than 7% of body and tail lesions, which account for 30% of cases, will be resectable. The majority of lesions in the head should be approached surgically. This discrepancy is the result of earlier presentation of periampullary and head lesions secondary to bile duct obstruction.

Clinical Presentation

Patients with pancreatic adenocarcinoma most often are first seen with vague abdominal pain and weight loss. Obstructive jaundice is a frequent accompaniment to lesions in the head of the gland. A painless, dilated, palpable gallbladder (Courvoisier's sign) may accompany distal common bile duct obstruction. Anorexia, weakness, altered bowel habits, and pruritis also may be present. Back pain is frequent and is often an ominous sign of unresectability. Depression and psychoses also have been noted with a greater than expected frequency. Physical examination is otherwise unremarkable, and a palpable mass is the exception.

Diagnosis

CT is essential for evaluation of pancreatic malignancy. Ideally, contrast enhanced, three-phase, dynamic thin-section CT should be performed, as it allows evaluation of the entire pancreas, adjacent blood vessels and organs, as well as regional and hepatic metastases (Figs. 24-13 and 24-14). MRI offers little advantage over CT in staging and judging resectability. Percutaneous transphepatic cholangiography (PTHC) and ERCP are rarely required but can provide important anatomic information about the common bile duct and may be therapeutic, because a biliary endoprosthesis can be placed for unresectable tumors. The routine use of preoperative biliary stents is contraindicated because of increased postoperative infections related to their use. Endoscopic ultrasound has shown great promise in the evaluation of resectability, but availability and expertise are limited. Laparoscopy also has been advocated for surgical staging before resection. Pancreatic cancers are staged according to the criteria set by the American Joint Committee on Cancer (Box 24-5).

Tumor markers may be helpful in differentiating benign from malignant pancreatic disease. The most useful is carbohydrate antigen (CA) 19-9 (elevated in 78% of patients with pancreatic cancer). Absolute levels predict unresectability because levels greater than 1000 units/mL have been associated with unresectable disease in 96% of patients. Additionally, serial postoperative levels predict recurrence before clinical and radiologic detection. Levels of CA 19-9 also may be elevated in carcinoma of the gallbladder, bile duct, colon and rectum, stomach, liver, lung, and ovary. Benign disorders including pancreatitis, hepatitis, and cirrhosis also may cause elevated CA 19-9 levels. CEA and CA-125 may be elevated in as many as

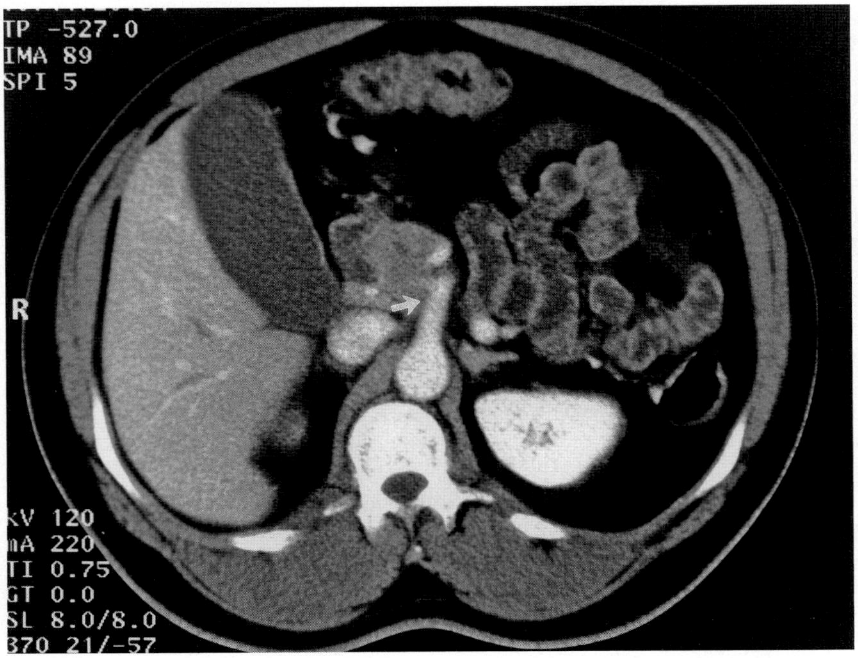

FIGURE 24–13 Computed tomography scan of adenocarcinoma of the head of the pancreas. Encroachment on superior mesenteric artery (*arrow*) is demonstrated. Notice dilated gallbladder resulting from biliary obstruction.

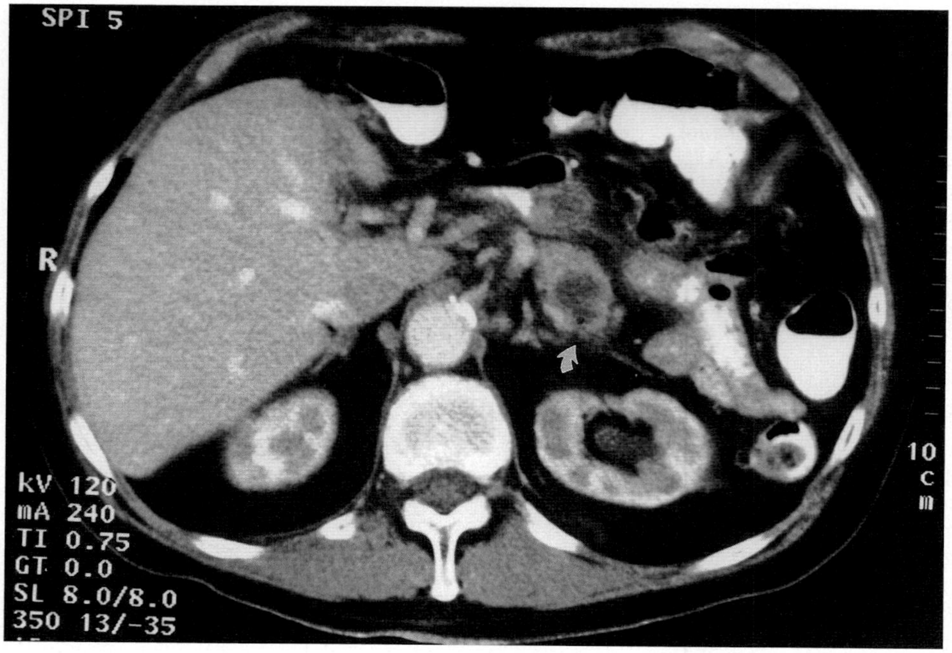

FIGURE 24–14 Computed tomography scan of adenocarcinoma of the body of the pancreas (*arrow*).

50% of patients with pancreas cancer but are far less specific and therefore not useful markers. Other serologic markers with limited availability and utility include DU-PAN-2, α-fetoprotein (AFP), and pancreatic oncofetal antigen (POA).

Management

All patients with potentially resectable pancreatic tumors should receive surgical evaluation. Initial diagnostic laparoscopy is helpful in diagnosing the 10% to 20% of patients with peritoneal spread and liver metastases not seen on preoperative imaging. However, it may not be necessary in those patients in whom other pathology, such as intestinal or biliary obstruction, must be addressed. Proceeding directly to laparotomy is warranted in this group. Pancreaticoduodenectomy (Whipple's procedure) is the most common operation performed for pancreatic cancer. Traditionally this entailed resection en bloc of the distal stomach, duodenum, gallbladder, distal common bile duct, and the neck, head, and uncinate process of the pancreas (Fig. 24-15). A duodenum-preserving modification has gained popularity because of reduced complications such as the dumping syndrome and marginal ulceration. No difference in recurrence or survival compared with that with the standard Whipple operation has been shown. Reconstruction of gastrointestinal tract continuity can be accomplished by several configurations, with few data to support superiority of one method over another (Fig. 24-16). Body and tail lesions should be treated with a distal pancreatectomy and splenectomy. Before any resection, the liver and local and regional lymph nodes should be carefully inspected. Any abnormal nodes or lesions should be sampled with biopsy and analyzed by intraoperative frozen section. Resection should be abandoned if extrapancreatic disease is identified. Sparse data exist to suggest any benefit to resection once the cancer has spread beyond the confines of the gland. Only rarely is resection advocated in this situation, but it may be of some benefit in alleviating pain and obstruction.

Pancreatic resection is still a formidable undertaking, but in experienced hands, the operative mortality is less than 5%. Pancreatic stump leaks approach 15% regardless of the method of reconstruction, with overall postoperative complications near 30%. However, resectable cancer in the head of the gland has a 5-year survival approaching 25% and median survival of 15 months, compared with the rare 5-year survival and 6- to 9-month medial survival in unresected cases. Cystadenocarcinoma, serous or papillary type, is diagnosed in about 10% of resected tumors and carries a much better prognosis than the more common ductal carcinoma because of the less aggressive nature and lower propensity for early metastasis.

Obvious unresectable lesions on preoperative imaging should be sampled by percutaneous, endoscopic, or laparoscopic techniques to establish a tissue diagnosis. Percutaneous biopsy is not recommended for lesions thought to be resectable on preoperative imaging studies. Pain may be controlled with oral analgesics but also may require more-invasive measures such as percutaneous or operative celiac nerve ablation. Biliary obstruction can be

BOX 24–5 Pancreas Cancer Staging

Primary Tumor (T)

TX	Primary tumor cannot be assessed
T0	No evidence of primary tumor
Tis	Carcinoma in situ
T1	Tumor limited to pancreas, 2cm or less
T2	Tumor limited to pancreas, >2 cm
T3	Tumor extends into duodenum, bile duct, or peripancreatic tissue
T4	Tumor extends into stomach, spleen, colon, or adjacent large vessels

Regional Lymph Nodes (N)

NX	Regional lymph nodes not assessed
N0	No regional lymph nodes
N1	Regional lymph node metastasis
PN1a	Metastasis in single lymph node
PN1b	Metastases in multiple lymph nodes

Distant Metastasis (M)

MX	Distant metastasis not assessed
M0	No distant metastasis
M1	Distant metastasis

Stage Grouping

0	Tis	N0	M0
I	T1	N0	M0
	T2	N0	M0
II	T3	N0	M0
III	T1	N1	M0
	T2	N1	M0
	T3	N1	M0
IVA	T4	any	M0
IVB	any	any	M1

From American Joint Committee on Cancer: AJCC Cancer Staging Manual, 6th ed. New York, Springer-Verlag, 2004, with permission.

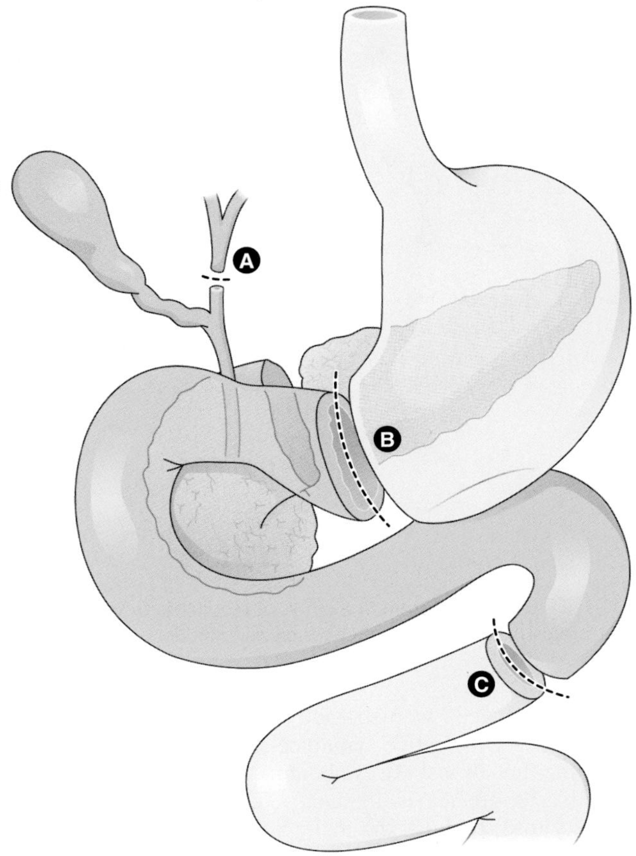

FIGURE 24–15 Whipple's operation. *A*, Transected common hepatic duct. *B*, Transected stomach. *C*, Transected jejunum.

managed with endoscopically placed stents, PTHC-placed drains, or surgical biliary/enteric anastomosis. Endoprostheses may require frequent reintervention and replacement because of obstruction, and percutaneous drains are often viewed as unsightly and difficult to manage by patients. The advantages of surgical intervention, internal drainage, and prolonged patency are often not realized because of the extremely poor survival. Occasionally surgery is required for duodenal, gastric, or colonic obstruction.

Results of adjuvant therapy have demonstrated no survival advantage when chemotherapy or radiation alone is administered after curative resection or for palliation of unresectable lesions. However, the combination of chemotherapy and external-beam radiation has shown a median survival benefit of 20 months versus 11 months when administered after a curative resection. This benefit has not been realized in unresected patients nor has a benefit been observed in ongoing investigations involving neoadjuvant therapy for pancreatic adenocarcinoma.

Acinar cell carcinoma is a rare variety of pancreas malignancy that usually is first seen late in its course, and the tumors are usually large. It should be managed in a fashion similar to that of the more common ductal adenocarcinoma.

Unusual Tumors of the Pancreas

Cystic Neoplasms; Serous and Mucinous Cystadenomas

The majority of cystic pancreas lesions are pseudocysts, but up to 10% are cystadenomas. They are often multilobulated and heterogeneous in appearance compared with pseudocysts. Benign lesions are indistinguishable from malignant cystic neoplasms of the pancreas in terms of clinical presentation, radiologic imaging, and gross appearance (Fig. 24-17). Cystadenomas have a predilection

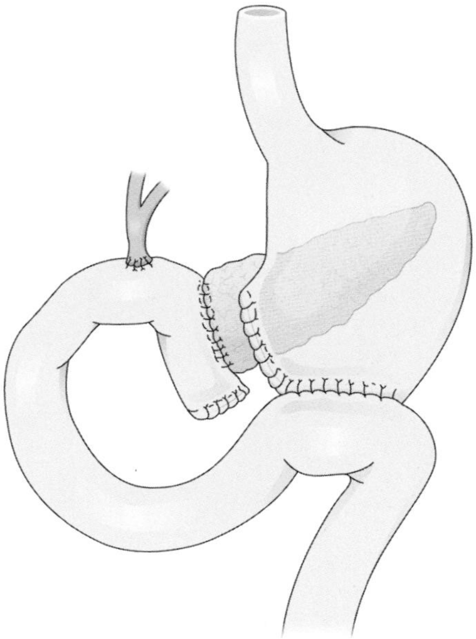

FIGURE 24–16 A common method of reconstruction of gastrointestinal continuity after pancreaticoduodenectomy.

for middle-aged women and have vague abdominal symptoms. Obstructive jaundice is rare. Serous cystadenomas are almost always benign, whereas the mucinous type has a greater malignant potential. Because of the inability to distinguish the malignant from benign variants, resection is recommended for all cystic neoplasms of the pancreas with the expectation of complete cure and infrequent recurrence in the majority of patients.

Solid and Cystic (Papillary Cystic) Neoplasms of the Pancreas

These lesions occur with greatest frequency in female subjects from 10 to 40 years old. They have a heterogeneous histologic appearance consisting of microcystic, papillary, and solid components, and contain frequent areas of cystic degeneration and hemorrhage (Fig. 24-18). They tend to grow large before detection and arise predominantly from the body and tail. Local invasion is frequent, despite the benign nature of these lesions. Complete resection is curative, and long-term survival is expected in the majority of patients. Resection is recommended for all of these lesions.

Intraductal Papillary Mucinous Tumors of the Pancreas

Intraductal papillary mucinous tumor (IPMT) is a recently described entity also known as mucinous ductal ectasia, intraductal mucin hypersecreting tumor, mucinous villous adenomatosis, mucinous papillary cystic tumor, and mucin-producing tumor. Unlike other cystic pancreatic neoplasms, IPMT is usually symptomatic in the form of chronic pancreatitis-like symptoms or recurrent bouts of acute pancreatitis. However, patients are usually 20 to 30 years older than those with chronic pancreatitis and have no identifiable risk factors for pancreatitis. Steatorrhea,

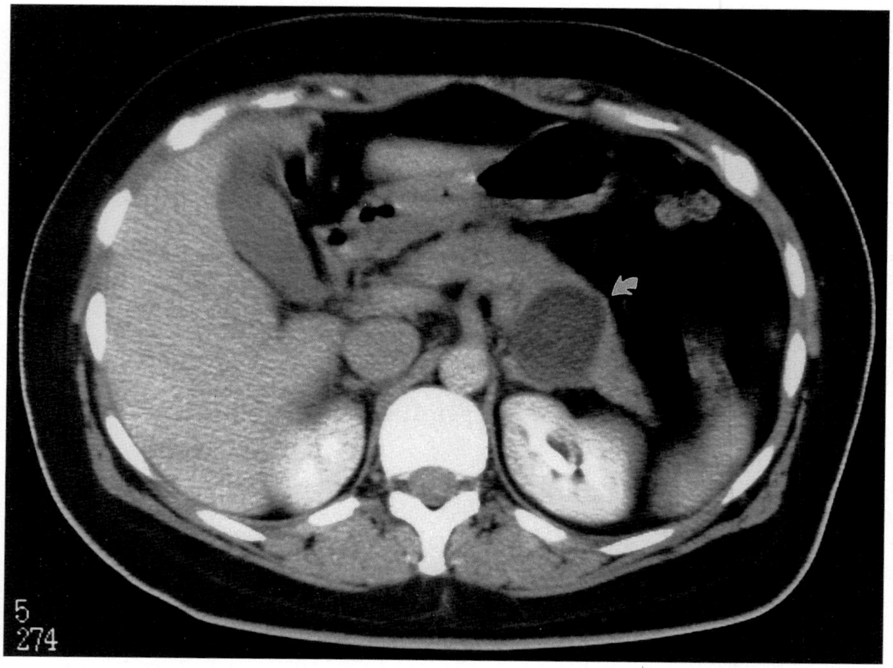

FIGURE 24–17 Computed tomography scan of a benign oligocystic serous cystadenoma of the tail of the pancreas (*arrow*).

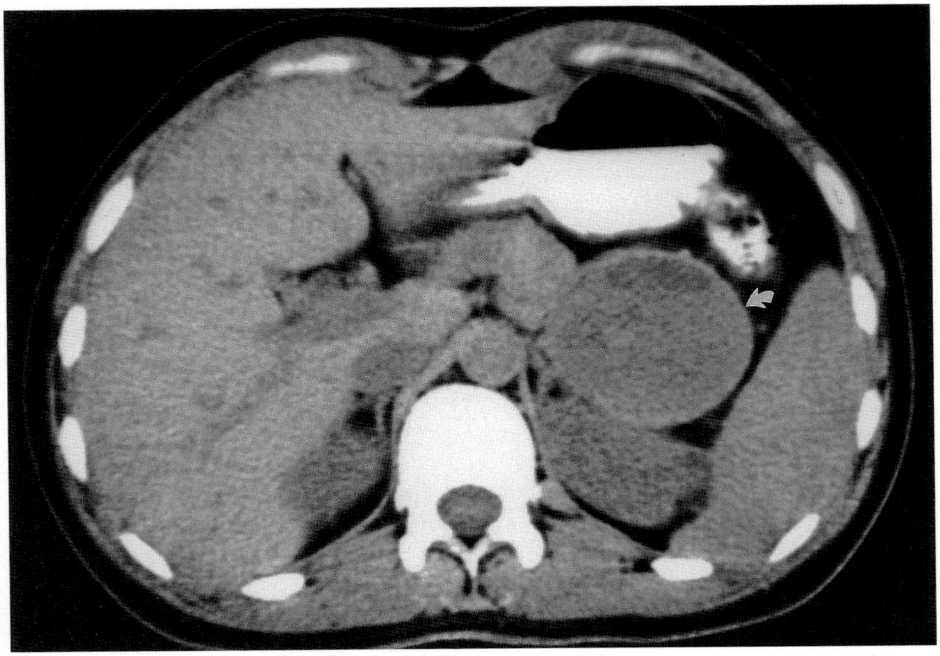

FIGURE 24–18 Computed tomography scan of a solid and cystic lesion in the tail of the pancreas (*arrow*).

diabetes, and unintentional weight loss are common. IPMT is usually first suspected when patients undergo CT for abdominal pain. ERCP demonstrates a dilated papilla (>30%) with a mucus-filled dilated main duct and frequent filling defects from papillomatous or malignant growths. Like other mucinous neoplasms of the pancreas, IPMT has the potential for malignant transformation. As many as 40% of patients will have an invasive malignancy at the time of resection. The remainder demonstrate areas of microcystic papillary atypia, dysplasia, or carcinoma in situ, confirming the malignant potential of IPMT. These changes are frequently multifocal.

Management of IPMT is surgical resection, but the procedure of choice is somewhat controversial. Most surgeons resect the area of primary ductal dilatation and, based on frozen section analysis of resection margins, extend the resection to include all areas of ductal atypia. Others recommend total pancreatectomy, based on the multifocal nature of IPMT. No consensus exists, but it is clear that patient age, medical condition, and psychosocial situation should be taken into account before a total pancreatectomy is performed for this tumor.

Lymphoma

Primary pancreatic non-Hodgkin's lymphoma is unusual and typically is first seen with weight loss, vague abdominal pain, and, rarely, gastric outlet obstruction or obstructive jaundice. It may be suspected on CT scan when a soft-tissue mass in the pancreas is present with peripancreatic lymphatic enlargement. Unfortunately, it is often indistinguishable from other pancreatic masses including carcinoma and pancreatitis. Percutaneous biopsy should be performed when it is suspected, and bone marrow biopsy and radiographic staging are necessary in confirmed cases. Laparoscopic or conventional surgical biopsy may be required if percutaneous methods fail to yield a diagnosis. Combination chemotherapy appears to be the preferred treatment in confirmed cases of pancreatic lymphoma, with long-term remissions expected after chemotherapy alone. Endoscopic or percutaneous biliary decompression and gastroenterostomy are occasionally required, but surgical resection confers no advantage in the treatment of pancreatic lymphoma.

Endocrine Tumors of the Pancreas

Insulinoma

Insulinoma is the most common endocrine tumor of the pancreas. It is characterized by Whipple's triad: fasting hypoglycemia that induces symptoms, blood glucose levels less than 50 mg/dL, and relief of symptoms after glucose administration. Hypoglycemic symptoms result from the autonomous secretion of insulin from the tumor. Ninety percent of insulinomas are benign, and these tumors are usually small (<2 cm), solitary, and evenly distributed throughout the pancreas. In the multiple endocrine neoplasia syndrome 1 (MEN-1), insulinomas will be multiple in up to 16% of patients. The diagnosis is made when 72-hour fasting insulin levels are greater than 25 microunits/mL in the face of hypoglycemia and an insulin-to-glucose ratio greater than 0.4 after an overnight fast. Proinsulin and C-peptide also are usually elevated. Many of these tumors are small enough to escape radiologic detection. Operative intervention in suspected cases should consist of thorough mobilization and palpation of the entire pancreas. Intraoperative ultrasound has improved the ability to detect evasive lesions. Small benign insulinomas are usually amenable to enucleation, but larger lesions may require distal pancreatectomy or, very rarely, pancreaticoduodenectomy, depending on their location in the gland. If the tumor cannot be identified during surgery, a distal pancreatectomy can be performed to be certain the patient does not have nesidioblastosis or islet cell hyperplasia. Malignant insulinoma and accessible metastases should be resected when possible. Tumor debulking also has some utility in reducing hypoglycemic symptoms. Diazoxide, thiazide diuretics, and octreotide have all been shown to be useful in patients with unresectable or residual disease.

Gastrinoma

Gastrinomas are rare nueroendocrine tumors of the pancreas that occur most frequently in the third to fifth decades of life with a male predominance. The 1955 description of two patients with gastric hypersecretion, florid peptic ulceration in unusual locations, and the presence of a pancreatic islet cell tumor secured the names of Drs. Zollinger and Ellison to the syndrome. More than half of all gastrinomas are located in the pancreas, approximately 40% in the duodenal wall, and fewer than 5% in the stomach or extraintestinal site (biliary system, omentum, ovary). Nearly 90% are found in the "gastrinoma triangle" bounded by the junction of the cystic duct and common bile duct cephalad, the junction of the second and third portions of the duodenum inferiorly, and the junction of the neck and body of the pancreas medially. Autonomous gastrin secretion typically results in refractory and recurrent peptic ulcer disease, vomiting, and diarrhea. Seventy-five percent of gastrinomas occur sporadically, with an estimated 25% associated with the MEN-1 syndrome (hyperparathyroidism, pancreatic endocrine tumors, and pituitary tumors). Typically, 60% are malignant, but more recent series have demonstrated this percentage to be lower.

A fasting gastrin level greater than 1000 pg/mL in suspected patients is virtually diagnostic. However, many patients with a gastrinoma will have gastrin levels above normal but less than 1000 pg/mL. These patients should undergo gastric acid analysis, to be sure they are producing acid, and provocative testing to serve as a baseline. A basal acid output (BAO) greater than 15 mEq/hr (>5 mEq/hr if previous acid-reducing operations have been performed) and a BAO/MAO (maximal acid output) ratio greater than 0.6 support the diagnosis of gastrinoma. Intravenous secretin stimulation is the provocative test of choice. An absolute increase in serum gastrin of 200 pg/mL over the baseline gastrin level is diagnostic of gastrinoma.

Initial management of gastrinomas consists of control of gastric hypersecretion. The substituted benzimidazoles (proton-pump inhibitors) have made this task easier, although large doses may be required. Resection should be attempted in all cases if metastases have been excluded. Normalization of serum gastrin and cure in this selected group of patients approaches 33%. However, a larger group of patients will have unresectable, metastatic, or residual disease. Pharmacologic gastric acid control and octreotide will be sufficient to control the symptoms of most patients, but occasional acid-reduction operations will be required in noncompliant patients.

VIPoma

Vasoactive intestinal polypeptide (VIP) is the most likely islet cell tumor product responsible for the watery diarrhea, hypokalemia, hypochlorhydria (WDHH or Verner-Morrison) syndrome. Oversecretion of VIP results in a profuse secretory diarrhea (>3 L/day) and subsequent potassium loss and dehydration. A similar syndrome has been attributed to islet cell tumors secreting prostaglandin E_1. These tumors are frequently large and metastatic at initial evaluation. Careful surgical exploration and intraoperative ultrasound is warranted in cases of documented elevations of serum VIP. More than 50% of VIPomas are malignant. Selective venous sampling may be of value in localizing these lesions, but it is rarely used because selective arterial calcium injection has been demonstrated to be more accurate for localizing VIPomas. Treatment should first focus on replacing fluid deficits and correcting electrolyte abnormalities. Diarrhea is often dramatically improved with the administration of intravenous octreotide. If a solitary lesion is identified, surgical resection is recommended. In metastatic disease, patients can often be maintained in a relatively asymptomatic state with octreotide, and as many as 90% of patients will obtain remission of metastatic disease with streptozotocin and 5-fluorouracil.

Glucagonoma

The majority of glucagonomas are located in the body and tail of the pancreas and are large at the time of diagnosis. The majority are malignant and metastatic at exploration. Patients classically are initially seen with mild diabetes and a characteristic skin rash termed *necrolytic migratory erythema*. It is located in areas of local trauma and irritation such as the perineum, perioral area, legs, feet, and hands. Fasting serum glucagon levels usually exceed 500 pg/mL with accompanying elevations in basal insulin levels. Resection and debulking are recommended and improve the diabetes and rash. Octreotide has shown benefit in controlling the hyperglycemia and rash in patients with metastatic, unresected, and residual disease.

Somatostatinoma

This is a rare islet cell tumor producing vague symptoms; it is usually located in the head of the pancreas and frequently metastatic at presentation. A form exists with small duodenal tumors more amenable to cure. Symptoms are nonspecific but may include gallstones, steatorrhea, and diabetes related to the inhibitory effect of somatostatin on digestive organ motility and hormone secretion. Serum somatostatin levels are usually markedly elevated. Resection and debulking are indicated when feasible, but resection for cure is rare.

Nonfunctional Islet Cell Tumors

Nonfunctional islet cell tumors of the pancreas represent fewer than 25% of the endocrine tumors of the pancreas. They are usually located in the head of the pancreas, and 90% are malignant. Presentation is usually related to advanced malignancy, with vague abdominal pain, weight loss, and obstructive jaundice being common. Surgical resection and even debulking are generally recommended. Biliary decompression and gastric outlet obstruction frequently require surgical intervention. Five-year survival for all patients reaches 40%, as this is a relatively slow-growing neoplasm.

Suggested Reading

Balthazar EJ, Ranson JHC, Naidich DP, et al: Acute pancreatitis: prognostic value of CT. Radiology 156(3):767–772, 1985.

Baron TH, Morgan DE: Acute necrotizing pancreatitis. N Engl J Med 340(18):1412–1417, 1999.

Howare J, Idezuki Y, Ihse I, Prinz RA: Surgical Diseases of the Pancreas, 3rd ed. Baltimore, Williams & Wilkins, 1998.

Karne S, Gorelick FS: Etiopathogenesis of acute pancreatitis. Surg Clin North Am 79(4):699–710, 1999.

Prinz RA, Greenlee HB: Pancreatic duct drainage in 100 patients with chronic pancreatitis. Ann Surg 194:313–320, 1981.

Sarles H: Etiopathogenesis and definition of chronic pancreatitis. Dig Dis Sci 31:91–107, 1981.

Trede M, Carter DC (eds): Surgery of the Pancreas. London, Churchill Livingstone, 1993.

Yeo C, Cameron J. Lillemoe K, et al: Pancreaticoduodenectomy for cancer of the head of the pancreas: 201 patients. Ann Surg 221:721, 1995.

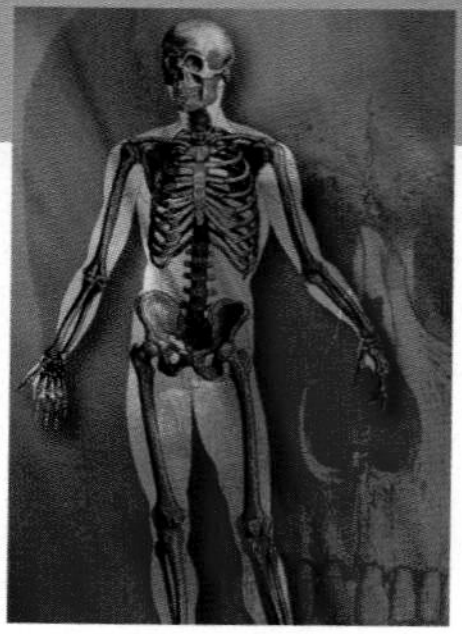

Chapter 25
Small Intestine

TAMARA J. INTNER, MD, EDWARD E. WHANG, MD, and STANLEY W. ASHLEY, MD

The small intestine is the principal site of digestion and absorption; thus it is the central component of the digestive system. It also contains the body's largest quantity of endocrine and immune tissue. Functionally, the intestine's capacity far exceeds demand, so that intestinal resection, used to treat many of the disease discussed in this chapter, is associated with little morbidity. The critical role of the small intestine becomes apparent, however, when, as a result of disease and/or resection, capacity does not meet demand, and the devastating disorder known as the short bowel syndrome results.

This chapter focuses on the anatomy, physiology, and surgical diseases of the jejunum and ileum. The duodenum is discussed elsewhere in the textbook.

Anatomy

Gross Anatomy

Demarcated proximally by the ligament of Treitz and distally by the ileocecal junction, the jejunoileal length averages 5 to 7 m in adults. No anatomic landmark defines the jejunoileal junction; the proximal two fifths is arbitrarily designated the jejunum, and the distal three fifths, the ileum. In general, the jejunum has a larger circumference and a thicker wall, and its mesentery contains more fat than that of the ileum.

The arteries to the jejunum and ileum arise from the superior mesenteric artery. The venous drainage occurs via the superior mesenteric vein. Lymph drains from the bowel to mesenteric lymph nodes and subsequently to the cisterna chyli, through lymphatic vessels coursing parallel to the arterial supply. The parasympathetic and sympathetic innervation to the small intestine is derived from the vagus and splanchnic nerves, respectively.

Microscopic Anatomy

The wall of the small intestine comprises four distinct layers: mucosa, submucosa, muscularis, and serosa.

The mucosa itself contains three layers: epithelium, lamina propria, and muscularis mucosa. The epithelium is exposed to the lumen and consists primarily of four types of cells: enterocytes, goblet cells, Paneth cells, and enteroendocrine cells. Finger-like projections of epithelium and underlying lamina propria form villi, which surround the crypts of Lieberkuhn. The epithelium of the small intestine is regenerating continuously, with new cells originating in the crypts, migrating up the villi, and ultimately being extruded at the villous tips. The total absorptive surface area of the intestine averages 200 to 500 cm^2. Three structural factors contribute to surface area expansion: (1) microvilli on the apical surface of enterocytes, (2) villi, and (3) **plicae circulares** (or **valvulae conniventes**), which are transverse folds of mucosa visible grossly and on radiographs.

The submucosa consists primarily of connective tissue and is the strongest layer of the bowel wall. The muscularis consists of an inner layer of circular muscle and an outer layer of longitudinal muscle. The serosa consists of visceral peritoneum that forms the outer surface of the intestine.

Physiology

Small intestinal function is governed by a complex network of neural and hormonal regulatory mechanisms. In many cases, the proximate regulatory signal consists of peptides generated within the intestine. Some of these "gut peptides" and their actions are described in Table 25-1. Specific aspects of intestinal physiology are summarized later.

Absorption and Digestion

Approximately 8 to 10 L of water, consisting of ingested water and salivary, gastric, biliary, pancreatic, and intestinal secretions, enter the intestine each day. Under normal conditions, only 0.5 L of this total escapes absorption in the small intestine to enter the colon. This efficient water absorption occurs passively, along concentration gradients generated by active solute transport.

Such solutes, including ions, nutrients, and vitamins, are absorbed through a variety of carrier-mediated mechanisms and, in some cases, through passive permeation via paracellular pores. Ingested carbohydrates, proteins, and fats are hydrolyzed to absorbable constituents within the intestinal lumen, largely through the action of digestive enzymes produced by the pancreas and enterocytes.

A detailed description of digestion and absorption is beyond the scope of this chapter, but knowledge of regional variation in absorptive capacity is relevant to understanding

TABLE 25–1 Examples of Hormones Produced by the Small Intestine

Hormone	Source	Action
Cholecystokinin (CCK)	Mucosa of proximal intestine	Stimulates gallbladder contraction, sphincter of Oddi relaxation, and pancreatic exocrine secretion
Secretin	S cells of proximal intestine	Stimulates pancreatic exocrine secretion
Motilin	M cells of proximal intestine	Activates migrating motor complex
Somatostatin (SMS)	D cells throughout gut mucosa	Inhibits motility, secretion, and release of other hormones
Peptide YY (PYY)	L cell of distal intestine	Inhibits motility and secretion
Glucagon-like peptide 2 (GLP-2)	L cell of distal intestine	Stimulates intestinal epithelial growth

possible sequelae of intestinal resection. Although most ingested nutrients are absorbed in the proximal jejunum, the entire small bowel has the capacity to absorb them, so that jejunal resection generally is well tolerated. In contrast, absorption of vitamin B_{12} and bile acids is limited to the distal ileum, so that ileal resection often results in anemia, malabsorption of fats and the fat-soluble vitamins A, D, E, and K, and the development of gallstones.

Motility

Small intestinal motility is the sum of several distinctive patterns of muscular contractions. The peristaltic reflex results in a series of contractions that are propagated in the aboral direction for 10 to 15 cm before abating. It is responsible for propelling ingested material through the intestine. In contrast, segmental contractions serve to promote mixing of intraluminal contents and their exposure to the absorptive mucosal surface. During interdigestive (fasting) periods, the migrating myoelectric complex (MMC) originating in the proximal duodenum initiates contractions that sweep throughout the entire intestine. These contractions are thought to expel residual debris from the intestine.

Immunology

The intestinal epithelium is the body's largest surface area exposed to the outside environment and its potentially noxious substances. Factors impeding proliferation of pathogenic bacteria within lumen and their translocation through the mucosa include (1) gastric acidity and proteolytic enzymes, (2) peristalsis, (3) intestinal flora, (4) rapid epithelial turnover, and (5) a well-developed intestinal immune system. Secretory immunoglobulin A (IgA) is the major immunoglobulin of the enteric immune system. Discrete aggregates of leukocytes exist in Peyer's patches, lymphoid follicles, and mesenteric lymph nodes. Individual leukocytes also exist in the lumen, epithelium, and lamina propria.

Impaired barrier function in critically ill patients has been hypothesized to allow the translocation of bacteria and their toxins or both from the intestinal lumen into the systemic circulation. This event may be a common denominator in the pathophysiology of sepsis associated with a wide range of critical illnesses, including pancreatitis, burn injury, and trauma.

Small-Bowel Obstruction

Mechanical small-bowel obstruction is the most frequently encountered surgical disorder of the small intestine. A wide range of conditions can lead to obstruction; postoperative adhesions are the most prevalent etiology in the general population (Table 25-2).

Pathophysiology

The obstructing lesion is classified by its anatomic relation to the bowel as intraluminal (e.g., foreign bodies, gallstones, or meconium), intramural (e.g., tumors, inflammatory strictures, or hematomas), or extrinsic (e.g., adhesions, hernias, or carcinomatosis).

With onset of obstruction, gas and fluid accumulate proximally within the intestinal lumen. Most of the gas originates from swallowed air, although some is produced within the intestine. The fluid consists principally of gastrointestinal secretions. As the bowel distends, intraluminal and intramural pressures increase, and the intestinal epithelium exhibits net fluid secretion, rather than net absorption. If the intramural pressure becomes high enough, microvascular perfusion to the intestinal wall is impaired,

TABLE 25–2 Most Common Etiologies of Small-Bowel Obstruction

Etiology	% of Cases
Adhesions	50–70
Malignacy	10–20
Hernia	10–20
Others	10

ultimately leading to **strangulation**, with intestinal ischemia and necrosis resulting.

With **partial small-bowel obstruction**, only a portion of the intestinal lumen is occluded, allowing passage of some gas and fluid. The progression of pathophysiologic events therefore occurs more slowly than with **complete small-bowel obstruction**, and development of strangulation is unusual.

In contrast, progression to strangulation occurs especially rapidly with **closed-loop obstruction**, in which a segment of intestine is obstructed both proximally and distally (e.g., volvulus). In such cases, the accumulating gas and fluid cannot be decompressed proximally or distally.

Differential Diagnosis

Small-bowel obstruction may be difficult to distinguish from **ileus**, in which intestinal distention is caused by impaired peristalsis rather than mechanical obstruction. **Postoperative ileus** is expected to occur after abdominal surgery and is not considered pathologic unless it persists beyond several days after surgery. Other causes of ileus include neurogenic (e.g., spinal cord injury), metabolic (especially hypokalemia), infectious (e.g., sepsis or intra-abdominal abscess), and pharmacologic (e.g., opiates and anticholinergics) factors.

Ileus is acquired and usually temporary if the primary inciting factor can be corrected. In contrast, **primary intestinal pseudo-obstruction** results from a congenital defect in either the innervation or the smooth muscle of the intestine, with defective peristalsis resulting. Both familial and sporadic forms of these disorders exist. Histologically indistinguishable defects occur as acquired abnormalities in association with connective tissue disorders (e.g., scleroderma and lupus), metabolic diseases (e.g., diabetes mellitus and amyloidosis), and neuromuscular diseases (e.g., muscular dystrophy).

Workup and Evaluation

The evaluation should focus on the following goals: (1) distinguishing mechanical obstruction from ileus, (2) determining the etiology of the obstruction, (3) discriminating partial from complete obstruction, and (4) discriminating simple from strangulating obstruction.

Important elements of the history include prior abdominal operations (suggesting the presence of adhesions) and underlying abdominal disorders (e.g., intraabdominal cancer or inflammatory bowel disease). The symptoms of small-bowel obstruction are abdominal pain (which is initially colicky but becomes continuous if bowel strangulation ensues), nausea, vomiting, and obstipation. Continued passage of flatus or stool or both 6 to 12 hours after onset of symptoms is more characteristic of partial than of complete obstruction.

The signs of small-bowel obstruction include abdominal distention (distention is most pronounced if the site of obstruction is the distal ileum; it may be absent if the site of obstruction is the very proximal jejunum) and hyperactive bowel sounds (hypoactive or absent with bowel strangulation). On examination, a meticulous search for hernias (particularly in the inguinal and femoral regions) should be conducted. The stool should be checked for gross or occult blood, suggestive of intestinal strangulation.

Laboratory findings reflect intravascular volume depletion and consist of hemoconcentration and electrolyte abnormalities. Marked leukocytosis and acidosis suggest strangulation.

The initial, and often sufficient, imaging test is the **abdominal series,** consisting of a supine radiograph of the abdomen, an erect abdominal film, and and erect chest film. The findings specific for small-bowel obstruction are the triad of dilated small-bowel loops (>3 cm in diameter), air/fluid levels seen on upright films, and a paucity of air in the colon (Fig. 25-1*A* and *B*). The abdominal series does have several limitations; it rarely reveals the etiology of obstruction, and it may not permit distinction between partial and complete obstruction and between mechanical obstruction and ileus. In some cases of obstruction, the intestinal lumen may be completely filled with fluid but no gas, thereby preventing visualization of air/fluid levels or bowel distention.

If diagnostic uncertainty exists, additional studies may be necessary. A contrast examination of the small bowel (**small-bowel series**) can be used to distinguish mechanical obstruction from ileus and partial from complete obstruction. In a **gastrointestinal upper GI** study, contrast is swallowed or instilled into the stomach through a nasogastric tube. In an **enteroclysis** study, contrast is instilled into the proximal jejunum via a long nasoenteric catheter. Enteroclysis, particularly if barium is used as the contrast agent, offers greater sensitivity than upper GI studies for detecting distal pathology. If intestinal perforation is suspected, then a water-soluble contrast agent, rather than barium, should be used.

Computed tomography (CT) scanning is indicated in selected cases of suspected bowel obstruction. A transition zone resulting from dilated bowel proximal to the site of obstruction, with decompressed bowel distally, is seen with mechanical obstruction but not with ileus. Extrinsic causes of obstruction (such as abscesses, inflammation, and tumors that are not seen on plain radiographs or contrast studies) can be identified. Signs of strangulation can be detected more readily than on other studies and include thickening of bowel wall, pneumatosis intestinalis (air in the wall of the bowel), portal venous gas, mesenteric haziness, and poor uptake of intravenous contrast into the bowel wall.

Treatment

Treatment begins with fluid resuscitation. Small-bowel obstruction is typically associated with a marked depletion of intravascular volume due to decreased oral intake,

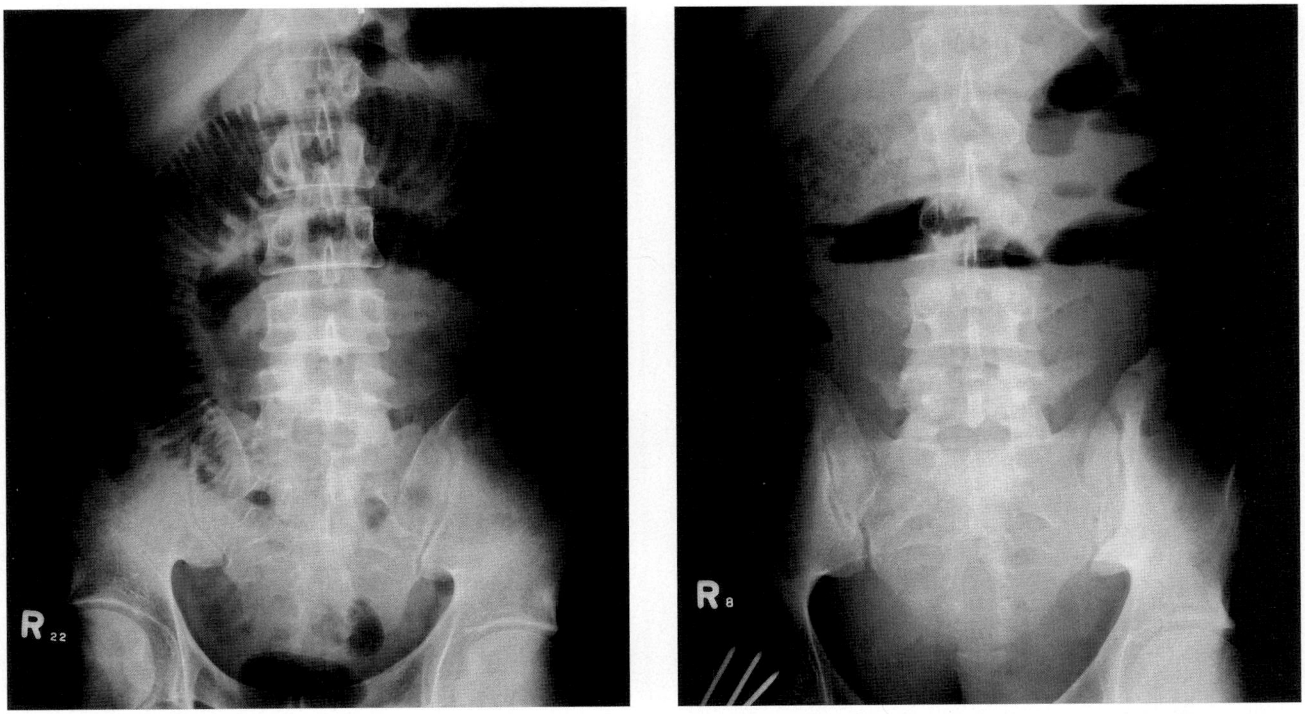

A B

FIGURE 25–1 Small-bowel obstruction. Radiographs taken with the patient in the supine (*A*) and upright (*B*) positions reveal the characteristic small-bowel dilation, air/fluid levels, and paucity of air in the colon.

vomiting, and sequestration of fluid in bowel lumen and wall. Isotonic fluid is given intravenously, and a Foley catheter is used to monitor urine output and thus adequacy of resuscitation. Central venous or pulmonary artery catheter monitoring may be necessary to assist with fluid management, particularly in patients with underlying cardiac disease. Broad-spectrum antibiotics are often administered, although no clear evidence suggests that they have efficacy in reducing infectious complications in this setting.

The stomach should be evacuated continuously of air and fluid by using a nasogastric tube. This maneuver decreases nausea, distention, and most important, the risk of vomiting and aspiration. Longer nasoenteric tubes were favored in the past but are used rarely today. They are associated with higher complication rates but no greater efficacy in decompression than nasogastric tubes.

The standard therapy for small-bowel obstruction, with the exception of specific situations described later, is expeditious surgery. The rationale for this approach is to minimize risk for bowel strangulation, which is associated with increased risk for perioperative morbidity and mortality. As the clinical signs of strangulation are difficult to detect before the onset of irreversible bowel ischemia, the goal to is operate before such signs become evident.

The specific procedure done varies with the etiology of obstruction. For example, adhesions are lysed, tumors are resected, and hernias are reduced and repaired. Regardless of the specific etiology, the affected intestine should be examined, and clearly nonviable bowel should be resected. Criteria for viability are normal color, peristalsis, and marginal arterial pulsations. Usually visual inspection alone is adequate in judging viability. In borderline cases, a Doppler probe may be used to check for pulsatile flow to the bowel, and intact perfusion can be verified by visualizing intravenously administered fluorescein dye in the bowel wall under ultraviolet illumination.

Exceptions to the rule of expeditious surgery for intestinal obstruction include partial small-bowel obstruction, early postoperative obstruction, inflammatory bowel disease, and carcinomatosis. Progression to strangulation is unlikely to occur with partial small-bowel obstruction, and an attempt at nonoperative resolution is warranted. Early postoperative obstruction is difficult to distinguish from the more common postoperative ileus. However, if complete mechanical obstruction is demonstrated in the postoperative period,

PEARLS FOR ROUNDS

Most common etiologies for small-bowel obstruction: adhesions, malignancy, hernia, inflammatory bowel disease, volvulus

Most common causes of ileus: neurologic injury/disease, hypokalemia, infection, opiates and anticholinergics, postoperative state

Management of small-bowel obstruction: fluid resuscitation, nasogastric tube, early surgery

Clinical indicators of obstruction with strangulation: steady pain, tachycardia, fever, absent bowel sounds, bloody stool, leukocytosis, acidosis

Most common indications for surgery in Crohn's disease: obstruction, perforation, bleeding, intractability

Factors preventing spontaneous closure of fistulas: malnutrition, sepsis, inflammatory bowel disease, cancer, radiation, obstruction of the intestine distal to the origin of the fistula, foreign bodies, high output, and epithelialization of the fistula tract

Causes of acute mesenteric ischemia: embolus, thrombus, vasospasm, venous thrombosis

Problems with prolonged total parenteral nutrition use: catheter sepsis, venous thrombosis, osteoporosis, cholelithiasis, kidney failure, liver failure, cost, increased mortality

expeditious surgery is still indicated. Obstruction due to inflammatory bowel disease usually responds to medical therapy. Obstruction occurring in the setting of carcinomatosis is a difficult issue, and its management must be tailored to individual patients.

Prognosis

Prognosis is related to the etiology of obstruction. After laparotomy, a 5% lifetime incidence of small-bowel obstruction due to adhesions is found. After surgery for small-bowel obstruction due to adhesions, the probability of recurrent obstruction ranges from 20% to 30%. The perioperative mortality rate for surgery for nonstrangulating small-bowel obstruction is less than 5%, with most deaths occurring in elderly patients with significant comorbidites. Mortality rates for surgery for strangulating obstruction range from 8% to 25%.

Instestinal Fistulas

A fistula is an abnormal communication between two epithelialized surfaces. The communication occurs between two parts of the GI tract or adjacent organs in an **internal fistula** (e.g., enterocolonic fistula or colovesicular fistula). An **external fistula** (e.g., enterocutaneous fistula or rectovaginal fistula) involves the skin or another external surface epithelium. Entercutaneous fistulas that drain less than 200 mL of fluid per day are known as **low-output fistulas** whereas those that drain more than 500 mL of fluid per day are known as **high-output fistulas**.

More than 80% of enterocutaneous fistulas represent iatrogenic complications that arise in the postoperative period as the result of enterotomies or anastomotic dehiscences. Spontaneous fistulas occur in the presence of underlying intestinal disease, such as Crohn's disease or cancer.

Pathophysiology

The manifestations of fistulas depend on which structures are involved. Low-resistance enteroenteric fistulas in which a significant portion of the small intestine is bypassed may result in malabsorption. Enterovesicular fistulas often result in recurrent urinary tract infections. The drainage from enterocutaneous fistulas is irritating to the skin and causes excoriation. The loss of enteric contents, particularly from high-output fistulas originating from the proximal small intestine, results in dehydration, electrolyte imbalances, and malnutrition.

Under ideal circumstances, fistulas close spontaneously. Factors inhibiting spontaneous closure include malnutrition, sepsis, inflammatory bowel disease, cancer, radiation, obstruction of the intestine distal to the origin of the fistula, foreign bodies, high output, and epithelialization of the fistula tract.

Workup and Evaluation

Postoperative enterocutaneous fistulas typically become evident between days 5 and 10 after surgery. Fever, leukocytosis, prolonged ileus, abdominal tenderness, and wound infection are the initial signs. The diagnosis becomes obvious when drainage of enteric material through the abdominal wound or through existing drains occurs. These fistulas are often associated with intraabdominal abscesses.

CT scanning is the most useful initial test. Leakage of enteral contrast from the intestinal lumen can be observed. Intraabdominal abscesses should be sought and drained percutaneously. If the anatomy of the fistula is not clear on CT scanning, an upper GI study with small-bowel follow-through is obtained to demonstrate the fistula's site of origin. This study also is useful to rule out the presence of obstruction distal to the site of origin. Occasionally, contrast administered into the intestine does not demonstrate the fistula tract. A **fistulogram**, in which contrast is injected under pressure through a catheter placed percutaneously into the fistula tract, may offer greater sensitivity in localizing the fistula origin.

Treatment

The treatment of enterocutaneous fistulas should proceed through an orderly sequence of phases.

1. Stabilization. Fluid and electrolyte resuscitation is begun. Nutrition is provided, usually through total parenteral nutrition (TPN). Sepsis is controlled with antibiotics and drainage of abscesses. The skin is protected with ostomy appliances or fistula drains.
2. Investigation. The anatomy of the fistula is defined by using the studies described earlier. A management plan is formulated.
3. Rehabilitation. Probability of spontaneous closure is maximized. Nutrition and time are the key components of this phase. Nutrition is given parenterally for fistulas originating from the proximal intestine, whereas enteral nutrition is used for distal fistulas. Two to three months is allowed for spontaneous closure. Fistulas that do not close during this period are unlikely to do so. The somatostatin analogue octreotide is sometimes used to reduce the volume of fistula output, although its administration is not associated with increased probability of spontaneous closure.

Finally, in the absence of spontaneous closure, surgery is performed. Because of dense adhesions, these operations can present formidable challenges. The operative strategy is to resect the fistula tract together with the segment of intestine from which it originates. Simple closure of the fistula opening is associated with high recurrence rates.

Prognosis

Enterocutaneous fistulas are associated with a 10% to 15% mortality rate, related mostly to sepsis or underlying disease. Overall, 50% of fistulas close spontaneously. Surgery for fistulas is associated with a greater than 50% morbidity rate, including a 10% recurrence rate.

Diverticular Disease

A Meckel's diverticulum, which is a remnant of the fetal omphalomesenteric (vitelline) duct, is the most common congenital abnormality of the GI tract, being present in approximately 2% of the population. It is classified as a "true" diverticulum, in that its wall consists of all four layers of the normal small intestine.

In contrast, the walls of acquired jejunoileal diverticula usually lack a muscular layer and consist of mucosa and submucosa alone. They are present in approximately 0.5% to 2% of the general population, and their prevalence increases with age.

Pathophysiology

Intestinal diverticula are asymptomatic until a specific complication arises. The most common complications of Meckel's diverticula in adults are intestinal obstruction and diverticulitis. The most common complication in children is bleeding. Obstruction is caused by volvulus of the intestine around the diverticulum, a phenomenon particularly likely to occur when the diverticulum is tethered to the abdominal wall by a duct remnant, or by intussusception of the diverticulum into the ileum. Diverticulitis is due to obstruction at the neck of the diverticulum and has a pathophysiology similar to that of appendicitis. Bleeding results from a peptic ulcer located in the intestinal wall opposite the diverticulum. Ulceration is the result of acid secretion by gastric mucosa that frequently occurs as ectopic tissue within a Meckel's diverticulum.

Jejunoileal diverticula can be associated with bacterial overgrowth, leading to vitamin B_{12} deficiency, megaloblastic anemia, malabsorption, and steatorrhea. They also can cause intestinal obstruction through intussusception or compression of adjacent bowel. Divertula located in the duodenum near the ampulla of Vater can obstruct the common bile duct, causing jaundice, or the pancreatic duct, causing pancreatitis.

Differential Diagnosis

Meckel's diverticulitis is often indistinguishable from **acute appendicitis** until surgery is performed. If the presentation is one of obstruction or bleeding, **intestinal neoplasms** should be considered.

Workup and Evaluation

Most intestinal diverticula are asymptomatic and are found incidentally during laparotomy for other reasons. Diverticula can be detected on contrast examination of the small bowel or enteroclysis. However, sensitivity is low; small diverticula are often missed. Meckel's diverticula containing ectopic gastric mucosa can be detected by radionuclide scanning with [99mTc]-pertechnetate, a radioisotope that is preferentially taken up by gastric mucosa. Bleeding caused by peptic ulceration due to a Meckel's diverticulum can be localized by angiography.

Treatment

Symptomatic Meckel's diverticula are treated with diverticular resection. If surgery is performed for hemorrhage, the segment of intestine containing the peptic ulcer is resected as well. It remains controversial whether asymptomatic Meckel's diverticula found incidentally at operation should be removed or left in situ. A rationale may exist for resection in children, who have a higher lifetime incidence of developing symptoms than do adults.

Asymptomatic acquired jejunoileal diverticula are left alone. Bacterial overgrowth is treated with antibiotics. Symptomatic diverticula are treated with segmental resection of the involved intestine.

Small-Bowel Neoplasms

The most common benign neoplasms occurring in the small intestine are adenomas, leiomyomas, and lipomas. The most common malignant neoplasms are adenocarcinomas, carcinoid tumors, lymphomas, and gastrointestinal stromal tumors (GISTs). Each of these lesions is quite rare. Although more than 90% of the mucosal surface area of the GI tract is found in the small intestine, only 2% of GI malignancies occur there.

Pathophysiology

Benign and malignant lesions of the small intestine tend to be asymptomatic until they become large. Symptoms are the result of bleeding into or partial obstruction of the intestinal lumen.

Proposed explanations for the low frequency of neoplasms in the small bowel relative to that in the colon include (1) a lower concentration of bacteria in the small bowel, with the bacteria being responsible for metabolizing luminal material into carcinogenic substances; (2) rapid transit of chyme through the small intestine, limiting the contact time between carcinogens and the mucosa; (3) mucosal protection by secretory IgA; and (4) more effective apoptosis (programmed cell death), which acts to eliminate epithelial cells that develop genetic mutations.

Differential Diagnosis

Small-bowel neoplasms should be distinguished from other lesions producing chronic partial obstruction or bleeding, such as strictures associated with **radiation enteritis** and **Crohn's disease.**

Workup and Evaluation

Because of the lack of specific symptoms, most small-intestinal neoplasms are not diagnosed until they become large or, in the case of malignant tumors, advanced-stage disease ensues. They are often encountered incidentally during laparotomy for other reasons.

A contrast examination of the small intestine is the test of choice for diagnosing small-intestinal neoplasms. Enteroclysis is more sensitive than the upper GI with small-bowel follow-through, particularly for tumors located in the distal small intestine (Fig. 25-2). CT scanning has less sensitivity in detecting the primary tumor but is useful in staging malignant disease. Endoscopy can be used to visualize and take biopsies of lesions in the extreme proximal and distal intestine but is not applicable for most of the intestine, which is beyond the reach of the standard endoscope. Tumors associated with significant hemorrhage can be localized by angiography or radioisotope-tagged red blood cell scans.

Treatment

Symptomatic benign tumors of the small intestine are treated with resection of the segment of intestine containing the tumor.

Adenocarcinomas are most often found in the duodenum. Tumors in the periampullary region are treated with pancreaticoduodenectomy. Five-year survival rates after successful resection range from 50% to 60%.

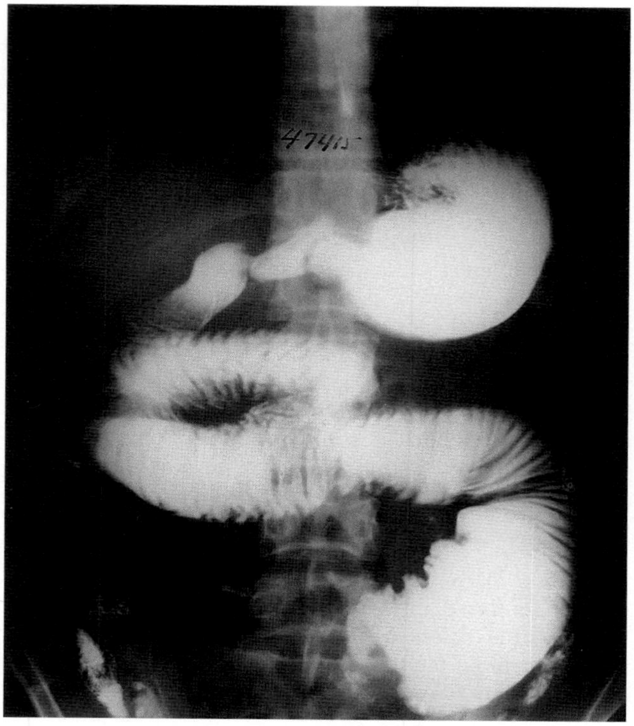

FIGURE 25–2 Jejunal adenocarcinoma. This contrast examination of the small bowel reveals a proximal intestinal obstruction due to an adenocarcinoma of the jejunum.

Adenocarcinomas located in the remainder of the small intestine are associated with a poorer prognosis and rarely are amenable to curative resection. For localized disease, segmental resection of the involved intestine and lymph node–bearing mesentery is performed and is associated with 5-year survival rates of only 5% to 30%. Usually resection is done merely to palliate obstructive symptoms. Chemotherapy is of no proven benefit.

GISTs are treated with wide local resection of involved intestine. In advanced disease, palliative resection is done to relieve obstruction or stop bleeding. For resected lesions, tumor size and mitotic index are the most important prognostic factors. The 5-year survival rate after surgical resection has been reported to range from 35% to 60%. Although standard chemotherapy is ineffective for GISTs, administration of imatinib, a tyrosine kinase inhibitor with potent activity against the KIT tyrosine kinase, leads to objective reductions in tumor volume in up to 60% of patients with GISTs.

Carcinoids are most commonly found in the appendix, where they are associated with a benign prognosis. Carcinoids located in the small intestine are more aggressive and usually are first seen with metastatic disease. If disease is localized, it is treated with wide local resection of

PEARLS FOR THE OR

Anatomy: jejunum is proximal two fifths of small intestine; ileum is distal three fifths. The jejunum has a larger circumference and a thicker wall, and its mesentery contains more fat than does that of the ileum. The strongest layer of the intestinal wall is the submucosa.

Complications of intestinal resection: anastomotic leak, fistula, stricture, vitamin B_{12} and bile salt malabsorption for ileal resection, short-bowel syndrome

Criteria for intestinal viability: (1) normal color, (2) peristalsis, and (3) marginal arterial pulsations. In borderline cases, use Doppler probe or visualize fluorescein dye in the bowel wall under ultraviolet illumination.

Meckel's diverticulum: Found in 2% of population, located within 2 feet of ileocecal valve, 2% symptomatic, 2 inches in length

Most common benign neoplasms of the small intestine: adenomas, leiomyomas, and lipomas. The most common malignant neoplasms: adenocarcinomas, carcinoids, lymphomas, gastrointestinal stromal tumors

Strategies for avoiding short-bowel syndrome: resect no more intestine than necessary, stricturoplasty, preserve colon, preserve ileocecal valve

the involved intestine, and the prognosis is excellent. Even in the presence of liver metastases, median survival time after diagnosis is 3 years. The tumor is moderately responsive to chemotherapy; doxorubicin, 5-fluorouracil, and streptozocin, alone or in combination, are used. Manifestations of carcinoid syndrome include diarrhea, flushing, hypotension, tachycardia, and fibrosis of the endocardium and valves of the right heart and result from the action of vasomotor mediators, of which serotonin, bradykinin, and substance P are candidates. Because these mediators undergo nearly complete metabolism during first passage through the liver, clinically evident carcinoid syndrome rarely occurs with intestinal carcinoids in the absence of hepatic metastases. Reducing the overall quantity of tumor cells by resecting metastases may ameliorate the vasomotor symptoms. Octreotide is the most effect pharmacologic agent for treating symptoms of carcinoid syndrome.

Lymphomas predominate in the ileum, which contains the greatest concentration of lymphoid tissue in the intestine. They are usually non-Hodgkin's B-cell lymphomas. Localized disease is treated with segmental intestinal resection. Diffuse disease is treated with chemotherapy rather than with surgery. Overall 5-year survival rates for patients with intestinal lymphoma range from 20% to 40%. For patients with localized disease amenable to surgical resection, the 5-year survival rate is 60%.

Mesenteric Vascular Disease

Mesenteric vascular disease can appear in one of two forms: acute mesenteric ischemia or chronic mesenteric ischemia.

Pathophysiology

Acute mesenteric ischemia is usually due to a sudden occlusion of the superior mesenteric artery or one of its branches by an arterial **embolus** or, less commonly, **thrombosis**. Mucosal sloughing occurs within 3 hours, and full-thickness infarction, within 6 hours of ischemia. If the arterial stenosis is incomplete, partial ischemia results, and progression to full-thickness infarction is delayed. Two other mechanisms can lead to acute mesenteric ischemia: **nonocclusive mesenteric ischemia** due to arterial vasospasm, typically occurring in critically ill patients being administered vasopressor agents; and **mesenteric venous thrombosis**, occurring in the setting of hypercoagulability.

Chronic mesenteric ischemia is the result of atherosclerotic disease of the mesenteric arteries. Generally, symptoms arise only after two or three of the main mesenteric vessels (celiac, superior mesenteric, and inferior mesenteric arteries) develop hemodynamically significant occlusive lesions. Superior mesenteric artery occlusion alone is enough to cause symptoms, however, if poor collaterals from the other vessels exist.

Differential Diagnosis

Acute mesenteric ischemia may resemble **intestinal obstruction with strangulation**. It may also be confused with other disorders causing poorly localized abdominal pain, such as **acute pancreatitis.**

Chronic mesenteric ischemia should be distinguished from other diseases causing vague abdominal pain and weight loss, such as **intraabdominal malignancies** and **peptic ulcer disease.**

Workup and Evaluation

Abdominal pain out of proportion to tenderness on examination is the hallmark of acute mesenteric ischemia. Severe, poorly localized abdominal pain is accompanied by varying degrees of nausea, vomiting, and diarrhea. Physical findings are characteristically absent early in the course of the disorder. With the onset of bowel infarction, abdominal distention, peritonitis, and passage of bloody stools occur.

Leukocytosis, acidosis, and elevations in amylase and creatine kinase (BB isoenzyme) are late findings; no specific laboratory tests indicate early reversible ischemia. Patients suspected of having acute mesenteric ischemia with peritonitis should undergo urgent laparotomy. If time permits, CT scanning can be used to rule out other possible etiologies for abdominal pain. Findings on CT suggesting intestinal ischemia include thickening of bowel wall, pneumatosis intestinalis, portal venous gas, mesenteric haziness, and poor uptake of intravenous contrast into the bowel wall. Angiography is diagnostic but is rarely obtained for acute mesenteric ischemia because of time constraints.

Chronic mesenteric ischemia begins insidiously. Postprandial pain is the most prevalent symptom, producing a characteristic "food-fear" and weight loss. These patients are often thought to have a malignancy and undergo an extensive workup before angiography, which is diagnostic, is done.

Treatment

By the time acute mesenteric infarction is diagnosed, intestinal infarction has usually already occurred, mandating urgent laparotomy. At operation, the bowel is assessed for viability. Criteria for viability were discussed in the bowel-obstruction section. Nonviable bowel is resected. If the bowel is ischemic but viable, then restoration of perfusion with embolectomy, thrombectomy, or aortomesenteric bypass is an option, if surgically feasible. If a question exists about the viability of large portions of the bowel, the operation is terminated, and reexploration is done 24 to 48 hours later to reassess viability.

Another option is thrombolysis, with thrombolytic agents instilled via a catheter placed percutaneously into the superior mesenteric artery. This approach is slow and must be abandoned if peritonitis develops. For nonocclusive mesenteric ischemia, infusion of the vasodilator papaverine via a catheter placed into the superior mesenteric artery is sometimes effective in restoring perfusion. For mesenteric venous thrombosis, anticoagulation is maintained for 3 to 6 months. Infarcted bowel must be resected regardless of the mechanism of ischemia, however.

For chronic mesenteric ischemia, surgical arterial reconstruction with bypass grafts to the superior mesenteric and celiac arteries is the standard treatment. Balloon angioplasty is another option, although experience with this approach is limited.

Prognosis

Mortality rates for patients with acute mesenteric ischemia range from 45% to 85%. Arterial reconstruction in this setting is associated with low patency rates. Mesenteric venous thrombosis is associated with a 30% mortality rate, with a 30% recurrence rate without long-term anticoagulation. Nonocclusive mesenteric infarction has a particularly poor prognosis, in part because of the serious illnesses characteristic of patients with this condition.

Surgery for chronic mesenteric ischemia carries a 5% to 10% operative mortality rate, with an 80% to 90% long-term patency rate for aortomesenteric bypass grafts.

Short-Bowel Syndrome

Intestinal resection is performed for many of the diseases discussed in this chapter and generally is associated with minimal morbidity. However, when extent of resection is great enough, a devastating condition known as the short-bowel syndrome may result. This disorder is characterized by insufficient intestinal absorptive capacity, manifested by intractable diarrhea, weight loss, dehydration, and malnutrition.

In adults, the most common etiologies of short-bowel syndrome are mesenteric ischemia, malignancy, and Crohn's disease. Seventy-five percent of cases result from a single massive intestinal resection. Twenty-five percent of cases result from the cumulative effects of multiple sequential intestinal resections. In pediatric patients, intestinal atresias, volvulus, and necrotizing enterocolitis are the most common etiologies.

The short-bowel syndrome is a major public health problem in the United States: between 10,000 to 20,000 individuals with this disorder are chronically dependent on TPN.

Pathophysiology

Resection of less than 50% of the small intestine is generally well tolerated. Clinically significant malabsorption occurs when more than 50% to 80% of the intestine is removed. Factors exacerbating malabsorption include diseased, rather than healthy, remnant intestine; loss of ileum rather than jejunum (the capacity for vitamin B_{12} and bile salt absorption is lost with ileal resection); loss of the colon (the colon has great capacity for water and electrolyte absorption); and loss of the ileocecal valve (the ileocecal valve delays intestinal transit, thereby prolonging contact time between nutrients and intestinal mucosa). Hypergastrinemia-associated gastric acid hypersecretion occurs after massive intestinal resection. The increased acid load in the intestine inhibits the function of digestive enzymes, most of which function optimally under alkaline conditions.

With time, **intestinal adaptation** occurs, resulting in a compensatory increase in the absorptive capacity of the remnant intestine. Changes in both morphology (e.g., increased villous height and crypt depth) and function are observed. The mechanisms underlying this phenomenon are incompletely understood; however, it is clear that the presence of luminal nutrients is required for adaptation to occur. Glucagon-like peptide 2, an intestinal growth factor secreted by the L-type enteroendocrine cells of the distal intestine, may be a key mediator of intestinal adaptation.

Treatment

For patients having undergone a massive intestinal resection, the initial treatment goals include replacing fluid and electrolytes lost in the severe diarrhea and providing nutrition with TPN. After the immediate postoperative period, enteral nutrition is gradually introduced. During the period of adaptation, which generally lasts 1 to 2 years, the relative amount of nutrition provided enterally is increased, while the amount provided parenterally is tapered. For the long term, patients are maintained on a stable regimen of both enteral and parenteral nutrition.

Useful pharmacologic adjuncts include histamine-2 or proton-pump inhibitors, to inhibit gastric acid hypersecretion, and antimotility agents.

TPN is lifesaving for patients with the short-bowel syndrome. However, prolonged TPN administration is associated with significant mortality rates (2% to 5% per year due to TPN-associated complications) and morbidity, including catheter sepsis, venous thrombosis, nutritional abnormalities, progressive kidney and liver failure, and osteoporosis. It also is expensive, costing between $50,000 and $100,000 per patient per year.

Because of the problems associated with TPN administration, other forms of therapy have been used. Various surgical strategies to slow intestinal transit or to attempt to augment surface area have received anecdotal experience. Their efficacy and safety are unproven, however. Intestinal transplantation has been performed but is associated with only a 50% 2-year survival and an even lower graft-survival rate. It remains risky and is not standard therapy. Pharmacologic means of increasing intestinal absorptive efficiency or stimulating intestinal regeneration have been reported, but remain experimental.

Suggested Reading

Dayton MT: Small bowel obstruction. In Cameron JL (ed): Current Surgical Therapy, 8th ed. St. Louis, Mosby, 2004, p 105.

Becker JM: Surgical therapy for ulcerative colitis and Crohn's disease. Gastroenterol Clin North Am 28(2):371, 1999.

Bickston SJ: Treatment of Crohn's disease at the turn of the century. N Engl J Med 339:401, 1998.

Mulvihill SJ: Gut hormones: Yesterday, today, and tomorrow. Ann Surg 225(2):143, 1997.

Vanderhoof JA, Langnas AN: Short-bowel syndrome in children and adults. Gastroenterology 113:1767, 1997.

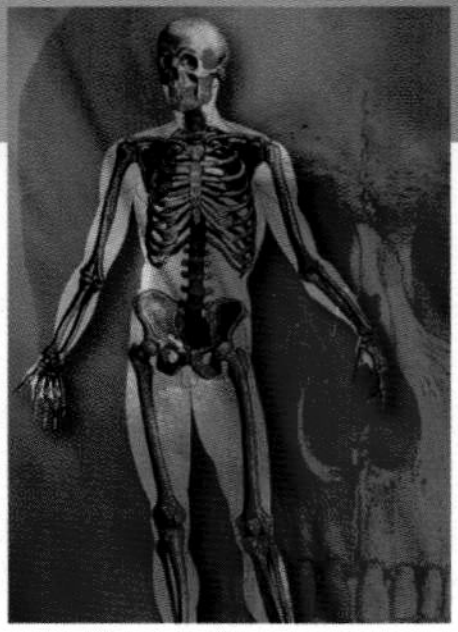

Chapter 26
Stomach and Duodenum

MERRIL T. DAYTON, MD

With its unique gastric mucosa, the stomach is a remarkable organ with the capability of concentrating hydrochloric acid 6 million-fold without autodigestion. That concentration of acid anywhere else in the body causes immediate injury. When mucosal defensive systems are injured or defective, the acid plays a role in peptic ulcer disease. An interesting phenomenon observed over the last 25-year period is that peptic ulcer disease has declined significantly. Nevertheless, gastric dyspepsia and problems associated with the stomach are the source of substantial human misery today, and more than $1 billion is spent each year on pharmacologic agents purchased to diminish pain associated with the stomach.

Although the stomach is not an organ critical for either digestion or life itself, it plays a very important role in increasing the efficiency of digestion. It acts as a storage tank and mixer to slowly meter out aliquots of grossly broken-down food to the duodenum to begin the process of digestion.

Surgical Anatomy

The stomach is a hollow expansile organ lying obliquely in the upper abdomen (Fig. 26-1). The stomach originates approximately 5 cm beyond the diaphragm, where the esophagus and its squamous epithelium are delineated from the origin of the stomach by the so-called Z line, which is made from columnar epithelium. The stomach is fixed at this point and is also fixed distally by the retroperitoneal duodenum. The distal stomach is separated from the duodenum by the circular pyloric muscle. The stomach is approximately the size of two cupped hands, but may vary tremendously, depending on the fed or fasting state and contractions. The stomach abuts a number of other organs in its position in the upper abdomen.

This saccular, hollow organ is composed of three different muscle layers, including an inner oblique muscle layer, a middle circular layer of muscle fibers, and an outer layer of longitudinal muscle fibers. The muscular wall of the upper stomach is much thinner than that of the lower stomach (antrum), which plays an important role in mixing. The oblique fibers in the upper stomach do appear to play some role in preventing acid reflux at the esophagogastric junction. The duodenum, like most hollow gastrointestinal (GI) organs, consists of an outer longitudinal and an inner circular muscle throughout. This configuration changes at the sphincter of Oddi, which is a muscular valve controlling evacuation of the ampulla of Vater. The duodenum consists of four portions. The first extends from the pylorus to the most superior portion of the duodenal bulb; the second portion of the duodenum is the descending portion, which appears primarily in a vertical configuration and contains the ampulla of Vater; the third is a transverse portion that crosses the spine and is often the area of injury in blunt abdominal trauma; and the final ascends up to the ligament of Treitz.

The cardia of the stomach represents the beginning of stomach and transition from esophagus to stomach (Fig. 26-2). A line drawn from the cardia in a horizontal fashion to the greater curve is the boundary line between the fundus and the body. The fundus is all gastric tissue above that horizontal line. The body is the portion from that line down to the incisura of the stomach, where it angulates. The area from the incisura to the pylorus represents the antrum. These zones are not clearly demarcated anatomically, but their demarcation is useful to the surgeon because of the concentration of cells in each of the areas with a specific function.

The body of the stomach contains most of the acid-secreting parietal cells and chief cells. Intrinsic factor also is produced in this region. The fundus is the portion of the stomach that can reflexively relax to accommodate food volume without increasing intragastric pressure. The antrum contains most of the G cells, which produce gastrin and thus make the stomach a hormonal organ as well. The mucosa of the fundus and body is characterized by multiple linear rugae, which represent substantial mucosal redundancy. The antral portion of the stomach is smooth and has very few folds. Similarly, the first portion of the duodenum is quite smooth, whereas the second, third, and fourth portions of the duodenum have redundant circular folds.

Blood Supply and Lymphatics

The stomach is one of the most richly perfused organs in the GI system. It is supplied by five arterial systems (Fig.

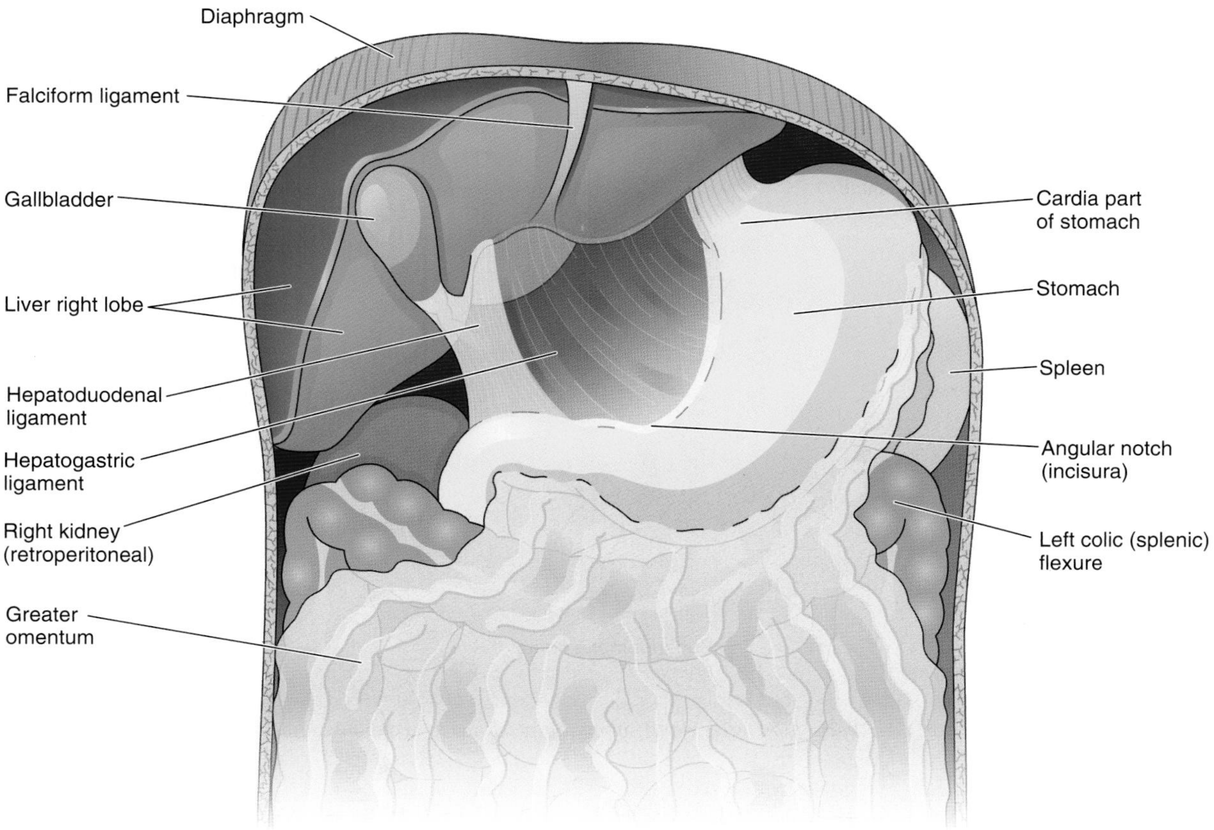

FIGURE 26–1 Oblique position of the stomach in the upper abdomen and relation to surrounding organs.

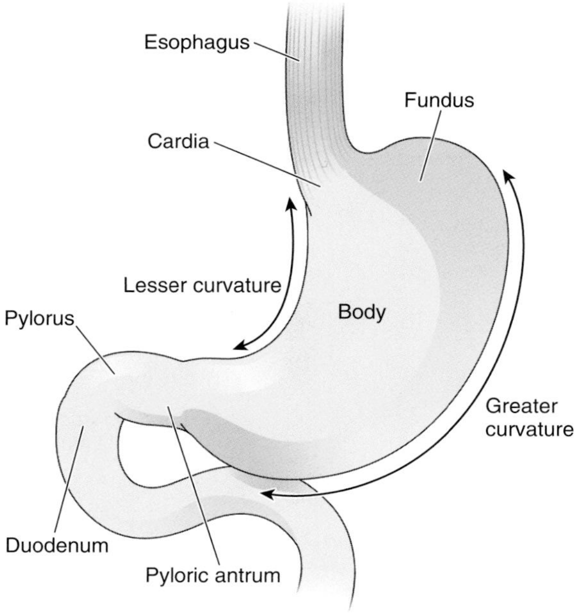

FIGURE 26–2 Anatomic regions of the stomach.

26-3), and thus gastric perfusion may be preserved even after ligation of four of its five arterial systems. The largest artery supplying the stomach is the left gastric artery, which is a branch of the celiac trunk. This artery anastomoses with the right gastric artery, which is a branch of the hepatic artery, to form a rich arcade of blood vessels supplying the lesser curve of the stomach. The greater curve of the stomach is perfused by the right gastroepiploic, which, in turn, is a branch of the gastroduodenal, and the left gastroepiploic, which is a branch of the splenic artery. Similarly, the proximal stomach and fundus area are perfused by short gastric arteries, which originate from the splenic artery. Venous drainage of the stomach parallels the arterial supply. The largest vein draining the stomach is the left gastric vein, which also is known as the coronary vein and becomes relevant during treatment of variceal bleeding from portal hypertension. The lymphatic drainage of the stomach also parallels gastric venous drainage. Because of a number of intramural communications, malignancies in the stomach often travel some distance from the primary tumor and necessitate a larger margin being required during surgical resection.

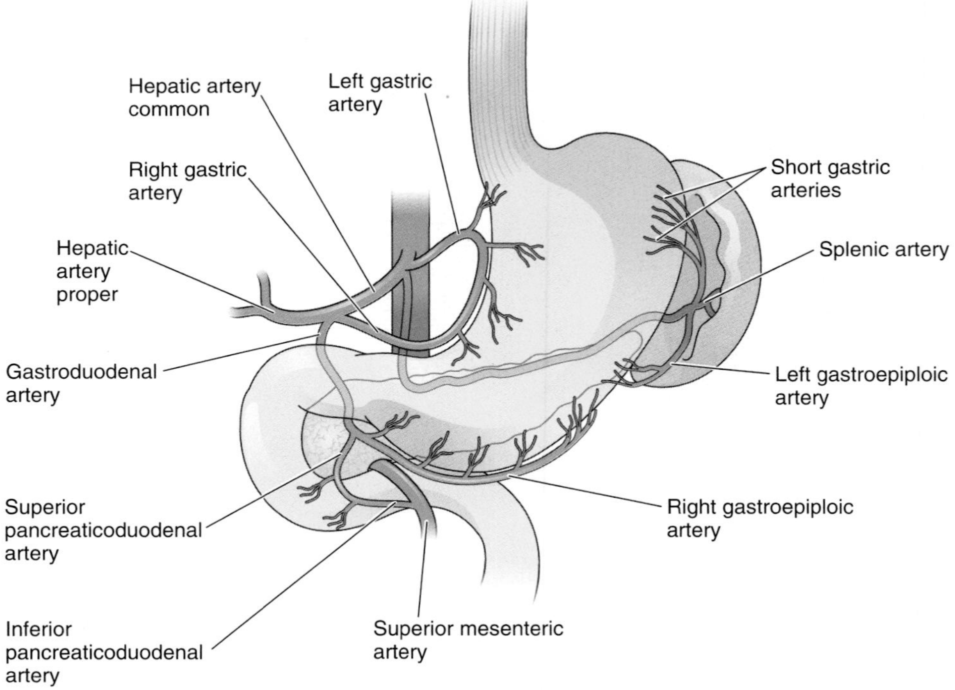

FIGURE 26–3 Arterial blood supply of the stomach and duodenum.

The blood supply of the duodenum is shared with the head of the pancreas. The vessels perfusing the duodenum are derived from superior, anterior, and posterior pancreaticoduodenal arteries, which arise from the gastroduodenal artery as well as inferior, anterior, and posterior pancreaticoduodenal arteries, which arise from the superior mesenteric artery. As noted earlier, venous drainage of the stomach and duodenum is through the portal system by way of the short gastric vessels, the gastroepiploics, splenic, and coronary vessels.

Nerve Supply

The nerve supply to the stomach and duodenum is primarily via parasympathetic and sympathetic nerves. The parasympathetic system is mediated primarily via the vagus nerves. The left and right vagus nerves descend on the lateral sides of the esophagus. As the vagus nerves descend into the abdomen, the left vagus nerve rotates to become the anterior vagus, and the right vagus nerve rotates to become the posterior vagus nerve (Fig. 26-4). The anterior vagus nerve sends a branch to the liver and gallbladder, whereas its distal members travel parallel to the lesser curve and give off multiple branches to the corpus. The distalmost fibers are known as the nerve of Latarjet and give off motor

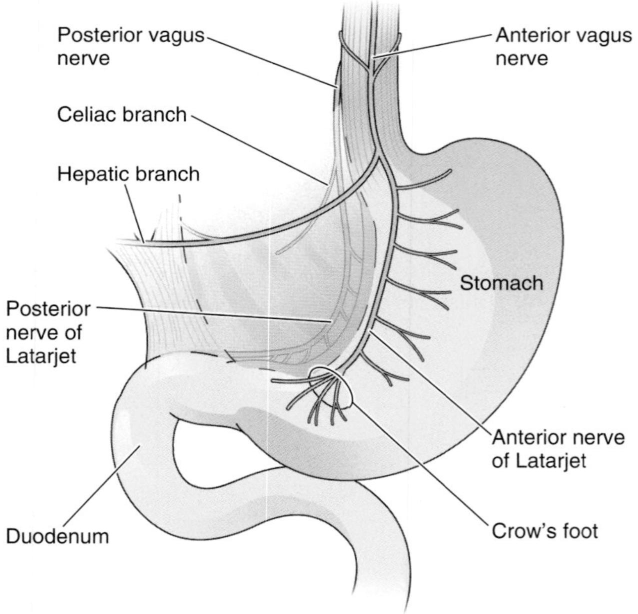

FIGURE 26–4 Vagal nerve supply to the stomach. Note the parallel anterior and posterior nerves of Latarjet.

branches to the distal stomach and pylorus, which help coordinate gastric emptying. The posterior vagus gives off branches to the celiac plexus and a posterior gastric branch.

The sympathetic nerves originate from spinal segments T5 through T10 and provide the route for pain perception. In general, the vagus nerve appears to stimulate stomach acid secretion and contraction, whereas the sympathetic system opposes it. This is most clearly manifested when a patient undergoes truncal vagotomy, and gastric atony or difficulty emptying gastric contents develops.

Microscopic Anatomy

The mucosa of the fundus region of the stomach consists primarily of columnar epithelium and mucus-producing cells. In the corpus of the stomach, oxyntic glands occur in large numbers. The surface of gastric mucosa is covered with mucus-producing columnar epithelial cells. These produce mucus as well as bicarbonate, which create an "unstirred layer," which is thought to be protective of the underlying epithelium. Parietal cells are found in the mid-portion of the oxyntic gland, whereas chief cells are located in the deeper portion. A constant migration of these cells occurs to the surface, with subsequent sloughing and renewal with newly growing cells. The antral region of the stomach has G cells present in large numbers. The gastrin glands are unique in that they are hormonally responsive cells and play an important role in stimulating acid secretion. Removal of the antral portion of the stomach is often done to treat intractable peptic ulcer disease.

Physiology

Hydrochloric Acid Synthesis

Gastric juice comprises a variety of products that play a role in initial breakdown of foodstuffs. Included are hydrochloric acid, pepsin, mucus, bicarbonate, and intrinsic factor. Acid secretion is produced by parietal cells, which number more than 1 billion. Basal acid secretion is 4 to 5 mEq/hr, whereas maximal acid secretory rate may approach 22 to 24 mEq/hr.

When each hydrogen ion is secreted, CO_2 derived from arterial blood is converted to bicarbonate and enters the interstitial fluid. This conversion is catalyzed by the enzyme carbonic anhydrase. Bicarbonate entering the bloodstream is directly proportional in amount to acid secreted. It is responsible for the alkaline tide that often occurs during acid secretion. The parietal cell contains receptors for three chemical agents: histamine, gastrin, and acetylcholine. Histamine occupying its receptor activates adenylate cyclase, which converts adenosine triphosphate (ATP) to cyclic adenosine monophosphate (AMP); this, in turn, activates protein kinase, which functions as a catalyst for protein phosphorylation (Fig. 26-5). Gastrin and acetylcholine, conversely, function primarily via a calcium calmodulin system, which stimulates phosphorylase kinase to stimulate acid secretion. Although histamine, acetylcholine, and gastrin all function by separate receptors and mechanisms to stimulate acid secretion, each of them functions by the mechanism of a specialized hydrogen-potassium pump as the final common pathway for acid production. This proton pump concentrates hydrogen ion and, by using ATP for energy, hydrogen ion is transported into the lumen while a potassium ion is exchanged for transport to the cell. It should also be noted that membrane receptors for the inhibition of acid secretion include receptors for somatostatin and prostaglandin. Histamine is produced by mast cells that lie in proximity to the gastric glands; acetylcholine is produced by the vagus nerve; and gastrin is produced by the hormonal gastrin G cells.

It also is notable that intrinsic factor is produced by the parietal cell. Chief cells, conversely, produce pepsinogen, which functions in the initial breakdown of proteins. Pepsinogen is converted to pepsin when the pH of the stomach decreases to less than 4.

Although it is an oversimplification of the physiologic process of acid secretion, it is generally useful to divide acid secretion into three phases: the cephalic phase, the gastric phase, and the intestinal phase. The cephalic phase is primarily under vagal control, but the gastric and intestinal phases are under hormonal control.

The cephalic phase is mediated by the vagus nerve in response to the sight, smell, and taste of food. When food is smelled, chewed, and spit out without swallowing, an immediate increase in acid production occurs in the stomach. The cephalic phase is able to influence gastric secretion in several ways. First, a direct cholinergic stimulation of parietal cells occurs; second, gastrin is released from the antrum by vagal stimulation; and third, vagal innervation sensitizes parietal cells to all stimuli.

The gastric phase is initiated by food arriving in the stomach and causing mechanical distention or chemical stimulation of the appropriate receptors. Proteins act to stimulate acid production, but foods entering the stomach also cause a buffering and elevation of the luminal pH, which acts as a powerful stimulant of acid production. This phase of gastric secretion is mediated by gastrin primarily and, to a lesser extent, by cholinergic stimulation of parietal cells.

The intestinal phase is the least understood phase of acid secretion but is thought to be mediated by an unidentified hormone, sometimes referred to as entero-oxyntin. This phase is initiated by the release of protein-rich food substances arriving in the proximal jejunum. Other proposed mediators for this effect include peptide YY, neurotensin, gastric inhibitory peptide, somatostatin, and secretin.

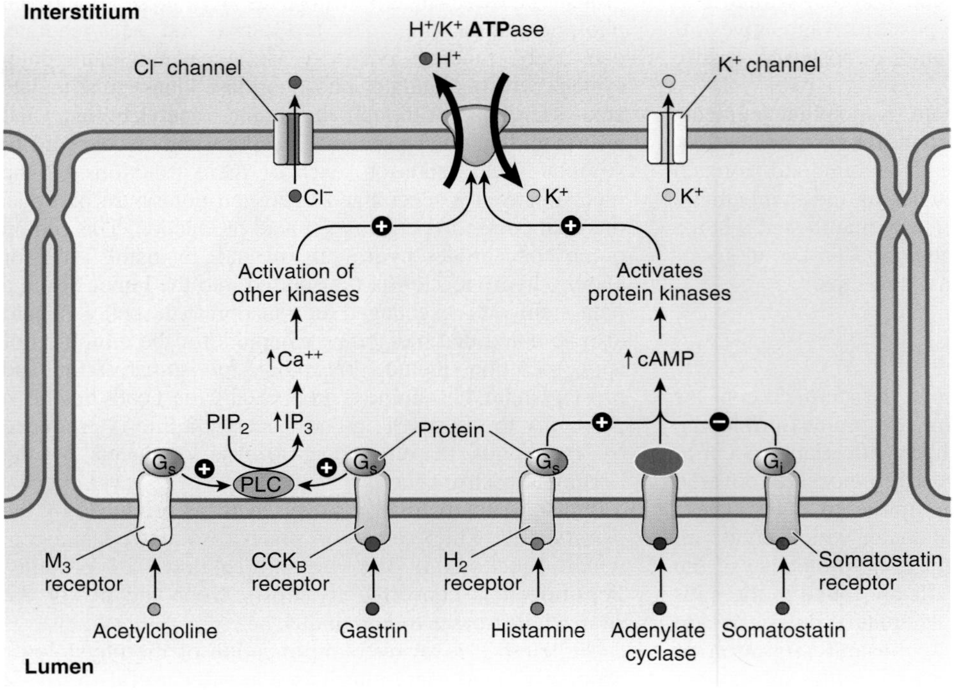

FIGURE 26–5 Histamine, acetylcholine, and gastrin all stimulate HCl secretion through separate receptor sites. However, the final common pathway for acid secretion is the hydrogen-potassium pump using adenosine triphosphatase.

Perhaps the most potent inhibitor of acid secretion is a pH of 2.5 or less. Thus vagal and local release of antral gastrin is blocked at pH of 2.5 or less, with the hydrogen ion causing its inhibition directly on the gastrin cell. In addition to acid, fat and hypertonic solutions in the duodenum may inhibit acid secretion. Hormonally, secretin is well known to inhibit gastric acid secretion, as does acidification of the duodenal bulb. Cholecystokinin released in the duodenum also may inhibit gastric secretion through gastrin inhibition and additional peptides vasoactive intestinal peptide (VIP), gastric inhibitory peptide (GIP), and somatostatin. Prostaglandin-E_2 also inhibits gastrin release and stimulates secretion of somatostatin, which is a known inhibitor.

A variety of mucosal defense systems are thought to be important in protecting the mucosa against hydrogen ion backdiffusion. Bicarbonate secretion by surface epithelial cells involves secretion of bicarbonate into a thin, unstirred layer of mucus coating the gastric mucosa. It is thought that a gradient is maintained because of the constant diffusion of bicarbonate, thus protecting the underlying mucosa. Because of the rich blood flow to gastric mucosa, injury rarely occurs. However, during times of shock or stress, sympathetic fibers may cause vasoconstriction of mucosal capillaries, which diminish flow to the mucosa and can be associated with stress erosions.

Prostaglandins are believed to increase gastric blood flow and simultaneously decrease acid secretion. For this reason, they are also thought to be protective. Inhibition of prostaglandin synthesis by nonsteroidal anti-inflammatory agents is also frequently associated with peptic ulcer disease. Counsel is often given to patients to avoid nonsteroidal anti-inflammatory agents during periods of ulcer healing.

Gastric Motility

Two motility types are found in the stomach: receptive relaxation and accommodation, which occur in the upper third of the stomach, and true peristalsis, which occurs in the lower two thirds of the stomach. Receptive relaxation is a unique motility form mediated by the vagus nerve; when food is consumed, the increasing volume stimulates inhibition of tonic contractions of the proximal stomach. Thus dilatation of the stomach begins with swallowing (receptive relaxation) and is completed with the presence of food in the stomach (accommodation). The second type of motility is associated with a myoelectric pacesetter, which is located high on the greater curve of the stomach. This pacesetter generates an electrical potential that occurs every 20 seconds and progresses distally. As the potential spreads from the pacesetter toward the pylorus, increased electrical activity results in peristaltic waves. As contractions of the antrum occur, the muscle strips foods down toward the pylorus, which simultaneously closes, thus resulting in most food being pushed back into the corpus.

A small amount may be metered out into the duodenum before closure of the pylorus. This results in a continuous mixing and churning, which breaks foods down, mixes them with acid and pepsin, and also combines them with mucus, a process termed *trituration*.

Obviously, the emptying of liquids occurs more quickly and efficiently than does that of solids. Patients who undergo a proximal gastric vagotomy obliterate the receptive relaxation motility form, resulting in accelerated liquid emptying associated with normal solid emptying. Truncal vagotomy, conversely, interrupts gastric emptying of solids because of the nerve of Latarjet being interrupted and causing problems with coordination of the antropyloric complex.

Duodenal Ulcer

Pathophysiology

Although peptic ulcer disease is less common than it was 25 years ago, duodenal and gastric ulcers continue to be a problem seen by gastroenterologists and surgeons. Surgery is required much less frequently than in the past, but an understanding of this disease is important for surgeons.

A simple way of thinking about the problem is that the inherent potential for injury to the lining of the stomach and duodenum is present simply because of the high concentrations of acid. To counteract that potential, a host of mucosal defensive factors is present. When those mucosal defensive factors are overcome, duodenal ulcers occur. Some of the causes of imbalance between the mucosa-threatening and the mucosa-protecting factors include an increase in acid production due to increased numbers of parietal cells, increased secretion per cell, increased basal acid secretion, or an increased acid response to meals.

A number of environmental factors also may play a role (such as nicotine, caffeine, alcohol, and salicylates). Recent evidence implicates the bacterium *Helicobacter pylori* as an etiologic factor. Some evidence exists that the inability of the duodenum to produce bicarbonate and mucus may play some role. What appears to be clear is that, in all of these cases, an injury occurs to the gastric mucosal barrier because of an imbalance in the gastric protective and aggressive factors. This results in hydrogen-ion back-diffusion into the mucosa, which results in injury to the tissues. This injury is initially superficial but, in time, erodes all the way to the muscularis propria (an "ulcer" extends to the muscularis propria, and an "erosion," into mucosa only).

Brief mention should be made of the large volume of work being done regarding the role that *H. pylori* plays in peptic ulcer disease. When Marshall initially suggested that bacteria could be causal in ulcer disease more than 15 years ago, great skepticism ensued. However, over time, it has become clear that this organism plays a very real role in duodenal ulcer disease, gastritis, and probably gastric ulcer disease, although that is less clear. Prospective, randomized studies now show that appropriate antibiotic therapy results in lower ulcer recurrence rates.

Differential Diagnosis

The pain of duodenal ulcers characteristically occurs in the upper abdomen, and any differential diagnosis must include other disease processes whose pain manifests in the epigastric region, primarily the organs perfused by the celiac axis and the embryologic foregut. Included in this are gastric ulcer, gastritis, biliary tract disease, pancreatic disease, and, much less commonly, certain types of liver disease. Also included in the differential diagnosis are neoplasms of the upper GI system, including gastric cancer, pancreatic cancer, and, less commonly, tumors of the biliary tree.

History and Physical Examination

The pain of duodenal ulcer is classically upper and midepigastric and is described as sharp, bright, and intense. Some patients describe the pain "as though a hot poker were being passed through the abdomen." Patients describe pain relief when eating a meal, drinking a glass of milk, or taking antacids. Pain often occurs late at night or early in the morning and is relieved only after eating breakfast. Duodenal ulcer tends to occur at a younger age than gastric ulcer, and men are more commonly affected than women are. The patient will often have a history of having taken commercially available antacids. No significant physical findings occur in a patient with duodenal ulcer disease, and even deep palpation does not reveal an increase in tenderness. Similarly, no specific laboratory values are helpful in the patient with duodenal ulcer disease. Occasionally, a picture of chronic anemia is seen, but that is such a nonspecific finding that it rarely leads immediately to the diagnosis of duodenal ulcer.

Imaging

The diagnosis of duodenal ulcer disease is usually made with barium contrast radiography or upper GI endoscopy. Clearly, endoscopy is the diagnostic procedure of choice because of its accuracy. However, the procedure is invasive, requires sedation, and does have a low, but real, morbidity. It also is more expensive than contrast radiography.

Barium upper GI studies are often used as a screening test for someone with dyspepsia. However, some studies show that up to 20% of duodenal ulcers may be missed by this diagnostic test. It also has associated radiation exposure, although it is small. When the ulcer is viewed, a defect projects beyond the level of the mucosa (Fig. 26-6). Similarly, obstruction is often associated with either scar formation or muscular spasm.

Endoscopy is able to diagnose between 90% and 95% of all lesions in the upper GI tract (Fig. 26-7). Most commonly,

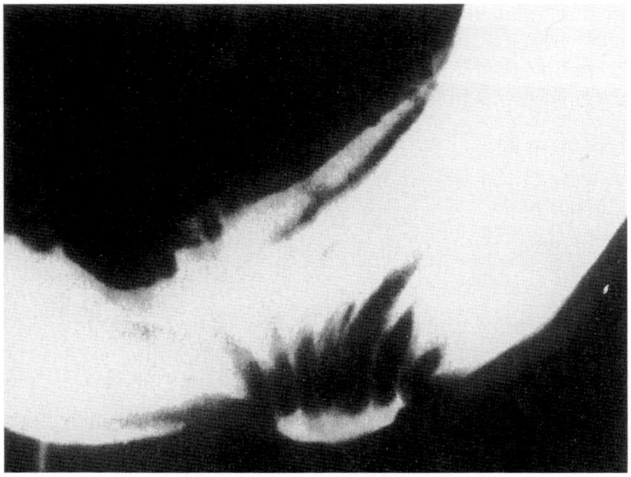

FIGURE 26–6 Barium upper gastrointestinal study showing a benign gastric ulcer. Note the smooth mucosal folds and projection of the ulcer crater outside the gastric lumen.

the duodenal ulcer is encountered in the bulb, which is that portion just beyond the pylorus. Ninety-five percent of all duodenal ulcers are found in that general area and demand that this area be carefully evaluated during the procedure.

Some controversy exists about which of these diagnostic modalities to use in a patient with symptoms of duodenal ulcer disease. However, most believe that if a patient has classic symptoms of peptic ulcer disease with food-relieved pain, endoscopy should be the first test. For the patient with vague, nonspecific dyspepsia, an upper GI barium study might be indicated as a screening test. The endoscopic appearance of a duodenal ulcer is characterized by a whitish, granular base with surrounding erythema and heaped-up mucosa. The ulcer often is sharply demarcated and looks as if it were punched out of the mucosa.

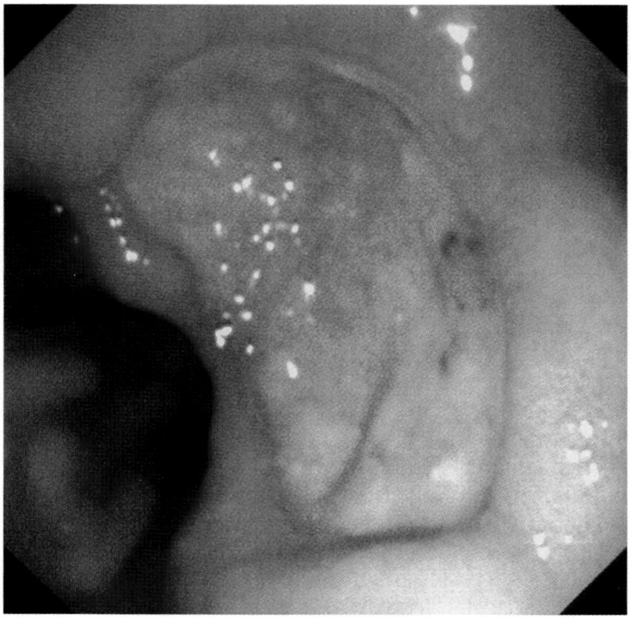

FIGURE 26–7 Endoscopic appearance of a large gastric ulcer. Note the radiating mucosal folds and whitish ulcer base.

Treatment Alternatives

Expectant

The natural history of duodenal ulcer is often contrasted with gastric ulcer to predict the course of a patient who has been recently diagnosed. Duodenal ulcers tend to be much more responsive to conservative pharmacologic treatment, especially when *H. pylori* is treated with antibiotics. Gastric ulcers, conversely, tend to be more refractory to conservative therapy and more often result in eventual surgical therapy.

Medical Treatment

A variety of pharmacologic agents have revolutionized the management of duodenal ulcers in the last 30 years. From the discovery of H_2 blockers in the early 1970s to the more recent development of proton-pump inhibitors, a wide array of pharmacologic agents is now available to the practicing surgeon and gastroenterologist.

Diet. Although dietary recommendations have been an important part of ulcer treatment in the past, more recent evidence suggests that diet plays little role in the healing of peptic ulcers. In the past, bland diets with milk and cream products were recommended. The only recommendations with regard to diet and other habits now include avoiding the use of alcohol products, caffeine, cigarette smoking, and nonsteroidal anti-inflammatory agents.

Antacids. Antacids were used extensively in the 1960s for the treatment of peptic ulcer disease. An obvious advantage of antacids is that, after administration, the patient senses almost immediate relief of ulcer pain. Antacids give more rapid pain relief than any other form of treatment. Based on acid levels during the course of a day, a regimen that was popular in the 1970s included administration of antacids 1 hour and 3 hours after meals and at bedtime. This regimen was shown to be very effective in healing ulcers but also was cumbersome, and compliance was very poor. Additionally, it was often associated with troublesome side effects of diarrhea. For this reason, antacids are largely used for symptomatic relief now and play a minor role in the actual treatment of peptic ulcer disease.

Sucralfate. Sucralfate is an interesting agent that has been added to the antiulcer armamentarium. It is aluminum sucrose sulfate and acts on a totally different principle than do antacids. This agent plays no buffering role and no neutralization role, but rather polymerizes in contact with acid and attaches to the ulcer itself, thus providing a barrier to further acid backdiffusion. The advantage of this medication is that very few side effects occur, other than constipation. It does not inhibit acid production, which results in normal flora in the gastric lumen and is relatively inexpensive. However, it is awkward to take, as it must be taken multiple times per day, does not offer immediate pain relief as antacids often do, and today plays a minor role in treatment of peptic ulcer disease.

Anticholinergic Medications. Anticholinergic medications can block the acetylcholine receptor on the parietal cell. However, in the past, agents such as atropine had so many side effects that patients refused to use them. More recent anticholinergics, which are selective and specifically block muscarinic receptors on the postganglionic nerves, have fewer side effects. However, because of the success of H_2 blockers and proton-pump inhibitors, anticholinergics such as pirenzepine are not commonly used today.

H_2 Blockers. The real revolution in the pharmacologic management of peptic ulcer disease began in the early 1970s with the development of cimetidine. This H_2 blocker was found to inhibit acid production by 60% to 65% with few side effects. It immediately became successful commercially and, at one time, was the most commonly prescribed medication in the world. Since then, a number of other H_2 blockers have been developed, including ranitidine, famotidine, and nizatidine (Table 26-1). These medications function by blocking the histamine receptor on the parietal cell and inhibit other forms of stimulated acid secretion. Initial H_2 blockers had q.i.d. drug dosage; but now, once-a-day or twice-a-day doses have become much more popular and are used routinely.

Proton-Pump Inhibitors. The most recent and most successful addition to antiulcer pharmacology is the family of proton-pump inhibitors (see Table 26-1). A hydrogen-potassium ATPase is responsible for the process whereby hydrogen ions are secreted into the lumen in exchange for potassium. The proton-pump inhibitors selectively block this hydrogen potassium pump and cause virtually complete cessation of acid production. As a result, ulcers heal rapidly, and symptomatic relief is sometimes dramatic. Most comparisons with H_2-receptor antagonists show that the proton-pump inhibitor is more effective in ulcer healing rates and pain relief. However, proton-pump inhibitors probably should not be used for long periods because of the hypergastrinemia that may result, as well as bacterial overgrowth in the stomach with no acid.

Prostaglandin Analogues. For several decades, scientists have known that some of the prostaglandins have direct effects on the gastric mucosa. Prostaglandins increase mucus and bicarbonate secretion and, at higher doses, actually inhibit acid production. As a result, researchers have developed misoprostol, which is now the only commercially available prostaglandin. This agent is now approved by the Food and Drug Administration for concomitant administration with nonsteroidal anti-inflammatory agents to protect against ulcer disease. The agent is infrequently used as first-line therapy for peptic ulcer disease because of the troublesome diarrhea associated with its administration.

TABLE 26–1 FDA-Approved H_2 Blockers and Proton-Pump Inhibitors

Drugs	Dose
H_2 Blockers	
Cimetidine	300 mg qid
Ranitidine	150 mg bid
Famotidine	20 mg qd
Nizatidine	300 mg qd
Proton-Pump Inhibitors	
Omeprazole	20 mg qd
Lansoprazole	15 mg qd
Rabeprazole	20 mg qd
Esomeprazole	20 mg qd
Pantoprazole	40 mg qd

Antimicrobial Therapy. Prospective randomized studies demonstrate that eradication of the organism *H. pylori* results in significant decreases in ulcer recurrence. The studies confirm that this agent is causal in duodenal ulcer disease and stress gastritis. The evidence of its implication in gastric ulcer disease is suggestive but less firm than the previously mentioned conditions. Studies show that a number of triple-agent regimens seem to be highly successful in eradicating the organism and thus diminishing ulcer recurrence. For example, a combination of bismuth, metronidazole, and amoxicillin will eliminate the organism in more than 90% of patients. Many regimens also include a proton-pump inhibitor or H_2 blockers, which seems to have increased the efficacy of therapy. Testing for *Helicobacter* should now be a routine part of conservative management of peptic ulcer disease. No patient should be referred for surgery without testing for this organism and, if it is present, being treated appropriately (Table 26-2).

Surgical Treatment

The majority of patients with duodenal ulcer disease will respond to pharmacologic treatment, and only a small

TABLE 26–2 Some FDA-Approved Regimens for *Helicobacter pylori* Treatment

Drug	Dose	Duration (days)
1. Ranitidine bismuth citrate	400 mg bid	14
(RBC) + clarithromycin	500 mg bid	14
then RBC	400 mg bid	14 additional days
2. Omeprazole	20 mg bid	10
+ clarithromycin	500 mg bid	10
+ amoxicillin	1 g bid	10
3. Omeprazole	40 mg qd	14
+ clarithromycin	500 mg bid	14
then omeprazole	20 mg qd	14 additional days
4. Lansoprazole	30 mg bid	10
+ amoxicillin	1 g bid	10
+ clarithromycin	500 mg tid	10

FDA, Food and Drug Administration.

percentage will require surgical therapy. It is estimated that 15% to 20% of people will have truly refractory disease and ultimately require surgical management. The classic indications for duodenal ulcer operation include intractability, perforation, hemorrhage, and obstruction. Because of the wealth of antiulcer medications now available, intractability is a much less common indication than in the past. However, obstruction, bleeding, and perforation appear to occur at about the same rates they did 25 years ago. Four operations are used in the treatment of duodenal ulcer disease.

Indications for Surgery

Intractability. In general, intractability refers to ulcer disease that will not respond to conservative management and requires surgical therapy. At one time, the definition of intractability was two failed 6-week courses of antacid or H_2-blocker therapy. However, the diagnosis is much more difficult to understand now, as patients will often be tried with H_2 blockers first, followed by sucralfate, followed by proton-pump inhibitors, and only after every medication available has been tried, is the patient deemed intractable. In general, however, any patient for whom two courses of optimal proton-pump inhibitor therapy and antibiotics have failed, and the symptoms recur, should be seriously considered for definitive operative therapy. In the absence of other ulcer-related complications, the operation of choice for treatment of intractability is proximal gastric vagotomy. Because of the low morbidity and low mortality associated with this operation, it should be the first-line choice for treatment of intractable ulcer disease. On occasion, vagotomy and antrectomy may be a better choice for the hard-driving, cigarette-smoking executive who is noncompliant. Disease in such a patient is likely to recur, and a gold standard operation should be used in that setting.

Hemorrhage. The incidence of bleeding associated with duodenal ulcer disease has not changed significantly in the past several decades. The patient with bleeding from a duodenal ulcer is first seen with hematemesis or melenic stools. Recognition of either of those signs of bleeding should result in prompt attention. Bleeding from an upper GI source demands that other causes be excluded including esophageal varices, gastritis, Mallory-Weiss tears, and carcinoma. Patients with peptic ulcer bleeding may have a history of ulcer disease, or they may have bleeding as their initial manifestation. Often a history of nonsteroidal anti-inflammatory medication is present.

Bleeding from an ulcer can vary from mild, chronic blood loss leading to anemia to truly life-threatening hemorrhage. In general, bleeding from duodenal ulcers will stop in the majority of patients (70% to 80%), so that operative intervention is usually not necessary.

Immediate attention should be given to diagnosing the source of bleeding. In this case, upper GI endoscopy is the diagnostic modality of choice. Initial management of the patient with an upper GI bleed depends on the degree of bleeding. If it is slow, chronic blood loss, the patient can be worked up electively. However, if the bleeding is rapid, characterized by hematemesis and melenic stools, the patient should be admitted to an intensive care unit (ICU) until the bleeding has stabilized. After admission to the unit, the patient should have placement of two large-bore IVs, an immediate check of the blood count, and blood should be typed and crossed to provide four units at all times for transfusion. Some benefit accrues from aspirating as much of the blood from the stomach as possible via irrigation of warm saline. Bleeding will usually cease with gut rest, IV hydration, and irrigation of the stomach. However, attention should be directed to a diagnostic procedure at this point. Upper GI endoscopy remains the procedure of choice in the patient with bleeding ulcers. During the course of endoscopy, the presence of blood in the stomach and an ulcer are strongly suggestive that the latter is the source of the bleeding, particularly with active oozing, clot on the ulcer, or a visible vessel. When an artery is visualized to be bleeding or oozing, endoscopic therapy may be instituted to attain hemostasis. This can be done through a variety of modalities including a heater probe, electrocautery, and epinephrine injections. If the endoscopist is unsuccessful in achieving hemostasis, the patient will probably require operative therapy.

General guidelines suggesting that operative therapy will likely be necessary include blood loss of more than 6 units, a visible vessel seen on endoscopy, rebleeding after initial hemostasis especially associated with hypotension, and continued bleeding (over a period of 3 to 4 days) that is slow but fails to cease.

The operation of choice for a bleeding duodenal ulcer depends on the scenario. In the patient with a rapid bleed who may be hypotensive, a pyloroplasty extended onto the bulb with oversewing of the ulcer and truncal vagotomy is appropriate. If the patient is more stable and has a history of peptic ulcer disease, vagotomy and antrectomy is a possibility after oversewing the ulcer. Occasionally, for more chronic blood loss, a highly selective vagotomy may be used. However, the operation most commonly used in this setting is vagotomy and pyloroplasty.

Perforation. Perforation of a duodenal ulcer constitutes a surgical emergency. The patient has the onset of abrupt, severe abdominal pain that is often described as boardlike rigidity of the abdomen. The hydrochloric acid and bacteria in contact with peritoneal surfaces cause an intense inflammatory reaction, which accounts for the pain. Shoulder pain is occasionally associated with the pain of perforation (Kehr's sign), and the abdomen will often be distended. Abdominal radiographs show free air under the diaphragm in 65% to 75% of patients and indicate the need for immediate laparotomy. Perforation most commonly occurs in the anterior portion of the duodenum, and more than 50% of patients have a history of some symptoms probably related to their peptic ulcer disease. Those patients who have a history of peptic ulcer disease should undergo a definitive antiulcer operation if no hypotension and no significant medical risk factors exist and if perforation is less than 6 to 8 hours old. In the absence of those criteria, the most commonly performed operation is to débride the ulcer at the perforation site, oversew it, and patch with omentum (Graham patch). Copious irrigation of the peritoneal cavity is indicated before closure. If required, a definitive antiulcer operation can be done at another time when the patient is stable and less contamination is present.

Obstruction. Obstruction occurs when an ulcer is strategically located in either the pylorus or prepyloric area, and substantial inflammation is found in the acute ulcer or scar formation in the chronic ulcer. Patients first seen with gastric outlet obstruction often have a metabolic alkalosis due to vomiting and loss of hydrochloric acid. Initial treatment of these patients with normal saline, nasogastric suction, and proton-pump inhibitors is usually indicated. If the obstruction is an acute one, very often the edema will resolve, and the patient will open up again. Some evidence supports upper GI endoscopy with hydrostatic dilatation of the narrowed pyloric channel. Approximately 40% to 50% of patients will open up and have a good result after dilatation. If the lesion is largely scar tissue, such dilatation is usually not successful. The surgical treatment of gastric outlet obstruction most commonly involves truncal vagotomy and antrectomy. Frequently, the patient has a large, floppy stomach, which takes a long time to begin contracting in a normal fashion. The clinician should anticipate the possibility of a prolonged course until the patient has resolution of this chronic ileus.

Surgical Procedures

Truncal Vagotomy and Gastroenterostomy. This operative procedure was used much more commonly in the past than it is today. In this operation, the vagus nerve is transected anteriorly and posteriorly as it passes through the diaphragm. An anastomosis between the jejunum and the greater curve of the stomach is then made, thus bypassing the ulcer disease in the duodenum. Virtually the only indication for this operation is a very high-risk patient with severe obstructive disease in the duodenum that would require a lengthy and bloody operation. The operation is seldom performed in the United States today.

Truncal Vagotomy and Pyloroplasty. In this operation, a truncal vagotomy is done, as described previously. Because the vagotomy interrupts not only secretory nerves but also motor nerves that innervate the antral pyloric pump, gastric stasis will develop if vagotomy is the only part of the procedure performed. As a result, a "drainage procedure" must be done. In this case, the drainage procedure most commonly used is a Heineke-Mikulicz pyloroplasty (Fig. 26-8). It should be noted, however, that for unique situations, two other types of drainage proce-

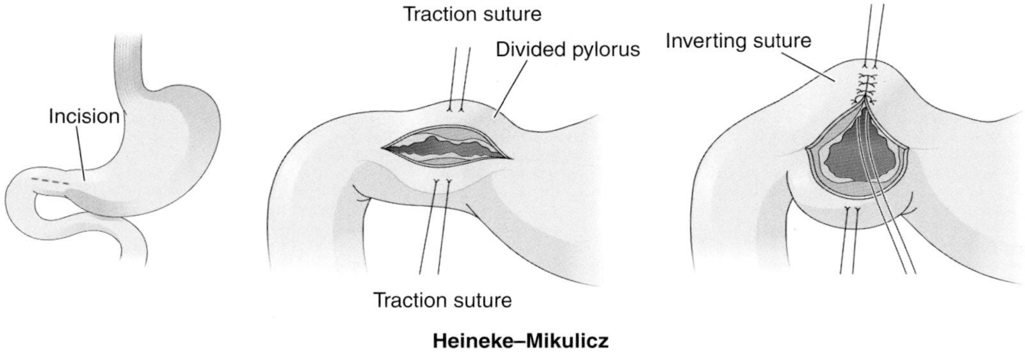

FIGURE 26–8 Heineke-Mikulicz pyloroplasty.

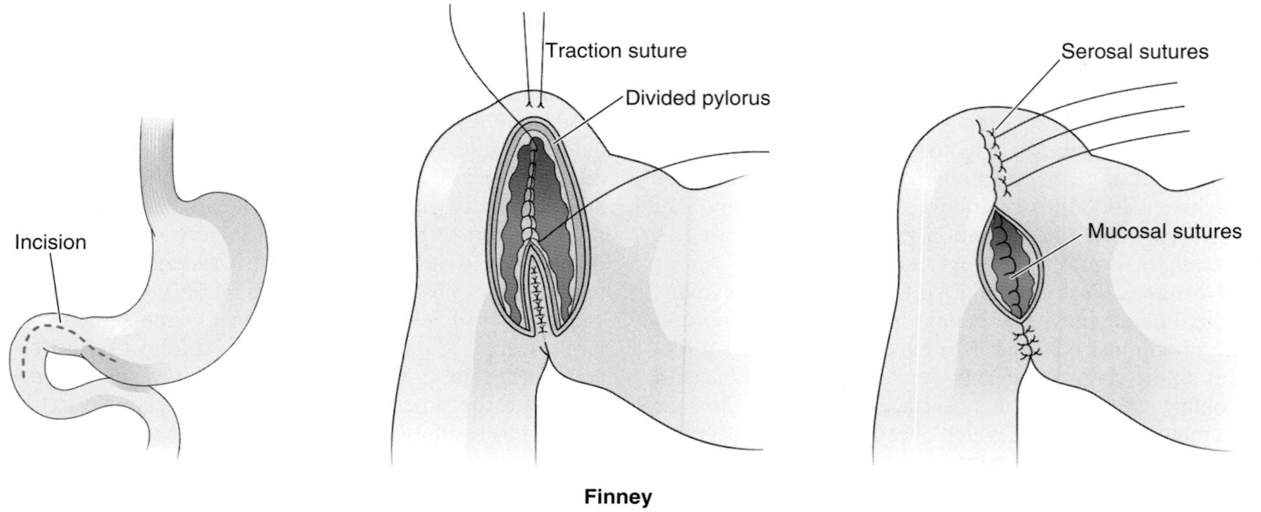

FIGURE 26–9 Finney pyloroplasty.

dures may be performed, including a Finney pyloroplasty (Fig. 26-9) and a Jaboulet gastroduodenostomy (Fig. 26-10). This operative procedure is rarely the procedure of choice for a patient with peptic ulcer disease. The operation has an ulcer recurrence rate of approximately 10% and is associated with a number of postpyloroplasty complications including dumping, diarrhea, and bloating (Table 26-3). This operation's greatest advantage is that it is technically easy and quick to perform. It is the ideal operation for the septic or unstable patient in the middle of the night for whom a quick procedure must be done. It also is often performed for high-risk patients for whom a quick, low-morbidity operation must be done.

Vagotomy and Antrectomy. Vagotomy and antrectomy is the gold standard operation with reference to ulcer recurrence. In this operation, truncal vagotomy is performed, as previously described. The lower third of the stomach is then removed, including all of the antrum, thus completely removing the gastrin G cells. Because this operation eliminates acetylcholine and gastrin input to acid

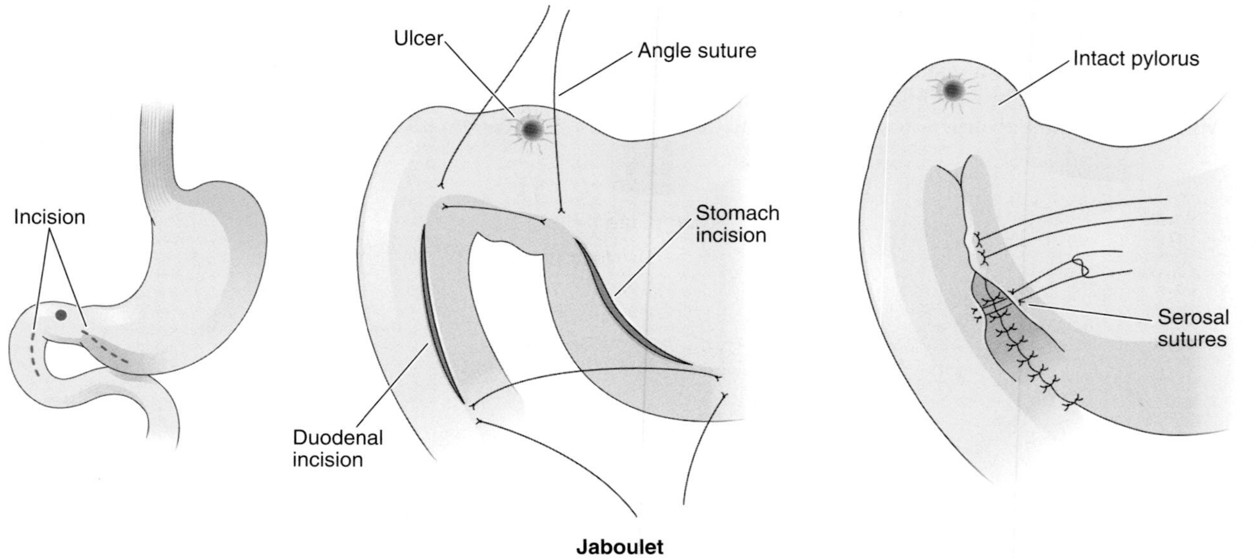

FIGURE 26–10 Jaboulet gastroduodenostomy.

TABLE 26–3 Three Most Common Operations for Treatment of Peptic Ulcer Disease

Operation	Technique	Advantages	Disadvantages	Uses
Vagotomy and antrectomy	Truncal vagotomy Remove antrum Billroth I or II hook-up	Gold standard for acid reduction Low ulcer recurrence (1%–2%)	High morbidity (dumping, diarrhea, alkaline reflux, afferent loop, etc.)	Refractory ulcer disease Distal peptic obstruction
Vagotomy and pyloroplasty	Truncal vagotomy Drainage procedure to prevent gastric stasis	Quick procedure in high-risk patient Technically easy	Moderately high morbidity High ulcer recurrence (10%–15%)	High-risk patients Contaminated field
Highly selective vagotomy	Cut nerves to acid-producing area of stomach Preserve motor nerve to pylorus (nerve of Latarjet)	Virtually no morbidity	High ulcer recurrence (15%–20%) Tedious, long operation	Intractable ulcer disease

production, it results in a 90% decrease in acid production. For this reason, ulcer recurrence rates range from 1% to 2% (see Table 26-3). After antrectomy, reconstruction can be done by using two common anastomoses: a Billroth I gastroduodenostomy (Fig. 26-11) and Billroth II gastrojejunostomy (Fig. 26-12). Rarely, a Roux-en-Y gastrojejunostomy is used as the reconstruction after a vagotomy and antrectomy (Fig. 26-13). However, the latter construction is often used as treatment for complications of vagotomy and antrectomy. Although vagotomy and antrectomy has a very low recurrent ulcer rate, it may be associated with a wide variety of postgastrectomy complications, which are discussed later in this chapter.

Proximal Gastric Vagotomy. This operation, which is also known as a highly selective vagotomy or parietal cell vagotomy, is performed by resecting only those nerves innervating the acid-secreting portion of the stomach in the fundus and corpus. The branch to the liver is left intact, as are the branches supplying the antropyloric pump (Fig. 26-14). The branches going to the antropyloric area are referred to as the nerve of Latarjet. This operation has the lowest morbidity of any acid-reducing operation, and the mortality is less than 0.5%. The only disadvantages of

PEARLS FOR ROUNDS

Two motility types occur in the stomach: receptive relaxation and accommodation in the fundus of the stomach, and true peristalsis in the antrum and pylorus.

Chronic infection with *Helicobacter pylori* is a risk factor for gastric carcinoma.

Indications for surgery for a duodenal ulcer include intractability, hemorrhage, perforation, and obstruction.

The early dumping syndrome refers to a complex of symptoms including tachycardia, diaphoresis, dizziness, lightheadedness, and weakness, which typically occur within 30 minutes of eating.

The key to management of stress erosion is prevention.

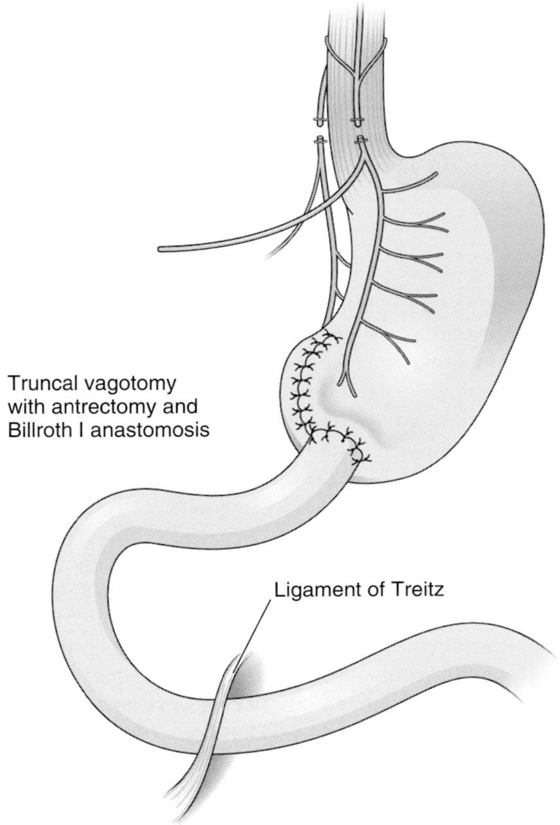

FIGURE 26–11 Reconstruction after antrectomy with a Billroth I gastroduodenostomy.

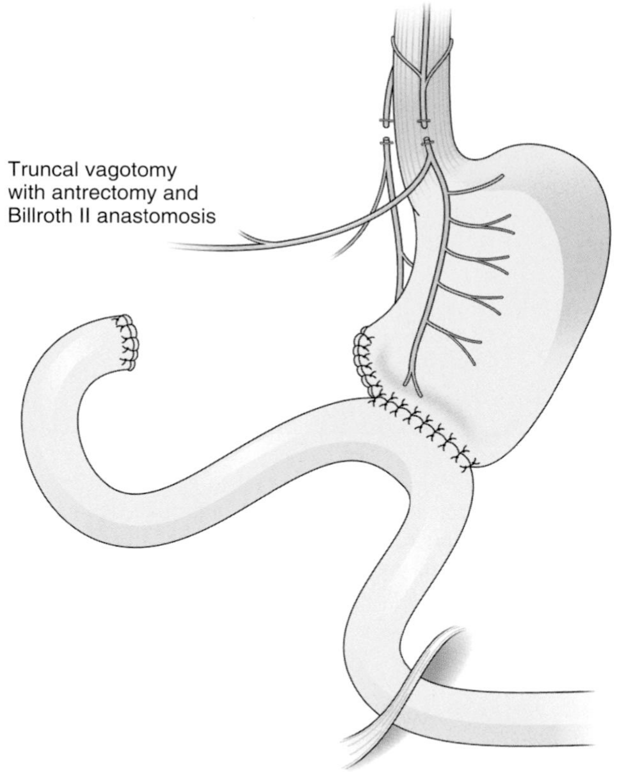

FIGURE 26–12 When gastric length is decreased after partial gastrectomy, Billroth II gastrojejunostomy is used.

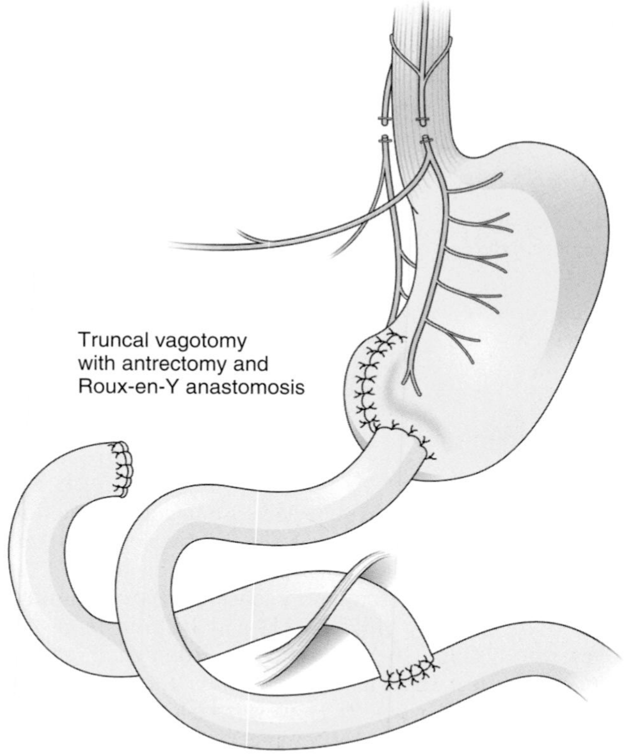

FIGURE 26–13 A Roux-en-Y gastrojejunostomy is occasionally used for reconstruction after partial gastrectomy.

this operation are a relatively high ulcer-recurrence rate, which approximates 15%, and the fact that it is technically tedious and somewhat more demanding. However, it does not have any of the postgastrectomy complications previously alluded to as side effects. It has become a common operation to treat intractable ulcers, as it has such low morbidity and, if ulcers do recur, they are successfully and rapidly treated with H_2 blockers or proton-pump inhibitors.

Newer Approaches. With the development of minimally invasive techniques via the laparoscope, some work has been done in performing a laparoscopic proximal gastric vagotomy. Other laparoscopic techniques include a truncal vagotomy of one of the two vagus nerves with a seromyotomy to eliminate any nervous connections on the anterior surface of the stomach. These procedures are limited primarily to highly skilled laparoscopic surgeons and are still finding their way into the mainstream of the antiulcer armamentarium. Nevertheless, it is reasonable to assume that over time, many more developments will be seen in this area.

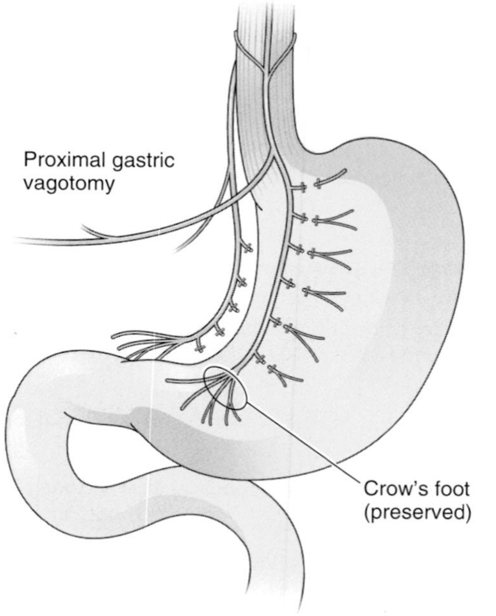

FIGURE 26–14 Highly selective or parietal cell vagotomy. Note preservation of the motor branches supplying the antropyloric region.

PEARLS FOR THE OR

No evidence indicates that a total gastrectomy confers any additional survival benefit over partial gastrectomy in gastric cancer.

Most surgeons agree that a 4- to 6-cm margin is necessary in gastric cancer because of submucosal spread of the tumor.

Vagotomy and antrectomy is the operation for duodenal ulcers with the lowest recurrence.

Truncal vagotomy and pyloroplasty is the ideal operation for the septic, unstable, or high-risk patient in whom a quick, low-morbidity procedure must be done for complications of peptic ulcer disease.

Newer approaches to duodenal ulcer include laparoscopic proximal gastric vagotomy and truncal vagotomy of the posterior vagus nerve with an anterior seromyotomy.

Gastric Ulcer

Pathophysiology

Gastric ulcers occur in an older age group than do duodenal ulcers. Patients tend to be in their late 50s or 60s, and gastric ulcers are uncommon before age 40 years. The pathophysiology of gastric ulcers tends to be somewhat different from that of duodenal ulcers. Duodenal ulcers tend to be characterized by excessive acid production overcoming the gastric mucosal defensive factors. A gastric ulcer usually occurs in the milieu of atrophic gastritis, hypochlorhydria, and what appears to be a defective barrier. Risk factors may include the presence of nonsteroidal anti-inflammatory medications for arthritis, steroid therapy, smoking, and prolonged alcohol use.

Other associated factors may include alterations in gastric motility. An amotile stomach with gastric stasis and food retention may result in increased gastrin release, which leads to increased acid secretion. Some evidence exists that *H. pylori* may play a role in gastric ulcers, but the evidence is not so clear cut as it is for duodenal ulcers and chronic gastritis. In general, gastric ulcers are less common than are duodenal ulcers.

Unlike duodenal ulcers that occur in the duodenal bulb 95% of the time, gastric ulcers can occur anywhere in the stomach. The most common location is on the lesser curve near the incisura. For many years, all gastric ulcers were treated similarly and thought to behave in a similar fashion. However, evidence now supports varied behavior, depending on the location of the ulcer. For example, the classic gastric ulcer on the lesser curve of the stomach in the body is usually a low-acid ulcer. However, those located in the prepyloric and pyloric regions are associated with high acid and behave more like a duodenal ulcer than a classic gastric ulcer. Gastric ulcers that are associated with concomitant duodenal ulcers also behave more like duodenal ulcers, whereas those high on the lesser curve near the cardia are frequently low-acid ulcers. The ulcers are classified according to location (Fig. 26-15).

Differential Diagnosis

Gastric ulcer is associated with epigastric pain and must be distinguished from duodenal ulcers, biliary tract disease, acute and chronic pancreatitis, and occasionally lesions in the liver. Distinguishing gastric ulcers from duodenal ulcers by symptoms is not easy, as a crossover in the symptoms often occurs.

Workup and Evaluation

History and Physical Examination

Symptoms of a gastric ulcer are often similar to those of duodenal ulcer, with a constant, unrelenting pain in the epigastrium, which may be described as burning or dull. The pain may be localized somewhat to the left of the midline and, in contrast to that of a duodenal ulcer, is

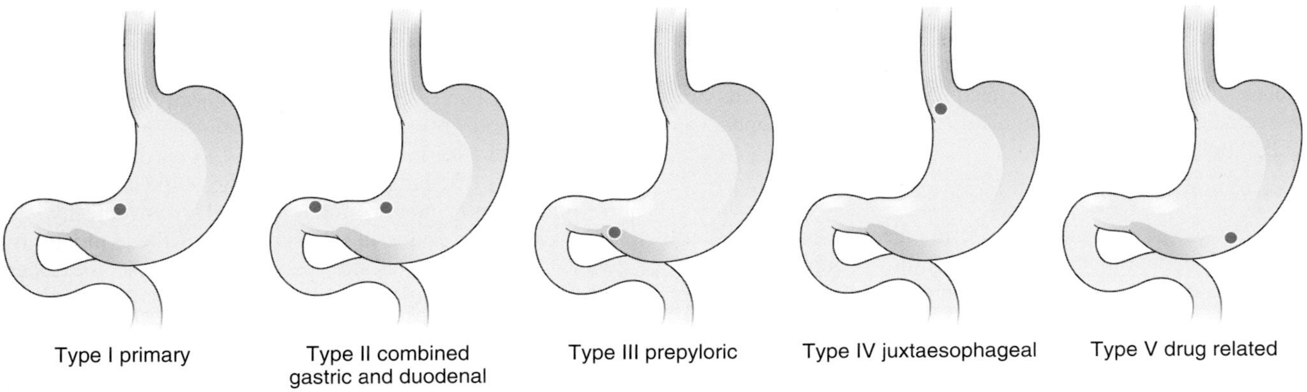

FIGURE 26–15 Characteristic location of gastric ulcers.

occasionally exacerbated by foods or liquid. This is particularly true when the liquids are hot or contain alcohol. Patients with gastric ulcer occasionally have early satiety, anorexia, and weight loss. Occasionally, the pain of gastric ulcer is relieved by eating or taking antacids.

Physical examination may show tenderness to deep palpation, but the physical examination is often normal. Occasionally, chronic anemia is detected, but, very often, laboratory studies are completely normal.

Imaging

The most common modality for diagnosing gastric ulcer is upper GI endoscopy. Endoscopy approaches 100% accuracy in diagnosing gastric ulcers. In addition, endoscopy is absolutely indicated if a gastric ulcer is diagnosed, because 5% to 10% of gastric ulcers have an associated malignancy. Thus the mere presence of a gastric ulcer is indication for endoscopy. During endoscopy, the patient is likely to have a 1-cm or larger defect on the lesser curve, with a white, fibrinous base and heaped-up edges with erythema. Biopsies should be taken of the periphery of the ulcer. The presence of an ulcer less than 1 cm in size carries a very small malignancy risk.

Barium contrast radiography of the upper GI system will diagnose more than 90% of gastric ulcers. The test is easy to perform, noninvasive, and associated with little discomfort, but if it indicates an ulcer in the stomach, the patient will require endoscopy anyway. For this reason, endoscopy is clearly the preferred diagnostic modality for gastric ulcers.

Treatment Alternatives

Expectant

Gastric ulcers tend to be larger than duodenal ulcers, and they are less likely to heal with conservative management. Ulcers do appear to have cycles of healing and recurrence. Because of the recurrent nature of gastric ulcers, they more frequently require operative therapy. Gastric ulcers may be associated with any number of complications including perforation, obstruction, malignant degeneration, and bleeding. Prepyloric ulcers and ulcers associated with duodenal ulcers bleed quite frequently. Massive bleeds are associated particularly with ulcers near the gastroesophageal (GE) junction.

Medical Treatment

Pharmacologic treatment of gastric ulcers is very similar to that of duodenal ulcers, except that they require more time to heal. Antacids may be used in the treatment of gastric ulcers but are associated with diarrhea and other side effects, and, because they require five to seven administrations per day, compliance tends to be very poor. For patients who are allergic to proton-pump inhibitors or H_2 blockers, sucralfate is sometimes successfully used in the treatment of gastric ulcers. Studies show that sucralfate is as effective as H_2 blockers in healing ulcers. Anticholinergics and prostaglandins also may be used in treatment of these ulcers; but, because of side effects and compliance problems, they are used much less frequently than H_2 blockers and proton-pump inhibitors. As pointed out earlier, when a patient is taking nonsteroidal anti-inflammatory medications for arthritis, misoprostol is often given concomitantly and has been shown to diminish the incidence of ulcers associated with those medications.

H_2-receptor blockers and proton-pump inhibitors are most commonly used in the treatment of gastric ulcers, and studies show that 80% of ulcers will heal within 6 to 8 weeks with H_2 blockers or proton-pump inhibitors. Unfortunately, a high recurrence rate is observed, and gastric ulcer patients require maintenance therapy for extended periods. Dietary prohibition plays little role in the treatment of gastric ulcers. Patients are instructed to avoid alcoholic drinks, caffeine-containing liquids and foods, and also are instructed to cease cigarette smoking during periods of attempted ulcer healing.

Patients who are found to be positive for *H. pylori* should also undergo a 2-week course of triple therapy before surgery should be considered. If the patient has *H. pylori* and undergoes a course of treatment, the ulcer recurrence rate after discontinuing therapy is only 20%.

Obviously, any patient taking nonsteroidal anti-inflammatory medication should cease it during treatment of gastric ulcers.

Surgical Treatment

Surgical treatment of gastric ulcers is dictated by the location of the ulcer. Gastric ulcers on the lesser curve in the corpus are usually associated with low acid production, and vagotomy is not required in the treatment. The operation of choice for gastric ulcer is a subtotal gastrectomy with elimination of the ulcer. Reconstruction is usually done by using a Billroth II reconnection (see Fig. 26-12). However, ulcers that occur in the prepyloric area and are associated with duodenal ulcers are high-acid ulcers, and treatment should include a vagotomy. The operation most commonly performed is vagotomy and antrectomy. Operations for gastric ulcers that occur on the lesser curve near the cardia are much more difficult. Because of the location, exposure tends to be poor, and performing a total gastrectomy is excessively aggressive in the treatment of these ulcers. In general, an attempt should be made to excise the ulcer and, if evidence of ulcers is noted in the distal stomach or duodenum, a vagotomy should be performed. If it is the impression of the operating surgeon that the ulcer is associated with achlorhydria, resection of the ulcer with primary closure is usually adequate therapy. Recurrence

BOX 26–1 Postgastrectomy Complications

- Alkaline reflex gastritis
- Postvagotomy diarrhea
- Dumping syndrome
- Afferent-loop syndrome
- Blind-loop syndrome
- Anemia
- Weight loss
- Gastric stump carcinoma
- Bezoar formation

rates after any of the operative procedures described tend to be less than 5%.

Postgastrectomy Complications. After vagotomy and antrectomy, most patients pass through a period of physiologic adjustment to the new anatomy. A host of symptoms including diarrhea, bloating, dumping, tachycardia, diaphoresis, and malaise have been described by patients (Box 26-1). In most patients, those symptoms disappear within 3 to 6 months of the gastrectomy if the patient is encouraged to eat small, frequent meals and to stay away from glucose-rich foods. However, 5% to 6% of the patients have persistent postgastrectomy complications. A brief discussion of those complications is appropriate.

Dumping. The dumping syndrome refers to a complex of symptoms including tachycardia, diaphoresis, dizziness, light-headedness, and weakness after eating. These symptoms occur within 30 minutes after the patient eats. The symptoms seem to be a combination of GI and cardiovascular symptoms. Symptoms are thought to be worse when liquids or sugar-rich foods are consumed during the meal. Symptoms may become severe enough to prevent the patient from eating. Dumping is poorly understood but is thought to be caused by osmotic changes that occur in the duodenum when a highly osmolar load pulls fluid from the vascular system into the duodenum, associated with the release of vasoactive substances.

The second type of dumping has been described as occurring a few hours after eating and is thought to result from inappropriate insulin release after eating a meal with high sugar concentrations. As mentioned earlier, most patients with the dumping syndrome will have resolution over the period of 3 to 6 months after the operation. However, for those patients who have severe, unrelenting dumping syndrome, surgical relief includes conversion of the Billroth I or II to a Roux-en-Y gastrojejunostomy. It should be emphasized that the vast majority of patients with dumping will not require an operation and can resolve their symptoms by eating six small meals, staying away from high-sugar foods, and drinking small amounts of liquids with their meals.

Postvagotomy Diarrhea. A small fraction of patients will have an intractable diarrhea that does not improve in the months after surgery. The cause of the diarrhea remains unknown. The patient with this syndrome will have multiple, watery bowel movements daily. They often are explosive and come without warning and with poor ability of the patient to control them. Dietary modification can manage diarrhea in most of these patients. The use of loperamide and fiber-bulking agents will often substantially improve this condition. In addition, cholestyramine has been successful in treating a number of these patients. If medical therapy fails, however, and the patient remains severely symptomatic, the operation of choice is to construct an antiperistaltic, 10-cm segment of jejunum and to reverse the segment 100 cm distal to the ligament of Treitz.

Afferent-loop Syndrome. Afferent-loop syndrome occurs exclusively in patients after a Billroth II anastomosis and is the result of mechanical obstruction of the afferent limb near its attachment to the stomach. The complication is characterized by explosive vomiting of clear, bilious fluid after a large meal. It is thought that after eating, the afferent limb fills with bile and pancreatic juice and that, only as pressure builds to push open the occluded area, does the explosive vomiting occur. Closely related to afferent-loop syndrome is blind-loop syndrome, which is characterized by a massive overgrowth of bacteria in the afferent limb, resulting in malabsorption and anemia. The latter complication can often be treated successfully with antibiotics. The diagnosis of the afferent-loop syndrome can be made by barium study in which little barium enters the afferent limb. It also may be seen on a hepatobiliary iminodiacetic acid (HIDA) scan, and occasionally with ultrasound demonstration of the large, distended afferent limb. Most patients with this complication will require an operation that usually results in reanastomosis of the jejunal limb, such that no twisting or kinking occurs. Occasionally, a Billroth II can be converted to a Billroth I anastomosis, but, in general, the approach is simply to redo the Billroth II anastomosis with precautions to make sure the afferent limb undergoes fixation at different locations to prevent twisting or kinking.

Alkaline Gastritis. Alkaline gastritis occurs more commonly with the Billroth II anastomosis. Bile and pancreatic juice from the afferent limb enter the stomach and are activated by foods. They then cause hyperemia and erosions of the stomach that can affect the lower stomach or the entire stomach, even extending into the esophagus. Patients complain of bilious vomiting, weight loss, and epigastric pain, which is made worse by eating. Although some question the existence of this disease because some asymptomatic patients have hyperemia and erosions after this connection, most believe that the entity exists. Medical therapy uniformly is unsuccessful in treating this condition.

Attempts at antacid administration, acid-blocking medications, and sucralfate have been unsuccessful. Surgical management of this lesion consists of conversion of a Billroth II to a Roux-en-Y gastrojejunostomy. It is critical that the jejunojejunostomy be performed 40 to 60 cm distal to the anastomosis so that duodenal contents cannot travel up the Roux-en-Y limb.

Weight Loss. Weight loss after gastric resection is a function of the size of the gastric resection, the type of vagotomy, and whether the pylorus is preserved. Most patients will lose a moderate amount of weight after major gastric resection and will plateau at a new weight. It was this observation that led to gastric stapling for morbid obesity. In most cases, once the patient reaches the new plateau, no additional concerns exist about malnutrition. Occasionally, significant weight loss occurs and may require tube feeding or, in rare cases, total parenteral nutrition (TPN). However, most adjust over time to the new anatomy.

Anemia. An iron-deficiency anemia not infrequently occurs after a major gastric resection. This is thought to be related to the decrease in acid, which makes absorption of dietary iron more difficult in the ferric state. Rarely, a B_{12} or folate deficiency is found. More commonly, it is an iron-deficiency anemia, and patients should be supplemented with ferrous iron.

Stress Gastritis

Stress gastritis, as the name implies, occurs in patients undergoing tremendous injury, trauma, or stress to the body. Because of our knowledge of high-risk clinical scenarios that predispose to stress erosions, they occur less frequently now than they did in the past, because prophylaxis is instituted immediately in high-risk patients. Nevertheless, an understanding of this condition is critical to surgeons who take care of septic, traumatized patients who are at risk.

Pathophysiology

Stress erosions are small punctate defects in the mucosa associated with a number of conditions including trauma, sepsis, burns, neurologic injury, hepatic dysfunction, massive transfusion requirements, and extended ICU stays. Unlike ulcers, erosions extend into the mucosa but not into the muscularis propria. They tend to be much smaller than ulcers, they are rarely painful, and they bleed more commonly. The pathogenesis of these small mucosal defects is not well understood, but current theories suggest that mucosal ischemia and vasoconstriction associated with trauma cause the mucosal barrier to be compromised, which in turn results in hydrogen ion backdiffusion, which results in tissue injury and compromise of the metabolic functions of the mucosa. Indeed, the permeability of gastric mucosa is increased and the ability of the tissues to buffer acid is compromised, leading to further injury. Some stress ulcers are associated with neurologic trauma (Cushing's ulcers), whereas others are associated with major burns (Curling's ulcers). Mucosal erosions similar to stress erosions also are seen in patients who drink large amounts of alcohol or take salicylates.

Differential Diagnosis

Patients with stress erosions usually are initially seen with upper GI bleeding. The differential includes duodenal and gastric ulcers, diffuse gastritis, bleeding varices, Mallory-Weiss tears, and bleeding from tumors.

Workup and Evaluation

Most patients with stress erosions have low-grade bleeding before major bleeding. The bleeding usually occurs 4 to 5 days after the traumatic injury, and, in most cases, bleeding stops spontaneously. However, occasionally the bleeding can become massive and may be associated with hypotension and projectile hematemesis. The physical examination usually reveals the significantly traumatized patient who is quite often desperately ill from the injury. Otherwise, the physical examination is not particularly helpful. Laboratory tests also are usually not helpful, except occasionally a low hematocrit will be detected. The most important diagnostic modality is upper GI endoscopy. Indeed, barium studies not only cannot make the diagnosis but often confuse angiography, if needed. On endoscopy, the patient is seen to have multiple, shallow mucosal defects of 2 to 3 mm with oozing (Fig. 26-16).

Treatment Alternatives

Expectant management of stress erosions is usually uniformly unsuccessful. Because of probable mucosal ischemia and injury to the barrier in the presence of acid, injury will recur and lead to bleeding unless something is done. Fortunately, with medical management, surgery can virtually always be avoided. Resuscitation of the patient should begin immediately. IV hydration with blood replacement (if hypovolemia is associated with the bleeding) is imperative. Hemostasis should be optimized by correcting all clotting abnormalities. If stress or unresolved infection is the source of the erosions, management of those primary problems is imperative before the erosions can be successfully treated. Lavage of the stomach with warm normal saline also may be implemented if bleeding has already occurred.

The key to management of this problem, however, is prevention. Our understanding of stress erosions now mandates that when a patient at high risk for stress erosions is identified, attempts must be made to increase the pH of the intraluminal gastric contents. Studies have demonstrated that if the pH of the luminal contents can be kept above 4, which is the pKA at which pepsinogen is activated, stress erosions virtually never occur. This can be accomplished with

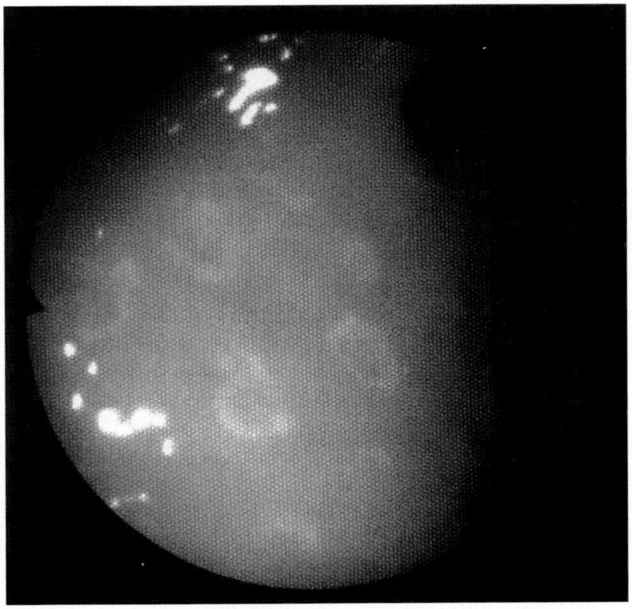

FIGURE 26–16 Stress erosions seen on endoscopy. Note the flat, superficial, multiple lesions with white bases.

proton-pump inhibitors, H_2 blockers, antacids, or a combination of these. If prophylaxis was not accomplished and bleeding is ongoing, occasionally the administration of pitressin can help stop bleeding. However, careful management of high-risk patients should rarely result in the need for pitressin. In 5% to 10% of patients with bleeding from stress erosions, the erosions will continue to bleed despite optimal attempts to control the pH. In the presence of ongoing bleeding that fails to cease, a patient must be taken to the operating room. In most cases, a generous gastrotomy is done, associated with evacuation of large amounts of clot from the gastric lumen. A careful search is then made for oozing from specific erosion sites. Usually, oversewing specific bleeding sites with suture will result in cessation of bleeding. This may require oversewing multiple lesions. If any question exists about acid production, vagotomy and pyloroplasty may accompany the oversewing of individual bleeders. Occasional vagotomy with partial gastrectomy may be required, and rarely, even total gastrectomy may be the life-saving operation in the presence of diffuse, massive bleeding that cannot be controlled by oversewing.

Neoplasms of the Stomach

Adenocarcinoma

One of the interesting epidemiologic phenomena of the last 30 years has been the decrease in the incidence of gastric cancer in the United States. Approximately 21,500 new cases of gastric cancer are diagnosed each year, with 13,000 deaths resulting each year from this disease. The reasons for the decrease in gastric cancer rates are probably related to lifestyle and dietary changes, but the exact cause has not been identified. The incidence and death rate for adenocarcinoma of the stomach vary widely in different parts of the world. In the United States, it accounts for 2% to 3% of all cancer deaths, whereas in Japan, it causes between 40% and 50%. Eighty percent of patients with this malignancy will undergo operation, with only 40% of those tumors being resectable for cure. Of those that are resectable for cure, approximately one third will survive for 5 years. Overall 5-year survival for all patients with this disease is 21%. This stands in contrast to the Japanese experience, in which 70% of all gastric cancers are early tumors, and surgical resection is associated with an 85% 5-year survival.

Pathophysiology

The pathophysiology of gastric carcinoma remains unclear. A number of risk factors have been implicated in the carcinogenesis. A high percentage of gastric carcinomas occur in a milieu of atrophic gastritis with hypoacidity. Patients with pernicious anemia have an increased risk of developing gastric cancer. Approximately 7% to 10% of gastric ulcers are associated with an adenocarcinoma. A number of dietary factors play some role in the development of cancer, including foods that have been smoked, pickled, and are extremely spicy. A final risk factor is thought to be chronic infection with *H. pylori*. Undeveloped countries have a high incidence of *H. pylori* infection and also have an associated high incidence of gastric cancer rates. In more developed countries, however, where the prevalence of *H. pylori* infection is lower, gastric cancer incidences are decreasing. A final risk factor that has been identified is the development of gastric cancer in the gastric stump 15 years after previous gastric surgery, perhaps because of chronic bilious reflux and irritation.

Certain gastric polyps also are associated with the development of gastric cancer. The two commonest polyp types seen in the stomach are hyperplastic polyps and adenomatous polyps. Hyperplastic polyps account for the majority of gastric polyps, occurring in 80% of patients who have gastric polyps. However, these polyps are thought to have no malignant potential and rarely are symptomatic. Occasionally, vague abdominal discomfort is associated with them, and if they bleed or cause symptoms, endoscopic removal should be carried out. Adenomatous polyps, conversely, have approximately a 15% risk of cancer development, particularly when they are larger than 2.5 cm. The symptoms with adenomatous polyps are virtually identical to those of hyperplastic polyps, but the mere presence of adenomatous polyps in the stomach is indication for removal. Some adenomatous polyps can be removed endoscopically; but if they are sessile and broad based, occasional wedge resection is required to remove an adenomatous polyp.

Histologically, two types of adenocarcinoma are seen in gastric cancer: diffuse and intestinal. The diffuse type has a genetic association and is associated with blood group A. Young and middle-aged patients are usually diagnosed with the disease, and it begins in the body or cardia of the stomach. The tumor cells are poorly differentiated and often have signet ring cells. The prognosis is very poor with this type of lesion. The intestinal type is seen most commonly in older patients and is usually seen in the distal stomach. The cell types are better differentiated and are thought to have a somewhat better prognosis. Grossly, three types of cancers are encountered: polypoid, ulcerative, and infiltrating. The latter type often involves the entire stomach, giving it a leathery, hard appearance. This condition is known as *linitis plastica* and is thought to be surgically incurable.

For many years, gastric adenocarcinomas occurred principally in the distal stomach. However, over the last 15-year period, a significant increase in proximal gastric carcinomas has been noted. Now, approximately 40% involve the proximal stomach, and 40%, the distal stomach, with about 15% manifesting diffuse involvement.

Staging of gastric cancer is through a tumor/node/metastasis (TNM) classification, as seen in Box 26-2. Five-year survival rates vary according to depth of tumor penetration, nodal involvement, and presence or absence of metastases.

BOX 26-2 TNM Classification for Gastric Carcinomas

Primary Tumor (T)

T0	No evidence of primary tumor
T1	Tumor invades submucosa
T2	Tumor invades muscularis propria
T3	Tumor penetrates serosa
T4	Tumor invades adjacent structures

Regional Lymph Nodes (N)

N0	No regional lymph node metastasis
N1	Metastasis in 1–6 regional lymph nodes
N2	Metastasis in 7–15 regional lymph nodes
N3	Metastasis in >15 regional lymph nodes

Distant Metastasis (M)

M0	No distant metastasis
M1	Distant metastasis

Differential Diagnosis

The differential diagnosis of gastric cancer involves virtually anything that can be associated with epigastric pain. Included in that category are benign peptic ulcers of the stomach and duodenum, chronic pancreatitis, gallbladder disease, and left liver lesions. Similarly, distal esophageal lesions, such as esophageal ulcers, may occur with pain in this region.

Workup and Evaluation

The symptoms of early gastric cancer are vague and quite nonspecific. Unfortunately, most lesions are advanced and have metastasized to lymph nodes by the time they are diagnosed. The patient may have unanticipated weight loss, early satiety, loss of appetite, and mild dyspepsia. Very proximal cancers may even be associated with dysphagia. As the lesion becomes more advanced, vomiting may occur, and even hematemesis is rarely seen. If metastasis has occurred, the symptoms may be a function of carcinomatosis, including abdominal distention, ascites, jaundice, bowel obstruction, and nodules in the pouch of Douglas, which are referred to as *Blumer's shelf*. Similarly, the physical examination with early gastric cancer is unrevealing. Occasionally, with advanced carcinoma, abdominal distention, an ascitic fluid wave, a palpable umbilical mass (Sister Mary Joseph sign), a palpable supraclavicular node (Virchow's node), or jaundice is detected on physical examination. Unexplained weight loss is usually a harbinger of advanced disease. No laboratory tests are diagnostic of gastric cancer, although patients will occasionally have anemia or guaiac-positive stools. With advanced liver metastases, alteration in liver enzymes may be seen.

The definitive diagnosis of gastric cancer is usually accomplished by upper GI endoscopy (Fig. 26-17). Patients with early satiety, weight loss, and abdominal pain should undergo esophagogastroduodenoscopy. At that time, a biopsy can be performed of any lesion encountered. Particularly in the face of a gastric ulcer, biopsies should always be taken to rule out the presence of concomitant malignancy. Endoscopy is thought to be 95% accurate in making the diagnosis of gastric cancer. Because of the high incidence of gastric cancer in Japan, aggressive public screening probably accounts for the high percentage of early cancers seen in published series from that country. A relatively low incidence of gastric cancer in the United States makes mass screening prohibitive.

In a patient with abdominal pain that is less clear cut, a screening upper GI barium study may be obtained. When air contrast is used, about 90% of gastric tumors will be diagnosed. Lesions such as ulcerations, masses, and rigidity of the gastric wall all argue for gastric cancer. However, even if the upper GI barium study is suggestive of a tumor, endoscopy still must be done to confirm the diagnosis in most cases.

CT scan is not used as a primary diagnostic modality but is used to help stage the patient. If the lesion is large

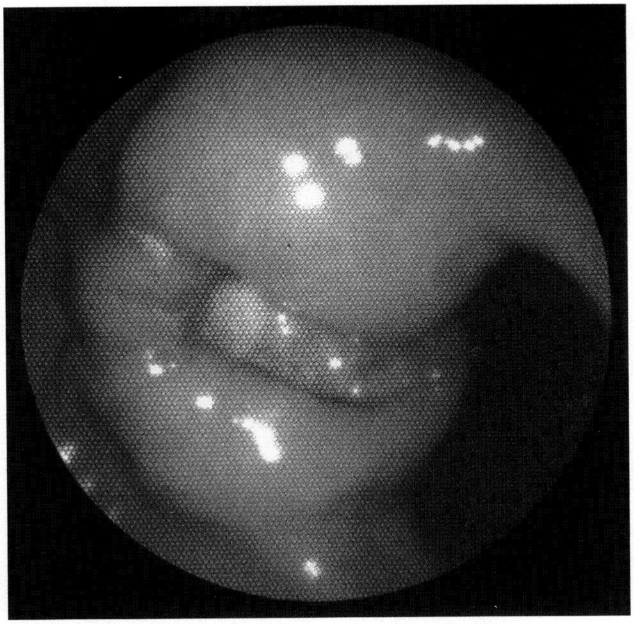

FIGURE 26–17 Endoscopic appearance of a moderate-sized gastric cancer. Note the ulcerated polypoid mass.

enough, it can be diagnosed occasionally during routine CT scanning for nonspecific symptoms. Endoscopic ultrasonography has proven valuable in staging low rectal cancers. It also shows some promise in determining depth of penetration in gastric tumors and even possible node involvement. However, more experience with this modality must be accrued before it can be used routinely.

Treatment Alternatives

Surgery is the only therapeutic modality with curative potential in gastric cancer. Unfortunately, cures represent a minority in this aggressive form of malignancy. Nevertheless, the surgeon should be aggressive at working up, staging, and operating on patients who have any chance of cure. The obvious aim of the operation is to remove not only the primary lesion but also any additional lymphatic drainage sites. These sites may include lymph nodes above the pylorus in the region of the porta hepatis, below the pylorus, near the pancreatic head, near the left gastric artery, and in the splenic hilum. The appropriate operation depends on the location and nodal involvement. A number of controversies regard surgical treatment of gastric cancers, which include whether the surgeon should do a partial gastric resection or total gastrectomy, whether an extensive lymphadenectomy should be done, what is an adequate proximal and distal margin, should the spleen be routinely removed, and implications of adjacent organ involvement.

In general, no evidence suggests that a total gastrectomy confers any additional survival benefit over partial gastrectomy. Similarly, although some evidence in the Japanese literature indicates that aggressive lymphadenectomy improves survival, studies in the Unites States and Western Europe have not confirmed those results. It is possible that the difference may be accounted for by the high percentage of early cancers in Japan. Most surgeons agree that a 4- to 6-cm margin is necessary in gastric cancer because of submucosal spread of the tumor. Similarly, little convincing evidence suggests that a routine splenectomy should be done during gastrectomy and adjacent organs should not be removed unless directly involved by tumor. Adenocarcinomas of the distal stomach are best treated by extensive distal gastrectomy with omentectomy. Reconstruction can be by gastroduodenostomy or, more frequently, by gastrojejunostomy, depending on whether tension occurs at the anastomosis. Large carcinomas arising in the corpus of the stomach should be treated with total gastrectomy with omentectomy and harvesting of perigastric lymph nodes.

Adenocarcinomas near the GE junction are always difficult management challenges and usually involve a proximal gastrectomy with esophagogastrostomy. However, if the tumor at the GE junction spreads into the esophagus, occasionally an esophagogastrectomy is required. This may involve resecting the tumor, making certain that all gastric margins are free, opening the right chest to remove the esophagus, and then pulling the stomach into the chest to do an esophagogastrostomy. Surgical management of linitis plastica also is quite controversial. Some surgeons believe that a total gastrectomy will give the patient some palliation. However, others think that because this is an incurable cancer, gastrectomy is not indicated and is palliative at best. The prognosis of gastric carcinoma after surgery obviously depends on the depth of penetration of the gastric wall and the presence or absence of lymph node or distal metastases. Early cancers, which are confined to the mucosa without positive lymph nodes, have a 90% 5-year survival. Unfortunately, they represent a very small minority of all resectable gastric cancers. As the tumors become increasingly invasive, including muscularis propria involvement and lymph node metastases, the prognosis becomes worse, so that 5-year survival of patients undergoing curative resection ranges between 30% and 40%.

Chemotherapy in the treatment of gastric carcinoma has been disappointing at best. The agents most commonly used are 5-fluorouracil (5-FU), mitomycin-C, and doxorubicin. Response rates are usually partial and range from 20% to 30%. Complete response is quite rare. Combination therapy with these three agents also has been attempted, and a response rate of 33% has been seen, with complete responses in 12% of patients. Similarly, radiation therapy has not been demonstrated to significantly help 5-year survival in patients with this disease. Clearly, a need exists for more effective chemotherapeutic agents in a disease in which the majority of patients are first seen with node-positive disease.

Lymphoma

Lymphoma of the stomach may occur as isolated gastric disease or as a manifestation of diffuse lymphoma. Unfortunately, more commonly, the disease is not isolated to the stomach. More than 50% of all GI lymphomas occur in the stomach, and non-Hodgkin's lymphomas account for 5% to 10% of malignant gastric tumors. If the diagnosis of gastric lymphoma is made and no systemic disease is encountered, the patient is considered to have a gastric lymphoma. Gastric lymphomas occur in elderly patients in their 60s or 70s, and symptoms are vague and nonspecific. Vague abdominal pain, weight loss, early satiety, anorexia, and nausea are quite common. Bleeding and anemia also are seen in 40% to 50% of patients. The diagnosis of gastric lymphoma is usually made with endoscopy, in which a mass is encountered during the diagnostic procedure. Biopsies of this mass usually confirm the presence of lymphoma, although occasionally the lesion may be submucosal, and a biopsy may return normal gastric mucosa. With a diagnosis of gastric lymphoma, a complete workup for staging should be accomplished including CT scan of chest and abdomen, bone marrow biopsy, and biopsy of any peripheral lymph nodes that may be enlarged.

Treatment of gastric lymphoma depends on whether it is a primary gastric lymphoma or whether the stomach is secondarily involved. In patients who have primary gastric lymphoma, a gastrectomy involving the portion of the stomach involved is indicated. A radical resection is not indicated, as the patient will almost certainly undergo chemotherapy and even possibly radiation therapy to treat any additional residual disease. If diffuse disease is encountered during the workup, it is usual to administer chemoradiation alone without surgical resection. A small risk for perforation exists as the tumor cells necrose in response to the chemoradiation. The prognosis of primary gastric lymphoma is much better than that of gastric adenocarcinoma, with 40% to 50% of patient surviving for 5 years.

Gastrointestinal Stromal Tumors

Approximately 3% of gastric malignancies are GI stromal tumors (GISTs). They appear as a mass encountered in the stomach during routine upper GI endoscopy. Biopsy often reveals normal gastric mucosa, as these tumors arise from the muscle wall of the stomach. By far the most common mesenchymal tumor is a leiomyoma. These tumors may grow rapidly and often umbilicate because of central necrosis. Because of the umbilication, they will bleed, thus leading to their detection. A wedge resection of the gastric wall is usually required to resect any small GIST, as a malignant potential exists. Any lesion known to be a gastric GIST should be treated with en bloc resection of the tumor and any involved structures. Obviously, a more radical resection is usually required with this tumor. Prognosis is a function of tumor size and involvement of adjacent organs. Lymph node involvement is uncommon with gastric GIST, as metastasis more commonly occurs by hematogenous routes.

Duodenal Neoplasms

Neoplasms of the duodenum are quite uncommon and, when they occur, are often associated with familial adenomatous polyposis. The most common adenomatous tumor occurring in this region is villous adenoma of the duodenum. These patients are initially seen with vague upper GI symptoms including epigastric pain, weight loss, jaundice, and, occasionally, melena or anemia. Eighty percent are periampullary in location, and 60% to 70% are benign. Likelihood of malignancy is a function of polyp size, with larger polyps being associated with invasive cancer. Most benign polyps can be treated with transduodenal submucosal excision. However, if high-grade dysplasia or invasive carcinoma is found, pancreaticoduodenectomy is required. Duodenal adenocarcinoma is a rare tumor, and most patients have weight loss, abdominal pain, and occasional bleeding. The diagnosis is made with upper GI endoscopy in which a biopsy of the mass reveals the presence of an adenocarcinoma. Because of its location at an important alimentary intersection in which the pancreatic head and duodenum share a common blood supply, a pancreaticoduodenectomy is indicated. Five-year survival after pancreaticoduodenectomy for this lesion is 20% to 30%.

Gastrinomas of the duodenum are also rare but, when present, are often associated with the Zollinger-Ellison syndrome. These gastrin-producing tumors are occasionally diagnosed because of the presence of virulent peptic ulcer disease. The majority of tumors occur in the gastrinoma triangle, which includes the head of the pancreas and the second portion of the duodenum. Patients usually have intractable ulcer disease, and the diagnosis is confirmed by a fasting serum gastrin of more than 100 pg/mL or an abnormal secretin stimulation test that results in a gastrin of more than 200 pg/mL. Preoperatively, the tumors can occasionally be localized by using selective portal venous sampling, but, in most cases, a visual search during laparotomy is required. Most commonly, a single, small tumor is found in the duodenal wall and is resected with any involved nodes. Up to 50% involve regional lymph nodes, and 5% to 8% may have associated liver metastases.

Suggested Reading

Barksdale AR, Schwartz RW: Current management of perforated peptic ulcer. Curr Surg 57:594–599, 2000.

Charr FK, Leung WK: Peptic ulcer disease. Lancet 360:633–641, 2002.

Csendes A, Maluenda F, Braghetto et al: Prospective randomized study comparing three surgical techniques for the treatment of gastric outlet obstruction secondary to duodenal ulcer. Am J Surg 166:45–49, 1993.

Cushieri A, Fayers P, Fielding D: Chemoradiotherapy after surgery compared with surgery alone for adenocarcinoma of the stomach or gastroesophageal junction. N Engl J Med 345:725–730, 2001.

Ohmann C, Imhof M, Roher HD: Trends in peptic ulcer bleeding and surgical management. World J Surg 24:284–293, 2000.

Taylor TV: Current indications for peptic ulcer surgery. Curr Pract Surg 7:131–134, 1995.

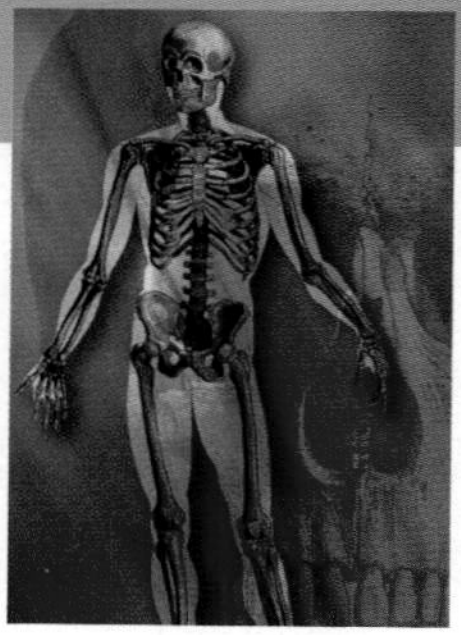

Chapter 27

Esophagus

JONATHAN F. FINKS, MD, and JOHN G. HUNTER, MD

Surgical Anatomy

The esophagus is a 30-cm-long muscular tube connecting the oropharynx with the stomach. It traverses three body compartments: the neck, the mediastinum, and the abdomen. The esophageal inlet is marked by the cricopharyngeal muscle (the upper esophageal sphincter), which is approximately 15 cm from the incisors. The gastroesophageal (GE) junction, in health, lies 40 to 45 cm from the incisors. Lesions of the esophagus are referenced by their position in the esophagus (proximal, middle, distal) and by their depth, as measured in centimeters from the incisors (Fig. 27-1).

The cricopharyngeus muscle is composed of striated muscle and is capable of voluntary contraction. Over the next 40% of the esophagus, the skeletal muscle is gradually replaced by smooth muscle (Fig. 27-2). The esophagus has no serosa, except over the final 2 to 3 cm, which reside in the abdomen and are covered by the visceral peritoneum. The outer layer of the esophagus consists of longitudinal muscle. Beneath the longitudinal muscle is a layer of circular muscle. The submucosa is richly innervated and contains a vascular plexus that extends the length of the esophagus. The esophageal mucosa is very loosely applied to the circular smooth muscle and is easily dissected away. The esophagus is lined by squamous epithelium, which is

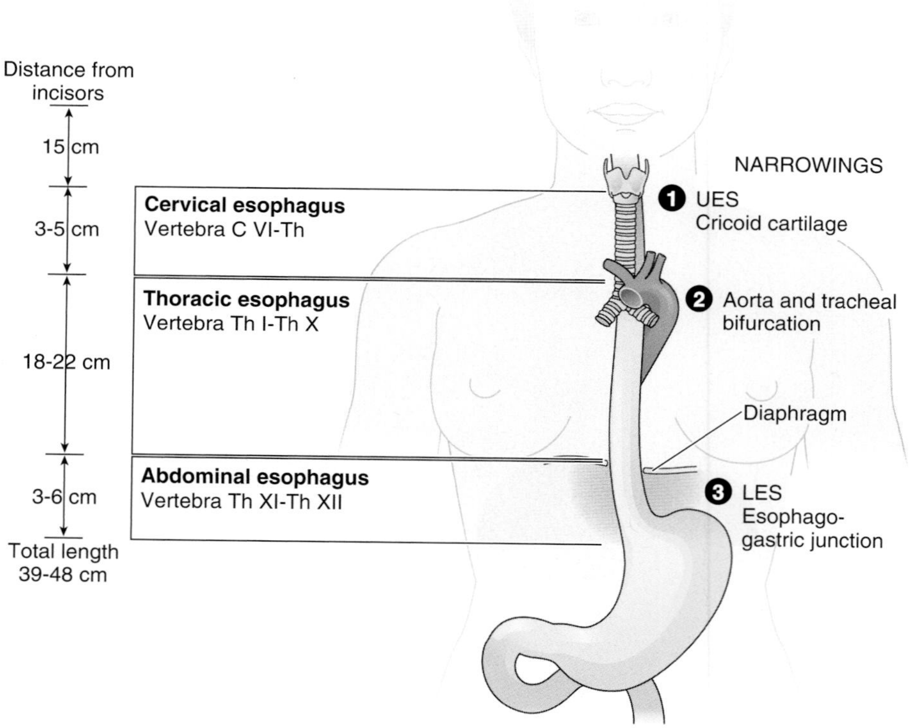

FIGURE 27–1 The esophagus is divided into three regions: the cervical esophagus, the thoracic esophagus, and the abdominal esophagus. The esophagus is narrowed in three regions, at the upper esophageal sphincter (UES), at the aorta, and at the lower esophageal sphincter (LES).

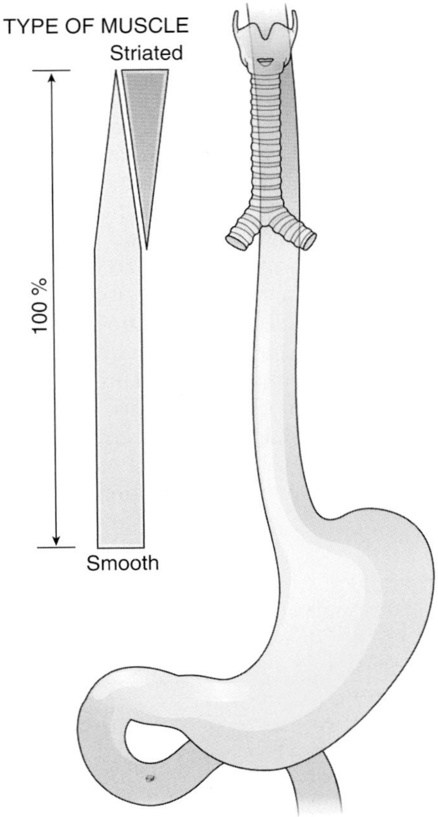

FIGURE 27–2 At the upper esophageal sphincter, striated muscle predominates, but below the tracheal bifurcation, the esophageal is composed entirely of smooth muscle.

PEARLS FOR ROUNDS

GERD
Complications of gastrointestinal reflux disease (GERD) include esophageal stricture, aspiration pneumonia, Barrett's esophagus, and esophageal adenocarcinoma.
Treatment options for GERD include dietary/lifestyle modifications, medical therapy with protein-pump inhibitors (PPIs), and surgical fundoplication, usually performed laparoscopically.

Achalasia
The diagnosis of achalasia requires the finding of aperistalsis on an esophageal-motility study.
Treatment options for achalasia include botulinum toxin (Botox) injection, pneumatic esophageal dilation, and surgical therapy with esophageal myotomy, usually performed laparoscopically.

Esophageal Cancer
Adenocarcinoma is now more common than squamous cell cancer in the United States.
Evaluation should include barium swallow as the initial study, followed by upper endoscopy to confirm the diagnosis; computed tomography and endoscopic ultrasonography are useful studies for staging the cancer.

resistant to the mechanical and thermal trauma of eating and drinking. The upper esophageal sphincter (UES) is anatomically definable and under voluntary control. The lower esophageal sphincter (LES) is indistinguishable from the smooth muscle above it but reacts independently to neurohumoral stimuli.

The blood supply of the esophagus comes from the neck, chest, and abdomen. The primary blood supply in the neck is the inferior thyroid artery. In the chest, arterial inflow comes primarily from the bronchial arteries and venous drainage to tributaries of the azygos vein. In the abdomen, several small ascending vessels from the celiac axis region supply the GE junction and distal esophageal body. Because of the rich intramural blood flow, mobilization of part of the esophagus from its attachments will not devascularize it. As long as the inferior thyroid artery is intact, the middle and distal esophagus can be mobilized without causing ischemia.

Lymphatic drainage of the esophagus is similar to arterial inflow. The distal esophagus is drained by lymphatics to celiac lymph nodes. The midesophagus drains to lymph nodes in the mediastinum and peritracheal region. The proximal esophagus drains into cervical lymph nodes. Given the extensive submucosal lymphatic plexus, esophageal cancer may be found in drainage regions far from the primary cancer.

The esophagus travels in the posterior mediastinum, behind the trachea and behind the heart. In the sagittal plane, it follows the curvature of the thoracic spine. In the coronal plane, the esophagus is midline in the neck but deviated toward the right chest by the aortic arch. Thus the midesophagus is best accessed through the right chest for esophagectomy. The distal esophagus curves to the left and passes through the diaphragm at an oblique angle. Operations involving the distal esophagus are best reached through the left chest or through the abdomen.

As the esophagus passes through the diaphragmatic hiatus into the abdominal cavity, it is accompanied by the anterior and posterior vagus nerves. The anterior (left) vagus nerve is intimately attached to the distal esophagus, whereas the posterior (right) vagus nerve often pulls away from the esophagus as it passes through the hiatus. Along the thoracic esophagus, the left and right vagi often separate into multiple nerve fibers, and then recondense into two nerve trunks on entering the abdomen.

Physiology

Food and saliva are moved through the esophagus by well-ordered segmental contractions of the esophageal body, a process known as *peristalsis*. Primary peristalsis is initiated by a voluntary swallowing effort. The first event in swallowing is the simultaneous relaxation of the upper and lower esophageal sphincters (Fig. 27-3). The constrictor muscles of the pharynx propel the food bolus into the esophageal body. The LES remains relaxed as the peristaltic wave propels the bolus through the lower esophagus and into the stomach. After the passage of the peristaltic wave, a period of hypercontraction of the lower esophagus occurs. Esophageal distention or the presence of a noxious stimulus in the esophagus, such as gastric acid, will elicit a peristaltic wave that is initiated at the point of stimulation. These waves are under involuntary control and are termed *secondary peristalsis*. *Tertiary peristalsis* describes high-pressure, segmental contractions of the esophageal body that are not peristaltic. These contractions may cause chest pain and are ineffective at propelling food in an orderly fashion. Tertiary contractions are more common in the elderly and are often associated with esophageal motility disturbances.

The LES is characterized by its physiologic function, because an anatomic sphincter is hard to recognize. Under resting conditions, the LES generates a pressure that is 15 to 35 mmHg above the pressure recorded in the stomach. This pressure gradient is important for protection against gastroesophageal reflux (GER). The high-pressure zone of the LES measures 4 cm in length and spans the crural portion of the diaphragm. Typically 2 to 3 cm of the LES reside in the abdomen, and 1 to 2 cm are found above the diaphragm. The LES relaxes with swallowing to allow the passage of food and postprandially to allow the venting of gas from the fundus of the stomach. This reflex, which is triggered by distention of the fundus, is known as a transient lower esophageal sphincter relaxation (TLESR).

The LES also is susceptible to a wide variety of humoral and pharmacologic influences. Relaxation of the sphincter

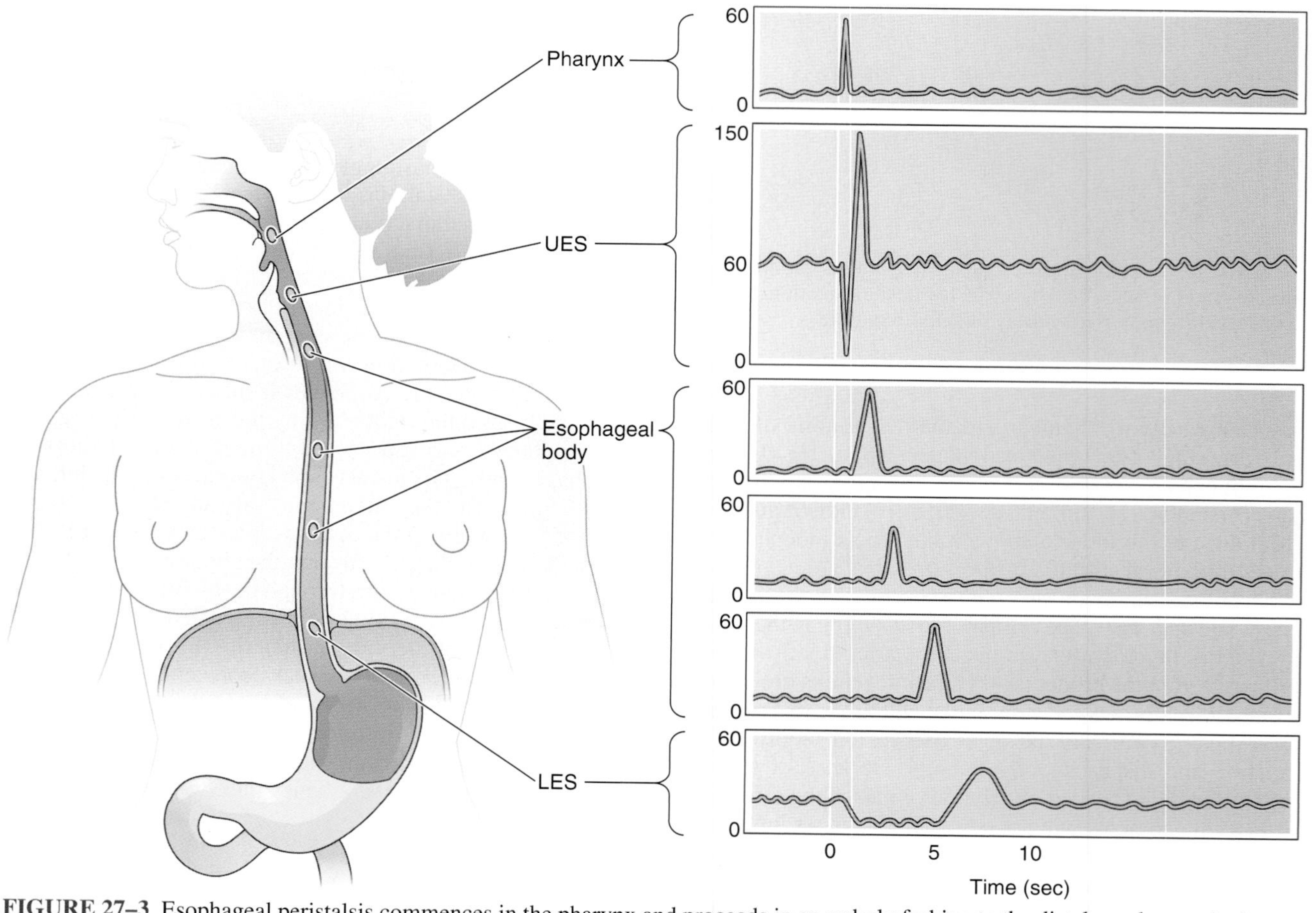

FIGURE 27–3 Esophageal peristalsis commences in the pharynx and proceeds in an orderly fashion to the distal esophagus. At the initiation of swallowing, the lower esophageal sphincter (LES) relaxes. After the passage of the food bolus, a period of hypercontractility occurs in the LES.

is mediated by nitric oxide (NO) and vasoactive intestinal peptide (VIP), whereas active contraction may be mediated by NO inhibition or acetylcholine (Fig. 27-4). Gastrin also will augment LES resting tone. Normally, food in the stomach increases gastrin and acetylcholine release, which increases LES tone. Unfortunately, many enjoyable foods (chocolate, wintergreen), as well as alcohol, caffeine, and nicotine, can decrease LES resting tone, leading to GER. Medications such as calcium channel blockers and long-acting nitrates also will reduce LES tone, as can high progesterone levels associated with pregnancy.

Disorders of the Esophagus

Gastroesophageal Reflux Disease

Epidemiology

Gastroesophageal reflux disease (GERD) is the most common chronic disease of the gastrointestinal (GI) tract. Nearly 40% of Americans are affected monthly, whereas 7% to 10% experience daily symptoms of GERD. Most people with GERD treat themselves with over-the-counter medications. In the United States, an estimated $10 billion is spent annually for medications to treat symptoms of this disease, making GERD the most common and the most expensive GI disorder in North America today.

Symptoms of GERD

Although GERD may be defined by the presence of excessive gastric acid in the esophagus or esophageal injury, it is most commonly defined by the presence of esophageal reflux symptoms.

Esophageal (Typical) Symptoms. Heartburn is the most common symptom of GERD. Its frequency defines the prevalence of the disease, and the ability to eliminate this symptom determines the effectiveness of GERD therapy. Heartburn, or pyrosis, is the sensation of substernal burning pain that usually ascends from the epigastrium and spreads to the upper chest, neck, and jaw.

Regurgitation is a sensation of swallowed food returning to the mouth. Regurgitation may originate from the stomach in patients with GERD and hiatal hernia, or it may stem from the esophagus, as in patients with achalasia. Esophageal regurgitation occurs immediately after swallowing and yields completely undigested food, whereas gastric regurgitation is delayed and consists of partially digested food.

Heartburn and regurgitation typically occur in the postprandial period and can be exacerbated by bending over, straining, or lying in the recumbent position. Intake of large meals of fatty food and alcohol often precede reflux episodes. These episodes also may be nocturnal, causing sleep disturbance.

The physiologic response to acid reflux is excessive salivation (**waterbrash**). Irritation of the posterior pharynx frequently causes chronic sore throat, hoarseness, or a sensation of a foreign body (**globus hystericus**). Esophageal injury, peptic stricture, and neoplasms can induce **dysphagia**, a sensation of food lodged in the distal

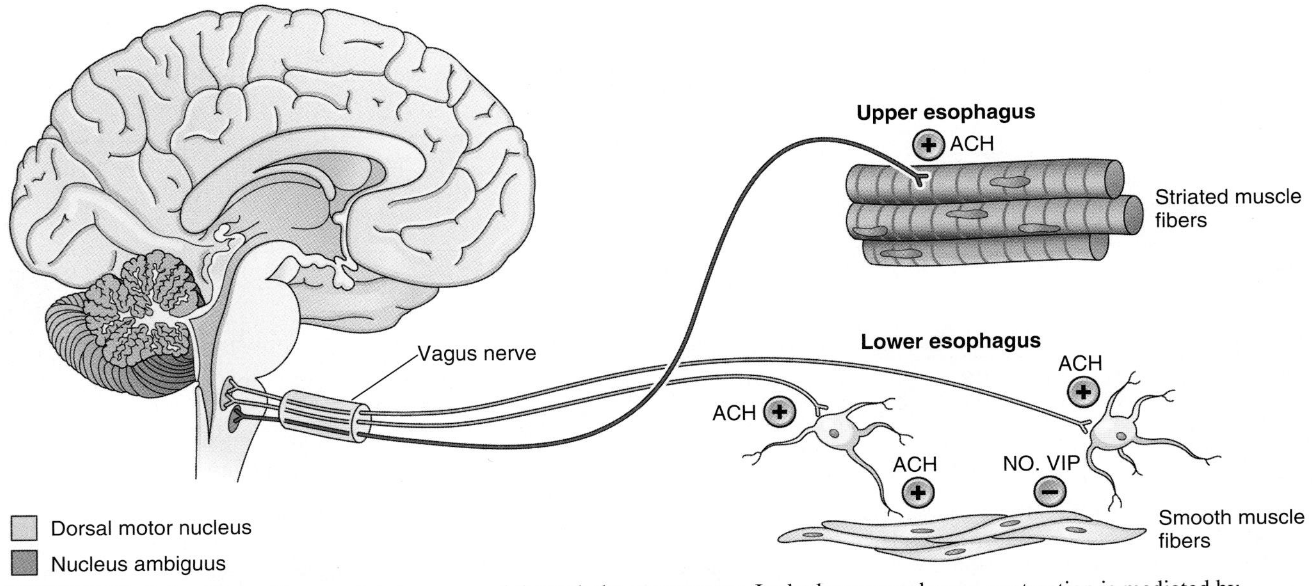

FIGURE 27–4 Esophageal innervation is conveyed through the vagus nerve. In the lower esophagus, contraction is mediated by acetylcholine, and relaxation of the lower esophageal sphincter is mediated by nitric oxide.

esophagus, often referred to the region of the sternal notch.

Extraesophageal (Atypical) Symptoms. Extraesophageal symptoms include those that arise from the oropharynx, airway, and respiratory tree. These symptoms include chronic cough, wheezing, choking, hoarseness, halitosis, and dental erosions. They are nonspecific and may indicate other disease processes, including cancer of the larynx, airway, or esophagus. A thorough search for a malignant source for these atypical symptoms must be undertaken when evaluating a patient with suspected GERD. Finally, steroid-dependent asthma and aspiration pneumonia are often the result of occult gastroesophageal reflux.

Pathophysiology

GERD may be defined as the pathologic excess of a normal physiologic process, the reflux of gastric contents into the distal esophagus. Normally when acid is refluxed during a TLESR, a secondary peristaltic wave will quickly clear the acid bolus from the esophagus. Successive wet swallows of saliva deliver sodium bicarbonate to the distal esophagus, thereby neutralizing the remaining acid (Fig. 27-5*A*).

In some instances, esophageal injury occurs as a result of conditions that impair the normal response to reflux. In patients with **xerostomia** (associated with Sjögren's syndrome or prior head and neck radiation), impaired salivation may allow acid-induced esophageal injury because of inadequate bicarbonate buffering (Fig. 5*B*). Disorders of esophageal peristalsis, such as **achalasia** and **scleroderma**, may render the esophagus incapable of clearing gastric acid after a reflux episode. Some degree of esophageal motility dysfunction is frequently associated with the complications of GERD, including Barrett's esophagus (BE) and esophageal stricture.

The Lower Esophageal Sphincter. Incompetence of the LES can lead to GERD, yet most patients with symptomatic heartburn do not manifest LES incompetence. Rather, the most common mechanism of GERD is excessive frequency or duration of the TLESRs, which often is seen clinically as excessive belching.

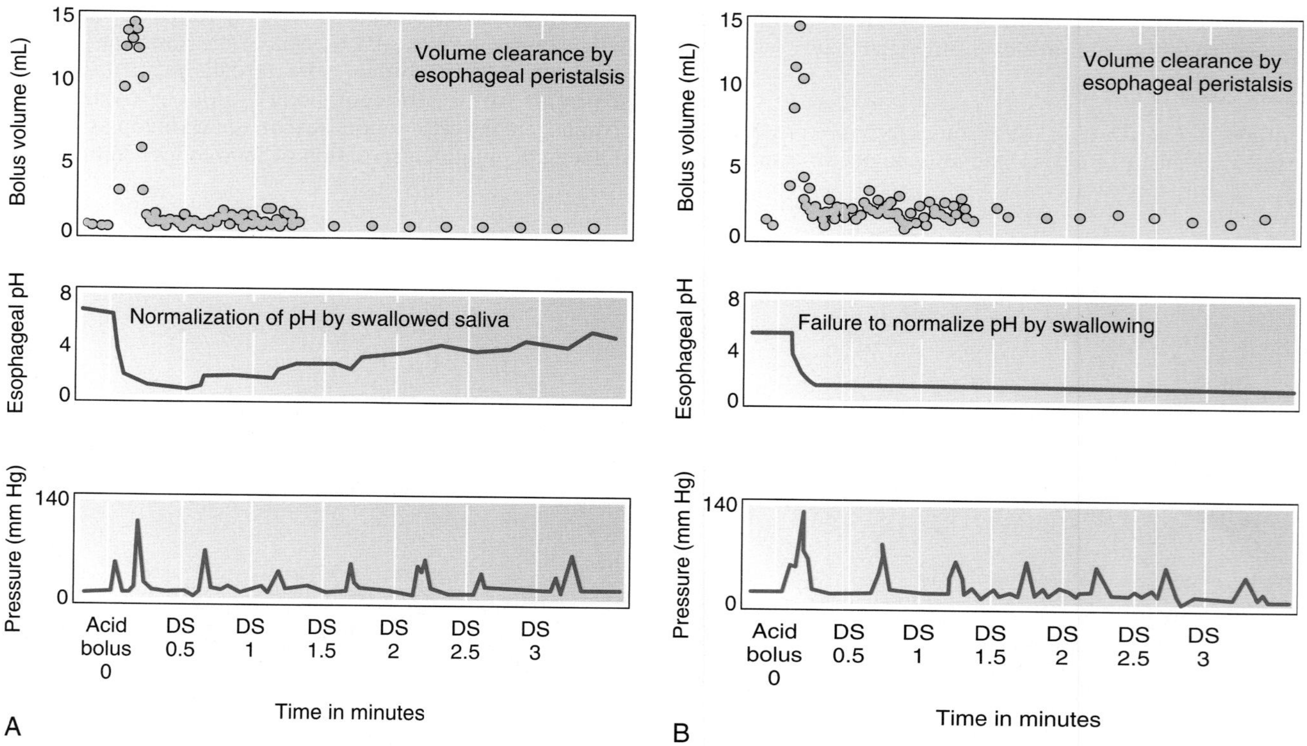

FIGURE 27–5 Esophageal acid clearance is a two-step process. *A*, An aliquot of hydrochloric acid placed in the distal esophagus is rapidly cleared by esophageal peristalsis, but pH is not normalized until a series of dry swallows brings bicarbonate-rich saliva to the distal esophagus. *B*, If saliva is aspirated from the pharynx and not swallowed, the pH in the distal esophagus does not neutralize with repetitive dry swallows. (Adapted from Helm JF, Dodds WJ, Pelc LR, et al: Effect of esophageal emptying and saliva on clearance of acid from the esophagus. N Engl J Med 310:284, 1984, with permission.)

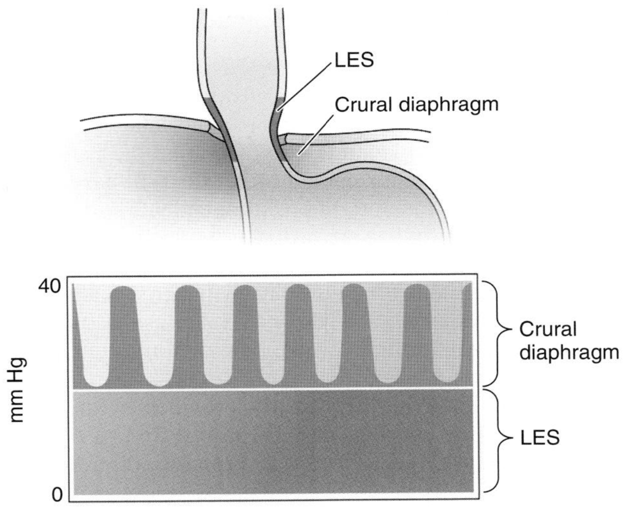

FIGURE 27–6 The normal antireflux barrier protects against gastroesophageal reflux by the combined actions of the crural diaphragm and the lower esophageal sphincter (LES). The LES provides tonic contraction, whereas the crural diaphragm provides maximal contraction amplitude during inspiration, when the transdiaphragmatic pressure is at a maximum. (Adapted from American College of Gastroenterology's Slide Lecture Program: An Update on GERD, 1996, with permission.)

Hiatal Hernia. Probably the most important pathophysiologic factor in severe GERD is hiatal hernia (HH). Hiatal hernias are common and often asymptomatic. They can promote GERD, however, by separating the two components of the reflux barrier (LES and the crural diaphragm), which work in concert to prevent reflux (Fig. 27-6). Normally, the crural diaphragm contracts during inspiration, helping to close the GE junction when the pressure gradient across the diaphragm is greatest. Once stretched by the herniated stomach of a patient with a HH, the crural diaphragm cannot provide adequate pressure to prevent the siphoning of gastric contents into the herniated stomach. These gastric contents can trigger frequent TLESRs, releasing a toxic refluxate into the distal esophagus. Finally, migration of the GE junction into the chest results in loss of the normally acute cardioesophageal angle (angle of His). This angle is a necessary component of the flapper-valve mechanism whereby pressure in the fundus of the stomach leads to pinching of the GE junction (Fig. 27-7).

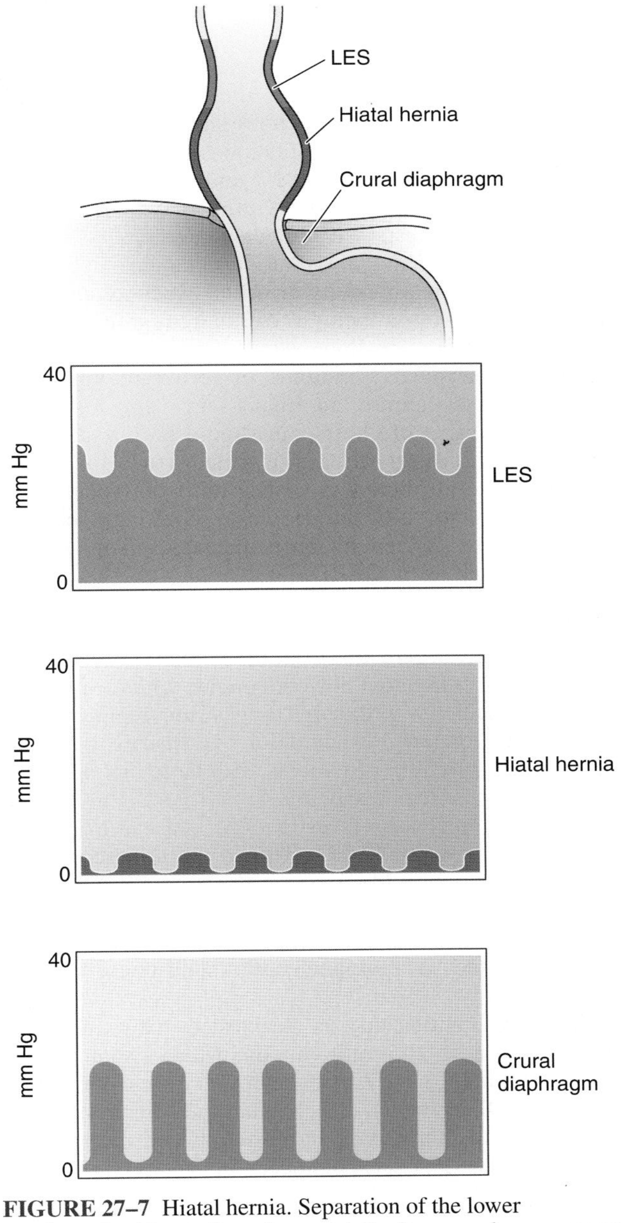

FIGURE 27–7 Hiatal hernia. Separation of the lower esophageal sphincter from the crural diaphragm reduces pressure at the gastroesophageal junction, promoting gastroesophageal reflux. (Adapted from American College of Gastroenterology's Slide Lecture Program: An Update on GERD, 1996, with permission.)

Gastric Emptying Disorders. Several conditions are associated with impaired gastric emptying, including previous vagotomy, diabetes mellitus, and pyloric channel ulceration. Poor gastric emptying can promote GERD through chronic gastric dilation, which leads to distortion of the GE orifice. In addition, the body and fundus of the stomach in patients with impaired emptying are often full of undigested food. Failures of LES function in these patients can lead to significant reflux events.

Differential Diagnosis of GERD

Heartburn and acid regurgitation remain the most common clinical manifestations of GERD, although up to two thirds of patients also may exhibit extraesophageal symptoms as well. When heartburn or regurgitation is the main symptom, specificity for GERD is high (89% and 95%, respectively). In most patients, the diagnosis of reflux may be established by an appropriate response to medical therapy.

The differential diagnosis of dysphagia is wider and includes esophageal motility disorders, such as achalasia, or obstruction by a benign or malignant esophageal lesion. A barium swallow usually differentiates these conditions. Atypical symptoms of reflux require more thorough investigation to make the diagnosis. An esophageal origin of chest pain should be pursued only after ischemic heart disease is ruled out. Hoarseness should not be attributed to GERD until the vocal cords are examined to rule out neoplasia. Similarly, chronic cough may be caused by bronchiectasis, neoplasm, or asthma, as well as by GERD.

Evaluation of GERD

The physical examination of an individual with GERD is usually normal. In about 50% of patients with esophagitis, however, tenderness of the high epigastrium region may be elicited. Laboratory examination is usually normal, although 20% to 30% of patients with large hiatal hernias will have iron deficiency anemia.

Five commonly used investigations assist in evaluation of the patient with GERD. Upper GI endoscopy and barium swallow provide important anatomic information. Foregut physiology is best evaluated with an esophageal motility study, 24-hour ambulatory pH measurement, and, when indicated, a radionucleotide solid-phase gastric-emptying study.

Upper GI endoscopy is performed with a flexible endoscope 8 to 10 mm in diameter. Esophagogastroduodenoscopy (EGD) can detect esophageal mucosal injury, including erosions (esophagitis) and strictures, as well as BE. With the endoscope in the retroflexed position, the endoscopist can assess the competency of the GE junction and the size of an HH. In addition, EGD will detect gastric anomalies such as gastritis, gastric ulcers, bezoars, and other features associated with gastric dysfunction. Overall, EGD is the single best test for making the diagnosis of GERD.

The **barium swallow** has little utility for making the diagnosis of reflux but is the first test one should order for the evaluation of dysphagia. Strictures of the esophagus and esophageal diverticula may be better assessed with barium swallow than with upper endoscopy. Even in the absence of a stricture, a video esophagram is a valuable test before antireflux surgery to assess swallowing function, HH size, and esophageal length. It is the *road map* for the esophageal surgeon.

A **24-hour ambulatory pH study** can be helpful in making the diagnosis of GERD. Gastric acid is normally present in the esophagus less than 4% of a 24-hour period. Greater exposure times are considered diagnostic of GERD. In addition to confirming abnormal esophageal acid exposure, the pH study can determine the pattern of reflux. Individuals with frequent TLESRs will have reflux predominantly in the upright position. Patients with resting LES dysfunction will have reflux in both the supine and upright positions. The 24-hour pH study is not necessary to make the diagnosis of GERD in all patients but is very helpful in patients who do not manifest esophageal mucosal damage on EGD or whose symptoms are entirely extraesophageal.

An **esophageal motility study** provides a functional evaluation of the esophageal body and LES. This test can help distinguish GERD from primary disorders of esophageal motility. A motility study also allows assessment of esophageal contractility, which may be important when planning an antireflux operation, because inadequate peristaltic strength may inhibit passage of a food bolus through a 360-degree fundoplication.

A **gastric-emptying study** is indicated for patients with symptoms suggestive of delayed gastric emptying, such as early satiety, nausea, and vomiting. These tests are performed by administering a known quantity of radiolabeled solid food and observing the rate of emptying on a gamma camera. Normally, 50% of a meal is emptied within 75 minutes. Patients with severe emptying disorders usually have half-emptying times more than twice normal. These patients deserve special consideration before performing an antireflux operation. Medical therapy with prokinetic agents, a gastric-emptying procedure, or occasionally even gastrectomy may be warranted in patients with gastric-emptying disorders and GERD.

Treatment of Gastroesophageal Reflux Disease

Lifestyle Modifications. The treatment of GERD starts by eliminating those agents that exacerbate it. Restriction of alcohol, cigarettes, caffeine, and fatty foods is a must, as is avoidance of eating within 2 hours of bedtime. Weight loss should be encouraged. In some cases, sleeping with the head of the bed elevated 30 degrees is helpful.

Medical Therapy. Medical treatment of GERD starts with over-the-counter medications, including antacids and alginates, which coat the inflamed esophagus. Antacids have the advantage of instantaneous action and the disadvantage of a short duration of relief.

Histamine-2–receptor antagonists, such as nizatidine and famotidine, block one of the three stimuli to acid secretion at the level of the parietal cell. These agents improve esophageal healing in up to 60% to 80% of patients after 12 weeks of use but provide long-term heartburn control in only 50% to 60% of individuals with GERD.

Prokinetic agents work by enhancing foregut motility or augmenting LES pressure or both. Metoclopramide stimulates smooth muscle contraction by inhibition of dopamine receptors. It is only marginally effective and limited by its side-effect profile. Cisapride, which stimulates acetylcholine release, has proven effective in relieving GERD symptoms but has been removed from the market because of cardiovascular side effects. Other promotility agents such as domperidone, erythromycin, and the selective 5-HT4 partial agonist tegaserod are currently under investigation.

Proton-pump inhibitors (PPIs), such as omeprazole and pantoprazole, are the most effective medications for the treatment of GERD. They work by blocking the sodium/potassium adenosine triphosphatase (ATPase) in the parietal cell. PPIs are 80% effective at maintaining remission in individuals with severe GERD. In combination with a prokinetic agent, they may be effective in 90% of individuals. Thus the majority of patients with GERD may be effectively managed with conservative measures and medical therapy. The therapy is life-long, however, and requires escalated dosing in up to 50% of individuals.

Surgical Therapy. Antireflux surgery and medical therapy with PPIs have both proven effective in treating GERD. In the only randomized controlled trial, omeprazole treatment (20 mg daily) was compared with open antireflux surgery for patients with erosive esophagitis. At 3-year follow-up, the rate of treatment failure was lower in the surgical group. However, when the omeprazole dose was adjusted to 40 to 60 mg daily, the difference was no longer statistically significant.

Patient Selection. The Society of American Gastrointestinal Endoscopic Surgeons (SAGES) defined the indications for surgery, as listed in Box 27-1. Despite the effectiveness of medical therapy, many patients with chronic GERD prefer surgical treatment, with a one-time cure, to the persistent need for medication. Some patients will have persistent symptoms despite maximal medical therapy. The most common "breakthrough" symptom in these patients is "volume reflux," or regurgitation.

The most difficult part of surgical decision making is deciding which patients will benefit from an antireflux procedure. The first step is to prove the diagnosis of GERD. If erosive esophagitis, peptic stricture, or BE is seen on endoscopy, the diagnosis is made. Visible esophageal injury is often absent in patients receiving effective medical therapy or those with primarily extraesophageal symptoms. In these patients, ambulatory 24-hour pH studies must be performed. Once the diagnosis is confirmed, esophageal function must be studied with an esophageal motility study and a videoesophagram. The former determines whether adequate peristalsis exists in the esophagus to propel food through a complete (Nissen) fundoplication. When esophageal peristalsis is absent (e.g., scleroderma) postoperative dysphagia can result, and these patients may benefit from subtotal fundoplication.

Operative Technique. Since Rudolph Nissen's original description of the GE fundoplication procedure, several variations of this operation have been proposed. Belsey described an anterior 270-degree fundoplication through a left thoracotomy. When an abdominal approach is used, most surgeons prefer the 360-degree Nissen fundoplication. A variety of partial fundoplications are popular in Europe,

BOX 27–1 Indications for Surgery

Surgical therapy should be considered in those individuals with documented GERD who

- Have had medical management that failed *or*
- Opt for surgery despite successful medical management (due to lifestyle considerations including age, time, *or* expense of medications, etc.) *or*
- Have complications of GERD (e.g, Barrett's esophagus; grade III or IV esophagitis) *or*
- Have medical complications attributable to large hiatal hernia (e.g., bleeding, dysphagia) *or*
- Have " atypical" symptoms (asthma, hoarseness, cough, chest pain, aspiration) and reflux documented on 24-hour pH monitoring.

PEARLS FOR THE OR

Anatomy
Rich submucosal vascular plexus allows for long-segment mobilization of the esophagus with low risk of causing ischemia. Extensive submucosal lymphatics allow cancer spread to remote lymphatic drainage basins.

Nissen Fundoplication
Fundoplications should be short (2 cm) and floppy, requiring mobilization of the short gastric vessels and performance of the wrap around a dilator (>50F) to ensure maximal floppiness.

Heller Myotomy
Myotomy involves complete division of the fibers of the lower esophageal sphincter and should be 6 to 8 cm in length, including 2 cm onto the cardia of the stomach. Partial fundoplication (Dor or Toupet) is performed to prevent gastroesophageal reflux disease after myotomy.

Esophagectomy
A gastric conduit is preferred for esophagectomy in adults, whereas an isoperistaltic left colon segment is the best esophageal replacement in children. The blood supply for the gastric conduit is based on the right gastroepiploic artery, which must be carefully preserved during mobilization of the stomach.

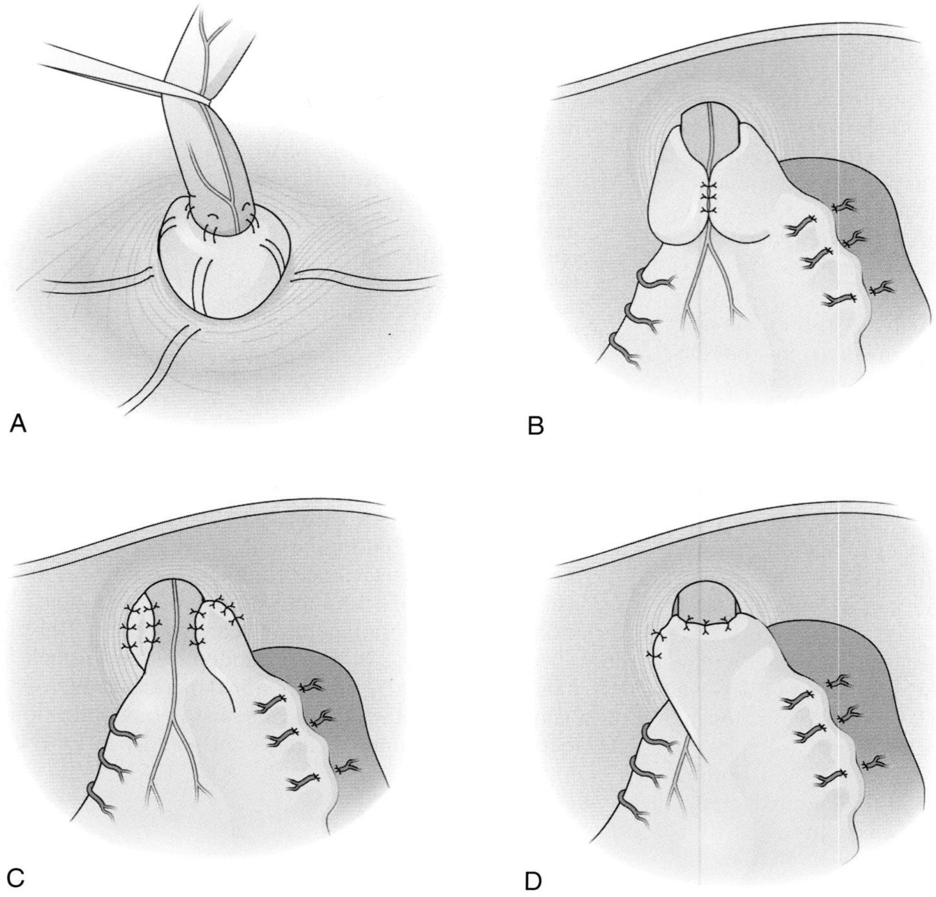

FIGURE 27–8 The four fundoplications most commonly performed. *A*, The Belsey procedure is a 270-degree anterior fundoplication performed through the left chest. *B*, The "floppy" Nissen fundoplication involves thorough mobilization of all fundus attachments from the left diaphragm and the spleen, followed by a 360-degree wrap. *C*, The Toupet fundoplication usually includes mobilization of the fundus followed by a 270-degree wrap. *D*, The Dor fundoplication incorporates an anterior 180-degree wrap and does not require fundic mobilization.

including the posterior 270-degree (Toupet) and the anterior 180-degree (Dor) fundoplications (Fig. 27-8).

The advent of laparoscopic Nissen fundoplication in the early 1990s reignited interest in the surgical approach to GERD therapy, which had fallen out of favor with gastroenterologists because of the effectiveness of antisecretory medications. This approach applies the same principles of the open operation but with considerably less postoperative pain, shorter hospital stays, and faster recovery times.

Nissen Fundoplication Technique. Access to the upper abdomen is achieved through either a midline incision or five laparoscopic trocars evenly spaced about the upper abdomen. The left lobe of the liver is retracted out of the way. Dissection of the esophagus starts by division of the phrenoesophageal ligament, usually above the hepatic branch of the anterior vagus nerve. The anterior aspects of the diaphragmatic crura are then easily visualized. Dissection proceeds posteriorly along the left and right crura until they meet behind the esophagus. The short gastric vessels are then divided, and the posterior attachments of the stomach to the diaphragm are taken down to expose the base of the left crus of the diaphragm. A Penrose drain is placed behind the esophagus under direct vision. The GE junction is retracted inferiorly, and all esophageal attachments are taken down to mobilize 2 to 3 cm of esophagus into the abdomen. The diaphragmatic crura are then reapproximated behind the esophagus with interrupted sutures. After the diaphragm is closed, the fundus of the stomach is pulled behind the esophagus from the left to the right. A large dilator (56 to 60F) is passed transorally into the stomach. Diaphragmatic closure is checked with the dilator in place. Two or three interrupted nonabsorbable sutures are then used to sew the stomach to itself, usually including a bit of esophagus. The dilator is important here to maintain the "floppiness" of the fundoplication. Generally, the fundoplication should be no longer than 2 cm. Creating a short, floppy fundoplication is essential to prevent dysphagia.

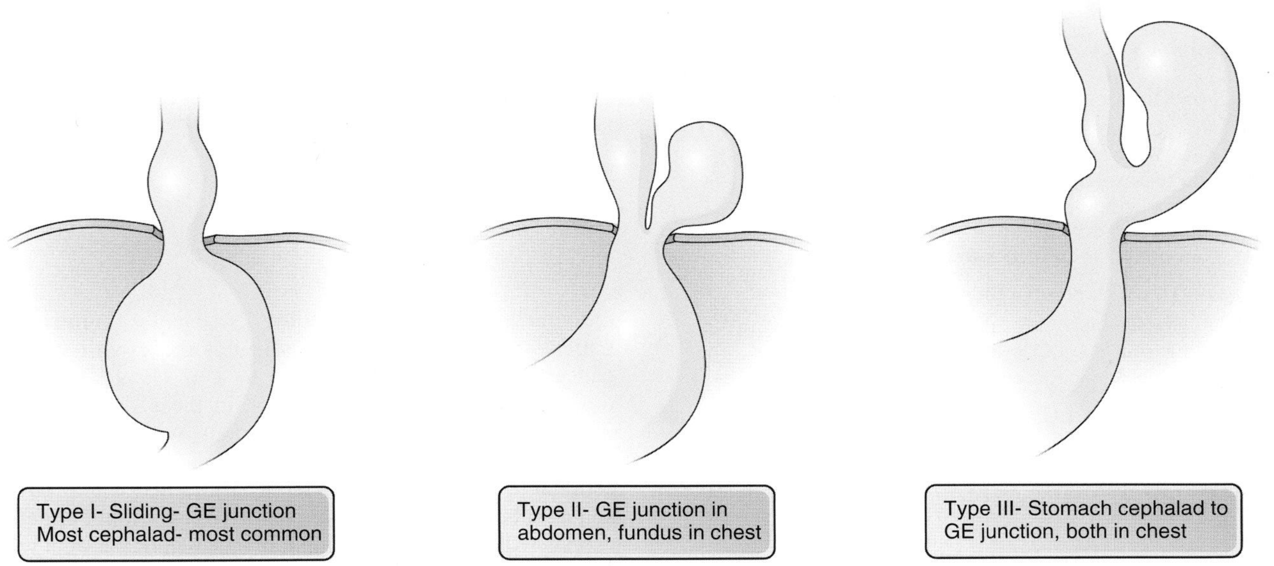

FIGURE 27–10 Three types of hiatal hernias are found. Type I is the sliding hernia, type II is the true paraesophageal hernia, and type III is the mixed hiatal hernia, the most common paraesophageal hernia.

low-grade dysplasia, yearly surveillance is warranted because of the increased risk of cancer development. Low-grade dysplasia is diagnosed by the loss of nuclear polarity and mature organization of the Barrett's epithelium. High-grade dysplasia (or carcinoma in situ) has the appearance of carcinoma but without the invasive characteristics. When high-grade dysplasia is detected, pathologic examination of the adjacent esophagus reveals invasive cancer in up to 40% of individuals. For this reason, acceptable-risk patients with high-grade dysplasia should undergo esophagectomy.

Effective therapy for GERD may prevent the progression of BE, but few data exist as to whether effective medical or surgical therapy reduces the incidence of adenocarcinoma developing in a Barrett's segment. Whether BE should be an independent indication for fundoplication remains controversial. Furthermore, no convincing evidence suggests that surgery prevents the development of cancer in a patient with BE.

Esophageal Carcinoma

Two distinct histologic types of esophageal carcinoma exist: squamous cell carcinoma, which may be found anywhere in the esophagus, and adenocarcinoma, which is typically located in the distal esophagus. Occasionally adenocarcinomas of the gastric cardia will extend above the GE junction in patients without GERD or BE.

Worldwide, squamous cell carcinoma of the esophagus is more common than adenocarcinoma, particularly in Asia, Africa, and portions of the Middle East. In Western countries, however, esophageal adenocarcinoma now predominates. In developing countries, diet has been implicated as a causative factor in the development of squamous cell carcinoma, whereas tobacco and alcohol use are the most prominent risk factors for this cancer type in the Western world. Esophageal adenocarcinoma is seen in patients with a long-standing history of GERD or BE and has been linked with obesity.

The most common symptom of esophageal carcinoma is dysphagia. Weight loss also is common. Other symptoms, such as dyspnea, hoarseness, and chest pain, are less common and usually signal advanced disease.

Workup and Evaluation

For the patient with dysphagia, the initial test should be a barium swallow. Esophageal carcinoma will appear as an irregular stricture or ulceration in the esophageal body. Endoscopic biopsy confirms the diagnosis. Once the diagnosis is obtained, cancer staging is next, by using a combination of chest and abdominal computed tomography (CT), as well as endoscopic ultrasound (EUS). EUS can help determine the depth of tumor invasion and detect lymph node involvement. Lymph node metastases can be confirmed by EUS-guided fine-needle aspiration. Positron-emission tomography (PET) has proven to be a useful adjunct in identifying lymph node and distant metastases not detected by CT or EUS. Finally, laparoscopy or thoracoscopy or both may be used to sample suggestive lymph nodes when treatment protocols will be affected by lymph node status. After these studies, a clinical stage can be assigned (Box 27-2 and Table 27-1).

BOX 27–2 Components of TNM Classification for Esophageal Cancer

Primary Tumor (T)

TX	Primary tumor cannot be assessed
TO	No evidence of primary tumor
Tis	Carcinoma in situ (high-grade dysplasia)
T1	Tumor invades lamina propria or submucosa
T3	Tumor invades adventitia
T4	Tumor invades adjacent structures

Regional Lymph Nodes (N)

NX	Regional lymph nodes cannot be assessed
N0	No regional lymph node metastasis
N1	Regional lymph node metastasis

Distant Metastasis (M)

MX	Presence of distant metastasis cannot be assessed
M0	No distant metastasis
M1	Distant metastasis

Treatment Planning

Treatment of patients with esophageal cancer starts by assessing their ability to withstand aggressive surgical treatment. Esophageal cancer patients are often quite debilitated from comorbid disease and, more important, from malnutrition. Therapy begins by addressing their nutritional needs. For patients who are not candidates for surgery on the basis of tumor stage (stage IV) or systemic illness, the ability to swallow can best be restored by deployment of an expandable metal stent in the distal esophagus. For patients undergoing preoperative chemotherapy and radiation, the best method of nutritional support is placement of a nasojejunal feeding tube. If the esophagus is completely obstructed, a laparoscopic or open gastrostomy or jejunostomy may be necessary before planning definitive therapy.

Definitive treatment of esophageal cancer is dependent on tumor stage. The histologic type of esophageal cancer does not influence treatment and has little influence on outcome. Esophagogastrectomy is usually curative in patients with stage I disease, whereas those with stage II cancer have a cure rate of 10% to 40% (Box 27-3). The only contraindication to resection in these patients is an excessively high operative risk. Patients with clinical stage III are cured infrequently (~15%), but the risk of esophagogastrectomy is moderate (mortality, 4% to 10%), so patients with a reasonable operative risk should undergo esophageal resection. The median survival of patients with stage IV disease is less than 6 months. Palliation of dysphagia is the primary goal in treating these patients.

TABLE 27–1 Staging of Carcinoma of the Esophagus by TNM Classification

Stage Grouping	T	N	M
0	Tis	N0	M0
I	T1	N0	M0
IIA	T2	N0	M0
	T3	N0	M0
IIB	T1	N1	M0
	T2	N1	M0
III	T3	N1	M0
	T4	Any N	M0
IV	Any T	Any N	M1

BOX 27–3 Five-year Survival from Esophageal Cancer as a Function of Stage

Stage 0	>95%
Stage I	50%–80%
Stage IIA	30%–40%
Stage IIB	10%–30%
Stage III	10%–15%
Stage IV	<5%

Palliation of Esophageal Cancer

Expandable metal stents have gained in popularity for palliation of unresectable disease because they are immediately effective and provide a larger lumen than do plastic stents, allowing a wider range of foods to be eaten. Laser recanalization of the esophageal lumen or catheter-based radiation therapy (brachytherapy) may be useful for tumor ingrowth through the stent interstices.

Neoadjuvant and Adjuvant Therapy

The value of preoperative chemotherapy and radiotherapy for esophageal cancer is controversial. In nonrandomized trials, it was demonstrated that preoperative radiation and chemotherapy resulted in complete tumor regression in up to 25% of patients. However, the use of preoperative chemoradiotherapy regimens has been investigated in several randomized controlled trials with disappointing results. To date, no survival advantage has been demonstrated with preoperative therapy. In young patients with bulky (stage III) disease, preoperative chemoradiotherapy may aid in resection by shrinking the tumor preoperatively, but it does not improve survival. Postoperative adjuvant therapy may be beneficial in patients with positive resection margins but is of little benefit in patients with no residual disease.

Surgical Therapy for Esophageal Cancer

With a malnourished patient, operation should be delayed 4 to 6 weeks to establish an anabolic state. In patients who undergo preoperative chemoradiation therapy for a bulky disease, operation should be delayed for 6 to 8 weeks after completion of treatment. In well-nourished patients with early-stage disease, surgery should proceed without delay.

Ivor-Lewis Esophagogastrectomy

The most common operation performed for cancer of the mid-distal esophagus is the Ivor Lewis esophagogastrectomy, performed through two incisions, a midline laparotomy and a right thoracotomy. With this two-field approach, the patient is placed supine, and the abdominal portion of the operation is performed first.

The abdomen is first inspected for the presence of metastases to the liver and celiac lymph nodes. The stomach is then completely mobilized from all attachments, starting at the GE junction and proceeding inferiorly. The left gastric artery is divided, as are the short gastric vessels and the left gastroepiploic artery. The right gastroepiploic artery *must* be carefully preserved, as this provides the majority of blood flow to the stomach when it is advanced into the chest. The right gastric artery may be divided if necessary for mobilization of the pylorus. A pyloroplasty or pyloromyotomy may be performed to prevent gastric stasis. The duodenum is mobilized from the retroperitoneum with a wide Kocher maneuver. The distal esophagus is then mobilized through the hiatus, which is widened to allow passage of the stomach.

Generally, the stomach is brought into the posterior mediastinum, but it also may be advanced to the neck through a substernal route if the esophagus is to be left in place. At this point, the stomach may be "tubularized" by dividing along the lesser curvature with a stapler, or it may be left intact. The abdomen is then closed, and the patient is rolled into the right lateral position for thoracotomy.

A standard right lateral thoracotomy is performed through the fifth or sixth thoracic interspace. The lung is deflated and retracted anteriorly. The esophagus is easily visualized in the posterior mediastinum, covered by a layer of parietal pleura. Lymph nodes adjacent to the esophagus are removed en bloc with the body of the esophagus. The esophagus is removed from its position in the posterior mediastinum, the vagus nerves are divided, and the stomach is advanced up through the diaphragmatic hiatus. The esophagus is divided 10 cm above the highest portion of the tumor. In a patient with BE, it is critical that the proximal margin of resection be clear of tumor and Barrett's epithelium. A two-layer anastomosis is then performed in the upper chest, by using nonabsorbable sutures. The anastomosis can be protected from reflux and leakage by wrapping a tongue of stomach around it. Once the anastomosis is complete, a nasogastric tube is placed through it, two chest tubes are placed, and the thorax is closed. Competency of the anastomosis is tested with a barium swallow after 5 to 7 days, and a soft diet is then started.

Transhiatal Esophagectomy

The transhiatal approach to esophagectomy avoids a thoracotomy and involves a cervical anastomosis. The patient is placed supine, and a midline laparotomy is performed. Gastric mobilization is performed, as described previously. After the esophageal hiatus is opened, dissection along the esophagus proceeds cephalad, first sharply, under direct vision, and then bluntly, by using tactile feedback provided by the surgeon's fingertips. Large vessels may be palpated and controlled with clips (Fig. 27-11).

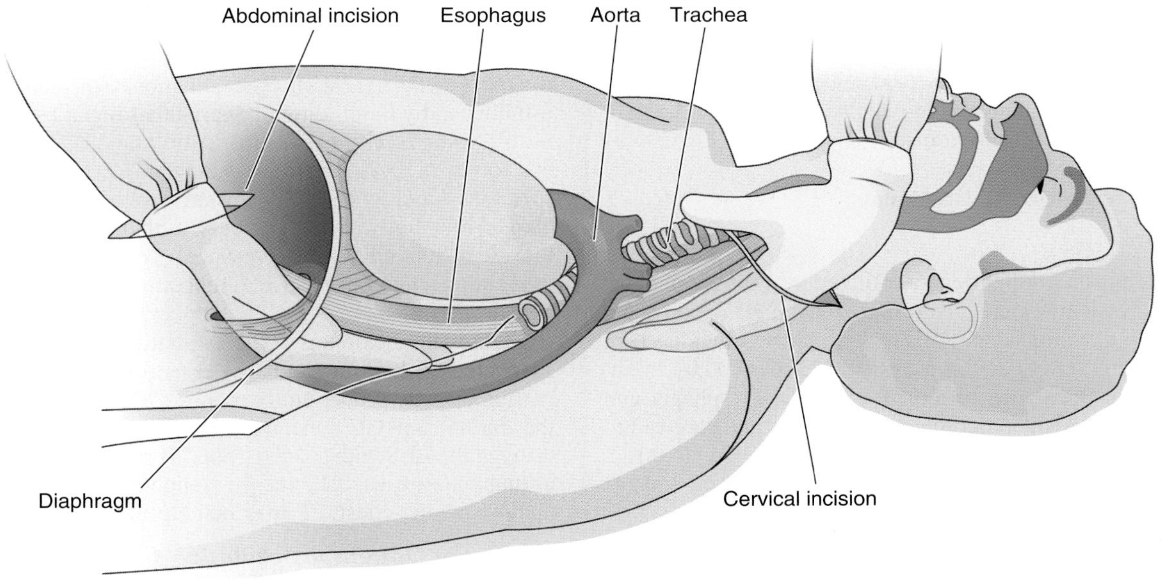

FIGURE 27–11 Transhiatal esophagectomy is performed with dissection along the esophagus by using tactile sensation, working from the abdomen and from the neck.

Cervical dissection begins through a left neck incision that exposes the esophagus in the prevertebral region. A drain is placed around the esophagus, and blunt dissection proceeds inferiorly with tactile control until the dissection from below is encountered, at which point the esophagus can be removed. The esophagus is retracted into the abdomen with a cloth tape sewn to the proximal resection margin. The tape is then attached to the proximal stomach, which is pulled back up through the tunnel into the neck. The stomach is tacked to the prevertebral fascia, and a two-layer anastomosis between the proximal esophagus and the stomach is fashioned, as previously described. A drain is placed in the neck, and both incisions are closed.

Transhiatal or Transthoracic Esophagectomy?

The Ivor-Lewis esophagectomy offers better lymph node clearance and a heartier anastomosis. The cervical anastomosis of a transhiatal approach is more prone to ischemia (greater reach for the stomach), with resultant leak or stricture. Cervical leaks, however, are much easier to manage than are those in the chest, which can be disastrous. Lymph node clearance is more complete with the transthoracic approach, but this has not translated to improved survival in randomized controlled studies. Perioperative morbidity, particularly the rate of pulmonary complications, is lower with the transhiatal approach.

Follow-up of Patients with Esophageal Cancer

Evidence-based guidelines for the follow-up of esophageal cancer do not exist. It is clear, however, that most recurrences occur within 2 years of resection. Typical follow-up includes an annual CT scan of the chest and upper abdomen for 5 years after esophagectomy. Endoscopy is reserved for the investigation of symptoms.

Esophageal Motor Disorders

Achalasia

Achalasia is an idiopathic motor disorder of the esophagus, characterized by aperistalsis of the esophageal body and impaired relaxation of the LES. The reported incidence of achalasia in Western countries is 0.4 to 1.1 per 100,000/year, with a peak incidence in the fifth decade. Dysphagia and regurgitation are the predominant symptoms and can lead to weight loss and pulmonary complications. In addition, achalasia is associated with a 16-fold increased risk of esophageal cancer.

Chagas' disease is a related disorder endemic to Central America and parts of South America. It results from infection with the parasite *Trypanosoma cruzi* and, like achalasia, involves degeneration of the myenteric plexus neurons. Clinically, Chagas' disease is indistinguishable from achalasia, and the treatment is identical.

Pathophysiology. Achalasia is associated with dysfunction of the myenteric plexus of the esophagus. Histologically, this plexus is replaced with dense lymphocytic infiltration and a loss of ganglion cells. A selective loss of inhibitory neurons occurs, with sparing of the stimulatory cholinergic innervation. This leads to failure of the LES to relax with swallowing.

Clinical Presentation. The most frequent findings in patients with achalasia are dysphagia, regurgitation, and weight loss. Nearly all patients with achalasia have one or all of these findings. Noncardiac chest pain and heartburn are reported by half of all individuals with achalasia, often leading to the incorrect diagnosis of GERD.

Differential Diagnosis. For patients with dysphagia, it is important to rule out **pseudoachalasia**. More than half of the cases of pseudoachalasia are caused by tumors of the cardia or GE junction. Other causes are lesions that result in extrinsic compression of the GE junction, such as tumors of the left lobe of the liver or diaphragm, bulky lymph node disease from lymphoma or metastatic cancer, and aortic aneurysms. Pseudoachalasia also may occur as part of a paraneoplastic syndrome in the absence of external compression. Scleroderma may mimic achalasia symptoms, as can certain neurologic disorders, such as Parkinson's disease.

Evaluation of Achalasia. The first study for a patient with dysphagia is a barium swallow. The characteristic appearance of a dilated esophagus with a "bird's beak" taper of the distal esophagus is suggestive of the diagnosis (Fig. 27-12). The diagnosis of achalasia is established by the finding of aperistalsis on an esophageal-motility study. High pressure, simultaneous contractions are found in 10% (vigorous achalasia), whereas 90% of patients have weak or absent contractions in the esophageal body. Most patients with achalasia have an elevated resting LES pressure (>25 mmHg), with associated incomplete LES relaxation (nadir pressure, >10 mmHg).

EGD is the next step in the evaluation of a patient with suspected achalasia and is essential for ruling out malignancy. A proper study requires a retroflexed view of the cardia and GE junction. The endoscope should pass through the LES with an easy "pop." If passage is obstructed, a malignant cause should be sought. EUS, as well as abdominal and chest CT, may be helpful in this situation.

Treatment Options in Achalasia

Medical therapy of achalasia is targeted at decreasing LES pressure to allow the esophagus to empty. Calcium channel

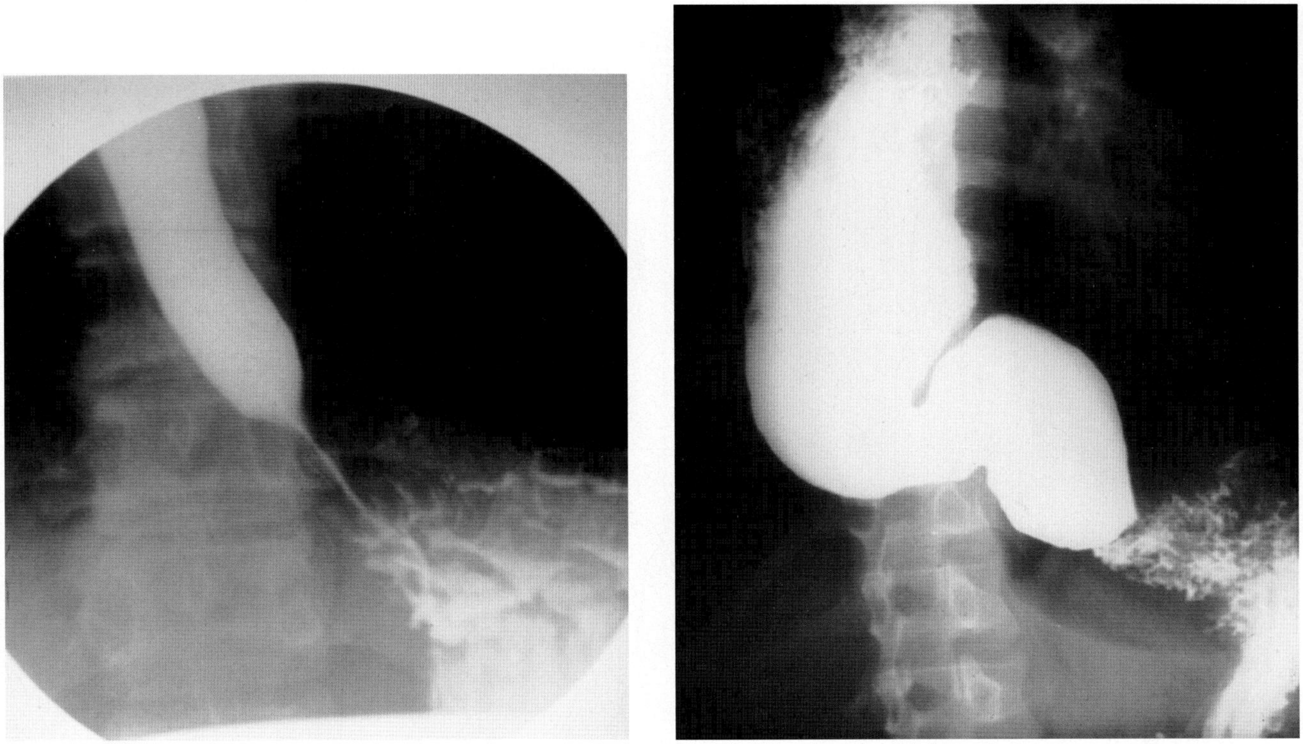

A B

FIGURE 27–12 The characteristic radiologic finding of achalasia is the bird's beak esophagus. The esophageal body may be normal in caliber (*A*), or it may be grossly dilated with a sigmoid appearance to the esophagus (*B*).

blockers and nitrates have been used with little success. They are reserved for patients with mild symptoms or those unable to tolerate invasive procedures.

Balloon Dilation. Pneumatic dilation is designed to rupture the fibers of the LES and is performed by rapid inflation of a 3- to 4-cm balloon in the distal esophagus under fluoroscopic guidance. A postprocedure barium swallow is necessary to rule out esophageal perforation, which occurs in 4% to 7% of patients. Most series report good to excellent results at 2-year follow-up in 65% to 80% of patients, but more than half will require repeated dilation. One long-term series reported a 50% remission rate at 12 years with a median of four treatments. The best results are seen in patients older than 40 years and in those with postdilation LES pressure less than 10. In patients with a tortuous, or sigmoid, esophagus, it may be difficult to place the balloon dilator safely.

Botulinum Toxin (BOTOX). BOTOX blocks release of acetylcholine at the neuromuscular junction and may be injected directly into the LES with endoscopic guidance. Symptom relief is seen in 70% to 100% of patients at 1 month. However, most patients require repeated injections by 6 to 9 months, and 1-year remission rates are low (~30%). In addition, the response to repeated injections is limited by antibody formation. BOTOX treatment is safe and is typically reserved for the elderly patient who is not a good risk for surgery.

Surgical Management. Surgical treatment of achalasia involves division of the fibers of the LES, a procedure first described in 1913 by Ernest Heller. The operation may be performed by using an abdominal or thoracic approach. The laparoscopic approach has largely replaced both laparotomy and thoracotomy for performance of an esophagomyotomy. To ensure that sphincter division is complete, it is recommended that the myotomy be 6 to 8 cm in length and extend at least 2 cm below the LES onto the anterior surface of the stomach. An adequate Heller myotomy should decrease the resting pressure of the LES to less than 10 mmHg.

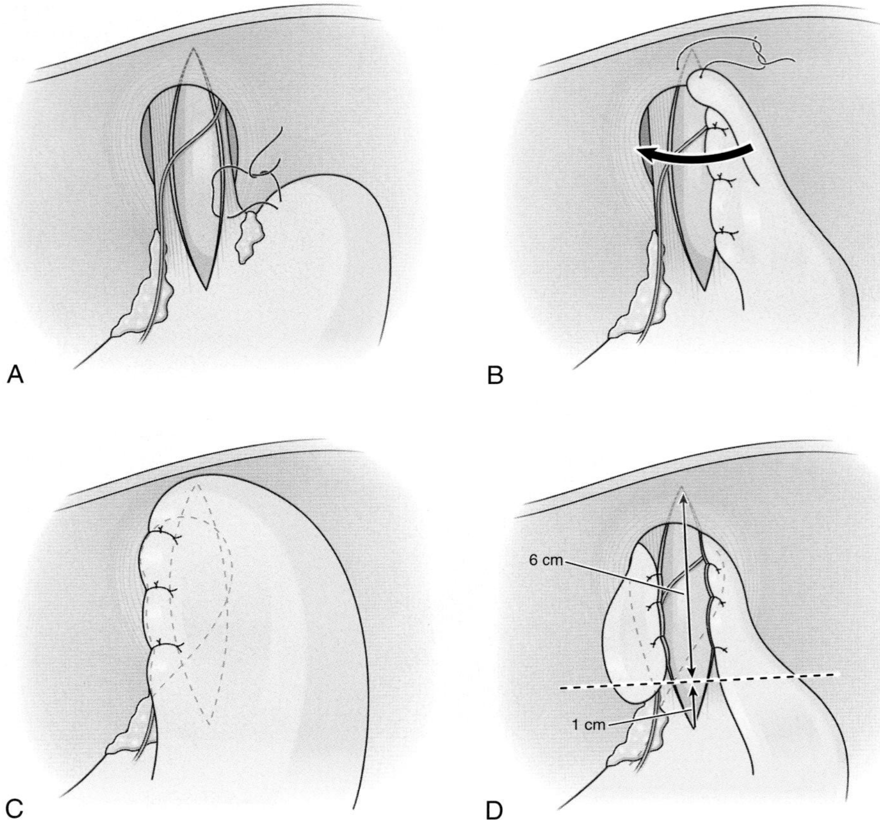

FIGURE 27–13 Abdominal Heller myotomy is performed by dividing the lower esophageal and proximal gastric musculature. *A–C*, An anterior fundoplication (Dor) covers the exposed esophageal mucosa. *D*, A posterior fundoplication (Toupet) holds the myotomy open. (Adapted from Hunter J, Trus T, Branum G, Waring J: Laparoscopic Heller myotomy and fundoplication for achalasia. Ann Surg 225(6):655–664, 1997, with permission.)

Complete division of the LES will lead to GERD in 40% of patients with achalasia if they are followed up long enough. For this reason, a partial fundoplication is recommended to help prevent postoperative reflux. The two partial fundoplications most commonly used are an anterior (Dor) 180-degree fundoplication or a posterior (Toupet) 270-degree fundoplication (Fig. 27-13). Both types of fundoplication appear nearly equivalent in their function. Even after fundoplication, 10% to 15% of patients may demonstrate subjective and objective findings of gastroesophageal reflux. A complete (Nissen) fundoplication is not recommended, however, given the risk of dysphagia.

Outcomes of Heller Myotomy. Laparoscopic Heller myotomy and fundoplication is the treatment of choice for patients with achalasia, offering durable symptom relief in 85% to 95% of patients. Even with a massively dilated or tortuous esophagus, Heller myotomy provides relief in 75% of patients. Rarely, esophagectomy may be necessary in patients with refractory dysphagia after Heller myotomy. Often these patients have associated peptic strictures of the esophagus, the consequence of post-myotomy GERD.

Spastic Disorders of the Esophagus

The most common of these rare disorders is *diffuse esophageal spasm* (DES), characterized by chest pain, dysphagia, and episodes of high-amplitude aperistaltic contractions that alternate with normal peristaltic contractions. Long esophageal myotomy has been advocated as treatment for this condition, but the outcomes are not sufficiently convincing to make a recommendation for surgical treatment of DES.

In patients with *hypertensive LES*, resting LES pressure is elevated (>45 mmHg), while esophageal body function remains normal. In these patients, pseudo-achalasia should be ruled out with a CT scan. Otherwise, treatment options are the same as those for the patient with achalasia.

Nutcracker esophagus is characterized by chest pain, in conjunction with high-amplitude peristalsis and normal LES function. Most commonly, this finding is associated with GERD, and treatment should address the reflux symptoms rather than the motility findings.

Esophageal Diverticula. These conditions are divided into traction and pulsion diverticula. Traction diverticula occur in the midesophagus, usually associated with a chronic inflammatory disorder such as tuberculous lymphadenitis. The sclerotic process *pulls* the esophageal wall into the form of a diverticulum. Once common, traction diverticula are now relatively rare. Pulsion diverticula result from esophageal motility disorders and occur above the upper and lower esophageal sphincters.

Zencker's Diverticulum. This diverticulum is a protrusion of the pharyngeal mucosa between the inferior pharyngeal constrictor and the cricopharyngeus muscle. The Zencker's diverticulum extends into the prevertebral space and is easily diagnosed on a barium swallow. Patients with a Zencker's diverticulum may be initially seen with cervical dysphagia, frequent aspiration events, and troublesome halitosis.

The Zencker's diverticulum is *always* associated with cricopharyngeal achalasia, a hypertensive, nonrelaxing UES. Treatment of the Zencker's diverticulum must include myotomy of the UES. This is usually accomplished through a left cervical incision. A small diverticulum may be suspended against the prevertebral fascia, but larger diverticula are usually excised by placing a surgical stapler across the neck of the diverticulum, with an esophageal dilator in place to preserve the caliber of the upper esophageal inlet. This treatment is successful in greater than 90% of patients with symptomatic Zencker's diverticulum. Effective endoscopic techniques for treatment of these diverticula also have been developed and are gaining in popularity. However, they do not treat the underlying motility disorder.

Epiphrenic Diverticulum. Patients with epiphrenic diverticula often complain of regurgitation or chest pain associated with food stuck in the diverticular sac. Management of the epiphrenic diverticulum should include treatment of the associated esophageal-motility disorder. Diverticulectomy is generally performed in association with Heller myotomy (in the patient with achalasia) or long esophageal myotomy (in the patient with DES). A laparoscopic or thoracoscopic approach is usually chosen, depending on the location of the diverticulum.

Esophageal Perforation

Esophageal perforation may be spontaneous (Boorhaave's syndrome), traumatic, or iatrogenic. Spontaneous esophageal perforation is associated with forceful prolonged retching. The clinical presentation is usually the development of acute systemic toxicity, chest pain, and pleural effusion after a spell of violent and extended vomiting. The diagnosis is established by performing a water-soluble contrast radiograph. If the perforation is fresh (<24 hours), thoracotomy and a repair of the perforation with chest drainage is generally successful. Usually, the repair is buttressed with pericardium or pleura.

When the perforation is more than 24 hours old, primary repair usually fails. Several alternative approaches have been described. Esophageal exclusion involves ligation of the GE junction with a suture or division with a stapler. A gastrostomy tube is placed for nutrition, and a cervical esophagostomy (spit fistula) is performed to drain the saliva. Esophageal exclusion is accompanied by chest-tube drainage. This radical procedure requires a subsequent esophageal reconstruction with stomach or colon interposition. Other treatments include the placement of a large T-tube at the site of the esophageal perforation with chest drainage, or the immediate resection and reconstruction of the lower esophagus.

Iatrogenic perforation of the esophagus has been associated with numerous endoscopic and surgical procedures, including stent placement and endoscopic sclerotherapy. If a water-contrast barium swallow and chest CT demonstrate a contained leak, treatment may be restricted to the use of antibiotics. When the leak extends into the chest cavity or abdomen or is associated with systemic toxicity, repair or exclusion must be used as described earlier. Perforation of the esophagus from blunt or penetrating trauma is diagnosed and managed in the same way as other forms of perforation.

Caustic Esophageal Stricture

Various substances may cause extensive damage to the esophagus when ingested. The alkali, or lye, stricture is usually associated with the ingestion of liquid drain cleaner and may be fatal. In survivors, a long stricture will develop. This condition is particularly prominent in the pediatric population or is associated with suicide attempts in adults. Esophageal dilation is primary therapy for these strictures but may result in perforation.

In the pediatric population, colon interposition is generally used for esophageal replacement because it is a better-size match to the esophagus than is the stomach, and it can be brought high into the neck without vascular compromise. It also is used in adults when gastric injury, cancer, or prior surgery precludes the use of a stomach conduit. The best colonic segment to use for esophageal reconstruction is the left colon, brought to the neck in an isoperistaltic fashion with blood supply from the left colic artery. The marginal artery of Drummond nourishes the transverse colon in the new location (Fig. 27-14). The right colon has a less-reliable blood supply and is a poor size match for the upper esophagus, but it may be used when a marginal artery is absent in the left

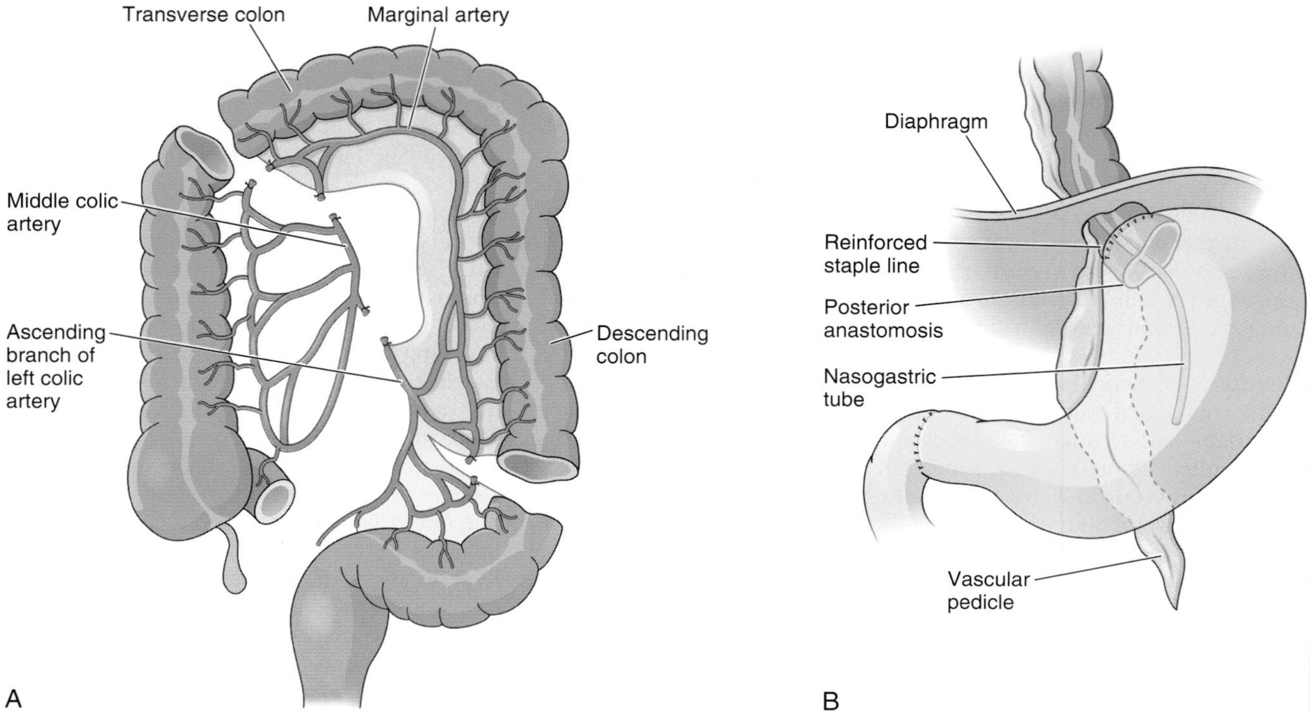

FIGURE 27–14 *A*, The best segment of colon to use for esophageal replacement is the left colon, which requires an intact marginal artery to supply the transverse colon, which is advanced into the neck. *B*, The completed colon graft includes an anastomosis in the neck, an anastomosis in the stomach, a pyloroplasty, and a colonic anastomosis.

colon. Antiperistaltic left colon grafts based on the middle colic artery may be used in desperate circumstances, but they tend to function more poorly than isoperistaltic grafts.

Suggested Reading

Balaji NS, Peters JH: Minimally invasive surgery for esophageal motility disorders. Surg Clin North Am 82(4):763–782, 2002.

DeMeester SR, DeMeester TR: Columnar mucosa and intestinal metaplasia of the esophagus: Fifty years of controversy. Ann Surg 231(3):303–321, 2000.

Enzinger PC, Mayer RJ: Esophageal cancer. N Engl J Med 349(23):2241–2252, 2003.

Hunter JG, Pellegrini CA (eds): Surgical Clinics of North America: Surgery of the Esophagus. Philadelphia, WB Saunders, 1997.

Pearson FG, Hiebert CA, Deslauriers J, et al: Esophageal Surgery. New York, Churchill Livingstone, 1995.

Spiess AE, Kahrilas PJ: Treating achalasia: from whalebone to laparoscope. JAMA 280(7):638–642, 1998.

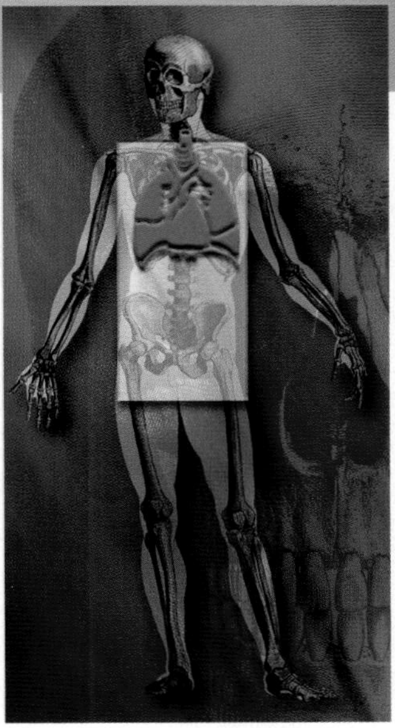

SECTION VII

CARDIOTHORACIC

Chapter 28

Disorders of the Trachea, Chest Wall, Pleura, Mediastinum, and Lung

HAROLD L. LAZAR, MD

Thoracic Surgery Incisions

The most frequently used incision for thoracic surgical procedures is the posterolateral thoracotomy (Fig. 28-1). This incision provides good exposure for all types of pulmonary and esophageal surgery, as well as access to the mediastinum for resection of mediastinal masses. The patient is placed in a lateral position on the operating table, and a soft roll is placed beneath the axilla. The lower leg is flexed to a 70-degree angle, and the upper leg is extended straight, with a pillow placed between the knees. The hips are stabilized with adhesive tape. The lower arm is placed on a padded armboard, and the upper is draped above it, with pillows between. The incision extends from a point lateral and posterior to the nipple to a fingerbreadth below the tip of the scapula and extends upward between the scapula and the spine. The subcutaneous tissues and the latissimus dorsi muscles are divided; usually an attempt is made to preserve the serratus anterior muscle. The ribs are counted, and the appropriate interspace is selected. For upper lobe lobectomies and pneumonectomies, the 4th or 5th interspace is selected. For lower and middle lobe lobectomies, the 5th or 6th interspace provides excellent exposure. Esophageal resections are usually approached from the 6th or 7th interspace. The chest may be entered by resecting a full rib or merely dividing it posteriorly (shingling). When a lung biopsy or an excision of a pulmonary nodule is required, a limited lateral incision may be all that is required. In a lateral muscle-sparing thoracotomy incision, the latissimus and serratus muscles are mobilized and retracted rather than divided.

The anterolateral thoracotomy incision is used less frequently. It is best used for lung biopsies and quick access to the chest and mediastinum in trauma cases. The median sternotomy incision is most popular for cardiac procedures. However, it also frequently is used for resection of bilateral pulmonary nodules and metastases, and resection of bilateral bullous disease. The axillary incision is best used for first-rib resections, thoracic sympathectomy, and resection of apical blebs. The anterior median sternotomy (Chamberlain procedure) involves removing a portion of the costochondral cartilage to gain access to the aortopulmonary nodes on the left, and to the anterior, mediastinal, and inframammary nodes on the right. It is especially useful for demonstrating mediastinal involvement with lung neoplasms and performing biopsies of mediastinal masses. The cervical mediastinoscopy incision allows sampling of the right paratracheal nodes. A curvilinear incision is made just above the thoracic inlet, and the pretracheal fascia is entered. A mediastinoscope is inserted, and nodal tissue is then sampled.

Trachea

Anatomy

The superior portion of the trachea receives its blood supply from the inferior thyroid artery. The middle and lower segments of the trachea receive blood flow from numerous sources, including the subclavian, intercostal, internal mammary, and bronchial arteries. Because the blood supply to the trachea comes mainly from end vessels and segments, it is important not to devascularize it by total circumferential dissection. Because the blood vessels enter the trachea laterally, it is best to dissect in an anterioposterior plane. This makes it easier to obtain more length during reconstructive procedures, especially when the trachea must be separated from the esophagus.

Primary Neoplasms of the Trachea

Adenoid cystic carcinoma and squamous cell carcinoma are the two most common neoplasms and comprise three

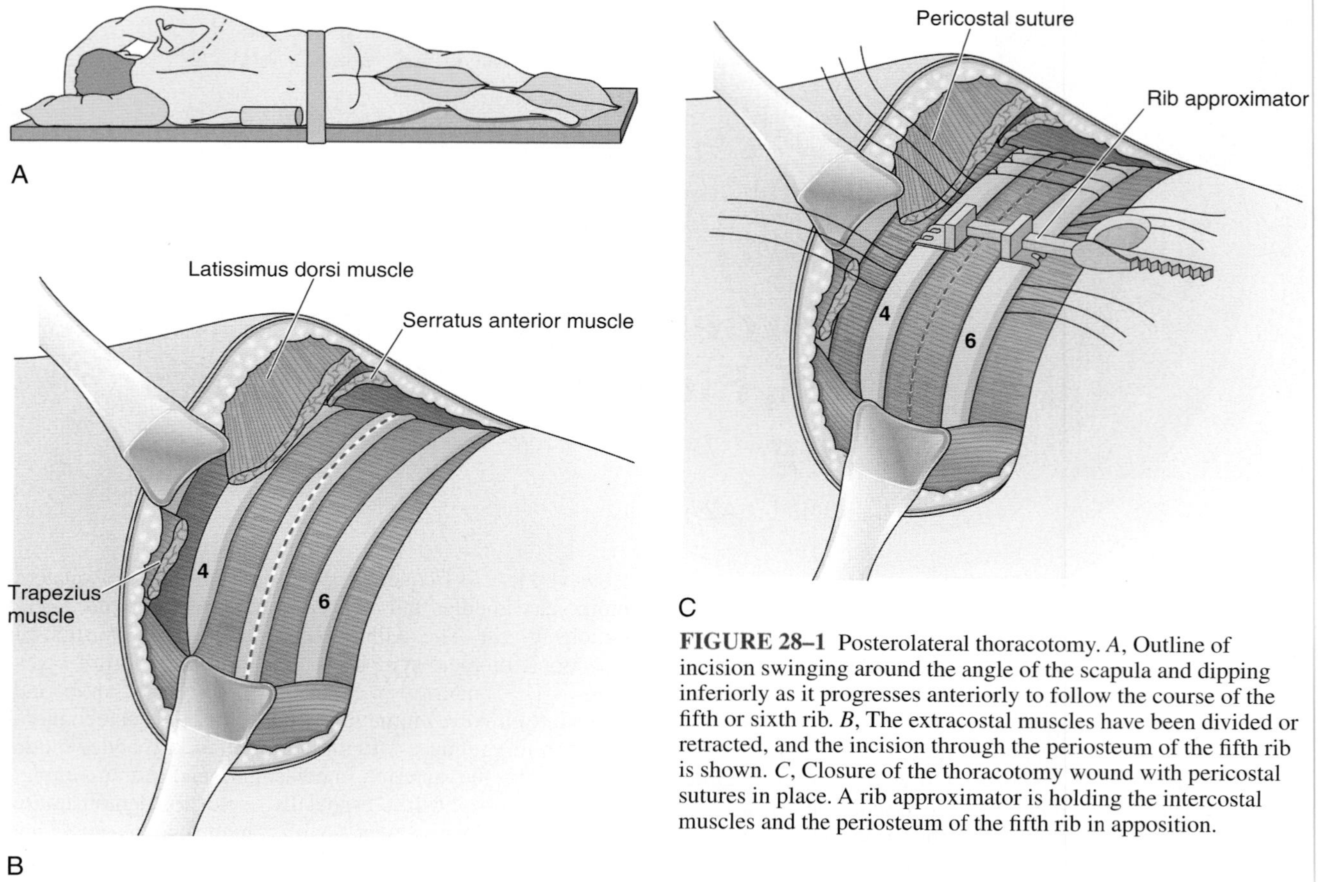

FIGURE 28–1 Posterolateral thoracotomy. *A*, Outline of incision swinging around the angle of the scapula and dipping inferiorly as it progresses anteriorly to follow the course of the fifth or sixth rib. *B*, The extracostal muscles have been divided or retracted, and the incision through the periosteum of the fifth rib is shown. *C*, Closure of the thoracotomy wound with pericostal sutures in place. A rib approximator is holding the intercostal muscles and the periosteum of the fifth rib in apposition.

fourths of all primary tracheal tumors. Adenoid cystic carcinoma is a slowly growing tumor, which tends to displace mediastinal structures rather than invade them directly. Perineural and submucosal spread is very common. The lung and bone are the most common sites for distant metastases. Squamous cell carcinoma of the trachea has numerous presentations. It may be well localized, ulcerated, or diffuse, involving the entire length of the trachea. Pulmonary and mediastinal involvement may already be present in nearly one third of patients who have this lesion.

Surgical resection is the best method for treating primary tracheal neoplasms. However, approximately one fourth of patients have tumors that are too extensive for surgical management. These patients are best treated with radiation therapy and a tracheostomy for airway protection, when necessary. In a large series of patients surviving surgical resection, 70% were alive without evidence of recurrent tumor; 40% of these had squamous cell carcinoma, and 75% had adenoid cystic carcinoma. All patients underwent postoperative radiation therapy, which has been shown to improve survival and decrease local recurrence.

Postintubation Tracheal Injuries

The most common indication for tracheal reconstruction involves a postintubation injury. Edema and circumferential erosion of the tracheal wall may occur even after only 48 hours of endotracheal intubation. Patients usually initially have dyspnea on exertion, wheezing, and stridor after extubation. Resection of the involved obstructing segments and tracheal reconstruction is the treatment of choice. If the patient's overall condition will not permit a reconstruction, bronchoscopic dilatation, reinstitution of a tracheostomy, or placement of a Silastic T tube that stents the airway may result in good palliation. The most important treatment of postintubation injury lies in its prevention. The use of large-volume, low-pressure cuffs that better conform to the shape of the trachea has resulted in a dramatic decrease in the incidence of postintubation injuries.

Tracheal Reconstruction

Before performing a tracheal resection, the surgeon must accurately determine the amount of trachea to be resected and the amount of normal tissue that is available for reconstruction. Anesthetic induction is obtained with an inhalation technique. Dilatation may be necessary so that the endotracheal tube can provide adequate ventilation during the procedure. Although the endotracheal tube may not be placed through the stricture or lesion, adequate ventilation of the distal lumen can still be obtained. High-frequency jet ventilation may be especially helpful for these cases. An anterior collar incision is used for lesions of the upper half of the trachea, whereas lesions of the lower half of the trachea are best approached through a posterolateral thoracotomy in the fourth interspace. When performing an upper tracheal reconstruction, as much as 4 cm of trachea may be safely resected without tension. If tension is present despite flexion of 35 to 45 degrees, a laryngeal release may be performed in which the larynx is mobilized by dividing the thyrohyoid muscles, the thyrohyoid membrane, and the superior cornua of the thyroid cartilage. Tracheal reapproximation is achieved with absorbable suture material. Every effort is made to extubate the patient after the procedure. A suture is placed from beneath the chin to the anterior chest wall to keep the neck in flexion for several days to minimize tension on the anastomosis. In performing lower tracheal resections, as much as 3 cm of trachea can be safely removed without tension. A maneuver that has been helpful in decreasing tension on the anastomosis involves dissecting the hilar contents of the lung and dividing the attachments around the carina. A pleural or pericardial fat flap is often used to decrease the incidence of anastomotic complications.

Tracheostomy and Cricothyroidotomy

The most common indication for tracheostomy in practice today is in those patients who will require prolonged mechanical ventilation. Other common indications include obstructing upper airway tumors, patients with chronic neurologic disorders who cannot clear their secretions or are at high risk for aspiration, and patients undergoing major head and neck resections. A short incision is made over the second tracheal ring (Fig. 28-2). The platysma is divided, and the midline fascia is entered. Occasionally, the thyroid isthmus should be divided. The trachea is entered between the second and third rings. The previous endotracheal tube is removed as the tracheostomy tube is inserted. If the tracheostomy is placed above the second ring, erosion into the first ring may result in damage to the cricoid cartilage. Low placement of the tracheostomy tube may result in a fistula between the trachea and innominate artery. With this complication, the patient has exsanguinating hemorrhage through the tracheostomy tube. When this occurs, immediately inflating the endotracheal tube to attempt to tamponade the artery may be lifesaving. The patient should be taken immediately to the operating room, where a median sternotomy incision with an extension into the right neck provides good exposure of the innominate artery and trachea. The innominate artery is oversewn at the bifurcation of the subclavian and carotid branches. A nonabsorbable suture is used to close the tracheal fistula. Muscle is placed to buttress the suture line.

Recently, the technique of percutaneous tracheostomy was developed. A transtracheal guide wire is placed in the trachea. The tracheal opening is progressively dilated until an adequate-sized tracheostomy tube can be inserted. The advantage of this technique is that it can be easily done at the bedside with a local anesthetic.

A cricothyroidotomy is an alternative to a tracheostomy. In this technique, after a skin incision over the thyroid cartilage, the cricothyroid membrane is punctured and, after progressive dilatation, a tracheostomy tube is inserted. One of the disadvantages of this technique is the increased risk for vocal cord injury.

Sternum and Chest Wall

Anatomy

The chest wall consists of the sternum, 10 pairs of ribs and their costal cartilages, 2 pairs of ribs without cartilages (floating ribs), and 12 thoracic vertebrae. Each intercostal space consists of 3 layers of muscles: the external, internal, and transversus thoracic muscles, and a vein, artery, and nerve that course along the lower edge of each rib. This anatomic fact is of importance when performing a thoracentesis or inserting a thoracostomy tube.

Congenital Deformities: Pectus Excavatum

Pectus excavatum is the most common congenital deformity of the sternum. The depression starts just above the xiphoid and continues to the sternomanubrial junction. The first and second ribs, along with their corresponding costal cartilages, are usually not involved. The vast majority of patients are asymptomatic; however, nearly a third may have frequent lower respiratory tract infections and asthma. The primary indication for surgical intervention in these patients is the desire for cosmetic improvement. Respiratory insufficiency with exercise limitation and recurrent pulmonary infections also are indications for surgical intervention. Surgery should be performed before the child reaches school age (5 years old) to minimize the psychological impact of the deformity. The best cosmetic results also are achieved in this age group because the deformity is usually limited to the costal cartilages, with minimal rib involvement.

The repair of a pectus excavatum involves the following principles (Fig. 28-3).

1. A midline incision (or a transverse inframammary incision in girls) is made, and the pectoralis muscle is reflected laterally to expose all the costal cartilages.
2. The deformed costal cartilages on both sides of the sternum are resected subperichondrially for the full extent of the deformity. The remaining perichondrium

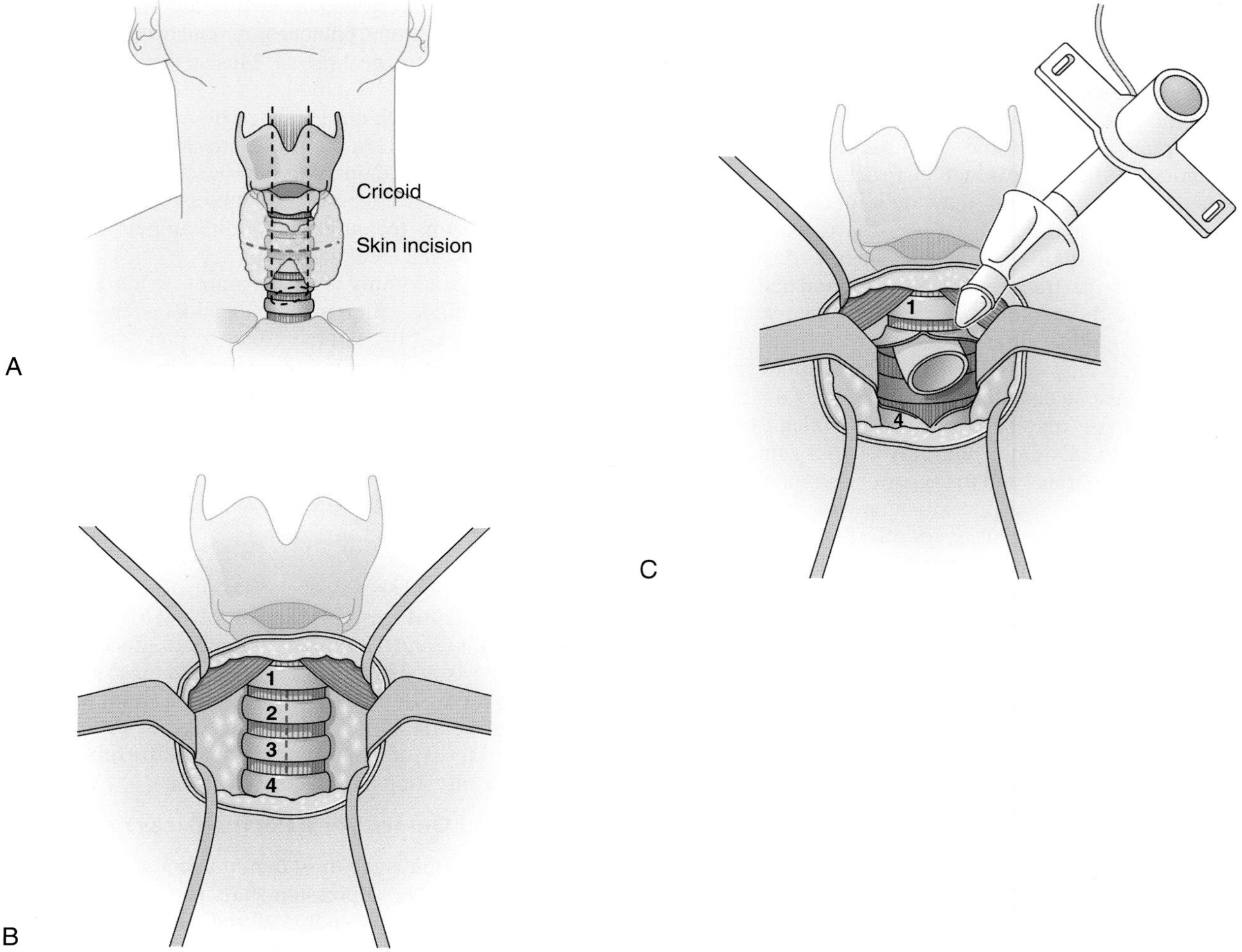

FIGURE 28–2 Technique of tracheostomy. *A*, An endotracheal airway is in place. With the patient's neck extended and centered in the midline, a short horizontal incision is made over the second or third tracheal ring after the level of the cricoid cartilage has been carefully palpated. The first and fourth tracheal cartilages are numbered. *B*, Following horizontal division of the platysma, the strap muscles are separated in the midline, the cricoid is identified, and the thyroid isthmus usually is divided and sutured to allow easy access to the second and third tracheal rings. The second and third rings are incised vertically. Occasionally an additional partial incision of the fourth ring is necessary. *C*, Smooth thyroid pole retractors are used to spread the opening in the trachea. The endotracheal tube is withdrawn to a point just above the incision. The tracheostomy tube is introduced with a small amount of water-soluble lubricant and with its large-volume cuff collapsed. The endotracheal airway is not removed until it is demonstrated that the tracheostomy tube is properly seated and permits suitable air exchange. Closure is made with simple skin sutures. The flange of the tracheostomy tube is both sutured to the skin and tied with the usual tapes around the neck. On a rare occasion when an airway cannot be established from above, an emergency incision may be necessary over the cricothyroid membrane for rapid establishment of a temporary airway. (From Grillo H: Tracheostomy and its complications. In Sabiston DC (ed): Textbook of Surgery. Philadelphia, WB Saunders, 1977, p 2058, with permission.)

will re-form new cartilages within several months in the correct anatomic position.

3. The sternum is separated from the xiphoid and intercostal bundles to help in its mobilization.
4. A transverse osteotomy is made on the posterior surface of the sternum through the sternomanubrial joint, allowing it to be lifted forward in its corrected position. This position is maintained by a bone graft that is wedged into the osteotomy.

This procedure is well tolerated and is associated with no mortality and minimal morbidity. The cosmetic results are excellent.

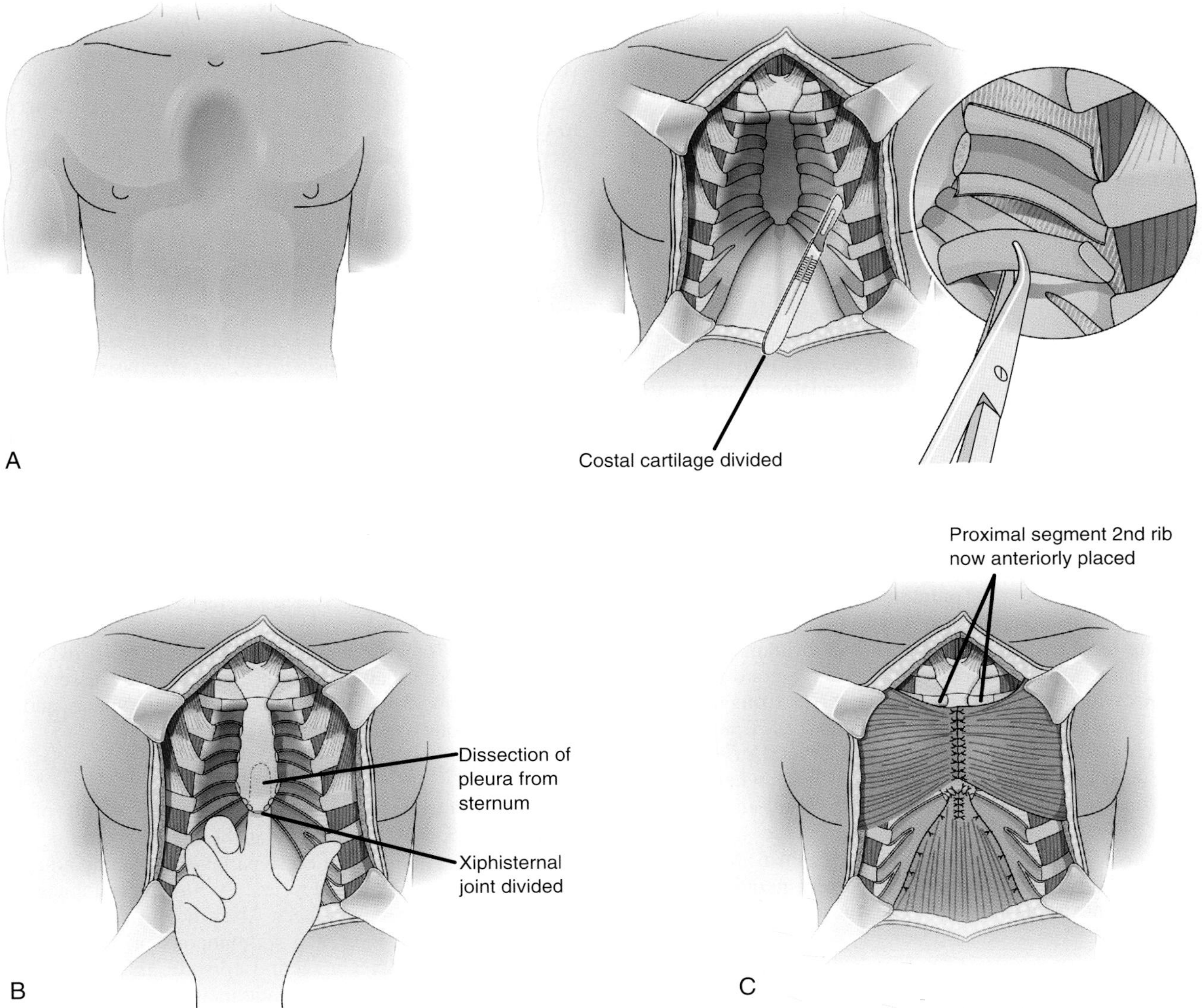

FIGURE 28–3 Repair of pectus excavatum. *A*, After exposure of the sternum, subperichondrial resection of all affected costal cartilages is performed. *B*, The xiphoid is excised, the sternum is freed from the substernal tissue and pleura using blunt dissection, a wedge osteotomy is created, and the sternum is displaced anteriorly. *C*, After placement of a substernal drain (not shown), the pectoral muscles are closed in the midline and the subcutaneous tissue and skin are closed in layers. (From Ravitch MM: Congenital deformities of the chest wall. In Sabiston DC (ed): Textbook of Surgery. Philadelphia, WB Saunders, 1997, p 1893, with permission.)

Tumors of the Chest Wall

The majority of chest-wall tumors are malignant. The most common include malignant fibrous histiocytoma (fibrosarcoma), chondrosarcoma, and rhabdomyosarcoma. Cartilaginous tumors (osteochondroma and chondroma) are the most common primary benign tumors.

Chest-wall neoplasms usually are first seen as slowly enlarging asymptomatic masses; however, with growth, they usually become painful. Pain is more commonly associated with malignant lesions. Magnetic resonance imaging (MRI) is helpful in visualizing the mass in different planes and distinguishing it from nerves and blood vessels. A computed tomography (CT) scan will help to determine whether metastatic lesions to the lung, liver, and kidney exist, as well as to regional lymph nodes. The only method of determining the diagnosis of a chest-wall lesion is by biopsy. An excisional biopsy rather than an incisional or needle biopsy should be done. This allows more accurate diagnosis of the lesion.

Wide resection of a primary chest-wall malignancy is the treatment of choice. At least a 4-cm margin of normal tissue on all sides should be obtained. The entire involved bone should be resected for high-grade malignancies. For rib neoplasms, the involved rib is removed in its entirety along with the costal arch for an anterior tumor, as well as the partial resection of two ribs above and below the tumor. For neoplasms involving the sternum and manubrium, the entire involved bone and bilateral costal cartilages are resected along with adjacent lung, thymus, pericardium, and chest-wall muscles.

Because wide resection is the mainstay for successful outcomes in the treatment of chest-wall neoplasms, dependable methods for chest-wall reconstruction are mandatory. Defects smaller than 5 cm anteriorly and 10 cm posteriorly, high on the chest wall, usually do not require reconstruction. All larger defects will require some type of reconstructive procedure. Stabilization of the bony thorax is best accomplished with prosthetic material. Soft tissue defects are best reconstructed with a muscle flap. When muscle flaps fail because of tension and necrosis, omentum can be mobilized from the abdomen. Although it has no structural stability of its own, it can be lifesaving in covering exposed large vessels, pulmonary parenchyma, and the myocardium.

Long-term survival of patients with primary chest-wall malignancies is dependent on the cell type and the extent of chest-wall resection. In a large series from the Mayo Clinic, the overall 5-year survival rate was 57%. Patients with chondrosarcomas had a 5-year survival of 96% after wide resection compared with only 70% when a local excision was performed. Patients with rhabdomyosarcoma had a 5-year survival of 70%; however, the survival rate was only 38% for patients with malignant fibrous histiocytoma. The development of a recurrent neoplasm had a poor prognosis, as only 17% of these patients survived 5 years.

The Pleura

Pneumothorax

A pneumothorax occurs when air enters the pleural space as a result of a pleural disruption. This disruption can be caused by a ruptured bleb, trauma, or an injured bronchus or esophagus. Pleural rupture results in entry but not exit of air in the pleural space. Inspiration results in a greater negative intrapleural pressure, thus further increasing the amount of air within the pleural space. During expiration, this results in a tension pneumothorax, which causes a shift of the mediastinum, which decreases venous return and results in a decreased cardiac output, cardiovascular collapse, hypoxemia, and cyanosis.

When the pneumothorax is small, the patients are asymptomatic. Patients with larger pneumothoraces will have diminished or absent breath sounds on the involved side. Cyanosis may be present, and a crunching sound (Hamman's sign) can be heard with mediastinal emphysema. Patients with a tension pneumothorax also may have neck-vein distention, and the trachea and cardiac apex are deviated toward the uninvolved side. Most pneumothoraces can be seen on a posteroanterior (PA) chest radiograph taken on inspiration. Air is seen as a hyperlucent space devoid of pulmonary markings in the periphery of the hemithorax. In patients thought to have a pneumothorax, but in whom no abnormalities are seen on an inspiratory chest radiograph, an expiratory film should be obtained. Expiration reduces lung volume and increases the radiographic density of the lung, thereby increasing the contrast between the lung and the air in the pleural space. In patients with bullous emphysema, it may be difficult to visualize a pneumothorax. Differentiating bullae from pneumothorax is critical because inserting a chest tube in a bulla can result in disastrous consequences. A CT scan is helpful in these patients because it visualizes the septae within the bullae, thus differentiating it from a pneumothorax. It is critical that after the lung is expanded, a repeated chest radiograph be obtained to rule out any other disease processes, including parenchymal masses, interstitial and parenchymal infiltrates, and pleural disease. In working up a patient for a pneumothorax, one also should consider and rule out other conditions that mimic this disease, including myocardial ischemia, acute aortic dissection, pulmonary embolism, spontaneous esophageal rupture, and a perforated peptic ulcer.

Primary Spontaneous Pneumothorax

Primary spontaneous pneumothorax is the result of a ruptured bleb, most commonly at the apices of the upper lobes. The vast majority of these patients are young adults; 85% are younger than 40 years. A higher incidence is found among cigarette smokers. After the initial episode, a 20% to 50% recurrence of a spontaneous primary pneumothorax occurs. After a second episode, the recurrence rate increases to 60% to 80%. Patients with large cysts tend to have a higher recurrence rate.

Secondary Spontaneous Pneumothorax

The most common etiology for a secondary spontaneous pneumothorax is chronic obstructive pulmonary disease (COPD). In contrast to primary spontaneous pneumothoraces, patients with a secondary spontaneous pneumothorax tend to be older (45 to 65 years) and have a higher morbidity and mortality because of its association with underlying pulmonary diseases. Other causes of a secondary spontaneous pneumothorax include malignant neoplasms and tuberculosis.

Management of Spontaneous Pneumothorax

A stable, small pneumothorax (<20%) in a patient who is asymptomatic is usually observed without any intervention.

These patients must, however, be monitored closely and have a repeated chest radiograph in 48 hours. Approximately 1.25% of all intrapleural air is absorbed daily from the pleural cavity; hence it will take weeks for the lung to expand fully. However, an increase in the size of the pneumothorax or the development of any symptoms is an indication for admission to the hospital and insertion of a thoracostomy (chest) tube. Although needle or small-catheter aspiration of a small to moderate pneumothorax is possible, several disadvantages of this technique exist. It is difficult to reexpand the lung fully, it cannot be used in patients with an active air leak, and it is unsuccessful in as many as 70% of patients. The most successful therapy for a pneumothorax is a thoracostomy tube. The tube is generally placed in the fourth or fifth intercostal space in the anterior axillary fold or the second or third interspace in the midclavicular line. A thoracostomy tube is successful because it results in complete re-expansion of the lung, resulting in adherence between the visceral and parietal pleurae. It also results in an inflammatory reaction, which obliterates the pleural space. In patients who are healthy and are compliant with instructions after the complete re-expansion of the lung, a Heimlich valve may be attached to the thoracostomy tube. The tube can then be removed in 3 to 4 days. Patients with significant underlying pulmonary disease, incomplete re-expansion of the lung, and a continuous air leak cannot be treated with this technique. Chemical pleurodesis is of limited value in treating patients with a primary pneumothorax. It should be considered only in those patients in whom surgery is contraindicated.

Surgical indications for patients with a spontaneous pneumothorax include a persistent air leak for more than 72 hours, a second recurrence, hemothorax, empyema, a previous contralateral pneumothorax, and bilateral simultaneous pneumothoraces. Patients with high-risk occupations, such as airline pilots and scuba divers, and individuals who live in remote areas should have surgery after the first episode. The surgical procedure consists of stapling the bleb tissue and performing a manual pleural abrasion to ensure adherence of the lung to the chest wall. In the open technique, a lateral or transaxillary incision is used. A median sternotomy may be used when bilateral pneumothoraces are present. Thoracoscopy also can be used to treat spontaneous pneumothoraces. However, no evidence exists that thorascopic surgery results in less operative pain and a shorter hospital stay. Furthermore, the recurrence rates appear to be significantly higher. After the open technique, a 97% to 99% success rate is noted. The success rate with the thorascopic technique is 92% to 94%.

Chylothorax

The presence of chyle in the pleural space is termed a *chylothorax*. The most common causes of a chylothorax are trauma and neoplasms. In addition to blunt and penetrating trauma, the duct can be injured during thoracic surgical procedures involving the aortic arch, the left subclavian artery, the esophagus, and during excision of mediastinal masses. More than 50% of chylothoraces in adults are secondary to neoplasms; the most common are mediastinal and retroperitoneal lymphomas. The diagnosis of a chylous effusion can be made by the color of the fluid and its contents. The fluid is milky and nonclotting and contains fat globules that stain with Sudan III. Most chylous effusions have a cholesterol-to-triglyceride ratio greater than 1. A triglyceride level of more than 110 mg/dL indicates a 99% probability that the fluid is chyle. With a triglyceride level less than 50 mg/dL, the probability is less than 5%. When a pleural effusion is diagnosed as a chylothorax, a chest tube should be inserted. The patient should receive either intravenous hyperalimentation or a diet with only medium-chain triglycerides. If the chest tube output is more than 1000 mL/day for longer than 7 days, the fistula is unlikely to close without surgical intervention. Approximately 50% of all patients will require surgical intervention. When a chylothorax is secondary to a lymphoma or other malignancies, the underlying neoplasm should first be treated with either radiation or chemotherapy. In planning the surgical approach, the chest is opened on the side of the effusion. The patient may be given 150 mL of cream 2 hours before the surgery so that the duct becomes engorged with chyle, and it is more easily found. It is often difficult to find the exact location of the fistula, but if possible, it should be ligated above and below the site of the tear. If no recognizable fistula is found, the thoracic duct should be ligated just above the diaphragm by ligating all tissue between the azygous vein and the aorta. A pleurodesis also is performed to prevent recurrent effusions. This procedure is successful in more than 80% of patients. No major side effects occur from ligating the thoracic duct.

Malignant Pleural Effusions

The most common cause of malignant pleural effusions is carcinoma of the lung in men and carcinoma of the breast in women. Other malignancies that are metastatic to the pleura include lymphomas and carcinoma of the ovary, kidney, colon, and prostate. Although a thoracentesis will result in immediate resolution of dyspnea, reaccumulation of fluid commonly occurs. Thoracostomy and chemical pleurodesis provide the most definitive therapy for malignant pleural effusions. A chest tube is inserted through the sixth or seventh intercostal space in the midaxillary line, and the effusion is completely drained.

Chemical pleurodesis will be effective only if the drainage is less than 150 mL/day. Currently, iodized talc is the most effective sclerosing agent and is successful in more than 80% of patients. The talc may be given as a slurry through the chest tube or insufflated under direct visualization by using video-assisted thoracoscopy. The most common side effects include pain and fever; however, talc microemboli, pneumonitis, and adult respiratory distress syndrome have all been described. The talc results in a dense fibrothorax, and this therapy is not recommended for benign disease or in young patients who may require a thoracic surgical procedure in the future.

When chemical pleurodesis is unsuccessful, pleurectomy and the insertion of a pleuroperitoneal shunt also may be considered. However, occlusion of the shunt occurs frequently, and pleurectomy is associated with increased morbidity and mortality in these debilitated patients.

Empyema

An empyema is the accumulation of purulent material in the pleural space. Empyemas are usually classified by three distinct phases: (1) the exudative or acute phase is characterized by pleural fluid, which has a low viscosity and cell count; (2) the fibrinopurulent or transitional phase is characterized by an increase in white blood cells and more turbid fluid; and (3) the organizing or chronic phase is characterized by viscous fluid and an organized pleural peel. The most common cause of an empyema is related to complications from a bacterial pneumonia. The second most common is as a complication from surgical procedures on the lung, mediastinum, or esophagus. Staphylococci, streptococci, and anaerobic organisms are the most common pathogens. Patients usually initially have pleuritic chest pain, fever, and shortness of breath. A chest film most commonly shows an area of parenchymal consolidation with a significant pleural effusion. Chest CT is very helpful in differentiating areas of consolidation from localized fluid collections. In the modern antibiotic era, it is rare for a patient to have an empyema necessitatis. In this condition, an undrained empyema finally erodes through the chest wall. The diagnosis of an empyema is made by aspirating pus from the pleural space. An empyema must be differentiated from a lung abscess. A lung abscess is surrounded by pulmonary parenchymal tissue and has no parietal pleural extension. An empyema requires immediate drainage, whereas a lung abscess may be treated with intravenous antibiotics. Insertion of a chest tube into a lung abscess can result in an empyema, pneumothorax, bronchopleural fistula, and hemorrhage. A CT scan is the diagnostic procedure of choice to help differentiate a lung abscess from an empyema.

Treatment of Empyemas

In the acute phase, the pleural fluid has a low viscosity and can easily be removed by thoracentesis. In addition, systemic antibiotics should be started. The combination of antibiotics and complete removal of all parapneumonic fluid is the key to preventing chronic empyema formation. A chest tube is used to evacuate more viscous collections and to drain large amounts of fluid. Loculated areas of fluid are best treated by drainage under CT scan guidance. It is important to remember that collections that cannot be aspirated by a syringe are unlikely to be drained by a chest tube. When thick, purulent material is drained with a chest tube, the tube can then be progressively withdrawn over several weeks as the cavity decreases in size.

By 6 weeks, the wall of an empyema cavity becomes organized and is unlikely to resolve by drainage alone. If the cavity is well localized, it can be treated by using a skin flap. A U-shaped flap of skin (Eloesser flap) is made parallel to the empyema cavity. A portion of two ribs is excised to allow adequate drainage. The top of the flap is turned down and tacked to the thickened pleura. The wound is changed daily with an antiseptic dressing. Ultimately, the cavity will granulate, with minimal deformity of the chest wall. This procedure is especially useful for critically ill, debilitated patients who cannot undergo a more extensive decortication procedure and who have large empyema cavities. A formal thoracotomy and decortication is indicated when the empyema results in a peel, which entraps a large portion of the lung and prevents re-expansion. This procedure should be done only when the empyema cavity has been drained and all underlying pneumonia has resolved.

Mesotheliomas

Mesotheliomas are primary tumors of the pleura that have been associated with long-term exposure to asbestos. They may be seen initially as either localized or diffusely spreading lesions and may be either benign or malignant. Most localized mesotheliomas are benign and constitute 10% of all mesotheliomas. Almost all diffuse mesotheliomas are malignant. Localized benign mesotheliomas are slow growing and are generally asymptomatic. They usually are seen as a localized mass on a chest radiograph and can be associated with hypoglycemia. The treatment of choice is complete surgical excision. Localized malignant mesotheliomas are usually symptomatic and appear with pleuritic pain, cough, dyspnea, and fever. Therapy consists of wide excision with adequate margins of pleura, lung, and chest wall, if necessary. Radiation therapy is indicated if complete resection is not possible. Incomplete resection results in a poor prognosis, with a median survival time of only 7 months.

Diffuse malignant mesotheliomas may involve the lung, pericardium, ribs, chest wall, and penetrate through the diaphragm into the peritoneal cavity. Patients usually have chest pain and dyspnea. The most common finding on a chest radiograph is a unilateral pleural effusion. Pleural thickening and nodularity also may be seen. The diagnosis is made by pleural biopsy. CT scans are helpful in determining the extent of the disease. No optimal treatment exists for malignant mesotheliomas. The vast majority of tumors are unresectable on presentation. Pleuropneumonectomy involves en bloc removal of the lung, pleura, pericardium, and diaphragm and has been associated with operative mortalities of 25% to 35%. This radical surgery has not affected overall survival, but, in some series, has been associated with longer recurrence-free survival. A combination of radiation and chemotherapy also is not curative but may result in better local control of the tumor. The prognosis for these tumors is poor. The average survival from onset of symptoms is 12 to 15 months, and from time of diagnosis, 8 to 10 months. Recently, 2-year survival rates as high as 48% have been reported by using a combination of extrapleural pneumonectomy and post-operative chemotherapy with and without radiotherapy. At present, however, drainage of effusions with and without pleurectomy and combinations of chemotherapy and radiation therapy are the most common methods to treat this highly malignant neoplasm.

Mediastinum

Because mediastinal tumors usually occur in characteristic locations, they are anatomically divided into anterior, middle, and posterior sections. In general, benign lesions of the mediastinum are asymptomatic. However, with the increased use of routine chest radiographs and the improved sensitivity of CT scans and MRIs, malignant mediastinal lesions are being found more frequently in asymptomatic individuals.

In general, the most common mediastinal masses are neurogenic tumors (21%), thymomas (19%), primary cysts (21%), lymphomas (13%), and germ-cell tumors (10%). They are more frequently found in the anterior mediastinum (54%) as opposed to the posterior (26%) or middle mediastinum (20%). Roughly, one third of all mediastinal masses are malignant. Anterior mediastinal masses are more likely malignant (59%), followed by middle mediastinal masses (29%) and posterior mediastinal masses (16%). Symptoms vary according to the histology of the mass and its location. In general, benign masses are asymptomatic. Tumors of the anterior mediastinum are more likely to cause symptoms than are those of the middle and posterior mediastinum. Symptoms can be related to the compression or invasion of mediastinal structures, such as the superior vena caval syndrome, Horner's syndrome, hoarseness, or chest-wall discomfort. Some mediastinal lesions produce hormones or antibodies that cause systemic symptoms such as Cushing's syndrome from ectopic adrenocorticotropic hormone (ACTH), wheezing from carcinoid tumors, thyrotoxicosis caused by mediastinal goiter, hypertension caused by pheochromocytoma, and hypercalcemia secondary to increased parathyroid hormone released from a mediastinal parathyroid adenoma.

Most mediastinal masses are discovered on routine chest radiographs. A CT scan with contrast is useful in all patients with a mediastinal mass. CT scan can predict the resectability of the mass, whether it invades surrounding structures including the chest wall, and whether it is a true mass or a collection of lymph nodes. MRI also is helpful in differentiating a mass from a cardiovascular structure such as an aneurysm or an anatomically aberrantly located vessel.

Serology may be helpful in some patients. Positive serologies for α-fetoprotein (AFP) and human chorionic gonadotropin-β (HCG-β) indicate a nonseminomatous germ-cell tumor, which is best treated with chemotherapy alone. Increased urinary excretion of vanillylmandelic acid and catecholamines is diagnostic of a pheochromocytoma.

Neurogenic Tumors

Neurogenic tumors are the most common mediastinal tumors and are located in the posterior mediastinum. They originate from the sympathetic ganglia (ganglioma, ganglioneuroblastoma, and neuroblastoma), and the intercostal nerves (neurofibroma, neurilemoma, and neurosarcoma). The majority of adult neurogenic tumors are benign, whereas they tend to be malignant in children. The most common presentation in an adult is that of an asymptomatic posterior mediastinal mass on a routine chest radiograph. Approximately 10% of these tumors have extensions into the spinal column (dumbbell tumors). A CT or MRI should be performed on all these tumors to look for evidence of intraspinous extension, which includes foramen enlargement, bony erosion, and intervertebral widening. Because the procedure of choice is a one-stage excision, it is important for the thoracic surgeon to know of any spinal involvement preoperatively so that a neurosurgeon will be present. The most common neurogenic tumors are neurilemoma and neurofibroma. Both are benign lesions arising from perineural cells. Surgical resection alone results in a cure. Neuroblastomas are highly invasive neoplasms that originate from sympathetic tissue. Most of these tumors occur in children and are already widely metastatic at the time of diagnosis. Multimodality therapy using surgical debulking, radiation therapy, and multidrug chemotherapy, as well as second-look explorations, offer the best chance for long-term survival.

Paraganglioma (Pheochromocytoma)

These rare tumors (<10% of all mediastinal tumors) can cause hypertension as a result of increased catecholamine production. Elevated urinary catechols and their metabolites (metanephrines and vanillylmandelic acid) are diagnostic. CT and metaiodobenzylguanidine (^{131}I-MIBG) scintigraphy are helpful in localizing the tumor in the mediastinum. Approximately 10% of these tumors occur as multiple lesions. Patients who have had an adrenalectomy for a pheochromocytoma and continue to have symptoms should undergo scanning of the mediastinum. Although 50% of tumors appear malignant by histologic criteria, metastatic disease develops in only 3%. Complete surgical resection is the treatment of choice.

Thymoma

The second most common mediastinal mass and the most common lesion of the anterior mediastinum is the thymoma. The most common syndrome associated with this tumor is myasthenia gravis, which occurs in 10% to 50% of patients and is characterized by weakness and fatigue of skeletal muscles. Other symptoms are related to tumor compression and include chest pain, dyspnea, hemoptysis, cough, and the superior vena caval syndrome. Histologically, thymomas are classified by the predominance of either epithelial or lymphocytic cells. However, the differential between benign and malignant disease is determined by the presence of invasion into adjacent structures and distant metastases. Stage I tumors are well encapsulated without evidence of gross or microscopic capsular invasion. Stage II lesions have pericapsular invasion into adjacent mediastinal fat, pleura, or pericardium. In stage III, the tumor invades adjacent organs, or intrathoracic metastases are present. In stage IV, extrathoracic metastases are present.

The primary therapy for thymomas is complete surgical resection whenever possible. Adjunctive radiation therapy is recommended for stage II and III disease. Chemotherapy is recommended for stage IV disease or when recurrent disease is not amenable to either surgery or radiotherapy. The prognosis for thymomas is closely related to their clinical stage. The 5-year survival ranges from 85% to 100% in stage I to 20% to 40% in stage IV.

Germ Cell Tumors

Germ cell tumors in the mediastinum are histologically identical to germ cell tumors arising from the gonads. However, they are considered primary mediastinal tumors because fewer than 5% show any testicular involvement. These tumors are found predominantly in the mediastinum and consist of tissue elements from all three embryonic layers. On occasion, the diagnosis can be made by the identification of well-formed teeth within the mass or evidence of bone or hair. Teratodermoid (dermoid) cysts are the simplest form and contain hair and sebaceous material. Teratomas are more complex histologically and contain bone, teeth, cartilage, thymus, lung, liver, or pancreas. The diagnosis is made at the time of surgery, at which time complete excision of these masses is curative.

Seminomas account for 50% of malignant germ cell tumors and occur most commonly in the anterior mediastinum. Malignant nonseminomatous tumors include choriocarcinoma, embryonal cell carcinoma, malignant teratoma, and endodermal cell (yolk-sac) tumors. The nonseminomas differ from seminomas in that they are more aggressive tumors with a poor prognosis, are rarely radiosensitive, and more than 90% produce either HCG-β or AFP. Seminomas are extremely radiosensitive and can be treated with radiation therapy or multiagent chemotherapy. The prognosis is excellent. In contrast, nonseminomas are highly invasive and have usually metastasized by the time the diagnosis is made. Multiagent chemotherapy is the only treatment available, and the overall prognosis is poor.

Lymphomas

Lymphomas usually occur in the anterior mediastinum or in the hilar regions of the middle mediastinum. CT and MRI are helpful in determining the extent of the disease and may differentiate other solid tumors from lymphomas, which comprise multiple enlarged lymph nodes. The surgeon's role in the treatment of lymphomas is to provide the clinician with an accurate histologic diagnosis, which is crucial in determining a treatment plan that consists of either radiation therapy, multiagent chemotherapy, or a combination of both.

Primary Carcinomas

Primary carcinomas comprise approximately 4% of all mediastinal masses. Their etiology is unknown, and they usually have extensive intrathoracic spread and distant metastases. Surgical excision is rarely possible, and the prognosis is poor.

Endocrine Tumors

Substernal mediastinal goiters are most commonly seen in the anterior mediastinum. Most of these tumors are adenomas and are contrasting/enhancing when visualized by CT scan. It is important to determine the presence of functioning cervical thyroid tissue before removal of these lesions. An asymptomatic mediastinal goiter need not be removed. These lesions are resected when they result in tracheal compression, causing cough, wheezing, and stridor. Although substernal extensions of a cervical goiter can usually be excised by using a cervical approach, the blood supply of a mediastinal goiter is derived from intrathoracic vessels, and therefore requires a median sternotomy or occasionally a posterolateral thoracotomy.

Patients with hypercalcemia after a cervical parathyroid exploration require mediastinal exploration. Approximately 80% of mediastinal parathyroid lesions are located in the anterior mediastinum and can be excised by using a partial sternal-splitting incision. Cryopreservation of the excised parathyroid gland is indicted if three or more glands had been excised during the initial cervical exploration.

Primary Cysts

Bronchogenic cysts are the most common primary cysts of the mediastinum. They are usually asymptomatic and located proximal to the trachea and bronchi. Symptoms occur because of enlargement and compression of the trachea or bronchi, superinfection, or very rarely, degeneration into a malignant lesion. For these reasons, surgical excision is recommended in all patients.

Pericardial cysts are the second most frequently encountered cysts within the mediastinum. They usually occur in the pericardiophrenic angles, more commonly (70%) on the right. They may or may not communicate directly with the pericardium. The CT appearance of a cystic mass with near-water attenuation values in the pericardiophrenic location is almost pathognomonic. Some cysts have been aspirated under CT guidance and monitored with serial CT scans. Surgical excision involves little morbidity and is indicated for diagnosis and to differentiate these cysts from malignant lesions.

Lung

Neoplasms of the Lung

Lung cancer is now the most common cause of death from a malignancy in both men and women. More important, the risk of death from lung cancer has increased steadily and shows no evidence of a plateau.

Pathology and Pathogenesis

The most important etiology in the pathogenesis of lung cancer is cigarette smoking. Even passive smoking, which accounts for 25% of lung cancer in nonsmokers, can increase the risk of cancer by 35% to 50% among nonsmokers.

Lung cancer can be divided into four major cell types: adenocarcinoma, squamous cell carcinoma, large cell carcinoma, and small cell carcinoma.

Adenocarcinoma is now the most frequent form of lung cancer (50%). Adenomas are usually peripheral and are not always associated with smoking. Adenocarcinomas may be subdivided histologically into acinar, papillary, and bronchoalveolar forms. Bronchoalveolar cancers may occur as a solitary pulmonary nodule or a diffuse infiltrative process and can be bilateral. Their prognosis is usually worse than that for other adenocarcinomas. Another form of adenocarcinoma is the "scar" carcinoma. These neoplasms usually arise in areas of previous areas of inflammation, healed infiltrates, granulomas, or tuberculosis. Their prognosis is usually better than that of other types of adenocarcinoma.

Squamous cell carcinoma is now the second most common type of lung cancer (30%). It is almost always related to cigarette smoking. These carcinomas originate centrally, grow toward the mainstem bronchus and pulmonary parenchyma, and include the regional, hilar, and mediastinal lymph nodes.

Large cell carcinomas occur as peripheral lesions. They rapidly invade the lung parenchyma and tend to metastasize early.

Small cell carcinomas are distinguished by the presence of cytoplasmic neurosecretory granules on electron microscopy. These neoplasms are almost always unresectable and tend to metastasize early to the liver, brain, bone, and adrenals.

Bronchopulmonary carcinoids are low-grade neoplasms, which also contain neurosecretory granules and may produce peptide hormones. Atypical carcinoids have frequent mitoses and may metastasize to regional lymph nodes in 10% to 15% of patients. In general, bronchial carcinoids have a much better prognosis than do other forms of lung cancer; the 5-year survival rate is 95% in patients with stage I disease.

Clinical Manifestations

Lung cancer may first be seen as an asymptomatic mass discovered on routine chest radiographs. However, the majority of patients have symptoms referable to their lung cancer. Centrally located lesions may be associated with cough, stridor, wheezing, hemoptysis, dyspnea, and chest pain. Peripheral tumors often are seen with pleuritic and musculoskeletal pain. Squamous cell tumors may undergo cavitation and occur as a lung abscess. Involvement of the recurrent laryngeal nerve is associated with hoarseness. Tumors arising from the endothoracic fascia of the lung apices (Pancoast tumor) may invade the eighth cervical and first thoracic nerves and the sympathetic chain and occur with arm and shoulder pain and Horner's syndrome (enophthalmus, ptosis, meiosis, and ipsilateral anhidrosis). Malignant pleural and parietal effusions result in dyspnea and arrhythmias. Tumors invading the right hilum and mediastinum can result in the superior vena caval syndrome. This is characterized by plethora, venous distention involving the arm and neck, and edema of the face, neck, and arms. Paraneoplastic syndromes are frequently associated with small cell lung cancer. These include hypercalcemia, neuropathies, myopathies, and hypertrophic pulmonary osteoarthropathy from ectopic production of parathyroid hormone (PTH), ACTH, antidiuretic hormone (ADH), and calcitonin.

Diagnosis and Staging

Staging of lung malignancies is extremely important because the staging determines prognosis and the selection of treatment protocols (Box 28-1).

The workup of all pulmonary malignancies begins with a chest radiograph. Pulmonary neoplasms may appear as a single solitary nodule, a pneumonic infiltrate, or a hilar mass. When dealing with a solitary pulmonary nodule, it is always important to attempt to obtain old films. The presence of a nodule of the same size on an old chest radiograph makes the diagnosis of a lung cancer very unlikely. Elevation of a diaphragm and the presence of a pleural effusion are ominous signs and usually are associated with unresectable tumors. CT scans have become an invaluable tool to stage lung cancers. They can detect enlarged hilar and mediastinal nodes and possible liver and adrenal metastases. However, no patient should ever be refused resectional therapy for a lung neoplasm on the sole basis of a CT finding without tissue confirmation. Bronchoscopy is helpful in determining the presence and extent of endobronchial lesions. Bronchial biopsy, brushings, and washing are used to make the histologic diagnosis of a lung cancer.

BOX 28–1 International TNM Staging System For Lung Cancer

Tumor (T)

TX Occult carcinoma (malignant cells in sputum or bronchial washing but tumor not visualized by imaging studies or bronchoscopy)

T1 Tumor 3 cm or less in greatest diameter, surrounded by lung or visceral pleura, but not proximal to a lobar bronchus

T2 Tumor > 3 cm in diameter, or with involvement of main bronchus at least 2 cm distal to carina, or with visceral pleural invasion, or with associated atelectasis or obstructive pneumonitis extending to the hilar region but not involving the entire lung

T3 Tumor invading chest wall, diaphragm, mediastinal pleura, or parietal pericardium; or tumor in main bronchus within 2 cm of, but not invading, carina; or atelectasis of obstructive pneumonitis of the entire lung

T4 Tumor invading mediastinum, heart, great vessels, trachea, esophagus, vertebral body, or carina; or ipsilateral malignant pleural effusion

Nodes (N)

N0 No regional lymph node metastases

N1 Metastases to ipsilateral peribronchial or hilar nodes

N2 Metastases to ipsolateral mediastinal or subcarinal nodes

N3 Metastases to contralateral mediastinal or hilar, or to any scalene or supraclavicular nodes

Distant Metastases (M)

M0 No distant metastases

M1 Distant metastases

Positron emission tomography (PET) has been useful in differentiating benign from malignant pulmonary nodules by demonstrating increased glucose metabolism in malignant cells. Cervical mediastinoscopy is recommended for biopsy of the lymph nodes in the right paratracheal region that are larger than 1 cm on CT scan. In patients with enlarged aortopulmonary nodes, a left anterior median sternotomy (Chamberlain procedure) is helpful in determining staging and operability. Thoracoscopy also can be helpful to confirm pleural invasion and the biopsy of subaortic, paraesophageal, carinal, and hilar lymph nodes.

Determination of Resectability

Because surgical excision offers the best hope for cure of lung cancer, it is imperative that indications and contraindications for surgical resection be accurately determined. Definitive contraindications for surgical resection in lung cancer include (1) distant metastases, (2) malignant pleural or pericardial effusion, (3) contralateral and extrathoracic adenopathy, and (4) involvement of the laryngeal nerve. Relative contraindications include poor pulmonary function (as described later) and the presence of T4 and N2 disease.

Surgical Procedures for Lung Cancer

The optimal surgical procedure performed for lung cancer must remove the entire tumor with adequate margins, while preserving the maximal amount of functional lung tissue. The most commonly performed procedure for lung cancer is a lobectomy. Segmentectomy and wedge resections are best performed for T1 lesions and in those patients with limited pulmonary reserve. Compared with lobectomy, a higher rate of local recurrence is associated with these procedures. A lymph node dissection may or may not be performed at the time of the resection. Although dissection of the mediastinal lymph nodes improves the accuracy of staging, it has no impact on patient survival.

Results of Surgical Resection for Lung Cancer

The treatment of choice for stage I lung cancer is a lobectomy. A wedge resection or segmentectomy can be performed for T1 lesions and in patients with poor pulmonary function, but, as noted earlier, local recurrence is higher. Overall, 5-year survival for patients with stage I disease is 70% to 85%. Patients with T1,N0 disease can expect a 5-year survival of 80% to 85%. The type of histology appears to have no effect on survival in this group.

Patients with stage II disease have 5-year survival rates of 40% to 50%. Postoperative radiation therapy has been shown to reduce the incidence of local recurrence, but does not affect overall survival.

For patients with stage IIIA disease who have T3,N0,M0 lesions, if the tumor has invaded the chest wall, a pulmonary and chest-wall resection offers the best chance for cure, which at 5 years is 40%. However, with N2 disease and chest wall involvement, the 5-year survival decreases to 25% to 30%. Resection for T3 disease with mediastinal involvement results in a much poorer prognosis, with only a 9% 5-year survival. The resectability of N2 disease remains controversial. When unsuspected N2 disease is found at the time of thoracotomy (negative preoperative CT scan), the treatment of choice is pulmonary resection combined with complete lymph node excision. Five-year survival rates as high as 25% have been reported in this group. The combination of T3 or T4 lesions with N_2 disease carries a very poor prognosis, and these patients are generally not considered surgical candidates. The presence of N2 disease by CT scan should always be confirmed histologically before embarking on a thoracotomy for a pulmonary resection. In general, the histologic confirmation of N2 disease preoperatively usually contraindicates a surgical resection. However, various neoadjuvant protocols may expand the role of surgical resection in this group of patients. One such protocol is from the Southwest Oncology Group (SWOG), which is randomizing patients with stage IIIA disease to either chemotherapy (cisplatin) and radiation therapy alone or chemotherapy and radiation therapy followed by surgical resection. To date, complete resection was achieved in 73% of patients, and the 2-year survival rate was 40%. A recent review of 15 trials of preoperative chemotherapy plus radiation therapy showed an overall 3-year survival of 25% to 30%; significantly improved from historical controls. The results of these trials are encouraging, but more data and 5-year outcomes will be necessary before drawing definitive therapeutic conclusions in patients with N_2 disease.

Patients with stage IIIB and IV disease are considered inoperable and are treated with combinations of chemotherapy and radiation therapy.

Management of Small Cell Lung Cancer

Small cell lung cancer has a dismal prognosis, with a 2-year survival of only 10%. The mainstay of therapy for these patients involves multiple chemotherapeutic agents. Occasionally, a patient with small cell lung cancer will have an isolated pulmonary nodule. An accurate histologic diagnosis is crucial because this diagnosis can be confused with a carcinoid tumor. With limited small cell lung cancer, combinations of chemotherapy and radiation therapy are instituted, followed by a repeated set of whole-body scans to exclude distant metastases. If none is found, surgical resection is performed. This is followed by postoperative radiation therapy and chemotherapy. Some small series have reported 5-year survival as high as 20% with this protocol.

Benign Tumors of the Lung

Benign tumors of the lung are usually asymptomatic and are first seen as peripheral lesions on routine chest radiographs. Whenever possible, a conservative pulmonary resection (wedge or segmentectomy) should be performed.

Hamartomas are the most common benign neoplasm of the lung. Most are asymptomatic and appear as a solitary pulmonary nodule on a routine chest radiograph. Histologically, they contain cartilaginous tissue and calcium deposits. The presence of "popcorn" calcification is pathognomonic for pulmonary hamartomas. Although these tumors are benign, malignant degeneration has been known to occur, and conservative surgical resection is considered the treatment of choice.

Bronchial adenomas are the second most common benign pulmonary tumor. The vast majority are carcinoids. In 10% to 15% of these tumors, atypical cells will be found, which are associated with a higher incidence of regional lymph node spread and a poorer 5-year survival. Conservative resection is the treatment of choice, except when a frozen section shows atypical cells with increased mitotic figures, at which time, a formal lobectomy and regional lymph node dissection is indicated.

Preoperative Evaluation of Pulmonary Function

Crucial to the successful outcome of all thoracic surgical procedures is the preoperative identification of patients who are at increased risk for pulmonary complications. In general, all patients in whom a pulmonary resection is planned should undergo pulmonary-function testing and measurement of arterial blood gases.

Pulmonary-function Testing

Several basic variables are involved in spirometry testing. The vital capacity (VC) is the maximal volume of air that can be exhaled after a maximal inhalation or the maximal volume that can be inhaled after a maximal exhalation. The FEV_1 is the volume of air expired in 1 second and tests maximal expiratory airflow. The FEV_1 is decreased in the presence of obstructive disease but may also be decreased in restrictive lung disease. For this reason, the FEV_1 also is related to the total exhaled VC. The ratio of FEV_1 to VC may be decreased in patients with airway obstruction but is normal in restrictive lung disease.

A single-breath carbon monoxide diffusion capacity test is rapid, simple, and a safe way to measure pulmonary diffusion capacity (DLCO). A reduction in DLCO is useful in detecting collagen diseases, sarcoidosis, infiltrative diseases, and emphysema. Arterial blood gases are useful in accessing oxygenation. Increased levels of P_{CO_2} (>45 torr) are associated with an increased incidence of postoperative pulmonary complications. Ventilation/perfusion (V/Q) scans help to measure the distribution of ventilation compared with blood flow in the various segments of the lung. In the presence of a large mass or an obstructing lesion, it can provide a more accurate estimation of the amount of normal-functioning lung that will remain after a pulmonary resection.

Preoperative Evaluation of Operative Risk

Patients found to have an FEV_1 of more than 0.8 L have a moderate risk of severe postoperative complications. The risk becomes prohibitive with an FEV_1 of less than 0.5 L. The presence of pulmonary hypertension and hypercapnia (P_{CO_2} >45) are relative contraindications to pulmonary resection. In certain instances, the results of spirometry testing and arterial blood gases are inconclusive in determining operability. In those instances, measurement of maximal oxygen consumption (MV_{O_2}) may be an important predictor of patient outcomes.

Suggested Reading

Adkins RB, Maples MD, Hainsworth JD: Primary malignant mediastinal tumors. Ann Thorac Surg 38:648–659, 1984.

Ginsberg RJ: Multi-modality treatment of resectable non-small cell lung cancer. Clin Lung Cancer 2:194–200, 2000.

Jamtaki A: A rational approach to total thymectomy in the treatment of myasthenia gravis. Ann Thorac Surg 24:120–130, 1977.

Landreneau RJ: Thorascopy for empyema and hemothorax. Chest 109:18–24, 1995.

Miyoshi S, Nakahara K, Ohnok S, et al: Exercise tolerance test in lung cancer patients: The relationship between exercise capacity and post-thoracotomy hospital mortality. Ann Thorac Surg 44:487–490, 1987.

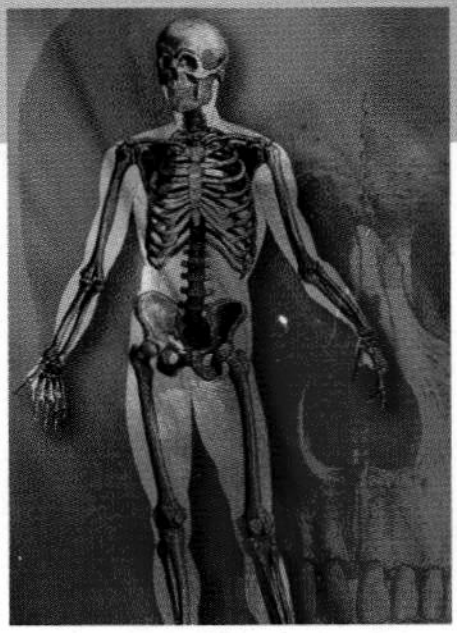

Chapter 29
Acquired Cardiac Disorders

RICHARD J. SHEMIN, MD, and ANTHONY DISCIPIO, MD

Surgical therapy for cardiac disease began in the 1930s and has enjoyed a dramatic increase over the last six decades. The initial procedures were performed to correct simple congenital cardiac anomalies. The advent of cardiopulmonary bypass (CPB) allowed surgeons to develop approaches to valvular heart disease, ascending and arch disease of the aorta, and coronary artery disease (CAD). Modern advances in diagnostic evaluation, intraoperative anesthetic management, conduct of CPB, myocardial preservation, and postoperative care have improved survival from cardiac procedures. In the United States alone, almost 300,000 cardiac procedures are performed annually, with mortality rates of 3% to 10%, depending on the procedure. The frontiers of surgical treatment continue to advance with new techniques in minimally invasive approaches to the heart, implantable portable cardiac-assist devices, transmyocardial laser revascularization, and robotic surgery.

Cardiac Anatomy

The heart consists of four chambers with two separate circulatory systems, the pulmonary circulation and the systemic circulation. Venous (deoxygenated) blood returns to the heart though the superior vena cava (SVC) and inferior vena cava, emptying into the right atrium. From there it passes through the tricuspid valve into the right ventricle (RV), which then pumps the blood to the pulmonary circulation through the pulmonic valve into the pulmonary artery. The main pulmonary artery bifurcates to the right and left as blood passes to the lungs, where it is oxygenated. Oxygenated blood returns from the lungs via the pulmonary veins into the left atrium (LA). The blood then passes through the mitral valve into the left ventricle (LV). The LV pumps blood through the aortic valve into the aorta, which then branches, distributing oxygenated blood through the systemic circulation (Figs. 29-1 and 29-2)

The cardiac valves develop in tandem, two valves between the atria and ventricles, and two valves between the ventricles and their respective circulatory systems. A fibrous skeleton exits through the heart in the region of the valves. The tricuspid valve, with three leaflets, and the mitral valve, with two leaflets, develop in conjunction with the RV and LV, respectively. These valves each are supported by a fibrous ring called the annulus. They structurally consist of leaflets that are tethered by chordae tendinae to muscular outgrowths of the ventricular wall called papillary muscles. These atrioventricular valves function in conjunction with the ventricular wall to prevent the regurgitation of blood into the atria during ventricular contraction. The aortic and pulmonic valves develop in the ventricular outflow tracts of the LV and RV, respectively. These valves are trileaflet valves attached to a fibrous annulus supported by the wall of the outflow tract. These valves prevent regurgitation of blood back into the ventricles after ventricular contraction has occurred (Figs. 29-3 and 29-4).

The blood supply to the heart comes from two major arteries, the right and left coronary arteries, which originate in the aortic root, just distal to the aortic valve. The left coronary artery consists of a short initial segment called the left main coronary artery, which bifurcates into the left anterior descending artery (LAD) and the left circumflex artery (LCx). The LAD gives off septal branches and lateral diagonal branches. The LCx branches to the obtuse marginal and posterolateral branches. The right coronary artery (RCA) branches to the acute marginal. The vascular dominance of the heart is determined by which system

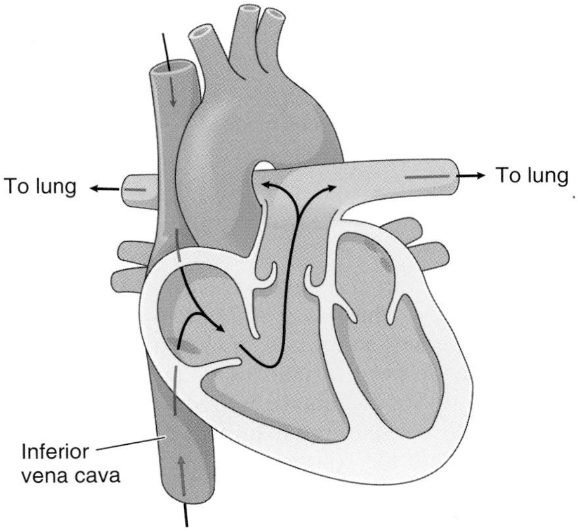

FIGURE 29–1 Blood flow through right heart.

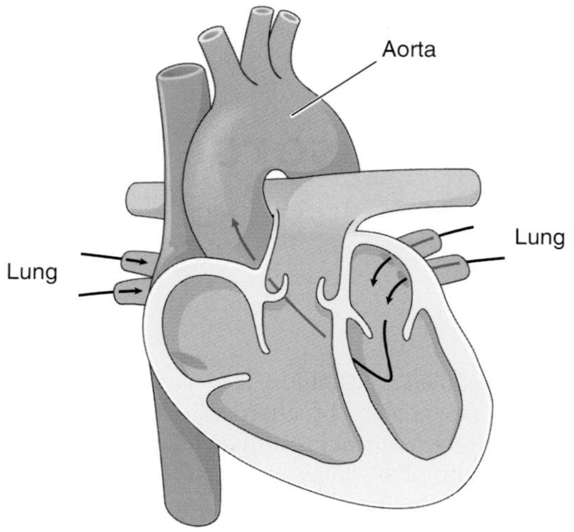

FIGURE 29–2 Flow of blood through the left heart.

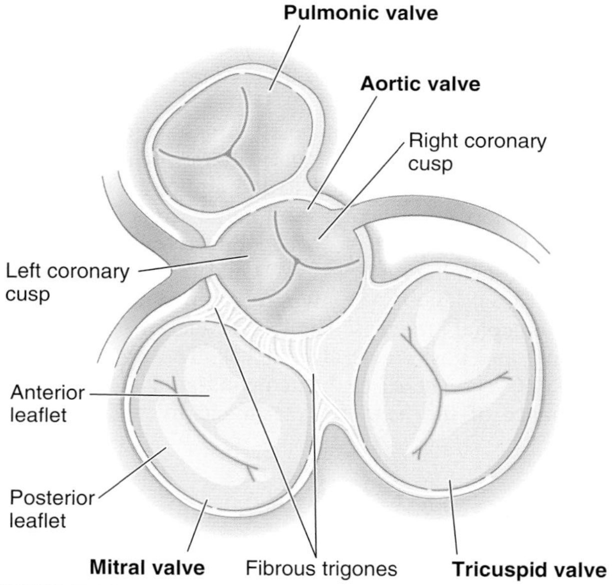

FIGURE 29–3 Fibrous skeleton of heart with relative positions of valves.

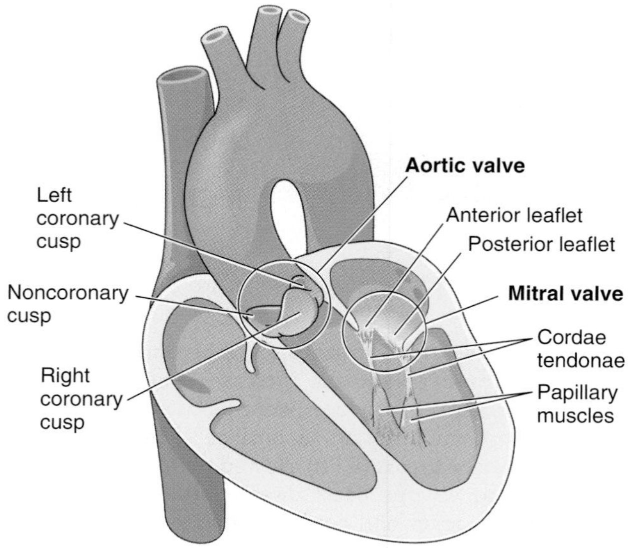

FIGURE 29–4 Relation of aortic and mitral valves.

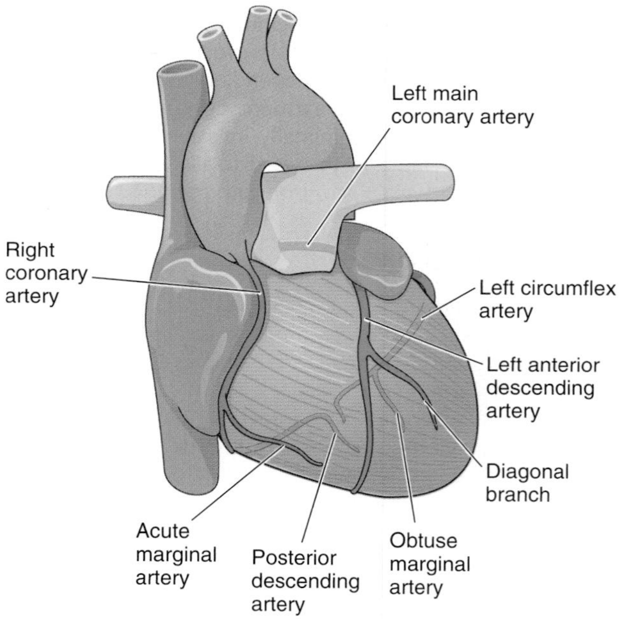

FIGURE 29–5 Coronary artery anatomy.

(right coronary or left coronary) gives rise to the posterior descending artery. Thus in a right dominant heart, the posterior descending artery is a branch of the RCA. The majority of hearts have a right dominant circulation, but left dominance or codominance is frequently seen. Blood returns from the myocardium mainly through the coronary veins draining into the coronary sinus and emptying into the right atrium (Fig. 29-5)

The conduction system of the heart is quite complex and not anatomically obvious. Cardiac contraction originates in the sinus node, which lies in the right atrium near the junction of the SVC. The interatrial conduction pathways are not well defined but loop around the fossa ovalis to the atrioventricular (AV) node, which lies in the right atrium adjacent to the tricuspid valve, at the apex of the triangle of Koch. The AV node connects to the ventricles through the bundle of His, which is situated in the membranous portion of the interventricular septum. The right bundle branch and the left bundle branch then carry the cardiac impulse to the ventricles.

Cardiac Physiology and Pathophysiology

The heart's function is to pump blood through two circuits. One circuit goes to the lungs to help eliminate carbon dioxide and take in oxygen. The other circuit receives this oxygenated blood and pumps it to the body. These circuits work in tandem and must pump equivalent amounts of blood to maintain normal homeostasis. The way we determine the adequacy of the heart's ability to pump is to look at the cardiac output.

The basic cardiac cycle consists of systole (contraction) and diastole (relaxation). To use the left heart as an example (Fig. 29-6), during diastole, the LV undergoes filling when the mitral valve opens and the LV relaxes. Ventricular filling is first passive, then active when the LA contracts. When diastole is complete, the LV undergoes isovolumetric contraction, closing the mitral valve and increasing ventricular pressure; this is the beginning of systole. When ventricular pressure exceeds aortic pressure, the aortic valve opens, and the ventricle ejects blood into the aorta, completing systole. As ejection is completed, the aortic valve closes, the LV relaxes, and diastole begins again.

Cardiac output is determined by Heart rate × Stroke volume, which is the volume of blood ejected with each ventricular contraction. However, because different body sizes do not all require the same cardiac output to maintain oxygen delivery, the cardiac index was developed to correct for this. Cardiac index is Cardiac output ÷ Body surface area, and the normal cardiac index is greater than $2 L/min/m^2$. Cardiac output can be affected only by altering the heart rate or the stroke volume. Stroke volume is altered by preload, afterload, and contractility. Therefore functionally, only four ways exist to affect the cardiac output: heart rate, preload, afterload, and contractility. The preload is ideally measured by the ventricular end-diastolic volume and refers to the volume loading of the ventricle. Afterload technically is the wall tension in the ventricle during contraction, but is often thought of simplistically as the pressure that the ventricle works against to eject blood. Contractility is a more nebulous term that is used to describe the inotropic state of the heart. Contractility is affected by many variables, including the energy state of the myocytes, and basically encompasses the heart's inherent ability to

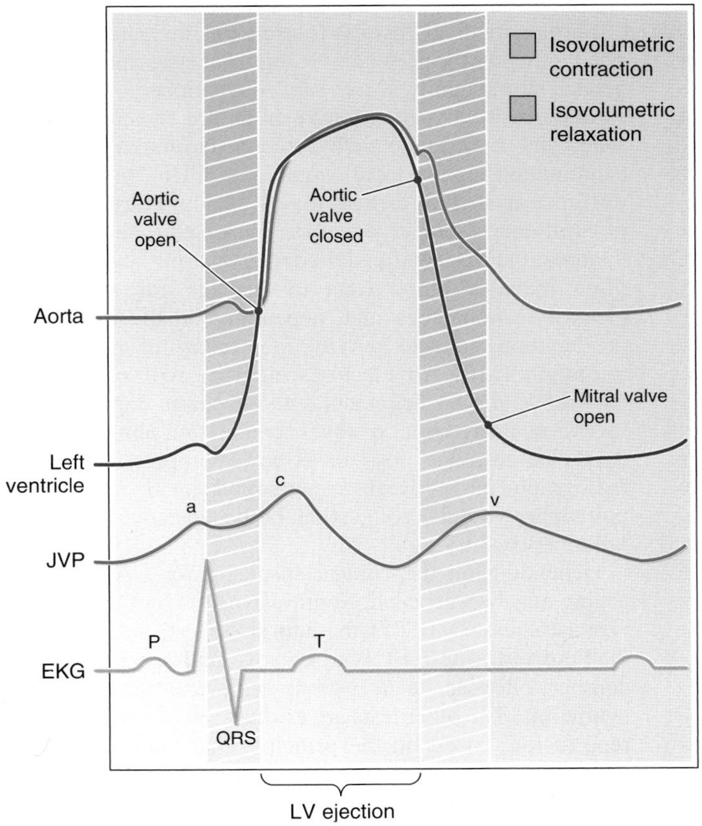

FIGURE 29–6 Wigger's diagram of the cardiac cycle.

contract effectively. These variables are intimately related to each other, but can be manipulated mechanically and pharmacologically.

Assuming that the hemoglobin and oxygen saturation remain constant, oxygen delivery is affected by changing cardiac output. Currently, cardiac output is monitored with the use of a pulmonary artery catheter with a thermodilution technique. The effectiveness of a cardiac contraction is measured by the ejection fraction, either with echo or angiographic techniques. Ejection fraction measures the percentage change in ventricular volume between ventricular diastole and end systole. Normally, the ejection fraction is more than 60%.

Most cardiac dysfunction results from either pressure or volume overload on the involved ventricle. Volume overloading results in ventricular distention and dilation, increased wall tension, increased myocardial oxygen demand, and decreased effective ventricular contraction. Pressure overloading results in concentric muscular hypertrophy of the ventricle, which requires increased pressure to maintain adequate ventricular diastolic filling, which in turn requires higher perfusion pressure to deliver blood flow to the myocardium. This causes increased myocardial oxygen consumption and finally results in decreased effective ventricular contraction. These dysfunctional states can result in decreased ejection fraction and congestive heart failure (CHF).

Cardiac dysfunction from ischemia, which is inadequate blood flow to cardiac muscle to meet metabolic demand, is not primarily a pressure or volume problem. However, once the heart loses contractile muscle secondary to ischemia and cell death, the ventricle begins to dilate and the ejection fraction decreases. This creates the physiology of a volume-overloaded heart, resulting in even worse cardiac function. Ventricular dilation also can cause valvular insufficiency of the involved AV valve, resulting in low output or pulmonary edema.

All causes of left heart failure eventually lead to increased hydrostatic pressure in the lungs as volume backs up in the pulmonary circuit, resulting in cardiogenic pulmonary edema, the clinical manifestation known as CHF causing shortness of breath and rales on pulmonary examination. Right heart failure causes backup of blood systemically into the venous circulation, causing pleural effusions, ascites, and ankle swelling, and can be the result of left heart failure, pulmonary disease with pulmonary hypertension, or a primary right heart problem.

Coronary Artery Disease

CAD is the leading cause of death in the United States. More than 500,000 people per year will die of complications related to CAD. The diagnosis and treatment of CAD began in the late 1950s with the birth of coronary angiography. Until then, CAD was an inferred diagnosis or a postmortem diagnosis. Coronary angiography gave us the definition of CAD-narrowing of one or more coronary arteries from atherosclerotic disease, which limits myocardial blood flow. Once the concept of stenotic CAD was established, a surgical approach to bypass the blockage was sought. The Cleveland Clinic reported the first early success with aortocoronary bypass in 1967, by using a reversed saphenous vein graft as the conduit to carry blood from the aorta into the coronary artery, bypassing the area of stenosis. This ushered in the modern therapy of CAD to reestablish blood flow to areas of the heart that have poor perfusion.

Presentation and Diagnosis

CAD most often is first seen with the symptom complex termed *angina pectoris*. Classically, this is pressure, usually associated with exertion, that lies in the chest and may travel to the jaw and left arm. Many variants of angina exist, and some diabetic patients may not feel any pressure or pain at all. Other symptoms that may be associated with angina are fatigue, shortness of breath, dyspnea on exertion, orthopnea, face or neck pain, and "indigestion" or dyspepsia. Usually, though, the symptoms are related to physical activity. Unstable angina is a many-faceted diagnosis but includes new-onset angina, angina at rest, crescendo angina, and postinfarct angina.

Further medical history is used to elucidate common risk factors for the presence of CAD: diabetes, smoking, age, gender, strong family history of CAD, peripheral vascular or carotid disease, hypertension, renal failure, hypercoagulable state, and hyperlipidemia/hypercholesterolemia. Physical examination may yield signs of CHF or valvular dysfunction such as arrhythmia, S_3 gallop, murmurs, rales or expiratory wheezes, cyanosis, increased jugular venous distention (JVD), and pedal edema. The initial evaluation often includes blood tests to evaluate for anemia or electrolyte imbalance and, depending on the manner of presentation, to rule out the possibility of myocardial infarction (MI). An electrocardiogram will often show changes in the ST segments with elevation, depression or inversion, arrhythmia, q waves, conduction abnormalities, axis changes, and loss of R-wave progression. Chest radiograph may reveal an enlarged heart shadow or pulmonary vascular congestion, both suggestive of cardiac failure (Box 29-1).

Depending on the clinical suspicion for CAD, further testing may be warranted. Noninvasive tests for CAD are the exercise stress test (ETT), thallium stress test, and persantine thallium test. The ETT is a sensitive and specific test for coronary disease in a patient with exertional anginal symptoms. The other tests are evaluations of perfusion and reperfusion, based on the principle that thallium can be delivered only to areas of the heart with blood flow. Thus if the heart becomes regionally ischemic with stress, then thallium uptake will be less in the ischemic area. If thallium

BOX 29–1 Risk Factors for Coronary Artery Disease

Positive family history
Smoking
Diabetes mellitus
Man or postmenopausal woman
Hyperlipidemia/hypercholesterolemia
Peripheral vascular disease or carotid disease
Hypertension
Renal failure
Hypercoagulable state
Age

reappears in that area when the stress is removed, then this indicates reperfusion. The one fault of this test is that global ischemia can be read as a false negative because the reduced uptake will be uniform throughout the heart.

Other noninvasive tests, which include cardiac echo and stress echo, can be used to assess the heart functionally. Regional wall-motion abnormalities seen on echo can be the result of ischemia or infarction. Echo can give a good estimate of ventricular function, regional wall motion, chamber size in systole and diastole, and valvular function. Stress echo can demonstrate areas susceptible to functional changes secondary to ischemia and can show how ischemic areas can improve with increased blood flow.

The sine qua non of the diagnosis of CAD, however, is still cardiac catheterization. Biplane coronary angiography involves sequential selective injections of radio-opaque contrast into the coronary arteries, while viewing the injections from multiple standardized views. A thorough coronary angiogram will image the left main, the left circumflex, the LAD, and the RCA, all in at least two planes. A stenosis of 50% or greater is considered significant to reduce blood flow through a coronary vessel during exercise, producing ischemia. An injection of contrast into the LV will help to estimate ventricular function by measuring the ejection fraction and noting regional wall-motion abnormalities. Simultaneously, hemodynamic measurements are performed to identify key variables, such as cardiac output and left ventricular end-diastolic pressure. The weakness of coronary angiography is that the views obtained are only two-dimensional. Because stenoses are often eccentric, angiography may underestimate or overestimate the degree of disease. Other adjuncts to cardiac catheterization now are direct angioscopy and intravascular ultrasound, a new modality of viewing CAD that is gathering momentum.

The result of stenotic CAD is MI, in which a region of the heart loses adequate blood supply and dies. MI is often associated with rupture of an atherosclerotic plaque and acute occlusion of the vessel when blood dissects into the wall of the plaque. Prolonged ischemia also can cause infarction without acute occlusion of the vessel when metabolic demands of the muscle far outstrip blood supply. Vessel occlusion in CAD is definitely associated with platelet activation, and antiplatelet therapy can help prevent infarction. Ischemia can be exacerbated by reperfusion of a chronically ischemic area, with resulting inflammation and cytokine release enhancing the insult. Sequelae of MI that are seen in patients who are candidates for surgical intervention are acute ventriculoseptal defect, acute mitral regurgitation with papillary muscle rupture, free-wall rupture of the ventricle, and ventricular aneurysm or pseudoaneurysm formation.

Treatment of Coronary Artery Disease

Once the diagnosis of CAD has been made, three main treatment options are available: medical therapy, catheter-based interventions, and surgical revascularization. It is important to note that all of these current treatments are palliative and not curative; they treat the symptoms but not the underlying disease process. Many outcome studies since the mid-1970s have examined the relative outcomes of these treatment options. Medical therapy versus surgical

PEARLS FOR THE OR

The stages of a standard operation for coronary bypass grafting can be divided into four quarters: (1) open the chest and harvest the conduit, (2) prepare for cardiopulmonary bypass, (3) form the bypass grafts, and (4) wean from cardiopulmonary bypass, and close the chest.

Usual preparation for cardiopulmonary bypass involves placement of cannulae into the arterial circulation and systemic venous circulation to flow blood to the body. Cardioplegia cannulae are inserted to flow preservative solution to the heart. Finally, the patient must be completely anticoagulated with heparin before cardiopulmonary bypass can be initiated.

The complications of cardiopulmonary bypass in general are emboli (either solid or air), aortic dissection, hypoperfusion, hyperperfusion, inflammatory response, thrombocytopenia, adult respiratory distress syndrome, and renal failure.

The conduction system of the heart crosses the interventricular septum adjacent to the aortic valve. This location is near the membranous septum, which lies under the commissure between the right and noncoronary cusps. Damage to the conduction system here with valve-replacement surgery can necessitate placement of a permanent pacemaker.

Mitral valve annuloplasty usually moves the posterior portion of the annulus toward the left ventricular outflow tract. One of the dangers of mitral valve repair is to move the anterior leaflet coaptation point too far into this outflow tract, thereby causing obstruction to the flow of blood from the ventricle. This is called *systolic anterior motion* of the *mitral* (SAM).

therapy was studied in the CASS (Coronary Artery Surgery Study), the Veterans Administration Cooperative Study, and the European Study. These studies defined those subgroups that receive longevity benefit from surgical therapy, separating the indications for surgery into two groupings: quality of life and longevity. The guiding principle of therapy is to escalate treatment until the patient is pain free, moving from medical therapy to surgery. However, identified left main coronary disease requires primary surgical therapy.

Medical therapy for CAD entails certain basic principles. Medications are given to dilate the coronary vasculature, reduce myocardial oxygen consumption, prevent further build-up of atherosclerosis, inhibit platelet activation and clot formation, and treat comorbid factors such as diabetes mellitus. Newer medications, such as angiotensin-converting enzyme (ACE) inhibitors, also are being used to aid in cardiac remodeling, reduce vascular inflammation, and perhaps stop the progression of atherosclerosis. CHF also requires treatment with additional medications, such as diuretics and inotropes. Medical therapy is effective for a large number of patients; however, it is often expensive and not without side effects.

Catheter-based interventions, such as percutaneous transluminal coronary angioplasty (PTCA) and intracoronary stents, are very effective methods of reestablishing coronary blood flow in selected patients, especially when combined with powerful new platelet inhibitors. PTCA was compared with surgery in a number of large randomized trials, such as the BARI (Bypass Angioplasty Revascularization Investigation). These trials demonstrated that multivessel angioplasty could produce a survival similar to that of surgery in selected patients. The best angioplasty results were in nondiabetic patients with discrete lesions amenable to this approach, although PTCA patients required more reinterventions, either repeated PTCA or crossover to bypass surgery. The use of stents has enhanced angioplasty results and reduced the number of interventions necessary to procure a favorable outcome. Continued improvement is noted in the results of catheter-based interventions, and the recidivism rate is decreasing.

The most recent advance in catheter-based intervention involves the use of "coated stents" to dilate coronary stenoses. Two stents have been approved for use in the United States. These stents are coated with tacrolimus or sirolimus, which inhibit tissue ingrowth into the stented region. These stents have been shown to reduce dramatically the incidence of in-stent stenosis, which was a primary cause of stent failure. However, they also have been associated with a slightly higher rate of acute stent thrombosis, and therefore require longer antiplatelet therapy.

The surgical intervention for coronary stenosis is the procedure known as CABG or coronary artery bypass grafting. Patients who experience a longevity benefit from CABG are those with left main stenosis greater than 50%, three-vessel disease (LAD, LCx, RCA) with reduced ejection fraction (<40%), and two-vessel disease with proximal LAD stenosis (>90%). All other patients do not have a survival benefit and receive quality-of-life improvement with freedom from angina, decreased medication requirements, decreased incidence of heart failure, reduction in risk of MI, and improved functional health. Because not all patients receive longevity benefit from CABG, the decision to operate must include a frank discussion of the risks and benefits of the procedure (Table 29-1).

TABLE 29–1 General Indications for Coronary Artery Bypass Grafting

Longevity	Quality of Life
≥50% stenosis of left main coronary	Class III or IV angina
Three vessel disease with reduced ejection fraction (<45%)	Unstable angina
90% proximal LAD stenosis with two-vessel disease	Postinfarct angina
CABG before aortic vascular procedure	Intolerance of antianginal therapy
	Failure of PTCA or Stent

LAD, left anterior descending artery; CABG, coronary artery bypass graft; PTCA, percutaneous transluminal coronary angiography.

Coronary Artery Bypass Grafting

Operations for CAD require a team approach involving many different disciplines. Anesthetic management plays a key role in safely anesthetizing a cardiac patient while preventing the onset of ischemia and maintaining adequate hemodynamics. A perfusionist oversees the CPB pump. This complex machine allows the heart to stop for a portion of the operation while maintaining oxygenated blood flow to the remainder of the body, removing CO_2, maintaining volume balance, and intermittently perfusing the heart with a cardioplegia solution to maintain diastolic arrest. The surgical team consists of highly trained nursing personnel who assist in maintaining the flow of the operation while the surgeon and the assistant focus on the technical maneuvers of performing the operation.

A significant amount of planning goes into the performance of CABG. The decision points for CABG are (1) selection for operation, (2) preop evaluation of comorbidities, (3) type of operation/selection of vessels to be grafted, (4) selection of conduit, (5) manner of myocardial preservation, and (6) adjunctive therapies.

Patient selection is an important part of the preop evaluation. The patient plays a key role in making the decision for medical or surgical therapy, especially if the indications for surgery relate to quality of life rather than

BOX 29-2 Risk Factors for Poor Outcome with CABG

Age
Poor ventricular function or CHF
Emergency/urgent operation
Renal failure/dialysis
Diabetes mellitus with sequelae
COPD
Cerebrovascular disease
Peripheral vascular disease
Morbid obesity
Prior cardiac surgery
Calcified aorta
Concomitant valve surgery
Female patient

CABG, coronary artery bypass graft; CHF, congestive heart failure; COPD, chronic obstructive pulmonary disease.

to longevity. Comorbidities that have a negative impact on outcome from CABG are age, poor ventricular function or CHF, cerebrovascular disease, renal failure, diabetes with sequelae, chronic obstructive pulmonary disease (COPD), morbid obesity, peripheral vascular disease, and prior cardiac operation. The urgency of the operation also affects outcome, with the worst outcome in emergency operations and the best in elective procedures (Box 29-2).

Once the patient is selected, a few options exist for how the revascularization can be done: (1) standard CABG with beating-heart cardiopulmonary bypass (CPB), (2) median sternotomy off-pump CABG (OPCAB), and (3) on-pump (Heartport) or off-pump minimally invasive (small incision) CABG (MIDCAB). Given the goal of total revascularization, targets for bypasses are selected based on angiographic appearance, stenosis greater than 50%, size of vessel, and quality of outflow. The choice of operation depends primarily on the patient's anatomy and the surgeon's level of comfort with each procedure.

Available conduits for CABG can be split into arterial and venous. Arteries that have been successfully used for conduit are the internal mammary artery (IMA), also called the internal thoracic artery (ITA), the radial artery, the gastroepiploic artery, and the inferior epigastric artery. Good evidence indicates that the best patency rates are obtained with ITA grafts, especially to the LAD distribution, and growing evidence suggests that the radial artery may have better long-term patency than the vein. Other arterial conduits are more difficult to harvest and may have other problems, which limit patency. The stalwart vein conduit has always been the reversed greater saphenous vein. Vein also can be obtained from the lesser saphenous system, the arms, and can be used as homologous tissue transplant with cryopreserved vein. No artificial (man-made) conduit material has been successful in coronary grafting (Figs. 29-7 and 29-8)

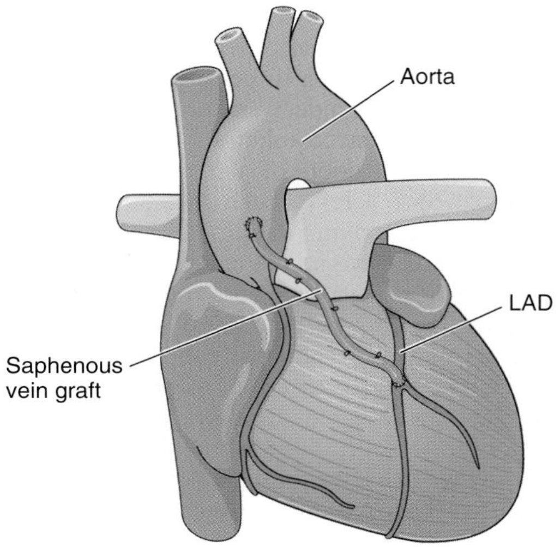

FIGURE 29–7 Reversed saphenous vein graft from the aorta to the left anterior descending coronary artery.

Myocardial preservation techniques vary greatly from surgeon to surgeon and patient to patient. The basic principle is that the heart is ischemic until revascularized and that the duration of ischemia should be as short as possible. If the CPB machine is used, the options include (1) on CPB with a beating heart, (2) intermittent cross-clamp, (3) fibrillatory arrest and no cross-clamp, and (4) cross-clamp with antegrade, retrograde, or combined cardioplegia. The cardioplegia solution is a buffered high-potasium electrolyte solution to induce and maintain diastolic arrest

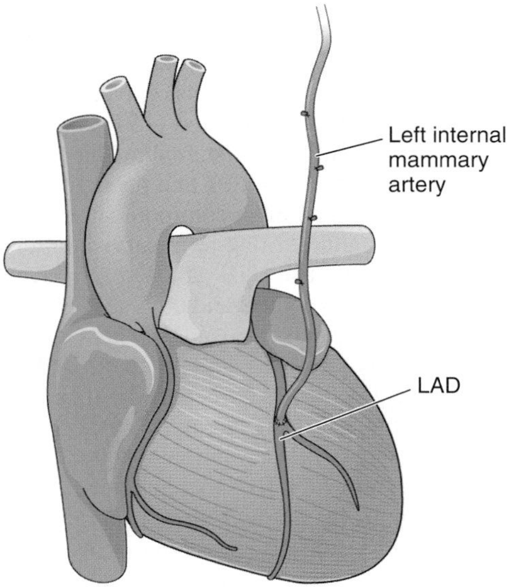

FIGURE 29–8 Internal mammary artery anastomosed to the left anterior descending coronary artery.

of the heart, protecting the myocardium during the ischemic surgical interval and providing a bloodless, still surgical field for the surgeon to perform optimal surgery. The many variations include warm or cold, crystalloid, blood, or substrate enhanced solutions. Sometimes factors such as severe calcification of the ascending aorta or mobile atheromatous debris in the ascending aorta will prohibit safe cross-clamping, thus forcing the decision on myocardial preservation to no-clamp techniques.

Depending on the patient's condition, certain interventions can be performed to improve outcome. Patients with severe preop ischemia or poor ventricular function can have an intra-aortic balloon pump (IABP) placed preoperatively. If a region marked for revascularization cannot be revascularized, transmyocardial laser revascularization can be performed. Vessels that have diffuse calcification or atheromatous debris can have the atheromatous core removed (i.e., endarterectomy) and then grafted. These are just a few of the adjunctive therapies available to improve the results of CABG. New therapies with angiogenesis and stem cells are under investigation.

The operation itself consists of four essential stages. The first stage is harvesting of the conduit. The second stage is preparation for CPB, with insertion of cannulae. The third stage is on-bypass time, with a subset of that being ischemic or cross-clamp time. The actual revascularization is performed during this stage. The final stage is closing and consists of reversal of anticoagulation, decannulation, and closure of the chest.

Outcomes of Coronary Artery Bypass Grafting

The outcomes of CABG have been widely studied since the initial randomized trials in the 1970s. For all patients in the United States who undergo CABG only, the average mortality is about 2.7% (from the Society of Thoracic Surgeons Database). Complications of the procedure include stroke (1% to 2%), atrial fibrillation (15% to 30%), bleeding requiring reoperation (2%), sternal/mediastinal infection (0.5% to 1%), renal failure (1%), and pneumonia/respiratory failure (2% to 5%). The most common cause of death after CABG is cardiac failure. Long-term survival after CABG is about 88% at 5 years and 75% at 10 years. Freedom from angina is about 80% at 5 years and 60% at 10 years. Freedom from MI is greater than 95% at 5 years. Finally, overall functional status is greatly improved after CABG, although this is intimately related to freedom from angina. Up to 10 years after the return of angina, about 50% to 60% of patients will be free of reintervention of any kind (Box 29-3).

Graft patency after CABG also has been evaluated. For saphenous vein grafts, about 10% will be occluded within the first 3 months, and after that, about 40% to 60% are patent at 10 years. Internal thoracic artery (same as the internal mammary artery) grafts have a much better patency, especially when anastomosed to the LAD system: approximately 97% are open at 3 months with about 90% open at 10 years. Internal thoracic artery-to-LAD grafts have been shown to improve overall survival in CABG patients. Radial artery grafts are showing good patency rates when used to bypass very obstructed arteries (>75% occlusion). The problem with all data for graft patency rates is that repeated cardiac catheterization does not occur unless the patient is symptomatic, so clinically silent graft occlusions are not detected. The causes of graft occlusion are multifactorial and include technical problems, intimal hyperplasia, in-graft atherosclerosis, and progression of native arterial disease. The use of postoperative aspirin, lipid-lowering agents, and smoking cessation are the standard of care after surgery to prolong graft patency and delay progression of atherosclerotic disease.

BOX 29-3 Complications of Coronary Artery Bypass Graft

- Death
- Myocardial infarction
- Bleeding requiring transfusion
- Bleeding requiring reoperation
- Infection (superficial or deep)
- Stroke
- Atrial fibrillation
- Ventricular arrhythmia
- Renal failure
- Pneumonia/respiratory failure
- Other organ failure

Valvular Heart Disease

Valvular heart disease should be understood as a mechanical problem that creates a pathophysiologic state. The important factors related to a patient's valvular disease can be remembered in the context of a generic framework. With the points of this framework, a valvular lesion can be accurately described and understood. These points are anatomic location, valvular pathology, etiology, pathophysiology, and functional status and symptoms (Table 29-2).

Valvular diseases can be identified by history, physical examination, and imaging tests. Many patients with valvular disease are initially seen with symptoms of fatigue, dyspnea, angina, syncope, arrhythmia, or CHF. A complete history for valvular disease should include a precise description of the timing of the onset of symptoms and the functional status of the patient. Physical examination of any patient with suspected valvular disease includes pulse examination, auscultation of the lungs for rales, palpation of the precordium for changes in the position of the ventricular impulse, auscultation of the precordium for murmurs, and examination for signs of CHF (i.e., JVD, pedal edema, liver pulsations). A good examination can usually identify the suspected lesion.

TABLE 29–2 Basic Valvular Lesions

Anatomic Location	Valvular Pathology	Etiology	Pathophysiology	Functional Status/Symptoms
Aortic valve	Stenotic	Rheumatic, senile calcific, bicuspid	Pressure overload on LV with concentric hypertrophy	Angina, syncope, CHF
Aortic valve	Regurgitant	Rheumatic, Annulo-aortic ectasia, Marfan, endocarditis, aortic dissection	Volume overload on the LV with dilation	Fatigue, dyspnea, exercise intolerance, CHF
Mitral valve	Stenotic	Rheumatic, senile calcific, congenital	Pressure load on LA, pulmonary vasculature and RV Dilation of LA and pulmonary hypertension + or – RV failure	Dyspnea, CHF, hemoptysis, thromboembolism, atrial fibrillation, cachexia
Mitral valve	Regurgitant	Ischemic, rheumatic, connective tissue disease, cardiomyopathy, endocarditis	Volume overload on LA and pulmonary vasculature, progressive LV dilation	Dyspnea, fatigue, CHF

LV, left ventricle; LA, left atrium; RV, right ventricle; CHF, congestive heart failure.

Further testing in patients with valvular disease includes chest radiograph to identify cardiac calcification, signs of pulmonary edema, cardiomegaly, or changes in the mediastinal silhouette. An electrocardiogram (ECG) is often helpful to demonstrate ischemia, previous infarction, axis changes, arrhythmia, or signs of hypertrophy. Laboratory investigations would include complete blood count (CBC) to identify anemia, blood urea nitrogen (BUN) and creatinine to identify renal problems, liver-function tests in patients with suspected right heart failure, blood cultures in patients with suspected endocarditis, albumin to measure nutritional status, and possibly arterial blood gas to evaluate pulmonary function.

The mainstay imaging test for valvular heart disease is two-dimensional echocardiography with Doppler and color flow imaging. This test can be performed either by transthoracic or transesophageal routes. This test can describe the anatomic appearance of all the valves, can calculate the functional surface area of the valves based on flow and velocity of flow through the valve, can evaluate for chamber hypertrophy or dilation, can assess biventricular function, and can estimate pulmonary artery pressures. Men who are older than 35 years and women older than 45 years should undergo cardiac catheterization before valve surgery. Cardiac catheterization can reveal CAD, measure pressure gradients across valves, measure chamber pressures during the cardiac cycle, and measure cardiac output. Nuclear imaging studies can be useful to evaluate for regional ischemia or to quantitate ventricular function.

Aortic Valve Disease

Aortic Stenosis

The aortic valve is a trileaflet valve positioned between the LV and the aorta. Its main function is to prevent regurgitation of blood into the LV after systole. Stenotic lesions of the aortic valve can be either supravalvular, valvular, or subvalvular; rarer is obstruction of the LV outflow tract by obstructive muscle hypertrophy. The normal surface area of an aortic valve is 3 to 4 cm^2. Stenosis, or obstruction to flow, is usually thought to be hemodynamically significant when the surface area is functionally less than 1 cm^2. The most common causes of valvular aortic stenosis (AS) are rheumatic fever, senile calcific degeneration, calcific aortic stenosis, and stenosis of a congenitally bicuspid aortic valve.

In aortic stenosis, the underlying physiology is related to increased pressure workload on the LV over a prolonged period. The increased pressure workload induces muscular hypertrophy, resulting in concentric hypertrophy of the ventricle. This hypertrophy results in a number of changes, including increased LV diastolic filling pressure, increased myocardial oxygen consumption and, over time, progressive LV dysfunction. It is important to remember that aortic stenosis is a flow-limiting lesion. Thus cardiac output is somewhat fixed, thereby preventing the heart from responding to body demands for increased cardiac output.

Patients with untreated critical AS are at risk for sudden death, usually related to hypotension and myocardial

PEARLS FOR ROUNDS

The indications for coronary artery bypass graft (CABG) can be split into categories of longevity and quality of life. Left main stenosis greater than 50%, three-vessel disease with ejection fraction less than 45%, and two-vessel disease with 90% proximal left anterior descending artery stenosis all improve longevity in surgically treated patients as compared with medically treated patients. Problems such as angina (which limits normal activities), unstable angina, postinfarct angina, intolerance of medical therapy for angina, and failure of percutaneous intervention are all indications for CABG, which improves quality of life.

The classic symptoms of aortic stenosis can help to predict the natural history of the disease if left untreated. Angina is associated with a 5-year average survival. Syncope is associated with a 3-year average survival. Congestive heart failure has the worst prognosis, with a 2-year survival.

Valve choice is a difficult problem. Mechanical valves are durable and have excellent hemodynamic properties; however, they require life-long anticoagulation. Tissue valves do not require anticoagulation; however, they are not as durable, and the patient may be faced with the prospect of reoperation when the valve fails. Therefore the patient's long-term expected survival is balanced with the risk of coumadin versus reoperation.

Prolonged anticoagulation with coumadin may carry significant problems, such as a 1% to 2% per year risk of thromboembolic or bleeding complications, and this effect is additive over a patient's lifetime. Coumadin is not good for the very elderly (older than 85 years), patients who are noncompliant or who will not maintain medical follow-up, patients with underlying progressive liver disease, patients with significant intracranial pathology, patients with a known bleeding disorder, or patients with medical illnesses that may require other surgical procedures.

ischemia. Patients with AS depend on increased preload for adequate filling of the LV and some measure of increased aortic pressures to maintain adequate coronary perfusion. These patients have problems when they vasodilate (either reducing preload or blood pressure) or develop tachycardia or atrial fibrillation. Decreased blood pressure causes decreased coronary perfusion, which quickly progresses to myocardial ischemia. The ischemia causes LV dysfunction, which then leads to further hypotension, ischemia, and eventual death. Tachycardia and atrial fibrillation can both decrease diastolic filling of the LV, resulting in hypotension as well.

The natural history of AS shows a long latency period between the development of stenosis and the onset of symptoms. The classic symptoms of AS are angina, syncope, and CHF. These symptoms have been used to prognosticate survival if AS is untreated. Angina has a 5-year survival, syncope has a 3-year survival, and CHF has a 2-year survival. Patients without symptomatic AS and greater than 1.0-cm^2 valve area can be monitored with 6- to 12-month examinations and echocardiograms. Arrhythmias should be promptly treated and followed up. Otherwise little role exists for medical therapy in AS.

Patients with critical AS (<0.75 cm^2 valve area and/or valvular gradient >50 mmHg) and symptoms of AS should be considered for surgical intervention. Asymptomatic patients with critical AS who show evidence of LV dysfunction or exercise intolerance also should be considered for surgery. Men older than 35 years and women older than 45 years should undergo preoperative cardiac catheterization to evaluate for the presence of CAD and quantify the severity of the AS.

Interventions for AS include balloon valvuloplasty, ultrasonic decalcification of the valve, and valve replacement. Balloon valvuloplasty has shown poor long-term results with calcific AS in adults, with rapid restenosis. However, it can provide immediate improvement in patients in cardiogenic shock or who are not candidates for surgical therapy. Valve decalcification is unsatisfactory in most patients and frequently results in valvular insufficiency and restenosis. The most durable outcome is obtained by aortic valve replacement.

The first decision to be made in valve-replacement surgery is what type of valve replacement to use. The options are the following:

- mechanical valve
- stented bioprosthetic (tissue) valve
- stentless bioprosthetic valve
- homograft valve
- pulmonary autograft valve

The factors considered in deciding between the types of prosthesis are desire for or contraindications to prolonged anticoagulation, age of the patient, size of the aortic root, and patient preferences. One special circumstance is women of childbearing age who wish to have children in the future; these women should not have a valve replacement requiring anticoagulation because of risks to the fetus and risks of thromboembolic and bleeding complications in the mother. The rules are as follows:

- Mechanical valves require prolonged anticoagulation but do not degenerate.
- Porcine aortic valves do not require anticoagulation but degenerate over time, usually 25% at 10 years and 50% at 15 years.
- Pericardial tissue valves only have 10% degeneration at 10 years.
- The patient should be left with the lowest residual gradient possible.
- Stentless tissue valves and mechanical valves have the lowest transvalvular gradients.
- Homograft and autograft procedures may have better durability, but the operative procedure is much more complex.

TABLE 29–3 Choice of Valve Replacement

Valve	Pro	Con
Tissue	Low thromboembolic rate	Degenerate over time, requiring replacement
Mechanical	Very durable	Higher rate of thromboembolic complication, require lifelong anticoagulation

In general, older patients (older than 70 years) are recommended for tissue valve replacement because the risk of thromboembolic problems and bleeding complications from anticoagulation can outweigh the risk of reoperation for valve degeneration. Younger patients are recommended to have mechanical valve replacement or tissue valve replacement with a homograft or pulmonary autograft (Tables 29-3 and 29-4).

The operation for aortic valve replacement requires CPB, aortic cross-clamping, adequate myocardial preservation, thorough débridement of the aortic valve, precise placement of sutures to secure the valve replacement, and adequate de-airing of the aorta and LV. The aortic-valve operation can be approached through a complete median sternotomy, a partial median sternotomy, or a right parasternal approach. Recently some evidence has accumulated that the two latter "minimally invasive" approaches may have some benefits in terms of pulmonary function, postoperative pain, and speed of postoperative functional recovery. The risks of aortic valve surgery include stroke, distal embolization, poor myocardial preservation, injury to main coronary arteries, arrhythmia, complete heart block, paravalvular leak, bleeding, and infection.

The operative mortality associated with aortic valve replacement is 2% to 7%, but is higher in patients with ventricular dysfunction or concomitant CAD. The 5-year survival after valve replacement is better than 85%. Almost all surviving patients undergo dramatic improvement in hemodynamics, with regression of LV hypertrophy over time and marked improvements in functional status.

TABLE 29–4 Types of Prosthetic Valves

Valve Type	Category	Example
Mechanical	Caged ball	Starr Edwards
	Tilting disk	Medtronic Hall
	Bileaflet	St. Jude
Tissue	Stented	Hancock Porcine Valve
		CE Bovine Pericardial
	Stentless	Toronto SPV
	Aortic homograft	

Aortic Regurgitation

Aortic regurgitation (AR) or insufficiency occurs when the aortic valve allows blood to leak back into the LV at the end of systole. The most common causes of AR are rheumatic disease, congenitally bicuspid aortic valve, annuloaortic ectasia, infective endocarditis, Marfan syndrome, aortic dissection, and degeneration of a bioprosthetic aortic valve. In general, these disease processes result in leaflet weakness or prolapse, leaflet scarring or degeneration, or aortic dilation at the sinotubular ridge, annulus, or both.

AR creates a volume overload in the LV. This results in progressive ventricular dilation and eventual dysfunction, leading to irreversible cardiac dysfunction. The eccentric hypertrophy of the ventricle creates increased wall tension (or afterload) on the LV, increasing myocardial oxygen consumption and thinning the ventricular wall thickness. As the ventricle continues to dilate, interstitial fibrosis of the myocardium occurs, resulting in irreversible myocardial dysfunction, eventually leading to chronic heart failure. Acute AR results on overwhelming volume overload on the ventricle with dramatic increasing in diastolic pressures, causing acute ventricular decompensation and the rapid onset of severe CHF.

Patients with chronic AR have a long latency period as the ventricular slowly dilates in response to progressive volume overload. These patients have fatigue, dyspnea, exercise intolerance, and CHF. Patients with acute AR are often first seen in extremis with severe CHF and cardiovascular collapse. Medical therapy for chronic AR includes afterload reduction with ACE inhibitors and antihypertensives, diuretic use to reduce volume overload, and prompt treatment of arrhythmias. Patients should be monitored every 6 months with examination and echocardiogram to assess symptoms, ventricular size, and ejection fraction. Patients with acute severe regurgitation require stabilization and immediate surgical intervention.

The timing of operation in chronic AR can be a difficult decision. The usual indications are severe regurgitation with symptoms, LV dysfunction, or excessive LV dilation. The risks of operation and valve replacement must be balanced against the risks of waiting too long and having irreversible LV dysfunction. Because the risks of surgery continue to improve, patients can be offered operation earlier, before the onset of LV dysfunction. Asymptomatic patients with evidence of LV dilation should be offered valve surgery.

Surgery for AR usually requires valve replacement. However, in cases of cusp prolapse and dissection, the valve can resuspended or repaired. Patients with aortic root dilation and normal annulus and leaflets can undergo replacement of the aortic root with implantation of the native valve into the prosthesis, reestablishing the geometry necessary for proper valve function and leaflet coaptation. The choice of valve replacement for AR is otherwise the same as that for AS. The surgical approach also is the same.

Long-term survival after surgical intervention is excellent in patients with preserved LV function and is associated with good functional status. Patients with significant LV dilation (>55 mm end-diastolic diameter) or severely reduced ejection fraction (<45% EF) do not see such an improvement in functional status or survival. These patients can continue to undergo progressive ventricular dilation and dysfunction, despite a competent aortic valve.

Mitral Valve Disease

Mitral Stenosis

The mitral valve is a bileaflet valve that prevents reflux of blood into the LA during LV systole. The valve mechanism should be thought of as a continuum between the annulus, valve leaflets, chordae tendinae, papillary muscles, and the LV wall. Any change in the function or configuration of these elements can cause mitral valve and ventricular dysfunction. Mitral stenosis (MS) is most commonly caused by rheumatic disease. Other causes include congenital MS, senile calcific disease, and connective tissue disorders. Left atrial myxoma and endocarditis with large vegetations can mimic MS. Rheumatic disease can cause scarring and retraction throughout the entire valve mechanism, including into the LV wall. The normal cross-sectional area of the mitral valve is 4 to 6 cm^2. Critical MS occurs with a valve area of 1.0 cm^2 or less. The pressure gradient across the mitral valve can be difficult to measure because it is highly dependent on flow across the valve, but is usually greater than 20 mmHg across a critical stenosis.

Pure MS is associated with pressure load on the LA and pulmonary vasculature. This can cause hypertrophy and dilation of the LA and lead to pulmonary hypertension that can approach systemic pressures. This pressure load through the LA and pulmonary vasculature leads to chronic CHF, LA dilation, chronic atrial fibrillation, and RV failure secondary to pulmonary hypertension. Often the LV assumes normal or small dimensions with a thin ventricular wall. The scarring of rheumatic disease through the subvalvular apparatus can cause decreased ventricular compliance and wall-motion abnormalities.

The primary presenting symptom of MS is dyspnea. Other common symptoms are hemoptysis, thromboembolism, and chest pain. Severe longstanding MS can result in biventricular failure with pulmonary edema, ascites, peripheral edema, hepatomegaly, and cachexia. The natural history of MS shows a long asymptomatic period, but rapid progression of disease once symptoms become apparent.

Medical therapy for MS includes diuretic therapy to treat pulmonary edema, treatment of atrial or ventricular arrhythmias, and often anticoagulation in patients with atrial fibrillation. In general, however, the treatment of MS requires an interventional approach.

The options for interventions include balloon valvuloplasty, closed mitral commisurotomy, open mitral commisurotomy, and mitral valve replacement. The decision for which intervention to carry out depends on (1) pathology of the valve and involvement of subvalvular apparatus, (2) degree of calcification present, (3) mobility of the valve leaflets, (4) age of the patient, and (5) need for prolonged anticoagulation. Scoring systems have been devised to predict the patient's suitability for balloon valvuloplasty and prognosis for restenosis. In selected patients, balloon valvuloplasty can yield excellent short-term and long-term results, particularly in patients looking to prolong the interval before valve replacement (i.e., women of childbearing age).

The modern surgical approach to MS is either open commisurotomy or mitral valve replacement. The mitral valve can be exposed by many different approaches: median sternotomy, partial median sternotomy, right thoracotomy, right anterior thoracotomy, or left thoracotomy. New techniques of cannulation for bypass, such as the Heartport system, have been devised to allow the mitral valve to be approached through a smaller incision. Open operation on the mitral valve requires CPB with arterial and usually bicaval venous cannulation, adequate myocardial protection, and adequate visualization. If the aortic valve remains competent, mitral operations can be performed without aortic cross-clamp under fibrillatory arrest with cooling. The valve is usually visualized through the LA by incision in the interatrial groove by the right pulmonary veins. The valve also can be approached via the RA through the interatrial septum.

Open commisurotomy involves incising the fused leaflets at the valve commissures as well as freeing adhesions in the subvalvular apparatus. The choice of valve replacement in the mitral position is essentially the same, although somewhat more limited, as that for aortic valve replacement, mainly mechanical valve or stented bioprosthetic valve. Some surgeons have reported early success with mitral valve homograft, although the data lack long-term follow-up. Mechanical valves in the mitral position have a higher rate of thromboembolic complications, presumably secondary to lower flow rates across the valve, and require increased anticoagulation. Tissue valves in the mitral position seem to degenerate at a faster rate than those in the aortic position and also can be associated with thromboembolic events. The risks of mitral valve replacement include stroke, peripheral emboli, bleeding, infection, arrhythmia, prolonged respiratory failure, perivalve leak, valve thrombosis, ventricular rupture, and persistent ventricular dysfunction.

Open commisurotomy carries a 1% to 2% mortality with a low rate of early restenosis at about 10% in 6 years. Mitral valve replacement carries a 2% to 10% mortality with good long-term results in patients with good LV function, normal RV function, and no CAD.

Mitral Regurgitation

In the United States, mitral regurgitation (MR) is probably the most common disease of the mitral valve. Any abnormality of the components of the mitral apparatus can lead to MR; these categories include leaflet problems, annular problems, chordae tendinae problems, papillary muscle problems, and ventricular wall problems. In general, the etiologies of MR can include rheumatic disease, mitral valve prolapse, congenital disorders, myxomatous degeneration, infective endocarditis, chronic or acute sequelae of ischemic heart disease, primary cardiomyopathy with ventricular dilation, and connective tissue disorders (Fig. 29-9)

Fundamentally, the pathophysiology of MR is volume overload on the LA and pulmonary vasculature with reduced forward cardiac output. During systole, the ventricle will initially eject some percentage of the stroke volume into the LA before the aortic valve opens and allows forward flow to the aorta. In the long term, this increases LV preload and increases LV end-diastolic volume, resulting in LV dilation. Acute and chronic severe MR lead to pulmonary hypertension and pulmonary edema. Initially, the LV improves the effectiveness of contraction, and the ejection fraction is increased to compensate for the regurgitant volume. However, the progressive dilation of the LV leads eventually to LV dysfunction and decompensation. Ischemic etiologies for MR exacerbate this cycle by quickening the progression to LV dysfunction. Acute severe MR can result in immediate decompensation and pulmonary edema because the LV cannot compensate for the decreased forward output or the regurgitant volume going backward into the pulmonary vasculature.

Acute severe MR often is first seen with cardiovascular collapse from reduced cardiac output and severe CHF. Chronic MR appears in a more insidious fashion, with increasing dyspnea and fatigue, which may not even be noticed by the patient. Patients can often compensate for their symptoms until congestive failure begins to develop from LV dysfunction. Those patients who have chronic MR related to ischemia usually see a more rapid progression of symptoms.

Therapy for acute severe MR is stabilization with inotropic support and usually an IABP. The goal is immediately to reduce afterload to enhance forward cardiac output. These patients invariably require urgent surgical intervention. Patients with chronic MR can be treated medically with afterload reduction with ACE inhibitors, diuretic therapy, and treatment of arrhythmias. Those patients with intermittent ischemic MR also should be treated for the ischemia. Patients with chronic MR can be monitored with examinations and echocardiography to assess a number of factors: (1) functional status and symptoms, (2) ventricular function, (3) presence or absence of associated CAD, (4) evidence of primary cardiomyopathy with ventricular dilation as cause of MR (these patients may not respond as well to surgical therapy), and (5) presence of other valvular lesions.

The indications for surgical intervention are currently in flux, especially with the advent of safe, reliable techniques for repair of the native mitral valve. Basically, patients with severe MR and LV dysfunction or symptoms should be considered for operation. Only those patients with a primary severe cardiomyopathy may not benefit from surgical treatment. As in aortic disease, patients being evaluated for mitral surgery should undergo cardiac catheterization to evaluate for concomitant CAD. The options for reparative treatment include ring annuloplasty, leaflet reconstruction with annuloplasty, and chordal reconstruction with neochordae, chordal shortening, or chordal transposition. If repair cannot be accomplished, then the valve must be replaced. It is important to

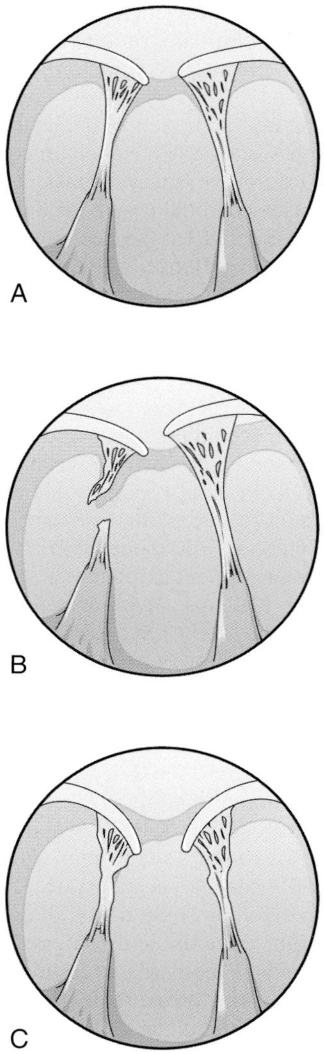

FIGURE 29–9 Mitral/ventricular complex. *A*, Annular or ventricular dilation. *B*, Chordal rupture. *C*, Myxomatous degeneration (floppy leaflets or chordae).

remember that valve replacement with MR should include preservation of the chordal structure in the ventricle. This helps to maintain normal LV function and geometry after valve replacement.

The operation and approach to the mitral valve for MR is the same as that for MS. Patients with concomitant CAD should undergo coronary artery bypass. Most valves with MR can be approached initially with the intent of performing a repair. Many factors affect the decision to repair a valve, including surgeon experience, valve pathology (posterior leaflet more amenable to repair than anterior leaflet), degree of annular calcification, leaflet mobility, and subvalvular involvement. The use of transesophageal echo to assess the valve repair intraoperatively is mandatory to achieve satisfactory results. Excessive (>2+) MR in the operating room after a repair would be considered a failed repair, and either that repair should be corrected or the valve should be replaced. Data from many centers show a 1% to 2% mortality with mitral valve repair, with excellent durability of the repair and freedom from reoperation. These patients also see a dramatic improvement in functional status. Mitral valve replacement for MR also can achieve similar results. Outcomes are not as good for either operation in patients with severe LV dysfunction or ischemic heart disease.

Tricuspid Valve Disease

The tricuspid valve is a trileaflet valve that prevents reflux of blood from the RV into the RA. Diseases of the tricuspid valve are less common than diseases of the left-sided heart valves. Tricuspid stenosis is usually secondary to rheumatic disease and almost always associated with MS. Tricuspid regurgitation (TR) can be secondary to RV dilation from pulmonary hypertension, infective endocarditis, carcinoid syndrome, or connective tissue disorders.

Tricuspid stenosis increases pressure in the RA and therefore increases the pressure in the systemic venous circulation. These patients are initially seen with fatigue, peripheral edema, hepatomegaly, and anasarca without pulmonary complaints. Because acquired tricuspid stenosis is usually associated with MS, these patients will not exhibit the symptoms of dyspnea or hemoptysis associated with classic MS. TR also is seen with signs and symptoms of elevated central venous pressures but is usually well tolerated unless other disease processes are involved, such as RV dysfunction, pulmonary hypertension, or left heart dysfunction.

The medical treatment of tricuspid stenosis is diuretic therapy and restriction of sodium intake. Surgical therapy involves open valve commissurotomy, opening the commissure between the anterior and septal leaflets, and freeing the subvalvular apparatus or tricuspid valve replacement. Often, this is part of a multivalve operation. Tricuspid valve replacement is usually performed with a bioprosthetic valve, because mechanical valves have a high rate of thromboembolic complications in the tricuspid position.

Medical treatment of TR is expectant unless the patient has pulmonary hypertension, RV dysfunction, or left heart dysfunction. Even then, the treatment of the primary problem treats the TR. Surgical therapy for TR associated with uncomplicated endocarditis can be as simple as merely excising the valve. In patients with a dilated RV and annulus causing TR, ring annuloplasty of the tricuspid annulus can greatly reduce the amount of regurgitation. Valve replacement for TR is reserved for patients with pulmonary hypertension and systemic problems related to increased central venous pressures. The major risk of tricuspid valve replacement or ring annuloplasty is damage to the AV nodal conduction system with the anatomic Triangle of Koch.

Aortic Dissection

Aortic dissection is a disease process in which the intima of the aorta literally tears, allowing entry of blood into the media of the aorta. Aortic dissection is associated with Marfan syndrome, connective tissue disorders, bicuspid aortic valve, trauma, aortic manipulation, or catheter injury. The dissection separates the intima from the adventitia of the aorta, creating a false channel of blood flow. Depending on the severity of the tear, the true lumen of the aorta can be totally occluded. Aortic dissection thus can be associated with aortic rupture, peripheral or organ ischemia due to flow occlusion, stroke, aortic valve insufficiency, and cardiac tamponade. Dissection usually is initially seen with chest pain and or back pain between the shoulder blades. Pain may be associated with limb ischemia, stroke, paralysis, anuria, abdominal pain, or tamponade. The diagnosis of aortic dissection can be suggested by history, physical findings of an aortic regurgitation murmur or posterior aortic murmur, widened mediastinum on chest radiograph, ischemia on ECG, or changes in pulse examination. The dissection can be imaged by the use of transesophageal echo, spiral CT scan, or MRI/magnetic resonance angiography (MRA). All three modalities are excellent.

Aortic dissection can be divided into two main groups, patients whose tear is in the ascending aorta distal to the aortic valve (Stanford type A) and patients whose tear is distal to the left subclavian artery in the descending aorta (Stanford type B). This distinction is important in deciding therapy. Type A dissections are treated surgically with excision of the tear and a portion of the ascending aorta, replacement with aortic graft, and repair or replacement of the aortic valve. The goals of surgical therapy are to remove the site of the intimal tear and to reestablish blood flow in the true lumen. Ascending dissection is treated operatively because of the risk of rupture into pericardium with resulting tamponade, risk of acute AR with onset of severe CHF and cardiovascular collapse, and risk of coronary ischemia with dissection into the coronary vessels. Uncomplicated type B dissection is treated

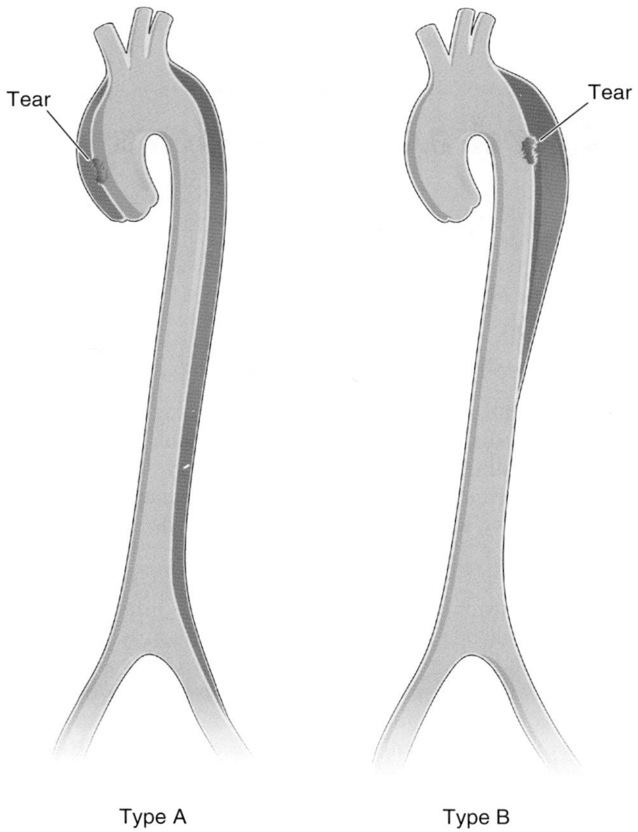

FIGURE 29–10 Aortic dissection (Stanford classification). Type A, Tear located in ascending aorta. Type B, Tear located in descending aorta.

medically with tight control of blood pressure by using β-blockers and afterload-reducing agents. β-Blockers are the primary therapy because they help to decrease the shear stress on the aortic wall. Complicated type B dissection may need to be treated surgically, either by aortic excision and graft replacement with necessary revascularizations or by refenestration of the false lumen to allow passage of blood back into the true lumen. Over time, uncomplicated type B dissections will become aneurysmal and may require resection and repair to prevent late rupture. This delayed operation, though, carries less risk than early operation at the time of dissection (Fig. 29-10).

Suggested Reading

Bonow RO, Carabello B, de Leon AC Jr: Guidelines for the management of patients with valvular heart disease: American College of Cardiology/American Heart Association Task Force on Practice Guidelines. Circulation 98:1949–1984, 1998.

Braunwald E, Zipes DP, Libby P: Heart Disease: A Textbook of Cardiovascular Medicine. Philadelphia, WB Saunders, 2001.

Eagle KG, Gayton RA, Davidoff R: ACC/AHA guidelines for coronary artery bypass graft surgery. Circulation 110(14):340–437, 2004.

Favaloro RG: Landmarks in the development of coronary artery bypass surgery. Circulation 98(5):466–478.

Kouchoukos NT, Blackstone EH, et al: Cardiac Surgery, 3rd ed. Philadelphia, Elsevier Science, 2003.

Shemin RJ: Randomized studies of coronary artery bypass grafting vs. medical or percutaneous catheter-based revascularization: A review. Adv Card Surg 11:1–34, 1999.

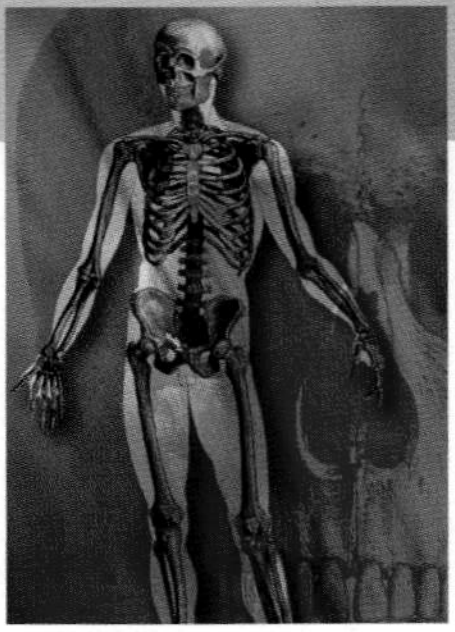

Chapter 30
Congenital Cardiac Disorders

OZ M. SHAPIRA, MD

Atrial Septal Defect

An atrial septal defect (ASD) is defined as an abnormal communication between the left and right atria, allowing shunting of blood between these two chambers.

Anatomy

Four anatomic types of ASD are found (Fig. 30-1):

1. The **ostium primum defect** is part of the spectrum of abnormalities of the atrioventricular (AV) canal septum.
2. The **ostium secundum defect** is the most common ASD and is located at the fossa ovalis.
3. The **sinus venosus defect** is either high (adjacent to the superior vena cava) or low (adjacent to the inferior vena cava) in the interatrial septum. A sinus venosus defect is usually associated with partial anomalous pulmonary venous return.
4. The **coronary sinus defect** with varying degrees of "unroofing" of the coronary sinus.

Pathophysiology

The physiologic mechanisms are similar in all types of ASD. The blood flow across ASDs is determined by the relative compliances of the right and left ventricles during diastole. In infancy, when the wall thickness of the right and left ventricles is similar, the flow across the ASD is low. However, as pulmonary vascular resistance decreases and becomes much lower than systemic vascular resistance, the wall of the left ventricle becomes much thicker and less compliant than that of the right ventricle, resulting in a significant left-to-right shunt. In adulthood, the difference in compliances usually becomes more pronounced as a result of processes that further decrease left ventricular compliance, such as myocardial ischemia or the presence of left ventricular hypertrophy secondary to hypertension or valvular disease. Thus an ASD with a small shunt early in life may not become clinically significant until the fifth, sixth, or seventh decade of life. Shunting is considered hemodynamically significant when the flow in the pulmonary circulation (Qp) is greater than or equal to 1.5 times the flow in the systemic circulation (Qs). Large left-to-right flow results in right ventricular volume overload, as well as varying degrees of pulmonary hypertension, leading to right atrial and right ventricular hypertrophy and dilation.

Evaluation

History and Physical Examination

Many patients are asymptomatic and are diagnosed when a murmur is discovered on routine physical examination. Typical findings include right ventricular uplift, a soft systolic murmur in the third intercostal space at the left sternal border, and wide fixed splitting of the second heart sound.

Infants with an ASD may first be seen with failure to thrive. Recurrent upper respiratory tract infections and pneumonia also are typical. The most common symptoms in children and young adults are those of congestive heart failure (CHF), including fatigue and dyspnea on exertion. Atrial and ventricular arrhythmias become more pronounced in the third and fourth decades of life. In up to 20% of patients, **Eisenmenger syndrome** will develop, characterized by severe pulmonary hypertension, reversed (right-to-left) shunt, right-sided heart failure, and cyanosis. Endocarditis is extremely rare in patients with ASD.

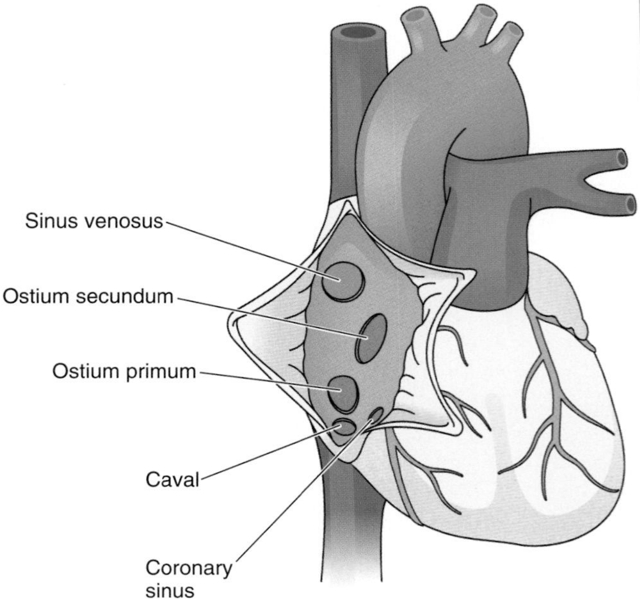

FIGURE 30–1 Types of atrial septal defects.

Electrocardiographic Studies

The electrocardiogram (ECG) typically shows right axis deviation, right ventricular hypertrophy, and conduction abnormalities, such as right bundle-branch block. Ostium primum defects are the only ASDs characterized by left axis deviation.

Imaging Studies

Plain films of the chest reveal right atrial and right ventricular dilatation and pulmonary artery enlargement. The diagnosis is confirmed by two-dimensional Doppler echocardiography. Cardiac catheterization is usually not necessary, but it is useful in patients who have severe pulmonary hypertension or in whom the anatomy is uncertain. Coronary arteriography is indicated only in patients who are older than 40 years or have multiple risk factors for coronary artery disease.

Treatment

Indications for Surgery

Spontaneous closure of a small ASD may occur during the first year of life but is rare after that time. Surgery is indicated in all symptomatic patients, as well as in asymptomatic patients who have an ASD that is larger that 1 or 2 cm, a (Qp/Qs) fraction that is greater that or equal to 1.5, and signs of right ventricular volume overload and pulmonary hypertension. The only contraindication for surgery is severe irreversible pulmonary hypertension (pulmonary vascular resistance exceeding 8–12 units/m^2).

Surgical Techniques

Surgery is performed with the use of cardiopulmonary bypass. The approach is through a median sternotomy, a right thoracotomy, a minimally invasive partial sternotomy, or subxiphoid incision. The ASD is closed either primarily with a continuous suture or with an autologous pericardial patch. In patients with a sinus venosus defect, baffling of abnormal pulmonary veins into the left atrium is required.

Complications and Outcome

The operative mortality rate is in the range of 0 to 1%. The frequency of major complications is in the range of 1% to 2%. In patients who undergo surgery early in life (before the development of CHF, atrial fibrillation, or pulmonary hypertension), long-term survival is equal to that of the healthy population. In one series with a 27-year follow-up, survival of patients who underwent surgery before they were 12 years old was 97%, whereas that of patients who underwent surgery after they were 40 years old was only 40%. These facts support an early and aggressive approach to the treatment of all patients who have ASD with a significant left-to-right shunt (Qp/Qs $\geq$ 1.5).

Total Anomalous Pulmonary Venous Return

Total anomalous pulmonary venous return (TAPVR) is a condition in which no direct communication exists between any of the pulmonary veins and the left atrium. The pulmonary veins drain either to a systemic vein or directly into the right atrium.

Anatomy

Darling and colleagues classified TAPVR into four types:

1. The **supracardiac type,** found in 40% to 45% of cases. The pulmonary veins drain into an ascending pulmonary vein that is connected to the innominate vein or the superior vena cava
2. The **cardiac type**, found in 20% to 25% of cases. The pulmonary veins drain directly into the right atrium or the coronary sinus.
3. In the **infracardiac type**, found in 20% to 25%, drainage is into an abdominal vein.
4. The **mixed type** is found in about 5% of cases.

Pathophysiology

The degree of cyanosis and severity of other symptoms are determined by the relative blood flows in the pulmonary and systemic circulation, which in turn are determined by three components: the degree of obstruction to flow in the anomalous connection, the degree of pulmonary hypertension, and the existence of an effective right-to-left shunt. Right-to-left shunting is almost always provided by a patent nonrestrictive foramen ovale. Significant venous obstruction is invariably accompanied by pulmonary arterial hypertension and is usually accompanied by systemic or supersystemic pulmonary arterial pressures. In the absence of pulmonary venous obstruction, an increase in pulmonary blood flow is associated with a low-compliance right ventricle, and this causes pulmonary arteriolar changes that lead to increased pulmonary vascular resistance and secondary pulmonary hypertension. Pulmonary vascular resistance and secondary pulmonary blood flow result in varying degrees of interstitial or alveolar pulmonary edema.

Without treatment, 80% of infants with TAPVR will die during the first year of life, with most deaths occurring during the first 3 months. However, 10% to 20% of patients who have nonobstructive connections without severe pulmonary hypertension survive to adulthood with minimal symptoms of heart failure, minimal cyanosis, and frequent respiratory tract infections.

Evaluation

History and Physical Examination

The severity of symptoms is directly related to the degree of obstruction of the anomalous connection. An infant with severe obstruction usually is first seen with respiratory distress, profound cyanosis, tachycardia, hypotension, and severe metabolic acidosis a few hours to several days after birth. In the absence of significant pulmonary venous obstruction, clinical manifestations are determined by the blood flow across the pulmonary circulation and the development of pulmonary hypertension. An infant with greatly increased pulmonary flow and severe pulmonary hypertension typically is initially seen in the first 1 to 2 years of life with symptoms of failure to thrive, right-sided heart failure, and intermittent cyanosis.

Laboratory Studies

Blood gas analysis shows arterial hypoxemia and metabolic acidosis.

Electrocardiographic Studies

An ECG is usually not helpful. In most patients with TAPVR, it shows right-axis deviation and right ventricular hypertrophy.

Imaging Studies

In patients with significant obstruction, plain films of the chest show a diffuse, bilateral, fine reticular pattern of interstitial edema without enlargement of the cardiac silhouette. In patients with hyperkinetic pulmonary circulation, plain films show prominent pulmonary vasculature and enlargement of the right atrium and right ventricle. In 90% of infants, the diagnosis is confirmed by two-dimensional Doppler echocardiography. Cardiac catheterization is rarely indicated in neonates but may be useful in older children or young adults.

Treatment

Indications for Surgery

TAPVR is the only congenital defect without any effective palliative medical treatment. Given the high rate of mortality in untreated cases, surgery in indicated whenever the diagnosis is made. Patients with severe obstruction during the first few hours of life should be transferred promptly to the operating room. Patients who do not have severe obstruction but have hyperdynamic pulmonary circulation should be scheduled for surgery early in infancy, to avoid the sequelae of cyanosis and pulmonary and right ventricular volume overload.

Surgical Techniques

TAPVR is corrected through a midline sternotomy incision, with the use of cardiopulmonary bypass. In many cases, the use of deep hypothermia and circulatory arrest is indicated to provide optimal exposure. The choice of operative technique is based on the type of defect, with a common goal of directing the pulmonary venous flow into the left atrium either by direct anastomosis between the anomalous connection and the left atrium or by various "baffling" techniques.

Complications and Outcome

Operative mortality and long-term survival rates are related to the degree of obstruction and pulmonary hypertension. In recent years, the operative mortality rate has decreased from 50% to 20% to 30% in neonates with severe obstruction. The rate is 5% to 10% in patients between ages 3 and 12 months, and it is lower than 5% in older children and young adults. Most patients have a good chance for long-term survival after a successful operation. In about 5% to 10%, recurrent pulmonary venous obstruction will develop. Patients undergoing late surgery may have progressive pulmonary hypertension despite a good repair.

Ventricular Septal Defect

Ventricular septal defect (VSD) is defined as an abnormal communication between the left and right ventricle. It may be an isolated anomaly or a component of a complex defect.

Anatomy

VSDs have been classified in various ways (Fig. 30-2). Because most VSDs are approached via the right side of the heart, a useful anatomic classification categorizes them into four groups, based on their involvement of the **atrioventricular canal;** the **muscular septum** (sinus septum); the **septal band** (proximal conoid septum or trabecula septomarginalis); and the **conoid septum** (infundibular septum, or parietal septum).

Pathophysiology

VSDs vary greatly in size, sometimes equaling or even exceeding the size of the aortic valve. VSDs that restrict the blood flow are called **restrictive VSDs,** whereas those causing no resistance to flow are called **nonrestrictive VSDs.**

In large nonrestrictive VSDs, the pressures in the right and left ventricles are equal. The flow across the VSD and therefore the relative flow in the pulmonary and systemic circulations (Qp/Qs) are determined by the relation between the pulmonary and systemic vascular resistance. Because pulmonary vascular resistance normally decreases shortly after birth, the flow in the pulmonary circulation increases, resulting in a Qp/Qs that exceeds 3.0. In small restrictive VSDs, the pressure in the right ventricle is only mildly elevated, and the Qp/Qs is usually less than 1.5. Medium-sized VSDs fall between these two categories, with a Qp/Qs in the range of 1.5 to 3.0.

Increased blood flow causes right and left ventricular volume overload, leading to biventricular enlargement and failure. Long-standing increased flow in the pulmonary circulation is associated with the development of pulmonary vascular disease. As pulmonary vascular resistance increases, the flow in the pulmonary circulation decreases. As a result, the shunt is smaller, and the patient may show

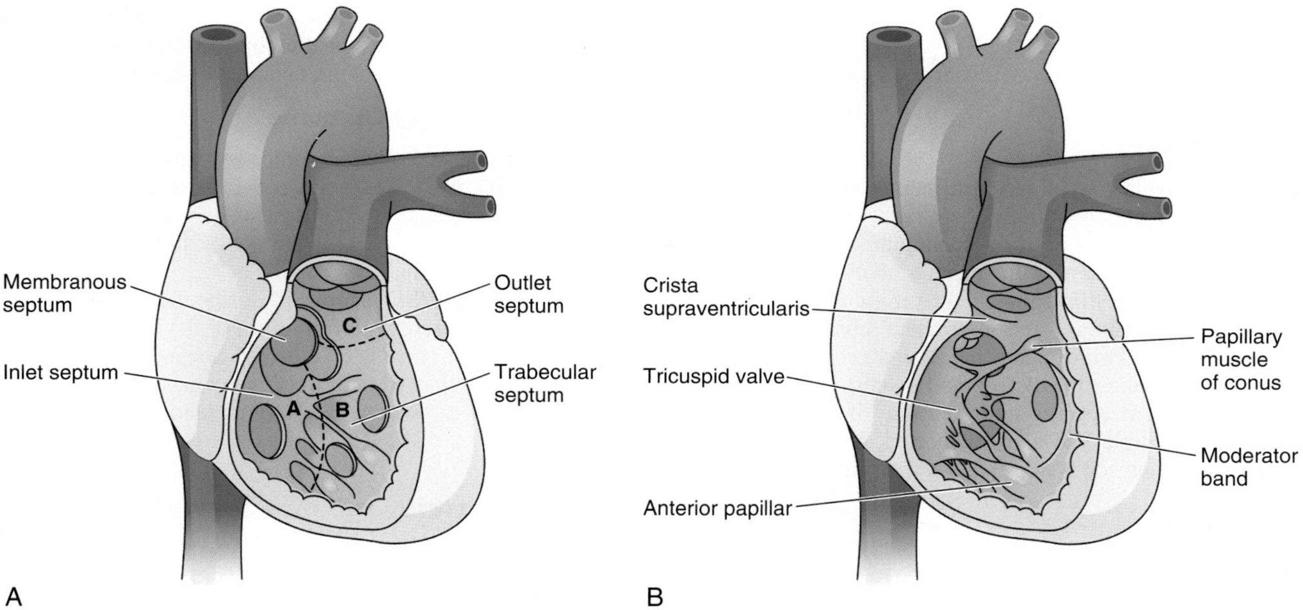

FIGURE 30–2 Classification of ventricular septal defects (VSDs). *A*, The intervening septum is commonly divided into inlet, trabecular, outlet, and membranous septum. *B*, VSDs are classified according to location within the septum. Membranous and perimembranous are the most common (70%). Other types include subarterial (in the outlet septum), inlet VSD (in atrioventricular canal), and muscular VSD. (Modified from Waldhausen JA, Pierce WS, Campbell DB (eds): Congenital heart disease. In Surgery of the Chest, 6th ed. Philadelphia, Mosby-Year Book, 1996.)

transient clinical improvement. However, changes in the pulmonary bed continue to develop, and eventually the pulmonary vascular resistance exceeds the systemic vascular resistance and results in reversed (right-to-left) shunt and **Eisenmenger's syndrome.** The patient then becomes cyanotic, with signs of severe right ventricular failure.

The chances that a VSD will spontaneously close are inversely related to the age of the patient. According to one study, the chances of spontaneous closure are 80% in patients at age 1 month, 60% at 3 months, 50% at 6 months, and only 25% at age 12 months. The likelihood of spontaneous closure also is related to the type of VSD.

Patients with a large VSD and a Qp/Qs exceeding 3.5 have about a 10% risk of dying during the first year of life of complications of CHF and recurrent infections. Patients who survive the first year will usually survive to the second or third decade of life and will die of complications of Eisenmenger's syndrome, including right-sided heart failure, hemoptysis, polycythemia, cerebral infarct, or abscess. Patients with Eisenmenger's syndrome rarely survive beyond age 40 years.

The risk of endocarditis in patients with VSDs is estimated to be 0.3% per year. In fewer than 5% of patients with VSDs will aortic insufficiency develop secondary to prolapse of the noncoronary cusp of the aortic valve.

Evaluation

History and Physical Examination

Patients with a small VSD have minimal or no symptoms and are usually diagnosed when a pansystolic murmur is found on routine physical examination.

Patients with a medium-sized VSD may be seen first during childhood or early adulthood and are usually physically small and underdeveloped. Those with severe pulmonary hypertension and minimal shunt have a quiet heart, with only a soft systolic murmur, no apical diastolic rumble, and no thrill. The precordium is not hyperactive. The left ventricle is of normal size, and the right ventricle is enlarged. In patients with a medium-sized VSD, the development of severe pulmonary hypertension and reduction of shunt may initially lead to clinical improvement, only to be followed by the development of cyanosis and right-sided heart failure.

Patients with a large VSD usually are seen in the first few months of life with symptoms of CHF, failure to thrive, and recurrent respiratory tract infections. Classic findings in these patients include the following: physical underdevelopment, tachypnea and pallor; elevated jugular venous pulse; bulging precordium with evidence of biventricular enlargement; and a palpable pansystolic thrill with a loud pansystolic murmur that is maximal at the third, fourth, and fifth left intercostal spaces.

Electrocardiographic Studies

The ECG typically shows biventricular enlargement and strain.

Imaging Studies

In patients with a small VSD, a plain film of the chest is normal. In patients with large shunt ratio, a plain film shows biventricular enlargement, prominent pulmonary vasculature, and pulmonary edema. In patients with Eisenmenger's syndrome, a plain film shows right ventricular enlargement, relatively clear lungs, and prominent central pulmonary artery branches. Two-dimensional Doppler echocardiography can fully visualize the defect and confirm the diagnosis. Cardiac catheterization is indicated only if the diagnosis is uncertain, multiple VSDs are suspected, or irreversible pulmonary hypertension is suggested by the clinical presentation.

Treatment

Indications for Surgery

Only 30% of patients with a VSD will require surgery during the first year of life. The need for prompt surgery depends on the severity and type of VSD.

Patients without severe symptoms can usually be treated medically, and in many cases, the VSD will close spontaneously during the first year of life. Those with medium-sized VSDs should undergo catheterization at the end of the first year. If the pressure in the pulmonary artery exceeds half of the systemic pressure, and the Qp/Qs is 2.5 to 3.0, surgery is indicated, because the defect is unlikely to close spontaneously, and the patient is at risk of developing pulmonary hypertension.

Patients with severe symptoms during the first 3 months of life should undergo surgery promptly. Surgery is recommended in patients with a large AV canal and conoventricular VSD, irrespective of age, because these patients are unlikely to experience spontaneous closure of the defect. A subpulmonary VSD should be repaired early to prevent secondary aortic insufficiency. Infants and children with a large VSD and elevated pulmonary resistance should be evaluated individually. Pulmonary vascular resistance should be evaluated individually. Pulmonary vascular resistance greater than 10 units/m^2 and a pulmonary-to-systemic vascular resistance ratio greater than 0.7 are considered contraindications to surgery.

Surgical Techniques

Surgery is performed via a complete or lower partial midsternotomy incision, with the use of cardiopulmonary bypass and cardioplegic arrest. The use of deep hypothermia and circulatory arrest may be indicated in neonates and small infants. Most VSDs are approached via the right atrium. The defect is closed with an autologous pericardium or Dacron patch, by using continuous or interrupted nonabsorbable sutures reinforced with Teflon felt. Care is taken to identify the area of the conduction system and to avoid damage to the tricuspid and aortic valves.

Complications and Outcome

The mortality rate in patients undergoing the repair of an isolated VSD is in the range of 0% to 2%. Operative mortality is unrelated to preoperative hemodynamics but is influenced by residual hemodynamically significant lesions and associated anomalies.

Patients whose VSD is repaired during the first or second year of life are cured, with full return of the hemodynamics to normal and a normal or close to normal life. Patients whose USD is repaired later in life may have arrhythmia or complications of severe and long-standing pulmonary hypertension.

Atrioventricular Canal Defect

AV canal defects represent a spectrum of defects originating from abnormal development of the embryologic AV canal septum (endocardial cushion).

Anatomy

The complete form of AV canal defect includes an ostium primum–type ASD, an inlet-type VSD, and abnormal mitral and tricuspid valves. The partial form of the defect is less severe and excludes some of these features. AV canal defects may be isolated or may be a component of a more complex anomaly, such as heterotaxia syndrome. In addition, many other cardiac anomalies that are not part of AV canal defects per se have been described in association with them.

Pathophysiology

In patients with AV canal defects, the clinical manifestations depend on the degree of atrial and ventricular left-to-right shunting and the degree of AV valve regurgitation. Patients with a large ventricular-level shunt have manifestations similar to those of patients with isolated VSD. These manifestations include accelerated development of pulmonary vascular disease because of the additional atrial-level shunt and AV valve regurgitation, both of which increase the degree of volume overload. Patients with partial AV canal defects are first seen later in life with manifestations similar to those of isolated ASD or isolated mitral or tricuspid valve regurgitation. A combination of ASD and AV valve regurgitation may result in increased volume overload with earlier symptoms of CHF.

Evaluation

History and Physical Examination

Infants with the severe form of AV canal defect usually are seen during the first few months of life with symptoms of CHF secondary to a large left-to-right shunt aggravated by

AV valve regurgitation. Pulmonary vascular occlusive disease tends to develop rapidly in these patients. Infants with less severe forms are seen later in life with milder forms of CHF, a murmur, or arrhythmias. Pulmonary vascular occlusive disease is less common.

Findings on physical examination include nonspecific signs of CHF, biventricular enlargement, a systolic flow murmur over the pulmonary valve, a widely split second heart sound, diastolic flow murmurs over the AV valves, and AV valve holosystolic regurgitation murmurs.

Electrocardiographic Studies

The ECG characteristically shows a right ventricular conduction defect, left anterior division block, left-axis deviation, and superior orientation with counterclockwise rotation of the QRS loop in the frontal plane.

Imaging Studies

A plain film of the chest reveals right atrial and ventricular enlargement, prominence of the right ventricular enlargement, prominence of the right atrial and ventricular enlargement, prominence of the right ventricular outflow tract (RVOT), and increased pulmonary vascular markings. Two-dimensional Doppler echocardiography is considered the standard for the diagnosis of all forms of AV canal defect. Cardiac catheterization is rarely necessary in infants younger than 6 months, but it may be indicated in patients older than 6 months, to evaluate the degree and reversibility of pulmonary vascular occlusive disease.

Treatment

Indications for Surgery

In symptomatic infants with complete or partial AV canal defect, surgery is indicated at the time of diagnosis. In asymptomatic patients with complete AV canal defect, surgery should be performed before the age of 6 months to prevent irreversible pulmonary vascular occlusive disease. In asymptomatic patients with partial AV canal defect, surgery is recommended later in life (at age 1 to 2 years). Long-standing AV valve regurgitation may induce degenerative changes in valve leaflets, and this may preclude future valve repair. Therefore surgery is indicated whenever AV valve regurgitation develops, even in otherwise asymptomatic patients.

Surgical Techniques

Surgery is performed via a midsternotomy incision, with the use of cardiopulmonary bypass and cardioplegic arrest. Complete repair by using a one-patch or two-patch technique is the procedure of choice. The approach to treating a partial AV canal defect is based on the specific defect. Valve repair is the procedure of choice for AV valve regurgitation. Valve replacement is rarely indicated as an initial procedure but may be necessary later.

Complications and Outcome

In patients with complete AV canal defects, the operative mortality rate is in the range of 5% to 10%. The risk of death is increased in patients seen during the neonatal period or who have associated anomalies or significant residual mitral valve regurgitation.

In patients with partial AV canal defects, the operative mortality rate is in the range of 1% to 3%. The risk of death is lower in older patients and in patients with an intact ventricular septum. It is higher in patients with residual mitral valve regurgitation.

A need for reoperation (mostly for mitral valve regurgitation) and the presence of pulmonary hypertension or arrhythmias compromise the long-term survival and quality of life. In one study, a 10-year survival of 90% was reported, with 78% of patients being in functional class I or II at the time of follow-up.

Tetralogy of Fallot

Tetralogy of Fallot (TOF) is one of the most frequent congenital heart anomalies. It consists of the combination of a VSD, infundibular pulmonary stenosis, right ventricular hypertrophy, and dextroposition of the aorta ("overriding" aorta). In its extreme form, TOF occurs with pulmonary atresia. The management and prognosis of TOF with pulmonary atresia are markedly different from those of other forms of TOF and are not discussed here.

Anatomy

Van Praagh and colleagues have suggested that the four components of TOF originate from a single defect, the abnormal development of the right ventricular infundibulum, which leads to the formation of malaligned conoventricular VSD, overriding of the aorta, and infundibular pulmonary stenosis. Right ventricular hypertrophy is secondary to RVOT obstruction.

Pathophysiology

The manifestations of TOF vary, depending primarily on the degree of RVOT obstruction and the systemic vascular resistance. The VSD is usually large and nonrestrictive, with the two ventricles functioning physiologically as a single chamber. In utero, with the ductus arteriosus still open, the defect has no effect on development of the infant. However, when the ductus spontaneously closes shortly after the infant's birth, the systemic vascular resistance decreases. Blood flow to the lung is limited and is dependent on the degree of RVOT obstruction. If the degree of obstruction is high, a significant right-to-left shunt will develop and will be seen with severe hypoxemia, cyanosis, and even acidosis shortly after birth. If the degree of obstruction is low or moderate, blood flow to the lungs may be adequate but is subject to changes in systemic vascular resistance. Decreased systemic vascular resistance will result in an increased right-to-left shunt (a "hypoxic spell") and vice versa.

The sequelae of long-standing hypoxemia include secondary polycythemia, hypervolemia, and hyperviscosity, and these lead to an increased incidence of cerebrovascular accidents and cerebral abscesses.

Without treatment, patients with TOF have a mortality rate of 30% at 6 months and 50% at age 2 years. Only 20% of patients will reach the age of 10 years, and 5% to 10% will reach the age of 20 years.

Evaluation

History and Physical Examination

The clinical picture varies, depending on the severity of the defect. Cyanosis, the hallmark of TOF, can be intense from birth, or it can be minimal and noticeable only during a hypoxic spell. Many infants frequently assume a squatting position to increase systemic vascular resistance and thereby increase the pulmonary blood flow.

Neonates and young infants are usually well developed, with a dusky complexion to severe cyanosis. Older children may be small for age and exhibit cyanosis and clubbing. A harsh systolic ejection murmur decreases or completely disappears during a cyanotic spell, reflecting decreased flow across the RVOT.

Laboratory Studies

Laboratory tests demonstrate arterial hypoxemia and secondary polycythemia.

Electrocardiographic Studies

The ECG shows right ventricular hypertrophy.

Imaging Studies

An initial plain film of the chest shows a diminished pulmonary vasculature, with absence of the pulmonary artery prominence. Later films show a typical boot-shaped silhouette of the heart, which results from the combination of right ventricular hypertrophy, overriding aorta, and an absent pulmonary artery prominence. Two-dimensional echocardiography is used to confirm the diagnosis and to search for other anomalies, with particular emphasis on additional VSDs and a patent ductus arteriosus (PDA). Cardiac catheterization is indicated if the diagnosis is uncertain, if the full anatomy is unclear, or if previous palliative surgery has altered the anatomy.

Treatment

Indications for Surgery

Because the mortality in untreated patients is so high, the diagnosis of TOF is an indication for surgery in the vast majority of patients. Complete repair (as opposed to palliative systemic-to-pulmonary shunt) is now advocated in most cases, because it minimizes secondary damage to other vital organs, obviates the need for a second operation, avoids the problem of distortion of the pulmonary artery, and is associated with a low operative mortality rate.

Surgical Techniques

The most common palliative procedure is a modified Blalock-Taussig shunt. A polytetrafluoroethylene (PTFE) graft is used to connect the subclavian artery to the pulmonary artery.

Complete repair is performed via a midsternotomy incision, with the use of cardiopulmonary bypass. Deep hypothermia and circulatory arrest may be indicated in neonates and small infants. The right ventricular infundibulum is opened longitudinally. Depending on the anatomy, the incision may be extended across the pulmonary valve to the main pulmonary artery. The VSD is closed with a Dacron patch, carefully avoiding the conduction system (Fig. 30-3). Resection of muscle to enlarge the RVOT is usually required only in patients who have severe right ventricular hypertrophy and do not undergo early surgery. The RVOT is reconstructed with an autologous pericardial patch (Fig. 30-4). Some surgeons prefer a transatrial repair.

Complications and Outcome

The operative mortality rate associated with an isolated primary repair, or a repair after a single systemic-to-pulmonary shunt is in the range of 0% to 6%.

Chances for long-term survival are good, with a 16- to 28-year survival rate of around 85%. Overall, 80% of patients who undergo repair resume a normal lifestyle, with normal intellectual development, exercise tolerance, and fertility rates. Reoperations are required in 7% to 10% of patients, most frequently because of residual or recurrent RVOT obstruction or residual VSD. Conduction abnormalities are common, and late arrhythmias are reported in 5% to 10% of patients. Cases of sudden death have been reported.

Patent Ductus Arteriosus

PDA is defined by a persistent postnatal communication between the main pulmonary artery and the aorta.

Anatomy

The ductus arteriosus is a normal structure in the fetus. It closes spontaneously after birth as a result of smooth muscle constriction mediated by various vasoconstrictors in response to an increase in oxygen tension. The ductus is functionally closed in 82% to 96% of neonates within 48 hours after birth. Anatomic closure with fibrosis is usually completed within 2 to 3 weeks. However, the ductal response is dependent on gestational age. Premature infants are less sensitive both to oxygen-induced vasoconstriction and to prostaglandin-mediated vasodilatation. The ductus arises intrapericardially from the main pulmonary artery or the proximal part of the left pulmonary artery and inserts extrapericardially into the descending aorta just distal to

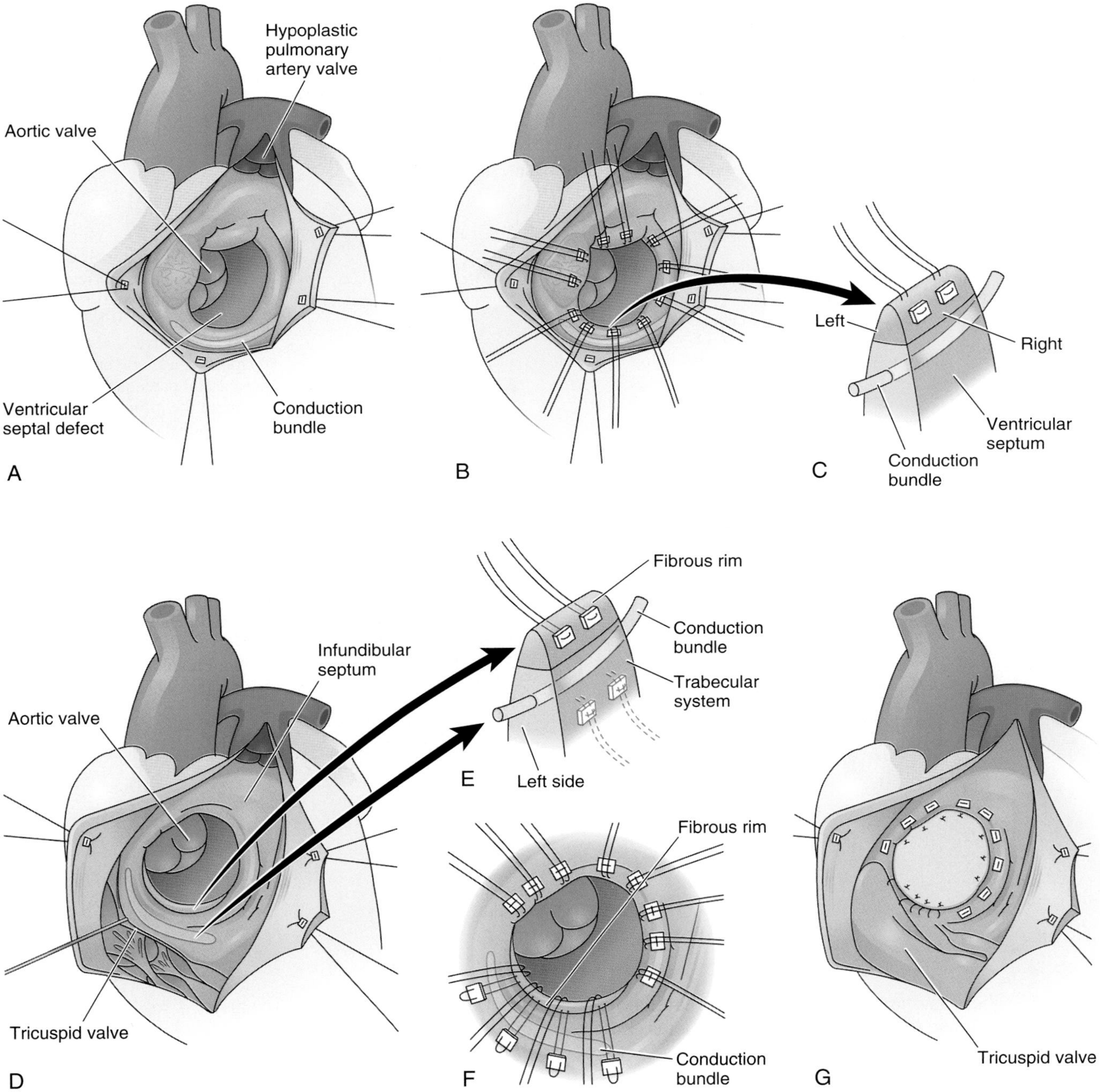

FIGURE 30–3 Repair of tetralogy of Fallot/closure of a ventricular septal defect (VSD) by using a Dacron patch. *A*, To improve exposure and access to the posteroinferior quadrant of the VSD, the parietal extension of the infundibular septum is partially incised. *B*, The malalignment VSD is closed. *C*, The posteroinferior limb of the trabecular septa marginalis is well developed, and the atrioventricular bundle is more deeply embedded within muscle and also more closely related to the left ventricular aspect of the septal crest. Sutures are placed safely within this muscle, avoiding encircling the crest of the ventricular septum. *D*, The posteroinferior limb of the septal band is hypoplastic and is reduced to a fibrous rim formed by the confluence of the aortic valve annulus and endocardial cushion tissue of the tricuspid valve, establishing aortic valve–tricuspid valve continuity. *E*, Because of the hypoplasia of the posteroinferior limb, the bundle of His is less deeply embedded and thus lies closer to the right ventricular surface of the septal crest. In this anatomic variant, the sutures are either anchored within the fibrous rim to avoid the bundle of His or placed approximately 5 mm from the ventricular crust. *F*, All interrupted sutures reinforced with pledgets are in place. *G*, The VSD is completely closed with a Dacron patch anchored with interrupted horizontal mattress sutures reinforced with Teflon pledgets. (Modified from Castaneda AR, Jonas RA, Mayer JE, Hanley FL: Cardiac Surgery of the Neonate and Infant. Philadelphia, WB Saunders, 1994.)

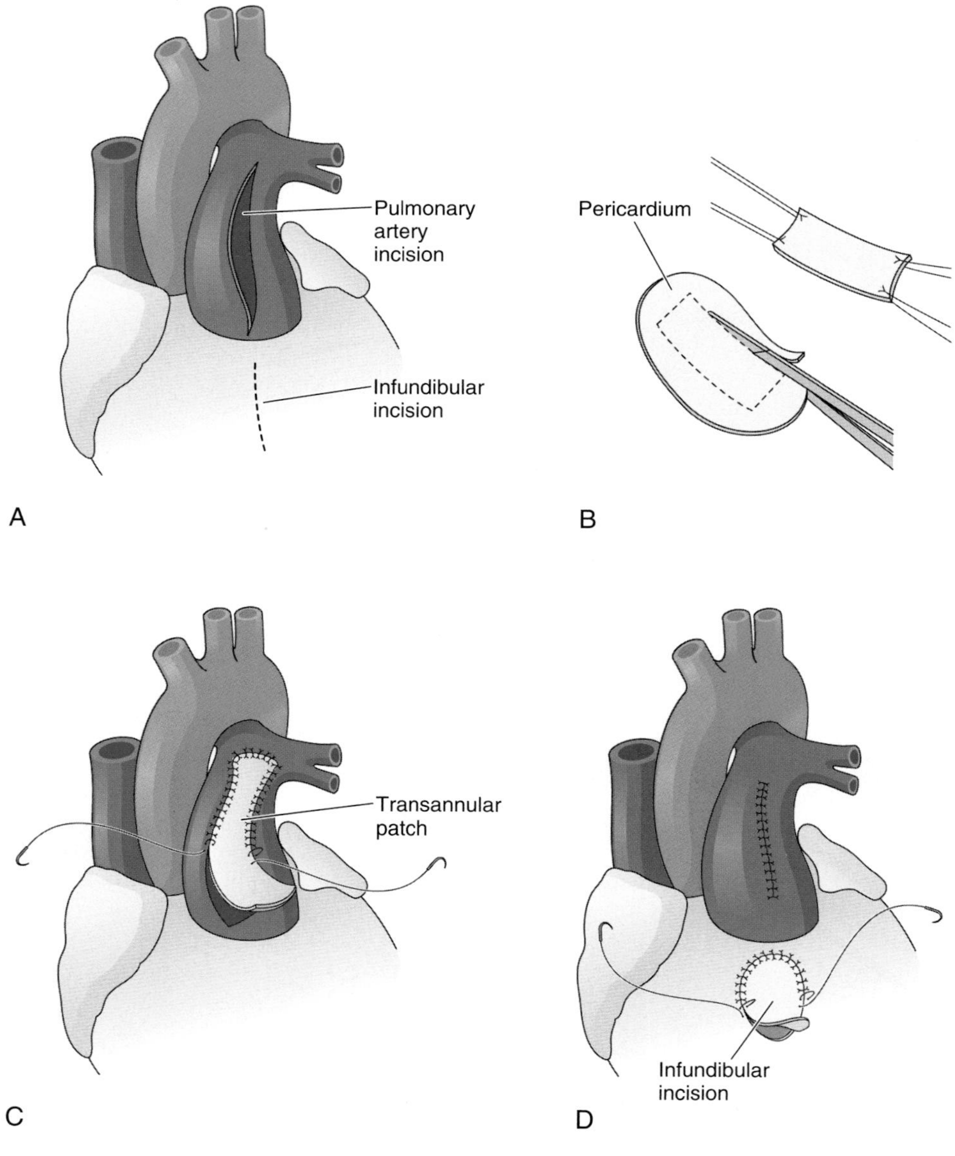

FIGURE 30–4 Repair of tetralogy of Fallot/correction of right ventricular outflow tract obstruction. *A–C*, When the pulmonary valve is severely dysplastic, a single autologous pericardial patch is used to augment the infundibulum, the pulmonary valve, and the main pulmonary artery. *D*, When the pulmonary valve is not dysplastic, pulmonary valvotomy and patch augmentation of the infundibulum are performed separately. (Modified from Castaneda AR, Jonas RA, Mayer JE, Hanley FL: Cardiac Surgery of the Neonate and Infant. Philadelphia, WB Saunders, 1994.)

the left subclavian artery. The left recurrent laryngeal nerve passes close to the aortic end of the ductus. Rarely, the ductus is absent, right-sided, or bilateral.

Pathophysiology

PDA allows arterial-level left-to-right shunt, the magnitude of which depends on the diameter of the ductus and the degree of pulmonary vascular resistance. Normally a decrease in resistance occurs after birth, and the shunt increases to its maximal level after 6 to 8 weeks, at which time symptoms of CHF develop. Because of underdeveloped vascular smooth muscle, pulmonary vascular resistance is lower in premature infants, and significant shunt may develop with severe CHF as early 24 to 48 hours after birth.

In some cases, the ductus closes spontaneously during the first few weeks of life. In other cases, infants with a medium-sized or large PDA are seen later in life with pulmonary vascular disease, pulmonary hypertension, and reversed (right-to-left) shunt with cyanosis.

Patients with PDA are at high risk for endocarditis. Infants who have a small restrictive PDA with insignificant shunt are asymptomatic but are still susceptible.

Aneurysmal dilatation is another potential complication of PDA reported in children and adults. Typical manifestations of ductal aneurysm include an asymptomatic mediastinal mass, respiratory distress secondary to bronchial compression, hoarseness from recurrent laryngeal nerve injury, and acute rupture or dissection.

The average life expectancy of untreated patients with PDA is 20 to 30 years. Eventually, 80% die of PDA-related complications, including CHF, endocarditis, and severe pulmonary hypertension.

Evaluation

History and Physical Examination

Small restrictive PDAs may be detected incidentally when a murmur is found on physical examination or when the patient has endocarditis later in life. Patients with large nonrestrictive PDAs are seen early in life with CHF. Those with medium-sized, well-compensated PDAs may appear later in life with CHF, failure to thrive, or Eisenmenger's syndrome.

Physical findings in infants with hemodynamically significant PDAs include bounding peripheral pulses with a large pulse pressure, tachycardia, tachypnea, poor tolerance to oral feeding, and a hyperdynamic precordium with a thrill and a systolic or continuous "machinery" murmur maximal in the pulmonary area and radiating toward the clavicle.

Electrocardiographic Studies

Results on ECG are nonspecific.

Imaging Studies

The diagnosis of PDA is usually established by two-dimensional Doppler echocardiography. Cardiac catheterization is rarely indicated and is contraindicated in premature infants.

Treatment

Indications for Surgery

After the first few weeks of life, the likelihood that a large PDA will close spontaneously is low. Therefore symptomatic infants should be treated promptly. Asymptomatic infants should be scheduled for elective closure at age 3 months.

Surgical Techniques

Closure of the PDA can be performed percutaneously with catheter-based techniques by using coils or clamshell devices. Surgical closure of an isolated PDA is performed via a left posterolateral thoracotomy. The preferred technique to minimize recurrence is double ligation and division. In recent years, video-assisted thoracoscopic surgical closure has been used increasingly, with excellent results.

Complications and Outcome

In infants with an isolated PDA closure, the operative mortality rate approaches 0% in most recent series. Deaths are usually associated with coexistent congenital anomalies. Potential surgical complications include hemorrhage, pneumothorax, chylothorax, and recurrent laryngeal nerve injury. Patients resume normal life after early repair. Operative and long-term mortality rates are increased in patients who undergo surgical repair later in life or require more complex surgery because of the presence of a calcified ductus, an infected ductus, or severe pulmonary hypertension.

Transposition of the Great Arteries

Transposition of the great arteries (TGA) is a severe congenital cardiac anomaly in which the aorta arises anteriorly from the right ventricle, the pulmonary artery arises posteriorly from the left ventricle, and the atria and ventricles are concordant.

Anatomy

Transposition of the aorta and pulmonary artery is a result of an abnormal growth pattern of the subaortic and subpulmonary conus. In affected patients, the aorta and pulmonary artery are of equal size. The ventricles are morphologically abnormal, and anomalies of the atrioventricular valves are common.

In the most common variant of simple TGA, the left coronary artery originates from the left sinus and branches to the left anterior descending and circumflex arteries, whereas the right coronary artery originates from the right sinus.

About 70% to 75% of patients with TGA have an intact ventricular septum, and 30% have a VSD. All types of VSD have been observed with TGA.

The foramen ovale and the ductus are commonly patent, but they are usually small and do not allow adequate mixing.

Pathophysiology

Patients with complete TGA have parallel systemic and pulmonary circulations. Survival is therefore dependent on mixing between these systems. In most infants with simple complete TGA, very little mixing occurs because the foramen ovale is small and the ductus is closing. Thus infants are seen shortly after birth with intense cyanosis and cardiovascular collapse.

Infants with a large VSD or a large PDA are less cyanotic, but marked CHF and early pulmonary vascular obstructive disease develop. Physiologic mechanisms in infants with TGA, a large VSD, and LVOT obstruction are similar to those in infants with tetralogy of Fallot.

About 50% of untreated patients with TGA die during the first month of life, and 90% do not survive the first year of life. Patients with a large atrial communication (congenital or intervention-induced) survive longer, but only 50% survive more than 2 years.

Evaluation

History and Physical Examination

Patients usually are seen in the newborn period with severe cyanosis that does not respond to supplemental oxygen. The clinical status may deteriorate when the ductus arteriosus closes 24 to 48 hours after birth. Infants with a large VSD or PDA have symptoms of CHF, including tachycardia, tachypnea, and enlarged liver. Infants with a VSD and LVOT obstruction have signs similar to those in infants with tetralogy of Fallot.

Laboratory Studies

Blood gas analysis shows hypoxemia, metabolic acidosis, and hypercapnia in late stage.

Electrocardiographic Studies

The ECG shows normal sinus rhythm in most patients, but a few have coronary sinus rhythm. Right-axis deviation and a pattern of right ventricular hypertrophy and strain are common.

Imaging Studies

Two-dimensional Doppler echocardiography is the procedure of choice to establish an immediate diagnosis and to assist in bedside atrial balloon septostomy (**the Rashkind procedure**), which is used as a palliative measure before surgery. Cardiac catheterization is indicated only if the anatomy is not completely defined by echocardiography.

Treatment

Indications for Surgery

Because the mortality is high in untreated patients, surgery is indicated at the time of diagnosis.

Surgical Techniques

Surgical procedures may be palliative or reparative. The palliative procedure that is generally used today is the Rashkind procedure, which should performed immediately to allow 1 to 3 days of resuscitation before a reparative procedure is performed. Other palliative procedures are rarely indicated.

Reparative procedures are performed via a midsternotomy incision, with the use of cardiopulmonary bypass, deep hypothermia, and circulatory arrest. Reparative procedures are categorized by the level of repair. An arterial-level repair called the *arterial switch operation* is the procedure of choice for most patients with complete TGA and an intact ventricular septum (Fig. 30-5). An atrial-level repair, such as the Mustard operation or the Senning operation, has been used only in special circumstances in recent years. The Rastelli operation is performed in patients with TGA, VSD, and LVOT obstruction. Intraventricular repair is infrequently performed but may be used in patients with TGA and a very large VSD.

PEARLS FOR ROUNDS

In general, congenital heart defects should be repaired early to avoid pulmonary vascular occlusive disease, to prevent the consequences of severe right and left ventricular volume or pressure overload, and to reduce damage to other organs. Symptomatic patients should undergo surgical repair at the time of diagnosis, and asymptomatic patients should do so at the age of 6 to 12 months. Young age by itself does not add risk to surgery.

A shunt is considered hemodynamically significant when the flow in the pulmonary circulation is greater than or equal to 1.5 times the flow in the systemic circulation (that is, when $Qp/Qs \geq 1.5$).

If possible, a complete repair of any congenital anomaly should be attempted during initial surgery, because operative mortality and morbidity rates associated with complete repairs are low, additional procedures become unnecessary, and the adverse effects of continued abnormal physiologic mechanisms are prevented. Palliative procedures, such as systemic-to-pulmonary shunts and pulmonary artery banding, should be reserved for special circumstances.

Complications and Outcome

In patients undergoing an arterial switch operation, the overall operative mortality rate is about 5%. The rate in low-risk patients (those with TGA and intact ventricular septum or a single simple VSD and no associated anomalies) is 2% to 3%. The rate in high-risk patients (those with multiple VSDs, associated aortic coarctation or interruption, AV valve anomalies, or atypical coronary anatomy) is 10% to 15%. The 5-year survival rate is greater than 90%. Late mortality and morbidity are related mostly to coronary artery problems, residual defects, supravalvular pulmonary stenosis, and semilunar valve insufficiency.

Coarctation of the Aorta

Coarctation of the aorta (COA) is defined as narrowing of the lumen of the aorta, with obstruction to blood flow. COA accounts for 5% to 10% of cases of congenital heart disease and is found in 1 of every 3000 to 4000 autopsies.

Anatomy

Traditionally, COA is divided into two anatomic types, called the infantile type and the adult type. The division is arbitrary, with a spectrum in between. The **infantile type** is common in neonates and infants and is characterized by a long-segment hypoplastic aortic arch and isthmus and a large PDA in continuity with the descending aorta. Collateral intercostal vessels are not prominent, and severe

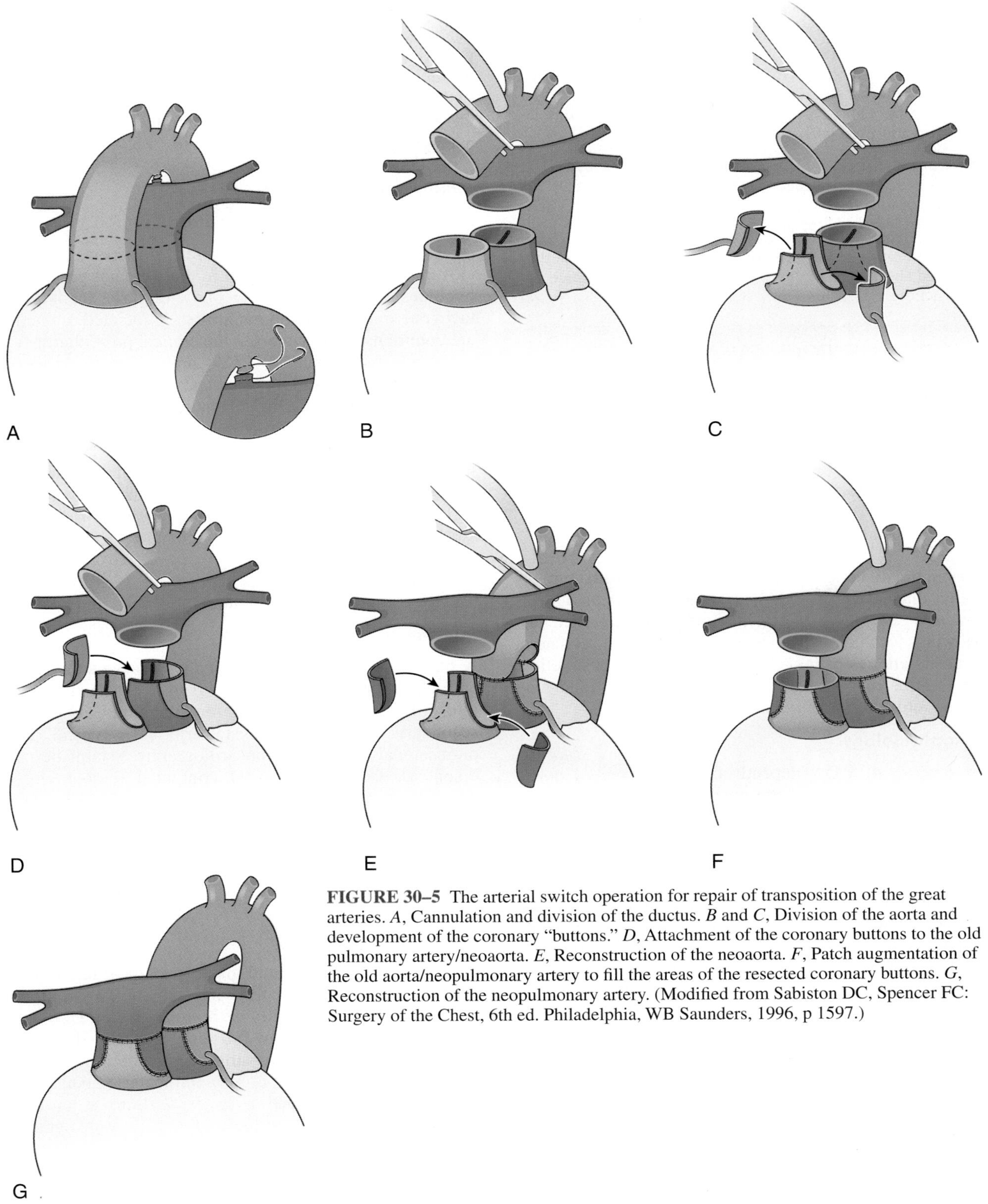

FIGURE 30–5 The arterial switch operation for repair of transposition of the great arteries. *A*, Cannulation and division of the ductus. *B* and *C*, Division of the aorta and development of the coronary "buttons." *D*, Attachment of the coronary buttons to the old pulmonary artery/neoaorta. *E*, Reconstruction of the neoaorta. *F*, Patch augmentation of the old aorta/neopulmonary artery to fill the areas of the resected coronary buttons. *G*, Reconstruction of the neopulmonary artery. (Modified from Sabiston DC, Spencer FC: Surgery of the Chest, 6th ed. Philadelphia, WB Saunders, 1996, p 1597.)

PEARLS FOR THE OR

The repair of most congenital cardiac anomalies requires the use of cardiopulmonary bypass and cardioplegic arrest. Deep systemic hypothermia (15°C to 18°C) and total circulatory arrest are frequently necessary to afford optimal exposure in neonates and small infants with complex anomalies.

Atrial septal defects (ASDs) and most ventricular septal defects (VSDs) are approached via the right atrium. ASDs can be closed with a continuous suture or with a patch. VSDs are almost invariably repaired with a patch.

Complete repair of tetralogy of Fallot includes closure of the VSD and elimination of the right ventricular outflow tract obstruction.

The arterial switch operation is the procedure of choice for most patients with transposition of the great arteries.

A resection with end-to-end anastomosis is the preferred technique for most patients with coarctation of the aorta.

In neonates, severe aortic stenosis is best managed initially with percutaneous balloon valvuloplasty. In older children, balloon valvuloplasty or surgical valvotomy should be attempted to allow growth of the aorta.

poststenotic dilatation is uncommon. The **adult type** is usually diagnosed in older children and adults and is characterized by a closed ductus and a discrete shelf-like narrowing located at the isthmus. Prominent collateral intercostal arteries develop secondary to aortic obstruction. Some degree of poststenotic dilatation is usual and may develop into a true aneurysm.

Pathophysiology

The severity of COA depends on the degree of aortic obstruction, the status of the ductus, and the presence or absence of associated anomalies.

Isolated mild to moderate obstruction may be well tolerated, even if the ductus is closed. Proximal aortic hypertension develops with compensatory left ventricular hypertrophy. With the development of significant collateral intercostal arteries, the gradient may diminish. Patients usually are first seen late in life with complications of long-standing hypertension. More severe obstruction will result in earlier development of left ventricular failure secondary to pressure overload.

Neonates with severe aortic obstruction may have minimal symptoms as long as the ductus is open. Even if the ductus is open, differential pressures and saturations still exist between the upper and lower parts of the body because of the lower pulmonary vascular resistance and the fact that the right ventricle contributes a significant portion of the lower body perfusion. When the ductus is closed, severe left ventricular pressure overload occurs, as well as lower body hypoperfusion, leading to CHF and acidosis, the severity of which depends on how developed the collateral circulation is and how quickly the ductus closes.

The mortality rate in untreated infants with symptomatic COA is high. In patients who survive to adulthood, the average age at death is 35 to 40 years.

Evaluation

History and Physical Examination

Infants with isolated COA, severe obstruction, and rapid closure of the ductus are seen in the neonatal period with hypotension, pulseless lower body, oliguria, tachycardia, tachypnea, and metabolic acidosis. Associated anomalies are common and may worsen the clinical presentation.

Infants with isolated COA and mild to moderate obstruction are well developed and asymptomatic and are diagnosed by the finding of systemic hypertension, a murmur on routine physical examination, or a pressure gradient between the upper and lower body.

Older children and adults have signs of long-standing hypertension, including headaches, epistaxis, heart failure, cerebrovascular accidents, and complications of aneurysm (such as rupture or dissection).

Electrocardiographic Studies

The ECG shows left ventricular hypertrophy and strain.

Imaging Studies

A plain film of the chest classically shows cardiomegaly and a "3"-shaped aortic contour from a coarctation in the midst of proximal and distal aortic dilatation. Rib notching secondary to dilated intercostal arteries is typical. Two-dimensional Doppler echocardiography establishes the diagnosis. Contrast-enhanced computed tomography or magnetic resonance angiography allows visualization of the coarctation. The gradient is most reliably measured by cardiac catheterization, although in most patients, this procedure is not necessary.

Treatment

Indications for Surgery

Symptomatic infants should undergo surgical repair at the time of diagnosis. Neonates with signs of cardiovascular collapse are treated initially with prostaglandin E_1 to keep the ductus patent and allow full resuscitation and recovery of all organ systems before surgical intervention.

Surgery is indicated in asymptomatic patients with significant COA, defined as a 50% decrease in aortic diameter or an upper-to-lower body pressure gradient exceeding 20 mmHg. The timing of surgery in asymptomatic patients is controversial. In the past, experts recommended that elective surgery be delayed until the patient reached at least age 10 years, thereby allowing the aorta to grow to the adult size and minimizing the risk of restenosis. However, the delay allowed complications of hypertension to develop in a significant number of patients, and in many cases, hypertension persisted despite a successful repair. Thus more recently, experts have recommended that elective repair be done when patients reach the age of 3 to 6 months or when COA is discovered if the patient is older than this. Elective surgery is not recommended before age 3 months, because of the possibility of active ductus remodeling.

Surgical Techniques

Several techniques are available for repair of COA, with the choice depending on the age of the patient and the surgical anatomy. The most common technique is resection of the narrow segment with end-to-end anastomosis (Fig. 30-6). Whether the type of suture material affects the rate of recurrence is unclear. Alternative techniques include patch aortoplasty and reverse subclavian artery flap. In older children and adults, a common approach consists of resection and reconstruction with interposition tube graft.

Complications and Outcomes

The operative mortality rate depends on the age of the patient, the surgical anatomy, and the presence of associated anomalies. In neonates, the rate is in the range of 5% to 10%. In infants who are older than 3 months and have isolated COA, the rate approaches 0%. Recurrent coarctation is still a significant problem in patients undergoing surgery during the neonatal period, although recent series have documented a 90% 5-year freedom from reoperation. In some patients, systemic hypertension persists despite successful technical repair, although persistence is less frequent with early repairs.

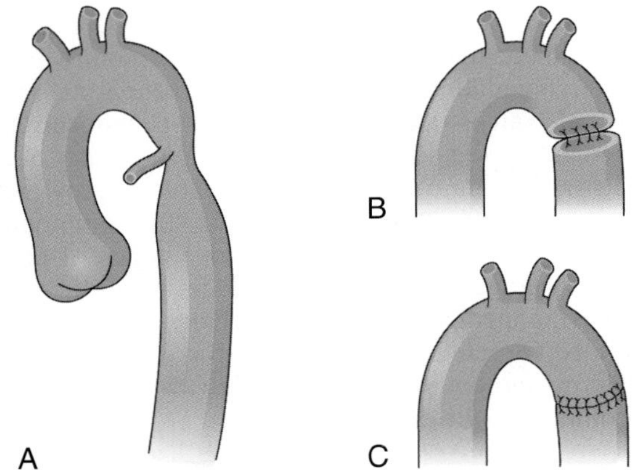

FIGURE 30–6 Repair of aortic coarctation with resection and end-to-end anastomosis. *A*, Neonatal aortic coarctation. *B*, After resection of the coarctation and the ductus arteriosus tissue, the transverse arch is incised to the origin of the left carotid artery. The descending aorta is incised posteriorly. *C*, Result after the extended end-to-end anastomosis.

Congenital Aortic Stenosis

Congenital aortic stenosis (AS) is defined as narrowing of the LVOT, with obstruction to blood flow. In its full spectrum, this is the most common congenital cardiac anomaly. The discussion here focuses on patients first seen in infancy who therefore have the more severe form of the disease.

Anatomy

Traditionally, congenital AS is categorized on the basis of the level of obstruction (Fig. 30-7). **Valvular AS** is usually associated with a unicuspid or bicuspid valve that is thickened and fibrotic, with myxomatous degeneration. **Subvalvular AS** may be organic, occurring secondary to a discrete subaortic membrane or long, tunneled, fibromuscular stenosis; or it may be dynamic, occurring secondary to a hypertrophied septum (idiopathic hypertrophic subaortic stenosis). **Supravalvular AS** may occur as an isolated form (sporadic or familial) or in association with peripheral pulmonary stenosis, elfin facies, and hypercalcemia (Williams' syndrome).

Pathophysiology

The pathophysiologic mechanisms are similar in all forms of congenital AS. Obstruction to blood flow leads to left ventricular pressure overload. This causes compensatory left ventricular hypertrophy with decreased left ventricular compliance. An increase in left ventricular end-diastolic pressure reduces the coronary perfusion pressure and thereby causes subendocardial myocardial ischemia and an increase in left atrial pressure. Systolic and diastolic left ventricular dysfunction will eventually lead to CHF. Arrhythmogenic foci may develop secondary to severe hypertrophy and patchy myocardial fibrosis.

Evaluation

History and Physical Examination

Valvular AS is three to four times more common in male than in female patients, and symptoms develop earlier in the presence of associated anomalies. Newborns with severe valvular AS have CHF at birth. Cyanosis may develop from a right-to-left shunt across a patent ductus. Symptoms worsen when the ductus closes, and cardiovascular collapse may develop. Typical findings on physical examination include a prolonged pulse with low pulse pressure (pulsus tardus and parvus), a systolic thrill, normal-sized heart, fourth heart sound, systolic ejection (crescendo-decrescendo) murmur, and midsystolic click.

Patients with moderate valvular AS have symptoms of CHF during the first few months of life. Patients with milder forms of AS are seen later in life with the classic

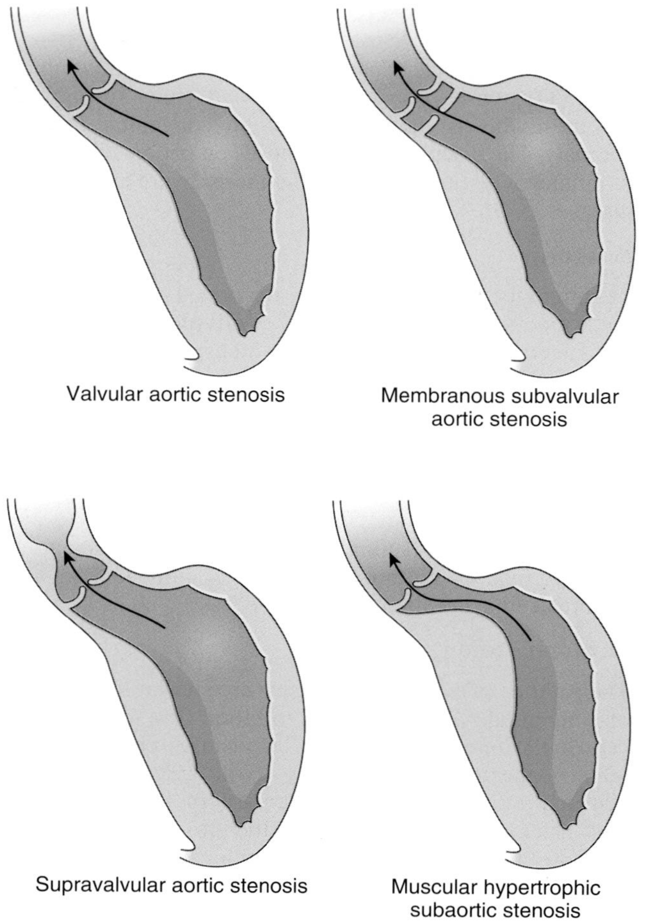

FIGURE 30–7 Anatomic classification of congenital aortic stenosis. (Modified from Sabiston DC, Spencer FC: Surgery of the Chest, 6th ed. Philadelphia, WB Saunders, 1996, p 1520.)

clinical triad of AS, including CHF, angina pectoris, or sudden death. Patients are also at high risk for infective endocarditis.

Patients with subvalvular AS infrequently are seen during the neonatal period. Symptoms usually appear during the first few years of life and are maximal during adolescence. Patients with supravalvular AS typically become symptomatic only as young adults.

Electrocardiographic Studies

The ECG typically shows left ventricular hypertrophy and strain.

Imaging Studies

In most cases, the diagnosis is confirmed by two-dimensional echocardiography, which defines the defect, allows functional assessment of the pressure gradient and valve area, and detects associated anomalies. The need for cardiac catheterization is controversial, although it may be useful not only for diagnosis but also for therapeutic purposes.

Treatment

Indications for Surgery

Neonates with severe AS should be treated promptly after adequate resuscitation. Prostaglandin E_1 is used to keep the ductus open. Older patients with AS should undergo surgery if they are symptomatic or if signs of physical examination suggest the presence of severe obstruction and the mean gradient across the valve is greater that 50 mmHg.

Surgical Techniques

In neonates with severe valvular AS, the procedure of choice is precutaneous balloon valvuloplasty. The short- and long-term results of this procedure appear to be equivalent to the results of surgical valvotomy. In older children, either percutaneous balloon valvuloplasty or surgical valvotomy can be performed, and either procedure will allow the aorta to continue growing and reach adult size before aortic valve replacement.

Operation for AS are performed via a midsternotomy incision, with the use of cardiopulmonary bypass and cardioplegic arrest. If valve replacement is indicated early in life, a variety of aortic annulus–enlarging procedures may be used to accommodate the largest valve possible and to minimize the need for a second replacement.

The choice of prosthetic valve in the pediatric population is important. Xenografts do not require anticoagulation but have a rapid rate of structural valve deterioration that necessitates early repeated replacement. Mechanical valves are durable but require long-term anticoagulation. Patients with xenografts and mechanical valves are at high risk for endocarditis. Replacement of the aortic valve with a pulmonary autograft (Ross procedure) may allow the valve to grow with the patient, although an allograft in the pulmonary position may be replaced. Distinct advantages of using pulmonary autografts or aortic allografts as aortic valve substitutes in pediatric patients include superb hemodynamic performance, lack of need for continued anticoagulation, and low risk of prosthetic valve endocarditis and thromboembolic complications.

Discrete subaortic membrane is approached and resected via the aortic valve, with care not to injure this valve, the anterior leaflet of the mitral valve, or the membranous septum. Either a ventricular patch septoplasty or the Konno operation can be used to repair tunneled fibromuscular subaortic stenosis. Various aortoplasty patch techniques are available for repair of supravalvular AS.

Complications and Outcome

The operative mortality rate associated with percutaneous balloon valvuloplasty or surgical valvotomy in neonates is relatively high (in the range of 10% to 45%) because patients frequently have associated anomalies and usually are in poor preoperative clinical condition. The results associated with either of these procedures in older infants are better, with mortality rates that approach 0% in children older than 1 year. However, follow-up studies of patients up to 20 years after valvuloplasty show that a second valve replacement is required in 35% to 40% of patients.

The operative mortality rate associated with elective repair of discrete subaortic stenosis, discrete supravalvular stenosis, or isolated aortic valve replacement in children approaches 0%. The rate increases in complex repair of tunneled subaortic stenosis, annular enlargement procedures, or procedures to repair diffuse supravalvular stenosis and may reach as high as 30% to 40%.

Hypoplastic Left Heart Syndrome

Hypoplastic left hear syndrome (HLHS) represents a group of congenital cardiac anomalies in which the left ventricle is severely underdeveloped or absent and in which blood flow in the left heart is severely limited by left-sided lesions, such as aortic stenosis or atresia and mitral stenosis or atresia.

HLHS is encountered in 1 of every 2500 births in the United States and is the fourth most common cardiac anomaly in patients with heart disease during the first year of life. It is also the most common single-ventricle defect. It accounts for 1.5% to 4.0% of congenital cardiac anomalies and close to 25% of deaths related to congenital heart disease.

Anatomy

HLHS is classified into four categories, based on the morphology of the aortic and mitral valves. The categories, listed in order of frequency, are (1) **aortic stenosis and mitral stenosis,** (2) **aortic atresia and mitral atresia,** (3) **aortic stenosis and mitral atresia**, and (4) **aortic atresia and mitral stenosis.** The more severe forms of the disease are those that include aortic atresia, characterized by smaller or absent left ventricle and a very small (2–3 mm) hypoplastic ascending aorta.

Pathophysiology

In the normal fetus, blood is oxygenated in the placenta, and the right heart delivers 60% of the systemic output via the ductus, so that the fetus develops normally. However, after birth, the newborn's left heart is too small or absent and is unable to support the systemic circulation. Therefore blood returning from the lungs via the pulmonary veins crosses over to the right atrium via a patent foreman ovale or an ASD and arrives at the right ventricle. The right ventricle supports both the pulmonary and systemic circulations, with the systemic flow maintained through the patent ductus. Partial closure of the ductus results in a significant worsening of the neonate's condition. Complete closure of the ductus is incompatible with life in neonates who have HLHS. The relative flow between the systemic and pulmonary circulations depends on the relation between the systemic and pulmonary vascular resistance. Pulmonary vascular resistance normally decreases immediately after birth, compromising systemic flow. Studies show that the smooth muscle in the pulmonary arterioles is more sensitive to arteriolar O_2 concentration and pH. Thus mechanical ventilation that increases O_2 and pH will enhance pulmonary overflow and reduce systemic flow in neonates with HLHS.

If HLHS is not treated, many neonates will die within the first few days of life, and 95% will not survive beyond the first month. Rarely, a patient with HLHS, a large PDA, and balanced pulmonary and systemic circulations will survive to the age of 5 to 10 years but will die of pulmonary vascular occlusive disease.

Evaluation

History and Physical Examination

Neonates with HLHS within 24 hours of their birth usually have restricted blood flow across the interatrial septum. However, most patients have normal Apgar scores and are seen a few days after birth as the ductus closes. Findings on physical examination are nonspecific and include respiratory distress, tachycardia, tachypnea, mild cyanosis, and signs of cardiovascular collapse. Palpation reveals a prominent right ventricular and diminished or absent left ventricular apical impulse, a normal first heart sound, and a single second heart sound with increased intensity.

Electrocardiographic Studies

The ECG reveals right atrial and right ventricular enlargement.

Imaging Studies

Plain films of the chest are nonspecific and may show cardiomegaly and increased pulmonary vascular markings. The diagnosis is confirmed by two-dimensional Doppler echocardiography. In many patients, an in utero diagnosis is now obtained by prenatal ultrasound examination. Cardiac catheterization is not routinely necessary and is not advisable in most cases because the neonate is extremely ill.

Treatment

Indications for Surgery

Because untreated HLHS is almost always fatal, surgery is indicated in most cases. Some experts recommend neonatal heart transplantation, whereas others recommend staged reconstructive procedures moving toward a single-

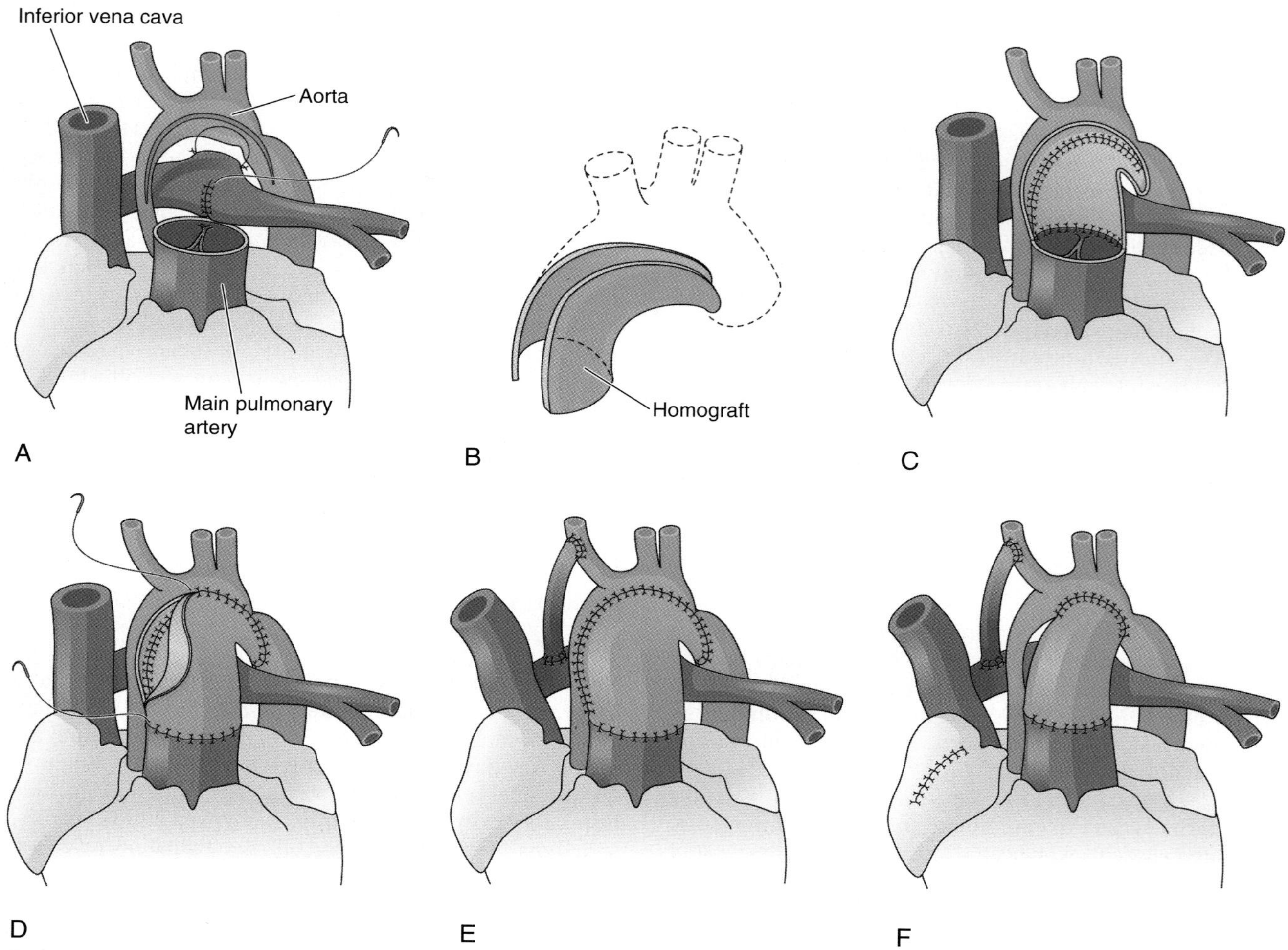

FIGURE 30–8 Norwood stage I procedure for repair of hypoplastic left heart syndrome. *A*, Incisions used for the procedure, incorporating a cuff of arterial wall allograft. The distal divided main pulmonary artery may be closed by direct suture or with a patch. *B*, Dimensions of the cuff of the arterial wall allograft. *C*, The arterial wall allograft is used to supplement the anastomosis between the proximal divided main pulmonary artery and the ascending aorta, aortic arch, and proximal descending aorta. *D* and *E*, The procedure is completed by an atrial septectomy and a 3.5-mm modified right Blalock shunt. *F*, When the ascending aorta is particularly small, an alternative procedure involves placement of a complete tube of arterial allograft. The tiny ascending aorta may be left in situ, as indicated, or implanted into the side of the neoaorta. (Modified from Castaneda AR, Jonas RA, Mayer JE, Hanley FL: Cardiac Surgery of the Neonate and Infant. Philadelphia, WB Saunders, 1994.)

ventricle physiology. Contraindications to surgical intervention include severe associated anomalies, serious chromosomal anomalies, poor ventricular function, and persistent multisystem organ failure despite adequate resuscitation. Severe tricuspid valve or pulmonary valve regurgitation is considered a contraindication to reconstructive surgery but not to heart transplantation.

Surgical Techniques

Adequate initial medical management is critical to the overall success of the surgery and includes the following: continuous intravenous administration of prostaglandin E_1 to ensure patency of the ductus; maintenance of balanced pulmonary and systemic vascular resistance by avoiding supplemental oxygen and respiratory alkalosis; and aggressive organ resuscitation.

Reconstructive procedures are usually performed in three stages as described Norwood and colleagues. Stage I (Fig. 30-8) is performed within 2 to 3 days of the patient's birth. Surgery is performed via a midsternotomy incision, with the use of cardiopulmonary bypass, deep hypothermia, and circulatory arrest.

- Stage I has three components: an atrial septostomy to allow unrestricted pulmonary venous return to the right atrium; association of the ascending aorta to the right ventricle, by using the proximal main pulmonary artery with patch augmentation of the ascending aorta and the aortic arch; and the construction of a PTFE shunt from the innominate artery to the right pulmonary artery to allow normal pulmonary vascular growth and development.

- Stage II, called the hemi-Fontan or bidirectional Glenn shunt, is performed when the patient is 6 months old. It involves interrupting the systemic-to-pulmonary shunt and connecting the superior vena cava directly to the right pulmonary artery.
- Stage III, called the Fontan operation, is performed when the patient is 1 to 3 years old and consists of connecting the inferior vena cava to the pulmonary artery, by using a variety of techniques.

Complications and Outcome

After the first-stage reconstruction, early and late mortality rates are now in range of 25% to 45% and 10% to 25%, respectively. After the Fontan operation, early and late mortality rates are 10% to 15% and 5% to 10%, respectively. The operative mortality rate associated with heart transplantation in patients with HLHS is in the range of 20% to 30%. However, because of the lack of donors, many patients die while awaiting transplantation. Allograft atherosclerosis is also a significant long-term problem. Thus overall mortality associated with transplantation is similar to that associated with the three-stage reconstruction.

Suggested Reading

Castaneda AR, Jonas RA, Mayer JE, et al (eds): Cardiac Surgery of the Neonate and Infant. Philadelphia, WB Saunders, 1994.

Kouchoukos NT, Blackstone EH, Doty DB, et al (eds): Kirklin/Barratt-Boyes Cardiac Surgery, 3rd ed. New York, Churchill Livingstone, 2003.

Zeevi B, Keane JF, Perry SB, et al: Invasive catheter techniques in the management of critical aortic stenosis in infants. In Jacobs ML, Norwood WI (eds): Pediatric Cardiac Surgery. Stoneham, MA, Butterworth-Heinemann, 1992.

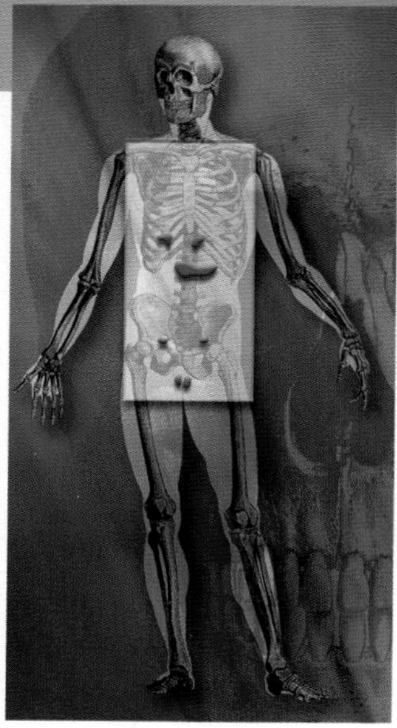

SECTION VIII

ENDOCRINE

Chapter 31

Thyroid

ANN T. SWEENEY, MD, and ROBERT M. BEAZLEY, MD

Overview

Embryology

During the third or fourth week of embryologic development, the thyroid gland appears as an endodermal proliferation in the floor of the pharynx at the base of the tongue. During its descent in the neck as a bilobate diverticulum from the foramen cecum, the thyroid gland acquires parafollicular cells. As the gland descends anterior to the hyoid bone and thyroid cartilage, the thyroglossal connection to the foramen cecum usually obliterates.

The two lateral thyroid lobes are connected medially by an isthmus. The thyroid gland becomes attached by connective tissue to the underlying trachea and is invested by a thin fibrous capsule that penetrates the gland and is responsible for the gland's typical pseudolobular surface texture.

The thyroglossal duct is usually completely reabsorbed. However, in about one third of patients, the distal portion remains and forms the **pyramidal lobe**. In a small percentage of patients, midline remnants of the thyroglossal duct lead to ectopic thyroid rests or thyroglossal duct cysts, which may be lined with thyroid cells. On occasion, a thyroglossal duct cyst may become infected or develop into papillary thyroid carcinoma.

Failure of the thyroid to descend into the neck may result in a **lingual thyroid** that serves as the patient's only functioning thyroid tissue.

Anatomy

The **arterial blood supply** of the thyroid gland arises from two major sources: the **inferior thyroid artery**, which originates from the thyrocervical trunk, and the **superior thyroid artery**, which is the first branch of the external carotid artery (Fig. 31–1). Occasionally, the **lowest thyroid artery** (thyroidea ima) will arise from the innominate artery or the aorta and enter the isthmus of the thyroid. The blood supply to the thyroid gland is abundant (4–6 mL/min/g) and exceeds the renal blood flow (3 mL/min/g). In hyperthyroidism, a marked increase in blood flow occurs, with rates that may even exceed 1 L/min/g. This increase is frequently associated with an audible bruit or a palpable thrill.

The **venous drainage** of the thyroid is variable and is accomplished by a network of thin-walled veins on the thyroid capsule. In general, the capsular network empties into three venous pedicles: the **superior thyroid vein** at the superior pole drains into the internal jugular vein; the **inferior thyroid vein or veins** that arise from the lower pole empty into the jugular vein or the innominate vein; and a variously present **middle thyroid vein** enters directly into the jugular vein. If the thyroid gland is enlarged and retrosternal, the inferior thyroid veins and the recurrent laryngeal nerve may look similar, so care must be taken to differentiate among them during surgery.

Lymphatic drainage within the gland is copious and may track bilaterally across the isthmus. The regional lymph nodes are located in the central neck between the carotid arteries and consist of the prelaryngeal, pretracheal, and paratracheoesophageal groups. **Prelaryngeal lymph nodes** lie superior to the isthmus. An enlarged prelaryngeal node that is occasionally associated with thyroid cancer is known as the **delphian lymph node** because it may predict carcinoma within the thyroid gland. **Pretracheal lymph nodes** are found inferior to the isthmus, and they drain into the anterior and superior mediastinum. Lymph from the central and lower portions of the thyroid lobes normally flows to the **paratracheoesophageal lymph nodes**, which lie lateral and deep to the thyroid gland and are intimately associated with the recurrent laryngeal nerve. The upper pole areas usually drain into the lateral neck nodes.

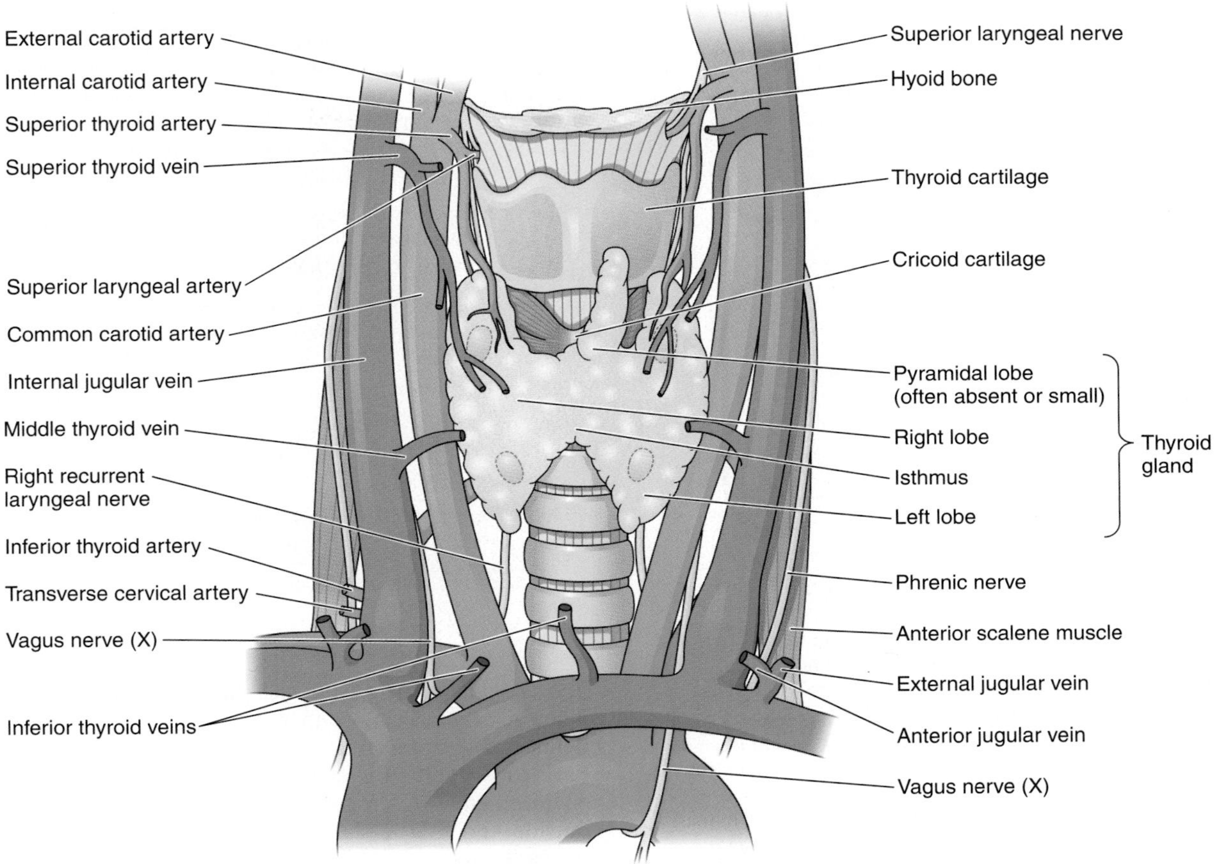

FIGURE 31–1 Anatomic structures of the neck, specifically those in the region of the thyroid gland. Note the anatomic location of the parathyroid glands and the recurrent laryngeal nerve. The nerve to the left of the vagus nerve is the phrenic nerve.

Physiology

Thyroid Hormones

The **parafollicular cells (C cells)** of the thyroid gland synthesize and secrete **calcitonin** hormone, the physiologic role of which in humans is unclear. Calcitonin acts as a potent inhibitor of bone reabsorption when it is administered in high concentrations.

The **thyroid cells** synthesize and secrete **thyroxine** (T_4, or tetraiodothyronine) and **triiodothyronine** (T_3). These two hormones are biologically active and play an important role in health and disease.

Role of T_4 and T_3 in the Pituitary-Hypothalamic Feedback System

T_4 and T_3 influence the secretion of **thyroid-stimulating hormone** (TSH), which is a pituitary hormone, and **thyrotropin-releasing hormone** (TRH), which is a hypothalamic hormone. These and other hormones are involved in the pituitary-hypothalamic feedback system.

TSH is a glycoprotein that is secreted by the anterior pituitary and is composed of alpha and beta subunits. TSH is secreted in response to TRH and T_3 levels within the pituitary. Pituitary T_3 is derived primarily from local deiodination of T_4 and to a lesser extent from the peripheral circulation. T_3 directly inhibits the synthesis and release of TSH in the classic negative-feedback control of hormone secretion. TRH produced in the hypothalamus also is under negative-feedback control by thyroid hormone levels. T_4 and T_3 feed back in a negative loop on the pituitary and hypothalamus to regulate the production of TSH and TRH (Fig. 31–2).

TSH regulates thyroid function by binding to TSH receptors on the basolateral membrane of follicular cells. The TSH receptor is a member of the G protein–coupled

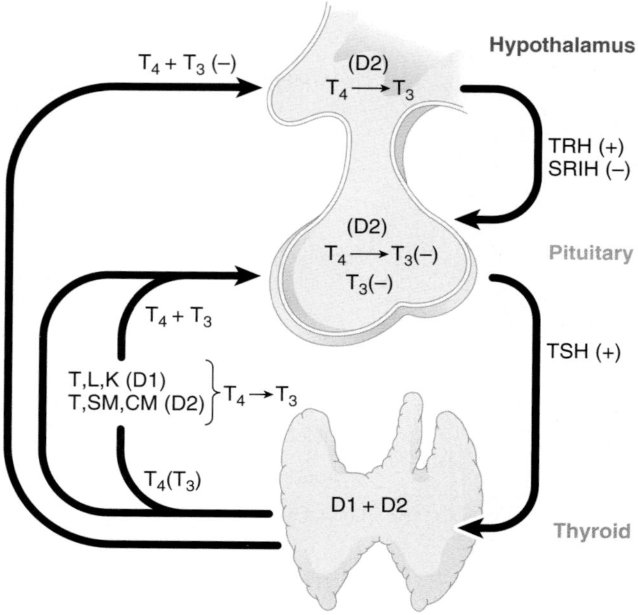

FIGURE 31–2 The role of thyroxine (T_4) and triiodothyronine (T_3) in the regulation of thyrotropin-releasing hormone (TRH) and thyroid-stimulating hormone (TSH). Thyroidal T_4 must be converted to T_3 to produce its effects. This conversion may take place in the thyroid (T), liver (L), and kidney (K) and is catalyzed either by the propylthiouracil-sensitive iodothyronine 5′-deiodinase (D1) or by the propylthiouracil-insensitive iodothyronine 5′-deiodinase (D2). D2 is present in the human pituitary, central nervous system, thyroid (T), and skeletal muscle (SM) and may be present in the cardiac muscle (CM). Somatotropin release – inhibiting hormone (SRIH) also is called somatostatin. (Modified from Larson PR, Davis TF, Hay ID: The thyroid gland. In Wilson JD, Foster DW, Kronenberg HM, Larson PR (eds): Williams Textbook of Endocrinology, 9th ed. Philadelphia, WB Saunders, 1998.)

receptor family and is composed of three domains. The binding of TSH to its receptor activates adenylate cyclase and phospholipase C pathways of intracellular signaling and thereby leads to thyroid hormone synthesis.

Classification of Thyroid Diseases

Thyrotoxicosis is defined as the clinical syndrome of hypermetabolism that occurs in association with elevated serum concentrations of T_4 and T_3. **Hyperthyroidism** is one major form of thyrotoxicosis and is due to increased hormone production and release from the thyroid gland. However, the terms *hyperthyroidism* and *thyrotoxicosis* are clearly not synonymous (Table 31–1).

The term *goiter* is derived from the Latin *guttur* (throat) and is used to refer to a swelling or enlargement of the thyroid gland. The swelling is called an **endemic goiter** when it occurs in more than 10% of the population in a defined geographic area. Characteristically, endemic areas have low levels of dietary iodine intake, high levels of environmental goitrogens, or both. Goiters that occur outside endemic areas are classified as **nonendemic** or **sporadic goiters** and include a variety of **benign thyroid conditions** seen in the developed world, such as Graves' disease, Hashimoto's thyroiditis, DeQuervain's thyroiditis, Riedel's thyroiditis, and most thyroid nodules.

Malignant thyroid conditions include papillary thyroid carcinoma, follicular thyroid carcinoma, Hürthle cell carcinoma, medullary thyroid carcinoma, anaplastic carcinoma, and malignant lymphoma of the thyroid.

PEARLS FOR ROUNDS

Patients with Graves' disease for whom surgery is indicated include those with very large glands who cannot be treated adequately with radioactive iodine and those who are allergic to thionamides or whose hyperthyroidism cannot be controlled with these drugs.

Thyrotoxic patients who are to be treated surgically should be adequately treated first with antithyroid medication (thionamides) to render them euthyroid.

Patients who require an emergency thyroidectomy and are thyrotoxic should be treated preoperatively for 5 days with dexamethasone, iopanoic acid, propanolol, and propylthiouracil.

Ionizing radiation is associated with the development of thyroid cancer, and the majority of radiation-induced tumors are of the papillary type.

Five prognostic factors for patients with thyroid cancer include metastases, age, completeness of surgery, and invasiveness of the tumor.

Graves' Disease

Graves' disease is a form of hyperthyroidism that occurs predominantly in females (female-to-male ratio of 7:1) and most frequently has its onset during the third and fourth decades of life. The disease is classically associated with goiter, ophthalmopathy, and dermopathy, but all three manifestations are not always present.

Etiology and Pathogenesis

Clearly a familial predisposition exists to acquiring Graves' disease, and genetic factors are known to play a significant role in disease pathogenesis.

Hyperthyroidism occurs as a result of TSH-receptor stimulation by TSH-receptor autoantibodies called thyroid-stimulating immunoglobulins (TSIs). Overstimulation leads

TABLE 31–1 Examples, Causes, and Mechanisms of Thyrotoxicosis

Examples	Causes and Mechanisms
Thyrotoxicosis with Hyperthyroidism	
Graves' disease*	Abnormal thyroid stimulation; production of antibodies to the thyroid-stimulating hormone (TSH) receptor
Toxic adenoma*	Intrinsic thyroid autonomy; point; mutation of the TSH receptor
Toxic multinodular goiter*	Intrinsic thyroid autonomy; point mutation of the TSH receptor
Hyperemesis gravidarum	Production of thyroid stimulators; high levels of chorionic gonadotropin
Iodine-induced hyperthyroidism	Iodine excess (from iodine, iodine-containing drugs, and radiographic contrast agents); thyroid autonomy
Lithium-induced hyperthyroidism	Possible thyroid autonomy.
Struma ovarii	Intrinsic thyroid autonomy; presence of toxic adenoma in an ovarian dermoid tumor
Thyroid carcinoma	Intrinsic thyroid autonomy; foci of functional autonomy
Trophoblastic tumor	Production of thyroid stimulators; high levels of chorionic gonadotropin
TSH hypersecretion	Presence of thyrotroph adenoma or thyrotroph resistance
Thyrotoxicosis without Hyperthyroidism	
Silent thyroiditis*	Inflammatory disease; release of stored thyroid hormone
Subacute thyroiditis*	Inflammatory disease; release of stored thyroid hormone
Thyrotoxicosis factitia*	Intake of exogenous source of thyroid hormone (medication or food)
Drug-induced thyroiditis	Inflammatory reaction associated with use of drugs such as amiodarone and interferon alfa; release of stored thyroid hormone
Infarction of thyroid adenoma	Inflammatory reaction; release of stored thyroid hormone
Radiation thyroiditis	Inflammatory reaction; release of stored thyroid hormone

* Common examples.
Data from Braverman LE, Utiger RD: Introduction to thyrotoxicosis. In Braverman LE, Utiger RD (eds): Werner's and Ingbar's The Thyroid, 7th ed. Philadelphia, Lippincott, 1991, with permission.

to an increase in the synthesis and secretion of thyroid hormones and to an increase in growth of the thyroid gland.

The reason for the generation of TSH-receptor antibodies is unclear, but infectious and environmental agents and stress-related immune suppression are possible underlying mechanisms. The causes of eye and skin manifestations of Graves' disease also are unclear. The manifestations may result from the cross-reaction of TSI with TSH receptors on fibroblasts in the orbital tissue and dermis. This interaction stimulates the elaboration of numerous cytokines and causes the fibroblasts to produce glycosaminoglycans. The mechanical changes caused by the accumulation of glycosaminoglycans and edema in tissues are recognized clinically as Graves' ophthalmopathy and dermopathy.

Evaluation

History and Physical Examination

Graves' disease often is first seen with various general symptoms and signs of thyrotoxicosis (Box 31–1). Hypertension, cardiac failure, and exacerbation of angina pectoris also may be noted, particularly in older patients with preexisting cardiac disease.

In Graves' disease, the thyroid gland is typically diffusely enlarged and may vary in consistency from soft to firm. A bruit or thrill indicative of hypervascularity may be apparent over the gland. An enlarged pyramidal lobe is often palpable.

Patients with Graves' disease may exhibit mechanical changes in the orbit (orbitopathy), including exophthalmos and proptosis. These changes can lead to complications that vary in severity from mild congestion (with chemosis, conjunctivitis, and periorbital swelling) to corneal ulceration, optic neuritis, optic atrophy, exophthalmic ophthalmoplegia, and orbital herniation. Rapidly progressive exophthalmos is termed malignant exophthalmos. Graves' eye disease also affects the extraorbital muscles, causing inflammation, muscle enlargement, and subsequent muscle fibrosis, and sometimes resulting in diplopia and impaired extraocular muscle movements.

The dermopathy associated with Graves' disease typically occurs over the dorsum of the feet or pretibial regions and is characterized by raised, thickened, hyperpigmented areas that have the appearance of an orange peel. The lesions may be pruritic and associated with nonpitting edema.

BOX 31–1 Clinical Manifestations of Thyrotoxicosis

Symptoms
- Anxiety
- Excessive sweating
- Fatigue
- Heat intolerance
- Hyperdefecation
- Irritability
- Menstrual irregularity
- Palpitations
- Shortness of breath
- Sleeplessness
- Weight loss

Signs
- Bounding pulse
- Elevated systolic blood pressure
- Fine, silky hair
- Fine tremor of the hands and tongue
- Hyperkinesis
- Hyperreflexia
- Onycholysis
- Proximal muscle weakness
- Stare, lid lag, and infrequent blinking
- Tachycardia
- Warm, moist, smooth skin

Laboratory and Imaging Studies

Undetectable levels of TSH and elevated levels of circulating free T_4 and T_3 concentrations are consistent with the diagnosis of Graves' disease and other forms of thyrotoxicosis. Occasionally, only T_3 levels are elevated; this is called T_3 toxicosis. In Graves' disease, a radioactive iodine uptake (RAIU) scan will characteristically demonstrate diffuse, elevated radioisotope uptake.

Differential Diagnosis

Thyrotoxicosis in association with goiter and infiltrative ophthalmopathy is virtually diagnostic of Graves' disease. In a patient with these features, an RAIU scan is rarely indicated.

A symmetrical goiter, particularly in the presence of a bruit, most likely represents Graves' disease, but rare causes of this presentation include a TSH-secreting adenoma and conditions associated with trophoblastic stimulation of the thyroid gland (conditions such as hydatidiform mole and choriocarcinoma). A palpable single nodule may indicate a toxic adenoma, whereas multiple nodules suggest a multinodular goiter. A tender thyroid gland in a patient with an antecedent viral illness is suggestive of subacute thyroiditis, whereas a small, firm nodular gland suggests chronic thyroiditis. Absence of a palpable gland raises the possibility of ingestion of exogenous thyroid hormone (thyrotoxicosis factitia) or, more rarely, an ectopic source of thyroid hormone (struma ovarii).

Hyperthyroidism, except in cases of iodine-induced hyperthyroidism, is associated with an elevated RAIU level. In contrast, thyroiditis caused by excessive release of stored hormone is associated with a subnormal RAIU level (uptake usually <1%). In patients with ectopic thyroid tissue, such as struma ovarii, increased uptake will be exhibited in the ovaries.

Treatment

All patients with Graves' disease require treatment with antithyroid drugs. In some cases, thionamides are used as first-line therapy to induce remission of the disease. In other cases, they are used as short-term therapy to control the symptoms of disease before radioactive iodine (RAI) treatment or surgery.

Nonsurgical Treatment

Thionamide Therapy. Drugs that are helpful in the treatment of Graves' disease include propylthiouracil (PTU), methimazole, and β-adrenergic–receptor antagonists (β-blockers). β-Blockers are useful as adjunct agents, because they help reduce many of the clinical manifestations of excessive sympathetic stimulation, such as tremor, palpitations, and anxiety.

In patients who are compliant, thionamide therapy generally is highly effective in controlling hyperthyroidism.

Groups in whom treatment with a thionamide alone is most likely to induce a spontaneous remission are children, adolescents, and patients with small goiters and mild hyperthyroidism. An increase in the long-term remission rate has been observed when patients are treated with thionamides for a longer period, so most thyroid specialists advocate therapy for at least 1 year.

Radioactive Iodine Therapy. RAI therapy has been used to treat hyperthyroidism since the 1940s, and many physicians prefer to use it to treat older patients with Graves' disease. It also is used to treat toxic multinodular goiters and toxic solitary adenomas and to ablate residual thyroid tissue or malignant tissue after near-total thyroidectomy for thyroid cancer. RAI therapy is absolutely contraindicated during pregnancy, because it may precipitate fetal hypothyroidism.

In patients scheduled for RAI therapy, a thionamide is initially used to reduce the thyroid hormone level. After the thionamide is withheld for 4 to 5 days, RAI is administered orally in the form of sodium iodide I 131 (^{131}I).

Although the goal of RAI therapy is euthyroidism, hypothyroidism often results and is dose dependent. Follow-up at 1 year after RAI shows that permanent hypothyroidism occurs in at least 50% of patients given high doses, whereas follow-up at 25 years shows that permanent hypothyroidism occurs in at least 25% of patients given lower doses. Therefore all patients treated with ^{131}I require long-term follow-up. No evidence suggests that RAI therapy increases the risk of developing cancer.

Surgical Treatment

The primary goal of surgery is to cure hyperthyroidism by reducing the amount of functioning thyroid mass. The size of thyroid mass to be retained is based on the size of the hyperplastic gland.

Indications for Surgery. Because pregnant women cannot undergo RAI therapy, surgery is indicated for all pregnant women who are allergic to thionamides or whose hyperthyroidism cannot be controlled with these drugs. Surgery also is indicated for nonpregnant patients who are allergic to thionamides or RAI, have a large goiter that causes airway compression or dysphagia, or prefer surgery to the use of other therapies.

Preoperative Preparation. Thyrotoxic patients who are scheduled for elective thyroidectomy should be treated initially with thionamides to render them euthyroid or at least bring their hyperthyroidism under control before surgery. β-Blockers should be used to decrease adrenergic signs and symptoms. For 7 to 10 days before surgery, oral potassium iodide should be given, in the form of either a saturated solution of potassium iodide or Lugol's solution (which contains 7 mg/drop).

For patients who require emergency thyroidectomy, preoperative treatment for 5 days with betamethasone (0.5 mg every 6 hours), iopanoic acid (500 mg every 6 hours), and propranolol (40 mg every 8 hours) has been demonstrated to be a safe and effective regimen to prevent postoperative thyrotoxic crises.

Surgical Techniques. The majority of thyroidectomies can be done through a low transverse collar incision (Kocher incision). Subplatysmal skin flaps are raised superiorly to the top of the thyroid cartilage, inferiorly over the sternoclavicular heads, and laterally to the medial borders of the sternocleidomastoid muscles.

Most surgeons divide the strap muscles vertically in the midline and elevate them from the underlying thyroid capsule by blunt dissection and lateral traction. After the upper pole of the thyroid gland is exposed, the superior thyroid artery and vein are ligated in continuity, with attention to avoid damaging the external branch of the superior laryngeal nerve. Freeing the upper pole facilitates mobilization of the lateral and posterior aspects of the thyroid lobe and identification of the inferior thyroid artery lateral to the thyroid gland.

The recurrent laryngeal nerve as it crosses the inferior thyroid artery medially near the thyroid capsule is identified. From this point, the recurrent nerve is carefully traced to its entry into the cricothyroid membrane while it is being separated from the overlying thyroid gland. In this same area, the superior parathyroid gland may be encountered, usually within a 1-cm radius of the junction of the inferior thyroid artery and recurrent nerve. Every effort should be made to preserve parathyroid tissue.

At this point in the operation, inferior and posterior venous branches to the thyroid gland can safely be managed. The isthmus is divided between clamps, and the thyroid lobe is sharply elevated from the underlying trachea. If a pyramidal lobe is present over the anterior trachea and larynx, it should be removed, because it may be a source of recurrent hyperthyroidism.

In patients with Graves' disease, the most frequently performed surgical procedure is a bilateral subtotal thyroidectomy. This requires that the described procedure be repeated on the opposite lobe. An alternative for treating Graves' disease is to perform a total lobectomy on one side and a subtotal resection on the opposite side (Dunhill procedure), leaving a slightly greater and more easily manageable remnant of tissue.

Complications. Because of the slight edema that is associated with intubation, a nerve injury may not be apparent at the time of extubation but may be suggested by the deterioration of the patient's voice over the next 12- to 24-hour period. Intraoperatively, it is helpful to stimulate the recurrent nerve with a nerve stimulator and to palpate a muscle twitch in the larynx. Then if the patient is hoarse postoperatively, the surgeon is assured that the nerves are electrically intact. With injury to the external branch of the superior laryngeal nerve, patients may experience early tiring of the voice and subtle changes in voice quality, particularly for high-pitched notes. This injury can be devastating for singers and public speakers. Thus during surgery, every effort should be made to identify and avoid the nerve as it courses in or near the vascular pedicle to the thyroid gland. Transient nerve palsy occurs in as many as 3% to 5% of patients, with recovery of nerve function taking from a few days to 4 months. Permanent nerve injury occurs in 1% or fewer patients.

Hypoparathyroidism can result from injury to or excision of the parathyroid glands. During surgery, these glands should be identified and every effort made to protect the delicate blood supply to them, which, in 30% of the patients, arises directly from the thyroid capsule. It is important to autotransplant parathyroid glands that appear to be compromised or are likely to be removed with the procedure. Transient hypoparathyroidism occurs in 3% to 5% of patients and requires the administration of activated vitamin D and supplemental calcium in the immediate postoperative period. Permanent hypoparathyroidism occurs in fewer than 1% of patients.

In the postoperative period, patients must be closely monitored to identify hemorrhage and airway obstruction. In patients with expanding wound hematomas, increasing symptoms of pain are occasionally followed by hoarseness and rapidly developing signs of airway obstruction, distress, and stridor. Suspected hemorrhage is effectively managed by removing the sutures, opening the wound, and evacuating the hematoma immediately (even at the bedside, if necessary). Occasionally, airway obstruction results from subglottic or supraglottic edema. This problem can be treated with conservative measures, such as the use of humidified oxygen and intravenous corticosteroids.

Thyroiditis

Thyroiditis is defined as an inflammatory condition involving the thyroid gland. Several forms exist and are described later. Patients with thyroiditis often are initially seen with diffuse enlargement of the thyroid gland.

Hashimoto's Thyroiditis

Hashimoto's thyroiditis commonly occurs in young to middle-aged women and is responsible for approximately 60% of the cases of hypothyroidism in the United States.

Evaluation

Hashimoto's thyroiditis is a chronic autoimmune-mediated form of thyroiditis that may be seen in association with other autoimmune diseases, such as pernicious anemia, vitiligo, alopecia areata, and Addison's disease. Findings include a bilateral, diffuse, firm goiter; lymphocytic infiltration of the thyroid gland; and the presence of antithyroid antibodies in the serum.

Treatment

Surgery is infrequently necessary in the management of Hashimoto's thyroiditis. However, it may be indicated for cosmesis, to alleviate airway obstruction, or to exclude the diagnosis of thyroid cancer. Total or near-total thyroidectomy is the preferred procedure.

DeQuervain's Thyroiditis

DeQuervain's thyroiditis, or **subacute granulomatous thyroiditis**, is a transient inflammatory condition of the thyroid. Patients commonly experience phases of thyrotoxicosis and hypothyroidism before euthyroidism is restored.

Evaluation

DeQuervain's thyroiditis often follows a flulike illness or upper respiratory tract infection. The thyrotoxic phase begins after thyroid follicular cell damage, is characterized by the breakdown of thyroglobulin and release of stored thyroid hormone, and lasts only until thyroid hormone stores are depleted. Although thyroid hormone levels and the erythrocyte sedimentation rate are elevated, the RAIU level is low, because thyroid hormone synthesis is not increased. During this phase, the thyroid gland is almost always tender to palpation. The thyrotoxic phase usually resolves after a few months. A hypothyroid phase then follows and also resolves spontaneously within a few months.

Treatment

Although the use of nonsteroidal anti-inflammatory agents will alleviate symptoms of inflammation in most patients, some may require treatment with corticosteroids. Subacute thyroiditis is not considered a surgical disease.

Riedel's Thyroiditis

Riedel's thyroiditis is a rare disease that also is called **Riedel's struma** and **fibrous thyroiditis** and may be seen in association with other fibrosclerotic conditions, such as sclerosing cholangitis and retroperitoneal fibrosis. A goiter is usually found fixed to the surrounding tissue and occasionally extending into the adjacent lateral neck structures.

Fine-needle aspiration (FNA) or true-cut biopsy will usually provide a tissue diagnosis, but open biopsy is occasionally required. Because of the intense fibrous reaction, the surgeon is not able to perform safely much more than an isthmusectomy. Surgical resection should be avoided, because it is associated with high morbidity and mortality rates.

Acute Suppurative Thyroiditis

Acute suppurative thyroiditis is a rare inflammatory condition that is usually caused by bacteria but may be due to fungi or parasitic organisms.

Infection may seed the thyroid gland through hematogenous spread from a distant site (pyelonephritis) or via the lymphatics as a consequence of a local infection such as pharyngitis or mastoiditis. Pyriform sinus fistulas, persistent thyroglossal duct cysts, and penetrating trauma also have been reported as sources of infection.

Evaluation

Typical symptoms of thyroiditis include fever, chills, sore throat, dysphagia, dysphonia, and the abrupt onset of anterior neck pain, which may radiate to the ear or mandible. The thyroid gland is warm and tender to palpation and usually appears to be bilaterally or unilaterally enlarged. The overlying skin may be erythematous.

In most cases, laboratory studies reveal leukocytosis with a leftward shift, and thyroid-function tests yield normal results. FNA of the lesion should be followed by Gram staining and culture to determine the cause of infection and the type of antibiotic to be given. The presence of purulent material is diagnostic of suppurative thyroiditis.

Treatment

Therapy consists of parenteral antibiotics and surgical drainage of the lesion.

Nodular Thyroid Disease

Thyroid nodules are clinically common and occur in 5% to 10% of adults. Autopsy reports indicate that either solitary or multiple nodules are present in up to 50% of individuals. Nodular thyroid disease may be either multinodular or uninodular.

Multinodular Goiter

Multinodular goiter has a marked female predominance, is found more frequently in areas where goiter is endemic, and is generally slow growing and of long-standing presence.

Etiology and Pathogenesis

A multinodular goiter can be classified as nontoxic or toxic, based on its functional status. A **nontoxic** or **diffuse multinodular goiter (simple goiter)** is defined as a thyroid enlargement that is not caused by autoimmune thyroid disease, thyroiditis, or neoplasia and is not associated with clinical or biochemical evidence of thyroid dysfunction. A **toxic-multinodular goiter** is characterized by excess secretion of thyroid hormone and may arise from a long-standing simple goiter. This transition from nontoxic to toxic goiter involves the development of functional autonomy within the thyroid gland (i.e., independence from the actions of TSH). Scattered foci of autonomous activity are evident on thyroid scans early in the disease process.

Multinodular goiters may evolve secondary to iodine deficiency or exposure to naturally occurring goitrogens. They also may occur in a familial pattern or sporadically. An inherent growth potential of different populations of thyroid cells is thought to play a major role in the pathogenesis and development of multinodular goiters. Recent studies indicate that the rate of malignancy in patients with a multinodular goiter is 25% to 60% of that in patients with a solitary nodule. To rule out the possibility of cancer, a dominant thyroid nodule within a multinodular goiter should be evaluated in the same manner as a solitary nodule.

Evaluation

History and Physical Examination. The symptoms and signs of multinodular goiter depend on the size and location of the goiter and on the functional status of the thyroid gland.

Patients may complain of chest tightness, urge to cough, hoarseness, and the sensation of a foreign body in the throat. In patients with multinodular goiter, exposure to excess iodine may lead to thyrotoxicosis (jodbasedow phenomenon). Therefore patients may display symptoms and signs of hyperthyroidism. Toxic multinodular goiter in the elderly is often heralded by the onset of atrial fibrillation or even heart failure as a result of autonomous hyperfunctioning nodules.

Exophytic growth of the goiter may be accompanied by only cosmetic changes, or it may cause tracheal and esophageal compression that results in airway problems and dysphagia. Retrosternal extension of the goiter may cause partial superior vena cava obstruction and result in congestion of the face and dilatation of cervical veins when the arms are elevated (Pemberton's sign).

Careful examination of the thyroid gland is an important part of the evaluation of nodular disease. The gland may be more easily palpated if the examiner faces the patient, rather than standing behind him or her. Locating the cricoid cartilage is a key initial step, because the isthmus of the thyroid lies just below it. The isthmus can be examined by placing the thumb in the horizontal position on the inferior portion of the cricoid cartilage. When the patient swallows, the thumb passes easily over the isthmus. The lobes of the gland can be palpated by placing two fingers of the right hand medial to the sternocleidomastoid muscle and along the lateral aspect of the trachea and asking the patient to swallow as the examiner massages the trachea with the fingers. After the thyroid is examined, the lymph nodes on both sides of the neck should be evaluated. The examiner must define the consistency and size of each thyroid lobe, the margins of the gland, the presence of nodules, the extent to which the gland extends below the clavicle or sternum, and the extent to which the trachea is displaced or deviated.

Laboratory Studies. An undetectable or low TSH concentration suggests autonomously functioning nodules. Therefore if the TSH is elevated, the diagnosis is more likely to be Hashimoto's thyroiditis than multinodular goiter.

Imaging and Other Studies. Ultrasonography may be used to evaluate further the nature of the multinodular gland and to determine how many nodules are present and whether they are solid or cystic. However, it not possible to rule out malignancy based on the sonographic appearance of the thyroid nodule. FNA is indicated if findings include a dominant nodule, a nodule with rapid growth, or a solitary solid nodule. Isotope imaging provides information concerning whether a nodule is hyperfunctioning ('hot,' or autonomously functioning), hypofunctioning ('cold'), or eufunctioning, and it also may reveal the anatomic extent of the goiter.

In patients who are hoarse or have had previous thyroid surgery, laryngoscopy is indicated. In patients in whom physical examination suggests the presence of tracheal deviation, compression, or extension into the mediastinum,

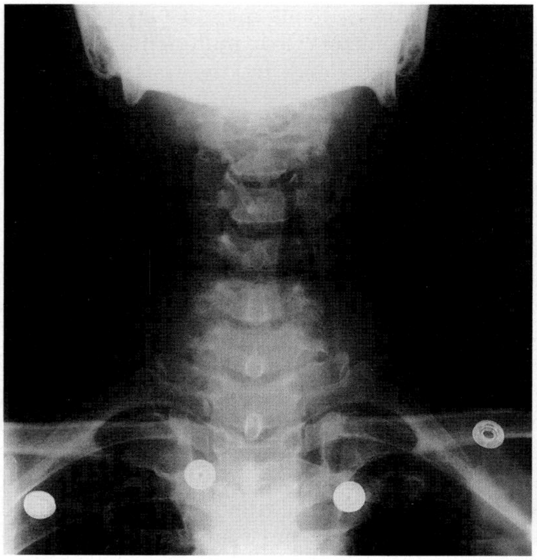

A

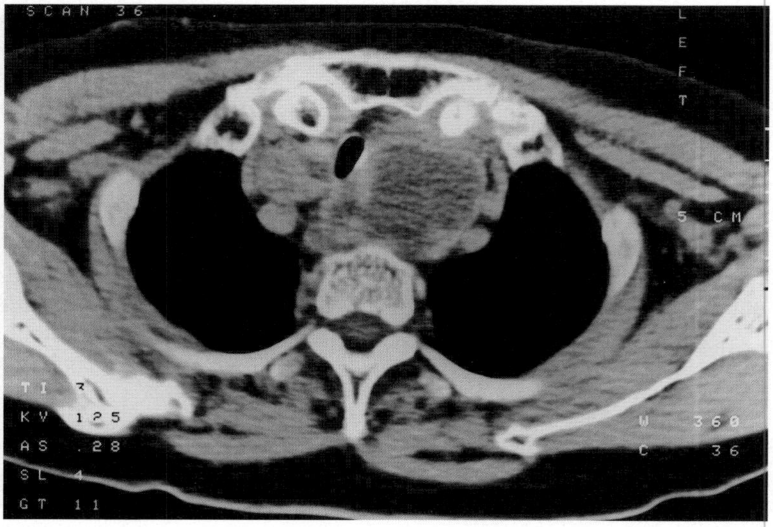

B

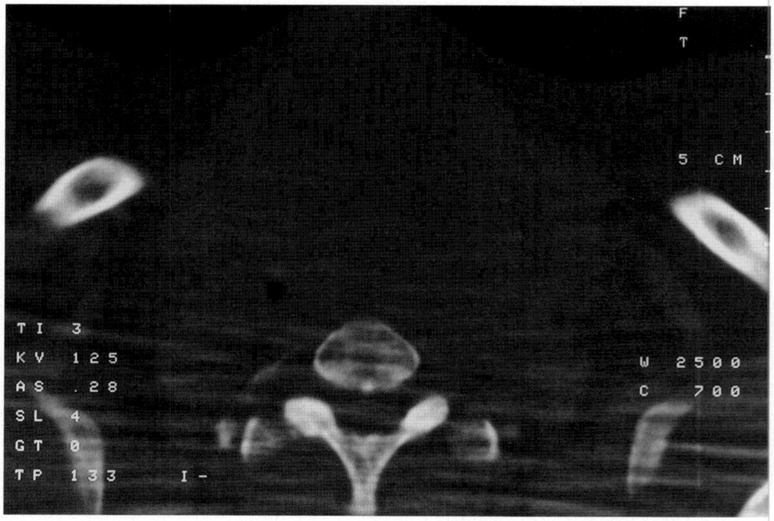

C

FIGURE 31–3 Patients with multinodular goiters. *A*, Anteroposterior radiograph showing displacement of the trachea to the left by a lower neck mass, causing increased density over the lower cervical region. *B*, Axial computed tomography (CT) scan showing a large multinodular goiter of varying tissue attenuation with tracheal compression and retrosternal extension. *C*, Axial CT scan showing marked tracheal displacement and compression by a large goiter.

radiographs or computed tomography scans may be helpful (Fig. 31-3).

Treatment

Because toxic multinodular goiter results from autonomous production of thyroid hormone, spontaneous remissions will not occur with this entity, as they do with Graves' disease. Therefore either RAI therapy or surgery is necessary. RAI therapy using ^{131}I is the treatment of choice for elderly patients with multiple medical problems. Thyroidectomy is the best choice for patients who are younger or have a large toxic goiter.

A large nontoxic goiter associated with airway compromise or substernal extension also is best treated surgically. However, if surgery is contraindicated, large doses of ^{131}I can successfully reduce the size of the goiter.

RAI therapy and surgical procedures for multinodular disease are similar to those outlined above for Graves' disease. If the multinodular goiter is confined to one thyroid lobe, a total lobectomy and isthmusectomy on the affected side should be performed. If it is not confined to one lobe, either a bilateral subtotal thyroidectomy or a bilateral total thyroidectomy can be performed.

Solitary Thyroid Nodule

The solitary thyroid nodule is a relatively common medical problem, occurring most frequently in regions that are nonendemic for goiters. In a large population study in Framingham, Massachusetts, clinically apparent nodules were found in 6.4% of women and 1.5% of men, but fewer than 5% of these lesions ultimately proved to be malignant.

Risk Factors for Thyroid Cancer

Age, gender, family history, and a history of thyroid irradiation are factors that affect the risk for developing thyroid cancer.

The occurrence of thyroid nodules increases with age. A thyroid nodule in a child is relatively rare and is twice as likely to be malignant as is one in an adult. The rate of thyroid cancer is twice as high in male as in female subjects, particularly in individuals who are younger than 30 years or older than 60 years. The rate of thyroid cancer also is increased in patients with a family history of papillary or medullary thyroid carcinoma.

A history of exposure to ionizing radiation to the head and neck region is associated with an increased incidence of thyroid nodules and cancer. Almost 80% of children diagnosed with thyroid cancer in the 1960s had been previously exposed to radiation. In most regions of the world, the incidence of childhood thyroid cancer is much lower today, because radiation therapy is infrequently used in children. New nodules in those previously exposed to either high-dose or low-dose radiation are malignant in 20% to 50% of cases.

Evaluation

History and Physical Examination. A thorough history should be taken, and patients should be asked specifically about risk factors for cancer as well as about symptoms of hypothyroidism, hyperthyroidism, dysphagia, and hoarseness. The sudden onset of hoarseness may indicate infiltration of the recurrent laryngeal nerve by a malignant nodule.

The physical examination should be directed toward determining whether the thyroid lesion is truly a solitary nodule or whether it is a dominant nodule in a patient with multinodular goiter. Differentiation is not always possible clinically, and as many as 50% of patients initially deemed to have solitary nodules will be found either by diagnostic tests or at surgery to have a multinodular gland. In addition to evaluating the character of the gland, the clinician should evaluate the size and consistency of the nodule and determine whether the nodule is adhering to the surrounding tissues. The neck should be carefully evaluated for the presence or absence of lymph nodes, particularly on the involved side.

A fixed hard mass, cervical lymphadenopathy, and symptoms of airway obstruction or vocal cord paralysis are strongly suggestive of thyroid cancer.

Laboratory Studies. Serum should be sent to determine the TSH level. Depending on the clinical situation, measurements of T_4, T_3, and antithyroid antibodies also may be helpful. A nodule in the setting of hypothyroidism likely represents a component of Hashimoto's disease, whereas one occurring in the setting of hyperthyroidism may represent a benign toxic adenoma.

Fine-Needle Aspiration Biopsy and Imaging Studies. Currently, FNA biopsy is the key component for the workup thyroid nodules and is considered the gold standard for diagnosing thyroid cancer. The rate of false-positive results associated with FNA biopsy is 0 to 1%, and the rate of false-negative results is usually 1% to 2%, so FNA biopsy is an excellent diagnostic test for selecting patients who may have cancer and require surgery. An individual who is adept at FNA biopsy should perform the procedure, and only an experienced cytopathologist should evaluate the specimen.

Some physicians will obtain radioisotope scans before FNA biopsy. However, the consensus of the American College of Physicians and the American Thyroid Association is to proceed with an FNA biopsy as long as the TSH level is normal. Ultrasound examination is helpful for determining the presence of other nodules in the thyroid and for documenting lesion size and consistency (solid or cystic). When nodules are difficult to palpate, ultrasound-guided FNA biopsy will improve the yield of diagnostic tissue.

The initial FNA biopsy results dictate the next step in patient management (Fig. 31–4). In patients who have a follicular neoplasm, especially if the serum TSH value is low, a radionuclide scan is indicated. If the scan shows a hyperfunctioning nodule, the patient is monitored clinically and evaluated for hyperthyroidism. If the scan shows a hypofunctioning or eufunctioning nodule, the patient is treated surgically or medically.

Treatment for Benign Solitary Thyroid Nodule

In patients who have a benign solitary thyroid nodule, clinical observation or treatment with levothyroxine (T_4) is indicated.

Treatment for Suspected or Confirmed Malignant Solitary Thyroid Nodule

Surgical Biopsy and Frozen-section Examination. In about 25% to 35% of thyroid lesions, the FNA findings will be read as suggestive. Many of these lesions will be interpreted as follicular neoplasms, with approximately 20% ultimately proving to be malignant carcinomas

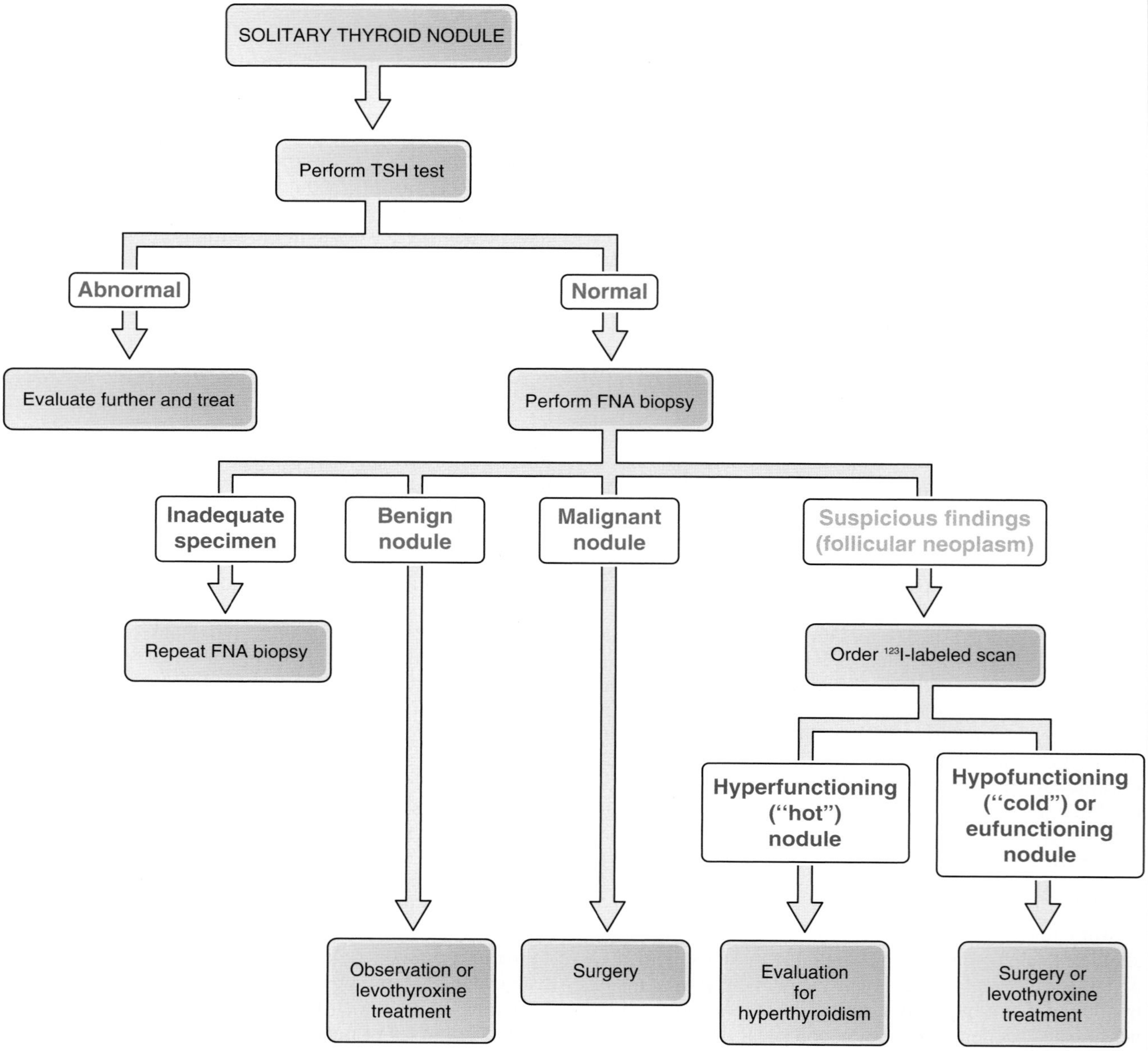

FIGURE 31–4 Algorithm for evaluating a solitary thyroid nodule. Note that a eufunctioning nodule may require further evaluation with a thyroxine (T_4) or triiodothyronine (T_3) suppression scan. TSH, Thyroid-stimulating hormone; FNA, fine-needle aspiration. (Modified from Singer PA, Cooper DS, Daniels GH, et al: Treatment guidelines for patients with thyroid nodules and well-differentiated thyroid cancer. Arch Intern Med 156:2167, 1996, with permission.)

(usually follicular or Hürthle cell carcinomas), and the majority proving to be benign colloid or follicular adenomas.

The diagnosis of follicular thyroid carcinoma is essentially impossible to make on the basis of cytologic findings alone, because the criteria for diagnosis include the findings of capsular and blood vessel invasion or distant metastases. Therefore in patients with suspected follicular thyroid carcinoma, surgical biopsy is usually indicated. Although some centers advocate frozen section to assist with the diagnosis, the vast majority of centers do not find frozen-section diagnoses to be reliable.

PEARLS FOR THE OR

The pyramidal lobe is a remnant of the thyroglossal duct.

The arterial blood supply of the thyroid arises from two major sources: the inferior thyroid artery, which originates from the thyrocervical trunk, and the superior thyroid artery, which is the first branch of the external carotid artery.

A delphian lymph node is an enlarged prelaryngeal node that is occasionally associated with thyroid cancer.

Venous drainage includes the superior and middle thyroid veins, which empty into the internal jugular vein, and the inferior thyroid vein, which also empties into the jugular vein or the innominate vein.

In contrast to follicular thyroid carcinoma, papillary thyroid carcinoma is readily diagnosed on the basis of cytologic findings, which may include overlapping nuclei, nuclear grooves, nuclear inclusions (Orphan Annie nuclei), clear ground-glass nuclei, or psammoma bodies. Most pathologists believe that the accuracy of FNA exceeds that of frozen section in the diagnosis of papillary thyroid carcinoma.

Thyroid Lobectomy and Isthmusectomy. If a surgical biopsy is indicated, the standard procedure consists of a thyroid lobectomy and isthmusectomy. Some surgeons will leave a small remnant of thyroid tissue to preserve the parathyroid gland after identifying and safely tracing the recurrent laryngeal nerve through its course to the cricothyroid membrane.

If tissue examination rules out cancer in the resected lobe and no detectable disease is present in the unresected lobe, additional surgery is not required. However, if disease is detected in the unresected lobe, additional surgery should be considered, even if the findings in the resected lobe are benign.

Near-total or Total Thyroidectomy. If a resected lesion is determined to be follicular thyroid carcinoma, near-total or total thyroidectomy is indicated. Some surgeons perform one of these procedures in all patients with follicular tumors to avoid a second operation should carcinoma be detected.

If a resected lesion is determined to be a small (≤1 cm) and well-differentiated papillary thyroid carcinoma and if no obvious abnormality is detected in the contralateral lobe, a lobectomy and isthmusectomy may be sufficient surgical treatment. However, if the resected lesion is a larger papillary thyroid carcinoma, many surgeons advocate near-total on total thyroidectomy. Several arguments are in favor of this approach. First, papillary thyroid cancer may be multifocal and bilateral. Second, the removal of all functioning thyroid tissue permits postoperative use of total-body ^{131}I scanning and ^{131}I therapy if necessary. Third, after all functional thyroid tissue has been removed, post-treatment monitoring of thyroglobulin levels in the absence of antithyroid antibodies is possible. Fourth, thyroidectomy reduces the incidence of local recurrence of tumor, perhaps at the cost of postoperative hypoparathyroidism (occurring in 1% to 2% of patients) and laryngeal nerve injury (occurring in 1%).

Postoperative Radioactive Iodine Therapy. At many medical centers, ^{131}I ablative therapy is administered postoperatively in all patients who have malignant lesions larger than 1 cm and are at high risk for recurrent disease (Fig. 31–5). The ^{131}I therapy will destroy any remaining thyroid tissue and thereby increase the sensitivity of

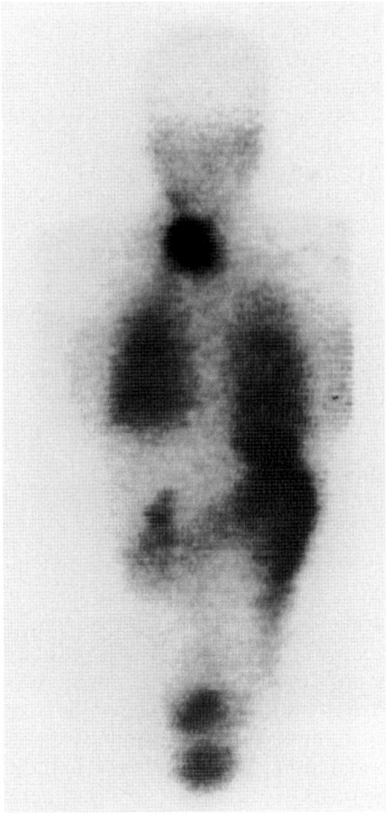

FIGURE 31–5 Sodium iodide I 131 (^{133}I) scan after thyroidectomy for papillary thyroid carcinoma. Intense uptake in the area of residual cervical thyroid tissue and diffuse bilateral uptake by lung metastases are evident. The gastrointestinal uptake is consistent with normal secretion of radioactive iodine. (Courtesy of Victor Lee, MD, Boston Medical Center, Boston, Massachusetts.)

subsequent ^{131}I total-body scans and the specificity of thyroglobulin measurements. Most important, ^{131}I therapy has been shown to decrease recurrence and mortality rates in those at high risk for recurrent disease.

Follow-Up Treatment and Monitoring. Because well-differentiated cancers contain TSH receptors and cancer growth is at least partially TSH responsive, patients are routinely given suppressive doses of levothyroxine after RAI treatment.

Thyroid Cancer

Thyroid cancer is rare. In the United States, it accounts for only 1% of cancers and 0.5% of cancer-related deaths. Worldwide, the annual incidence of thyroid cancer ranges from 0.5 to 10 cases per 100,000 population. Despite its infrequent occurrence, thyroid cancer is the most common malignant endocrine disorder and is responsible for more deaths than all other endocrine cancers combined.

The five types of thyroid cancer that have the highest incidence are the papillary, follicular, Hürthle cell, medullary, and anaplastic types. Papillary and follicular thyroid carcinomas are referred to as differentiated forms of thyroid cancer.

Rare types of thyroid cancer include malignant lymphoma of the thyroid and metastases to the thyroid from breast cancer, colon cancer, melanoma, or renal carcinoma.

Papillary Thyroid Carcinoma

Papillary thyroid carcinoma (PTC), the most common form of thyroid carcinoma, accounts for 80% of differentiated thyroid cancers. The disease occurs predominantly in women (female-to-male ratio of 3:1) and has a peak incidence in the third and fourth decades. It arises from follicular epithelial cells, grows slowly, and is associated with a favorable prognosis.

Etiology

PTC is more common in iodine-rich areas and has been noted to increase in incidence after the establishment of iodine prophylaxis in regions with endemic goiter and iodine deficiency. Ionizing radiation is associated with the development of thyroid cancer, and about 85% of radiation-induced tumors are of the papillary type.

Papillary carcinomas are occasionally familial and are found in association with dominant hereditary gastrointestinal polyposis, Cowden disease, Gardner's syndrome, and familial polyposis.

Evaluation

History and Physical Examination. A thyroid nodule discovered incidentally on routine physical examination is often the initial clue to the diagnosis of PTC. Occasionally, enlarged cervical lymph nodes are the presenting feature of the disease. In rare instances, distant pulmonary metastases are detected before the primary tumor.

Laboratory and Other Studies. The initial evaluation is the same as that described earlier for a solitary thyroid nodule. The diagnosis is ultimately made from a cytologic specimen obtained by FNA biopsy.

Cytologic Findings. Papillary cancers are typically non-encapsulated, well-demarcated lesions. They may be cystic. Microscopically, the lesions are characterized by papilliform axial fibrovascular stroma arranged in a branching or treelike pattern. Large overlapping nuclei with loose chromatin, cytoplasmic inclusions (Orphan Annie nuclei), longitudinal nuclear grooves, and clefts are all classic cytologic features of papillary carcinoma. About 50% of papillary carcinomas contain psammoma bodies or laminated calcifications thought to represent remnants of infarcted papillae.

Treatment and Prognosis

For treatment, see the section entitled Treatment for Suspected or Confirmed Malignant Solitary Thyroid Nodule.

Several prognostic scoring systems have been proposed to predict the aggressiveness of thyroid lesions and provide the clinician with treatment decision guidelines.

The TNM system is a widely used international classification system for staging various types of cancer on the basis of three components: the primary tumor (T); the regional lymph node involvement (N); and metastasis (M) (Table 31–2). Based on this system, a worse prognosis is observed in patients who are older than 45 years at first treatment, have a tumor that is larger than 4 cm, and show evidence of invasion of the thyroid capsule and distant metastases. Although a retrospective analysis found that this system is suitable for predicting age-related rates of

TABLE 31–2 Fluid Compartment

Stage	Age of Patient and Description*
Stage I	Younger than under 45 years with any T; any N; MO. Older than 45 years with T1; NO; MO.
Stage II	Younger than 45 years with any T; any M; M1. Older than 45 years with T2 or T3; NO; MO.
Stage III	Older than 45 years with T4 or N1; MO.
Stage IV	Older than 45 years with any T; any M; M1.

* T refers to the extent of the primary tumor. T1 is <1 cm; T2 is 1–4 cm; T3 is >4 cm; and T4 indicates invasion of the thyroid capsule. N refers to the absence (NO) or presence (N1) of regional lymph node involvement. M refers to the absence (MO) or presence (M1) of distant metastatic lesions.

death caused by cancer, it is less accurate for predicting recurrence-free survival.

The Mayo Clinic devised a prognostic scoring system that is called the **MACIS system** and includes five weighted variables: **metastases** (scored as +3.0 if distant metastases are present); **age** (scored as +3.1 if the patient is 39 years old or younger, or calculated by multiplying the number of years by 0.08 if the patient is older than 39 years); **completeness of surgery** (scored as 0 if tumor resection was complete or scored as +1.0 if it was incomplete); **invasiveness of the tumor** (scored as 0 for no invasion or as +1.0 for local invasion); and **size of the tumor** (calculated by multiplying the number of centimeters by 0.3).

Based on MACIS scores, the 20-year survival rates in patients with papillary carcinoma are as follows: 99% for scores under 6; 89% for scores from 6 to 6.99; 56% for scores from 7 to 7.99; and 24% for scores of 8 or more.

Follicular Thyroid Carcinoma

In the United States, follicular thyroid carcinoma (FTC) accounts for about 10% of all thyroid cancers. The worldwide incidence of this carcinoma has decreased over the last 75 years as a result of the institution of iodination, but the disease continues to be prevalent in geographic regions of endemic goiter.

Like PTC, FTC arises from follicular epithelial cells, occurs predominantly in women (female-to-male ratio of 3:1), grows slowly, and has a favorable prognosis. On average, patients with follicular cancer are older than those with papillary cancer. The mean age for follicular cancer is older than 50 years.

Unlike PTC, FTC is not commonly associated with regional lymph node and contralateral involvement. Follicular cancer metastasizes via the bloodstream to the lungs, bone, and liver, and occasionally, to the brain. Between 5% and 20% of patients with FTC have distant metastases on presentation. Spinal cord involvement may occur as a result of bony metastases. The tumor cells are osteolytic, so metastases may not be detected with conventional bone scans.

Evaluation

History and Physical Examination. Like patients with PTC, patients with FTC often have a painless, solitary thyroid nodule. In contrast to those with PTC, patients with FTC often do not have associated cervical lymphadenopathy. Hoarseness, dysphagia, cough, and dyspnea suggest advanced disease. Symptoms of hyperthyroidism may be present if a functioning metastatic follicular carcinoma is in the lung or elsewhere.

Laboratory and Other Studies. The initial evaluation is the same as that described earlier for a solitary thyroid nodule.

Cytologic Findings. Cytologic examination of aspirate from the FNA biopsy is unable to differentiate a malignant follicular neoplasm from a benign follicular adenoma. The cytology report typically indicates the presence of a follicular neoplasm or microfollicular adenoma with scant colloid in nodules suggestive of a follicular malignancy. FTC will ultimately be found in 5% to 20% of these suggestive nodules. Demonstration of capsule invasion or angioinvasion is needed for a definitive diagnosis, and this information can be gleaned only by surgical removal of the nodule and subsequent detailed pathologic analyses.

FTCs have a follicular differentiation pattern, but they lack the characteristic features of PTCs (ground-glass nuclei, well-formed papillae, and psammoma bodies). FTCs are usually encapsulated, and invasion of the capsule and blood vessels is the major feature that distinguishes them from follicular adenomas. Based on the degree of invasion, these tumors are classified as either minimally invasive carcinoma or widely invasive carcinoma. The tumor growth pattern may vary from a macrofollicular pattern with good differentiation to a solid pattern with marked areas of poor differentiation and atypia.

Treatment and Prognosis

For treatment, see the section entitled Treatment for Suspected or Confirmed Malignant Solitary Throid Nodule.

To predict the aggressiveness of FTC, the Mayo Clinic has devised a simplified scheme using three risk factors: **age** older than 50 years, marked **angioinvasion**, and **metastatic disease** at diagnosis. Patients who have none or one of these risk factors have 5-year and 20-year survival rates of 99% and 86%, respectively. Patients who have two or three of these risk factors have 5-year and 20-year survival rates of 47% and 8%, respectively.

Hürthle Cell Carcinoma

Hürthle cell carcinoma accounts for fewer than 5% of all thyroid cancers. It is seen more frequently in women than in men and has its peak incidence in the fifth and sixth decades. Roughly one third of affected patients have a history of radiation exposure, and no other predisposing risks factors have been identified.

Evaluation

Hürthle cell carcinoma is classified by the World Health Organization as a variant of follicular carcinoma. Hürthle cells are large, polygonal thyroid follicular cells with abundant granular cytoplasm and numerous mitochondria. Hürthle cell carcinoma is defined as an encapsulated group of follicular cells made up of at least 75% Hürthle cells.

Unlike the common benign Hürthle cell adenomas, the rare Hürthle cell carcinomas demonstrate capsular invasion, vascular invasion, or invasion of the surrounding adjacent tissues. Therefore the diagnosis cannot be made by cytologic examination alone. Because of the need for extensive histologic evaluation, frozen section does not play a major role in the diagnosis or clinical management.

Treatment and Prognosis

Total or near-total thyroidectomy is usually indicated. If cervical lymph nodes are involved, biopsy should be performed with resection if the biopsy is positive. Hürthle cell carcinomas generally do not concentrate ^{131}I, so RAI therapy is not routinely used. However, because the tumor has been reported to produce thyroglobulin, use of ^{131}I may be helpful in some individuals.

The 10-year mortality rate for Hürthle cell carcinoma ranges from 20% to 35%, depending on the extent of disease at the initial diagnosis and on whether complete tumor resection is possible.

Medullary Thyroid Carcinoma

Medullary thyroid carcinoma (MTC) accounts for about 5% to 10% of thyroid cancers and may be sporadic or familial.

Etiology and Pathogenesis

Three autosomal dominantly inherited familial forms of MTC have been described: **multiple endocrine neoplasia type IIa** (MEN type IIa), **multiple endocrine neoplasia type IIb** (MEN type IIb), and **familial medullary thyroid carcinoma** (FMTC). Patients with MEN type IIa have MTC, pheochromocytoma, and parathyroid hyperplasia. Those with MEN type IIb generally have MTC, pheochromocytoma, and mucosal neuromas (especially around the lips and mouth); often have a marfanoid habitus; occasionally have intestinal ganglioneuromas; and lack parathyroid hyperplasia. MTC has close to 100% penetrance in both of these MEN syndromes. Patients with FMTC have MTC but lack other features of the MEN syndromes.

Various mutations in the *RET* proto-oncogene are responsible for familial forms of MTC. This proto-oncogene is localized to chromosome 10 and codes for a tyrosine kinase receptor. Almost 100% of patients with MEN type IIb have demonstrated germline mutations in codon 918 (exon 16), and 85% of patients with MEN type IIa have mutations in codon 634 (exon 11). Most kindreds with FMTC also have detectable mutations in codon 634 (exon 11).

MTC develops from the parafollicular cells (C cells) of the thyroid. These cells are located in the upper one third of the thyroid lobe and are responsible for synthesizing and secreting calcitonin. The C cells are derived from neural crest cells and are part of the amine precursor uptake and decarboxylation (APUD) system of neuroendocrine cells. Thus MTC may have histologic features of other neuroendocrine tumors, such as carcinoid and islet cell tumors.

MTC is multicentric in many patients and is often bilateral in patients with FMTC. The tumor frequently metastasizes to regional lymphatics of the neck and mediastinum, and it also may metastasize to lung, liver, bone, and brain.

About 80% of observed MTC is of the sporadic variety. Sporadic MTC occurs more often in women than in men, and it typically is first seen in the fifth and sixth decades. The most common presentation is of a solitary nodule, and the nodule is usually located in the upper portion of a thyroid lobe. Approximately 50% of patients will have clinically detectable cervical lymph node involvement, 15% will have symptoms related to airway or esophageal compromise, and 5% will have distant metastases.

Evaluation

In patients without a family history of MTC, the diagnosis of this carcinoma is made with FNA biopsy. The accuracy of FNA biopsy is 50% to 80% without immunocytologic stains but is even higher with stains. Some investigators recommend that calcitonin measurements be routinely performed in all individuals with nodular goiters so that cases of MTC will not be missed, but this recommendation is controversial.

Cytologic evaluation of MTC typically demonstrates sheets of spindle-shaped pleomorphic cells without follicular development. These findings may be initially misdiagnosed as anaplastic carcinoma. Occasionally, red cytoplasmic granules are visualized, and the stroma often stains positive for amyloid. Immunocytologic stains are positive for calcitonin.

Once the diagnosis is established, it is important to determine whether the lesion is sporadic or a component of a syndrome. Pheochromocytoma is found in about 50% of patients with MEN type IIb and is often bilateral. Failure to recognize and treat pheochromocytoma before surgery for MTC could have catastrophic consequences. Therefore a 24-hour urine sample should be collected and assessed for catecholamines, metanephrines, and vanillylmandelic acid. Screening tests for the presence of *RET* mutations also should be performed.

If the patient demonstrates a germline mutation, then total thyroidectomy should be scheduled. In addition, the patient's first-degree relatives should undergo genetic screening. If these relatives demonstrate germline mutations in the *RET* proto-oncogene, they should undergo total thyroidectomy as soon as they reach age 5 years or at the time of diagnosis if they have already reached this age.

Treatment and Prognosis

Regardless of whether the MTC is sporadic or familial, total thyroidectomy should be performed to allow sampling of the central compartment from the innominate vessels to the hyoid bone and laterally to the carotid arteries. In patients with MEN type IIb and primary lesions that are larger than 2 cm, sampling of lateral neck nodes should be considered. If the lateral nodes yield positive results, the surgeon should perform a functional or modified neck dissection that spares the jugular vein, the sternocleidomastoid muscle, and the accessory nerve. No effective adjuvant therapy is known for MTC, so thorough and exact surgery is required.

Postoperatively, patients should be monitored for recurrent disease by measuring basal or stimulated serum calcitonin levels. Carcinoembryonic antigen levels also may be used as a marker for recurrent disease. Generally, the carcinoembryonic antigen level is higher in more malignant MTC, whereas the calcitonin level is higher in more differentiated MTC.

The overall prognosis of patients with MTC is intermediate between well-differentiated thyroid cancer and the poorly differentiated variants of thyroid cancer. The 10-year survival rate is 65%. Independent predictors of outcome include local tumor invasion and calcitonin immunostaining. Patients without local tumor invasion have much higher survival rates. Patients whose tumors retain more than 50% calcitonin staining also have higher survival rates.

Anaplastic Carcinoma

Anaplastic carcinoma accounts for fewer than 5% of all thyroid cancers. The incidence is highest in regions of endemic goiter, and the mean age of patients at the time of diagnosis is 65 years. Anaplastic carcinoma frequently arises in the background of well-differentiated thyroid cancer or benign thyroid tumors. In more than 90% of cases, either local or distant metastases are evident on initial presentation. The disease is the most aggressive form of thyroid cancer and is universally fatal.

Evaluation

History and Physical Examination. Patients with anaplastic carcinoma commonly are first seen with shortness of breath, dysphagia, hoarseness; pain, cough, and hemoptysis. Unlike patients with differentiated forms of thyroid cancer, these patients frequently also have constitutional symptoms of disease, such as weight loss and fever. Examination commonly reveals a fixed, hard, asymmetrical thyroid gland with associated cervical lymphadenopathy. Other signs indicative of tracheal invasion and compression may include tracheal deviation, stridor, and vocal cord paralysis. With retrosternal extension of the mass, Pemberton's sign may be present.

Imaging Studies. Computed tomography or magnetic resonance imaging studies of the neck will provide information regarding the location, extent of tumor involvement, and presence of vascular invasion. It is not unusual for anaplastic carcinoma to invade the jugular veins, carotid arteries, and larynx.

Cytologic Findings. The diagnosis is often suspected clinically and confirmed by FNA biopsy. Cytologic examination characteristically demonstrates pleomorphic cells that are medium to large in size, have prominent nuclei, and show evidence of mitosis. Multinucleated giant cells containing abnormal mitotic figures are frequently encountered, as are malignant-appearing spindle cells. Sarcomatous changes also may be present.

Treatment and Prognosis

Within a year of diagnosis, the majority of patients will die as a result of either strangulation from local tumor invasion or distant metastases. The median survival from the time of diagnosis is 3 to 7 months, and the 1-year and 5-year survival rates are 20% to 35% and 5% to 10%, respectively.

Total thyroidectomy does not prolong survival, except in patients with small lesions confined to the thyroid gland. Conventional doses of radiation therapy and chemotherapy have not been shown to prolong survival. Combination treatment with doxorubicin and hyperfractionated radiation therapy improves the local response rate and prolongs the median survival rate to about 1 year.

Malignant Lymphoma of the Thyroid

Malignant lymphoma accounts for fewer than 5% of all thyroid cancers. It occurs more frequently in women than in men and has a peak incidence in the seventh decade. An association between thyroid lymphomas and chronic lymphocytic thyroiditis has been recognized for many years.

Evaluation

History and Physical Examination. Most patients have a long-standing history of Hashimoto's thyroiditis. Malignant lymphoma is characterized by a rapidly enlarging, painless goiter or mass that is occasionally associated with hoarseness, dysphagia, and dyspnea. On palpation, the mass is firm and may be fixed to surrounding structures. About 50% of patients have cervical lymph node involvement.

Cytologic Findings. Thyroid lymphomas are derived from B cells, and the majority are of the diffuse large cell type or follicular cell origin. The prognosis is more favorable for follicular tumors than for diffuse large cell or immunoblastic lymphomas. FNA biopsy typically demonstrates an abundant infiltration of lymphoid cells.

Treatment and Prognosis

The treatment of thyroid lymphoma is somewhat controversial and depends largely on the extent of disease. Patients with disease localized to the neck (stage I or II) may be treated with surgical resection followed by local radiation therapy and chemotherapy. Those with more advanced disease (stage III or IV) are usually treated with external radiation therapy and chemotherapy, although patients occasionally respond well to external radiation therapy alone. Aggressive surgical debulking of large thyroid lymphomas is not feasible.

The overall survival rate is 50% to 70%. The overall prognosis of patients with MTC is intermediate between well-differentiated thyroid cancer and the poorly differentiated variants of thyroid cancer. The 10-year survival rate is 65%. Independent predictors of outcome include local tumor invasion and calcitonin immunostaining. Patients without local tumor invasion have much higher survival rates. Patients whose tumors retain more than 50% calcitonin staining also have higher survival rates.

Suggested Reading

Mazzaferri EL, Kloos RT: Clinical review 128: Current approaches to primary therapy for papillary and follicular thyroid cancer. J Clin Endocrinol Metab 86(4):1447–1463, 2001.

Schlumberger MJ: Papillary and follicular thyroid carcinoma. N Engl J Med 338(5):297–306, 1998.

Sherman SI: Thyroid carcinoma. Lancet 361(9356):501–511, 2003.

van Heerden JA: Endocrine surgery. J Am Coll Surg 186(2):141–148, 1998.

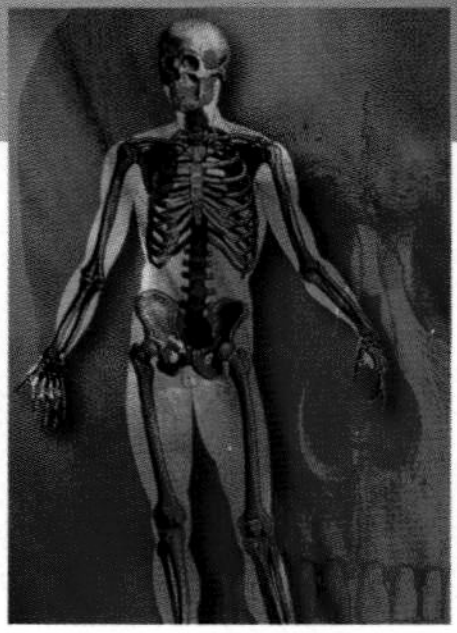

Chapter 32
Parathyroid Glands

ANN T. SWEENEY, MD, and ROBERT M. BEAZLEY, MD

Overview

Embryology and Anatomy

The parathyroid glands are small (averaging 6 × 3 × 2 mm), weigh from 30 to 40 mg, are located adjacent to the thyroid gland, and have an ovoid shape and soft consistency. Because the parathyroid tissue has a tan or yellow color, it sometimes looks like fatty tissue. However, parathyroid tissue will sink in normal saline solution, whereas fatty tissue will float.

Most individuals have four parathyroid glands (two associated with each lobe of the thyroid). However, the total number varies from two to six, with autopsy series reporting five or six parathyroid glands in 5% of individuals.

Embryologically, the **superior parathyroid glands** are derived from the fourth branchial pouch, so they may be located anywhere between the upper border of the larynx and the lower pole of the thyroid. In 80% of individuals, however, they are found behind the upper lobe of the thyroid, at the level of the cricoid cartilage and about 1 cm above the junction of the inferior thyroid artery and recurrent laryngeal nerve (Fig. 32-1). Ectopic superior glands are generally found within the surgical capsule of the upper pole of the thyroid gland.

The **inferior parathyroid glands** may be located anywhere from the angle of the jaw to the pericardium. The long migration of the inferior glands during embryologic life accounts for this variability. The inferior glands develop with the thymus and descend caudally through the neck from the third branchial pouch. If the thymus fails to descend, the glands will be located at the level of the thyroid cartilage. If the glands fail to dissociate from the thymus during their descent, they will be carried with the thymus into the thorax and be found in the superior mediastinum. In 61% of individuals, the inferior parathyroid glands are posterior or lateral to the lower poles of the thyroid (see Fig. 32-1). The majority of ectopic inferior parathyroid glands are located within the thymus, either in the lower neck or inside the mediastinal thymus.

The parathyroid glands usually receive their **arterial blood supply** from the **inferior thyroid arteries.** Occasionally, however, they receive it from the **superior thyroid arteries** or from longitudinal anastomoses between the inferior and superior thyroid arteries. **Venous drainage** occurs through the thyroid plexus of veins located on the anterior surface of the thyroid gland and trachea.

A thorough knowledge of the anatomic relation between the **recurrent laryngeal nerve** and the inferior thyroid arteries, parathyroid tissue, and thyroid tissue is essential for preventing complications of parathyroid and thyroid surgery. The complications of thyroidectomy include injury to the recurrent laryngeal nerve and injury of the parathyroid glands or the blood supply to these glands. The parathyroid glands are more likely to be injured during a total thyroidectomy than during a subtotal thyroidectomy, because the posterior portion of the thyroid (the thyroid bed) is preserved in the subtotal operation.

Physiology

The parathyroid glands are responsible for the synthesis and secretion of **parathyroid hormone** (PTH). This hormone and the **activated form of vitamin D** (called 1,25-dihydroxyvitamin D or $1,25[OH]_2D$) play critical roles in the maintenance of **calcium homeostasis** (Fig. 32-2). The ionized calcium concentration is of vital physiologic importance to a number of cellular functions, including intracellular signaling, cell movement, enzymatic activity, neurohumoral activation, and excitation-contraction coupling. PTH maintains the ionized calcium concentration in the serum by acting directly on the bones and kidneys and by acting indirectly (via $1,25[OH]_2D$) on the small intestines.

PTH is an 84-amino-acid polypeptide that is synthesized within the chief cells of the parathyroid glands. The secretion of PTH is tightly controlled in a negative-feedback loop by the ionized calcium concentration in serum. Any decrease in this calcium concentration results in an increase in PTH secretion. The increase in PTH stimulates osteoclastic bone resorption and causes an increase in the flow of calcium from the bones into the blood. This promotes renal 1α-hydroxylation of 25-hydroxyvitamin D (25[OH]D), and the activated vitamin D then increases intestinal calcium absorption and renal calcium resorption.

Vitamin D synthesis occurs in the skin through exposure to sunlight. When the immediate precursor of cholesterol, 7-dehydrocholesterol, is exposed to ultraviolet light, it is

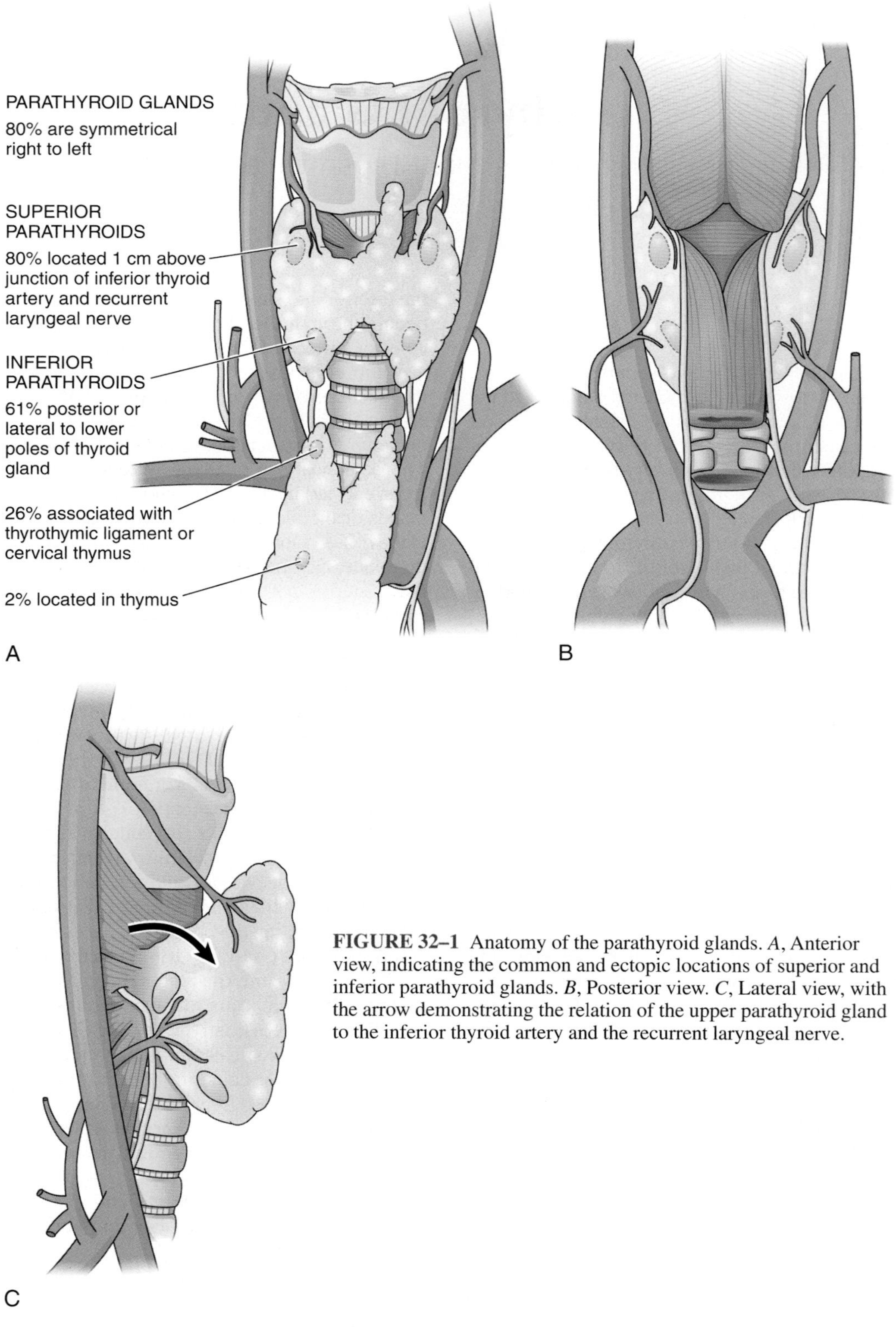

FIGURE 32–1 Anatomy of the parathyroid glands. *A*, Anterior view, indicating the common and ectopic locations of superior and inferior parathyroid glands. *B*, Posterior view. *C*, Lateral view, with the arrow demonstrating the relation of the upper parathyroid gland to the inferior thyroid artery and the recurrent laryngeal nerve.

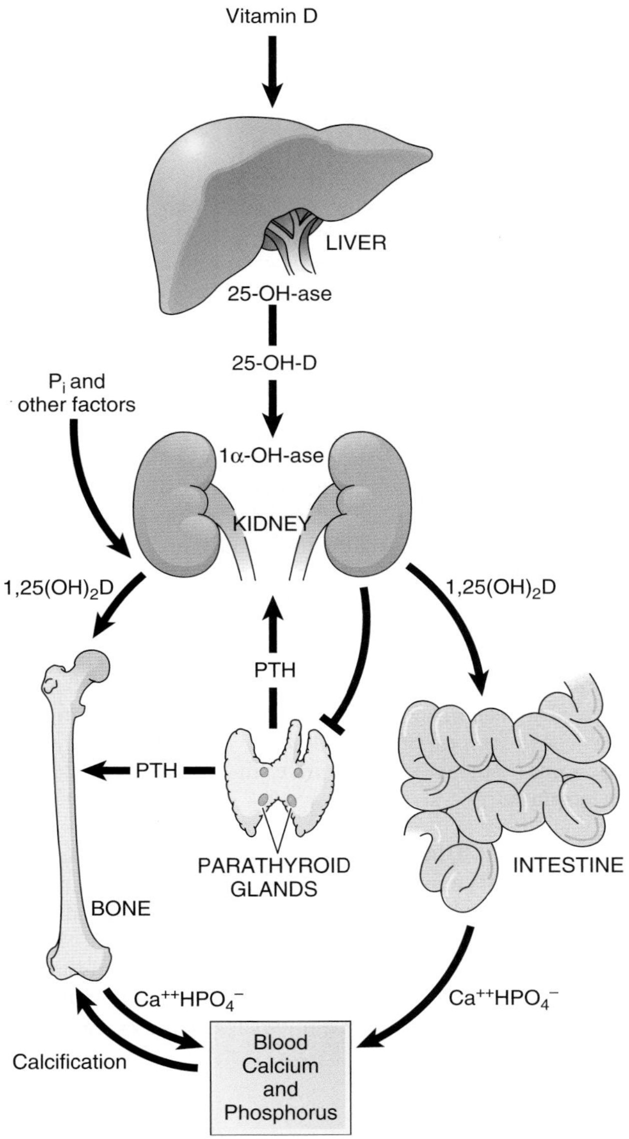

FIGURE 32–2 Metabolism of vitamin D and biologic action of 1,25-dihydroxyvitamin D, or 1,25(OH)$_2$D. PTH, parathyroid hormone. (Modified from Holick MF: McCollum Award Lecture, 1994: Vitamin D: New horizons for the 21st century. Am J Clin Nutr 60:619–630, 1994, with permission.)

converted to previtamin D$_3$. Previtamin D$_3$ is then thermally isomerized to produce vitamin D$_3$ and translocated from the skin to the circulation. Within the circulation, vitamin D is bound to vitamin D–binding protein. Vitamin D circulates to the liver and kidneys to undergo two successive hydroxylations, first to 25(OH)D in the liver and then to 1,25(OH)$_2$D in the kidneys. The activated form, 1,25(OH)$_2$D, increases intestinal calcium absorption, promotes mineralization of bones by calcium and phosphorus, and enhances PTH-mediated bone resorption. The synthesis of 1,25(OH)$_2$D also is strictly regulated. Increased serum concentrations of phosphorus impair renal 1α-hydroxylase activity and thereby decrease 1,25(OH)$_2$D production. In addition, elevated 1,25(OH)$_2$D levels inhibit PTH secretion.

Hyperparathyroidism

Primary Hyperparathyroidism

Primary hyperparathyroidism (PHPT) is defined as a hypercalcemic state caused by excessive secretion of PTH from one or more parathyroid glands. The disease occurs more frequently in women than in men and is most commonly seen in postmenopausal women. In the past, the disease was usually associated with "stones, bones, and abdominal groans" (see St. Goar, 1957). Today, however, it is often asymptomatic and in many cases is detected only through routine laboratory tests.

Etiology and Pathophysiology

In 80% of cases, PHPT is caused by a **solitary adenoma,** which is a collection of chief cells surrounded by normal tissue. The adenoma is found in only one parathyroid gland, and the remaining glands are normal. In 15% to 20% of cases, PHPT is caused by **four-gland hyperplasia.** This hyperplasia may occur sporadically or in association with **multiple endocrine neoplasia (MEN) types I and II.** In fewer than 1% of cases, PHPT is caused by **parathyroid carcinoma.**

Normally, an elevated calcium level would inhibit PTH secretion and would therefore be associated with a suppressed PTH level. In patients with a solitary adenoma, this normal feedback control of calcium is lost. In patients with four-gland hyperplasia, elevated calcium levels are due to an increased number of PTH-secreting cells, rather than to the loss of negative feedback control.

Evaluation

History. Obtaining an accurate and detailed history is essential in postmenopausal women and other patients in whom PHPT is suspected. Conditions associated with this disease include bone diseases, kidney stones, nephrocalcinosis, hypercalciuria, peptic ulcer disease, hypertension, endocrinopathies that are part of MEN syndromes types I and II, and radiation therapy during childhood. Because treatment with some agents (such as thiazides, lithium, vitamin A, and vitamin D) also can cause hypercalcemia, patients should be specifically asked about the use of drugs and vitamins.

Overt bone diseases, such as osteitis fibrosa cystica, were seen in up to 15% of patients with PHPT in the past but now are found in only 5%. Nephrolithiasis was seen in

PEARLS FOR ROUNDS

Primary hyperparathyroidism (PHPT) and malignancy account for 90% of hypercalcemic cases.

Classic radiographic manifestations of osteitis fibrosa cystica include subperiosteal resorption of the distal phalanges, a salt-and-pepper appearance of the skull, and tapering of the distal clavicles.

Primary hyperparathyroidism may occur in association with multiple endocrine neoplasia (MEN) I and IIA syndromes.

PHPT is caused by parathyroid carcinoma in fewer than 1% of cases.

up to 40% of patients but now is found in only 20%. Neuromuscular weakness, which was a common feature in the past and was attributed to type II muscle fiber atrophy, also is rarely seen today. This changing clinical profile of PHPT is attributed to early detection of the disease by the use of routine blood tests.

Physical Examination. Most patients are asymptomatic, but some have neuropsychiatric symptoms that include fatigue, depression, emotional lability, memory impairment, and sleep disturbances.

The results of physical examination may be unremarkable. The parathyroid glands are not usually palpable. If they are, this suggests parathyroid carcinoma. Band keratopathy, characterized by calcification in the lateral margin of the limbus, is a sign of PHPT but is rarely seen.

Laboratory Studies. Hypercalcemia in the presence of an elevated concentration of intact PTH is virtually diagnostic of PHPT. Laboratory studies usually demonstrate the following: a serum calcium concentration that is mildly elevated (mean, 11.1 mg/dL; normal, 8.5–10.3 mg/dL); a serum phosphorus concentration that is on the low end of normal (mean, 2.9 mg/dL; normal, 2.6–4.5 mg/dL); an intact PTH concentration that is elevated (mean, 60 mg/dL; normal, 15–60 mg/dL); and a 24-hour urine calcium excretion rate that is slightly elevated (~250 mg of calcium per gram of creatinine).

Imaging Studies. Classic radiographic manifestations of osteitis fibrosa cystica include subperiosteal resorption of the distal phalanges, a salt-and-pepper appearance of the skull, and tapering of the distal clavicles. Additional manifestations, which also can be seen on conventional radiographs, include brown tumors (collection of osteoclasts intermixed with poorly woven bone) and bone cysts.

PHPT causes selective cortical bone loss, and bone density measurements usually show reduced bone mass at the distal radius and hip.

Imaging studies that can be used to localize parathyroid adenomas include ultrasonography, computed tomography, magnetic resonance imaging, and scintigraphy. Technetium 99m sestamibi scanning, which has become the preferred imaging technique at many institutions, is a sensitive technique for locating parathyroid adenomas. The sestamibi is taken up by the parathyroid and thyroid glands, but it persists only in the parathyroid glands and allows them to be easily visualized (Fig. 32-3). This type of scanning has a success rate of 85% to100% in detecting parathyroid adenomas but is less sensitive in detecting four-gland hyperplasia.

Differential Diagnosis. Although many causes of hypercalcemia exist (Box 32-1), PHPT and cancer account for 90% of the cases. These two diseases are usually not difficult to distinguish. Most patients with PHPT demonstrate only mild hypercalcemia (with serum calcium levels that are ≤1 mg/dL above the upper limit of normal and are almost always <12 mg/dL), and a review of the

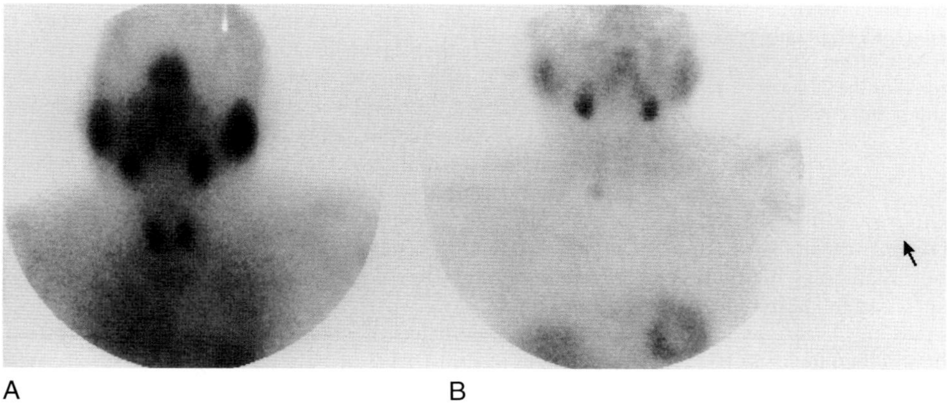

FIGURE 32–3 Sestamibi imaging in a patient with a parathyroid adenoma. *A*, Symmetrical early uptake is seen in the thyroid. *B*, The persistent right-sided activity on the delayed scan is caused by slower washout from the hyperfunctioning parathyroid adenoma.

BOX 32–1 Causes of Hypercalcemia

Cancer-related Causes

Hematologic cancers (leukemia, lymphoma, and multiple myeloma)
Humoral hypercalcemia of malignancy
Solid tumor metastases

Conditions Associated with Accelerated Bone Turnover

Hyperthyroidism
Immobilization
Vitamin A intoxication

Conditions Associated with Renal Failure

Aluminum intoxication
Milk-alkali syndrome

Parathyroid Hormone–related Causes

Familial hypocalciuric hypercalcemia
Primary hyperparathyroidism
Tertiary hyperparathyroidism
Treatment with hydrochlorothiazide or lithium

Vitamin D–related Causes

1,25-Dihydroxyvitamin D production in sarcoidosis and other granulomatous disease
Vitamin D intoxication

Other Endocrine Diseases

Addison's disease
Pheochromocytoma

laboratory profile may reveal long-standing mild hypercalcemia. Unlike patients with PHPT, patients with cancer appear ill and frequently have classic symptoms and signs of hypercalcemia. The cancer is usually not occult.

Hypercalcemia in the presence of an elevated PTH level is the biochemical hallmark of PHPT. However, a few other conditions may produce an identical biochemical profile and should be considered in the differential diagnosis. These include tertiary hyperparathyroidism, familial hypocalciuric hypercalcemia (FHH), and the use of medications such as lithium and thiazides. Tertiary hyperparathyroidism occurs in the setting of renal failure, when hyperplastic cells progress to monoclonal proliferation, and is discussed later in this chapter. FHH is an autosomal dominant disease characterized by moderate hypercalcemia and relative hypocalciuria. In FHH, an alteration in the set point for PTH secretion is found, so PTH continues to be secreted at higher calcium levels than normal. Obtaining a 24-hour urine sample to rule out FHH is essential, because FHH is a benign syndrome and does not require surgery. Lithium is known to alter the set point for PTH secretion and results in hypercalcemia in about 10% of patients. Long-term thiazide administration leads to a reduction in urinary calcium excretion.

PEARLS FOR THE OR

The superior parathyroid glands are derived from the fourth branchial pouch and may be located anywhere from the upper border of the larynx to the lower pole of the thyroid.

The inferior parathyroid glands are derived from the third branchial pouches and may be located anywhere from the angle of the jaw to the pericardium.

The inferior glands are most commonly located on the anterolateral or posterolateral surface of the lower thyroid gland.

The majority of ectopic glands are located within the thymus.

The parathyroids receive their blood supply primarily from the inferior thyroid arteries; however, sometimes anastomoses occur between the superior and inferior thyroid arteries.

Treatment

Indications for Surgery. Parathyroidectomy is the only curative treatment for PHPT. Because this disease is often asymptomatic, most endocrinologists are selective regarding which patients they refer for parathyroidectomy. Possible indications for the procedure are outlined in Box 32-2.

Surgical Techniques. Parathyroid surgery requires expertise in localizing ectopic parathyroid glands and in distinguishing a solitary adenoma from four-gland hyperplasia. If the disease is caused by hyperplasia, the surgeon can resect three and one-half of the parathyroid glands. Alternatively, the surgeon can perform a total parathyroidectomy with autotransplantation of a resected gland into the brachioradialis muscle of the nondominant forearm. If the disease is caused by a solitary adenoma, only the adenoma is excised.

Historically, parathyroid surgery required exploration to locate an adenoma or to find four glands in the case of hyperplasia. Today, with the use of technetium 99m sestamibi imaging, the location of an adenoma can be successfully predicted before surgery in about 85% of patients. In other cases, surgeons are able to perform radioisotope-guided parathyroidectomy by preoperatively administering sestamibi and using the gamma probe to plan the incision and to localize the adenoma.

With the use of modern chemiluminescence techniques, PTH can now be sampled and assayed during the intraoperative period. The half-life of PTH is short (3–5 minutes). When the intact PTH molecule is sampled 10 minutes after adenomectomy and assayed with a chemiluminescence technique, the results are usually available in less than

BOX 32-2 Possible Indications for Surgery in Patients with Primary Hyperparathyroidism

- Serum calcium level >12 mg/dL
- Marked hypercalciuria (>400 mg in 24 hr)
- Any overt manifestation of primary hyperparathyroidism (such as nephrolithiasis, osteitis fibrosa cystica, or classic neuromuscular disease)
- Marked reductions in cortical bone density
- Reduced creatinine clearance in the absence of another cause
- Age younger than 50 years

Data from National Institutes of Health: 1991 Consensus Development Conference Statement on Primary Hyperparathyroidism. J Bone Miner Res 4:283–291, 1991.

20 minutes. If the adenomectomy is successful, the PTH level will decrease 50% or more. This indicates that the diseased portion of the gland has been excised and that no additional exploration is required. If no decrease occurs or if an insufficient decrease in the PTH level is found, further exploration is needed to find an additional adenoma (which is present in 2% to 5% of cases) or to find previously unsuspected four-gland hyperplasia.

Box 32-3 shows the parathyroidectomy protocol used by Boston University Medical Center. The postoperative course is generally smooth, and patients are usually ready for discharge within 24 hours of surgery.

Complications. Hypocalcemia is the major postoperative complication and may occur in association with transient hypoparathyroidism or with the hungry-bone syndrome. Serum tests will differentiate the two. Hypoparathyroidism is characterized by hypocalcemia and hyperphosphatemia, whereas hungry-bone syndrome is characterized by hypocalcemia and hypophosphatemia.

Transient hypoparathyroidism occurs because it takes a short time for the normal glands to resume function after adenoma resection. If the patient is treated with oral calcium supplements (1500 to 2000 mg of elemental calcium), this problem usually resolves within a few days.

After a parathyroidectomy is performed in a patient who had overt bone disease caused by the prolonged skeletal effects of excessive PTH levels, the bones become "hungry" for calcium and phosphorus and will avidly take up these substances from the blood. Patients with hungry-bone syndrome require treatment with intravenous calcium (see Box 32-3).

A rare complication of parathyroid surgery is recurrent laryngeal nerve damage. This may cause hoarseness and a reduction in voice volume.

BOX 32-3 Parathyroidectomy Protocol

1. Determine baseline Chvostek score* and baseline serum levels of 25-hydroxyvitamin D, calcium, magnesium, phosphorus, and albumin before surgery.
2. Check the Chvostek score in the recovery room and recheck every 6 hr with vital signs.
3. Check serum levels of calcium, magnesium, phosphorus, and albumin every 6 hr until stable.
4. If the magnesium level is <1.5 mg/dL, administer two ampules of magnesium sulfate intravenously (provided that the creatinine level is <1.5 mg/dL).
5. Start giving calcium supplements (Tums), 500mg orally three times per day.
6. If the corrected calcium level is <8.5mg/dL, start giving calcitriol, 0.25 μg orally twice per day.
7. If the corrected calcium level remains <8.5mg/dL, increase the calcitriol dosage to 0.5 μg orally twice per day.
8. If the corrected calcium level is <8.0mg/dL, start an intravenous infusion of calcium gluconate, begin electrocardiography, and monitor the QTc interval. If the patient is symptomatic, give two ampules of calcium gluconate over 20 min and repeat until asymptomatic. Otherwise, mix 10 ampules in 1 L of normal saline and infuse over 10 hr.

*Chvostek's sign is elicited by lightly percussing the facial nerve ~2 cm anterior to the earlobe, just below the zygomatic process (Chvostek I) or between the zygomatic arch and the corner of the mouth (Chvostek II). The responses consist of twitching of the muscles supplied by the facial nerve and are graded as follows: +1 is twitching of the lip to the corner of the mouth; +2 is twitching of the angle of the mouth and the ala nasi; +3 is contraction of the orbicularis oculi; and +4 is contraction of all facial muscles innervated on the side being tested. The Chvostek I sign is due to direct mechanical stimulation of the facial nerve, whereas the Chvostek II sign is due to reflex stimulation.

Prognosis

If parathyroidectomy or adenomectomy is performed by an expert parathyroid surgeon, a successful resection can be expected in 95% of patients who have no previous history of neck surgery.

Some patients, although considered asymptomatic, may have subtle preoperative neuropsychological disabilities that are alleviated with parathyroid resection. In a survey of 104 patients who underwent surgery for PHPT, many patients reported a substantial improvement in their subjective health status after parathyroidectomy (see Burney et al., 1999). Interestingly, no difference in the level of improvement was seen in patients with high preoperative calcium levels versus those with low preoperative calcium levels.

A 10-year prospective trial in patients with asymptomatic PHPT demonstrated that parathyroidectomy resulted in normalization of biochemical parameters and an increase in bone density (12% at the lumbar spine and 6% at the hip).

Secondary Hyperparathyroidism

Etiology and Pathophysiology

Secondary hyperparathyroidism is an acquired disorder that is characterized by parathyroid hyperfunction and is caused by perturbations in the feedback system described earlier in this chapter. The disorder is encountered most frequently in patients with renal failure but also occurs in those with vitamin D deficiency and resistance.

In most patients with renal failure, some degree of hyperplasia of the parathyroid glands develops, and hypocalcemia is the major stimulus for this hyperplasia. In patients with chronic renal failure, hypocalcemia occurs because of phosphate retention. Hyperphosphatemia causes hypocalcemia through two mechanisms: it directly reduces the serum ionized calcium concentration, and it inhibits 1α-hydroxylase activity in the kidney and thereby impairs intestinal calcium absorption. As a compensatory mechanism, excessive PTH is secreted by hyperplastic parathyroid glands. With progressive renal failure, the PTH clearance decreases, and this further contributes to hyperparathyroidism.

Evaluation

The combination of hypocalcemia, hyperphosphatemia, and markedly elevated PTH concentration in a patient with chronic renal failure is diagnostic of secondary hyperparathyroidism. As a consequence of excessive PTH secretion and decreased production of activated vitamin D, patients may have excessive bone resorption (osteitis fibrosa cystica), defective bone mineralization (osteomalacia), bone pain, and pathologic fractures. Renal osteodystrophy is a term used to encompass these and other skeletal abnormalities associated with renal failure. Soft tissue calcification may be present, particularly if the calcium × phosphorus product is greater than 70. Vascular calcification also may be present, and in rare cases, this will lead to ischemic necrosis of the skin (calciphylaxis) and pruritus.

Treatment

Therapy is first directed toward maintaining the serum calcium and phosphorus levels within the normal range. If this is not feasible, then parathyroidectomy is usually required. In patients with secondary hyperparathyroidism, the specific indications for parathyroidectomy include intractable pruritus, progressive extraskeletal calcification, persistent hyperphosphatemia, severe bone pain or fractures, and the development of calciphylaxis.

Tertiary Hyperparathyroidism

Etiology and Pathophysiology

With prolonged hypocalcemia, parathyroid tissue may become autonomous and secrete extremely high levels of PTH (up to 10 times the normal amount), eventually leading to hypercalcemia. When high PTH levels and hypercalcemia occur in the setting of renal failure, the disorder is called tertiary hyperparathyroidism. Studies in humans and animals have demonstrated that PTH levels are nonsuppressble in tertiary hyperparathyroidism. Mechanisms proposed to explain this refractoriness include an increased number of parathyroid cells, alterations in the calcium-sensing mechanism, and abnormalities in the vitamin D receptor.

Evaluation

Because tertiary hyperparathyroidism evolves from secondary hyperparathyroidism, many of the skeletal and other manifestations are identical. Patients with tertiary hyperparathyroidism also have elevated calcium levels and therefore may complain of fatigue, memory loss, depression, and emotional lability.

Treatment

Cure of tertiary hyperparathyroidism requires surgical intervention to debulk the parathyroid tissue. Surgical treatment is indicated in symptomatic patients with persistently elevated PTH levels.

Parathyroid Carcinoma

Parathyroid carcinoma accounts for fewer than 1% of all cases of PHPT. In contrast to benign adenoma, which occurs most often in women (female/male ratio of 2.5:1), parathyroid carcinoma occurs with equal frequency in women and men. Parathyroid carcinoma has a peak incidence in the fifth decade and occurs earlier than benign adenoma.

Evaluation

Parathyroid carcinoma should be strongly suspected if a patient has a palpable neck mass, a serum calcium concentration that exceeds 14 mg/dL, a markedly elevated PTH level, and laryngeal hoarseness without a history of neck surgery.

In contrast to patients with benign PHPT, patients with parathyroid carcinoma usually have symptoms of severe hyperparathyroidism, have a much higher incidence of renal and bone disease, and are more likely to have a topical neck mass that can be detected on physical examination. Although the serum calcium level in patients with benign PHPT rarely exceeds 12 mg/dL, about 75% of patients with parathyroid carcinoma have a level that exceeds 14 mg/dL. One study reported that the intact PTH level was 2.8 times the upper limit of normal in patients with benign PHPT but was 10 times the upper limit of normal in those with parathyroid carcinoma.

Benign adenomas are reddish brown in color. In contrast, parathyroid carcinomas are white and hard, and they frequently infiltrate or adhere to adjacent structures. Characteristic histologic features of parathyroid carcinoma include a trabecular pattern, mitotic figures, thick fibrous bands, and blood vessel invasion.

Treatment

Treatment results are best with early diagnosis and en bloc wide excision of the carcinoma. Adequate resection should include the ipsilateral thyroid lobe, isthmus, and central lymph nodes. Involved structures should be removed, including the recurrent laryngeal nerve if it is infiltrated.

Chemotherapeutic agents such as dacarbazine, cyclophosphamide, and doxorubicin have been used to treat parathyroid cancer, but chemotherapy has met with limited success. Radiation therapy for inoperable disease is generally ineffective, although remissions have been reported with radiation therapy for recurrent disease.

Prognosis

The initial operation provides the best opportunity for cure. Unfortunately, recurrent hypercalcemia dictates the need for reoperation in up to 60% of patients. Multiple operations are required in the majority of patients and usually result in only temporary amelioration of symptomatic hypercalcemia. The 5-year survival rate after aggressive surgical therapy ranges from 50% to 69%.

Suggested Reading

Bilzekian JP: Primary hyperparathyroidism. In Favus MJ (ed): Primer on Metabolic Bone Disease, 4th ed. Philadelphia, Lippincott, 1999.

Holick MF: McCollum Award Lecture, 1994: Vitamin D: New horizons for the 21st century. Am J Clin Nutr 60:619–630, 1994.

Potts JT Jr: Diseases of the parathyroid gland and other hypercalcemic and hypocalcemic disorders. In Fauci AS, Braunwald E, Isselbacher KJ, et al (eds): Harrison's Principles of Internal Medicine, 14th ed. New York, McGraw-Hill, 1998, pp 2227–2247.

Silverberg SJ, Bilzekian JP: Extensive personal experience: Evaluation and management of primary hyperparathyroidism. J Clin Endocrinol Metab 81:2036–2040, 1996.

St. Goar WT: Gastrointestinal symptoms as a clue to the diagnosis of primary hyperparathyroidism: A review of 45 cases. Ann Intern Med 46:102–118, 1957.

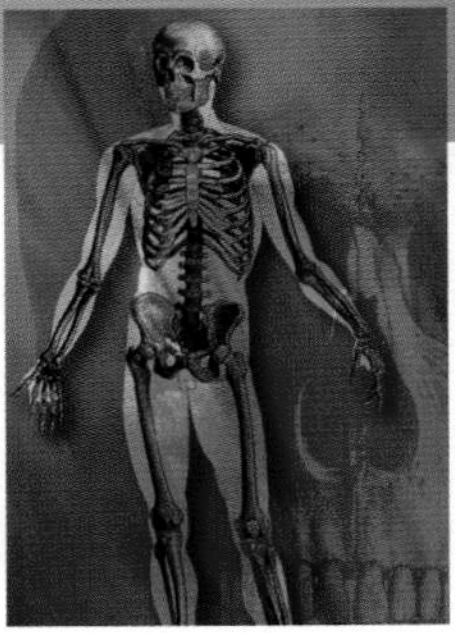

Chapter 33
Adrenal Glands

ANN T. SWEENEY, MD, and ROBERT M. BEAZLEY, MD

Overview

Embryology

The adrenal glands are paired suprarenal organs that are separated into two regions, the **adrenal cortex** and the **adrenal medulla.** These regions are derived from separate embryologic tissues and are distinct both structurally and functionally. The adrenal cortex is formed during the fourth and fifth week of gestation from coelomic mesothelial cells. The adrenal medulla and sympathetic nervous system develop from neural crest cells. As the neural crest cells migrate, some of them form the sympathetic ganglia along the aorta, and small groups of them detach to form glandular rests along the vertebral column. Although most of the rests regress, two groups of them do not. One group migrates, invades the adrenal cortex, and eventually forms the chromaffin cells of the adrenal medulla. The other group forms the organ of Zuckerkandl, which is located at the bifurcation of the aorta, close to the origin of the inferior mesenteric artery.

Anatomy

The adrenal glands are small, bilateral glands located above the kidneys in the retroperitoneal space between the eleventh thoracic and first lumbar vertebrae. Each gland is enclosed, along with a kidney, by perirenal fascia (Gerota's fascia) and is surrounded by fat. Each gland is covered by a fibrous capsule and measures about 3.0 × 5.0 × 0.5 cm. Although the average gland weighs 3 to 5 g, a gland may weigh up to 20 g at autopsy if the patient was under stress caused by a terminal illness.

The **right adrenal gland** is pyramid-shaped and lies in contact with the hemidiaphragm posteriorly, the right kidney inferiorly, the inferior vena cava anteromedially, and the right lobe of the liver anterolaterally. The **left adrenal gland** is slightly larger and is crescent-shaped. The left gland lies in contact with the hemidiaphragm posteriorly and is contiguous with the pancreas, splenic artery, and renal vein anteroinferiorly.

The adrenal glands have a generous **blood supply** (Fig. 33-1). For their size, they are one of the most vascular organs in the body, receiving an estimated 5 mL of blood per minute. The arterial supply is from three main sources: the **superior suprarenal artery,** which is a branch of the inferior phrenic artery; the **middle suprarenal artery,** which arises from the aorta; and the **inferior suprarenal artery,** which is a branch of the renal artery. These arteries form an arterial plexus and then enter a sinusoidal system that penetrates the cortex and medulla and ultimately drains into a central vein within each gland. The **right adrenal vein** is a short vein that exits the medial aspect of the gland and drains directly into the posterior aspect of the inferior vena cava. These features make the right adrenal gland particularly hard to catheterize. The **left adrenal vein** leaves the gland anteriorly and drains into the left renal vein.

Physiology

The adrenal cortex, which comprises the outer 80% of the adrenal gland by weight, is responsible for the synthesis of **steroid hormones derived from cholesterol.** Three functionally distinct zones are present within the adrenal cortex. The **zona glomerulosa** is the outermost layer and is responsible for the synthesis and secretion of **aldosterone.** The **zona fasciculata** is the middle layer and functions mainly to produce and release **cortisol.** The **zona reticularis** is the innermost layer and synthesizes and secretes **androgens** (adrenal steroids, or sex steroids).

Cortisol production is regulated by the **hypothalamic/pituitary axis** (Fig. 33-2). Corticotropin-releasing hormone (CRH), secreted by the hypothalamus, stimulates adrenocorticotropic hormone (ACTH) secretion by the anterior pituitary. ACTH stimulates the adrenal gland to produce cortisol, which in turn feeds back and inhibits ACTH and CRH.

Cortisol is referred to as a **glucocorticoid** because of its glucose-regulating properties, which include stimulating protein and lipid catabolism, increasing hepatic gluconeogenesis and glycogenesis, and decreasing peripheral uptake of glucose. Cortisol is essential to life in times of stress and critical illness. Under these circumstances, cortisol functions primarily to maintain cardiac output. This is achieved by supporting vascular tone, vascular permeability, and endothelial integrity and by maintaining the amount of total body water within the vascular compartment.

The adrenal medulla, which comprises the middle 20% of the gland, regulates the synthesis and secretion of

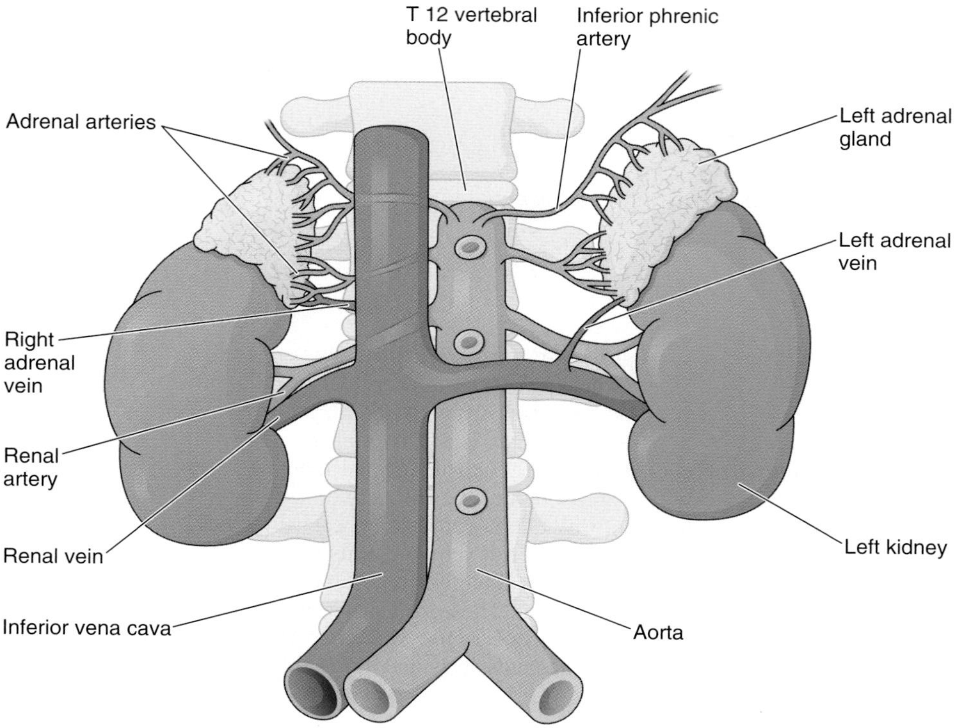

FIGURE 33–1 Anatomy of the adrenal glands.

catecholamines. Within the adrenal medulla are chromaffin granules, which are electron-dense membrane-bound vesicles that are similar in structure and function to secretory vesicles of neural and endocrine cells. The catecholamines are synthesized and stored within the chromaffin granules, and their production and secretion are regulated by the sympathetic nervous system. Acetylcholine released by preganglionic nerve endings is the main stimulus for catecholamine release.

Pheochromocytoma

Pheochromocytomas are catecholamine-secreting tumors that are derived from chromaffin cells. Most occur within the adrenal glands (**intra-adrenal pheochromocytomas**), but about 10% arise in and around the sympathetic ganglia outside the glands (**extra-adrenal pheochromocytomas** or **paragangliomas**). The term *pheochromocytoma* means dusky-colored tumor and refers to the appearance of the tumor cells when they are stained with chromium salts.

Pheochromocytomas affect the right adrenal gland more often than the left, and their incidence is slightly higher in female than in male subjects. Their peak incidence is between the third and fifth decades of life, and 10% of the tumors are malignant. Pheochromocytomas have been found in 0.1% of hypertensive patients. Although pheochromocytomas are rare, their diagnosis is important, because they may precipitate life-threatening hypertension or cardiac arrhythmias if they are not discovered and removed. Accurate diagnosis and treatment can lead to a complete cure.

The following **rule of tens** highlights some of the features of pheochromocytomas: 10% are extra-adrenal, 10% are malignant, 10% are bilateral, 10% are incidental, 10% occur in children, and 10% recur.

Etiology and Pathophysiology

Pheochromocytomas are found to occur in association with several familial disorders (Box 33-1). They occur in about 50% of patients with **multiple endocrine neoplasia (MEN) type IIa,** 50% of those with **MEN type IIb,** 1% of those with **neurofibromatosis type I,** and 20% of those with **von Hippel–Lindau disease.** The tumors occur bilaterally in 50% of the patients who have MEN syndromes that include pheochromocytomas.

The clinical manifestations of pheochromocytoma are due to excessive catecholamine secretion by the tumor. The biologic effects of catecholamines on the various tissues in the body are well known. Stimulation of α_1-adrenergic receptors results in elevated blood pressure, increased cardiac contractility, glycogenolysis, gluconeogenesis, and intestinal relaxation. Stimulation of α_1-adrenergic receptors results in an increase in heart rate and contractility.

In normal tissues of the adrenal medulla, catecholamine release is provoked by neural stimulation. Because pheochro-

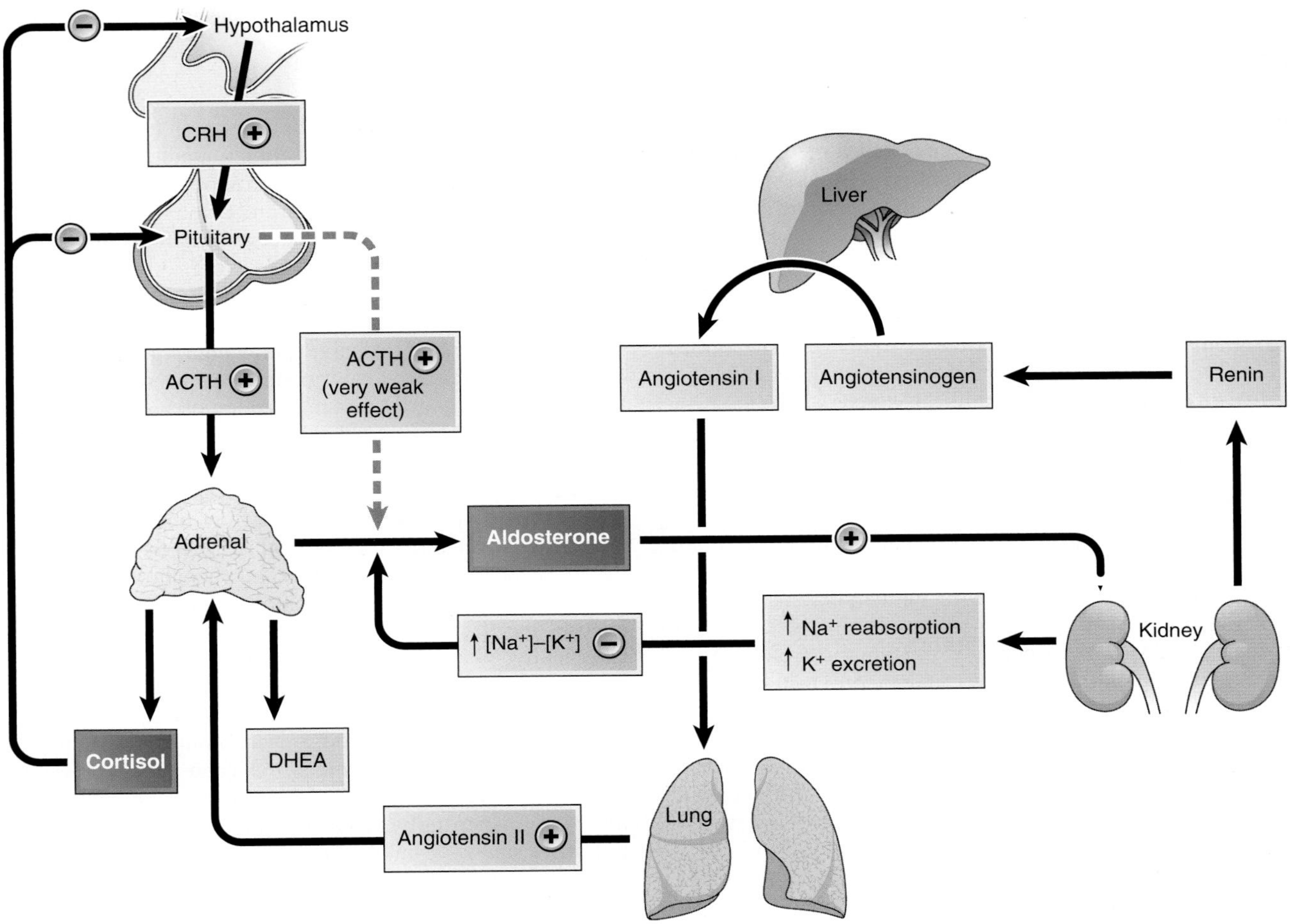

FIGURE 33–2 Regulatory systems for cortisol and aldosterone. CRH, corticotropin-releasing hormone; ACTH, adrenocorticotropic hormone; DHEA, dehydroepiandrosterone. (Modified from Brunt MJ, Melby JC: Adrenal gland disorders. In Noble J (ed): Primary Care Medicine, 2nd ed. St. Louis, Mosby, 1996, p 517.)

BOX 33–1 Components of Familial Syndromes in Which Pheochromocytoma Occurs

Multiple Endocrine Neoplasia (MEN) Type IIa
- Pheochromocytoma (in 50% of patients)
- Hyperparathyroidism
- Medullary thyroid carcinoma

Multiple Endocrine Neoplasia (MEN) Type IIb
- Pheochromocytoma (in 50% of patients)
- Hirschsprung's disease
- Intestinal ganglioneuromatosis
- Marfanoid habitus
- Medullary thyroid carcinoma
- Mucosal neuroma

Neurofibromatosis Type I
- Pheochromocytoma (in 1% of patients)
- Peripheral nerve tumors

Von Hippel–Lindau Disease
- Pheochromocytoma (in 20% of patients)
- Central nervous system hemangioblastoma
- Renal carcinoma
- Retinal angioma

mocytomas are not innervated, their catecholamine release is triggered by other means, possibly including changes in tumor blood flow and direct pressure on the adrenal gland. Factors reported to precipitate catecholamine discharge from a pheochromocytoma include childbirth; anesthesia induction; and use of radiographic contrast media, opiates, dopamine antagonists, catecholamine reuptake inhibitors (such as tricyclic antidepressants and cocaine), and cold medications.

Secretions of the normal adrenal medulla contain about 85% epinephrine. Although most pheochromocytomas secrete predominantly norepinephrine, familial pheochromocytomas typically secrete large amounts of epinephrine. This may explain normotensive or even hypotensive episodes in patients with familial pheochromocytomas.

Evaluation

History and Physical Examination

Patients with pheochromocytoma usually experience spells characterized by palpitations, headaches, and diaphoresis (the classic triad) in association with hypertension. The hypertension is paroxysmal in about 50% of patients, and the spells may vary in occurrence (ranging from once a month to several times a day) and in duration (ranging from seconds to hours).

The presence of the classic triad is 91% sensitive and 94% specific for the diagnosis of pheochromocytoma. In the absence of the classic triad and hypertension, the diagnosis may be excluded with close to 100% certainty.

In addition to the classic triad and hypertension, other symptoms and signs may include the following: nausea, weakness, anxiety, flushing, epigastric pain, flank pain, constipation, weight loss, postural hypotension, retinopathy, fever, pallor, tremor, arrhythmias, ileus, café au lait spots, and neurofibromas. It may be helpful to remember the "five Ps" that are manifestations of pheochromocytoma: palpitations, pain, pallor, perspiration, and pressure.

Laboratory Studies

A 24-hour urine sample should be sent to measure levels of total catecholamines, metanephrines, and vanillylmandelic acid (VMA). Elevated metanephrine levels are the most sensitive and specific findings, and elevated VMA levels are the least specific (with a false-positive rate of 15%). Optimally, urine should be collected during a crisis.

Blood tests may reveal hyperglycemia, hypercalcemia, and erythrocytosis. Tests for plasma levels of chromogranin A, an acidic monomeric protein that is stored and secreted with catecholamines, are reported to be 83% sensitive and 96% specific for detecting pheochromocytoma. Recent studies also indicated that the measurement of plasma metanephrine levels is a sensitive test and may be used in the future for diagnosing pheochromocytoma. Although provocative testing was used in the past, it is rarely performed today.

Imaging Studies

Imaging studies to localize the tumor or tumors should be performed only after biochemical studies confirm the diagnosis. About 90% of pheochromocytomas are intra-adrenal. Extra-adrenal pheochromocytomas develop in sympathetic ganglia and may occur anywhere from the base of the brain to the urinary bladder (Fig. 33-3); however, about 98% of them are located within the abdomen, either along the sympathetic chain or in the organ of Zuckerkandl. In approximately 1% of cases, paragangliomas are located within the thorax (specifically along the paravertebral sympathetic chain, intra-atrial septum, or glomus jugulare). Other rare locations include the bladder wall, spermatic cord, and vagina.

Magnetic resonance imaging (MRI) is preferable to computed tomography (CT) in detecting both intra-adrenal and extra-adrenal pheochromocytomas. MRI has a sensitivity of 100% in detecting intra-adrenal pheochromocytomas, does not require the use of contrast media, and does not expose the patient to ionizing radiation (Table 33-1). Classically, pheochromocytomas appear hyperintense on T_2-weighted MRI (Fig. 33-4). CT scanning can accurately detect 85% to 95% of adrenal masses but cannot always differentiate an adenoma from a pheochromocytoma.

A ^{123}I-metaiodobenzylguanidine scan (^{123}I-MIBG) is reserved for cases in which the diagnosis of pheochromocytoma is strongly suspected but MRI or CT scanning fails to visualize a tumor. The molecular structure of ^{123}I-MIBG resembles norepinephrine and concentrates in intra-adrenal or extra-adrenal pheochromocytomas. Its use should be considered in patients with familial syndromes, recurrent pheochromocytomas, or malignant pheochromocytomas.

Treatment

Surgical resection of the tumor is the treatment of choice and usually results in cure of the patient's hypertension.

Preoperative Preparation

Careful preoperative treatment with α-blockers and β-blockers is required to control blood pressure and prevent an intraoperative hypertensive crisis. From 7 to 10 days before surgery, α blockade with phenoxybenzamine should be started to allow expansion of contracted blood volume. Liberal salt intake should be encouraged. Only after α blockade is found to be working effectively should treatment with a β-blocker be initiated. If β blockade is started too early, unopposed α stimulation could precipitate a hypertensive crisis.

On the morning of surgery, the last doses of oral α-blockers and β-blockers should be given. An arterial line and a Swan-Ganz catheter should be placed, and cardiac

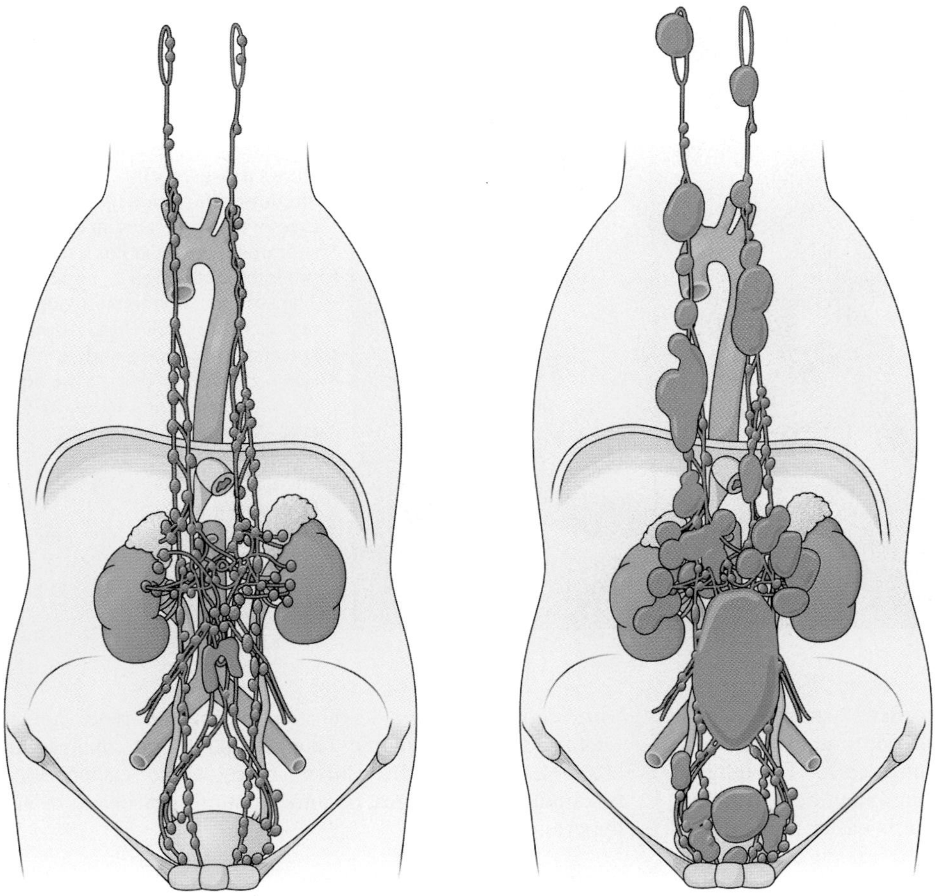

FIGURE 33–3 Sites of extra-adrenal pheochromocytomas. The pheochromocytomas (*right*) occur in sites containing chromaffin tissue in the newborn (*left*). (From Wilson JD, Foster DW, Kronenberg HM, Larsen PR (eds): Williams Textbook of Endocrinology, 9th ed. Philadelphia, WB Saunders, 1998; modified from Coupland RE: The Natural History of the Chromaffin Cell. London, Longmans, Green, 1965, pp 192–194.)

monitoring should be used. If bilateral resection is planned, “stress steroids” (hydrocortisone) should be administered to compensate for the fact that cortisol output will be suppressed.

Surgical Techniques

Although an anterior midline approach was used in the past, laparoscopic adrenalectomy is now the procedure of choice for treating solitary intra-adrenal adenomas that are smaller than 8 cm. The laparoscopic procedure involves the use of four instrument ports and is usually performed with the patient in the lateral position. On the right side, the triangular ligament must be moved to allow the liver to be retracted to the patient’s left. For a left adrenal lesion, the splenorenal ligament is incised to permit the spleen to rotate medially. Both maneuvers reveal the underlying adrenal

TABLE 33–1 Accuracy of Three Imaging Techniques in the Localization and Diagnosis of Pheochromocytoma*

Technique	Sensitivity	Specificity	Positive Predictive Value	Negative Predictive Value
Computed tomography	98%	70%	69%	98%
Magnetic resonance imaging	100%	67%	83%	100%
MIBG nuclear scanning	78%	100%	100%	87%

*Data are based on a pheochromocytoma prevalence rate of 38% in a selected group of 104 patients. The study included 30 intra-adrenal tumors and 10 extra-adrenal tumors.

MIBG, Metaiodobenzylguanidine.

Data from Gifford RW, Manger WM, Bravo EL: Pheochromocytoma. Endocrinol Metab Clin North Am 23:398, 1994.

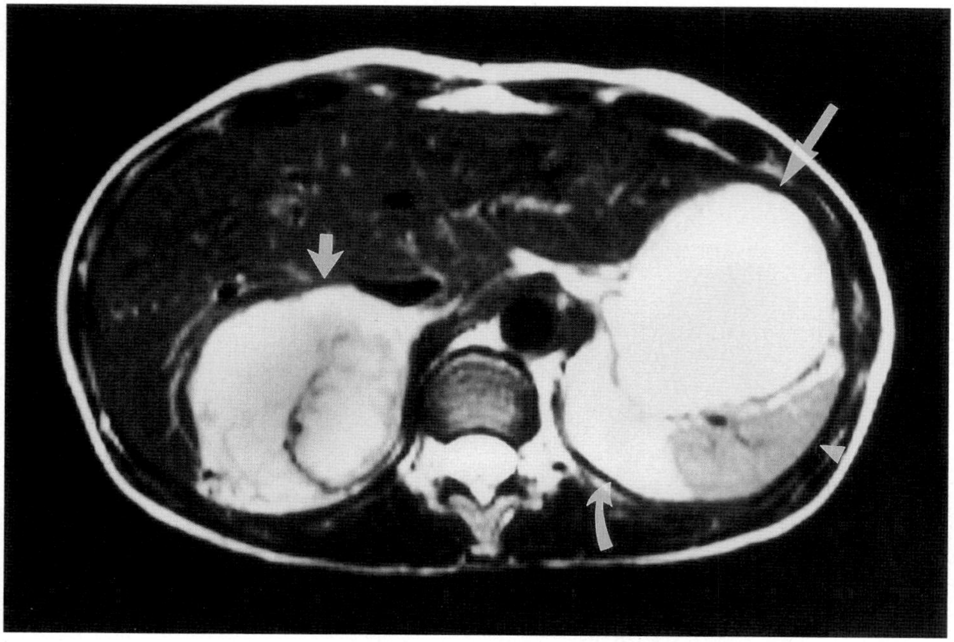

FIGURE 33–4 Magnetic resonance imaging (MRI) scan of a pheochromocytoma. The T_2-weighted axial abdominal MRI shows a large, well-circumscribed mass (*short arrow*) that is located in the right suprarenal area and has a predominantly high T_2 signal. The structures on the left side represent stomach (*long arrow*), spleen (*arrowhead*), and fat (*curved arrow*). (From Sweeney AT, Malabanan AO, Blake MA, et al: Megacolon as the presenting feature in pheochromocytoma. J Clin Endocrinol Metab 85(11): 3968–3972, 2000. Copyright 2000, The Endocrine Society.)

gland, and modern optics permit excellent anatomic visualization. When dealing with a pheochromocytoma, the surgeon should obtain vascular control early. The adrenal vein on the right is extremely short and may be a technical challenge, but blood pressure control is easier after venous ligation. Surrounding fibrovascular attachments are managed with cautery and clip ligation. The blood pressure will fluctuate less with the laparoscopic approach than with the open approach. If the pheochromocytoma is in the adrenal gland, the entire gland should be resected. If the tumor is malignant, it is important to remove as much of it as possible. Bilateral procedures may be performed if the patient is turned and reprepared.

Complications and Follow-up

Hypotension commonly occurs after adrenalectomy but can be effectively treated with a 0.9% intravenous saline or colloid solution. Two weeks after surgery and then once a year for the next 5 years, a 24-hour urine sample should be collected and sent for measurement of total catecholamines, metanephrines, and VMA. Studies indicate that if the levels of these substances have returned to the normal range, the survival rate of patients will approach that of age-matched controls.

Prognosis

The patient's blood pressure usually normalizes before discharge. Complete resection of a pheochromocytoma will cure hypertension in about 75% of patients. In the remainder, continued hypertension may be due to the resetting of baroreceptors, an accidental ligation of the renal artery, established hemodynamic changes, structural changes in blood vessels, altered sensitivity of vessels to vasopressors, functional renal changes, or coincident primary or secondary hypertension.

PEARLS FOR ROUNDS

Pheochromocytomas occur in association with several familial disorders including multiple endocrine neoplasia IIa (MEN-IIa), MEN-IIb, von Hippel–Lindau, and neurofibromatosis.

Rule of 10s for pheochromocytoma: 10% bilateral, 10% occur in children, 10% extra-adrenal, 10% malignant, 10% incidental, and 10% recur.

A unilateral aldosterone-producing adenoma (APA) is the most common type of primary aldosteronism and is treated with surgical removal.

Adrenal venous sampling is considered the gold standard for differentiating a unilateral APA from primary adrenal hyperplasia.

Specific signs of Cushing's syndrome include central obesity, proximal muscle weakness, wide purple striae, spontaneous ecchymoses, and facial plethora.

Patients with adrenocortical carcinoma (ACC) have a poor prognosis, with a 5-year survival of less than 50%.

Complete surgical resection is the only effective and potentially curative treatment for ACC.

The surgical mortality rate is less than 2% to 3% with an experienced surgeon and anesthesiologist. The 5-year survival rate is greater than 95% in patients with nonmalignant pheochromocytomas but is less than 50% in those with malignant pheochromocytomas.

Primary Aldosteronism

Primary aldosteronism is also called **primary hyperaldosteronism** or **Conn's syndrome.** The disorder is caused by the renin-independent overproduction of aldosterone and is characterized by the presence of hypertension, hypokalemia, and metabolic alkalosis. Numerous subtypes of primary aldosteronism include the following: **unilateral aldosterone-producing adenoma** (unilateral APA), which accounts for nearly 65% of cases; **idiopathic hyperaldosteronism** (IHA), which accounts for nearly 35% of cases; and **unilateral primary adrenal hyperplasia** (unilateral PAH), **aldosterone-producing carcinoma** (a form of adrenocortical carcinoma [ACC]), and **glucocorticoid-remediable aldosteronism** (GRA), each of which accounts for fewer than 1% of cases.

Evaluation

History and Physical Examination

Patients with aldosteronism have hypertension and may have a history of episodic or easily provoked hypokalemia. Physical examination may be unremarkable except for the presence of grade II retinopathy. Patients with hyperaldosteronism are often asymptomatic. Patients with hypokalemia may experience cramping, muscle weakness, headaches, palpitations, polydipsia, polyuria, nocturia, or a combination of these. Clinical signs include mild to severe hypertension, and fundoscopy may reveal group 1 or 2 hypertensive changes. Laboratory features may include hypokalemia, metabolic alkalosis, hypomagnesemia, and impaired glucose tolerance.

Laboratory Studies

Plasma aldosterone and renin levels should be measured. The finding of an aldosterone/renin ratio that exceeds 20:1 suggests the diagnosis of primary aldosteronism. The diagnosis can be confirmed by using a salt-loading test to demonstrate that plasma or urine aldosterone levels are insuppressible. In this test, aldosterone levels are measured after the patient is given 2 L of intravenous saline solution over a 4-hour period. A plasma aldosterone concentration exceeding 10 ng/dL or a 24-hour urinary tetrahydroaldosterone level exceeding 65 μg is consistent with insuppressible aldosterone secretion.

Measurement of plasma 18-hydroxycorticosterone, the immediate precursor of aldosterone, may assist in the differential diagnosis (Table 33-2). An 18-hydroxycorticosterone level greater than 100 ng/dL is highly suggestive of either APA or PAH.

TABLE 33–2 Accuracy of Various Techniques in the Differentiation of Aldosterone-producing Adenoma, Primary Adrenal Hyperplasia, and Idiopathic Hyperaldosteronism

Technique	Accuracy
Adrenal venous sampling	95%
Computed tomography or magnetic resonance imaging of adrenal glands	75%
Measurement of 18-hyroxycorticosterone: Level >100 ng/dL in APA and PAH	80%

Data from Melby JC: Diagnosis of hyperaldosteronism. Endocrinol Metab Clin North Am 2:252, 1991.

Imaging Studies

After biochemical confirmation of aldosteronism, either CT scanning or MRI can be performed to detect an adrenal abnormality. These imaging studies are only 75% accurate in differentiating an adrenal adenoma from hyperplasia. On the one hand, if the imaging study reveals a unilateral nodule that has an appropriate signal and is larger than 1 cm, this is considered sufficient evidence of unilateral APA. On the other hand, what appears to be an adenoma that is smaller than 1 cm may actually represent a small area of hyperplasia. Therefore if the abnormality is small, adrenal venous sampling should be performed.

Adrenal Venous Sampling

Considered to be the gold standard for differentiating unilateral APA from PAH, adrenal venous sampling has a reported accuracy rate of 95%. The procedure involves sampling aldosterone concentrations from the right and left adrenal veins via a catheter. Obtaining the samples is difficult and requires a highly skilled and experienced angiographer. The right adrenal vein may be particularly difficult to catheterize because it enters the inferior vena cava posteriorly at an acute angle. If a unilateral APA is present, a suppressed aldosterone level will be noted on the contralateral side.

Treatment

In patients with primary aldosteronism, the goal of treatment is to prevent morbidity and mortality associated with hypertension and hypokalemia. The method of treatment depends on the disease subtype.

Patients with IHA should be treated medically. Spironolactone, an aldosterone antagonist, is considered first-line therapy. The results of unilateral or bilateral adrenalectomy in patients with IHA have been disappointing, because hypertension subsides in only one third of cases.

The treatment of choice for patients with unilateral APA, PAH, or aldosterone-producing carcinoma is unilateral complete adrenalectomy, performed through either a laparoscopic approach or a posterior abdominal approach. The laparoscopic approach is associated with a shorter hospital stay and less morbidity. The posterior abdominal approach entails a lengthier recovery time and is associated with lateral wall abdominal laxity. With unilateral adrenalectomy, the intraoperative administration of "stress steroids" is usually not necessary. Hypokalemia typically resolves rapidly, but hypertension may take longer (1 to 3 months). In cases of APA, the response of the patient to spironolactone is predictive of the response to surgery.

Prognosis

The long-term cure rate for hypertension is 50% to 70% for patients with APA. Persistent hypertension may be associated with the resetting of baroreceptors, coexisting essential hypertension, functional and structural changes within the kidneys, and structural changes within the blood vessels. The following factors are associated with an increased postoperative risk of persistent hypertension: male sex, age older than 50 years, and preoperative hypertension that lasted more than 5 years.

PAH treated surgically generally has a good prognosis. Patients with IHA have a good prognosis if their hypertension is adequately treated. Patients with ACC have a poor prognosis. The prognosis for GRA is good when it is treated with low doses of dexamethasone. Dexamethasone suppresses ACTH production and reverses the syndrome.

Cushing's Syndrome

Cushing's syndrome is a form of **hyperadrenocorticism.** In 10% of affected patients, the excess in cortisol is due to a cortisol-producing adrenal adenoma. Because this tumor is monotropic and secretes only cortisol, the predominant clinical manifestations are those of cortisol excess and not androgen excess. Like cortisol-producing adrenal adenomas, adrenal carcinomas are examples of non–ACTH-dependent causes of hyperadrenocorticism.

Hyperadrenocorticism also can be due to ACTH-dependent causes. These include ACTH-secreting tumors (Cushing's disease), other pituitary tumors, and ectopic ACTH production from a neoplasm (typically a bronchial carcinoid or small cell lung cancer).

Evaluation

History and Physical Examination

Patients with Cushing's syndrome may have a history of easy bruising, back pain, and height loss (signs of compression fractures); osteopenia or osteoporosis; decreased libido; oligomenorrhea; or depression. Specific signs of Cushing's syndrome include central obesity, proximal muscle weakness, wide purple striae, spontaneous ecchymoses, and facial plethora. Other physical findings may include moon facies, florid complexion (due to telangiectasia), buffalo hump, supraclavicular fat pads, and thin skin.

Laboratory Studies

Laboratory tests often demonstrate hypokalemic alkalosis and hyperglycemia.

The 1-mg overnight dexamethasone suppression test is a good screening test for Cushing's syndrome. After a dose of dexamethasone is given at 11 PM, a serum sample is collected at 8 AM, and the cortisol level is measured. In healthy individuals, the dexamethasone suppresses the cortisol production, causing the plasma cortisol level to decrease to around 5 μg/dL or lower (Fig. 33-5). In patients with Cushing's syndrome, the cortisol level is not suppressed. The next step is to collect a 24-hour urine sample to measure the levels of creatinine, 17-ketosteroids, and free cortisol. If the patient's cortisol level was not suppressed in the dexamethasone test and the level of free cortisol in the urine is elevated, the diagnosis of Cushing's syndrome is confirmed. At this point, a serum sample should be obtained to measure the

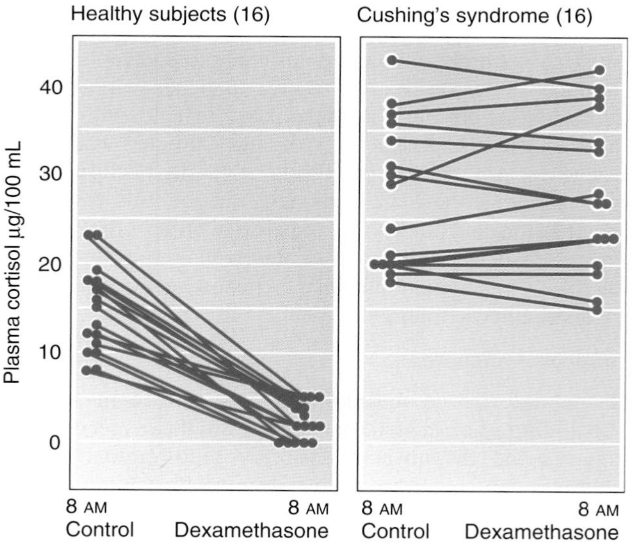

FIGURE 33–5 Results in the overnight dexamethasone suppression test. Cortisol is initially measured at 8 AM. After a 1-mg dose of dexamethasone is given at 11 PM, a serum sample is collected at 8 AM the next morning, and the cortisol level is measured. In healthy subjects, the dexamethasone suppresses the cortisol production, causing the plasma cortisol level to decrease. In patients with Cushing's syndrome, the cortisol level is not suppressed. (From Melby JC: Assessment of adrenocortical function. N Engl J Med 285:737, 1971, with permission.)

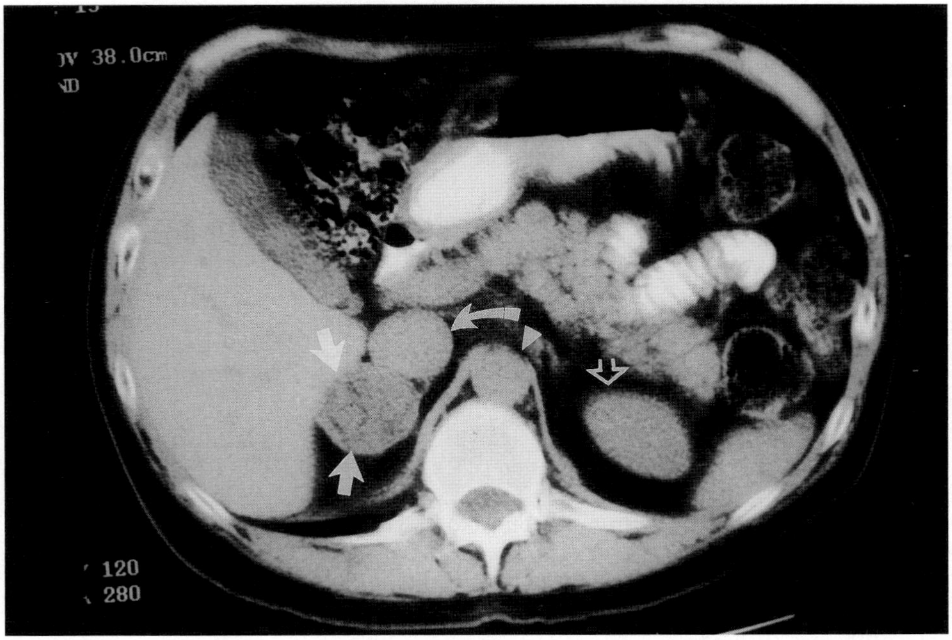

FIGURE 33–6 Computed tomography scan of a suprarenal mass in a patient with Cushing's syndrome. This axial abdominal view shows a well-circumscribed, 2 × 2-cm suprarenal mass (*short arrow*), the inferior vena cava (*curved arrow*), aorta (*arrowhead*), and kidney (*open arrow*).

ACTH level. If the ACTH is suppressed, the results are consistent with the diagnosis of non–ACTH-dependent Cushing's syndrome.

Imaging Studies

Either CT scanning (Fig. 33-6) or MRI can be useful in evaluating patients with Cushing's syndrome. MRI may be more helpful in distinguishing a malignant lesion from a benign lesion.

Treatment and Prognosis

The treatment of choice is a unilateral complete adrenalectomy. Laparoscopic adrenalectomy is the preferred method for smaller tumors. An open surgical approach is required for larger tumors and for carcinomas. Patients with Cushing's syndrome usually have profound suppression of the hypothalamic/pituitary/adrenal axis and require glucocorticoid replacement for months after resection of the tumor.

In patients with a cortisol-secreting adrenal adenoma, the cure rate is close to 100%. In those with ACC, the stage of the tumor determines the prognosis. However, the cancer patients tend to have recurrences that do not respond to radiation therapy or chemotherapy. Medical therapy with mitotane, an adrenal enzyme inhibitor, is often needed to control the level of cortisol.

Adrenal Incidentaloma

Incidentally discovered **adrenal masses** have become increasingly common as the result of technologic advances in imaging techniques such as CT scanning and MRI. Autopsy studies have demonstrated a 2% to 15% incidence of adrenal masses.

Classification

Adrenal masses can be classified as nonfunctioning masses or hyperfunctioning masses. **Nonfunctioning masses** include benign adenoma, hematoma, myelolipoma, cyst, neurofibroma, ganglioneuroma, teratoma, metastatic carcinoma, and primary malignancy. **Hyperfunctioning masses** include pheochromocytoma, masculinizing tumor, feminizing tumor, nodular hyperplasia, congenital adrenal hyperplasia, and masses associated with primary aldosteronism and Cushing's syndrome.

PEARLS FOR THE OR

The adrenal glands, along with the kidney, are enclosed by Gerota's fascia and are surrounded by fat.

The arterial blood supply to the adrenal glands is from three main sources: the superior suprarenal artery, which is a branch from the inferior phrenic artery; the middle suprarenal artery, which arises from the aorta; and the inferior suprarenal artery, which is a branch from the renal artery.

The right adrenal vein is short, exits the medial aspect of the glans, and drains directly into the inferior vena cava.

The left adrenal vein leaves the gland anteriorly and drains into the left renal vein.

Evaluation

The first priority in evaluating an adrenal mass is to determine whether the mass is hyperfunctioning and whether it is malignant.

History and Physical Examination

The history and physical examination should focus on the signs and symptoms of adrenal hyperfunction (see the earlier discussions of pheochromocytoma, primary aldosteronism, and Cushing's syndrome) and of cancer (see the later discussion on ACC). Details should be obtained regarding weight loss, bone pain, and smoking history. Primary adrenal cancer is quite rare, but other cancers (particularly lung cancer) may metastasize to the adrenal glands.

Laboratory Studies

The patient should be screened for pheochromocytoma and Cushing's syndrome by collecting a 24-hour urine sample and measuring the levels of catecholamines, VMA, metanephrines, and free cortisol. If the patient is hypertensive, serum samples should be tested for renin and aldosterone levels. The serum dehydroepiandrosterone sulfate (DHEAS) level also should be measured to exclude a virilizing tumor.

Imaging Studies

The size of the adrenal mass is an important factor in determining the probability of malignancy. The risk of cancer is significantly higher when the mass is larger than 6 cm.

Certain imaging features are characteristic. With CT scanning, the finding of a uniform fat attenuation indicates a mass with a high fat content and is consistent with the diagnosis of myelolipoma. On an unenhanced CT scan, the typical benign adenoma is smooth, round, and homogeneous; is under 4 cm in diameter; and has a low-density value (<10 Hounsfield units). On MRI, adenomas appear isointense with the liver on T_2-weighted images.

Pheochromocytomas may be bilateral, variable in size, and cystic or hemorrhagic; and they usually appear hyperintense on T_2-weighted MRI. Metastases to the adrenal gland may be unilateral or bilateral; are usually irregularly shaped and nonhomogeneous; have a higher density than adenomas on an unenhanced CT scan (>10 HU); and may have an intermediate to high signal intensity on T_2-weighted MRI. ACCs also appear irregular in shape, are usually larger than 4 cm in diameter, have high unenhanced CT attenuation values (>10 HU), and may have an intermediate to high signal intensity on MRI.

Treatment and Follow-up

For nonfunctioning adrenal lesions that are larger than 4 cm and for all hyperfunctioning lesions, surgical resection is indicated. The presurgical treatment and preparations will depend on the tumor function.

For nonfunctioning adrenal lesions that are smaller than 4 cm, imaging should be repeated at 3 months and at 12 months. If the lesion increases by more than 1 cm in diameter, surgical resection is indicated. If no change in size or in function test results is seen at 12 months, no further follow-up is indicated.

Adrenocortical Carcinoma

Adrenocortical carcinoma (ACC) is a rare, aggressive cancer with an estimated incidence of 1 case per 2 million people per year. The ACC is hyperfunctioning in 50% to 70% of patients and nonfunctioning in the remainder. Hyperfunctioning ACC can be seen in association with isolated Cushing's syndrome (40% of cases), concomitant Cushing's syndrome and virilization (22%), isolated virilization (22%), feminization (2%), and hypertension (10%).

The age of the patient when ACC is diagnosed varies from 6 months to 72 years, with a median age of 40 years. The majority of patients with hyperfunctioning ACC are female (female/male ratio of 2.5:1), whereas the majority of patients with nonfunctioning ACC are male.

Evaluation

History, Physical Examination, and Laboratory Studies

The key to successful management of ACC is early detection. However, the adrenal gland is a deep-seated, relatively inaccessible organ, and tumors often remain silent until symptoms are produced from advanced malignancy, a large mass, or hormonal excess. Moreover, hyperfunctioning tumors do not produce early signs and symptoms, because malignant cells are highly inefficient in synthesizing steroids, and a large mass is required to elevate steroid levels.

The mean duration of symptoms reported for patients with nonfunctioning and hyperfunctioning tumors is 9 months. In patients with nonfunctioning tumors, the three most common presenting features are pain, a palpable abdominal mass, and metastases. Fatigue, weight loss, and fever also may be present. In patients with hyperfunctioning tumors, the manifestations vary but may include those associated with virilization, feminization, or Cushing's syndrome. The hormonal presentation also varies (Table 33-3), but laboratory findings most commonly include elevated levels of testosterone and DHEAS in serum, as well as elevated free cortisol and 17-ketosteroids in urine. A 17-ketosteroid concentration that exceeds 20 mg per milligram of creatinine is strongly suggestive of ACC. All hirsute female patients should have their serum testosterone and DHEAS levels screened to exclude a virilizing tumor.

Imaging Studies

ACC characteristically has high attenuation values (>10 HU) on unenhanced CT and shows even higher values

TABLE 33–3 Functional Status of 105 Adrenocortical Carcinomas, Based on the Measurement of Steroids in Plasma, Urine, or Both

Functional Status and Steroids Secreted	Number (Percentage) of Tumors
Nonfunctioning tumors	**22 (21%)**
Hyperfunctioning tumors	**83 (79%)**
Glucocorticoids and androgens	35 (42%)
Glucocorticoids	34 (41%)
Androgens	8 (10%)
17-Hydroxyprogesterone	2 (2%)
Aldosterone	1 (1%)
Glucocorticoids and 17-hydroxyprogesterone	1 (1%)
Glucocorticoids, 17-hydroxyprogesterone, and aldosterone	1 (1%)
Glucocorticoids, androgens, and estradiol	1 (1%)
Estradiol	0

Data from Luton JP, Cerdas S, Billaud L, et al: Clinical features of adrenocortical carcinoma, prognostic factors, and the effect of mitotane therapy. N Engl J Med 322:1195–1201, 1990.

(>40 HU) 30 minutes after an intravenous contrast medium is administered. On T_2-weighted MRI, lesions are of high to intermediate intensity. Typically, lesions associated with ACC are irregularly shaped, heterogeneous, and larger than 4 cm in diameter (Fig. 33-7). Often unilateral evidence of invasion or local metastases exists.

Treatment and Follow-up

Complete surgical resection is the only effective and potentially curative treatment for ACC. Adjuvant radiation therapy is not beneficial. Although postoperative therapy with mitotane is controversial, some experts recommend it because it has been reported to prolong survival. Mitotane treatment is begun immediately after surgery. Side effects of mitotane include nausea, vomiting, anorexia, rash, diarrhea, lethargy, sedation, dizziness, ataxia, gynecomastia, and leukopenia.

Imaging studies should be performed at 3-month intervals to assess the recurrence or progression of disease. Patients with hyperfunctioning tumors should have appropriate follow-up laboratory studies. In the case of recurrent disease, surgery is the best option.

Prognosis

The prognosis depends on the tumor stage (Table 33-4) and the patient's age at presentation. Based on a study of 156 patients with ACC, 5% of patients are initially seen in stage I, 48% in stage II, 25% in stage III, and 22% in stage IV (see Icard et al, 1992). Common sites of metastases in stage IV patients include the liver, lung, lymph nodes, and bone. Survival rates are significantly lower for patients who are older than 40 years and have distant metastases at the time of diagnosis. Studies have revealed no statistically significant difference in survival with regard to functional status or weight of tumors.

Mitotane begun immediately after surgery may delay or prevent recurrence in patients who have undergone a

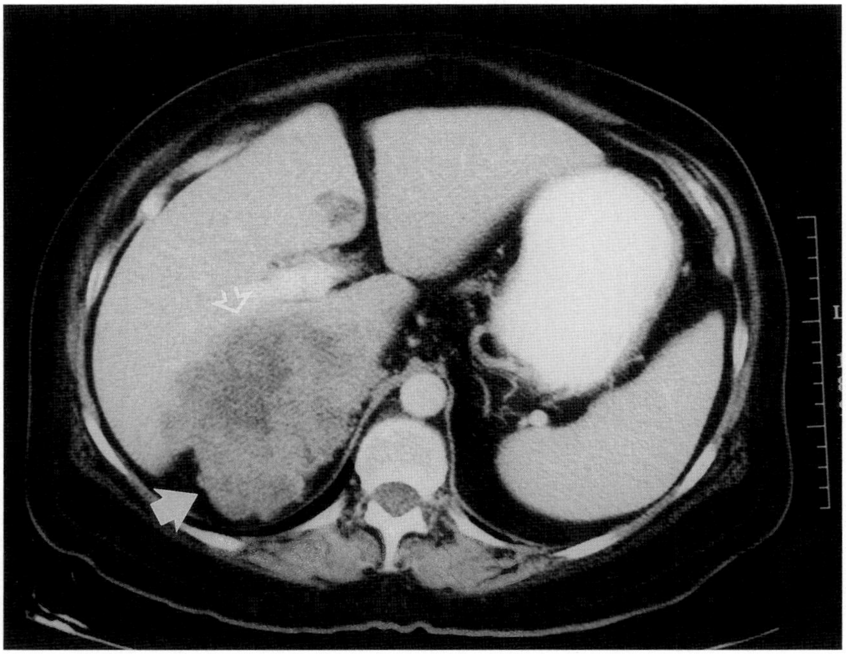

FIGURE 33–7 Computed tomography scan of an adrenocortical carcinoma. This view of the upper abdomen was obtained after an intravenous contrast medium was administered. It shows a 10 × 9-cm heterogeneously enhanced mass (*short arrow*) in the right suprarenal area. The mass is invading the neighboring liver parenchyma (*open arrow*).

TABLE 33–4 Staging Systems for Adrenal Carcinoma

Stage	Description
Stage I	T1 with N0 and M0
Stage II	T2 with N0 and M0
Stage III	T1 or T2 with N1 and M0; or T3 with N0 and M0
Stage IV	Any T, any N, M1; T3, T4, N1

T refers to the extent of the primary tumor; T1 is <5cm with no invasion; T2 is >5cm with no invasion; T3 is any size, including local invasion but not involving adjacent organs; and T4 is any size, including local invasion and involving adjacent organs. N refers to the absence (N0) or presence (N1) of regional lymph node involvement. M refers to the absence (M0) or presence (M1) of distant metastatic lesions.

Data from Henley DJ, van Heerden JA, Grant CS, et al: Adrenal cortical carcinoma: A continuing challenge. Surgery 94:926–931, 1983.

primary tumor resection. Studies have shown that the median survival time after diagnosis of ACC ranges from 14.5 to 36 months in adults who are treated with surgery and chemotherapy versus an average of 3 months in those who are not treated.

Suggested Reading

Avisse C, Marcus C, Patey M, et al: Surgical anatomy and embryology of the adrenal glands. Surg Clin North Am 80:403–415, 2000.

Barzon L, Boscaro M: Diagnosis and management of adrenal incidentalomas. J Urol 163:398–407, 2000.

Ganguly A: Primary aldosteronism. N Engl J Med 339:1828–1833, 1998.

Icard P, Chapois Y, Andreassian B, et al: Adrenocortical carcinoma in surgically treated patients: A retrospective study on 156 cases by the French Association of Endocrine Surgery. Surgery 112:972–979, 1992.

Ng L, Libertino JM: Adrenocortical carcinoma: Diagnosis, evaluation, and treatment. J Urol 169:5–11, 2003.

Pacak K, Linehan WM, Eisenhofer G, et al: Recent advances in genetics, diagnosis, localization, and treatment of pheochromocytoma. Ann Intern Med 134:315–329, 2001.

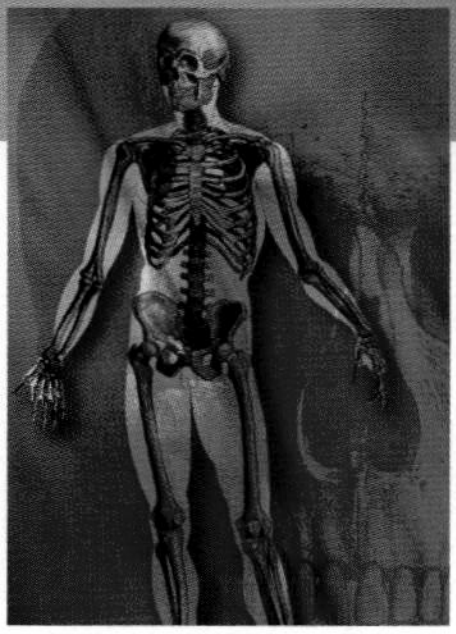

Chapter 34
Pituitary Gland

ANN T. SWEENEY, MD, and ROBERT M. BEAZLEY, MD

Overview

Embryology and Anatomy

The pituitary gland is divided structurally and functionally into two lobes. The **anterior lobe (adenohypophysis)** is derived from Rathke's pouch, which is an evagination from the floor of the embryologic oral cavity. The **posterior lobe (neurohypophysis)** is formed from a diverticulum that originates from the floor of the third ventricle and joins Rathke's pouch.

The pituitary gland weighs about 0.5 g, measures 13 × 10 × 6 mm, and is located within the **sella turcica** (Turkish saddle) in the sphenoid bone at the base of the skull. The sella is partially covered by an extension of the dura mater called the sellar diaphragm. A small hole in this diaphragm allows the **pituitary stalk** to pass through. The **optic chiasm** is located slightly anterior to the pituitary stalk and just above the diaphragm. Any sellar lesion that extends upward may easily compress the optic chiasm and cause visual field abnormalities. Lateral to the sella are the cavernous sinuses containing the **internal carotid artery** and **cranial nerves III, IV, V, and VI** (Fig. 34-1). Thus lateral extension of a pituitary tumor may cause cranial nerve palsies. Inferior to the pituitary is the **sphenoid sinus,** which is sometimes invaded by aggressive pituitary tumors.

The rate of **blood flow** to the anterior pituitary (0.8 mL/g/min) is higher than the rate of blood flow to any other tissue in the body. Arterial blood is supplied from two major sources. One is the **superior hypophyseal artery,** which is a branch of the internal carotid artery and the hypothalamic-pituitary-portal circulation. The other is **the inferior hypophyseal artery,** which supplies blood to the posterior pituitary (Fig. 34-2).

Physiology

The anterior pituitary is responsible for the synthesis of six major hormones, whereas the posterior pituitary is responsible for the storage of two additional hormones.

Cell Types, Hormones, and Hormone Regulation

As shown in Table 34-1, five distinct cell types produce trophic hormones in the anterior pituitary: **corticotrophs** produce **adrenocorticotropic hormone** (ACTH); **gonadotrophs** produce **follicle-stimulating hormone** (FSH) and **luteinizing hormone** (LH); **lactotrophs** produce **prolactin** (PRL); **somatotrophs** produce **growth hormone** (GH); and **thyrotrophs** produce **thyroid-stimulating hormone** (TSH).

Each anterior pituitary hormone is part of a tightly regulated system in which either stimulatory or inhibitory influences are exerted by the **hypothalamus** and in which feedback occurs from the organs affected by the hormone.

The hypothalamus synthesizes various **hypophysiotropic hormones,** each of which is necessary for the synthesis and secretion of a particular anterior pituitary hormone (see Table 34-1). The hypophysiotropic hormones are released into the portal vascular system and circulate through the pituitary stalk to the anterior lobe. Any disruption of the pituitary stalk leads to a reduction in the ACTH, FSH, LH, GH, and TSH levels; however, it leads to an increase in the serum PRL levels because the portal system carries an inhibitory factor (dopamine) that controls PRL secretion.

The communication between the hypothalamus and the posterior pituitary is physical, rather than chemical. The cell bodies of the supraoptic nuclei and paraventricular nuclei of the hypothalamus synthesize **antidiuretic hormone (ADH)** and **oxytocin,** respectively. Each of these hormones travels down its own tract to reach the posterior pituitary.

Anterior Pituitary Hormones

Growth Hormone. GH, also called somatotropin, is a large polypeptide composed of 191 amino acids. GH secretion is stimulated by growth hormone–releasing hormone (GHRH) and is inhibited by a hormone called somatostatin or GH release–inhibiting hormone (GIH). GH is released in a pulsatile fashion. After it binds to receptors on liver cells, it stimulates hepatic production of insulin-like growth factor 1 (IGF-1), a substance that mediates many of the biologic actions of GH.

GH is essential for normal linear growth. It also acts as an insulin antagonist and promotes protein synthesis from amino acids. The secretion of GH increases in response to physical stress, hypoglycemia, and exercise. In children, a deficiency of GH leads to short stature, whereas an excess

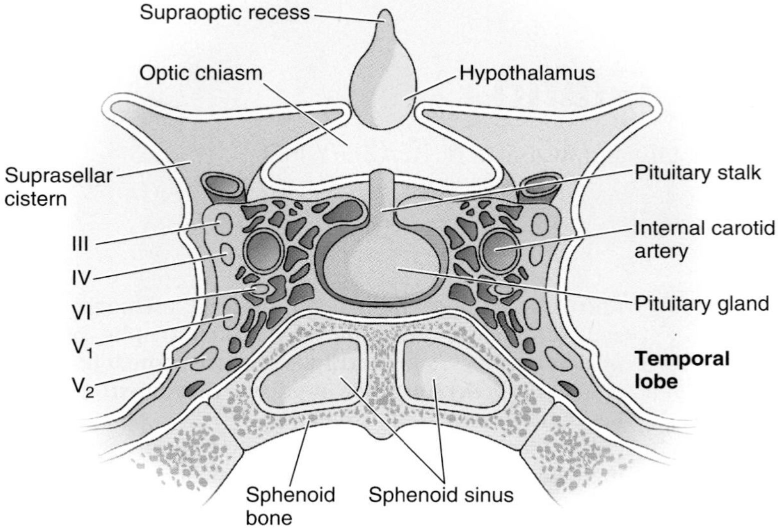

FIGURE 34–1 The pituitary fossa and its anatomic relations seen in coronal orientation. The pituitary gland is bordered laterally by the cavernous sinuses containing the internal carotid artery and cranial nerves III, IV, V1, V2, and VI. The optic chiasm resides immediately above the pituitary gland and is separated by a cistern filled with cerebrospinal fluid. (Adapted from Lechan RM: Neuroendocrinology of pituitary hormone regulation. Endocrinol Metab Clin North Am 16:477, 1987.)

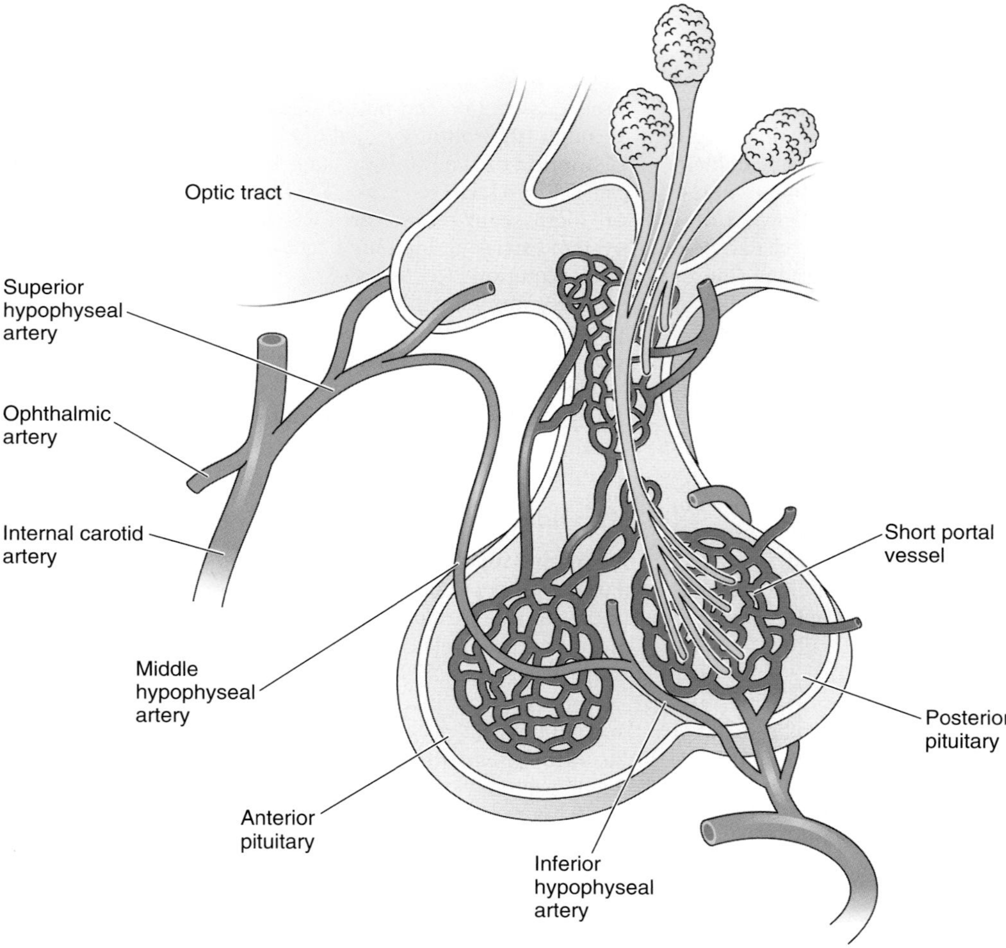

FIGURE 34–2 Vascular system of the pituitary gland. (Adapted from Lechan RM: Neuroendocrinology of pituitary hormone regulation. Endocrinol Metab Clin North Am 16:477, 1987, with permission. Originally adapted from Gay VL: The hypothalamus: Physiology and clinical use of releasing factors. Fertil Steril 23:50, 1972.)

TABLE 34–1 Anterior Pituitary Hormones and the Hypothalamic Hormones That Are Involved in Their Regulation

Pituitary Cells	Anterior Pituitary Hormones	Regulatory Hypothalamic Hormones
Corticotrophs	Adrenocorticotropic hormone (ACTH, or corticotropin)	Corticotropin-releasing hormone (CRH)
Gonadotrophs	Follicle-stimulating hormone (FSH, a gonadotropin) and luteinizing hormone (LH, a gonadotropin)	Gonadotropin-releasing hormone (GnRH) and luteinizing hormone–releasing hormone (LHRH)
Lactotrophs	Prolactin (PRL, or lactotropin)	Prolactin-inhibiting factor (PIF)
Somatotrophs	Growth hormone (GH, or somatotropin)	Growth hormone–releasing hormone (GHRH) and growth hormone release–inhibiting hormone (GIH, or somatostatin)
Thyrotrophs	Thyroid-stimulating hormone (TSH, or thyrotropin)	Thyrotropin-releasing hormone (TRH)

of GH before closure of the epiphyseal plates causes gigantism. In adults, an excess of GH causes acromegaly (Fig. 34-3).

Adrenocorticotropic Hormone. ACTH, also called **corticotropin,** is a 39-amino-acid polypeptide that regulates glucocorticoid production by the adrenal glands. ACTH secretion is influenced by a hypothalamic hormone called **corticotropin-releasing hormone** (CRH) and by adrenal production of **cortisol.** When cortisol levels are adequate, they feed back negatively on the pituitary and hypothalamus to reduce ACTH and CRH production. ACTH secretion follows a diurnal rhythm, with peak levels occurring in the early morning and trough levels occurring in the late afternoon. Factors other than CRH that increase ACTH production include severe stress, trauma, illness, fever, and hypoglycemia.

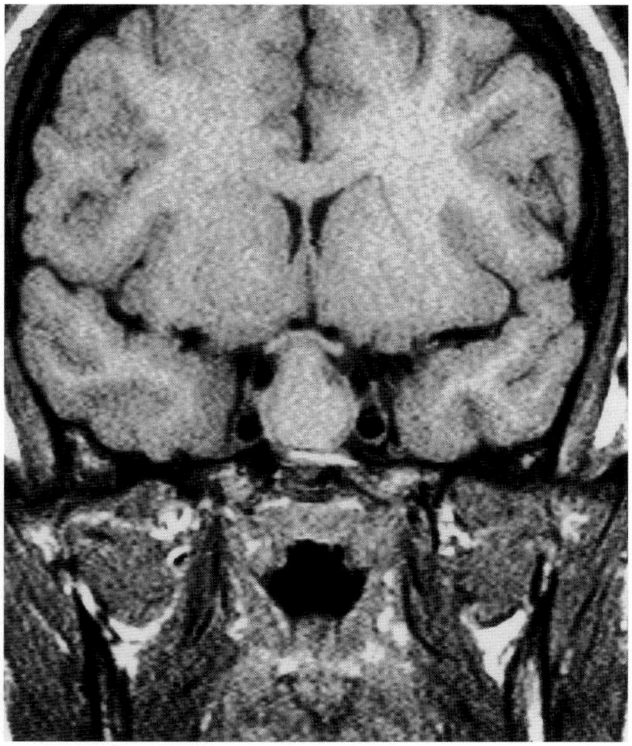

FIGURE 34–3 A patient with acromegalic features and markedly elevated levels of insulin-like growth factor 1 (IGF-1). This coronal T1-weighted magnetic resonance imaging scan through the pituitary fossa demonstrates a large pituitary mass displacing the optic chiasm superiorly.

Thyroid-stimulating Hormone. TSH, also called **thyrotropin,** is a glycoprotein consisting of an α subunit and a β subunit. The α subunit is like that found in FSH, LH, and human chorionic gonadotropin (hCG), but the β subunit is unique. TSH regulates the synthesis, storage, and release of **thyroid hormones** (T_4 and T_3) and thereby affects the size of the thyroid gland. **Thyrotropin-releasing hormone** (TRH) secreted by the hypothalamus stimulates the pituitary to release TSH. Thyroid hormones feed back in a negative loop on the pituitary and hypothalamus to regulate TSH production. TSH levels are highest in the early morning.

Thyroid failure leads to a TSH increase that is characteristic of primary hypothyroidism. Secondary hypothyroidism, which is rare, results from a failure of the pituitary to release an adequate amount of TSH and may be due to the presence of a pituitary tumor or infiltrative disease.

Prolactin. PRL is a 198-amino-acid polypeptide that is necessary for lactation. During pregnancy, elevated estrogen levels stimulate replication and growth of the pituitary lactotrophs, and this leads to a progressive increase in PRL secretion, with PRL levels reaching their peak (100 to 300 ng/mL) at term. Elevated estrogen levels that are present during pregnancy prevent PRL from acting on the breast, so lactation does not occur until estrogen levels decrease at childbirth.

Unlike other pituitary hormones, PRL is under tonic inhibitory control. Dopamine is normally released by the hypothalamus and acts as a **prolactin-inhibiting factor** (PIF). Any disruption of the pituitary stalk by a tumor or infiltrative disease may lead to low levels of all of the anterior pituitary hormones except PRL. Two hypothalamic factors, TRH and somatostatin, act to increase PRL secretion. This is an important point and explains why patients with primary hypothyroidism and acromegaly may have concomitant hyperprolactinemia. Medications that may cause hyperprolactinemia include estrogens, phenothiazines, tricyclic antidepressants, metoclopramide, cimetidine, methyldopa, reserpine, and cocaine.

Follicle-stimulating Hormone and Luteinizing Hormone. FSH and LH, also called **gonadotropins,** are glycoproteins that have identical α subunits but different β subunits. **Gonadotropin-releasing hormone** (GnRH), which is secreted in a pulsatile fashion by the hypothalamus, regulates the secretion of FSH and LH.

In women, a complex negative feedback system involving estradiol and progesterone helps regulate the cyclic secretion of FSH and LH that is necessary for the follicular and luteal phases of the menstrual cycle. An increase in LH (and, to a lesser extent, in FSH) occurs just before ovulation. FSH stimulates growth of the granulosa cells of the ovarian follicle and regulates aromatase, the enzyme responsible for the synthesis of estradiol. LH stimulates the ovarian theca cells to produce androgens, which then diffuse into the granulosa cells, where they are converted to estrogens.

In men, LH stimulates testosterone production by the testicular Leydig cells. FSH and testosterone together promote spermatogenesis by the seminiferous tubules.

Posterior Pituitary Hormones

Antidiuretic Hormone. ADH, also called **vasopressin,** is synthesized within the magnicellular neurons of the hypothalamus as a prohormone complex and is transported via terminal axons to the posterior pituitary. The prohormone complex is then cleaved to yield ADH and its carrier protein, neurophysin. ADH conserves water by concentrating the urine. ADH binds to the vasopressin V_2 receptor in the renal distal tubule and enhances hydrosmotic flow. This helps maintain stable plasma osmolality and volume. An increase in plasma osmolality above 285 mOsm provokes ADH secretion and results in a decrease in urinary water loss. In contrast, a reduction in plasma osmolality leads to a decrease in ADH secretion.

Oxytocin. Like ADH, oxytocin is synthesized within the magnicellular neurons of the hypothalamus and is then transported via terminal axons to the posterior pituitary, where it is cleaved from neurophysin. Oxytocin stimulates uterine contractions during pregnancy, and it triggers milk let-down during lactation.

Classification of Pituitary Tumors

Pituitary tumors, which account for 15% of all intracranial tumors, are classified by size and function. Pituitary tumors smaller than 10 mm are called **microadenomas,** whereas those 10 mm or larger are called **macroadenomas.** About 30% of pituitary tumors do not cause classic hypersecretory syndromes and are therefore called **nonfunctioning pituitary adenomas.** About 60% are **hyperfunctioning pituitary adenomas,** and these occur in the following order of frequency: prolactinomas, GH-secreting adenomas, ACTH-secreting adenomas, and TSH-secreting adenomas.

Hyperfunctioning Pituitary Adenomas

Prolactinomas

Prolactinomas, or **prolactin-secreting adenomas,** account for about 60% of all hyperfunctioning pituitary tumors. The size of a prolactinoma correlates well with the level of hormone secretion. Macroadenomas cause high PRL levels, whereas microadenomas are associated with lower PRL levels. Most macroadenomas (60%) are found in men, whereas the majority of microadenomas (90%) are found in women.

Evaluation

History and Physical Examination. Small prolactinomas may produce only hypogonadism, whereas large prolactinomas may cause hypogonadism, headaches, visual compromise, and loss of other hormone function. The hypogonadism associated with hyperprolactinemia is due to the inhibition of GnRH by high PRL levels.

In women, the signs of hyperprolactinemia, such as amenorrhea, galactorrhea, and infertility, are more likely to result in an earlier diagnosis. Although manifestations of sexual dysfunction, such as impotence, loss of libido, and infertility, are present in the majority of men with macroadenomas, they account for only 15% of presenting signs and symptoms in these men. More research is needed to determine whether tumors in men show more aggressive growth than do those in women.

Laboratory and Other Studies. PRL levels associated with a prolactinoma are usually higher than 100 ng/mL. Hyperprolactinemia may occur with hypothyroidism, renal failure, antidopaminergic drugs, or pregnancy, and all of these causes should be excluded. If the PRL level is elevated in the absence of known physiologic, pathologic, or pharmacologic factors, magnetic resonance imaging (MRI) studies with views of the pituitary fossa are indicated, and formal visual field testing should be performed. The characteristic visual field defect present is bitemporal hemianopsia.

Treatment and Prognosis

Medical therapy with a dopamine agonist, such as bromocriptine or cabergoline, is the preferred treatment for prolactinomas. Dopamine agonists inhibit the secretion and synthesis of PRL and impair lactotroph proliferation and growth. About 80% to 90% of patients with microadenomas and 60% to 75% of those with macroadenomas will respond to treatment with dopamine agonists. Surgery is considered second-line therapy for those who fail to respond. Surgery is associated with a 55% response rate in patients with microadenomas and a 75% response rate in those with macroadenomas.

Growth Hormone–secreting Tumors

About 20% of all hyperfunctioning pituitary tumors are GH-secreting pituitary adenomas, and 75% of the GH-secreting tumors are macroadenomas.

Evaluation

History and Physical Examination. GH hypersecretion in adults results in acromegaly, an insidious and progressively debilitating disease that is characterized by acral and soft tissue overgrowth, generalized visceromegaly, arthropathy, carpal tunnel syndrome, chronic pain, and disfigurement. Headaches, visual defects, and hypopituitarism occur secondary to tumor expansion.

The coarse features that are characteristic of acromegaly progress slowly, so the diagnosis is often delayed. If acromegaly is suspected, a detailed history should be obtained with an emphasis on acral enlargement and increases in shoe and hat size. A comparison of earlier photographs may provide helpful clues.

Classic findings on physical examination include frontal bossing, widely spaced teeth, prognathism, hypertension, cardiomegaly, carpal tunnel syndrome, skin tags, hypertrichosis, and increased heel-pad thickness. Patients often have a warm, doughy handshake. Visual field defects also are often present, because the majority of GH-secreting tumors are macroadenomas when diagnosed.

Patients with acromegaly are at increased risk for cardiovascular disease, hypertension, obstructive sleep apnea, and colonic polyps. The presence of skin tags seems to correlate with an increased prevalence of colonic polyps and perhaps an increased risk of colon cancer.

Laboratory Studies. Measuring the IGF-1 level is an excellent way to screen for acromegaly, because patients typically have an elevated level of this growth factor. Measuring the GH level after 100 g of glucose is given orally also is important. Patients with acromegaly often have GH levels that exceed 10 μg/L after a glucose load, whereas individuals without this disorder normally have levels less than 2 μg/L.

Imaging Studies. If laboratory results are suggestive of GH hypersecretion, an MRI with pituitary views should be obtained. In most cases, the tumors are found to be macroadenomas.

Treatment and Prognosis

Trans-sphenoidal adenomectomy is considered first-line therapy for patients with GH-secreting pituitary microadenomas and macroadenomas. After surgery, GH levels may normalize within hours and IGF-1 levels within 1 week. In about 15% of patients who undergo surgery, hypopituitarism develops. The cure rates after trans-sphenoidal resection for microadenomas and macroadenomas are 90% and 50%, respectively. Radiation therapy is often needed in those patients who are not cured by surgery. Acromegaly recurs after several years in about 5% to 10% of patients.

Somatostatin analogues are sometimes given preoperatively to patients with invasive macroadenomas. These agents also can be used for immediate relief of symptoms in patients who are awaiting surgery or have recurrent disease.

Adrenocorticotropic Hormone–secreting Tumors

Excessive secretion of ACTH by the corticotroph cells of the anterior pituitary results in Cushing's disease. The ACTH-secreting adenomas seen in patients with this disease account for about 15% of pituitary tumors. More than 90% of ACTH-secreting adenomas are microadenomas.

Evaluation

The clinical features of patients with Cushing's disease are identical to those of patients with Cushing's syndrome, and the initial steps in the diagnosis of the two are identical. Readers are referred to the section on Cushing's syndrome in Chapter 33 (p. 416) for a discussion of the history, physical examination, and laboratory studies, including a description of the 1-mg overnight dexamethasone suppression test, the low-dose dexamethasone suppression test (LDDST), and other diagnostic studies.

The LDDST is used as a screening tool. If the patient's cortisol level is not suppressed by this test and if the level of free cortisol in a 24-hour urine sample is elevated, the next step is to measure the ACTH level. A suppressed ACTH level is consistent with the diagnosis of non–ACTH-dependent Cushing's syndrome. A normal or elevated ACTH level suggests ACTH-dependent pituitary disease (Cushing's disease), in which case, administration of the high-dose (8-mg) dexamethasone test (HDDST) is helpful. In patients with pituitary tumors, feedback inhibition is maintained, although at a higher set point. Therefore when the HDDST is given, pituitary tumors will demonstrate feedback inhibition with suppressed ACTH production and with serum cortisol levels that decline to less than 50% of baseline.

Treatment and Prognosis

Trans-sphenoidal adenomectomy is the treatment of choice for patients with ACTH-secreting pituitary adenomas. Transient adrenal insufficiency will occur postoperatively and usually requires glucocorticoid-replacement therapy for 1 year.

In patients with microadenomas, the surgical cure rate ranges from 75% to 90%. In those with macroadenomas, surgical failure is more common. If surgery is not successful, a second operation generally results in a 75% cure rate. The mortality rate is less than 1%, and the morbidity rate is low when adenomectomy is performed by experienced surgeons.

Thyroid-Stimulating Hormone–secreting Tumors

TSH-secreting adenomas are exceedingly rare and account for fewer than 1% of pituitary tumors. The majority of TSH-secreting tumors are macroadenomas.

Evaluation

History and Physical Examination. Patients with TSH-secreting tumors are clinically hyperthyroid and therefore show classic signs of thyrotoxicosis, including tachycardia, bounding pulses, diffuse goiter, tremor, hyperreflexia, and warm, moist skin. Unlike patients with Graves' disease, patients with TSH-secreting tumors do not have ophthalmopathy or pretibial myxedema. Because TSH-secreting tumors are usually large, they generally cause visual field defects.

Laboratory Studies. Thyroid-stimulating immunoglobulin (TSI) is not detected in patients with TSH-secreting adenomas. Although TSH is detectable, the level is often less than 10 μU/mL. The TSH is thought to have enhanced bioactivity.

Like patients with pituitary resistance to thyroid hormone, patients with TSH-secreting adenomas have TSH levels that are detectable despite elevated thyroid hormone levels. To differentiate the two conditions, α-subunit levels can be measured. These levels are often markedly elevated in patients with pituitary macroadenomas. However, when the α-subunit levels are analyzed, it is important to consider the gonadal axis of the patient and to keep in mind that FSH, LH, TSH, and hCG all share a common α-subunit. Postmenopausal women have elevated α-subunit levels because of elevated FSH levels.

Imaging Studies. A discrete pituitary adenoma, usually a macroadenoma, can be seen on MRI.

Treatment and Prognosis

Surgical removal of the tumor is considered first-line therapy but achieves a cure in only about 50% of cases. Because many of the tumors are large and locally invasive, complete resection may be dangerous and impractical. The combination of surgery and radiation therapy produces a cure in up to 90% of patients. In addition, adjuvant medical therapy with octreotide, a somatostatin analogue, has been shown to be efficacious in reducing TSH and thyroxine levels.

> **PEARLS FOR THE OR**
>
> The cavernous sinus borders the pituitary gland and contains the internal carotid artery and cranial nerves III, IV, V, and VI.
>
> The blood supply to the pituitary is maintained by the superior and inferior hypophyseal arteries.
>
> The surgical cure rate for a patient with acromegaly due to a macroadenoma is 50%.

Nonfunctioning Pituitary Adenomas

Nonfunctioning pituitary adenomas account for 30% of all pituitary adenomas. The majority of them are of gonadotroph origin and secrete intact gonadotropins and their α and β subunits. The intact gonadotropins are secreted inefficiently, and the α and β subunits are secreted discordantly.

Evaluation

History and Physical Examination. Because nonfunctioning pituitary adenomas do not cause hypersecretory syndromes, they are often not detected until they are large enough to produce symptoms by their mass effects. The two most common complaints are headaches and visual problems. About 60% of patients with nonfunctioning pituitary adenomas have visual field defects, which indicate compression of the optic chiasm. These patients also have manifestations of pituitary insufficiency, which result from compression or destruction of the normal pituitary gland. GH is the first anterior pituitary hormone that is lost as a result of compression or destruction. The next hormones to be lost are gonadotropins, TSH, and ACTH (in that order). In a study of 26 patients with clinically nonfunctioning adenomas, almost all were GH deficient, 96% had central hypogonadism, 81% had secondary hypothyroidism, and 62% had adrenal insufficiency (see Arafah, 1986).

Laboratory and Imaging Studies. In the presence of a pituitary mass found on MRI, an elevated level of intact FSH or free α subunit suggests a nonfunctioning pituitary adenoma. Clearly, in postmenopausal women or patients with primary gonadal failure, these findings are not reliable. The adenoma has to be quite large to interfere with TSH and ACTH secretion.

Treatment and Prognosis

In an asymptomatic patient with a tumor smaller than 10 mm (microadenoma), surgery is not recommended, because the tumor may be an incidentaloma. Instead, observation and follow-up imaging studies are advised to determine whether the tumor is growing.

In a patient with a tumor of 10 mm or more (macroadenoma), trans-sphenoidal surgery performed by an experienced neurosurgeon is the only effective way to reduce the tumor size, alleviate the symptoms caused by mass effects, and suppress the secretion of α subunit. After trans-sphenoidal surgery, vision improves in 70% of patients who had preoperative visual field defects, and manifestations of hypopituitarism also may subside. According to one study, 60% of premenopausal women and 32% of men showed recovery of gonadal function, 57% of patients showed recovery of thyroid function, and 38% of patients showed recovery of adrenal function.

Close postoperative observation is advised, because about 15% of tumors will recur within 5 or 6 years. Postsurgical MRI scans are recommended at 1-year intervals for 5 years and at 2-year intervals thereafter.

Craniopharyngiomas

Craniopharyngiomas account for 3% to 5% of all intracranial neoplasms and are derived from remnants of Rathke's pouch. Most craniopharyngiomas are suprasellar, but 15% are intrasellar. The tumors primarily affect children, although a bimodal distribution occurs, with an early peak between the ages of 5 and 10 years, and a second (smaller) peak between the ages of 50 and 60 years. In most cases, the tumors contain calcium, are cystic or partially cystic, and are lined with squamous epithelium.

Evaluation

History and Physical Examination. Children often are first seen with signs of increased intracranial pressure, including headache, vomiting, and papilledema secondary to hydrocephalus. About 60% have visual field defects. Manifestations of hypopituitarism include short stature (in 10% to 20% of patients), delayed sexual development (in 20%), and diabetes insipidus.

About 80% of adults have visual complaints, and often an additional 10% will have visual field abnormalities evident on formal visual field testing. Headaches and personality changes are commonly reported, with an incidence of 40% and 25%, respectively. Manifestations of pituitary insufficiency include hypogonadism (in 35%), hyperprolactinemia (in 30%), and diabetes insipidus (in 15%). In rare cases, aseptic meningitis occurs secondary to leakage of cyst contents into the cerebrospinal fluid.

Imaging and Other Studies. Calcification in a granular or curvilinear pattern is usually evident on lateral skull films or computed tomography scans. Perform a complete assessment of the hypothalamic-pituitary axis, as often hypofunction of one or more hormones is found. Blood should be sent for FSH, LH, either testosterone or estradiol (depending on the sex of the patient), TSH, free T_4, cortisol, and prolactin levels. Consider an insulin tolerance test.

PEARLS FOR ROUNDS

Prolactin levels associated with a prolactinoma are usually greater than 100 ng/mL.

Medical therapy with a dopamine agonist (bromocriptine or cabergoline) is the preferred treatment for prolactinomas.

Measuring the insulin-like growth factor (IGF-1) level is the best screening test for acromegaly.

Trans-sphenoidal adenomectomy is the preferred first-line therapy for patients with acromegaly.

Treatment and Prognosis

Complete surgical resection is not always possible, and when it is done, it sometimes results in major functional deficits. A more conservative approach is often taken and involves limited resection followed by radiation therapy. The risk of radiation damage to the hypothalamus, pituitary, and optic nerve is relatively low after conventional fractionated radiation (doses to total of 4500 rad). Visual impairment ranges between 1% and 1.5%. A common deficit seen regardless of treatment modality is mild impairment in manual dexterity. The intelligence quotients of the surgical and radiotherapy groups remain within normal limits.

Central Diabetes Insipidus in Postoperative Patients

Central diabetes insipidus develops in about 5% of patients who have undergone trans-sphenoidal surgery. About 50% of affected patients experience a spontaneous resolution of the condition within a few days, and 30% have unremitting diabetes insipidus. The remaining 20% demonstrate a triphasic response that is associated with injury of the pituitary stalk. In phase 1, polyuria has an abrupt onset and persists for a few days. In phase 2, symptoms of the syndrome of inappropriate antidiuretic hormone (SIADH) begin. This is because acute injury and impaired blood flow to the pituitary stalk cause the posterior pituitary to become necrotic and release its stored vasopressin in an uncontrolled manner. The SIADH phase lasts for 5 to 10 days, during which time the patient's water intake should be carefully controlled. In phase 3, when the posterior pituitary is depleted of all ADH, permanent diabetes insipidus ensues.

In patients who have undergone trans-sphenoidal surgery, the fluid intake and output should be carefully monitored, and the serum and urine osmolality levels should be checked every 12 hours. The diagnosis of diabetes insipidus is made if the serum osmolality is more than 300 mOsm but the urine osmolality is less than 100 mOsm. Initially, a single dose of desmopressin should be given parenterally, and the urinary output should be carefully monitored. Every 24 hours, desmopressin should temporarily be withheld, because in 50% of cases, the diabetes insipidus will be transient, and in 20% of cases, it may transition into SIADH as part of the triphasic response.

Suggested Reading

Arafah BM: Reversible hypopituitarism in patients with large nonfunctioning pituitary adenomas. J Clin Endocrinol Metab 62(6):1173–1179, 1986.

Biller BK, Daniels GH: Neuroendocrine regulation and diseases of the anterior pituitary and hypothalamus. In Fauci AS, Braunwald E, Isselbacher KJ, et al (eds): Harrison's Principles of Internal Medicine, 14th ed. New York, McGraw Hill, 1998, pp 1972–1999.

Freda PU, Wardlaw SL: Clinical review 110: Diagnosis and treatment of pituitary tumors. J Clin Encrinol Metab 84(11):3859–3866, 1999.

Shimon H, Melmed S: Management of pituitary adenomas. Ann Intern Med 129:472–481, 1999.

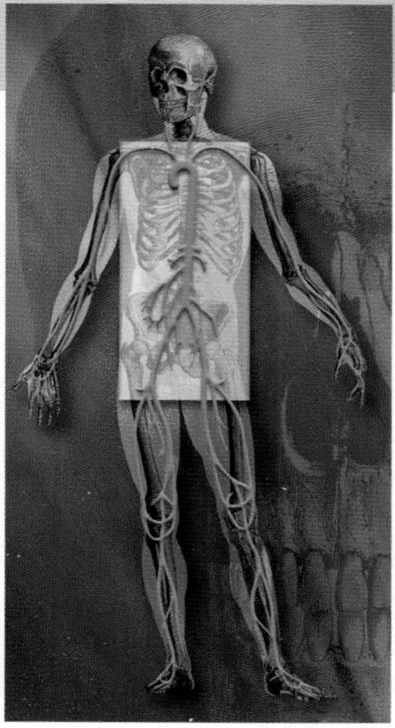

SECTION IX

VASCULAR

Chapter 35

Lymphatic and Venous Systems

NANCY L. CANTELMO, MD, and JAMES O. MENZOIAN, MD

Lymphatic System

The primary functions of the lymphatic system are the transport of proteins and fluid from the extracellular space into the venous system and the removal of bacteria and foreign materials. Failure of this system results in lymphedema, manifested by swelling and skin changes. Lymphedema has been a difficult management problem for physicians for a number of reasons. The lymphatic system is not readily seen and not easily imaged. The signs of lymphedema usually take years to develop, and the problem is difficult to treat. Recently increased interest has been seen in lymphedema, generated by new insights into its pathophysiology and further experience with treatment of this difficult problem.

Anatomy

The three major components of the lymphatic system are the capillaries, the collecting vessels, and the lymph nodes. The specialized lymph capillaries differ from vascular capillaries in three ways: the lymphatic endothelial junctions are both open and closed, their basement membrane is very scant or absent, and anchoring fibers hold the lymphatic capillaries open, in the face of higher interstitial pressure.

The lymphatic channels are composed of three layers, as in the vascular system: adventitia, media with smooth muscle, and intima. These channels also contain valves, but more numerous than those in the venous system. Lymphatic channels accompany the venous system in almost all parts of the body, except the central nervous and the skeletal systems. In the lower extremity, a superficial lymphatic system is found on the medial side of the leg and a deep subfascial system, with little communication between the two. The lymph channels from the lower extremities and intestines converge to form the cysterna chyli, adjacent to the aorta, and enter the bloodstream by way of the thoracic duct near the junction of the left subclavian and jugular veins. Lymph from the left upper extremity and left head and neck joins the thoracic duct, whereas the right upper extremity and right side of the head and neck drain into the venous system in a number of right thoracic ducts.

The lymphatic organs, concerned with filtration and immunologic function, consist of lymph nodes interspersed at various sites along the lymphatic channels, the spleen, the thymus, and tonsils. The microscopic anatomy of a lymph node consists of several afferent channels bringing lymph into the node along the convex upper surface. The lymph percolates through the inner nodal sinus and exits from the hilum via a single efferent channel. About 500 to 1000 nodes are found in the human lymphatic system and are generally not palpable in the healthy state.

Physiology

The lymphatic system acts as a fine tuner of the microenvironment of the capillaries and interstitial space. The regulation of fluids and proteins between the vascular, lymphatic, and interstitial systems is based on the hydrostatic and oncotic pressures of the various compartments. The net efflux of fluid from the vascular capillaries normally exceeds the net influx from the interstitial space. The lymphatic system removes this excess fluid from the interstitial space in the balance of the normal physiologic state.

Lymphatic fluid is propelled cephalad toward its connections to the venous system by the intrinsic contractions of the lymph channels. The numerous valves present in the channels maintain the position of the lymph on its ascent. Although other forces such as muscular contraction, coughing, and straining contribute somewhat, it is primarily the intrinsic contractions that serve to move the lymphatic fluid. In contradistinction to the vascular system, the lymphatic macrosystem is not filled with a constant column of lymph. Approximately 2 to 2.5 L/day is transported through the lymphatic system. A direct relation exists between the force of the intrinsic contractions and the volume of lymph in the system.

A dynamic process exists whereby the interstitial space is nourished by the various molecules and respiratory gases as they travel from the vascular and into the lymphatic system. The special structure of the lymphatic capillary wall with its scant basement membrane and endothelial cell gaps permits the entry of cells and protein molecules into the lymphatics. A large proportion of intravascular proteins are thought to circulate each day through this blood/interstitial space/lymphatic continuum. The specific protein content of lymphatic fluid varies with its location; extremity lymph may be relatively low in protein (0.5 g/dL), whereas postprandial lymph along the intestines may be visibly white with chylomicrons containing fat and protein.

The lymphatic organs filter and collect bacteria, foreign proteins, and cells. The complex process of immunoreactivity is initiated, as macrophages, lymphoid cells, chemoattractants, and growth and necrotic factors intermingle.

In addition to acting as a filtering waystation on the lymphatic transport system, nodes may also impede the flow of lymph. When nodes are swollen with fluid or cells, atrophic, or absent, lymph flow may be obstructed, back up into the tissue, and cause lymphedema.

Pathophysiology

The accumulation of fluid in the interstitial spaces is called *edema*. Venous hypertension from obstruction or valvular incompetence causes localized edema as interstitial fluid floods the interstitial spaces, and a similar backup occurs on a larger scale with cardiac failure. Impedance to flow in the lymphatic system along with an accumulation of edema fluid laden with protein causes a condition called *lymphedema*. Protein-rich interstitial fluid, containing more than 1.5 g/dL, is characteristic of lymphatic obstruction, as compared with fluid of other etiologies, which contains typically less than 1.0 g/dL of protein.

The disruption of lymphatic flow and the development of refractory edema are the hallmarks of chronic lymphedema. This edema is nonpitting and brawny in nature.

Lymphedema may be caused by developmental abnormalities of the lymph vessels or acquired obstruction of the lymphatic system. Causes of obstruction may be infection, tumor invasion, trauma, surgical excision, or irradiation.

Clinical Classifications

Primary Lymphedema

Primary lymphedema is divided into *congenital* (onset before age 1 year), either nonfamilial or familial (Milroy disease), and *praecox* (onset from ages 1 to 35 years), also with subgroups of nonfamilial and familial (Meige disease). A third division of primary lymphedema is called *tarda* (onset after age 35 years).

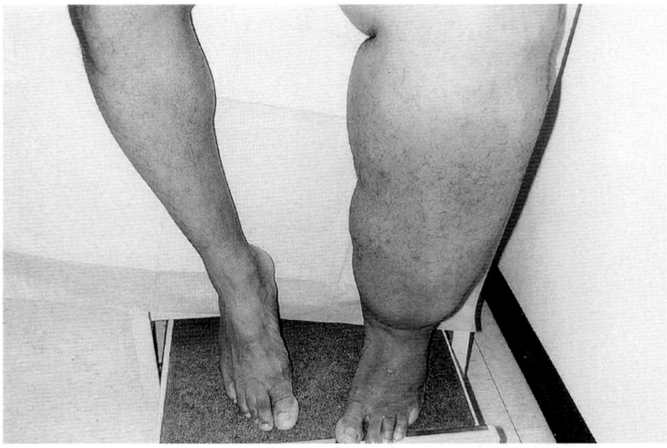

FIGURE 35–1 A 30-year-old man with lymphedema involving his left lower extremity.

Primary lymphedema is rare and occurs most frequently in girls. It has been further anatomically characterized into distal obliteration (80% of cases and usually bilateral), proximal obliteration (10% of cases and usually unilateral), and congenital hyperplasia (10%, mostly bilateral and greater in male than in female patients).

Secondary Lymphedema

Obstructive injury to the lymphatic system is the cause of secondary acquired lymphedema. In Europe and North America, the most common cause is surgical excision and irradiation, as part of cancer therapy. Worldwide, the most frequent cause is the parasitic infection, filariasis. Other causes include infection from bacteria or fungi, tumor invading the lymphatics or lymphoproliferative disease, and lymphedema secondary to trauma. Figure 35-1 shows a patient with chronic lymphedema.

Clinical Presentation and Differential Diagnosis

The causes of extremity edema can be divided into systemic or regional. The systemic etiologies include major system failures, such as cardiac, renal, or hepatic, as well as hypoproteinemia and hypothyroid myxedema. In addition to lymphedema, other regional causes of edema include acute venous thrombophlebitis, chronic venous insufficiency, congenital vascular malformation, and arteriovenous fistula. Infection, drug dependence, and trauma, including snake or insect bites, are included in the differential diagnosis.

As in the approach to all clinical problems, a careful history and physical examination are the cornerstones of diagnosis. A family history of extremity edema may suggest a familial lymphedema. A teenage girl with no other apparent cause of edema may have a primary lymphedema. History of travel to a tropical area may lead to a diagnosis of secondary lymphedema.

The hallmark of the clinical diagnosis is a painless swelling of the leg that is slow to develop. Swelling usually starts distally, involving the ankles, and causes a "tree-trunk" appearance. Edema of the dorsum of the foot produces a characteristic "buffalo hump." Squaring of the toes is identified as *Stemmer's sign*. As the disease progresses and is more chronic, the edema assumes a nonpitting characteristic due to fibrosis of the tissues.

Skin of chronic lymphedema has a "pigskin" appearance. Superficial excoriation and chronic dermatitis are common, but ulcers are rare, in contrast to a venous hypertensive etiology. Small, draining vesicles and a wartlike character to the skin of a patient may be seen with chronic lymphedema. Frequent complications include bacterial or fungal infections. Rarely, chronic long-standing lymphedema develops into a lymphangiosarcoma.

Diagnostic Tools

After a complete history and performing a physical examination, the direction of further investigation is usually suggested. Routine laboratory tests will be helpful in consideration of systemic etiologies. If a local cause of systemic swelling is not indicated, additional tests may be needed. Because venous hypertension is more common than lymphatic disease, tests such as duplex Doppler insonation will usually make the diagnosis of venous insufficiency or obstruction. Computed tomography (CT) is useful in the evaluation of malignancy, and magnetic resonance imaging (MRI) is helpful in the diagnosis of vascular malformation.

The most widely used test in the evaluation of lymphedema is lymphoscintigraphy. The test is performed on a supine patient, who receives a web-space injection of a radiocolloid. The patient exercises the extremity, and a gamma camera is used to image the patient over a number of hours. A normal lymphoscintogram (Fig. 35-2) will essentially rule out the diagnosis of lymphedema. The lymphoscintigraphic patterns of primary and secondary lymphedema may be similar, including delay in lymph transit and abnormal distribution. An abnormal study also may be obtained in patients with chronic venous insufficiency due to either venous or lymphatic edema.

Contrast lymphangiography is a study rarely used since the development of lymphoscintigraphy. It involves the direct cannulation of a lymph channel, or, more commonly, the subepidermal injection of contrast material and conventional radiographic imaging. This technique provides a more detailed visualization of the lymphatic channels, especially in the body cavities (Fig. 35-3)

Nonoperative Management of Chronic Lymphedema

The goal of treatment in chronic lymphedema is reduction of the size of the involved extremity. In more than 90% of cases, this may be achieved with conservative, nonoperative management. If treatment is begun early in the course of the disease, it may be possible to reduce the limb to its normal size. After the fibrosis of chronic lymphedema is established, reduction to normal size is rarely possible, but major improvement is usually achievable.

A program of complex physical therapy has remained the mainstay of treatment for much of the world. The components of such treatment consist of elevation, specialized massage, called manual lymphatic drainage (MLD), wrapping, exercise, and meticulous skin care. Another treatment, particularly in the United States, is the use of specialized sequential pumps to reduce the edema fluid from the extremity.

During the course of therapy and after the treatment goal has been achieved, support systems must be used continuously to maintain limb size in the ambulatory or upright patient. One type of support is elastic graduated-support stockings, in which the pressure is greatest distally and lessens proximally. These stockings are available in various sizes, are fitted to the specific patient, and are available in various lengths. Another method of compression consists of the nonelastic support of a device with Velcro straps, which maintain the compressive pressure on the extremity and may be easier to apply than the elastic stockings for some patients.

Operative Management of Chronic Lymphedema

Excisional Surgery

Nonoperative treatment is the therapy of choice and helpful to the vast majority of patients, but a very small number may require operative management if conservative therapy fails. The most effective and long-lasting surgical procedure for chronic lymphedema is staged subcutaneous excision between flaps. This is performed in two parts, first on the medial side, and 3 months later on the lateral side of the extremity. It consists of raising flaps and removing the subcutaneous tissue below the flaps, with excision of some redundant skin and closure of the wounds. After a postoperative course of bed rest, elevation, and suction drainage, elastic stockings are used on a regular basis when the patient is ambulatory.

Two other techniques have been used in the past but have not proven as effective. Total subcutaneous excision also is known as the Charles procedure. It involves cutaneous and subcutaneous excision with skin-graft closure of the extremity. The result of this very extensive excision may sometimes be cosmetically inferior to the original appearance of the leg.

A buried dermis flap also is called the Thompson procedure; it seeks to provide an excisional as well as physiologic solution to the difficult problem of chronic lymphedema. Tissue is resected between flaps, and, in addition, part of the flap is de-epithelialized and buried in

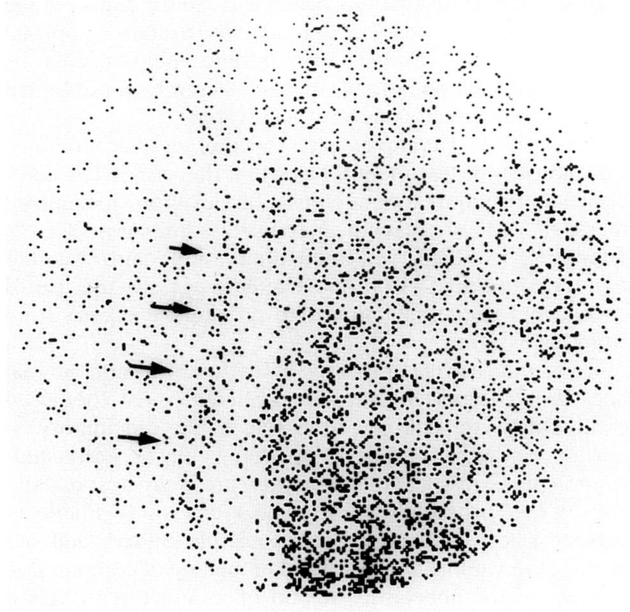

A

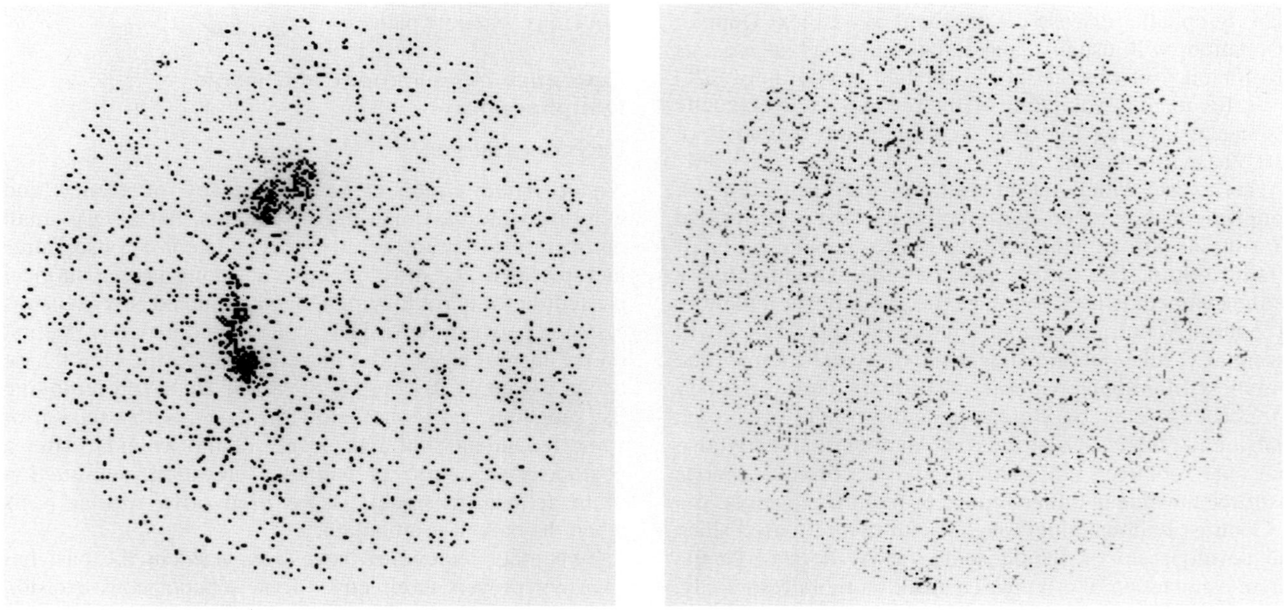

B

FIGURE 35–2 Lymphoscintogram of the patient in Fig. 35-1. Radioactive ^{99m}Tc-sulphur colloid is injected intradermally into the dorsum of each foot at the base of the first and second toes. Images are then obtained at various levels of the extremities. *A*, A well-formed lymphatic channel in the right extremity (*arrows*), abnormal flaring of the lymphatics in the left extremity, and no well-defined lymphatic channel. *B*, Well-defined radioactive uptake in the lymph nodes in the right groin, but no concentration of radioactivity in the left groin.

the muscle in an effort to establish lymphatic connections in the muscle. These connections have not been clearly demonstrated, and it is thought the excisional portion if the surgical procedure is responsible in large part for successful results.

Lymphatic Reconstruction

The more recently developed microvascular techniques have led surgeons to attempt direct lymphatic anastomosis with two kinds of procedures. One surgical technique

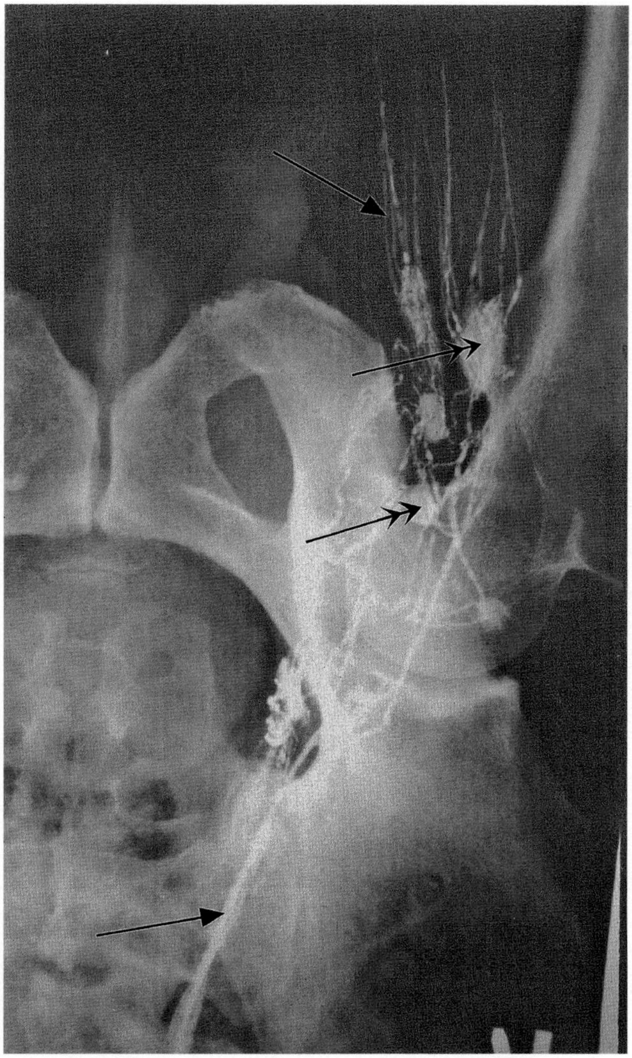

FIGURE 35–3 This is a normal lymphangiogram, showing lymphatic channels (*single arrows*) and lymph nodes (*double arrows*).

involves ipsilateral thigh lymphatic-to-saphenous vein anastomoses on one extremity in an attempt to drain the lymph locally directly into the venous system in the thigh. Another surgical procedure involves the cross-pelvis lympholymphatic anastomosis of lymphatic channels from one involved leg to those of a normal leg for the treatment of unilateral lymphedema. These procedures are technically demanding, and results have been difficult to assess.

Indirect techniques also have been described; they attempt to provide lymphatic drainage, without using direct anastomosis of lymphatic channels. In an attempt to provide drainage to affected lymph nodes, ileum (denuded of its mucosa) or omentum is sewn over the transected nodes. These procedures remain unproven in their efficacy.

In all of the treatment techniques described for this difficult and disabling disease, the result remains palliation, not cure. Although the majority of patients will benefit from conservative and nonoperative treatment, a few patients will require surgical procedures. Further investigation is needed to develop more efficacious and more widely applicable surgical techniques for the treatment of chronic lymphedema.

Venous System

The veins in the lower extremities consist of a superficial system and a deep system, connected by a communicating system of veins called *perforator veins* (Fig. 35-4).

The Superficial System of Veins

The venous system begins at the cutaneous microcirculation, where it can be differentiated from the arterial system by the ultrastructure of the walls. A parallel network of arterioles and venules is present in the papillary dermis, from which capillary loops arise and connect to the postcapillary vessels in the deeper layers of the dermis and fat. Venules in the deep layer of the skin drain into small veins of the foot and are the first vessels in which valves can be identified.

In the lower extremity, the superficial venous system consists of a large number of cutaneous and subcutaneous veins. These veins run between the skin and fat and are known as the *saphenous veins*. The greater saphenous vein originates from the dorsal arch and medial marginal veins of the foot. The vein then curves medially and ascends in the leg 2 cm from the edge of the tibia. Accompanied by the saphenous nerve, it crosses the knee in a more superficial plane and continues in a straight course to enter the femoral canal at the fossa ovalis, 2 to 4 cm lateral and to 1 to 2 cm below the tubercle of the symphysis pubis. Duplication of the greater saphenous vein occurs in 10% to 37% of the population, with the two limbs often joining in the thigh within 10 cm of the knee joint. Occasionally the greater saphenous vein will not terminate at the femoral vein but will continue beyond it, crossing the inguinal ligament to terminate in a cutaneous vein.

The lesser saphenous vein originates from the lateral marginal vein and runs between the lateral malleolus and the Achilles tendon. It ascends in the leg in the subcutaneous tissues and enters the deep fascia at varying levels in the leg. Its most distal portion is subcutaneous and is subject to varicose formation. It travels in close proximity to the sural nerve and enters the popliteal vein between the two heads of the gastrocnemius muscle, usually 3 cm above the popliteal fossa. The lesser saphenous vein may join the superficial femoral vein in the thigh, or it may communicate with the greater saphenous vein in the midthigh or at the level of the knee.

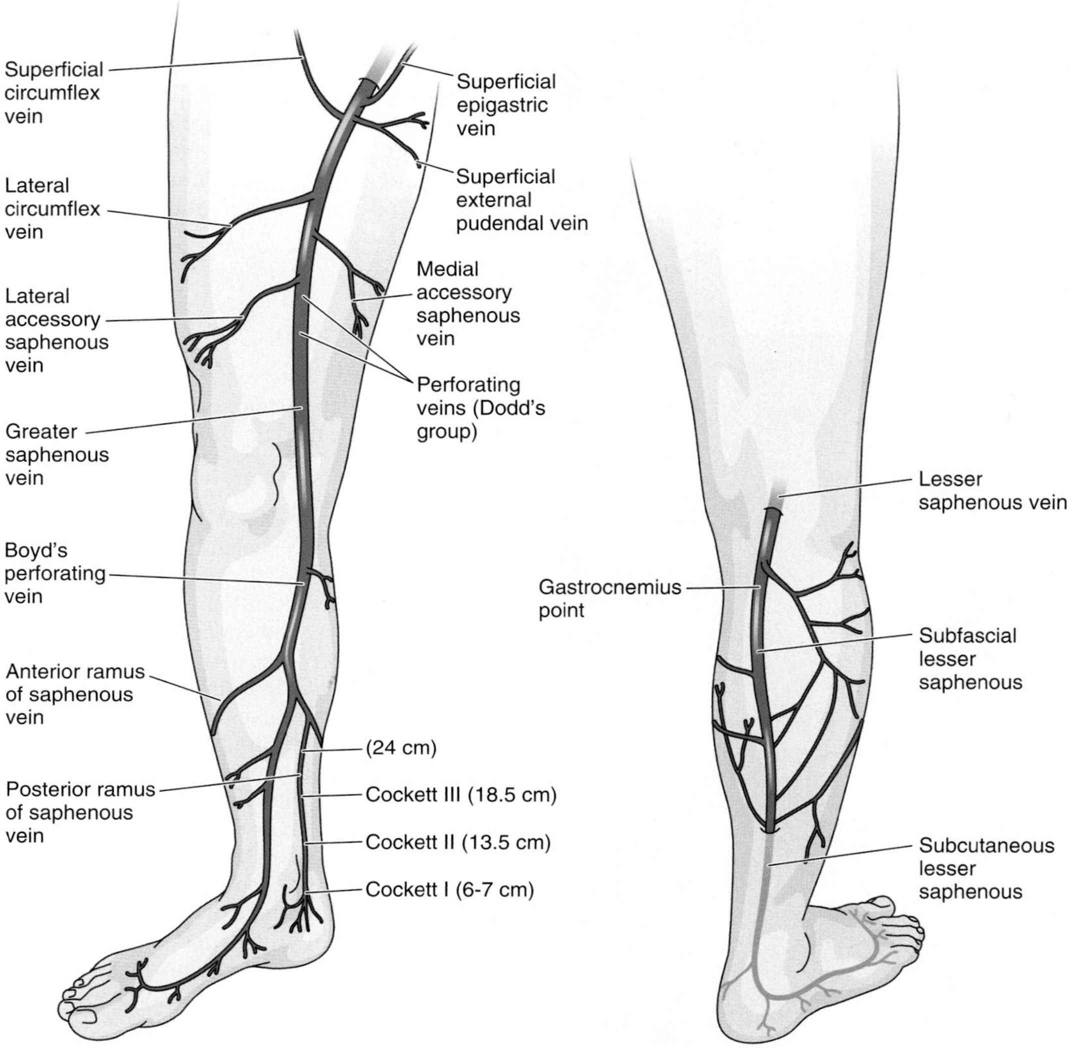

FIGURE 35–4 The normal anatomy of the superficial and perforator veins of the lower extremity.

The Deep System of Veins

The deep system starts with the intermetatarsal veins, which unite in the foot to form the deep plantar arch. Three separate veins emerge from the dorsal arch. The anterior tibial vein arises from the dorsal arch and runs medial to the hallucis longus extensor to enter the leg under the flexor retinaculum. The posterior tibial vein is formed by the junction of the medial and lateral plantar veins; it crosses the ankle inferior to the medial malleolus. The peroneal vein forms at the level of the lateral malleolus from the junction of the anterior and posterior tibial veins.

The deep veins of the leg emerge from the foot as two or three vena comitantes, with various ramifications, traveling with the arteries bearing the same name. They unite proximally into single trunks, which join at different levels. The anterior tibial vein forms the popliteal vein, which ascends behind the knee and then joins the common tibioperoneal trunk, most often as a double system of veins. In the thigh, the popliteal vein drains into the superficial vein at the adductor canal and travels posterior to the artery, not uncommonly as a double system. It is joined below the inguinal ligament by the deep femoral or profunda femoral vein, which drains the muscles of the thigh. As it crosses the inguinal ligament, it becomes the external iliac vein and receives many branches from the deep iliac circumflex, the epigastric, and the obturator veins. The internal iliac vein joins it to form the common iliac vein, which joins its

PEARLS FOR ROUNDS

The lymphatics are a unidirectional, closed-loop system, which returns fluid and protein that have traveled from the vascular capillaries into the interstitial space and back to the venous system. The thoracic duct of the lymphatic system enters the vascular system at the junction of the left subclavian and jugular veins. A number of lymphatic ducts enter the venous system on the right side.

Primary lymphedema is characterized as congenital (younger than 1 year at onset), praecox (1–35 years), or tarda (older than 35 years). Secondary lymphedema is the result of obliterative cancer therapy in Europe and North America and most commonly is caused by filariasis worldwide.

Duplex ultrasonography can provide both anatomic and physiologic information relevant to venous function. It is the most widely used modality to evaluate the venous system and to determine treatment.

counterpart from the other leg to form the inferior vena cava. The left iliac vein is longer and often compressed by the right iliac artery against the fifth lumbar vertebra, often forming adhesive bands that may contribute to a higher incidence of thrombosis on the left side.

The Perforating Veins

The perforating veins provide a communication between the deep and superficial systems in the leg. Some connect the superficial veins directly to the posterior tibial vein on the medial aspect of the leg (Fig. 35-5). Others are indirect perforators connecting the superficial and deep system through muscular veins. To reach the deep veins, the perforators must pierce the deep fascia of the leg. During their intrafascial course, the perforators take a horizontal or slightly upward course. This anatomic relation between the perforating veins and the fascia may play a role for normal emptying of perforating veins into the deep system.

Physiology

The venous system in the lower extremity has the function of returning blood to the heart against gravity and serving as a capacitance reservoir capable of storing varying amounts of blood, as dictated by posture and systemic hemodynamic considerations. This active system requires energy. Contractions of calf muscles eject and propel blood into the thigh and pelvis and eventually to the heart, facilitated by abdominal and thoracic musculature. Bicuspid valves are present in all three venous systems. These valves ensure forward flow, prevent reflux, and are essential for normal venous function.

Venous Hemodynamics

The propulsive energy required for blood flow in the veins of the lower extremity is imparted by several muscular pumps: the heart, the muscles of the leg and foot, and the

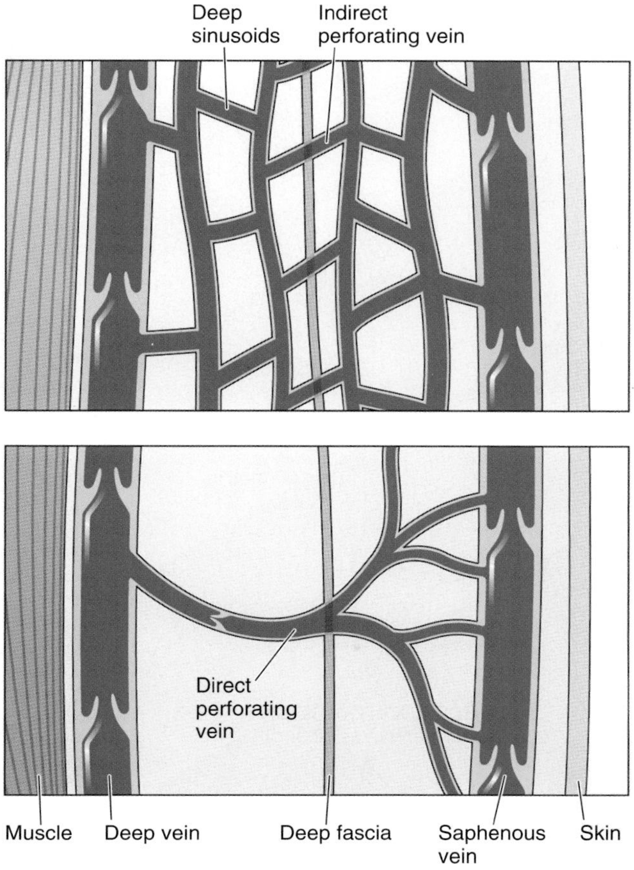

FIGURE 35–5 The perforator venous system.

thoracoabdominal muscles. The pumping action of the heart generates the energy to deliver blood to all body organs, including the lower extremities. It also provides some of the energy required to return the blood to the heart (referred to as "vis-a-tergo"). The contraction of foot and leg muscles also provides energy for venous return and helps propel blood into the thigh and pelvis (Fig. 35-6). In addition, excursion of the abdominal and thoracic walls during breathing creates pressure gradients between the chest and abdomen and generates energy (vis-a-fronte), which further facilitates the flow of blood into the right side of the heart.

Venous Pressures

Venous pressures are influenced by several interacting factors, including the extent to which the vein is filled, vasomotor tone, posture, and muscle activity. When partially collapsed, veins are able to accommodate a relatively large volume of blood with minimal change in venous pressure. The ability of the venous system to adjust its capacitance in response to changes in systemic hemodynamics or pharmacologic alterations in vascular tone provides an

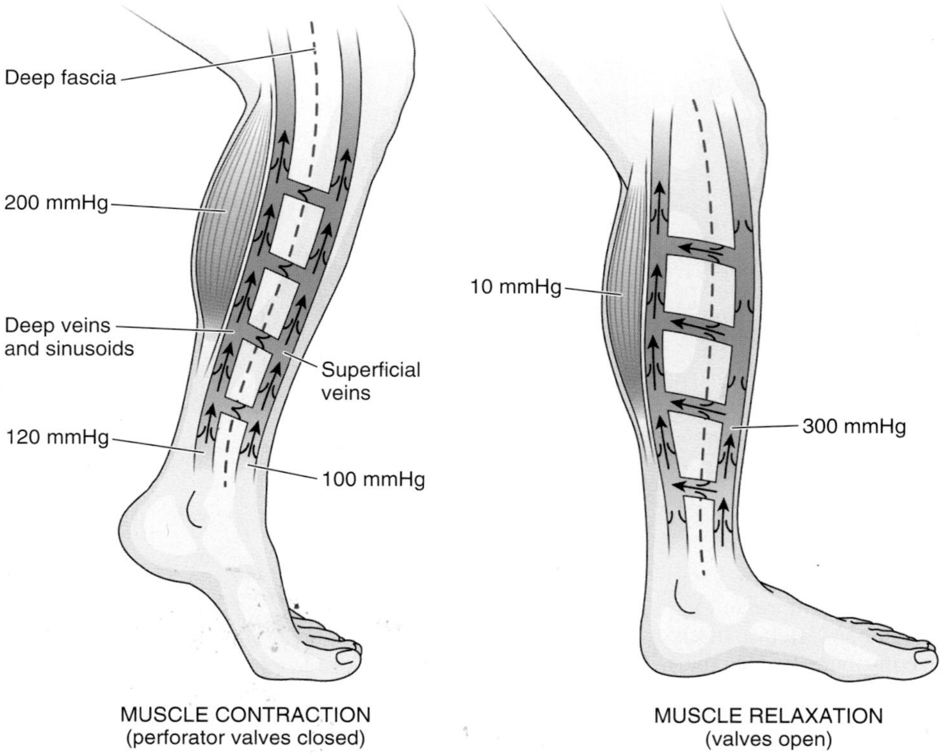

FIGURE 35–6 The action of the calf-muscle pump and venous flow during calf-muscle contraction and muscle relaxation.

important buffer function during manipulation of cardiac preload and filling pressures.

In the supine position, the net driving energy generates a venous pressure that averages 10 to 15 mmHg at the ankle and 0 to 5 mmHg at the level of the right atrium. When one assumes the upright position, about 250 mL of blood shifts into each of the two lower extremities, and the calf volume increases by 2% to 3%. As blood fills the veins, the hydrostatic pressure generated by the weight of the column of blood increases, and venous pressure at the ankles increases to 50 to 70 mmHg in the sitting position and 90 to 110 mmHg in the standing position.

The Calf Muscle Pump

In the standing position, the energy required to return blood to the heart from the leg is substantial. When standing still, this energy is supplied solely by the dynamic pressure generated by the heart (vis-á-tergo) and thoracoabdominal muscles (vis-á-fronte). With ambulation, venous return is greatly facilitated by the pumping action of the muscles in the foot and calf. Contraction of the muscles in the calf exerts pressure up to 200 mmHg on the intramuscular veins in that compartment. With this pressure, blood is squeezed out of the soleus/gastrocnemius sinusoids and deep veins and propelled into the tibial veins. In addition, the contractions of the leg muscles continue to propel the blood up the leg. With muscle contraction, the venous valves open to allow blood to flow up the leg. The valves in the perforating veins close to prevent blood from being propelled backward into the superficial system.

During muscle relaxation, pressure in the muscular compartments decreases, allowing blood flow from the capillaries and deep veins into the soleus sinusoids. Valves in the perforating veins open, and blood flows out of the superficial system into the deep system. With a single step, pressure in the saphenous vein decreases to about 45 mmHg, and within 20 to 30 seconds, a return is seen to the starting pressure of 80 to 90 mmHg. After 8 to 10 contractions of the calf muscles, most of the venous blood is evacuated from the leg, and venous pressure at the ankle decreases to about 20 mmHg. This is referred to the ambulatory venous pressure (AVP). Failure of the AVP to remain low is referred to as *venous hypertension* and is thought to be the underlying hemodynamic abnormality leading to chronic venous insufficiency.

Clinical Testing of the Venous System

The two major abnormalities of the venous system that can lead to clinical problems are venous valvular insufficiency and venous obstruction. Venous insufficiency can be either from some congenital abnormality causing valvular incompetence or from previous deep venous thrombosis (DVT)

PEARLS FOR THE OR

The treatment of choice for chronic lymphedema is conservative and nonsurgical, consisting of elevation, massage, compression, exercise, and skin care. Surgical procedures are rarely performed.

The venous system is composed of three anatomic parts: deep veins and superficial veins, as related to muscle fascia, and perforating veins, which connect these two systems.

Most patients with chronic venous insufficiency and venous ulcers have a mixture of superficial, deep, and perforating vein incompetence.

resulting in valvular incompetence. Previous DVT also can cause venous obstruction by fibrosis of the involved vein. Four methods of studying venous hemodynamics exist: (1) direct measurements of venous pressure, (2) contrast venography, (3) plethysmography, and (4) duplex ultrasound evaluation, the most commonly used modality.

Ambulatory Venous Pressure

The oldest method of assessing AVP involves the placement of a needle in a vein on the dorsum of the foot and connecting it to a pressure transducer. Pressures are then recorded with the patient in an upright position and then during various maneuvers, such as doing tiptoes in place to mimic walking. If the calf-muscle pump is functioning and if no valvular incompetence or venous obstruction exists, the venous pressure should decrease. The AVP is the lowest pressure achieved after exercise. This test has the disadvantage of being an invasive procedure and has been largely replaced with newer noninvasive methods.

Ascending and Descending Venography

X-ray–opaque contrast material can be injected directly into the venous system while radiographic images are obtained. This provides good anatomic detail and also can be used to assess the presence of venous valvular incompetence. If contrast is injected into the common femoral vein, and the patient is in an upright position, the contrast, which is heavy, will fall to the level of the first competent venous valve. The degree to which the contrast column falls can be a measure of the degree of valvular incompetence. Direct contrast venography is helpful, but again is less used and has been largely replaced by noninvasive techniques.

Plethysmography

This method is a measure of changes in blood volume. It can be performed in a variety of ways including air-plethysmography, strain-gauge plethysmography, and photo-plethysmography. Each of these methods has the ability to measure changes in blood volume, either at a small point in the skin (photo) or as a change in blood volume of the calf in response to a variety of maneuvers such as calf contractions, leg elevation, and leg dependence while recording changes in blood volume. These methods are accurate, quantitative, noninvasive, and can provide useful information about venous valvular function and venous obstruction.

Duplex Ultrasound

This is currently the most widely used method to assess venous function. Duplex scanning combines Doppler with B-mode ultrasound, making it possible to visualize veins and simultaneously to assess their degree of reflux. By using a variety of maneuvers including the Trendelenburg position, the Valsalva maneuver, and manual compression, one can accurately quantitate venous reflux in the deep, superficial, and perforating systems and determine velocity and direction of blood flow. Duplex ultrasound also can provide very accurate assessment of venous obstruction and DVT.

Diseases of the Venous System

Varicose Veins

Varicose veins are distended, elongated, tortuous superficial veins with incompetent valves. They are called primary varicose veins when they develop spontaneously without antecedent history of DVT. Primary varicose veins tend to be familial and involve predominantly the greater saphenous vein and its tributaries. Secondary varicose veins usually occur as a result of DVT. The prevalence of varicose veins is in the range of 20% to 70% among adults in industrialized nations but appears to be less prevalent in less technologically advanced populations. The prevalence is generally higher in women and increases with age. Varicose veins are associated with parity, family history of varicose veins, obesity, sedentary lifestyle, and occupations requiring prolonged sitting or standing.

Pathological evaluations of varicose veins reveal that the collagen content of primary varicose veins is less than that of normal veins. This results in a disruption of the normal architecture of the vein wall and produces disorganization of the smooth muscle layer. Primary varicose veins show no evidence of infection or signs of antecedent thrombophlebitis. When secondary varicose veins occur after DVT, fibroblasts, mast cells, and polymorphonuclear leukocytes invade the wall, and the occluded lumen is usually restored by a combination of thrombus retraction and recanalization.

Pathophysiology of Varicose Veins. Many theories exist as to the etiology of varicose veins, but none appear to offer the complete story. Numerous studies have demonstrated that a variety of factors may be causative, such as biochemical, epidemiologic, genetic, and anatomic factors, but it seems plausible that the pathogenesis is multifactorial. Perhaps genetic factors establish the potential for developing varicose veins, while subsequent events and exposures to other factors dictate their occurrence and severity. Primary biochemical or anatomic abnormalities in the vein wall may provide a necessary but not solely sufficient condition for the evolution of varicosities. Subsequently, other factors, some of which are related to lifestyle, may trigger the formation of varicose veins.

Evaluation and Treatment of Varicose Veins. Patients with varicose veins usually complain of pain or are concerned about the cosmetic effect of their varicose veins. The pain is usually described as a heavy, achy feeling, especially in warm weather, at the end of the day, or in association with the menstrual period. The pain is usually due to pronounced venodilatation. Many have relief from their symptoms with the use of elastic support stockings. It is important for the stockings to be custom fitted with graduated compression, measured in mmHg, with higher compression distally. Ill-fitting stockings with inadequate compression are uncomfortable, and patients usually abandon their use. Devices are available to help patients put on stockings, such as zippers or Velcro, which may enhance compliance.

Significant and symptomatic varicose veins should be evaluated with duplex ultrasound. This test should evaluate all three venous systems. The patency and valvular competency of the deep system is determined. The greater and lesser saphenous veins are then evaluated for patency and for the presence of significant valvular reflux along the course of the vein and at the junction with the deep system at the saphenofemoral or saphenopopliteal junction. The presence of valvular reflux with reversal of flow in the perforating veins also is determined.

If one of the major axial superficial veins, the greater or lesser saphenous, is found to have valvular incompetence, surgery is usually the treatment of choice. The surgical options include (1) removal of the saphenous vein, with ligation of major branches at the junction with the deep system, called stripping and ligation; (2) ligation of the lesser saphenous vein at the saphenopopliteal junction; and (3) endovenous ablation of the greater and/or lesser saphenous vein by using radiofrequency or laser energy. The newer endovenous procedure involves percutaneous introduction of the catheter distally into the saphenous vein under ultrasound guidance, gradually pulling the energized catheter back so as to injure the venous intima, which will eventually close the vein to venous blood flow. This often can be a less-invasive procedure than stripping and ligation.

If the axial saphenous veins have competent valves and are without reflux by duplex examination, the symptomatic branch varicosities may be surgically removed, leaving the saphenous veins intact. These branches may be removed by small incisions over the veins with serial removal (phlebectomy) or by subcutaneous excision with a powered device and transillumination of the veins through the skin.

Sclerotherapy injection is another technique to obliterate blood flow through smaller, nonaxial veins. A number of sclerosant solutions are available for use. The solution is injected directly into the vein, which causes intimal injury, fibrosis, and shut-down of the vein. Sclerotherapy may be used on branch varicosities of the saphenous system, or smaller veins, such as reticular or spider veins. Reticular veins are usually smaller than 3 mm and often not protruding through the subdermal tissue where they occur. Spider veins or spider telangiectasias are dermal structures, often of cosmetic concern. They are treated with sclerotherapy directly into the small vein lumen, or by extrinsic laser, obliterating them through the skin.

Chronic Venous Insufficiency

Chronic venous insufficiency (CVI) is a syndrome that results primarily from valvular incompetence or venous outflow obstruction or both in the lower extremity and evolves into a characteristic clinical picture. Initially ankle swelling and discomfort occur. Edema and pain worsen as the disease progresses, and the skin in the so-called "gaiter" area (a bandlike area in the vicinity of the malleoli) becomes inflamed, hyperpigmented, and develops eczematoid changes. Eventually subcutaneous fibrosis (lipodermatosclerosis) and skin ulcerations may develop. Recurrent cycles of ulceration and healing are not unusual. It is estimated that approximately 5 million people in the United States exhibit some evidence of CVI, and one in a hundred have had or have a venous ulcer.

Pathophysiology of CVI. It is well established that CVI can occur as a consequence of DVT. The many changes that occur in the vein once a thrombotic process has occurred are well documented and include venous obstruction, recanalization, valvular destruction, loss of vein wall distensibility, fibrosis, and intense inflammation. It is unclear that CVI is strictly a consequence of DVT, because many patients with CVI have no demonstrable evidence of previous thrombosis. In these patients, primary valvular incompetence, leading to reflux and venous hypertension, could be an alternative cause of CVI. One problem, however, is that some patients with varicose veins have significant venous reflux and venous hypertension without developing any changes characteristic of CVI. Why some patients with venous insufficiency only have varicose veins and in others, CVI develops, remains a mystery and the subject of numerous research investigations.

Edema/Lipodermatosclerosis. Patients first seen with edema and or lipodermatosclerosis are best treated with elastic compression therapy. This will help to reduce the edema and may minimize the progression of the severe fibrosis associated with CVI. In some patients, the use of external compression pumps also can be of great benefit.

Patients must be educated about the reasons for the swelling and fibrosis, so that they may be more involved in their care. Simple measures such as keeping their legs elevated when sitting for prolonged periods or taking time out during the day to get their legs elevated can be very beneficial.

Ulceration. The treatment of patients with CVI and leg ulcers is one of the most difficult, time-consuming, expensive, and often frustrating clinical problems encountered in vascular disease. The fact that the average venous ulcer takes many months to cure and that the recurrence rate is very high, approaching 75% in some series, speaks to the complexities of treating this very difficult clinical problem for both the patient and the clinician. The cornerstone of therapy is external compression to both minimize and treat the problem of edema. Markedly swollen tissue in any setting is difficult to heal, with edema fluid preventing vascular penetrance of the affected area to assist with healing. In addition, the local treatment of the ulcer itself and the treatment of any associated cellulitis and frank infection are essential. In the absence of frank purulence, fever, elevated white blood cell (WBC) count, or obvious cellulites, chronic ulcers are not routinely cultured, because it is well known that they are colonized with many bacteria, and antibiotic treatment is not indicated. A number of options exist for treating venous ulcers. One method is application of a topical hydrocolloid gel pad applied directly to the ulcer bed followed by compression, and another is the application of medicated layered dressings, which include external compression.

Noninvasive duplex evaluation of the venous system is recommended at some time during the healing process to determine the venous pathophysiology causing the ulcer or CVI. Surgery might be indicated to correct the venous abnormality and to diminish the likelihood of ulcer recurrence and symptoms of CVI. If the saphenous system is found to be incompetent, removal or obliteration of the saphenous system is recommended. If the perforating veins are found to be incompetent, these veins are ligated, either directly through the skin, or endoscopically. Most patients with CVI and venous ulcers have a mixture of sites of venous incompetence, involving various components of the superficial, perforating, and deep systems. Repair of deep-system incompetence is often difficult, but in some circumstances, direct valve repair can be done. In some patients, repair is not possible because of severe scarring, and transplanting a segment of axillary vein with an intact competent valve into the superficial femoral or popliteal vein might be possible. A small number of patients with CVI do not have reflux disease, but rather have severe venous outflow obstruction from thrombosis. These patients may be treated with venous bypass procedures to alleviate the outflow obstruction.

Suggested Reading

Clement DL: Venous ulcer reappraisal: Insights from an international task force. J Vasc Res 36(suppl) 1:42–47, 1999.

Gloviczke P, Yao JST (eds): Handbook of Venous Disorders, 2nd ed. Guidelines of the American Venous Forum. London, Arnold Publishers, 2001.

International Society of Lymphology: The diagnosis and treatment of peripheral lymphedema: Consensus document of the International Society of Lymphology. Lymphology 36(2):84–91, 2003.

Menzoian JO, Arbid EJ, Phillips TJ, et al: Venous system of the lower extremities: Physiology and pathophysiology. In Sidawy AN, Sumpio BE, DePalma RG, (eds): The Basic Science of Vascular Disease. Armonk, NY, Futura Publishing, 1997, pp 385–406.

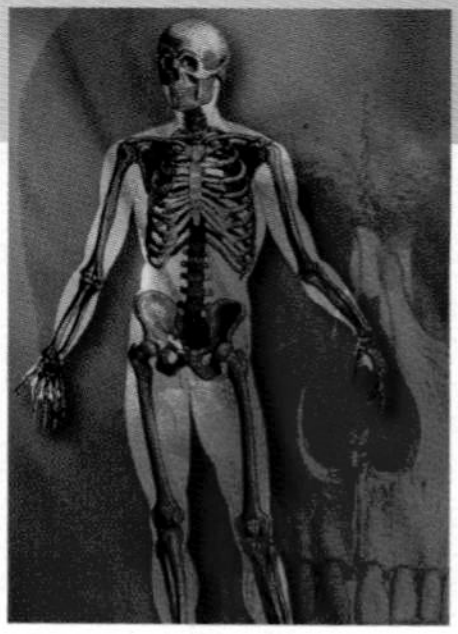

Chapter 36

Deep Venous Thrombosis and Pulmonary Embolism

JOHN J. RYAN, MD, and WILLARD C. JOHNSON, MD

Deep venous thrombosis (DVT) refers to blood clotting in the deep veins of the calf, thigh (femoral or popliteal veins), the iliofemoral venous system, or a combination of these. It is a common condition in a hospital setting and is frequently underdiagnosed. DVT may lead to serious sequelae including the postphlebitic syndrome and potentially fatal pulmonary embolism (PE). Pulmonary emboli, it is estimated, account for 3% of surgical inpatient deaths and are probably the most preventable. Although it is recognized that PE may result from thrombosis of the axillary-subclavian system, the vast majority of PE results from thrombosis in the deep venous system of the lower limb, especially of the iliofemoral component.

On a surgical service, the development of DVT is most commonly seen in patients undergoing major pelvic and abdominal surgery or major orthopedic procedures, especially of the hip, pelvis, and lower limbs. Prophylaxis is important and greatly reduces the incidence of DVT and PE in elective surgery of this type. In addition, patients undergoing prolonged immobilization and multiple trauma patients benefit from such prophylaxis. The clinical presentation of DVT and PE is nonspecific, and a high index of diagnostic suspicion is required. However, clinical findings supported by appropriate investigations can yield a high degree of diagnostic accuracy and prevent major morbidity and mortality.

Deep Venous Thrombosis

Pathophysiology

In the 1840s, the Prussian pathologist Rudolf Virchow first associated thrombosis in the deep venous system of the lower limbs with fatal PE, as evidenced at autopsy. *Virchow's triad* refers to those predisposing conditions whereby venous thrombosis is enhanced (i.e., stasis, vascular injury, and increased coagulability of the blood). Although our knowledge and understanding of this process has greatly increased since the time of Virchow, it remains accurate to classify predisposing factors to the development of DVT under these headings (Box 36-1).

In health, frequent contractions of the muscles of the lower limbs (activity) enhance the venous return to the right heart. The backpressure of the venous column of the lower limbs is reduced greatly by the interposition of venous valves, which effectively prevent reflux during times of muscular relaxation. Immobility (prolonged bed rest, surgical procedures, long airplane journeys, etc.) results in reduction or loss of the activity of the muscle pump, leading to venous stasis. This may lead to venous thrombosis, which may be confined to the small sinusoidal veins of the muscles of the calf, may involve the calf veins themselves, or may propagate to include the femoral, popliteal, and iliofemoral veins. Certain patients may be more prone to the development of DVT because of the presence of so-called procoagulant (thrombophilic) abnormalities of the plasma (e.g., Leiden factor V, protein C

BOX 36-1 Predisposing Conditions for Development of DVT

Stasis	– Prolonged bed rest
	– Postoperative, especially abdominal, pelvic and orthopedic procedures
	– Multiple trauma
	– Paralysis
	– Long airplane journeys
	– External venous compression (e.g., tumor, popliteal artery aneurysm, pregnancy)
Vein wall injury	– Trauma
	– In-dwelling catheter
	– Thrombophlebitis
	– History of previous thrombosis
Altered coagulability (thrombophilia)	– Leiden factor V carriers
	– Protein C deficiency
	– Protein S deficiency
	– Antithrombin III deficiency
	– Hyperhomocysteinemia
	– Dysfibrinogenemia
	– Malignancy
	– Oral contraceptives
Other	– Obesity
	– Nephrotic syndrome
	– Bechet's syndrome
	– Congestive cardiac failure
	– Varicose veins

deficiency, protein S deficiency, antithrombin III deficiency, hyperhomocysteinemia, and dysfibrinogenemia). In addition, obesity, the presence of malignancy, and the use of the oral contraceptive pill all increase the propensity to DVT formation. It is estimated that 80% of young patients who experience recurrent DVT have an identifiable procoagulant factor present. The risk of developing DVT is proportional to the number of clinical and laboratory risk factors, in addition to the type and length of surgical procedure involved. Therefore it is possible to identify clearly a subset of patients who are at greatest risk for the development of DVT and who therefore would derive the greatest benefit from prophylaxis.

Diagnosis

DVT, sometimes referred to as phlebothrombosis, may be entirely asymptomatic. The degree of symptoms exhibited may not necessarily correlate with the extent of DVT formation. Patients with a personal or family history of DVT are obviously at high risk. Calf pain or painless swelling of the ankle, especially if unilateral, may be the earliest presentation of DVT formation. Calf tenderness may be found, but this is not confirmatory. Homans' sign refers to calf pain elicited on forced dorsiflexion of the ankle. Originally thought to be diagnostic of DVT, it is unfortunately no more than 50% sensitive and specific. It is therefore not useful in the diagnosis of DVT. Conversely, massive swelling of the leg and thigh may indicate complete iliofemoral thrombosis. DVT is not necessarily totally occlusive. The first indication of the formation of DVT may be the effects of pulmonary embolization, including chest pain, tachypnea, dyspnea, or sudden cardiovascular collapse. The clinician must attempt an accurate diagnosis in any patient in whom a DVT is suspected, as failure to diagnose and treat may have serious sequelae. Long-term anticoagulation without confirmatory evidence of DVT or PE or both carries significant morbidity. Therefore it is important to arrive at a reasonably confident diagnosis before institution of long-term therapy.

Venography has been considered the "gold standard" for the diagnosis of DVT; however, in hospital practice, this is not generally the first investigation. Venography, although accurate, carries a small risk of vascular injury, contrast reaction, and anaphylaxis. In addition, it is invasive and cumbersome and may place a heavy demand on hospital resources. It is possible that magnetic resonance venography will become the investigation of choice when it is generally available. Noninvasive tests for the diagnosis of DVT include continuous wave Doppler, duplex ultrasonography, radioiodine-labeled fibrinogen scanning (no longer available, as fibrinogen may be a carrier of blood-borne viruses), and venous impedance plethysmography. Continuous-wave Doppler examination elicits the characteristic phasic venous flow and detects changes in flow as a result of augmentation (inspiration and calf pressure). This test can be performed at the bedside and can examine the femoral vein at the groin, the popliteal vein, and the posterior tibial vein behind the medial malleolus. The continuous-wave Doppler technique is highly operator dependent. This technique investigates flow and lacks visualization. Therefore partially occlusive thrombus or recanalized thrombus may be missed. This may be a significant disadvantage, especially in the patient in whom PE is suspected.

Duplex ultrasonography combines the flow information of the Doppler examination with B-mode ultrasonography, thereby adding anatomic characteristics of the vessel to the investigation. It is possible by this method to differentiate fresh thrombus from old, organized thrombus. The diagnostic accuracy of this investigation is therefore superior. Again, however, the accuracy is strictly operator dependent. An experienced operator, however, can elicit diagnostic accuracy with sensitivity and specificity in excess of 95%. Duplex ultrasonography, in practical terms, has therefore become the investigation of choice and, when combined with clinical assessment of the patient, can be highly accurate in the diagnosis of DVT. One significant exception to this, however, is where the diagnosis of isolated iliac vein thrombosis is suspected, and in this setting, plethysmography may be particularly useful. In everyday practice, the clinical suspicion of DVT can be satisfactorily confirmed by duplex ultrasonography in experienced operator hands.

More recently, magnetic resonance venography has been found to be valuable in the diagnosis of proximal venous thrombosis, in particular, in the iliac veins and in the inferior vena cava. It is highly sensitive and superior to duplex scanning in these locations. The presence of metallic implants and the inability of certain patients to tolerate the claustrophobic aspect of the test limit its application in some patients.

Measurement of D-dimer has been used in patients with suspected DVT. When a clot (thrombus) forms, soluble fibrinogen is cleaved to form insoluble fibrin. Plasmin lysis of cross-linked fibrin generates the fragment D-dimer. Elevated D-dimer levels are thus found in patients who have DVT/PE. Elevated D-dimer levels also are found in a variety of other conditions (i.e., abdominal aortic aneurysm, trauma, recent surgery, sickle cell crisis, disseminated intravascular coagulation [DIC], arterial thrombosis, pregnancy, and inflammatory states). Therefore the specificity of elevated D-dimer levels in DVT/PE is low. However, the absence of elevated D-dimer levels may be valuable in the exclusion of DVT as a likely diagnosis because of its high sensitivity and corresponding negative predictive value.

Treatment

Patients who are undergoing procedures that are known to pose a high risk for DVT formation should be protected with either low-dose heparin (5000 units subcutaneously every 12 hours starting before incision) or calf-compression devices intraoperatively and postoperatively until ambulation occurs. Low-molecular-weight heparins also can be used effectively. These modalities are known to reduce the perioperative incidence of DVT formation.

In patients in whom the diagnosis of DVT is established, anticoagulation is the treatment of choice. Once the diagnosis is made, the patient is given a bolus of intravenous heparin (100 units/kg) and maintained on a heparin drip (usually 1000 units/hr) with the objective of establishing an activated partial thromboplastin time (aPTT) approximately twice normal. At the same time, oral anticoagulation is begun, by using warfarin (Coumadin). This is continued for a minimum of 3 months. Comparative data indicate that effective treatment is achieved on reaching an International Normalized Ratio (INR) of 2.0 to 3.0. Heparin is discontinued once an adequate level of anticoagulation on warfarin is established. Some controversy persists with regard to the need for anticoagulation when the DVT is confined to the calf veins. Calf-vein thromboses do not characteristically embolize to a significant extent. However, it is known that small-vein thrombosis in the calves may propagate in 6% to 30% of cases in postoperative and hospitalized patients. Additionally, even calf-vein thrombosis can result in deep-vein valve destruction, increasing the risk of the postphlebitic syndrome and embolization. If such patients are not treated with anticoagulation, it is recommended they be monitored with venous duplex imaging until full activity is resumed after discharge.

In the absence of a contraindication, all patients with femoral-popliteal venous thrombosis should be treated with anticoagulation or clot lysis. Anticoagulation is instituted to prevent clot propagation and embolization. Anticoagulation per se does not result in lysis of established clot. In the absence of a contraindication to thrombolysis, some authorities recommend lytic infusion (tissue plasminogen activator, streptokinase, urokinase) until resolution of the thrombus occurs, followed by oral anticoagulation. The use of lytic agents may be prohibited in the early postoperative period. In patients in whom an absolute contraindication exists to anticoagulation or thrombolysis, or in those patients who, despite adequate anticoagulation, continue to propagate clots and embolize, treatment is by percutaneous placement of a vena cava interruptive device or filter (Fig. 36-1).

Occasionally, massive swelling of the entire lower limb is seen with generalized pallor (so-called "milk leg" or phlegmasia alba dolens). When total venous outflow occlusion occurs, the skin becomes congested and cyanotic (blue). This limb-threatening condition is referred to as phlegmasia cerulea dolens (painful blue leg). This is an emergency condition that, left untreated, will lead to venous gangrene and amputation. Thrombolysis (catheter directed) is the treatment of choice. Operative intervention may be necessary where lysis is contraindicated. This may take the form of either femoral thrombectomy or crossover outflow establishment to the opposite limb by using either saphenous vein or a prosthetic conduit. Anecdotally, these procedures have been limb saving.

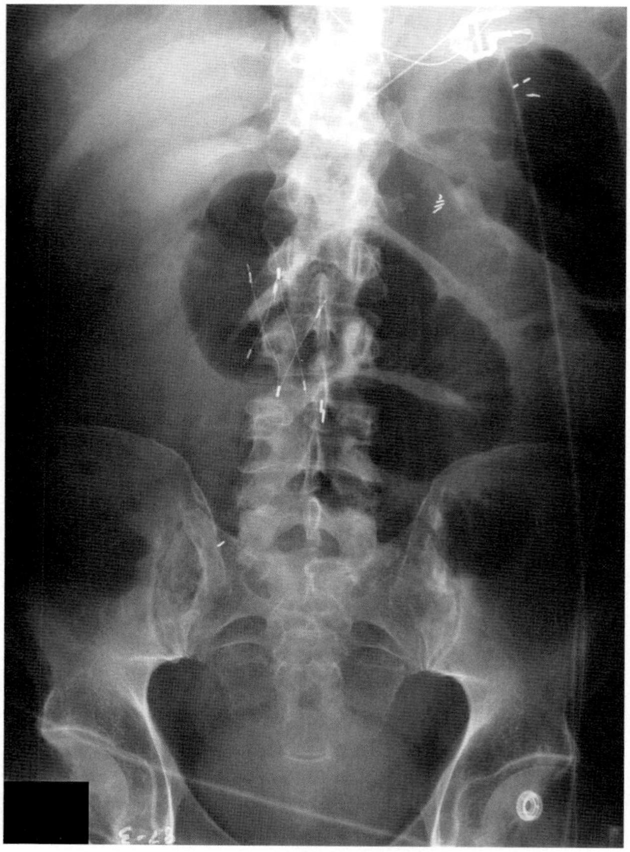

FIGURE 36–1 Vena cava filter overlying third lumbar vertebra.

Pulmonary Embolism

Pathophysiology

The vast majority of venous thrombi that embolize to the pulmonary circulation arise from the deep veins of the thigh and pelvis. Fewer than 5% of pulmonary emboli arise from other sources, including the axillary-subclavian venous system. Untreated, clinically apparent PE has a mortality rate of 30% to 35%. A treated PE has a mortality rate of 2% to 5%.

DVT limited to the veins of the calf typically does not place the patient at high risk for PE, whereas up to 40% of patients with proximal DVT will have PE. The pathophysiologic effects of such emboli and the clinical expression of such changes will vary greatly, but will

PEARLS FOR ROUNDS

The majority of cases of deep vein thrombosis (DVT) are *asymptomatic.*

DVT occurs frequently in patients undergoing orthopedic, abdominal, and pelvic surgery.

Younger patients in whom DVT develops will often have a predisposition to hypercoagulopathy.

Pulmonary embolism should be high on the differential diagnosis in any postoperative patient experiencing respiratory symptoms or sudden collapse.

depend ultimately on the pre-embolic pulmonary status of the patient and the magnitude of the embolism itself. Smaller emboli may pass through the right heart and the pulmonary outflow tract and result in minor and transitory occlusion of the lesser pulmonary vasculature. Larger emboli, having passed through the right heart and major pulmonary veins, may obstruct middle-order venous outflow tracts, leading to interrupted pulmonary perfusion despite adequate ventilation, and, if unresolved, may lead to localized pulmonary infarction. Pulmonary infarction is, however, uncommon because of the "collateral" blood supply of the bronchial arteries to the lung tissue. More significant emboli may result in major pulmonary artery obstruction leading to acute hypoxemia and cardiopulmonary instability or collapse. Massive PE may totally occlude the main pulmonary artery outflow tract, leading to sudden death.

Significant PE, therefore, results in pulmonary shunting because of the ventilation/perfusion mismatch. The pulmonary cross-sectional area affected, although ventilated, has decreased or absent alveolar/arteriolar gas exchange. If this area is large enough, a resultant oxygen desaturation of arterial blood will occur, as well as a variable hypoxemia. When hypoxemia exists, the degree of reduced oxygenation roughly correlates with the extent of embolism, as judged by ventilation/perfusion (V/Q) scanning and measurement of pulmonary artery pressures. Other clinical situations seen in the hospital setting may, however, result in a similar pathophysiologic disturbance and are important to keep in mind. These include pneumothorax, massive lung collapse, and significant atelectasis. Significant and repeated pulmonary emboli can result in increased pulmonary vascular resistance, leading to pulmonary hypertension. Smaller and nonrepetitive emboli may resolve totally over time (usually 7 to 10 days), through natural fibrinolysis. The so-called paradoxical embolization occurs in a patient with an embolus and in whom an atrial or ventricular septal defect exists, thereby permitting passage of the embolus to the left heart and the resultant peripheral arterial embolic presentation.

Diagnosis

PE must be considered in the differential diagnosis in any patient with cardiopulmonary symptoms and signs who is postoperative, or who has undergone prolonged bed rest, or in whom other risk factors for the development of venous thrombosis are present. The commonest symptoms of PE include dyspnea, chest pain (pleuritic), hemoptysis, palpitations, and mental confusion. The commonest signs include tachypnea, tachycardia, signs of right heart strain, auscultatory crepitations (rales), hypotension, cyanosis, pleural friction rub, and fever. In addition, clinical evidence of DVT in the lower limb should be sought (swelling and Doppler-wave examination at the bedside). Chest radiograph, electrocardiogram, and arterial blood gases should be examined to rule out other causes of such a clinical presentation (myocardial infarction, pneumothorax, cardiac tamponade, massive atelectasis, and pulmonary collapse), which may, in themselves, exhibit findings supportive of the diagnosis of PE.

Chest radiograph should be performed in all cases of suspected PE and, indeed, in all patients with acute onset of the clinical presentation described earlier. Findings indicative of significant embolism include prominent central pulmonary outlines and enlargement of the hilum. Alternatively, chest radiograph may demonstrate diminished pulmonary markings, particularly in a pleural-based wedge-shaped area (Westermark's sign). Pleural effusion may be evident and supportive of a recent PE, but is not specific.

All patients should undergo arterial blood gas analysis. The typical pattern seen in patients with PE demonstrates reduced partial pressure of oxygen (resulting from V/Q mismatch), reduced partial pressure of carbon dioxide (resulting from tachypnea), and reduced oxygen saturation levels of the blood. As stated earlier, the degree of hypoxia on blood gas measurement does correlate with the extent of embolism. The presence of a normal blood gas pattern, however, does not rule out PE. The Prospective Investigation of Pulmonary Embolism Diagnosis study reported that 38% of patients without previous cardiopulmonary disease and in whom a PE was demonstrated, had an arterial blood gas pattern with a partial oxygen pressure greater than 80 mmHg on room air.

Electrocardiography (ECG) should be performed on all patients in the first instance to rule out a primary cardiac event or dysrhythmia. Conversely, ECG findings of right heart strain and ischemia support the diagnosis of PE. Traditionally, the $S_1\ Q_3\ T_3$ pattern was described on the ECG of patients undergoing PE, but this was found to be present in only a minority of such patients.

In these patients and in the setting of urgent presentation of possible PE, Doppler-wave ultrasound assessment at the bedside may reveal the presence of iliofemoral or femoropopliteal thrombosis, which will increase the likelihood of PE and warrant acute heparinization, thus giving the

PEARLS FOR THE OR

Most deep vein thromboses (DVTs) in the surgical patient occur on the OR table.

Prophylaxis is critical in prevention of DVT/pulmonary embolism (PE).

Subcutaneous heparin (5000 units), given *before* surgery and continued (twice daily) postoperatively until full mobilization is achieved, is effective. Alternatively, low-molecular-weight heparin may be used to the same effect.

Intermittent calf-compression devices also are effective in prevention of DVT.

patient the advantage of early anticoagulation. The treatment of DVT and PE with heparin, followed by a minimum of 3 months of long-term oral anticoagulation after discharge with warfarin is essentially the same. If duplex ultrasound and the operator expertise are available for performing this test, the diagnosis may be further enhanced.

In practice, chest radiograph, ECG, and arterial blood gas analysis will neither confirm nor eliminate the diagnosis of PE with certainty, although the absence of other causes of the presenting symptoms makes the diagnosis more likely. Where the diagnosis remains probable, the patient is given anticoagulation with heparin and sent for confirmatory tests such as the V/Q scan, CT angiogram of the chest, or pulmonary angiogram. The V/Q scan consists of two components, the first of which is a perfusion scan performed by the injection of radioisotope into the venous circulation, resulting in "visualization" of the pulmonary vasculature in several planes. Emboli may result in loss of perfusion in one or more areas. The absence of any perfusion defect makes the diagnosis of PE extremely unlikely. The opposite, however, is not necessarily true. That is, a positive scan (i.e., the presence of perfusion defects) also may result from other causes such as chronic pulmonary disease, atelectasis, and pneumothorax. It is obvious, therefore, that the diagnostic yield of an abnormal perfusion scan is greatly enhanced in the presence of a normal chest radiograph. The ventilation scan is performed by the inhalation of radioactive aerosols and comparison of the resulting radioactive image with the perfusion scan, looking especially for a V/Q mismatch. The V/Q scan is most accurate in those patients in whom clearly a V/Q mismatch is found, indicating a high probability of PE, or in whom no defect is seen, indicating a low probability. In a large number of patients, the scan results are indeterminate.

Pulmonary angiography has remained the gold standard for the diagnosis of PE. However, it is probably unnecessary to subject these patients to pulmonary angiography if the presence of DVT is demonstrable. Occasionally, however, it will be necessary to perform pulmonary arteriography in those patients in whom DVT cannot be demonstrated and in whom a definitive diagnosis is required. Pulmonary angiography yields the greatest sensitivity and specificity in the diagnosis of PE, but is associated with a 5% morbidity rate and a less than 1% mortality rate. Computed tomographic angiography (CTA) has been described recently as having sensitivity and specificity equivalent to pulmonary angiography and, where available, may replace pulmonary angiography in these patients (Fig. 36-2). CTA is becoming, in certain centers, the first-line modality for imaging PE. Previous concerns regarding the use of CTA for the accurate diagnosis of peripheral (smaller) PE have been overcome by the introduction of multidetector-row spiral CT. As this technology has become more widely available, and because it is cost effective, this noninvasive technology appears to be surpassing all other imaging modalities for the accurate detection of central and peripheral PE.

Treatment

In the first instance, treatment is supportive, with the aim of maximizing resuscitation. Depending on the patient's condition, this may consist of intravenous fluid administration and face-mask oxygenation. Alternatively, a patient initially seen with acute respiratory insufficiency may require immediate endotracheal intubation.

Heparinization is the mainstay of treatment for PE. In the normal-sized adult patient, 10,000 units of heparin is administered intravenously as a bolus, followed by an infusion rate of 1000 to 1500 units/hr, with the objective of maintaining the aPTT in the two- to three-times-normal range. The rate of infusion required to reach this goal may vary considerably, even among patients of similar body mass. Occasionally, in a patient with preformed antibodies to heparin, acute thrombocytopenia will develop, necessitating discontinuation of the heparin. It is important to reach the desired therapeutic range of anticoagulation as quickly as possible to limit the patient's vulnerability to a second and potentially fatal embolus.

Warfarin (Coumadin) therapy is begun the same day as heparin, with the objective of achieving the desired prolongation of the PT, as measured by the INR. This should be in the range of 2.5 to 3.0. Oral anticoagulation with warfarin is continued for a minimum of 3 months. Depending on the patient's history and risk factors for recurrent embolization, this period may be prolonged. Patients with recurrent DVT or PE may require lifetime anticoagulation. Patients are monitored on an outpatient basis with weekly measurements of the INR by the anticoagulation clinic.

Massive PE presenting as cardiovascular collapse may be treated by thrombolysis therapy or by suction or open pulmonary embolectomy. Catheter-directed tissue plasminogen activator (tPA) given at a rate of 100 mg over a

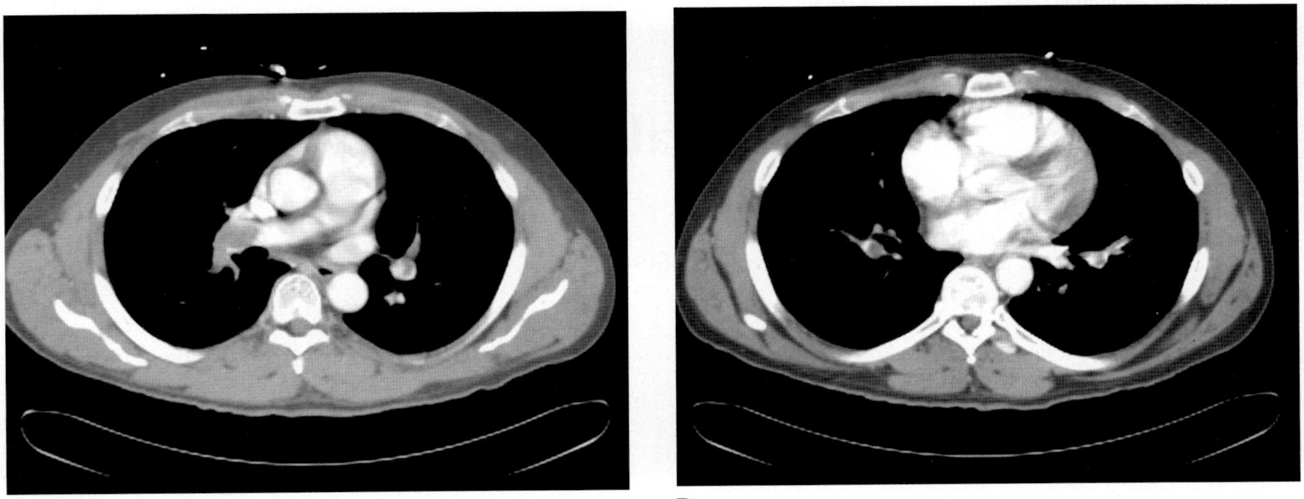

A B

FIGURE 36–2 Computed tomography angiograms. *A*, Central pulmonary emboli. *B*, Segmental pulmonary emboli.

2-hour period has been used in the emergency setting and has been shown to be effective in achieving the dissolution of clot with minimal residual pulmonary damage. In critical circumstances, and where lysis therapy is either contraindicated or unavailable, emergency sternotomy with pulmonary embolectomy may save lives.

Some patients experience further embolic events despite adequate anticoagulation. In other patients, anticoagulation may be absolutely contraindicated (e.g., recent intracranial hemorrhage). For these patients, the best alternative may be the transvenous placement of an inferior vena cava filter device (see Fig. 36-1). These devices are usually permanent, but temporary (retrievable) devices are available. The device is placed under fluoroscopic guidance into the inferior vena cava below the level of the renal veins. Typically, this is performed by an interventional radiologist, and the placement of the device is fairly straightforward and can even be performed at the bedside.

Suggested Reading

Benjamin ME, Sandager GP, Cohn EJ Jr, et al: Duplex ultrasound insertion of inferior vena cava filters in multitrauma patients. Am J Surg 178:92–97, 1999.

Carson JL, Kelley MA, Duff A, et al: The clinical course of pulmonary embolism. N Engl J Med 326:1240–1245, 1992.

Comerota AJ: Acute deep venous thrombosis. In Gloviczki P, Yao JST (eds): Handbook of Venous Disorders. London, Chapman and Hall, 1999, pp 243–259.

Comerota AJ, Aldridge SC: Thrombolytic therapy for acute deep vein thrombosis. Semin Vasc Surg 5(2):76–84, 1992.

Gillies TE, Ruckley CV, Nixon SJ: Still missing the boat with fatal pulmonary embolism. Br J Surg 83:1394–1395, 1996.

Goldhaber SZ: Contemporary pulmonary embolism thrombolysis. Chest 107:455–515, 1995.

Lensing AWA, Prandoni P, Prins MH, Buller HR: Deep vein thrombosis seminar. Lancet 353:479–485, 1999.

Manganelli D, Palla A, Donnamaria V, et al: Clinical features of pulmonary embolism: Doubts and certainties. Chest 107:25S–32S, 1995.

O'Donnell JA, Hobson RW: Comparison of electrical and impedance plethysmography: calibration of an impedance rheograph. J Surg Res 24:459–464, 1978.

Quiroz R, Schoepf UJ: Spiral CT for pulmonary embolism: The paradigm has shifted. Am Heart Hosp J 1:281–288, 2003.

Rosendaal FW: Risk factors for venous thrombosis: prevalence, risk and interaction. Semin Haematol 34:171–187, 1997.

Stein PD, Atanasoulis C, Alavi A, et al: Complications and validity of pulmonary angiography in acute pulmonary embolism. Circulation 85:462–468, 1992.

Stein PD, Goldhaber SZ, Henry JW: Alveolar-arterial oxygen gradient in the assessment of acute pulmonary embolism. Chest 107:139–143, 1996.

Stein PD, Goldhaber SZ, Henry JW, et al: Arterial blood gas analysis in the assessment of suspected acute pulmonary embolism. Chest 109:78–81, 1996.

Tai NRM, Atwal AS, Hamilton G: Modern management of pulmonary embolism. Br J Surg 86:853–868, 1999.

Wells PS, Anderson DR, Rodger M, et al: Evaluation of D-dimer in the diagnosis of suspected deep-vein thrombosis. N Engl J Med 349:1227–1235, 2003.

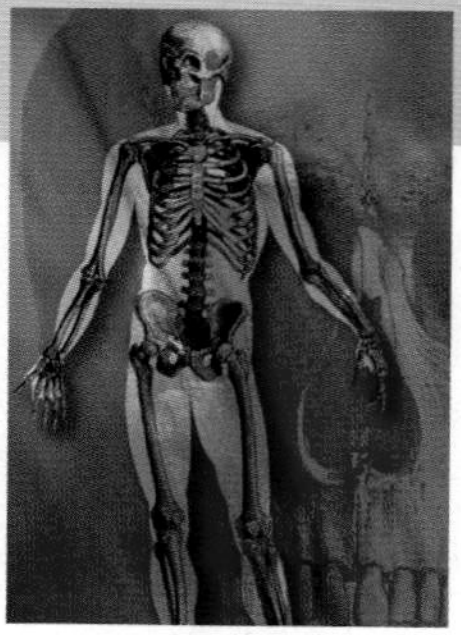

Chapter 37

Peripheral Arterial Occlusive Disease

WILLARD C. JOHNSON, MD

As of the year 2004, nearly 15% of America's population was older than 65 years, and the high prevalence of arterial occlusive disease in this group of approximately 35 million people leads to many patients seeking relief of their symptoms. Peripheral arterial occlusive disease is defined as arterial occlusive disorders affecting all areas of the body other than the heart. This chapter focuses on the care of patients with disorders of the lower extremities, kidneys, and gastrointestinal tract.

Lower Extremity Ischemia

Arterial occlusive disease of the lower extremities occurs more commonly in patients who smoke and have hypercholesterolemia. Focal lesions of atherosclerosis develop in areas more prone to endothelial injury, such as an arterial bifurcation or areas of posterior fixation where shearing forces and turbulent flow are the highest. The site of an arterial stenosis or occlusion may vary with age, as young symptomatic patients (45–55 years old) tend to have a stenosis that begins at their aortoiliac bifurcation, whereas patients from 55 to 70 years old have superficial femoral artery (SFA) occlusive disease, frequently starting at Hunter's canal, and patients older than 70 have tibial/peroneal occlusive disease (Fig. 37-1). In diabetic patients, tibial occlusion tends to develop at a much younger age. The reason for this observation is not clear and may be variable in an individual diabetic patient. Aortoiliac occlusive disease is commonly referred to as "inflow" obstruction of flow to the groin, whereas femoropopliteal disease is referred to as "outflow" obstruction with reference to the groin.

A basic understanding of the physics of blood flow is helpful to the understanding of arterial occlusive disease. Flow within an artery with a stenosis is governed by the Poiseuille equation:

$$Q = (P_1 - P_2)R^4/\mu L$$

where Q is the flow, $P_1 - P_2$ represents the pressure gradient between two different points, R is the radius of the stenotic area, μ is the viscosity of blood, and L is the length of the stenosis. In addition, sequential arterial obstructions within the same artery provide further resistance to flow, such that each obstruction is additive.

Arterial stenosis and obstruction enhance the development of collateral vessels from existing smaller arteries. Small arterial branches above and below the obstruction anastomose to provide an autogenous bypass around the occlusion. However, collaterals take time to develop, and their presence provides evidence of a chronic obstructive lesion. In patients who are first seen with acute arterial obstructions, adequate collaterals have not had time to develop and thereby the patient has more severe symptoms of ischemia.

Vascular Examination

The major component to the vascular examination is the pulse examination of the femoral, popliteal, and pedal vessels. (The popliteal is best felt with slight passive flexion of the knee and gentle bimanual finger pressure in the popliteal fossa.) Of importance is the integrity of the skin of the distal lower leg, foot, and toes. *Dependent rubor,* signified by the foot turning red when the patient goes from a lying to a sitting position suggests long-term, significant arterial occlusive disease and represents an increase in the number of capillaries present. Capillary refill should be present in all toes with chronic insufficiency; if refill is not present, the arterial occlusive disease is either acute or very severe.

Doppler Examination

The small hand-held Doppler machine/probe (cost, ~$300) provides a great deal of information about the arterial occlusions with little added time investment during the physical examination. For the ABI (ankle/brachial systolic pressure index), one places a blood pressure cuff at the ankle and listens over the dorsalis pedis/posterior tibial artery for a good signal, then inflates the cuff until the flow is obliterated (ankle systolic pressure) and compares this pressure with the highest brachial pressure.

Further refinement in the Doppler assessment is achieved by placing the cuff on the calf, low thigh, and high thigh (while listening at the dorsalis pedis/posterior tibial [dp/pt]), which determines the systolic pressure at those sites. This will allow the examiner to determine the site of arterial occlusion and whether multiple sites are present. Diabetic patients may have a falsely elevated ABI or

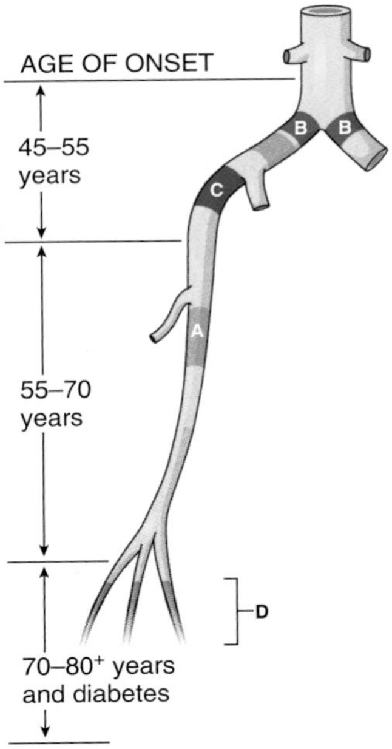

SITES OF OCCLUSION

DOPPLER		A	B	C	A+B or A+C	D
HTBI	1.0	1.0	0.7	0.7	0.7	1.0
LTBI	1.0	1.0	0.7	0.7	0.7	1.0
CBI	1.0	0.7	0.7	0.7	0.3	0.4
ABI	1.0	0.7	0.7	0.7	0.3	0.4
TYPICAL PATIENT COMPLAINTS	None	Calf claudication	Impotence, hip claudication	Thigh claudication (not impotent)	Rest pain	Diabetic toe necrosis

FIGURE 37-1 Patterns of arterial occlusive disease.

noncompressible pedal arteries from the calcification present in their vessels.

With chronic ischemia, the ABI is usually 0.7 ± 0.2 for patients with claudication, 0.4 ± 0.1 for rest pain, and 0.3 ± 0.1 for tissue necrosis. For acute ischemia, the ABI is usually 0.0 – 0.2.

Tissue Oxygen Measurements

Transcutaneously, the partial pressure of oxygen ($tcPo_2$) can be measured in the subcutaneous tissue of the body. The normal value is more than 60 mmHg. However, with arterial occlusive disease, a decrease occurs in the $tcPo_2$. A level greater than 30 mmHg suggests that adequate oxygenation exists for spontaneous healing, whereas levels less than 20 mmHg suggest that vascular reconstruction will be required to relieve rest pain or to heal areas of tissue loss. The $tcPo_2$ measurements are particularly helpful in diabetic patients with calcified vessels who may have a fictitiously elevated ABI from their vessel calcification. The $tcPo_2$ level also will aid in the treatment of diabetic foot ulcers, where healing may be expected from proper local foot care if the $tcPo_2$ is greater than 30.

Angiography

Angiography is indicated when operative or interventional treatment is planned. A good history and physical examination with ABIs will usually ensure a correct diagnosis, so diagnostic angiography is not indicated. Conventional angiography requires the placement of a catheter into the arterial system and injection of contrast to provide visualization of the arterial tree. Magnetic resonance angiography (MRA) and spiral computed tomography (CT) with IV contrast are now used frequently to visualize the arterial system, as they have less morbidity and are less expensive than conventional angiography.

Claudication

Vascular claudication is a symptom of muscle pain when walking, which disappears when one stops walking and remains standing. Claudication is the earliest sign of chronic arterial occlusive disease and may remain mild for many years or be progressive in severity, resulting in critical ischemia (i.e., rest pain or skin necrosis). Although "neurologic claudication" from spinal stenosis also may occur with walking, it does not disappear when one remains standing, but usually requires sitting or recumbency for pain relief. Neurologic claudication is usually bilateral and involves hips and buttocks.

The location of the muscle pain when walking is very helpful in determining the site of arterial occlusive disease:

- Calf pain, SFA stenosis/occlusion.
- Thigh pain, external iliac stenosis/occlusion.
- Hip/buttock pain, common iliac or aortic stenosis/occlusion
- Impotence, bilateral stenosis/occlusion of internal iliac artery or aortobilateral common iliac stenosis/occlusion. The *Leriche syndrome* consists of impotence with bilateral hip and thigh claudication, sometimes labeled "three-legged claudication."

PEARLS FOR ROUNDS

The five Ps of acute arterial occlusion are pain, pallor, pulselessness, paresthesia, and paralysis.

Ankle/brachial systolic pressure index values: claudication, 0.5 to 0.9; chronic rest pain, 0.3 to 0.5; tissue necrosis, 0.2 to 0.4; acute rest pain, 0.0 to 0.3

Six-hour rule: Nerve ischemic injury begins after 6 hours of no blood flow. Thus to avoid paresis and neuritic pain, revascularization must be completed within 6 hours after an acute arterial occlusion.

During the vascular physical examination, record how far (in feet) the patient can walk before the pain begins, onset of claudication, and the maximal walking distance (MWD) the patient can walk before he or she must stop for relief. To get accurate information, it may be appropriate during the evaluation for the examiner to walk with the patient and record these distances.

Infrequently, on physical examination of a symptomatic patient, a palpable pedal pulse may be present and confusing to the examiner. In this situation, the patient must be reexamined immediately after exercising to determine whether the pulse has disappeared. It should disappear with vascular claudication but remains present in patients with neurologic claudication. However, in general, patients with calf claudication have absent pedal and popliteal pulses, whereas for thigh or hip claudication, the femoral pulse is absent. The ABI is usually 0.7 but may vary from 0.5 to 1.0.

Treatment of Claudication

The natural history of claudication, in most patients, does not progress to a stage of critical ischemia. In patients followed for 5 years, only 5% to 10% will require bypass surgery or amputation, and those patients are most often those who have not done appropriate risk modification.

The initial treatment for a patient is *education* about risk factors (e.g., the need to stop smoking, to get the cholesterol level back to normal, and lose weight if obese). Note that a significant reduction in the serum cholesterol levels may lead to a regression of some arterial stenoses. Walking exercises are very important, and a daily program will usually lead to a 200% increase within 2 months in the distance one can walk. The exercise program frequently recommended is to walk in one direction as far as one can, even if the muscles are beginning to hurt, until the patient must stop—then rest, and when the pain disappears, continue to walk again until the need to stop again arises. At this point, the patient should note the distance walked and return home at a comfortable pace. The program is undertaken twice a day. Improvement is easily measured by the increase in walking distance away from the starting point.

This exercise has two benefits: first, the muscle pain (ischemia) liberates vascular growth factors that lead to collateral arteries enlarging and growing, and second, it allows "conditioning" of the muscles to tolerate less blood flow (as do the muscles in long-distance runners). The exercise program must be maintained if maximal walking distance is to be achieved; if the program is stopped, the onset of claudication will occur at a shorter distance.

Some pharmacologic agents may help. Pentoxifylline (Trental), the first medication approved for the treatment of claudication, reduces blood viscosity by changing the red blood cell wall rigidity of newly formed red cells. Although pentoxifylline has a statistical benefit as compared with placebo, the average increase in walking distance is only about 30 yards and thus may not be of clinical significance. However, each patient's response is variable, some patients being helped more than others. Overall, only about 50% of patients are helped, and because it is hard to determine which patient will improve, a trial of 4 months of treatment may be appropriate. Most clinicians believe that pentoxifylline should be started only if an exercise walking program has been unsuccessful. Celestozol (Pletal), introduced in 1999, also has shown some benefit in randomized studies. Its comparative efficacy to pentoxifylline is unknown, and because it has more side effects and a cost disadvantage, celestozol should probably be a second-line treatment agent. In general, all claudicant patients probably should be taking aspirin (325 mg/day) to reduce the risk of thrombosis of the stenotic arteries in their legs, as well as for their possible coronary and cerebral vascular benefits.

Percutaneous angioplasty (PTA)/stenting or bypass surgery should be advised only after a risk-modification program and exercise walking program have failed. Many vascular surgeons believe that operations for claudication relief should not be performed in patients who continue smoking or who have elevated cholesterol levels. Patients with "inflow disease," aortoiliac occlusive disease, probably have a lower threshold for intervention, as PTA/stent treatment has a reasonable benefit for minimal risk and may have similar short-term functional patency as a bypass procedure. Aortofemoral or femorofemoral and femoropopliteal bypasses, either prosthetic or vein, should be reserved for special situations, such as employment (the mailman) or quality-of-life enhancement (golfer, hunter, or others willing to risk losing the leg to walk better).

Critical Ischemia

Critical ischemia is defined as arterial occlusive disease that renders the leg at risk for major amputation. This is manifested by postural rest pain (i.e., pain that usually occurs with recumbency and is relieved with standing [the hydrostatic driving pressure provides more flow when standing]), constant toe/foot pain, or loss of skin integrity of the toes, heel, or foot and an associated absence of pedal pulses and an ABI less than 0.4.

Patients with critical ischemia require vascular intervention and usually have two-segment arterial occlusive disease (i.e., aortoiliac plus SFA disease, or SFA plus popliteal occlusive disease). For those patients with aortoiliac occlusive disease and SFA occlusion, an "inflow procedure" may convert a patient with rest pain to one with only claudication, and no further interventional treatment may be required. However, for patients with tissue loss, both an inflow procedure and an outflow procedure may be necessary for healing of the foot lesion.

For patients with aortoiliac bilateral occlusive disease, the standard procedure is an aorta bifemoral bypass with either Dacron or polytetrafluoroethylene (PTFE) material (they have similar patencies of ~75% at 5 years). Aortofemoral bypasses are now being performed by using a laparoscopic approach or rarely an endovascular approach from the groin. In patients who are poor candidates for aortic level surgery, axillobifemoral bypasses are an acceptable alternative with only a slightly lower patency. For patients with unilateral iliac occlusive disease, a femorofemoral bypass (either Dacron or PTFE) will give good patency performance (70% at 5 years). For patients with a focal iliac stenosis, a PTA/stent may provide adequate inflow to the groin and have similar patency.

For patients with femoropopliteal occlusive disease, the vascular reconstruction can be more complex. For patients with a stenotic or occluded distal popliteal artery or proximal tibial occlusive disease (frequently in diabetes), a femoral to tibial or peroneal bypass with a vein conduit is optimal. The saphenous vein may be used in situ (the large vein anastomosed to the large artery, and the small end of vein anastomosed to the small artery) with valve lysis and branch ligation or a "reversed" vein where valve lysis is not required. Arm veins also may be used. The 5-year patency of vein bypasses to single tibial arteries is about 60%.

For patients with a patent popliteal artery and good tibial runoff, the options are more variable, with choices of an autologous bypass (reversed vein, in situ vein, arm vein) or a prosthetic bypass (PTFE, Dacron, human umbilical vein, or cryopreserved saphenous vein). In general, autologous veins are the bypass of choice, as their patency is better (Table 37-1); however, in some situations, a prosthetic bypass may be appropriate (i.e., no veins are available, a patient with coronary artery disease who may require future coronary revascularization so the saphenous vein is "banked" for future care, or a poor-risk patient in need of a "quick" operation). A vein cuff at the distal anastomosis of a PTFE or Dacron bypass may provide improved patency.

Long-term oral anticoagulation (warfarin), with or without aspirin, may enhance patency in patients with complex venous bypasses or prosthetic bypasses to the popliteal or distal vessels. In general, all patients who have received a bypass should be taking an antiplatelet agent such as aspirin to improve the patency of the bypass as well as to reduce the risk of a stroke or myocardial infarction (MI).

TABLE 37–1 Bypass Performance

Bypass	Material	5-year Assisted Primary Patency (%)
Ao-Fem-Fem	Dacron	80
	PTFE	80
Axillo Fem-Fem	Dacron	70
	PTFE	70
Fem-Fem	Dacron	75
	PTFE	75
Fem-Popliteal AK	Vein	75
	HUV	65
	PTFE	50
Fem-Popliteal BK	Vein	75
	HUV	60
	PTFE	40
Fem-tibial	Vein — in situ	60
	— reversed	60
	HUV	30
	PTFE	20

PTFE, Polytetrafluoroethylene; HUV, human umbilical vein; BK, below knee; AK, above knee.

The role of a lumbar sympathectomy, either operative, laproscopic, or percutaneously with chemicals, is not well defined, but usually is reserved for patients with rest pain or less than 1 cm of tissue loss in the foot in whom a bypass is a risky procedure. An increase in foot $tcPo_2$ with dependency may be a positive predictor of success with a sympathectomy.

Bypass Surveillance/Failure

Infrainguinal (Outflow) Bypasses

About 20% to 30% of vein bypasses are at risk for the development of a stenosis within the bypass itself. The stenoses frequently occur at the site of a valve or endothelial injury during the initial operation or from recurrent arteriosclerosis. These vein bypasses can frequently be salvaged with a focal repair, either operatively or angiographically, before bypass thrombosis occurs. Once a thrombosis occurs, with the associated endothelial hypoxic injury, long-term salvage of the bypass is poor. Hence a program of bypass surveillance has been developed to identify these "failing" bypasses. Patients are seen every 3 months during the first year, and thereafter, every 6 months. The patients are evaluated for recurrent symptoms, the ABI is checked, and most important, a duplex ultrasound of the entire bypass is performed, looking for stenotic areas, as identified by a focal increase in velocity of twofold or more as compared with adjacent areas.

Prosthetic femoral popliteal bypasses usually fail from intimal hyperplasia at the distal anastomosis of the bypass graft. Patients are prescribed aspirin to reduce this hyperplastic response. Bypass-surveillance programs are less successful in identifying a failing prosthetic bypass before it fails, but serial ABI measurements are helpful at times. Duplex ultrasound examinations are rarely helpful in the asymptomatic patient. If a prosthetic bypass is identified with an anastomotic stricture, operative angioplasty with a vein patch will usually provide enhanced patency. If the bypass has already occluded, one must reevaluate the indication for reoperation; if the patient's complaint is only claudication, nonoperative care may be the most appropriate treatment.

For patients with critical ischemia of the leg, thrombolysis of the bypass and operative correction of the stenotic segment with an extended bypass or angioplasty may help. If the ipsilateral or contralateral saphenous vein or arm veins are available, a new venous bypass may be the preferential bypass choice for new revascularization.

Inflow Bypasses

Aortofemoral, axillofemoral, femorofemoral bypasses that have a distal anastomosis in the groin are at risk for subsequent failure, and the cause is usually progressive arterial stenosis or occlusion in the superficial femoral or profunda femoral artery. Anastomotic hyperplasia is less frequently seen than with prosthetic femoropopliteal prosthetic bypasses. No formal surveillance program is endorsed for these patients, but they are advised to return when claudication returns or gets worse. Most of these patients are seen annually for pulse examination, detection of a pulsatile mass (anastomotic pseudoaneurysm), and ABI.

Acute Ischemia

Acute arterial ischemia of the lower leg is defined as an arterial occlusion occurring with acute symptoms and signs frequently referred to as the five Ps: pain, pallor, pulselessness, parathesia, and paralysis.

The etiology of an acute ischemic leg is usually embolic, from a myocardial thrombus (recent MI or chronic atrial fibrillation), fragments of an aortic aneurysm or an acute thrombosis of a previously stenotic arterial segment, or very rarely a "paradoxical" embolus from DVT via a cardiac shunt. An embolic event occurs suddenly without warning, whereas acute thrombosis is usually preceded by a history of claudication. Today, with the prevalent use of warfarin in patients with atrial fibrillation, and anticoagulation of patients with an MI, most acute leg ischemia is caused from the occlusion of a previously stenotic segment of the arterial system, such as the superficial femoral artery, external iliac artery, or common iliac artery. The "blue toe syndrome," which is manifested by a painful bluish mottling of the toes or feet, is usually caused by smaller emboli such as the thrombotic material inside an aortic aneurysm or a large ulcerative placque in the aortoiliac system.

The site of acute occlusion can be determined by the pulse examination: iliac occlusion if no femoral pulse is present, femoral occlusion if no popliteal pulse is present, or distal popliteal occlusion if no pedal pulse is present. Likewise, the "line of coolness" is as follows: a cool foot for popliteal occlusion, a cool lower leg for superficial femoral occlusion, and a cool thigh for common iliac occlusion or common femoral and profunda femoralis occlusion.

Early diagnosis and treatment are important to avoid an unsatisfactory outcome. For patients with pain, pallor, and pulselessness, with intact sensory and motor function, treatment is urgent heparinization (10,000-unit bolus and 1000 units/hr, to maintain a PTT of twice normal; the arterial vascular position (patient with the head and trunk elevated [i.e., heart ~40 cm above ankle]; nasal O_2 at 2 L/min, and possibly a trial of intravenous Dextran 40 if no contraindications exist). Heparin prevents propagation of the arterial occlusion by maintaining patency of vessels distal to the acute occlusion. If the patient improves, then treatment will depend on the etiology of the acute process (i.e., early embolectomy if an embolus, or semielective vascular bypass of an occluded artery that has recently thrombosed its stenotic segment).

For those patients with a decrease or loss in sensory or motor function of the toes/foot, a more urgent revascularization program is required before peripheral nerve ischemia develops. Successful treatment within 6 hours of onset will usually provide a good clinical outcome. Delayed successful revascularization may provide a viable foot, but the lower leg may be paretic and with severe neuropathy and its associated pain (causalgia) or numbness. Urgent treatment depends on the etiology of the occlusion; if it is an embolus, then an embolectomy via a femoral artery exploration with catheter extraction may be appropriate. However, for acute thrombosis of a stenotic arterial segment, the treatment program may be either intraarterial lytic therapy (tissue plasminogen activator [TPA]) with angiographic angioplasty and stenting or both, or emergency arterial bypass, such as would be performed for chronic ischemia.

In the urgent situation, when revascularization is successful, a risk exists for a reperfusion injury to the ischemic calf muscles and the development of a compartment syndrome, which may require fasciotomy. The diagnosis of a compartment syndrome is suspected because of pain in the calf, venous distention of the foot, a numb foot, and foot weakness, and confirmed by direct measurement of the pressure in the muscle compartment. If the acute arterial occlusion has been present for more than 6 hours, some surgeons will incise the fascia constricting the muscle groups of the lower leg, a prophylactic fasciotomy, at the time of successful revascularization of the extremities. Successful reperfusion also will liberate the products of anaerobic metabolism that have accumulated in the ischemic muscles; these are myocardial toxic and may produce a decrease in cardiac output. Such patients must be monitored very closely for such a possibility.

Renal Vascular Disorders

The two disorders that may be improved by renal revascularization are hypertension and chronic renal failure. Renal artery stenosis causes hypertension by activation of the renin-angiotension system. Renin is an enzyme produced in the juxtaglomerular cells of the afferent arterioles of the kidney and released into the renal veins in response to decreased renal blood flow. Renin acts on a plasma substrate to produce angiotensin I, which is converted to angiotensin II in the pulmonary circulation by an angiotensin-converting enzyme (ACE). This converting enzyme is inhibited by captopril. Angiotensin II both vasoconstricts and stimulates the release of aldosterone. Renal artery stenosis accounts for 7% of all hypertension and occurs more often in young individuals and in patients not well controlled with antihypertensive therapy. A bruit may be present in the epigastrium. The renal artery stenosis is most often caused by arteriosclerosis, but in young adults, fibromuscular dysplasia may be the etiology. The diagnostic evaluation of hypertension should include other surgically treated disorders such as primary hyperaldosteronism, pheochromocytoma, coarctation of the aorta, hyperthyroidism, Cushing's disease, and unilateral renal parenchymal disease (shrunken kidney); however, about 90% of all hypertension is "essential" (i.e., hypertension in the absence of an identifying cause).

The diagnostic evaluation should include a captopril radionucleotide renal scan, and if this is positive, then an MRA, which may identify a renal arterial stenosis. Chronic renal failure is usually caused from a primary intrarenal disorder; however, some patients also have an extrarenal contributing factor, a renal artery stenosis. These patients must be identified, as correction of the renal artery stenosis may avoid dialysis. It is generally recommended that all patients with a creatinine level greater than 2 mg have an MRA to evaluate the possibility of an associated renal artery stenosis.

Treatment of a renal artery stenosis has shifted during the past few years to a treatment program of primary angioplasty/stenting, as the mortality/morbidity is lower than that with direct aorto/renal revascularization. Success is highest for patients with a mid–renal artery stenosis, but ostial lesions also do respond to balloon angioplasty. Surgical revascularization by direct endarterectomy of the renal artery or bypass from the aorta to the distal renal artery is usually reserved for patients for whom angioplasty has failed or who are quite young with few operative risk factors. In some patients, the aorta may be heavily calcified, and the bypass is then performed by using the splenic or gastroduodenal artery as the site of inflow for the bypass. Some patients who are having an aortofemoral bypass will have an extra "limb" from their bypass extended to the distal renal artery at the time of revascularization for aneurysmal or occlusive aortic disease. Renovascular hypertension is improved in 80% to 90% of patients with successful revascularization achieved by either an operation or angiographic balloon angioplasty with or without stenting. Renal function is improved or stabilized in approximately 70% of patients with pretreatment renal insufficiency.

PEARLS FOR THE OR

Five factors for successful arterial reconstruction are good inflow, good outflow, good bypass or endarterectomy, good surgeon (operative technique), and an honest coagulation system.

Bleeding that does not stop in the OR rarely stops in the recovery room.

Never say "Oops," because patients under anesthesia remember such things.

Mesenteric Ischemia

Mesenteric arterial insufficiency may be seen as either an acute or chronic clinical problem. The cause of the acute ischemia is usually an embolus to the superior mesenteric artery (SMA), and because this embolus stops just beyond the orifice of the middle colic artery, the jejunum, ileum, and right colon are ischemic, whereas the transverse colon is frequently viable. In the acute situation, the diagnosis is often missed preoperatively (e.g., a patient is operated on for "an acute abdomen" of unknown etiology, and extensive gangrene of the bowel is found). Symptoms and signs that may suggest acute mesenteric ischemia are abdominal pain out of proportion to the degree of tenderness, unexplained acidosis, diffuse small bowel dilation, gas in the bowel wall on plain or CT film, and portal gas on plain film or CT. An MRA will confirm the diagnosis.

The natural history of acute mesenteric ischemia is bowel infarction and death, if it is untreated. Even with operative intervention, 50% to 75% of patients die because of a delayed diagnosis with massive infarction, or a profound reperfusion injury to the heart and lungs if revascularization is successful.

Treatment of acute mesenteric arterial insufficiency is early operation and revascularization if part of the bowel is still viable. This revascularization may include embolectomy of the SMA or bypass from the aorta to the SMA. At the same operation, resection of the clearly infarcted bowel also is performed. Questionable segments of bowel are left behind, and the patient is reexplored 24 hours later (a "second look") to remove any remaining necrotic bowel. Most often, when the bowel has been resected, reanastomosis is not performed, and the patient is left with a small bowel stoma and distal mucous fistula, which can be closed at a later date. Postoperatively, some of these patients will have a "short gut" syndrome and may need temporary or permanent IV hyperalimentation to maintain their weight.

In some patients, nonocclusive mesenteric arterial ischemia develops from a low-flow circulatory state associated with impaired cardiac function, cardiogenic shock, and occasionally from the splanchnic vasoconstrictive effects of digitalis or other vasopressors used to support the failing heart. These patients require treatment of their cardiac status and possibly angiography-directed SMA perfusion of a vasodilator (papaverine) before any operative intervention. Surgery is delayed for about 2 hours after SMA infusion has started, to determine the status of bowel viability.

Chronic mesenteric ischemia usually presents as postprandial pain (intestinal angina), associated with weight loss (i.e., the patients tend not to eat because of the fear of abdominal discomfort). On physical examination, a bruit may be heard in the epigastrium. Blood supply to the gut is normally by the celiac, SMA, and inferior mesenteric arteries, and because of the good collateral connection of these three major vessels, the clinical syndrome of chronic mesenteric ischemia is usually not seen until two or three of these vessels are stenotic or occluded. The diagnosis is usually supported by an MRA, but an angiogram is usually required to formulate a treatment plan. PTA/angioplasty is now being advocated for treatment of chronic mesenteric ischemia. Operative treatment usually consists of a bypass from the supraceliac aorta to either or both the celiac and SMA arteries. The bypass is most often performed with Dacron or PTFE, but some surgeons prefer a saphenous vein bypass, whereas others perform a direct aortic endarterectomy. Bypass surgery is quite successful, with weight gain and relief of postprandial pain in 90% of patients.

Suggested Reading

Dutch Bypass Oral Anticoagulation or Aspirin (BOA) Study Group: Efficacy of oral anticoagulants compared with aspirin after infrainguinal bypass surgery: A randomized trial. Lancet 355:346–351, 2000.

Johnson WC, Lee K, with members of the Veterans Affairs Cooperative Study #141: Comparative evaluation of saphenous vein, PTFE, and human umbilical vein for femoral popliteal above-knee bypasses. J Vasc Surg 32:268–277, 2000.

Rodriguez-Lopes JA, Werner A, Ray L, et al: Renal artery stenosis treated with stent deployment: Indications, technique, and outcome for 108 patients. J Vasc Surg 29:617–624, 1999.

Timaran CH, Prault TL, Stevens SL, et al: Iliac artery stenting versus surgical reconstruction for TASC type B and type C iliac lesions. J Vasc Surg 38:272–278, 2003.

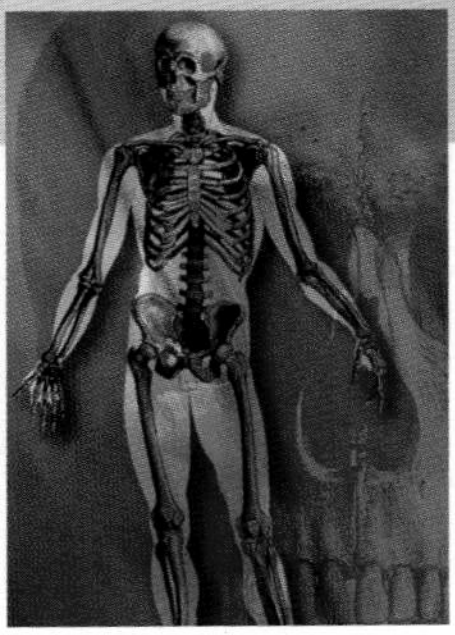

Chapter 38

Aneurysms

FADY HADDAD, MD, MARYANN BARRY, RN, and
JAMES O. MENZOIAN, MD

Abdominal Aortic Aneurysm Disease

An abdominal aortic aneurysm (AAA) is a localized irreversible arterial dilatation that increases the diameter of the abdominal aorta by at least 50%. The normal diameter of the abdominal infrarenal aorta is approximately 2 cm; therefore by definition, an AAA has a diameter of 3 cm or more. AAAs are the thirteenth leading cause of death in the United States, claiming 15,000 lives per year. The incidence is increasing because of an aging population and better screening (Fig. 38-1).

Rupture of the aneurysm is the primary cause of death associated with an AAA. Because an AAA is seldom symptomatic before rupture, investigation is necessary for timely diagnosis and operative repair. Elective surgical repair provides better clinical outcomes and may reduce the 80% to 90% mortality rate associated with AAA rupture. If a person with an AAA lives long enough, rupture of the AAA is inevitable.

Pathogenesis/Etiology

The exact pathogenesis of AAA disease is not known. AAAs originate from a weakening of the elastic fibers in the tunica media of the arterial wall. As a result, the vessel dilates and the wall tension increases. No unified concept of the pathogenesis of AAA development has yet emerged; however, several factors appear to have an important role in the development of AAAs; they include degenerative changes in the structural matrix of the aortic wall, enzymatic and cellular factors, hypertension, predisposition of the abdominal aorta to atherosclerotic changes, gender of the patient, familial clustering, race, and genetics.

Course

Lacking precise data on the natural history of AAAs, many investigators have focused on the relation of aneurysm size and expansion rate to the risk of rupture (Fig. 38-2). Large aneurysms, those more than 5 to 6 cm in diameter, tend to expand more rapidly than small ones. Unfortunately, it is impossible to predict the rate of expansion of an AAA in any one patient; some aneurysms remain stable for years and then expand rapidly. Aneurysm growth rate is predicted neither by size nor by previous growth rate. It is known, however, that AAA expansion rates increase as a function of the size of the aneurysm. Because all AAAs are potentially lethal and rates of expansion and frequency of rupture are unpredictable, most vascular surgeons recommend repair for all symptomatic or ruptured AAAs and for all AAAs 5 cm in diameter or larger, provided that coexisting conditions do not preclude repair.

Incidence

Accurate incidence data for asymptomatic AAA in the community are sparse and unreliable, as valid incidence estimates can be obtained only by screening a defined population for a second time. The reported incidences of asymptomatic AAA in the literature vary between 1.0 and 117.2 per 100,000 person years. All studies report sharp increases in the age-adjusted incidence of AAA in recent years, resulting perhaps from the increased use of ultrasound. The risk factors most strongly associated with AAA are smoking, race, and male gender. Abdominal/flank pain and

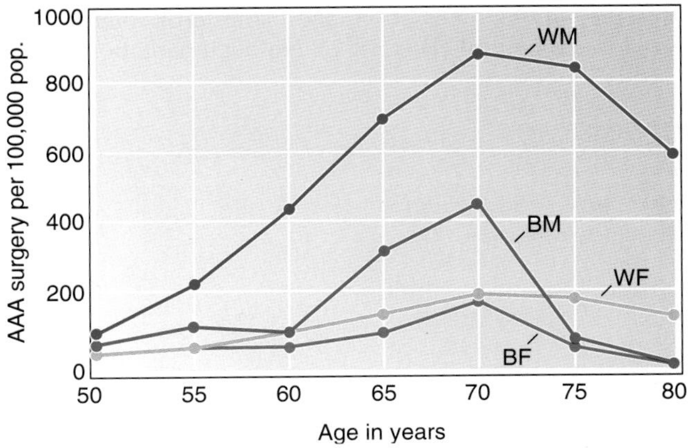

FIGURE 38–1 Age-specific rates of abdominal aortic aneurysm surgery in Massachusetts from 1984 through 1988. (Adapted from LaMorte WW, Scott TE, Menzoian JO: Racial differences in the incidence of femoral bypass and abdominal aortic aneurysmectomy in Massachusetts: Relationship to cardiovascular risk factors. J Vasc Surg 21:422–431, 1995, with permission.)

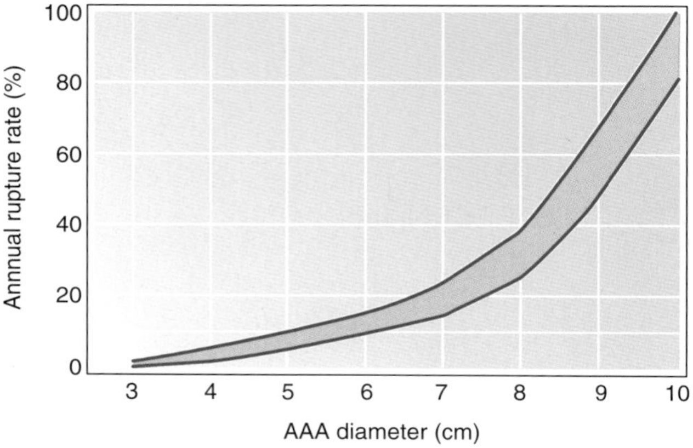

FIGURE 38–2 Estimated annual rupture rate based on abdominal aortic aneurysm diameter. The range is based on different published estimates. (Data from Samson LN, Cronenwett JL: Abdominal aortic aneurysms. In Zelenock GB (ed): Problems in General Surgery in Vascular Surgery, Vol II. Philadelphia, JB Lippincott, 1995, pp 385–417.)

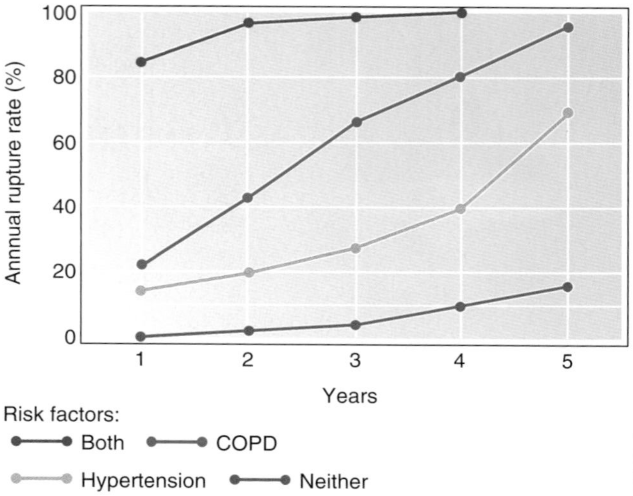

FIGURE 38–3 Predicted cumulative rupture risk for a 5-cm abdominal aortic aneurysm depending on the presence of risk factors. (Adapted from LaMorte WW, Scott TE, Menzoian JO: Racial differences in the incidence of femoral bypass and abdominal aortic aneurysmectomy in Massachusetts: Relationship to cardiovascular risk factors. J Vasc Surg 21:422–431, 1995, with permission.)

hypotension are the most common symptoms of rupturing or expanding (symptomatic) AAA. Most aneurysms (75%) are discovered when still asymptomatic, either as a pulsatile mass on physical examination or unexpectedly during the course of an evaluation for an unrelated condition.

Associated, Aggravating, and Ameliorating Factors

As no single etiology in the development of AAAs has emerged, at present no factors are known to help alleviate or aggravate the development of an AAA. The reduction and modification of risk factors, such as control of blood pressure, smoking cessation, and cholesterol control may prove to be helpful (Box 38-1). No documentation exists in the literature as to anything that a patient can do to aggravate or alleviate the development of an AAA. Factors that have been found to be independently predictive of AAA rupture include AAA size, hypertension, and chronic obstructive pulmonary disease (COPD) (Fig. 38-3).

BOX 38–1 Risk Factors for Aneurysm

- Age: usually >50 yr, mean age, 69 yr
- Male/female ratio, 4–5:1
- Family history of AAA
- Previous atherosclerotic disease
- Cerebrovascular disease
- Peripheral vascular disease
- Cardiovascular disease
- Hypertension
- Chronic obstructive pulmonary disease (COPD)
- Smoking
- Hypercholesterolemia
- Race; occurs more commonly in whites than blacks
- Certain genetic disorders (e.g., Marfan syndrome, Ehlers-Danlos syndrome)

AAA, Abdominal aortic aneurysm.

Physical Examination

The only physical-examination maneuver of demonstrated value for the diagnosis of an AAA is abdominal palpation to detect a widened or tender aorta. Palpation of the abdominal aorta is safe and has not been reported to precipitate rupture but unfortunately identifies only approximately 35% of AAAs.

An AAA, when palpable, is usually located to the left of the midline, above the umbilicus, in the epigastric area. The primary physical finding is a laterally expansile (throws the examining hands out laterally), pulsating abdominal mass in the epigastrium. It is the width, not the intensity, of the aortic pulsation that suggests the presence of an AAA.

Abdominal palpation may detect most aneurysms large enough to warrant surgery, but it cannot be relied on to exclude the diagnosis entirely. The sensitivity of abdominal palpation is reduced by abdominal obesity and by abdominal examination not specifically directed at measuring aortic width. Typical signs and symptoms of asymptomatic and symptomatic AAA are given in Box 38-2.

BOX 38-2 Signs and Symptoms of Abdominal Aortic Aneurysm

Patient may have one or more of the following:
- Asymptomatic AAA
  - Pulsatile abdominal mass
    - May or may not be present
    - Usually no other signs or symptoms
- Symptomatic AAA
  - Pulsatile abdominal mass
  - Back or flank pain
  - Abdominal pain
  - Hypertension
  - Decreased hematocrit
  - Pallor
  - Tachycardia
  - Diaphoresis
  - Oliguria
- Mottling of the lower extremities or abdomen or both
  - Umbilical or flank ecchymosis
  - Hemorrhagic shock/ circulatory arrest

PEARLS FOR ROUNDS

The primary cause of death of patients with an abdominal aortic aneurysm (AAA) is rupture.

AAA expansion rates increase as a function of the size of the AAA.

The most consistent results for monitoring growth of an AAA come from using the computed tomography scan.

The most common etiologies for thoracoabdominal aneurysm formation are atherosclerotic medial degeneration, followed by dissection.

Factors predicting neurologic complications after surgical repair of thoracoabdominal aneurysms are prior proximal aneurysm repair, presence of aortic dissection, duration of aortic cross-clamp time, oversewing of intercostal arteries, and hypotension.

Femoral and popliteal artery aneurysms account for 90% of peripheral aneurysms.

The mere presence of a popliteal or femoral aneurysm and not the size is an indication for surgical repair because of the high risk of thromboembolic complications.

Diagnosis

Diagnostic Tests

A plain abdominal radiograph will reveal an AAA only with a calcified wall of the abdominal aorta and is not very useful clinically. Abdominal ultrasound has a 95% to 100% specificity and sensitivity for AAA detection and is an inexpensive and noninvasive way to detect and accurately measure an AAA. Abdominal computed tomography (CT) has a sensitivity and specificity similar to those of abdominal ultrasound but, in addition, provides consistency for serial evaluations of AAAs. For this reason, most experts rely on CT measurement for serial studies rather than ultrasound measurement of an AAA. CT scans remove the limitations of ultrasound testing that is dependent on the expertise of the technologist and the poor visualization of the abdominal aorta caused by bowel gas. Furthermore, CT eliminates the variable size measurements of the AAA that occur, depending on the angle of insonation of the ultrasound probe.

Differential Diagnosis

Of patients with a pulsatile abdominal mass, the differential diagnosis can be an AAA or a tumor mass (a thin person with a mass may have aortic pulsations similar to an AAA; however, these tumors are rarely laterally expansile).

Of patients with abdominal or flank pain and hypotension, the differential diagnoses include an acute abdomen caused by a perforated peptic ulcer, diverticulitis, acute pancreatitis, or mesenteric ischemia; gastrointestinal bleeding; renal colic or infection; urinary tract obstruction; a leaking or enlarging AAA; thoracic aortic dissection or thoracic aneurysm with dissection into the abdominal aorta, a myocardial infarction, or a combination of these.

Follow-up and Treatment Plan

AAAs grow at widely varying rates. The initial growth rate of an AAA does not predict its subsequent growth rate. AAAs larger than 4 cm may be safely followed up by yearly ultrasound or CT scan. AAAs larger than 4 cm and smaller than 5 cm may be followed up with an ultrasound or CT scan every 6 months. AAAs 5 cm or larger have substantial risk of rupture and should be referred for surgical evaluation and repair.

Lifestyle changes such as smoking cessation, an exercise regimen, and a low-cholesterol diet should be encouraged. β-Blockers are advocated because some experimental evidence indicates that they may slow AAA expansion.

Surgical Repair of AAA

Traditional Open Repair

The "gold standard" for repair of an AAA involves the surgical placement of a vascular prosthesis within the lumen of the aneurysm via a midline or left retroperitoneal incision below the 12th rib. Elective repair of an AAA in this manner has an overall mortality rate of 1.4% to 7.6%, whereas the repair of a symptomatic AAA (patients with symptoms of acute expansion or rupture at the time of repair) has a less than 30% survival rate.

The basic principles of operative repair include proximal aortic control above the aneurysm as well as distal control below the aneurysm. The aorta is opened, and back-bleeding from lumbar arteries is controlled by direct suture repair.

Assessment of back-bleeding from the inferior mesenteric artery (IMA) is now undertaken. If brisk back-bleeding is present, it can be assumed that the IMA is well collateralized from the superior mesenteric artery and can be ligated. If no back-bleeding is present, probably the IMA has been chronically occluded and has not been important in providing flow the bowel. If very faint back-bleeding is noted, it must be presumed that the IMA was open and being fed directly from the aorta, and the IMA must then be reimplanted into the new aortic graft. A graft of synthetic material is then used to replace the diseased aorta. The proximal anastomosis is done to the "neck" of the aorta, which is the nonaneurysmal aorta just above the aneurysm. Once this is done, the distal end of the graft is sewn to the healthy aorta just below the AAA. If the AAA disease extends to the distal aorta, a bifurcated graft is sewn to both iliac arteries. Once flow is reestablished, the aneurysm sack is sewn over the synthetic graft to prevent erosion of the graft into the overlying bowel.

Endovascular Repair

Endovascular repair represents a relatively new procedure with favorable short-term results. Long-term results and evaluation of AAA repairs done in this manner are unavailable. Endovascular repair of an AAA involves the introduction of an endovascular stented graft into the abdominal aorta under radiographic guidance via an open femoral artery access. The endovascular stented graft is positioned in the abdominal aorta at the site of the aneurysm under fluoroscopic control and deployed to attach with the stents to the nondilated walls of the proximal aorta. The distal limbs of the graft are deployed in both the iliac arteries just proximal to the bifurcation into the external and internal iliac arteries. Decisions regarding the eligibility of patients to have an AAA repaired by a stented graft are based on the anatomy of the AAA, the patient's risk for conventional surgical repair, and the presence of coexisting medical problems, which could make the risk of conventional open operative repair prohibitive.

Morbidity and mortality are reduced with the use of an endovascular graft, rather than conventional open repair. Long-term abdominal CT surveillance of the grafts is necessary, looking for late problems with the endograft.

Thoracoabdominal Aneurysm

Classification

In 1986, Crawford classified thoracoabdominal aneurysms (TAAs) according to their extent. This classification carries an important prognostic and therapeutic impact. Type I TAA involves most of the descending thoracic and upper abdominal aorta. Type II involves the descending thoracic and most of the abdominal aorta. Type III involves the distal descending thoracic aorta and most of the abdominal aorta. Type IV involves most or the entire abdominal aorta including the visceral artery segment.

Etiology

The single most common etiology for TAA is atherosclerotic medial degenerative disease (82%), followed by dissection (17%). Other causes include Marfan syndrome, Ehlers-Danlos syndrome, mycotic aneurysm, and Takayasu aortitis. Hypertension is frequent in both dissecting and nondissecting TAA. Mycotic TAA presents a particularly challenging situation because of the dual goal of eradicating infection and providing arterial reconstruction.

Natural History

Only about one fourth of unoperated-on patients who have TAA are alive at 2 years. Conversely, patients who have undergone surgery for TAA have a 71% 2-year survival rate.

Cambria and others reported the rupture rate for degenerative TAA to be 12% at 2 years (18% for aneurysms >5 cm in diameter) and 32% at 4 years. The expansion rate for TAA is less than 5 mm/year. However, the larger the aneurysm, the higher the expansion rate. Rupture of TAA is almost uniformly fatal. Aneurysms smaller than 6 cm in diameter still have a 10% incidence of rupture. The size threshold recommended for surgery is 5 cm, especially for a type IV and dissecting aneurysms. A 6-cm threshold is used in many centers for types I to III.

Clinical Presentation

Asymptomatic presentation occurs in 43% of patients with degenerative TAA (much less in dissecting TAA). Pain is the most frequent complaint in symptomatic patients. It could be acute (expansion, rupture, or dissection) or chronic. Pain is located in the back, flank, or chest. Other less common symptoms may result from adjacent organ compression: hoarseness, cough, hemoptysis, dyspnea, and dysphagia. About 25% of patients will be operated on for urgent or emergency presentation. The typical patient will be in his 70s with diffuse atherosclerotic disease, hypertension, and a smoker, often with COPD. Cerebrovascular and lower extremity occlusive disease and visceral and renovascular disease could be associated with TAA.

Diagnosis

Accurate radiologic evaluation is essential for precise operative planning. A contrast-enhanced CT scan provides essential information including proximal and distal extent of the aneurysm, status of the visceral arteries, location and topography of the renal arteries, and size and perfusion of the kidneys. Standard contrast angiography is performed in all elective cases. It is particularly helpful in assessing the patency of intercostal vessels for reimplantation and the status of iliac arteries in cases in which retrograde aortic perfusion is planned. In patients with impaired renal function, a combination of nonenhanced CT scan and magnetic resonance angiography (MRA) can provide the necessary information without using nephrotoxic contrast material.

Treatment

Surgical repair with graft replacement is the only effective treatment for TAA. Nonoperative therapy is reserved for patients with prohibitive surgical risks or limited life expectancy. Emerging endovascular technology could offer an alternative in the treatment of TAA not involving the visceral vessels or critical intercostal vessels; a combination of open and endovascular approach in high-risk patients also is possible.

The basis of the surgical technique is the one described by Crawford in 1965, consisting of opening the aneurysm sac after cross-clamping the aorta and replacing the diseased segment with a graft. The major intercostal arteries and the visceral aortic segment will be included or reimplanted in the graft. Emphasis is made on operative expediency.

Exposure is achieved through a left TA incision. Adjunctive measures used for spinal protection include spinal drainage with or without epidural cooling (See also Neurologic Complications).

The anesthetic management plays a crucial role. Coordination between anesthesia and the surgical team is of utmost importance. Large-bore IVs in the upper extremities or neck are used for high-flow volume replacement. Arterial and Swan-Ganz monitoring is used. A double-lumen endotracheal tube is used in most cases. Transesophageal echocardiography is helpful in monitoring myocardial contractility and detecting early ischemia. A thoracic epidural catheter is used for perioperative pain management and possible spinal cooling. A lumbar intrathecal catheter can be used for cerebrospinal fluid (CSF) drainage.

Postoperatively the patient is maintained on mechanical ventilation for 24 to 48 hours. The same high level of monitoring is used in the postoperative period. Maintaining hemodynamic stability helps in avoiding major morbidities like cardiac or neurologic complications. Spinal drainage is maintained for about 3 days, because neuronal swelling and ischemia can occur during this period.

Postoperative Complications

Neurologic Complications

Second to mortality, this is the most dreaded and the most devastating complication of TAA repair. The reported incidence averages 13% in degenerative TAA and higher in dissecting aneurysm. This is, however, improving, and an incidence as low as 2% at discharge is being achieved. Factors predictive of neurologic deficit include prior proximal aneurysm repair, presence of aortic dissection, duration of aortic cross-clamp, extent of aorta replaced (highest with type II), oversewing of intercostal arteries, and hypotension and hypoxia.

Multiple surgical adjuncts that help to decrease this devastating complication include (1) maintaining adequate perfusion pressure to the spinal cord. This is done by having proximal aortic pressure in the 150 to 170 mmHg systolic range and decreasing CSF pressure with spinal drainage; (2) distal aortic perfusion during cross-clamp; and (3) spinal drainage. Other adjuncts that can increase neuronal tolerance to ischemia include hypothermia and pharmacologic agents such as steroids and barbiturates.

Pulmonary Complications

Respiratory failure is the most common complication after TAA repair. The incidence varies from 25% to 45%, depending on the definition. Predictive factors for this complication include cigarette smoking; baseline COPD; or cardiac, renal, or bleeding complications. Optimization of pulmonary function should be done preoperatively in elective cases. Intraoperatively, radial division of the diaphragm should be avoided when possible, replaced by a diaphragm-sparing technique.

Renal Insufficiency

Definition of postoperative renal failure varies according to the reports but is often referred to as a doubling of the baseline creatinine or a creatinine greater than 3 mg/dL. The incidence varies between 3.8% and 18%, with an average of 14.7%. Not all patients will require dialysis. Operative mortality is increased in these patients in whom renal failure develops. Etiologic factors include duration of renal ischemia, baseline renal dysfunction, and embolization during aortic manipulation, with preoperative renal failure being the most predictive. Serum creatinine has been found to correlate to some degree with perioperative mortality.

Measures taken to minimize this complication include

1. Limiting the use of preoperative nephrotoxic contrast agents
2. Intraoperative treatment of renal artery stenosis
3. Preoperative volume expansion and intraoperative use of mannitol
4. Minimizing renal ischemia time. Distal aortic perfusion with selective renal perfusion is controversial. Cold renal perfusion and mild systemic hypothermia can be protective
5. Postoperative low-dose dopamine (2–3 mg/kg/min)
6. Hemodialysis is better withheld unless absolutely necessary because of the potential for hemodynamic instability

Cardiac Complications

This is the second most common complication after respiratory failure. Based on a preoperative history of angina and or abnormal stress echocardiography and dipyridamole thallium scans, coronary revascularization may be necessary in some patients.

Measures that help to decrease cardiac complications include

1. Preoperative coronary revascularization when indicated
2. Preoperative intensive care setting with Swan-Ganz catheter placement and arterial monitoring to optimize myocardial performance. This is continued intraoperatively and postoperatively
3. Distal aortic perfusion (arterial-femoral bypass), in type I to II TAA, which helps decrease the left ventricular afterload during cross-clamping by controlling pump flow.

Bleeding Complications

Reoperation for bleeding is required in about 7% of cases. It is associated with higher perioperative mortality, up to 58% in some reports. The etiology is multifactorial and includes inadequate hemostasis, preoperative coagulopathy, coagulopathy secondary to hemodilution, hypothermia, and mesenteric and hepatic ischemia/reperfusion. Common sources of postoperative bleeding include splenic tears and unrecognized lumbar or intercostal back-bleeding.

Clinical Outcome

Survival at 5 years after surgery is around 60%. This is comparable to survival after elective AAA repairs. Most patients return to independent-living status. Cardiac events are the most common cause of late mortality. Patients with paraplegia or who are dialysis dependent have shorter survival.

PEARLS FOR THE OR

Most abdominal aortic aneurysms are found below the renal arteries.

No back-bleeding or brisk back-bleeding from the inferior mesenteric artery once the abdominal aneurysm is opened indicates that good collateral circulation to the left colon exists.

Endovascular repair of an abdominal aortic aneurysm requires frequent computed tomography or duplex evaluation, looking for late technical complications.

Spinal fluid drainage or spinal cooling or both have been shown to reduce the incidence of postoperative neurologic complications.

The most frequent complication after thoracoabdominal aneurysm repair is respiratory failure.

Femoral artery aneurysms are repaired by excision, and popliteal artery aneurysms are repaired by ligation and bypass.

Peripheral Arterial Aneurysms

Although less common than aortic aneurysms, peripheral aneurysms may cause significant morbidity. Death related directly to these aneurysms may occur; however, the more common complication is compromise of end-organ circulation from thrombosis or distal embolization. The most common etiology for true aneurysms is atherosclerotic. The anatomic locations of true aneurysms are, in descending order, popliteal, femoral, subclavian/axillary, and carotid. More distal extremity aneurysms are very rare and limited to small series.

Femoral and Popliteal Aneurysms

Incidence and Etiology

Most commonly, femoral and popliteal aneurysms are atherosclerotic in origin, except for rare degenerative disorders. Together, they account for more than 90% of peripheral aneurysms. Femoral aneurysms involve mainly the common femoral artery (CFA). The male-to-female ratio is 30:1. These may extend into the superficial femoral artery (SFA) or the deep femoral artery (DFA). A particular feature of popliteal and femoral aneurysms is their association with other atherosclerotic aneurysms, often aortoiliac. Femoral aneurysms are associated with another aneurysm in 95% of cases. Conversely, 3% of AAAs have an associated femoral aneurysm.

Popliteal aneurysms have a reported incidence of fewer than four cases in 100,000 hospitalized patients. Popliteal aneurysms are associated with another aneurysm in 78% of cases. About 50% of popliteal aneurysms are bilateral. Every patient with peripheral aneurysms should be screened for an aortoiliac aneurysm, which may be life threatening.

Natural History

Unoperated-on aneurysms carry a 40% to 50% incidence of complications, mostly thromboembolic. Profunda femoral aneurysms are more likely to rupture than are common femoral aneurysms. Thrombosis of a CFA aneurysm may be first seen with critical leg ischemia, because both SFA and PFA flows are interrupted. Unoperated-on popliteal aneurysms can lead to major complications, mainly thromboembolic. About one third of patients will have limb-threatening complications within 3 years. Rupture is rare but may occur. Other complications include pain from severe compression or popliteal vein thrombosis.

Clinical Presentation

Femoral aneurysms: The typical patient is a male in his seventh decade with risk factors for atherosclerosis. These may be asymptomatic in 40% of cases, with a palpable pulsatile mass, or more often, with local pain, compression symptoms, or distal ischemia. Thrombosis with acute ischemia occurs in 1% to 16%. "Blue-toe syndrome" or distal gangrene can be the presenting finding in 10%.

Popliteal aneurysms: The presentation can be on a spectrum from an asymptomatic pulsatile mass in the popliteal fossa in 45% of cases to severe limb-threatening ischemia from thrombosis or embolization. The majority of patients will have ischemic symptoms. Fewer than 5% of popliteal aneurysms will be seen initially with rupture.

Diagnosis

Most peripheral aneurysms are amenable to diagnosis by physical examination. Further diagnostic studies are used for confirmation and surgical planning. Ultrasound or CT scan easily diagnoses femoral and popliteal aneurysms. Arteriography is necessary only for imaging of run-off vessels and preoperative planning. Preoperative catheter-directed thrombolytic therapy could play a role in improving the run-off and thus improving chances of limb salvage in patients with thrombosis and embolization. MRA can be an alternative to conventional angiography.

Indications for Operation

Unlike that in AAA, size is not a major factor in assessing risks from these lesions. This is because of the high incidence of thromboembolic complications. For many surgeons, the mere presence of an aneurysm in the femoral and especially popliteal location is an indication for intervention. With femoral aneurysms, usually a diameter of 2.5 cm is accepted as a cutoff point for intervention, unless the patient is otherwise a high surgical risk. The limited literature regarding the natural history of non–operated-on femoral artery aneurysms suggests that limb-threatening complications from an asymptomatic lesion are very rare. Thus observing a small asymptomatic femoral aneurysm in a high-risk patient is not unreasonable.

For the popliteal aneurysm, the natural history is quite different. Non–operated-on asymptomatic aneurysms are invariably associated with a high incidence of ischemic complications. Consequently, symptomatic popliteal aneurysms should be repaired expeditiously and asymptomatic popliteal aneurysms repaired electively, unless the patient represents a very poor surgical risk.

Treatment

Femoral artery aneurysms are treated with resection and graft interposition. Popliteal aneurysms are treated with bypass with proximal and distal ligation, usually from the above-the-knee to the below-the-knee segment of the popliteal artery, by using autogenous vein. This is done through a medial or posterior approach. In the case of a large popliteal aneurysm with compression symptoms, resection may be appropriate, through a posterior approach. Preoperative or intraoperative lytic therapy may be beneficial in situations in which distal runoff and microcirculation is occluded from severe thromboembolization.

When a concomitant AAA and peripheral aneurysm are identified, the life-threatening AAA is usually operated on first, unless the peripheral aneurysm has already caused limb-threatening complications.

Results

When aneurysms are treated before thromboembolic events, results are usually excellent, with patency and limb-salvage rates of more than 90% at 5 years. Conversely, when thromboembolic complications have occurred, the patency and the limb-salvage rates decrease to 50% and 60%, respectively.

Tibial Artery Aneurysms

These are uncommon and often represent pseudoaneurysms secondary to infection or trauma. They may be asymptomatic or occur with distal embolization. Treatment options include observation, ligation, or bypass, depending on symptoms and the status of the other tibial vessels.

Upper Extremity Aneurysms

Subclavian/Axillary Aneurysms

Incidence and Etiology. These aneurysms are rare and represent only 1% of peripheral arterial aneurysms. They can be divided into proximal, mid, and distal subclavian or subclavian/axillary. The latter are by far the most common, usually nonatherosclerotic, related to thoracic outlet syndrome. The natural history is difficult to establish because of the rarity of the lesions and because the diagnosed cases are usually symptomatic. The primary complication is embolization, which usually occurs in younger people, more commonly in women, and is almost always associated with cervical ribs. The subclavian artery is compressed where it crosses the first rib, and this sometimes may result in poststenotic dilatation. Patients often are initially seen with distal embolization, manifested by punctuated digital or palmar tender lesions or loss of distal pulses. Angiography remains the most useful diagnostic test. It also allows preoperative planning.

Treatment. Small, asymptomatic aneurysms secondary to thoracic outlet syndrome can be treated with outlet decompression alone. In all other situations, the aneurysm must be excluded, and circulation restored. Thoracic outlet decompression should be done concurrently. This can be performed through a supraclavicular or axillary approach or a combination of both approaches. Decompression may include first-rib resection, or cervical-rib resection and anterior scalene decompression.

Results. Arterial reconstruction after subclavian-axillary resection has a very favorable outcome. Results are less favorable when the run-off has been occluded by embolization.

Hand Aneurysms

True aneurysms in this location are very rare. They are commonly associated with occupational trauma. The presentation is usually with a mass and pain. Distal embolization is less common. Diagnosis is usually made by palpation and is confirmed by ultrasound or CT scan. If not palpable, aneurysms are often diagnosed on angiograms done for distal embolization.

The most common entity is the hypothenar hammer syndrome, in which the ulnar artery becomes aneurysmal secondary to repetitive trauma. This occurs in its segment between Guyton's canal and the palmar aponeurosis, where the artery is superficial and anterior to the hook of the hamate. The most accepted treatment is aneurysm resection and microsurgical vein interposition. Surgery might not be required in asymptomatic thrombosed aneurysms.

Suggested Reading

Ailawadi G, Eliason JL, Upchurch GR Jr: Current concepts in the pathogenesis of abdominal aortic aneurysm. Vasc Surg 38:584–588, 2003.

Beebe HG: Lessons learned from aortic aneurysm stent graft failure; observations from several perspectives. Semin Vasc Surg 16:129–138, 2003.

Brewster DC, Cronenwett JL, Hallett JW Jr, et al, and Joint Council of the American Association for Vascular Surgery and Society for Vascular Surgery: Guidelines for the treatment of abdominal aortic aneurysms: Report to the subcommittee of the Joint Council of the American Association for Vascular Surgery and Society for Vascular Surgery. Vasc Surg 37:1106–1117, 2003.

Cambria R, Davidson JK, Zannetti S: Thoracoabdominal aneurysm repair: Perspectives over a decade with the clamp-and-sew technique. Ann Surg 226:294–305, 1997.

Ernst CB: Abdominal aortic aneurysm. N Engl J Med 328:1167–1172, 1993.

LaMorte WV, Scott TE, Menzoian JO: Racial differences in the incidence of femoral bypass and abdominal aortic aneurysmectomy in Massachusetts: Relationship to cardiovascular risk factors. J Vasc Surg 21:422–431, 1995.

Powell JT, Greenhalgh RM: Clinical practice: Small abdominal aortic aneurysms. N Engl J Med 348:1895–1901, 2003.

Sampson LN, Cronenwett JL: Abdominal aortic aneurysms. In Zelenock GB (ed): Problems in General Surgery. Vol II: Vascular Surgery. Philadelphia, JB Lippincott, 1995, pp 385–417.

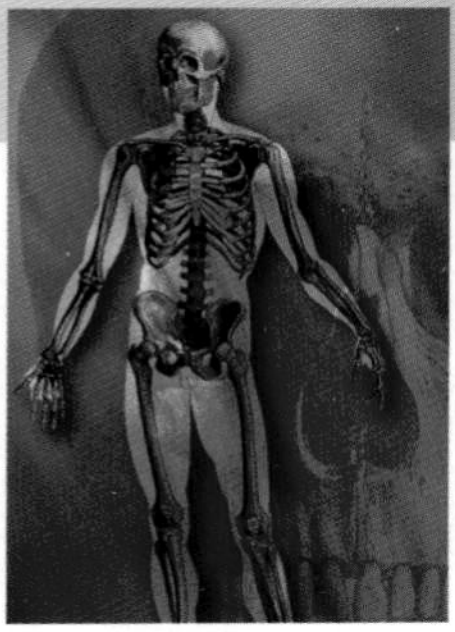

Chapter 39

Cerebrovascular Disease

NANCY L. CANTELMO, MD, BRIAN J. MARIEN, MD, and JAMES O. MENZOIAN, MD

Introduction

Stroke is one of the most urgent health concerns in the United States. It is the third leading cause of death, after heart disease and cancer, and the primary cause of adult disability. Each year, approximately 500,000 people have a stroke. Almost 150,000 will die as a result of the stroke, and the remaining 350,000 will be left with impairments, ranging from minimal to total disability. It is estimated that the annual costs, both direct and indirect, total $40 billion.

Stroke is a general, and somewhat imprecise, term that means a vascular injury to the brain. A stroke may be considered a brain infarct, in the same sense as a myocardial infarction—both result in tissue death. In the brain, however, an area of secondary injury may occur, called the ischemic penumbra. These brain cells surround those that have died and also become susceptible to injury by a series of chemical and electrical disturbances. The brain tissue in this area has the potential either of infarcting and causing further neurologic deficit or of recovering and causing symptomatic improvement.

The two major types of strokes are *hemorrhagic* and *ischemic*. A *hemorrhagic stroke* is caused by bleeding in the brain. An *ischemic stroke*, caused by an interruption of the blood supply to part of the brain, will result in a persistent neurologic deficit, which lasts longer than 24 hours. *Transient ischemic attacks (TIAs)* are ischemic neurologic deficits that last for less than 24 hours, and frequently for minutes. A *reversible ischemic neurologic deficit (RIND)* is defined as a neurologic deficit that lasts longer than 24 hours but resolves in a few days, much like a longer TIA. This term is now infrequently used, as it has no longer proven helpful to define this specific period.

Much of our information about the incidence of strokes comes from population-based studies, such as the Framingham Study, but exact etiologies are often difficult to ascertain. Hemorrhagic strokes account for about 20% of strokes and are usually caused by rupture of a cerebral aneurysm. They are described by the territory in which they occur, either subarachnoid or intracerebral. Each has a different presentation, but both are associated with headache, nausea and vomiting, and decreased level of consciousness.

The two major types of ischemic strokes are *thrombotic* and *embolic*. A thrombotic stroke occurs when thrombosis occurs within the brain vasculature, usually because of atherosclerotic disease. Embolic strokes are due to thrombi, platelets, fibrin, or cholesterol, which originate from the heart, aorta, or extracranial carotid arteries and travel to the large vessels of the brain. Another type of stroke, called a *lacunar* stroke, is related to ischemia of the smaller vessels of the brain, especially the penetrating vessels of the basal ganglia.

Epidemiology

A steady decrease has occurred in ischemic stroke over the past three decades, as has a marked improvement in stroke survival. Although not completely understood, it is thought to be attributed to better control of the risk factors causing stroke and improved management of the patients who have had strokes. Certain areas are recognized as having a higher stroke frequency and mortality, such as the southeastern United States, which is referred to as the "stroke belt." Racial differences also occur with stroke incidence and mortality. African-American men and women have an incidence and death rate more than twice that of the white population of the United States.

The incidence of stroke increases with age. A previous stroke or TIA increases the stroke risk significantly. Elevated blood pressure is an important risk factor for all types of stroke, but particularly for hemorrhagic and lacunar strokes. Heart disease is a risk factor, and atrial fibrillation is a particular risk factor for embolic stroke.

Anatomy

The circulation to the brain is divided into the anterior and posterior portions. The anterior circulation comprises the carotid arteries. The right common carotid artery originates from the innominate or brachiocephalic artery, the first branch of the aortic arch, as the innominate divides into the right common carotid and right subclavian arteries (Fig. 39-1). The left common carotid artery comes directly off the aortic arch as the second branch; the third branch is the left subclavian artery.

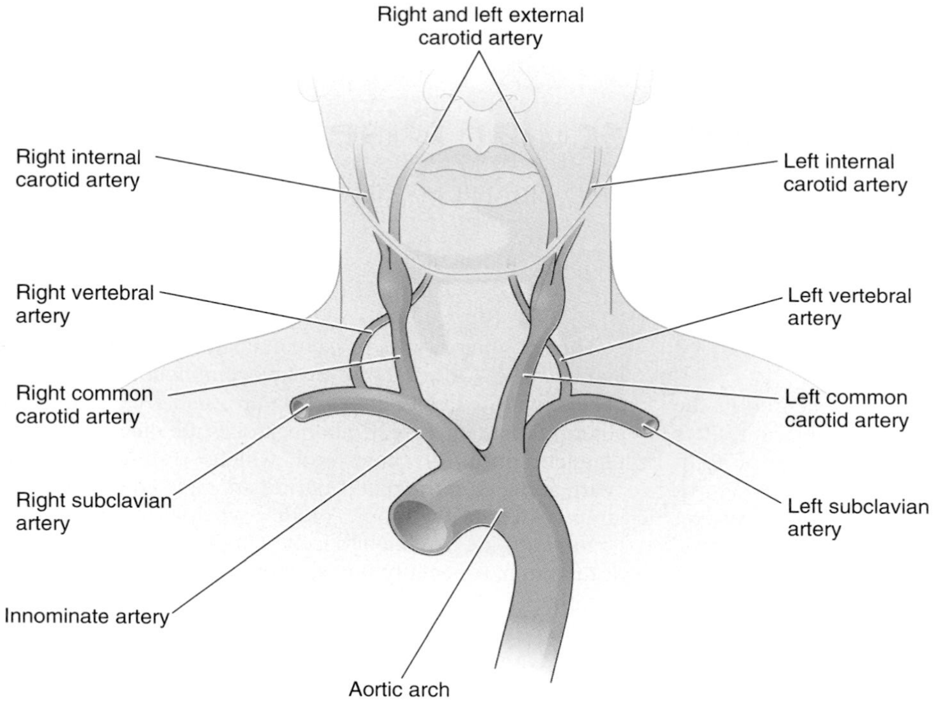

FIGURE 39–1 Circulation to the brain.

Each common carotid artery divides into the external and internal carotid arteries. The external carotid artery is located medially, and the internal carotid artery is lateral. The external has many branches that supply the head and neck. The internal carotid artery has no branches in the neck; its first major branch is the ophthalmic artery, located intracranially. The internal carotid artery bifurcates into the middle cerebral and the anterior cerebral arteries. The middle cerebral is larger and initially courses in a straighter direction than the anterior cerebral artery.

The right and left vertebral arteries begin the posterior circulation. They originate as the first branch of the subclavian artery and travel through the foramina of the cervical vertebrae. They join to form the basilar artery, which then gives rise to the right and left posterior cerebral arteries.

The circle of Willis is the connection between the anterior and posterior circulation and balances the inflow from the carotid and vertebral arteries to the anterior, middle, and posterior cerebral arteries. The anterior communicating artery connects the two sides of the anterior circulation, and two posterior communicating arteries form the posterior circulation. In only about 20% of people is the circle complete. Most individuals have hypoplasia of one or more segments, and about one fourth of people have hypoplasia or absence of one or both posterior communicating arteries.

Pathophysiology of Extracranial Cerebrovascular Disease

The most common mechanism of cerebral ischemia is emboli from an extracranial site. The emboli originate from a cardiac source, especially in patients with atrial fibrillation or valvular disease. The other main sources of emboli are the aorta arch or the carotid bifurcation, in association with an atherosclerotic plaque.

The atherosclerotic plaque is a complex of cholesterol and precipitated calcium salts, with an associated fibroblastic proliferation from an inflammatory response. This process, which occurs within the intima and media, undergoes structural remodeling during its interaction with the various aspects of the blood. The surfaces are frequently irregular, with ulcerated areas, into which thrombi and platelets may collect. Ulcerated plaques also may form when a hemorrhage occurs within the plaque. The thin fibrous covering over the intraplaque hemorrhage ruptures and releases emboli from the plaque, leaving a cavity behind (Fig. 39-2*A–C*).

Branches or arterial bifurcations are important sites of atheromatous plaque formation. The carotid bifurcation is the most important site in either the intracranial or extracranial circulation. Extensive research on the carotid bifurcation has elucidated factors of geometry, flow-velocity profiles, and wall-shear stress to be associated

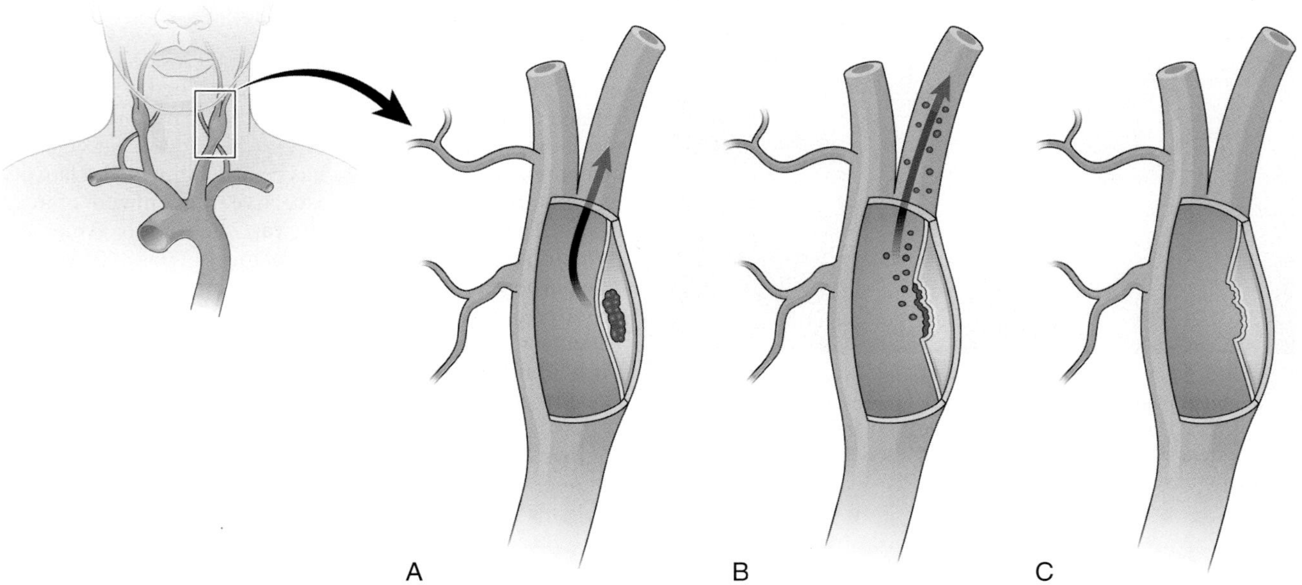

FIGURE 39–2 Extracranial cardiovascular disease. *A*, Plaque in carotid artery (yellow) with intraplaque hemorrhage (*black*) and thin fibrous cap. *B*, Ruptured intraplaque hemorrhage, releasing platelet emboli. *C*, Ulcerated plaque remaining after plaque rupture.

with plaque formation at specific areas within the carotid bifurcation. The slightly dilated section where the common carotid bifurcates into the internal and external carotid arteries is called the bulb. This bulb area, opposite the flow divider, is subjected to circular movement of blood and low sheer stress, where plaque proliferates.

A second, but far less frequent, cause of the focal neurologic symptoms of stroke or TIA is a hemodynamic change. Individuals with an incomplete or hypoplastic circle of Willis would seem to be at risk for underperfusion of areas of the brain with a decrease in systemic blood pressure. The brain, however, is protected by an autoregulatory compensation, which maintains cerebral perfusion within a wide range of systemic blood pressure fluctuation. This is the most likely reason that hemodynamic changes do not more frequently result in cerebral hypoperfusion and neurologic events.

Clinical Presentation

The middle cerebral artery, by reason of its anatomic relationship with the internal carotid artery, is the most frequent target of extracranial embolic disease. The clinical manifestations of a stroke or TIA involving the middle cerebral artery of the dominant hemisphere would be weakness or numbness in the contralateral face, arm, or leg and aphasia. The aphasia could be either an expressive problem with normal comprehension (Broca's aphasia), or a difficulty with both comprehension and expression (Wernicke's aphasia). A lesion of the nondominant hemisphere also would produce contralateral weakness or numbness. Comprehension would be normal, but the most common speech change would be a monotone expression.

Emboli from the left carotid artery to the left hemisphere might cause symptoms of paralysis of the right side of the body as well as aphasia, because the left hemisphere is dominant in most people. An embolus from the left carotid artery also might travel to the left ophthalmic artery, the first major branch of the internal carotid artery, and cause specific visual symptoms. Emboli to the eye may result in either transient or permanent retinal ischemia. Patients will often describe a "shade coming down" over one eye, loss of vision in one eye, or a specific field of vision being affected. These symptoms are recognized as a kind of TIA, specific to the eye, and are called *transient monocular blindness (TMB)* or *amaurosis fugax*, which is derived from the Greek for transient loss of vision. Cholesterol emboli, which originate from atherosclerotic plaques, may at times be visualized by funduscopic examination. These are called Hollenhorst plaques (Fig. 39-3).

Embolic symptoms of the ophthalmic artery are always ipsilateral to the source, whereas body symptoms will always be contralateral to the source of the emboli and the hemisphere affected. Major strokes may produce eye findings such as contralateral hemianopsia and eye deviation, but they result from an insult to brain tissue, rather than a transient ischemic event to the ophthalmic artery.

In addition to TIA and stroke, some other clinical situations are referable to the cerebrovascular circulation.

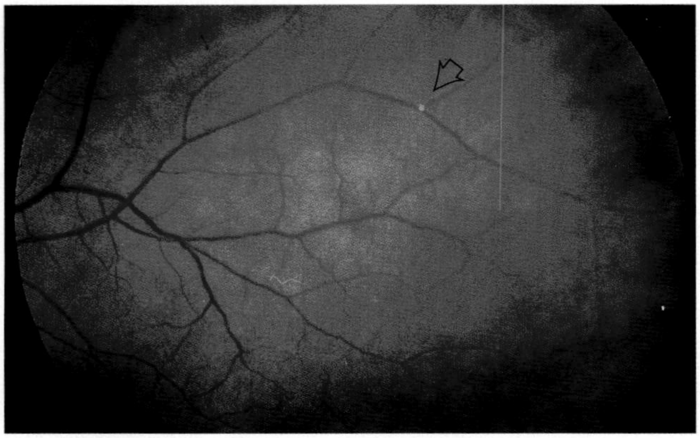

FIGURE 39–3 A funduscopic examination showing a Hollenhorst plaque, which appears as a bright spot in a branch retinal vessel. This small piece of cholesterol has embolized from a stenosis in the ipsilateral carotid artery by way of the ophthalmic artery to the retina.

One entity is called *crescendo TIAs*, and involves a series of TIAs that occur frequently and are usually not affected by anticoagulation. A *stroke in evolution* refers to a situation in which the symptoms of a stroke worsen, perhaps related to the penumbra effect or to repeated embolization. Symptoms that are nonlateralizing, such as syncope, dizziness, or ataxia, may be associated with the vertebrobasilar system of the posterior circulation and may be hemodynamic in origin. It also is possible that with a combined lesion of the anterior and posterior circulations, symptoms of the posterior circulation may be expressed.

A complete physical examination should include auscultation for bruits, indicative of a flow disturbance due to arterial stenosis. The best place to place the stethoscope on the neck is just below the angle of the mandible, in the region of the carotid bifurcation. The bell of the stethoscope is frequently more helpful than the diaphragm, and the patient may need to hold his or her breath. It is important to differentiate between a bruit and a transmitted murmur, by listening lower down on the neck and also auscultating the chest. A bruit that is heard bilaterally along the neck from the mandible to the clavicle and is accompanied by a heart murmur would most likely be a transmitted murmur.

The presence of a cervical bruit is recognized as a risk factor for stroke. Patients with bruits should undergo noninvasive testing to evaluate the degree of stenosis of the underlying carotid artery.

A TIA is recognized as a risk factor, or warning sign, for a stroke. However, only 30% to 50% of patients who have a stroke have had a prior TIA. A group of patients who have asymptomatic carotid stenosis, often identified by a cervical bruit, benefit from intervention for their disease.

Indications for Carotid Surgery

Symptomatic Carotid Stenosis

Therapeutic surgical intervention for atherosclerotic disease of the extracranial carotid artery has been considerably refined over the last half century and continues to evolve as more data become available. The efficacy of surgery for symptomatic carotid disease has been documented relatively recently by three large prospective randomized clinical trials. The most influential was the North American Symptomatic Carotid Endarterectomy Trial (NASCET). The purpose of the study was to determine whether carotid endarterectomy (CEA) reduced the risk of stroke among patients with symptomatic ipsilateral carotid artery stenosis. Fifty clinical centers throughout the United States and Canada participated. In total, 659 patients were identified to have between a 70% and 99% stenosis by cerebral angiography. The patients were subsequently randomized to either best medical therapy (n = 331) or CEA plus best medical therapy (n = 328). The trial was halted in February 1991 by a monitoring committee, which reported a statistically significant benefit of CEA over medical therapy alone. Life-table analysis demonstrated the risk of any ipsilateral stroke at 2 years of 26% versus 9% in the medical and surgical groups, respectively. This represented an absolute risk reduction of 17%.

The European Carotid Surgery Trial (ECST), a similar large multicenter prospective randomized clinical study, confirmed the results of the NASCET trial. Eighty centers throughout Europe participated. The 778 symptomatic patients were identified by cerebral angiography to have an ipsilateral carotid stenosis of 70% to 99%. Of these, 323 patients were randomized to the medical group, and 455 patients to the surgical group. A statistically significant benefit to surgery was identified. The 3-year risk of any death or stroke was 12.3% for surgery versus 21.9% for medical therapy.

The third large multicenter prospective randomized study was the Veterans Affairs Symptomatic Trial. Sixteen university-affiliated Veterans Affairs medical centers participated. The 189 men with angiographically documented symptomatic ipsilateral carotid artery stenosis greater than 50% were again randomized to either optimal medical therapy alone (n = 91) or CEA plus optimal medical therapy (n = 98). The study was discontinued early after reports of the NASCET and ECST demonstrated a statistically significant benefit to surgery. Nonetheless, this study confirmed the results of the prior trials, revealing a 7.7% versus a 19.4% risk of stroke or crescendo TIA in the surgical and nonsurgical patients, respectively. This represented an absolute risk reduction of 11.7%. Further analysis demonstrated an absolute risk reduction of 17.7% in 129 patients with a carotid stenosis greater than 70%.

The aforementioned clinical trials unequivocally demonstrated the therapeutic efficacy of CEA in selected patients. The present indication for CEA based on these studies includes a carotid stenosis of greater than 70% in patients who sustain ipsilateral hemispheric TIA, amaurosis fugax, RIND, or a mild nondisabling stroke. Other indications considered acceptable, although not yet supported by definitive clinical trials, include carotid stenosis of 50% to 69% in patients who (1) sustain similar neurologic events despite medical therapy, (2) have an associated contralateral carotid occlusion, or (3) display angiographic evidence of ulceration. However, the benefit of surgery will not be realized if the procedure-related complications and death are excessive. The perioperative combined morbidity and mortality should not exceed 5% for TIAs and 7% for ischemic stroke. Contraindications to CEA include TIA or stroke with less than a 50% stenosis, not receiving antiplatelet therapy, hemispheric cerebrovascular accident, and associated dense neurologic deficit, multi-infarct dementia, global cerebral ischemia, senile dementia, or Alzheimer's, hemorrhagic infarct, TIAs of the vertebrobasilar distribution, uncontrolled congestive heart failure, recent myocardial infarction, unstable angina, or advanced malignancy.

Asymptomatic Carotid Stenosis

Asymptomatic carotid artery stenosis is usually discovered by duplex ultrasonography performed to investigate a newly discovered carotid bruit, preoperative screen before coronary artery bypass grafting, or incidentally during evaluation of a contralateral symptomatic carotid lesion. Although asymptomatic carotid stenosis seems to imply a relatively benign pathologic diagnosis, it is the harbinger of a potentially unpredictable and catastrophic neurologic event.

Two large prospective randomized clinical trials demonstrated the efficacy of CEA in selected asymptomatic patients. The Asymptomatic Carotid Atherosclerosis Study (ACAS) was initiated to determine the efficacy of combining aggressive medical management and CEA in reducing the incidence of stroke in patients with asymptomatic carotid stenosis. Thirty-nine clinical centers throughout the United States and Canada participated. In total, 1662 asymptomatic patients with an internal carotid artery stenosis of 60% or greater were randomized. The trial was halted by the monitoring committee in December 1994, when it demonstrated a statistically significant benefit in the surgical group. The 5-year aggregate risk of ipsilateral stroke, any perioperative stroke, and death was 5.1% versus 11% in the surgical and medical groups, respectively.

The Veterans Affairs Cooperative Asymptomatic Trial was conducted to determine whether the addition of CEA to best medical management would result in fewer TIAs in patients with asymptomatic, hemodynamically significant carotid artery stenosis. Eleven Veterans Affairs Medical Centers participated. In total, 444 asymptomatic men with an angiographically documented 50% or greater internal carotid artery stenosis were randomized. A statistically significant benefit was derived from endarterectomy. The risk of all ipsilateral neurologic events was 8.0% in the surgical group versus 20.6% in the medical group.

These trials clearly demonstrate the efficacy of CEA in those patients who have an asymptomatic, hemodynamically significant internal carotid artery stenosis. It is hard to justify an operation for an asymptomatic lesion with an annual estimated stroke risk of 2% to 5% if the perioperative stroke and death rates exceed these percentages. Hence, endarterectomy should be performed only by experienced surgeons who have demonstrated a consistent performance record with minimal morbidity and mortality. Even though the aforementioned studies reveal a benefit of surgery in asymptomatic patients who have stenosis 50% to 60% or greater, most surgeons reserve operation for only good-risk patients with advanced stenoses of 80% or more.

Recurrent Carotid Stenosis

Carotid artery restenosis after endarterectomy has a reported range of incidence between 1% and 36%. The importance of identifying such lesions again relates to the risk of future stroke. The two distinct forms of restenosis are based on the temporal relation to the original operation. Early restenosis, generally occurring within 3 to 18 months after endarterectomy, is secondary to myointimal hyperplasia. The reported incidence in the literature ranges from 4% to 19%. Potential contributing factors to the development of early recurrence include continued cigarette smoking, female gender, age older than 65 years, primary arterial closure, and the use of distal tacking sutures.

Myointimal hyperplastic lesions are morphologically dissimilar to atherosclerotic plaques, in that the former are not prone to ulcerate, calcify, or have intraplaque hemorrhage. In addition, regression of this form of stenosis has been documented by serial noninvasive tests. The incidence of neurologic events, reportedly between 1% and 5%, appears to be lower when compared with an atherosclerotic lesion of the same luminal diameter. However, questions still remain whether these intimal hyperplastic lesions eventually degenerate into atherosclerotic plaques. As a result, controversy exists regarding appropriate management of this entity.

Therapeutic options include medical treatment with antiplatelet agents, reoperation using patch angioplasty, and endovascular techniques using balloon angioplasty and stent placement. Reoperation involves a marginally increased risk of perioperative neurologic events and cranial nerve injury. Endovascular techniques involve risks of carotid dissection, acute occlusion, stent deformation, air embolism, progressive stenosis requiring reoperation, and stroke. The Carotid Revascularization: Endarterectomy versus Stent Trial (CREST) is a multicenter study presently being conducted to compare reoperative versus endovascular treatment for early carotid restenosis. Reoperation for this entity presently may be considered in patients with symptomatic or high-grade lesions, who are at risk for carotid occlusion, and also those patients with persistent or progressive asymptomatic high-grade (>80%) stenoses. Endovascular therapy for such lesions should be used only for those patients enrolled in controlled clinical trials at this time.

In some centers in the United States and abroad, endovascular treatment is being used as the primary treatment for carotid stenosis. Indications vary from a difficult operative field, such as that resulting from prior radiation or a very high bifurcation, to use as standard treatment, in place of a routine CEA. As the standard treatment for carotid disease, the CEA is a durable procedure with low morbidity and mortality in experienced hands. The use of endovascular stenting to replace this procedure must be carefully considered.

Late restenosis, occurring more than 18 months after CEA, is usually secondary to atherosclerosis. The approximate incidence is reportedly 1% to 5%. The contributing factors for late restenosis include elevated serum cholesterol and primary arterial closure. The incidence of neurologic events and the indications for operation are therefore similar to those of primary atherosclerotic lesions. Again, a marginally increased risk of adverse perioperative neurologic events and cranial nerve injuries exists for reoperation. The American Heart Association Stroke Council consensus statement of 1989 stated that the acceptable stroke-death rate is 10% for operative therapy of carotid restenosis. The recommended procedure is redo endarterectomy and patch angioplasty.

Combined Carotid and Coronary Disease

Approximately 8% to 14% of coronary artery bypass graft (CABG) patients have a hemodynamically significant carotid stenosis, and nearly 40% to 50% of CEA patients have severe coronary artery occlusive disease. Stroke is one of the most devastating postoperative complications of CABG surgery. Therapeutic options for the cohort of patients with concomitant carotid and coronary disease include combined CABG/CEA performed under the same general anesthesia or staged CABG/CEA performed as separate procedures after a variable interval. The literature is highly controversial on this subject. Two recently published meta-analyses revealed conflicting results in regard to stroke and death in combined versus staged procedures. Therefore recommendations for either a combined or staged approach must be individualized. Most patients can safely undergo staged procedures without incurring an increased risk of perioperative neurologic complications. However, those patients who demonstrate unstable angina or high-grade left main coronary lesions associated with either symptomatic high-grade carotid stenosis, bilateral high-grade asymptomatic stenoses, or ipsilateral high-grade asymptomatic stenosis with contralateral carotid occlusion should be considered candidates for a combined procedure. A subgroup of patients who require emergency CABG may undergo a reversed staged approach, whereby the CEA is performed some time after CABG.

Surgical Procedure

The first successful surgical procedure on the extracranial carotid was reported by Eastcott, Pickering, and Robb in 1954. They performed a resection and primary anastomosis on a woman with TIAs. Other surgeons later reported cases that were performed before that of Eastcott, but his group is given the credit for the pioneering procedure. Currently the most commonly performed procedure is carotid endarterectomy, in which the carotid plaque, located at the carotid bifurcation, is removed from the wall of the artery, usually between the intima and media.

Preoperative evaluation of patients for carotid endarterectomy must include evaluation of their cardiac system, because many patients have atherosclerotic occlusive disease located in various arterial sites. A history, physical examination, and electrocardiogram will yield information necessary to decide whether further cardiac evaluation is needed.

Carotid endarterectomy may be performed by using either local or cervical block anesthesia or general endotracheal anesthesia. The major advantage of the awake patient, who is having the procedure under local or regional block, is the ability to perform continual neurologic examination, with the opportunity of evaluating the effects of surgical maneuvers by the patient's neurologic response. It also avoids the cardiodepressant effects that may be associated with general inhalational agents. The major benefit of the fully anesthetized patient is better control of the airway and ventilation and the lack of patient movement due to anxiety or discomfort.

The patient is positioned on the operating table with the neck slightly hyperextended and the patient's head turned in the opposite direction. The head of the table is slightly elevated.

Two incisions are commonly used: One is vertical and parallel to the sternocleidomastoid muscle, and the other is oblique or transverse, in one of the skin creases. After the skin incision, the subcutaneous tissue and fascia are dissected to the anterior border of the sternocleidomastoid muscle. The muscle is mobilized to expose the carotid sheath, which lies underneath. The contents of the carotid sheath are the carotid artery medially, internal jugular vein laterally, and vagus nerve posteriorly. The common facial vein, a large branch if the internal jugular vein, frequently marks the location of the carotid bifurcation. It is divided, and the jugular vein is retracted laterally to expose the carotid artery.

The common carotid artery is dissected and encircled with a silicone rubber (Silastic) tape. The carotid bifurcation is identified, and nerves to the carotid sinus, located at the bifurcation, are injected with lidocaine, to prevent sinus bradycardia. The internal carotid artery is dissected beyond the plaque, usually 3 to 4 cm beyond the bifurcation. The external carotid artery and its first branch, the superior thyroid artery, are dissected. All are encircled with Silastic loops. It is important to dissect carefully in the area of the bifurcation to avoid embolization of adherent thrombus or platelet material into the brain.

In addition to the vagus or tenth cranial nerve, the hypoglossal or twelfth cranial nerve is frequently encountered above the bifurcation. It innervates the tongue, and damage to this nerve will cause deviation toward the side of injury, and difficulty with speech and swallowing. In addition to the sternocleidomastoid muscle, the omohyoid muscle is identified inferiorly, and the digastric muscle is located superiorly. These muscles may be divided if further operative exposure is needed.

Cerebral Protection

Before occlusion of the arteries to perform the carotid endarterectomy, thought must be given to the maintenance of cerebral blood flow after it is interrupted on the side of the endarterectomy. A number of options exist. If the patient is awake, it is possible to assess his or her reaction to the cross-clamping of the carotid artery by asking for motor or speech responses.

If an altered response is elicited, a shunt may be placed. A shunt is a plastic tube that carries the blood from the common carotid artery below the operative site to the internal carotid artery distal to the arteriotomy, to maintain cerebral blood flow. A shunt placed in the situation of a neurologic deficit in an awake patient would be an example of selective shunting, performed only when the need has been demonstrated. Some surgeons choose to use a shunt during every carotid endarterectomy to give adequate protection and to avoid the use of some method of assessing cerebral ischemia. Those who selectively shunt believe that the shunt itself may introduce problems, such as intimal damage, particulate or air emboli, and diminished exposure to the internal carotid artery.

For those surgeons who use general anesthesia and selective shunting, other methods of assessing cerebral blood flow must be used. The measurement of internal carotid artery backpressure, also known as stump pressure, is one technique. This involves measurement of the pressure above the clamped internal carotid artery, as a reflection of perfusion in the circle of Willis. Various threshold lower limits have been suggested, ranging from 25 to 50 mmHg.

Electroencephalographic (EEG) monitoring during the carotid endarterectomy also is used by some surgeons. This involves the placement of leads before surgery, and either a technician who monitors the tracing during the case, or computer-assisted interpretation, to detect alterations in waveform or velocity. A drawback to this method is that EEG is sensitive to the electrical activity of the brain only at the surface.

Another intraoperative technique is transcranial Doppler (TCD), which measures intracranial flow velocity. A direct measurement of the ipsilateral flow velocity in the middle cerebral artery is made before and after carotid artery clamping. If the hemisphere has adequate circulation, a minimal change in flow velocity will result. A shunt may be needed if systolic flow velocity decreases to less than 60% of the baseline value. In addition to measuring flow velocity, transcranial Doppler also can detect emboli that might occur during the procedure, allowing the surgeon to alter technique. TCD also can demonstrate problems that might occur during shunting. The disadvantage of this technique is the need to maintain an intraoperative probe position on the patient during surgery, and the need for the presence of a technician to interpret the findings.

Before cross-clamping of the arteries, the patient is given systemic heparin, which is allowed to circulate. An arteriotomy is made from the common into the internal carotid artery, and if a shunt is elected to be used, it is inserted at this point. The actual endarterectomy is now performed. The plaque is dissected from the wall of the artery, ideally between the intima and media, at the level of the internal elastic lamina (Fig. 39-4). The plaque is removed first from the common carotid, where it is divided at the proximal end of the arteriotomy. It is next removed from the external carotid artery, by eversion of that vessel, and last from the internal carotid artery. The plaque usually feathers out as it ends in the internal carotid artery. Figure 39-5 shows a carotid plaque after the endarterectomy. After the plaque is removed and surface of the artery is cleaned of any loose debris, the artery is sutured closed, often using a patch to prevent narrowing. This patch may be made of vein or synthetic material. Some surgeons choose to patch all endarterectomy closures, whereas others will selectively use a patch only on smaller arteries.

Alternative invasive treatment of carotid stenosis includes endovascular stenting, as mentioned previously, and eversion endarterectomy. The later technique is favored by some centers over the open carotid endarterectomy. It involves an incision in the common carotid artery only, with removal of the internal carotid artery plaque blindly by dissecting around it and pulling it distally out of common carotid arterotomy.

Other Lesions of the Carotid Arteries

Aneurysms

Aneurysms of the extracranial carotid arteries are uncommon lesions associated with variable etiologies. Atherosclerosis is presently the most common cause of extracranial carotid

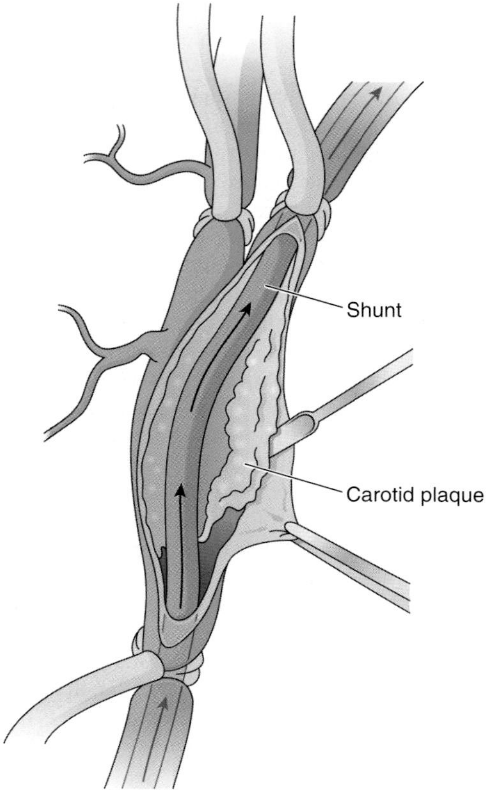

FIGURE 39–4 Carotid plaque (*yellow*) being dissected from the carotid artery with a shunt (*red*) in place for cerebral protection.

aneurysms. The incidence reported in the literature is between 0.1% and 2.0%. Clinical signs and symptoms associated with these lesions include a pulsatile neck mass, pain, dysphagia, hemorrhage, and cranial nerve dysfunction. Adverse neurologic events may be the result of thrombosis, embolization, dissection, or rupture. Other etiologies include infection, trauma, fibromuscular dysplasia (FMD), cystic medial necrosis, carotid artery angioplasty, previous carotid surgery, and Marfan syndrome. All patients, symptomatic and asymptomatic, once identified as having these lesions, should be referred for surgical intervention because of the extremely high risk of stroke.

Dissection

Extracranial carotid artery dissections can be of spontaneous, iatrogenic, or traumatic etiology. The exact incidence is unknown. Patients may experience headache, neck pain, syncope, tinnitus, blurred or lost vision, Horner's syndrome, cranial nerve dysfunction, transient ischemic symptoms, and the most frequent and severe manifestation, stroke. Fortunately, cerebral ischemic symptoms usually are preceded by neck pain, allowing prompt diagnosis and treatment, potentially averting a neurologic catastrophe. Angiography is considered the gold standard for diagnosis and usually reveals an origin of dissection 2 to 4 cm distal to the carotid bifurcation. A classic "string sign" is often present. Initially, the recommendation for therapy is anticoagulation for 3 to 6 months. Indications for surgical intervention include patients in whom symptoms of cerebral ischemia develop despite adequate anticoagulation. Lesions confined to the accessible portion of the extracranial artery circulation may be repaired by autogenous vein graft interposition or external carotid artery transposition. Occasionally, the dissection extends to the base of the skull. In this instance, ligation may be performed, provided the stump pressure exceeds 70 mmHg. Ligation plus extracranial/intracranial bypass should be entertained in those cases in which stump pressure is less than 70 mmHg.

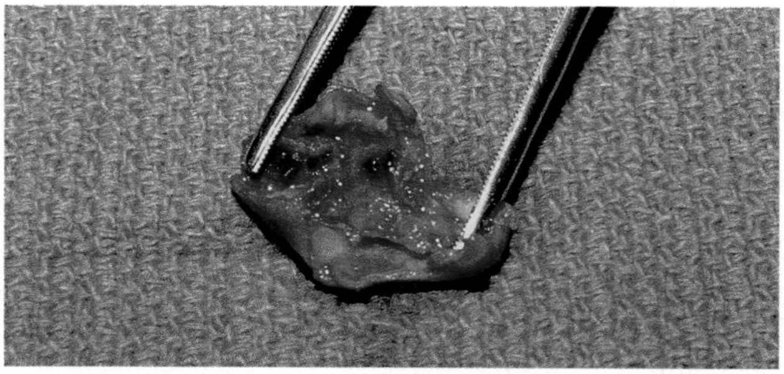

FIGURE 39–5 A pathologic specimen of the atherosclerotic plaque removed during carotid endarterectomy. Darkened areas represent formed clot in irregular ulcerated areas on the surface of the plaque.

Fibromuscular Dysplasia

Extracranial carotid artery FMD is a nonatherosclerotic angiopathy of unknown etiology. The internal carotid and vertebral arteries are usually the affected vessels in the cervical region. Approximately 30% of patients have intracranial aneurysms, 65% are bilateral, and 25% to 50% have associated atherosclerotic disease. Symptoms are similar to those of atherosclerotic carotid stenosis. However, caution must be exercised when attributing such symptoms solely to FMD, as patients commonly have other entities that may be the cause of cerebral ischemia. In addition, symptoms rarely recur and do not appear to be premonitory signs of impending cerebrovascular accident. The natural course of FMD may be extremely benign and therefore support these clinical observations. As a result, indications for operation are controversial. Intervention is clearly not indicated in asymptomatic patients. Virtually all symptomatic patients with FMD, unassociated with other lesions, can be managed nonoperatively without risk of serious neurologic sequelae. Rarely, patients who experience persistent symptoms with angiographic documentation of FMD or associated lesions deserve consideration for operative intervention.

Takayasu's Arteritis

Takayasu's arteritis is an inflammatory vasculopathy of unknown etiology affecting the aorta and its major branches. The disease occurs predominantly in women during the second or third decade of life. The inflammation affects all three layers of the vessel wall, resulting in stenosis, occlusion, aneurysm formation, or a combination of these. A wide variation in clinical course and prognosis has been reported. Unfortunately, stroke commonly is seen as the initial cerebrovascular event. Therefore symptomatic patients warrant prompt surgical treatment, and asymptomatic patients in whom hemodynamically significant stenoses of the innominate or carotid arteries or both develop should undergo prophylactic surgical intervention. The involvement of all layers of the vessel wall precludes standard techniques of endarterectomy or angioplasty or both. Bypass procedures are thus the recommended operative treatment for patients with Takayasu's lesions.

Radiation Arteritis

Radiation arteritis can induce accelerated atherosclerotic changes in the extracranial vessels after external cervical radiation. Hypercholesterolemia and hyperlipidemia have been reported to increase the risk of developing radiation-induced lesions. These changes tend to occur in regions of the extracranial circulation that are unusual for typical atherosclerotic lesions. A 30% incidence of moderate to severe lesions in patients who survived more than 5 years after cervical irradiation compared with 5.6% in nonirradiated age-matched controls has been reported. Surveillance duplex scanning should be used in all patients who survive beyond 5 years after radiation therapy to the cervical region. Patients with hemodynamically significant stenoses on noninvasive testing require preoperative angiography to evaluate the extent of the arteritis. The indications for surgery are essentially identical to those for asymptomatic and symptomatic carotid artery atherosclerotic occlusive disease. However, radiation-induced damage may preclude the ability to perform endarterectomy, and therefore bypass or the newer endovascular techniques may be required.

Carotid Body Tumors (Paragangliomas)

Carotid body tumors, also known as paragangliomas, are rare hypervascular neoplasms of neural crest origin located at the carotid bifurcation. These lesions occur sporadically in 90% of cases. Several investigators reported an association with hypoxemic stimuli, such as chronic obstructive pulmonary disease and living at high altitude. Familial cases account for nearly 10% and are transmitted in an autosomal dominant manner. Bilaterality occurs in only 5% of sporadic cases, but in upward of 30% in the familial form. Malignancy, defined by the presence of metastatic disease, has an incidence of between 2% and 9%. Most patients are initially asymptomatic. Eventually, an enlarging neck mass, pain, dysphagia, hoarseness, tinnitus, or syncope is seen. Approximately 1% to 5% of carotid body tumors are functional and thereby secrete catecholamines. These patients experience hypertension, headaches, palpitations, dysrhythmias, diaphoresis, and photophobia. Duplex scanning is the most widely used noninvasive diagnostic method for detection. Computed tomography (CT) and magnetic resonance imaging (MRI) are useful in defining the extent and relation to adjacent structures in the cervical region. Angiography and preoperative embolization remain essential in large paragangliomas to limit blood loss during resection. Surgical excision is the only curative therapy and therefore is indicated once the diagnosis is established. Perioperative stroke occurs in approximately 2% to 5% of patients. The greatest morbidity is due to cranial nerve injury, ranging from none to 40%, with one half resulting in permanent deficits. Patients with a prohibitive operative risk, terminal illness, or extreme age, however, may instead benefit from radiotherapy.

PEARLS FOR ROUNDS

Stroke is the third leading cause of death in the United States and the primary cause of adult disability.

The two major types of stroke are hemorrhagic and ischemic.

The circle of Willis connects the anterior and posterior circulation of the brain and balances the inflow from the carotid and vertebral arteries to the anterior, middle, and posterior cerebral arteries.

The most common mechanism of cerebral ischemia is emboli from an extracranial site.

Complications of Carotid Artery Surgery

Stroke

Cerebral infarction is responsible for the most devastating complication of carotid surgery. The American Heart Association established acceptable risks of perioperative stroke based on preoperative indications in patients scheduled for carotid endarterectomy as follows: asymptomatic stenosis, less than 3%; previous TIA, less than 5%; prior ischemic cerebral infarction, less than 7%; and recurrent carotid stenosis, less than 10%. The incidence of stroke must not exceed these estimates, or the benefit of carotid endarterectomy for such indications will not be achieved.

Perioperative stroke may be either ischemic or hemorrhagic. Ischemic cerebral infarction may be secondary to thromboembolic phenomena, clamp ischemia, arterial injury, or carotid thrombosis. Risk factors include ulcerated atheromatous plaques, preoperative TIAs or cerebral infarction, contralateral carotid occlusion, synthetic patch angioplasty, and primary closure. Neurologic events attributable to cerebral ischemia usually occur within 12 to 24 hours postoperatively. These patients require either emergency noninvasive duplex scanning or reoperation. A nonoperative course is indicated if technical error and carotid thrombosis can be reliably excluded by noninvasive studies. However, in the event that duplex scanning is unavailable or the aforementioned complications are identified, urgent reoperation is indicated. Reexploration, intraoperative angiography or duplex scanning, thrombectomy, and repair may be performed to correct the underlying pathology.

Hemorrhagic infarction is a rare and irreversible catastrophic event usually occurring after 24 postoperative hours. Risk factors include the hyperperfusion syndrome and administration of anticoagulants. Neurologic deficits appearing in this period require emergency CT scanning to exclude intracerebral bleeding. Duplex scanning or cerebral angiography should be performed if the CT scan is negative. Further management is dependent on results of these studies.

Cranial Nerve Injury

Iatrogenic cranial nerve injury is an uncommon event. The overall estimated incidence of symptomatic dysfunction, based on retrospective clinical studies, is between 2% and 8%. A prospective analysis reported an incidence of 16% after CEA; however, only 60% were symptomatic. Functional recovery usually occurs within 3 months, suggesting that intraoperative blunt trauma (i.e., retractor injury) is the most likely etiology. The frequency of injury to the vagus nerve or recurrent laryngeal branch of clinical significance is 5% to 7%. Dysfunction of these nerves results in ipsilateral vocal cord paresis. Most patients are symptomatic and experience some degree of hoarseness. However, patients may remain asymptomatic after unsuspected injury to these structures. Asymptomatic individuals who require surgery on the contralateral carotid artery as a staged approach are therefore at risk of developing total airway occlusion, should the contralateral vagus or recurrent laryngeal nerve also be injured. Laryngoscopy is thus recommended before staged contralateral surgical intervention. Detection of a dysfunctional vocal cord mandates rescheduling the operation until recovery is complete. Hypoglossal nerve injury occurs in approximately 4% to 6% of cases. Damage results in ipsilateral deviation of the tongue, uncoordinated mastication, and inarticulate speech. Injury to the superior laryngeal nerve, a 1% to 3% incidence, is almost always asymptomatic except for those patients who are vocalists or public speakers. These individuals may experience voice fatigability and the loss of high-pitched phonation. The incidence of marginal mandibular nerve damage is 1% to 3% and manifests as an ipsilateral nasolabial-fold droop. The glossopharyngeal nerve is rarely injured; however, if injured, it may be symptomatically the most serious of all cranial nerve deficits. Patients experience dyscoordinated oropharyngeal deglutition, resulting in aspiration. Enteral tube feeding or intravenous hyperalimentation is therefore required during the recovery phase, which typically lasts approximately 1 month. Occasionally, the greater auricular nerve or transverse cervical nerve is traumatized, manifested by paresthesias of the ipsilateral neck, lower face, and lower ear. In 0.5% to 1%, the spinal accessory nerve is damaged, resulting in an ipsilateral shoulder droop and weakness when turning the head to the contralateral side. Anecdotal reports exist of injury to the superior cervical sympathetic chain, causing an ipsilateral Horner's syndrome.

PEARLS FOR THE OR

The absolute risk reduction of a stroke after carotid endarterectomy in symptomatic patients is 17%.

The common facial vein frequently marks the bifurcation of the carotid artery in the neck.

Carotid artery dissection is treated with anticoagulation for 3 to 6 months.

Cranial nerve injury after carotid endarterectomy is uncommon and can occur in 2% to 8% of patients. Vagus, hypoglossal, and glossopharyngeal nerves are the nerves that can be injured.

Ipsilateral stroke after carotid endarterectomy should not occur in more than 2% to 3% of patients.

The major cause of death after carotid endarterectomy is myocardial infarction and occurs in 1% to 2% of patients.

Wound Hematoma

The incidence of cervical hematoma is surprisingly low despite the use of perioperative antiplatelet agents and intraoperative systemic anticoagulation. The risks of postoperative bleeding include tracheal, carotid artery, and cranial nerve compression. Airway obstruction, cranial nerve dysfunction, wound infection, and poor cosmesis may result. The identification of a large asymptomatic postoperative cervical wound hematoma requires urgent reoperation. In the event of acute airway obstruction, wound staples or sutures should be removed immediately at the patient's bedside to relieve tracheal compression. The patient must then be transported to the operating room for hemostasis and wound closure. A closed suction drain is routinely used after the hematoma evacuation and control of bleeding.

Hyperperfusion Syndrome

Chronic cerebral ischemia due to progressive carotid stenosis results in an altered autoregulatory state. Hyperperfusion may occur after surgical intervention restoring normal cerebral blood pressure and flow. The incidence is between 0.3% and 1%. Risk factors include a high-grade (>70%) stenosis, chronic ipsilateral hypoperfusion, poor collateral hemispheric flow, contralateral carotid occlusion, hypertension, preexisting ipsilateral cerebral infarction, and perioperative anticoagulation. The syndrome initially manifests as a severe headache, usually within 1 postoperative week. The headache may be followed by focal motor seizures. Intracerebral hemorrhage is the most catastrophic complication of the hyperperfusion syndrome.

Infection

Wound infection after cervical incisions is an extremely rare event as a result of a clean surgical field without bacterial contamination, abundant cervical circulation, and routine use of prophylactic antibiotics.

Pseudoaneurysm

The incidence of pseudoaneurysm formation after carotid surgery is extremely low. Approximately 50% are associated with the technique of patch angioplasty. False aneurysm development is most commonly attributed to infection or suture failure. Discovery requires reoperation and appropriate surgical repair.

Death

Myocardial infarction is the leading cause of early and late death after carotid surgery for atherosclerotic occlusive disease. A thorough preoperative cardiac evaluation is therefore mandatory, including history, physical examination, electrocardiography, and possibly exercise stress testing, persantine-thallium radionuclide perfusion scanning, dobutamine stress echocardiography, coronary angiography, or a combination of these, based on the initial assessment. A study from the Cleveland Clinic reported a 26% incidence of severe coronary artery disease discovered through angiography in patients under consideration for carotid endarterectomy. In addition, no clinical suspicion existed for 17% of those patients with surgically correctable coronary disease.

Suggested Reading

Ecker RD, Pickelman MA, Meissner I, Meyer FB: Durability of carotid endarterectomy. Stroke 34(12):2941–2944, 2003.

Menzoian JO: Presidential address: Carotid endarterectomy, under attack again! J Vasc Surg 37(6):1137–1141, 2003.

Naylor AR, Rothwell PM, Bell PR: Overview of the principal results and secondary analyses from the European and North American randomized trials of endarterectomy for symptomatic carotid stenosis. Eur J Vasc Endovasc Surg 26(2):115–129, 2003.

Wholey MH, Wholey M: Current status of cervical carotid artery stent placement. J Cardiovasc Surg 44(3): 331–339, 2003.

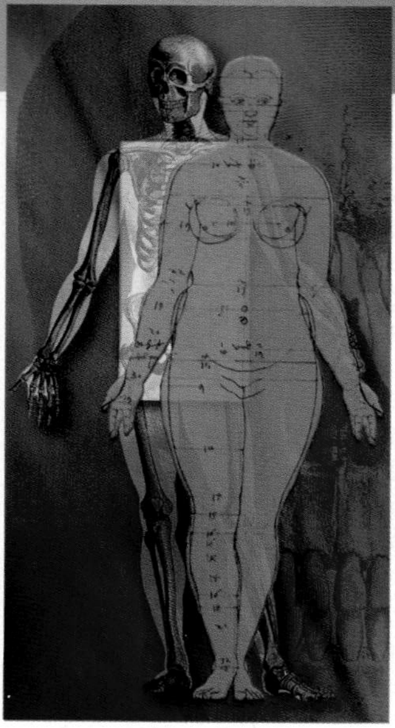

SECTION X

TUMORS AND ONCOLOGY

Chapter 40

Breast Cancer

MAUREEN T. KAVANAH, MD

The incidence of breast cancer in American women continues to remain the highest of all malignancies, with more than 211,000 new invasive cancers and 58,490 noninvasive cancers estimated for 2005 by the National Cancer Institute. Breast cancer remains the leading cause of cancer-related deaths among women between the ages of 20 to 59 years, and with 40,110 deaths estimated for 2005, it is second only to lung cancer as the cause of death of all cancers in women in the United States. The magnitude of the impact of this disease on society is even more significant because it affects not only the patient but also her family, her friends, and her caregivers.

It is most important to continue the basic science, translational, and clinical research efforts currently under way to change the course of this disease. Many areas need further improvement for patients to have the best chance for survival while maintaining their quality of life. The list is extensive, but some important areas include prevention or reduction in the risk of breast cancer, detection of cancer at the earliest stage possible, and better treatment modalities with improved outcomes and fewer toxicities. At the molecular level, we need to discover the scientific basis for understanding the biologic behavior of breast cancer.

Embryology

Each mammary gland develops as an ingrowth of ectoderm, which forms the ducts and alveoli. The mesenchymal layer forms the supportive connective tissue, which includes blood vessels and lymphatic channels. During early fetal development, mammary ridges extend from the axilla to the inguinal areas. Except for the mammary glands, most of these ridges regress; occasionally, accessory breast tissue remains and is clinically evident in the axilla. In some women, accessory nipples may be found anywhere along the "milk line." (Note: The presence of accessory axillary breast tissue is a developmental anomaly. During pregnancy, this tissue becomes prominent in response to the high levels of estrogen. Elective surgical resection can be performed postpartum and after lactational changes regress.)

Anatomy of the Breast

Breast tissue is bounded anteriorly by the superficial fascia and posteriorly by the deep layer of the superficial fascia, which is fused with the deep pectoral fascia of the pectoralis major, the serratus anterior, and the external oblique muscles. Cooper's ligaments are fibrous bands that extend from the deep fascia through the breast parenchyma to the superficial fascia and dermis, thereby providing support for the breast. In relation to the chest wall, breast tissue extends vertically from the level of the second rib to the sixth or seventh ribs. Clinically and during the performance of a mastectomy procedure, the corresponding landmarks are the inferior border of the clavicle and the top of the rectus sheath. Transversely, the breast tissue extends from the ipsilateral border of the sternum to the axillary extent of the gland, which is known as the tail of Spence. Breast cancer can occur anywhere within these boundaries, and, in the treatment of patients with invasive breast cancer, consideration must be given to this entire area at risk (Fig. 40-1).

The nipple and the areola are composed of lactiferous ducts, muscle fibers, and connective tissue. Accessory glands in the areola appear as small elevations on the surface known as Montgomery tubercles. Thick yellow or green secretions are often seen in association with these glands, and care must be taken to distinguish these physiologic secretions from an infection.

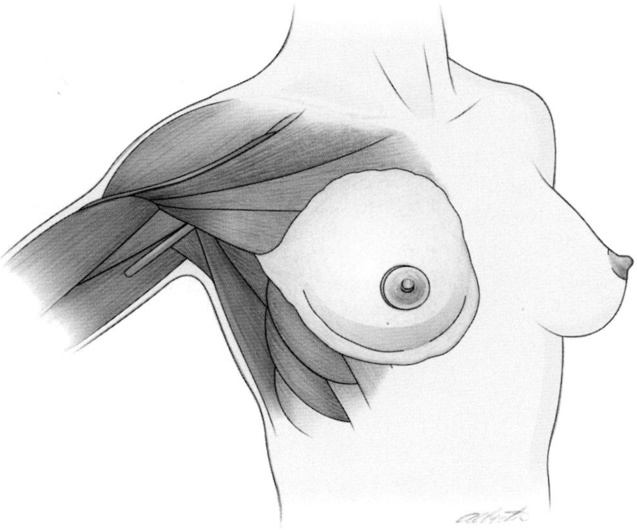

FIGURE 40–1 Approximate distribution of breast tissue on the anterior chest wall. Ductal tissue extends beyond the grossly observable limits of the breast. Posterior relationships are the pectoralis major muscle and the upper abdominal fascia. The lower portion of the breast lies over the deep abdominal and rectus fascia rather than the pectoralis major. (Adapted from Spratt JS, Donegan WL, Tobin G: Gross anatomy of the breast. In Donegan WL, Spratt JS (eds): Cancer of the Breast, 5th ed. Philadelphia, Saunders, 2002, pp 29–44.)

The principal blood supply is from branches of the internal mammary artery, branches of the posterior intercostal arteries, and branches from the thoracoacromial artery, including the thoracic, lateral thoracic, and pectoral branches (Fig. 40-2). Primary venous drainage of the breast is toward the axilla. Drainage of the thoracic wall is through the internal thoracic vein and posterior intercostal veins. Secondary drainage from the thoracic veins into the vertebral venous plexus of Batson provides the pathway for metastases of breast cancer to the skull, central nervous system, vertebrae, and pelvic bones (Fig. 40-3).

Sensory innervation is provided by the anterior and lateral cutaneous branches of the second through sixth intercostal nerves. Nipple sensation is derived mainly from the fourth thoracic nerve. Compression of these nerves as they pass through the underlying chest-wall structures will often cause pain to be referred to the breast. Teitze's syndrome refers to this occurrence at the level of the fourth interspace on the left side (Fig. 40-4).

Lymphatic drainage is extensive and in multiple directions, including to the skin and through internal mammary lymphatics into subclavian, deep cervical, and supraclavicular nodes and veins. The main lymphatic flow, however, is toward the axilla, where nodal groups have been identified according to their position with respect to the pectoralis minor muscle: level I nodes are located lateral to and below the lower border of the pectoralis minor muscle; level II nodes are located deep and posterior to the pectoralis minor muscle, and include Rotter's nodes, which are located between pectoralis major and minor muscles; and level III nodes are located medial to or above the upper border of the pectoralis minor muscle and include the subclavicular and supraclavicular nodes (Fig. 40-5).

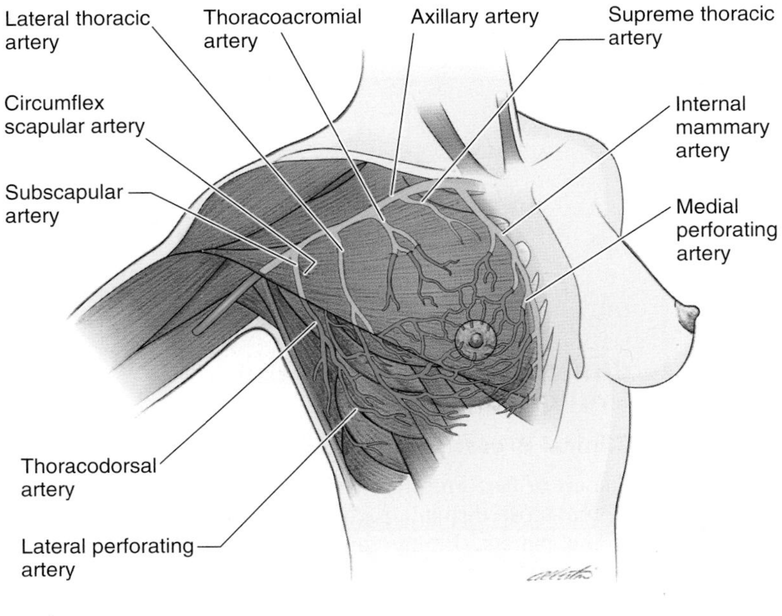

FIGURE 40–2 Arteries of the breast. The arteries have their origin from the internal mammary and axillary arteries. The medial half of the breast is supplied by anterior perforating branches of the internal mammary artery; the lateral half is supplied by the external mammary (lateral thoracic) artery from the axillary artery. Branches of the thoracoacromial artery penetrate the pectoralis major muscle and may enter the deep surface of the breast. (Adapted from Spratt JS, Donegan WL, Tobin G: Gross anatomy of the breast. In Donegan WL, Spratt JS (eds): Cancer of the Breast, 5th ed. Philadelphia, Saunders, 2002, pp 29–44.)

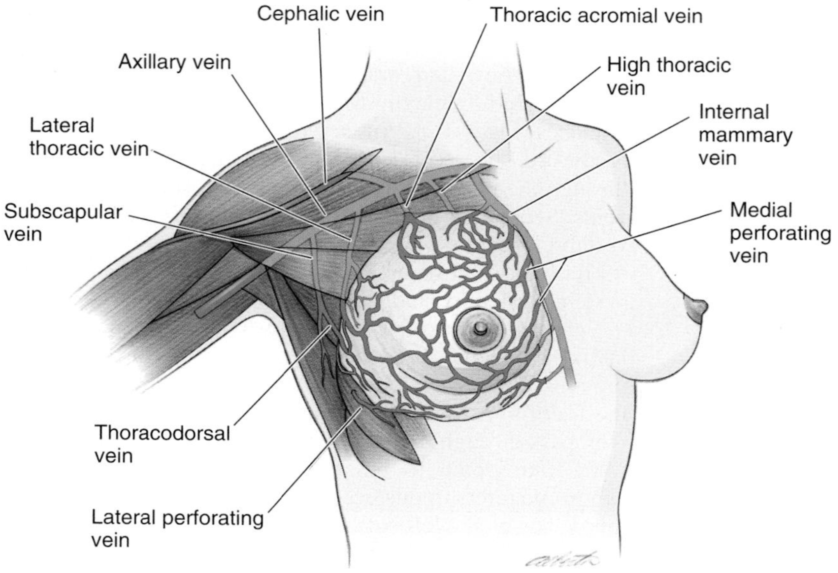

FIGURE 40–3 The venous drainage of the breast. (Adapted from Spratt JS, Donegan WL, Tobin G: Gross anatomy of the breast. In Donegan WL, Spratt JS (eds): Cancer of the Breast, 5th ed. Philadelphia, Saunders, 2002, pp 29–44.)

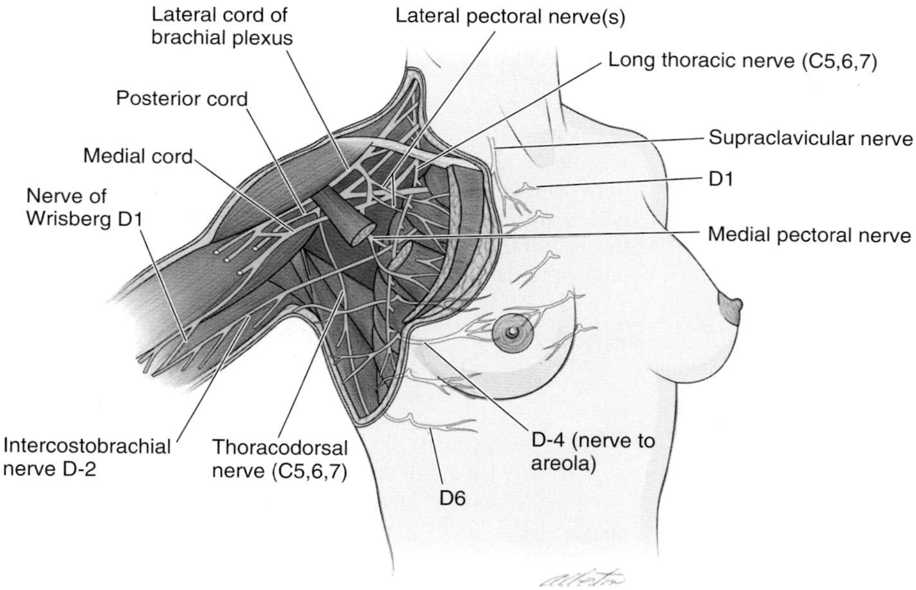

FIGURE 40–4 Major motor and sensory nerves relating to the breast and axilla. (Adapted from Spratt JS, Donegan WL, Tobin G: Gross anatomy of the breast. In Donegan WL, Spratt JS (eds): Cancer of the Breast, 5th ed. Philadelphia, Saunders, 2002, pp 29–44.)

Metastases from breast cancer occur through many of these pathways in a disorderly and unpredictable manner. Systemic spread may occur even when the axillary lymph nodes are pathologically negative for cancer. This occurs because lymph nodes do not trap all the cancer cells, and some cancer cells may pass through the lymph nodes. Other cancer cells spread directly through venous channels and into the systemic circulation.

Clinical Presentation and Evaluation

Clinical Breast Examination

The art of performing a clinical breast examination is one of the most difficult parts of the physical examination of the patient. Benign proliferative tissue is present in most American women, and changes occur frequently

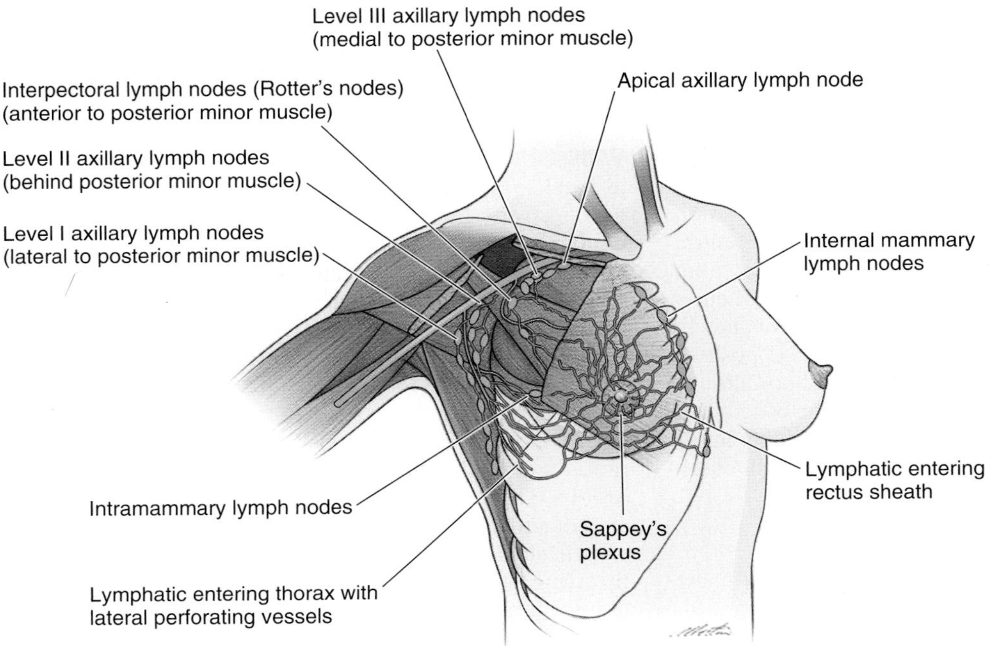

FIGURE 40–5 Lymphatics of the breast showing principal regional lymph node groups. Lymphatics drain to axillary and, to a lesser extent, the internal mammary nodes. Lymph nodes also may be found in the parenchyma of the breast (intramammary lymph nodes). For surgical purposes, the axillary nodes are divided into three levels. (Adapted from Spratt JS, Donegan WL, Tobin G: Gross anatomy of the breast. In Donegan WL, Spratt JS (eds): Cancer of the Breast, 5th ed. Philadelphia, Saunders, 2002, pp 29–44.)

throughout the menstrual cycle or under the influence of hormone replacement therapy. Differentiating proliferative or prominent glandular tissue from a hard or dominant lump can be challenging.

Any observations described by the patient, including skin changes, nipple discharge, and palpable abnormalities should be noted in the medical record, preferably with an anatomic sketch, and evaluated. The breasts should be carefully inspected, with the patient's arms extended overhead, and then with her hands on her hips, leaning forward, noting any evidence of skin retraction, edema (peau d'orange), erythema, nipple inversion, or changes in the skin of the nipple or areola. Palpation of the entire breast tissue is performed with the patient in the sitting and supine positions; palpation of the axillary, supraclavicular, and cervical lymph node areas is also performed with the patient sitting as well as supine. The findings of this examination are best documented in the patient's record on the anatomic drawing and with written observations. Any suggestive palpable mass should be shown to the patient so that she will be able to point it out to the consulting surgeon or radiologist.

Mammography, Ultrasonography, and Magnetic Resonance Imaging

Low-dose film/screen techniques deliver 0.1 cGy to the midbreast region per mammographic view. This small amount of irradiation has not been associated with an increased risk of breast cancer. The benefits of mammography in detecting small, nonpalpable, but curable cancers have far outweighed any potential risks.

Mammographic findings considered suspicious for malignancy include an irregular or new mass with or without microcalcifications; a cluster of microcalcifications, numbering at least five or six; or any change such as architectural distortion in a breast treated for breast cancer with conservative surgery and radiation therapy (XRT). Each of these mammographic abnormalities must be thoroughly evaluated pathologically.

Ultrasonography is not a screening test and has no role in the evaluation of the whole breast. When a patient is first seen with a palpable mass or when a mass is identified mammographically, ultrasonography may be used to try to differentiate between a solid and a cystic mass. On ultrasound evaluation, lesions that are complex or contain a solid component within a cystic structure are suspicious for an intracystic cancer, and surgical excision, not aspiration, should be performed. Ultrasonography is useful for needle biopsy procedures, placement of clips to mark the cancer site, and intraoperatively, for the surgeon to locate nonpalpable solid masses. Ultrasonography of the axilla is not routinely performed; however, there is an emerging role for performing ultrasound-guided biopsy on suspicious lymph nodes in patients with newly diagnosed breast cancer.

Magnetic resonance imaging (MRI) is helpful in selected patients with breast cancer, especially in delineating the extent of disease in patients with infiltrating lobular breast cancer. In some small reported series, unsuspected sites of multicentric cancers have been identified; however, many years of clinical experience has shown that these sites may be present as high as 30% of the time, and they do not require surgical resection. When patients with clinical or mammographically detected cancers (or both) are treated with breast-conservation surgery followed by XRT, these unsuspected multicentric sites of other cancer are well controlled. At this time, more investigative work must be done to determine whether MRI should be done as standard of care in patients newly diagnosed with breast cancer. To date, the false-positive rate is too high with many noncancer abnormalities identified by MRI. Potential areas for other investigations include standardization of technique, determining interpretation criteria, and reducing the costs of the technology while improving the specificity and sensitivity.

Screening for Breast Cancer

Clinical breast examination and conventional two-view mammography are complementary screening techniques. If either study identifies a suggestive finding, a biopsy is necessary. The current guidelines of the American Cancer Society concerning the frequency of performing these examinations as screening tests in asymptomatic women are as follows:

- breast self-examination monthly for all women starting at age 20 years
- clinical breast examination every 3 years at ages 20 to 39 years, and annually starting at age 40 years
- annual mammography starting at age 40 years

For women who are at increased risk for breast cancer, more frequent examinations may be recommended at the discretion of the physician and based on the difficulty of the clinical breast examination.

Diagnostic Evaluation

Clinical breast examination and screening mammography may identify suggestive lesions, but only the pathologist can diagnose a malignancy. Frozen-section histologic analyses of tissues are associated with few false-positive results; an occasional false-positive result occurs with cytologic analysis. False-negative results may occur more frequently, especially when the lesion is a ductal or lobular carcinoma in situ, atypical ductal hyperplasia, or sclerosing adenosis. The use of touch prep analysis, based on the biologic principle that tumor cells are loosely bound to each other and therefore are easily shed onto a glass slide, is highly accurate, especially with the availability of an experienced cytopathologist. In most cases, definitive cancer treatment recommendations should be made based on permanent pathology results confirming the presence or absence of invasive disease.

Fine-needle aspiration biopsy (FNAB) can be performed as an office procedure if the lesion is palpable. For nonpalpable lesions, it can be performed under ultrasound or mammographic guidance. The procedure is performed by using a 10-mL syringe and a 19- or 21-gauge needle. With sterile technique and using 1% lidocaine (Xylocaine) as local anesthetic (optional), the needle is passed into the lesion several times and at different angles, always maintaining negative pressure on the barrel of the syringe to suction the loosened cells into the syringe. The specimen is placed into cytologic suspension fluid right away and submitted for cytologic analysis. If the specimen is sufficient and positive for malignancy, immunohistochemical staining of the cells for estrogen and progesterone receptors can be performed.

Core needle biopsy (CNB) also is performed as an office procedure if the lesion is palpable. For nonpalpable lesions, it can be performed under ultrasound or stereotactic mammography guidance. Local 1% lidocaine anesthesia should be used, and the procedure performed by using sterile technique. Because tissue samples are obtained, histologic analyses are performed and can help determine if invasive cancer is present. Although multiple core biopsies will minimize the chance of a false-negative result, only a few well-targeted biopsies should be done to minimize the chances of disrupting the tumor and creating a hematoma or interfering with the pathologic measurement of the tumor size. This is not a therapeutic procedure. A clip may be placed at the radiographic site of the lesion so that the area can be identified if subsequent surgery is necessary. It is important to remember that the most accurate tumor measurements are made when the tumor is intact. If the tumor is removed in multiple pieces, only estimates of tumor size can be performed. With improvements in accuracy, only a few cores need to be taken, thereby preserving the tumor for definitive surgical resection and pathologic analysis.

The mammotome instrument cores the tissue into multiple fragments, and therefore its use imposes a limitation on the pathologic measurement of the size of the malignancy. In addition, margin status cannot be assessed with mammotome resections. This instrument may have a better role in the management of benign lesions (e.g., fibroadenomas in young women).

An excisional biopsy involves the complete removal of the lesion with a rim of normal-appearing surrounding breast tissue. On the day of surgery, is important to ask the patient to point out the palpable lump and to mark the site of the palpable lesion with a skin marker before the patient receives any premedication or anesthetic agent. For nonpalpable lesions, radiologic guidance can be provided with preoperative needle localization under mammographic or ultrasound guidance or intraoperative real-time images with ultrasonography.

At the time of excision, every effort should be made to orient the specimen anatomically for the pathologist by using sutures, surgical clips, or colored inks. If the lesion is proven to be malignant and the margins are labeled, the pathologist can identify which margin(s) is involved with cancer. This will avoid an excessive and unnecessary resection of a large amount of breast tissue at the time of reoperation if the patient is a candidate for the conservative breast surgery approach. Only the involved margin(s) will be reexcised rather than the entire tumor site. For the nonpalpable lesions, specimen mammography should be obtained immediately to confirm that the suggestive lesion is identified within the resected tissue. This specimen radiograph should be made available to the pathologist as an aid to identification of the location of the abnormality in the resected tissue.

For malignant lesions, pathologic analysis includes the measurement of the intact tumor size, including the invasive and noninvasive components, identification of any involved margins, the cell type, the histologic grade of the tumor, and the estrogen (ER) and progesterone (PR) hormone-receptor levels. Her-2/neu receptor status is requested only if the medical oncologist is considering the administration of trastuzumab as systemic therapy. In the future, other prognostic and predictive markers may be recommended.

Benign Breast Conditions

Many pathological entities are not associated with an increased risk for breast cancer. Some of the more frequently encountered lesions are fibrocystic disease, fibroadenomas, cysts, and ductal ectasia. Lesions seen with less frequency include papillomas, phylloides tumors, radial scars, and areas of sclerosing adenosis. Each entity is very briefly described. More-detailed information may be found in textbooks on breast disease and pathology.

Fibrocystic disease is a condition in which patients usually are symptomatic with pain, especially in the second half of the menstrual cycle. Clinically, multiple nodular densities are palpable. Symptom relief may be achieved with cold compresses, reduced caffeine intake, properly fitted bras, and occasionally, the use of anti-inflammatory agents.

Fibroadenomas are discrete round or ovoid solid rubbery lesions that grow under the influence of estrogen. They are the most common solid lesion in women younger than 40 years; however, it is important to remember that 5% of breast cancers also occur in this age range. Patients may choose to be followed up frequently if the clinical breast examination, breast imaging studies, and FNAB or CNB are all benign. The pathology must be consistent with a fibroadenoma and not just breast tissue. This is known as the "triple test." Surgical excision is appropriate for patients who choose not to undergo a long-term follow-up program, who do not mind a surgical scar, or who have a lesion larger than 2 cm. Surgical excision is important for lesions that increase in size, for women age 40 years and older, and for patients who fail the triple test.

Cysts are discrete lesions that, when distended, especially before the menstrual period, may suddenly feel quite hard. An ultrasound study will usually confirm this diagnosis. An aspiration can be performed for therapeutic management, especially if the lesion is large and painful. After aspiration, if the lesion completely disappears and the fluid is not bloody, no further testing is needed. Bloody fluid should be sent for cytology. An intracystic carcinoma or papilloma may be present, especially when the ultrasound study indicates a solid component within the cyst. In this case, aspiration should not be performed; a surgical consultation is needed. Surgical excision is recommended for cysts identified as complex or having a solid component on ultrasonography, cysts that recur after a few aspirations, and cysts that leave a palpable mass after fluid is aspirated.

Ductal ectasia refers to the presence of ducts ending in the areolar tissue rather than in the nipple. These are often associated with a discharge of thick yellow/green secretions. Differentiating these physiologic secretions from purulence is possible because of the absence of pain and cellulitis, which, when present, are more characteristic of an infection. Good hygiene is important to avoid secondary infections. Surgery is not indicated for this condition.

Papillomas may occur in any duct in the breast. Pathologic evaluation of the area immediately around these lesions is important to search for concomitant areas of atypical ductal hyperplasia, dysplasia, or carcinoma in situ. When they occur in major ducts close to the nipple, a spontaneous bloody nipple discharge is often the presenting sign. Surgical excision is recommended, and preoperative radiologic guidance with a ductogram is often very helpful. The role of ductal lavage is under study. To date, it has been able to detect cytologic abnormalities but has not improved the ability to detect cancer.

Phylloides tumors clinically resemble fibroadenomas; pathologically, however, they are distinguished by cellular proliferative activity of stroma and epithelium and compression of surrounding normal tissue. Complete surgical excision, including the surrounding compressed tissue with a margin of about 1 cm, is recommended to reduce the chance of local recurrence. Because of the high local recurrence rate of these lesions when they are larger than 3 cm, a prospective randomized controlled clinical trial is now testing the worth of postoperative radiation to the involved breast.

A malignant variant, termed *cystosarcoma phylloides,* is a very aggressive tumor. Metastatic spread is hematogenous rather than lymphatic. Treatment, therefore, includes a total mastectomy and aggressive chemotherapy; axillary lymph node dissection (ALND) is performed only for clinically enlarged lymph nodes.

Radial scars and areas of **sclerosing adenosis** clinically and radiographically mimic infiltrating cancers. Surgical excision is necessary to determine the correct histopathology. These lesions are benign and are not associated with an increased risk for breast cancer.

Carcinoma of the Breast

Incidence and Mortality

The lifetime risk of developing breast cancer was 1 in 13 during the 1970s. It is now 1 in 9 for white American women. The incidence of breast cancer in American women of black and Hispanic descent is lower than that of white American women, but in recent years, the rate of increase among black and Hispanic women has been increasing significantly. That of African-American women may soon approach the same level of occurrence as is found in white women. Although the incidence of breast cancer remains high, the mortality rate has decreased proportionately for both white and minority women; unfortunately, however, the 5-year survival rate for each stage of disease is lower for minority women as compared with white women.

Statistics from the National Cancer Data Bank, which receives information on the diagnosis, staging, treatment, and annual follow-up of all cancer cases (except for nonmelanotic skin cancers) from all tumor registries approved by the Commission on Cancer of the American College of Surgeons, provide an accurate monitoring of the impact of efforts directed at early detection and state-of-the-art treatment. With the advent of heightened screening programs during the last 10 years, an increasing downward shift has appeared in the stage of newly diagnosed breast cancer patients, and this has contributed to a lower mortality rate. In addition, improvements in survival have occurred in some subsets of patients as a result of systemic adjuvant therapy programs, the majority of which have been developed through clinical trials.

Clinical Trials

During the last 30 years, we have witnessed significant changes in the treatment of breast cancer. Almost all of these are a result of clinical research and large prospective randomized controlled clinical trials conducted at many institutions, both academic and community hospital based.

Justification for the "experimental" treatment arm or arms in these phase III trials has been based on smaller "pilot" studies that look promising but must be tested for reproducible results in a large group of consenting patients and by a large group of participating physicians before a new standard of care can be established. This is true for surgical procedures as well as for XRT, chemotherapy, and hormone therapy. The nonexperimental arm in these phase III studies is the current standard-of-care treatment practiced at the time the trial is designed and conducted.

In the area of drug development, a long sequence of scientific studies begins preclinically in the laboratory, testing the activity of the drug as well as the associated toxicities in tumor-bearing animals. Drugs are then selected for preliminary studies in patients who have recurrent cancers and for whom standard therapies have already failed. These patients do not meet the eligibility requirements of available phase II and phase III trials. These patients consent to participate in phase I trials, which try to determine the preliminary activity of the drug against the measurable cancer. If successful, phase II trials are conducted to try to determine the safety profile (i.e., the highest dosages providing significant tumor response with minimal or tolerable toxicities). Phase III trials are then conducted as adjuvant therapy for patients with presumed micrometastatic systemic disease or as treatment for patients with documented systemic recurrence. These phase III trials, therefore, usually compare the current or standard therapy with the newer experimental therapy.

These trials test more than the technical or medical aspects of treatment. Inherent in each trial are questions testing the current hypotheses on the biology of the cancer, whether it be of the primary tumor, of the regional or systemic metastases, or all three sites of disease. Incorporated in many of the trials, especially in the past 10 to 20 years, are basic science or translational studies trying to determine which potential prognostic or predictive markers are clinically relevant in determining tumor biology or response to treatment or both. New hypotheses are developed based on analyses of completed trials, and these formulate the basis for the design of newer trials.

Active participation in clinical trials is one of the best methods of continuing education for physicians treating patients with breast cancer. Presenting updated information and fully disclosing to the patient established treatment recommendations, or standard of care, and those that are investigational and have not yet been tested in comparative studies, allows the patient to make a truly informed consent. In addition, potential treatment benefits as well as risks and toxicities must be presented in writing to the patient. For clinicians, however, this may be challenging, because it requires time for keeping updated with the numerous clinical trials. These discussions are lengthy, and most patients usually require more than one discussion to assimilate and comprehend this information. It is usually helpful to include in these discussions interested and concerned family members or close friends who will be providing support for the patient during treatment planning and subsequent care.

Not all patients will be eligible for clinical trials. Trials are not always open for every subset of patients with breast cancer. When it is appropriate, however, patients should be given the opportunity to participate in a trial. We are already indebted to those who have participated in these trials; without them, we would have no results, and our treatments would not have become "state of the art." Minority women, however, have been very reluctant to participate in these trials, and they now should join in with the white women participants. This is becoming increasingly important as the increase in breast cancer incidence in minority women is approaching that of white women, and, unfortunately, their mortality from breast cancer remains comparatively higher.

Breast Cancer Risk Factors

As compared with women throughout the rest of the world, American women carry the highest lifetime risk of developing breast cancer (one of nine). It is strongly recommended that physicians and women follow the current guidelines of the American Cancer Society for breast cancer screening. There are identifiable risk factors that place some women at an even higher lifetime risk for breast cancer. Based on our present knowledge, the following are some of the more important factors that have been identified and recently validated as risk factors for breast cancer.

Genetic Factors

If a patient has a family history of breast cancer with a high incidence and distribution suggestive of an autosomal-dominant pattern of inheritance (e.g., maternal grandmother and mother), especially with an early stage of onset, or has bilateral premenopausal breast cancer, the term *hereditary breast cancer* is clinically suspected. A patient who has one or more first-degree relatives with breast cancer but does not have the other associations listed for hereditary breast cancer is identified clinically as having familial breast cancer. The best estimates at this time are that 5% to 10% of breast cancer patients may have a genetic mutation in *BRCA1*, *BRCA2*, or another as yet unidentified gene.

Two breast cancer–susceptibility genes have been mapped: *BRCA1*, located on chromosome 17q, has been identified in families with hereditary breast and ovarian cancer syndrome; and *BRCA2*, located on the q12-13 region of chromosome 13, has been identified in families with male hereditary breast cancer and prostate and pancreatic cancer. Routine genetic testing for these chromosome abnormalities is not recommended. In families with a history suggestive of increased genetic susceptibility to breast and these associated cancers, referral to specialists in counseling and, if decided on, genetic testing is now available in many medical centers.

Estimates of increased breast cancer risk may be made based on the first-degree relative's menopausal status at the time of her diagnosis and whether she had unilateral or bilateral breast cancer (Table 40-1).

TABLE 40–1 Increased Breast Cancer Risk Based on First-degree Relative's Characteristics

Menopausal Status	No. of Breast Cancers	↑ Risks	% Risk
Postmenopausal	Unilateral	1.5–2.0	15–20
Premenopausal	Unilateral	3.0	25–30
Postmenopausal	Bilateral	4.5	40–45
Premenopausal	Bilateral	9.0	>80

Age

The incidence of breast cancer continues to increase throughout life. An 80-year-old woman has twice the chance of having breast cancer as a 45-year-old woman.

Personal History of Breast Cancer

The lifetime risk for the development of a new primary contralateral breast cancer in a woman previously treated for breast cancer is 15% to 20% or even higher. Recent data from clinical trials in which patients with estrogen-receptor–positive breast cancers received adjuvant therapy with tamoxifen or anastrozole show a reduction in the occurrence of contralateral breast cancer by as much as 40% to 45%. Additional long-term follow-up data are needed to corroborate this result further and to determine the length of time for which this risk reduction occurs.

Prior Exposure to Ionizing Irradiation

Patients who received head and neck or chest irradiation have an increased risk for breast cancer. This includes patients treated for acne, postpartum mastitis, pulmonary tuberculosis, and breast cancer. Survivors of atomic bomb explosions also have an increased risk of breast cancer. Patients with Hodgkin's disease treated with total nodal or mantle irradiation have a greater than 30% chance of developing breast cancer. In this last group of patients, because of the dosages of irradiation already delivered to the breast tissue and spinal cord, the option of breast-conservation surgery with postoperative breast irradiation cannot be offered as a treatment. Screening for breast cancer in those patients who have survived Hodgkin's disease must begin around age 30 years because they are at above-average risk for developing breast cancer and at an earlier age.

Lobular Carcinoma in Situ

The natural history of this pathologic entity has led to its consideration as a marker of increased risk rather than as a precursor of invasive disease, although invasive lobular cancer has developed in some patients. Patients who have lobular carcinoma in situ (LCIS) have a more than 30% chance of developing breast cancer, and the subsequent invasive cancer has an equal chance of occurring in either breast. This invasive cancer is often ductal in origin. Treatment is therefore directed at risk reduction or "prevention" and must be directed at both breasts because both are at equal risk. Recent data from the first National Surgical Adjuvant Breast and Bowel Project (NSABP) Breast Cancer Prevention Trial P-I showed a significant benefit in 5-year risk reduction in women with LCIS who received tamoxifen, 20 mg daily, for 5 years. Long-term follow-up data will be important to determine the duration of this benefit. Under clinical trial investigation is the NSABP P-2 study, known as the STAR trial, which is a comparison of raloxifene and tamoxifen for risk reduction in postmenopausal women at increased risk, including women with LCIS. Premenopausal women are excluded from this study because of insufficient safety data on the use of raloxifene in these women. Outside of this trial, the Food and Drug Administration (FDA) has approved only of tamoxifen for LCIS, and this includes pre- and postmenopausal women. As far as surgery is concerned, some very preliminary data from some of the treatment trials suggest that invasive lobular cancer occurrence can be reduced if the site of the LCIS is resected as a lumpectomy. The current standard of care, however, does not incorporate these new findings, although this could change in the near future.

Atypical Ductal Hyperplasia

This pathologic entity may be hard to distinguish from ductal carcinoma in situ (DCIS). In addition, atypical ductal hyperplasia (ADH) may often be seen in association with DCIS. Depending on the difficulty of interpreting the lesion, a second pathologist's opinion may be advisable. In patients with ADH, the subsequent risk of breast cancer may be as high as 20% to 25%. Recent data from the NSABP Breast Cancer Prevention Trial P-I showed a significant benefit in 5-year risk reduction in favor of women who received tamoxifen, 20 mg daily, for 5 years. Long-term follow-up data also will be important in this group of women to determine the duration of benefit. The same additional comments with respect to LCIS apply to patients with ADH.

Child Bearing and Fertility

For women younger than 30 years, the risk of breast cancer decreases with decreasing age at the time of the first completed pregnancy. Recent data suggest that women who have their first completed pregnancy after age 30 years are at increased risk for breast cancer, and this risk may be higher than the risk for women who are nulliparous. Careful epidemiologic studies are needed to determine the magnitude of this breast cancer risk with respect to age of the patient at the time of her first live birth.

Menstrual History and Hormone Therapy

Early onset of menses, age 8 years or younger, is associated with an increased risk for breast cancer. Late onset of menses, age 14 years or older, is associated with a lower risk of breast cancer. Onset of menopause before age 45 years is associated with a lower risk of breast cancer. Menopause occurring at age 55 years or older is associated with an increased risk of breast cancer.

Although many studies and reports have been published, no convincing data now exist to indicate conclusively an adverse effect on breast cancer risk in women in the United States using oral contraceptives. Recent data from the Women's Health Initiative Study show an increased risk of breast cancer in women taking hormone replacement therapy.

PEARLS FOR ROUNDS

According to the American Cancer Society guidelines, annual screening mammography begins at age 40 years.

Lumpectomy is not appropriate for multicentric cancers, persistent positive margins, or patients who received prior radiation therapy to the breast.

Axillary node dissection is indicated if the sentinel node is positive or for axillary node recurrence after sentinel node surgery.

Chemotherapy before surgery is indicated for locally advanced and inflammatory breast cancer and for patients with matted axillary nodes.

Proven prognostic factors are tumor size; number of positive axillary lymph nodes; estrogen- and progesterone-receptor status; and age/menopausal status of the patient.

Calculating the Risk for Breast Cancer

The Breast Cancer Demonstration Project, sponsored by the American Cancer Society and the National Cancer Institute, enrolled 283,222 volunteer women between 1973 and 1980 in a 5-year mammography and clinical breast examination screening program. An analysis of the risk factors identified in the subset of women in this study in whom breast cancer developed was performed by Dr. Mitch Gail and others at the National Cancer Institute. This analysis has evolved into the development of a model, known as the Gail Model, for calculating breast cancer risk. This model was further modified by the statisticians for the NSABP Clinical Cooperative Group to include LCIS and to adjust for race-specific rates for invasive breast cancer. The model was then used as the basis for determining patient risk and eligibility for entry into the first Breast Cancer Prevention Trial, the NSABP-PI study.

Gail Model Variables

- age
- number of first-degree relatives with breast cancer
- nulliparity or age at first live birth

- number of breast biopsies
- age at menarche
- LCIS or ADH identified by biopsy

Breast Cancer Risk Reduction

This trial has now validated the Gail Model with prospective data. Because of the importance of this information, risk-assessment tools are now available through the National Cancer Institute for calculating 5-year and lifetime risks for breast cancer in American women age 35 years and older. A discussion about breast cancer risk can now be incorporated into medical practice. The FDA has now approved the use of tamoxifen for breast cancer risk reduction in women who are at the same level of risk as women who participated in the P-1 Trial. For all women, however, the risks of taking tamoxifen in terms of thromboembolic events and, to a lesser extent, the risk of endometrial cancer must be discussed and weighed against the potential benefits. Based on this risk assessment, eligible postmenopausal women are participating in the second NSABP Breast Cancer Prevention Trial P-2. Accrual has been completed, and results will be released when an important end point is reached.

Staging of Breast Cancer

The staging of breast cancer provides an objective measure for predicting survival, for comparison of outcomes of different treatment modalities, and for deciding on treatment recommendations. The tumor/node/metastasis (TNM) system was modified 2 years ago by the American Joint Committee on Cancer (AJCC) (Box 40-1). Initial pretreatment staging is based on clinical and pathologic examinations. The primary tumor (T) is determined by the pathologic measurement of the invasive disease; if multiple core biopsies have been performed, a significant understaging of the tumor may occur. Please note the descriptions in the categories T4a to d. Lymph node status (N) has now incorporated information about internal mammary, infraclavicular, and supraclavicular lymph nodes. In addition, a separate symbol is used when only sentinel node surgery is performed. A separate designation is used when the routine hematoxylin and eosin stains of the lymph-node sections are negative for metastatic spread, but the immunohistochemistry stain identified cancer cells. This finding now has no clinical relevance, and this latter method of staining is usually reserved for research purposes and not routinely performed.

Modifications of this system may be needed in the near future to account for extent of disease in patients with DCIS; for "estimates" of tumor size when multiple core needle-biopsy fragments are submitted and little or no tumor is found at the time of definitive cancer surgery; and when molecular tumor markers, histologic grade, or possibly genetic microarrays are shown in clinical outcome studies to have value as prognostic or predictive markers or both.

Common sites of systemic metastases include bones, liver, lungs, and brain. In patients with newly diagnosed invasive breast cancer, baseline evaluations for completing the staging include careful history, complete physical examination including a gynecologic examination, bilateral mammography, complete blood count, and liver-function tests. Additional studies on the liver are performed if hepatomegaly or abnormal liver-function tests are found or at the discretion of the medical oncologist. Bone scans are performed in patients with acute bone pain, advanced tumors, or in those with signs or symptoms suggestive of skeletal involvement. Bone scans alone are not always accurate, because some false-positive and some false-negative results may be found. Additional skeletal films may be needed to evaluate further areas of increased uptake on bone scan, because benign diseases also may be associated with bone scan "positivity." Site-selected skeletal films are important in patients with pain to determine whether a pathologic fracture is pending. In addition, because bone scans indicate only osteoblastic activity, patients with rapidly growing skeletal metastases may have mainly osteolytic activity, and therefore their bone scans may be "normal." Skeletal films will be important for identifying these lytic lesions in symptomatic areas. Computed tomography (CT) scans and MRI may be indicated to evaluate symptomatic areas further, especially when brain or spinal cord involvement is suspected. Some patients with stage II disease and many patients with stage III disease will have CT, MRI, or PET scans even when asymptomatic, and at the discretion of the medical oncologist or as part of a clinical trial protocol.

Prognostic and Predictive Factors

The currently accepted prognostic factors for breast cancer that reflect the aggressiveness of the tumor are the size of the primary tumor, the number of ipsilateral axillary lymph nodes involved with metastases, and the age and menopausal status of the patient. Based on clinical studies of the impact of treatment on the natural history of breast cancer and according to stage are the following proven predictive factors: estrogen-receptor status and amplification of the epidermal growth factor Her-2/neu as determined by fluorescence in situ hybridization (FISH) analysis. Many other potential prognostic or predictive markers or both are under clinical investigation, but validation studies in large numbers of patients are needed before any of these markers become incorporated into standard medical practice.

Clinical Pathologic Management of Breast Cancer

The treatment of breast cancer has always been based on the current beliefs in the principles of tumor biology. Over

BOX 40-1 Definition of TNM

Primary Tumor (T)

Definitions for classifying the primary tumor (T) are the same for clinical and for pathologic classification. If the measurement is made by physical examination, the examiner will use the major headings (T1, T2, or T3). If other measurements, such as mammographic or pathologic measurements, are used, the subsets of T1 can be used. Tumors should be measured to the nearest 0.1-cm increment.

TX	Primary tumor cannot be assessed
T0	No evidence of primary tumor
Tis	Carcinoma in situ
Tis (DCIS)	Ductal carcinoma in situ
Tis (LCIS)	Lobular carcinoma in situ
Tis (Paget's)	Paget's disease of the nipple with no tumor

Note: Paget's disease associated with a tumor is classified according to the size of the tumor.

T1	Tumor 2 cm or less in greatest dimension
T1mic	Microinvasion 0.1 cm or less in greatest dimension
T1a	Tumor more than 0.1 cm but not more than 0.5 cm in greatest dimension
T1b	Tumor more than 0.5 cm but not more than 1 cm in greatest dimension
T1c	Tumor more than 1 cm but not more than 2 cm in greatest dimension
T2	Tumor more than 2 cm but not more than 5 cm in greatest dimension
T3	Tumor more than 5 cm in greatest dimension
T4	Tumor of any size with direct extension to (a) chest wall or (b) skin, only as described below
T4a	Extension to chest wall, not including pectoralis muscle
T4b	Edema (including peau d'orange) or ulceration of the skin of the breast, or satellite skin nodules confined to the same breast
T4c	Both T4a and T4b
T4d	Inflammatory carcinoma

Regional Lymph Nodes (N)

Clinical Classification

NX	Regional lymph nodes cannot be assessed (e.g., previously removed)
N0	No regional lymph node metastasis
N1	Metastasis to movable ipsilateral axillary lymph node(s)
N2	Metastases in ipsilateral axillary lymph nodes fixed or matted, or in clinically apparent* ipsilateral internal mammary nodes in the *absence* of clinically evident axillary lymph node metastasis
N2a	Metastasis in ipsilateral axillary lymph nodes fixed to one another (matted) or to other structures
N2b	Metastasis only in clinically apparent* ipsilateral internal mammary nodes and in the *absence* of clinically evident axillary lymph node metastasis
N3	Metastasis in ipsilateral infraclavicular lymph node(s) with or without axillary lymph node involvement, or in clinically apparent* ipsilateral internal mammary lymph node(s) and in the *presence* of clinically evident axillary lymph node metastasis; or metastasis in ipsilateral supraclavicular lymph node(s) with or without axillary or internal mammary lymph node involvement
N3a	Metastasis in ipsilateral infraclavicular lymph node(s)
N3b	Metastasis in ipsilateral internal mammary lymph node(s) and axillary lymph node(s)
N3c	Metastasis in ipsilateral supraclavicular lymph node(s)

**Clinically apparent* is defined as detected by imaging studies (excluding lymphoscintigraphy) or by clinical examination or as grossly visible pathologically.

Pathologic Classification (pN)[a]

pNX	Regional lymph nodes cannot be assessed (e.g., previously removed, or not removed for pathologic study)
pN0	No regional lymph node metastasis histologically, no additional examination for isolated tumor cells (ITCs)

Note: Isolated tumor cells (ITCs) are defined as single tumor cells or small cell clusters not greater than 0.2 mm, usually detected only by immunohistochemical (IHC) or molecular methods but which may be verified on H&E stains. ITCs do not usually show evidence of malignant activity (e.g., proliferation or stromal reaction).

pN0(i –)	No regional lymph node metastasis histologically, negative IHC
pNo(i +)	No regional lymph node metastasis histologically, positive IHC, no IHC cluster greater than 0.2 mm
pN0(mol -)	No regional lymph node metastasis histologically, negative molecular findings (RT-PCR)[b]
pN0(mol +)	No regional lymph node metastasis histologically, positive molecular findings (RT-PCR)[b]

[a]Classification is based on axillary lymph node dissection with or without sentinel lymph node dissection. Classification based solely on sentinel lymph node dissection without subsequent axillary lymph node dissection is designated (sn) for "sentinel node," (e.g., pN0 [i +] [sn]).
[b]RT-PCR, reverse transcriptase/polymerase chain reaction.

pN1	Metastasis in one to three axillary lymph nodes, and/ or in internal mammary nodes with microscopic disease detected by sentinel lymph node dissection but not clinically apparent**
pN1mi	Micrometastasis (greater than 0.2 mm, none greater than 0.2 mm)
pN1a	Metastasis in one to three axillary lymph nodes

BOX 40-1 Definition of TNM (*cont'd*)

pN1b Metastasis in internal mammary nodes with microscopic disease detected by sentinel lymph node dissection but not clinically apparent**

pN1c Metastasis in one to three axillary lymph nodes and in internal mammary lymph nodes with microscopic disease detected by sentinel lymph node dissection but not clinically appararent** (If associated with greater than three positive axillary lymph nodes, the internal mammary nodes are classified as pN3b to reflect increased tumor burden)

pN2 Metastasis in four to nine axillary lymph nodes, or in clinically apparent* internal mammary lymph nodes in the absence of axillary lymph node metastasis

pN2a Metastasis in four to nine axillary lymph nodes (at least one tumor deposit greater than 2.0 mm)

pN2b Metastasis in clinically apparent* internal mammary lymph nodes in the absence of axillary lymph node metastasis

pN3 Metastasis in 10 or more axillary lymph nodes, or in infraclavicular lymph nodes, or in clinically apparent* ipsilateral internal mammary lymph nodes in the presence of one or more positive axillary lymph nodes; or in more than three axillary lymph nodes with clinically negative microscopic metastasis in internal mammary lymph nodes; or in ipsilateral supraclavicular lymph nodes

pN3a Metastasis in 10 or more axillary lymph nodes (at least one tumor deposit greater than 2.0 mm), or metastasis to the infraclavicular lymph nodes

pN3b Metastasis in clinically apparent* ipsilateral internal mammary lymph nodes in the presence of one or more positive axillary lymph nodes; or in more than three axillary lymph nodes and in internal mammary lymph nodes with microscopic disease detected by sentinel lymph node dissection but not clinically apparent**

pN3c Metastasis in ipsilateral supraclavicular lymph nodes

**Clinically apparent* is defined as detected by imaging studies (excluding lymphoscintigraphy) or by clinical examination.

***Not clinically apparent* is defined as not detected by imaging studies (excluding lymphoscintigraphy) or by clinical examination.

Distant Metastasis (M)

MX Distant metastasis cannot be assessed

M0 No distant metastasis

M1 Distant metastasis

STAGE GROUPING

Stage 0	Tis	N0	M0
Stage I	T1*	N0	M0
Stage IIA	T0	N1	M0
	T1*	N1	M0
	T2	N0	M0
Stage IIB	T2	N1	M0
	T3	N0	M0
Stage IIIA	T0	N2	M0
	T1*	N2	M0
	T2	N2	M0
	T3	N1	M0
	T3	N2	M0
Stage IIIB	T4	N0	M0
	T4	N1	M0
	T4	N2	M0
Stage IIIC	AnyT	N3	M0
Stage IV	AnyT	Any N	M1

*T1 includes T1mic

Note: Stage designation may be changed if postsurgical imaging studies reveal the presence of distant metastases, provided that the studies are carried out within 4 months of diagnosis in the absence of disease progression and provided that the patient has not received neoadjuvant therapy.

From American Joint Committee on Cancer (AJCC): AJCC Cancer Staging Manual, 6th ed. New York, Springer-Verlag, 2002, with permission.

the years, changes have occurred in these beliefs, initially through large retrospective studies and more recently through the conduct of prospective randomized controlled clinical trials. Research studies are under way to understand further the biologic behavior of breast cancers at the molecular level. Now the scientific basis for breast cancer treatment is the pathologic extent of the tumor, the hormone-receptor analysis results, and the presence of Her-2/neu amplification.

A multidisciplinary team approach including the surgical oncologist or general surgeon, the plastic surgeon, the radiation oncologist, and the medical oncologist is important for treatment planning. After a careful physical examination of the patient and review of the pathology slides and breast imaging studies, recommendations can be made in a unified manner and should be without any apparent competing conflicts. Alternative choices in treatment should be presented without bias and clearly indicate potential risks and benefits. For some patients, meeting with all of these consultants in one visit is preferred. For many, however, individual doctor's visits allow less confusion and more time for thorough discussions about treatment benefits and risks. When appropriate and if available, clinical trials should be presented so that patients can make a truly informed decision about their treatment.

Ductal Carcinoma in Situ: Stage 0

With more widespread use of breast cancer screening and improved mammographic techniques, DCIS now accounts for 20% or more of newly diagnosed breast cancers. About 5% of the cases are initially seen with a palpable mass; most of these tumors appear mammographically as an area of clustered microcalcifications. Pathologically all the cancer cells are confined to the ducts, with no invasion of the basement membrane. Histologic patterns include solid, cribriform, or papillary types; comedonecrosis may or may not be present.

Treatment is directed at reducing the risk of an invasive cancer recurrence. Two prospective randomized controlled clinical trials by the NSABP, B17 and B24, have provided data to support breast-conservation surgery and XRT for many of these patients. If a patient has extensive DCIS, a total mastectomy remains the best treatment. Although an axillary lymph node assessment is not indicated in noninvasive disease, in patients with extensive DCIS in which microinvasion may be present or has been identified, a limited ALND or a sentinel lymph node biopsy may be appropriate. At this time, insufficient data exist to identify a subset of patients who do not need XRT after a lumpectomy. Currently, under the auspices of the Radiation Therapy Oncology Group (RTOG), this issue is being tested in a large-scale multi-institutional prospective randomized controlled clinical trial.

The NSABP B24 trial has shown an additional benefit of tamoxifen in reducing ipsilateral invasive breast cancer recurrence to 2.6% and the incidence of contralateral breast cancer occurrence by 47%. These benefits were seen in patients with DCIS with positive estrogen receptors. Currently both the RTOG 9804 trial and the NSABP B35 trial are investigating tamoxifen or anastrozole in patients with DCIS treated with breast conservation; in the RTOG trial, patients with certain tumor characteristics and resection margins are randomized to receive XRT or no XRT. In NSABP B35, all patients receive XRT. No established prognostic or predictive factors now exist for local recurrence in DCIS. Under investigation are margin status, tumor size, the presence of comedonecrosis, histologic grade, Her-2/neu amplification, and estrogen-receptor status.

Stage I and Stage II Breast Cancer: Surgical Management

The primary surgical treatment of T1 and T2 breast cancers has changed considerably throughout the past 30 years as a result of large-scale prospective randomized controlled clinical trials. Prior to the 1980s, patients were treated with the Halsted radical mastectomy or even more extensive surgical procedures, which included the resection of supraclavicular and internal mammary lymph nodes. These operations were based on the light-microscopy work of Virchow and other pathologists, suggesting that breast cancer spreads in an orderly fashion from one tissue plane and lymph node chain to the next, and that the surgical resection should extend to one area beyond the last known area involved with cancer.

These hypotheses and others have been challenged and changed through the work of many investigators in the United States, Canada, and Europe. Data from the NSABP B-04 trial indicated that for patients with T1 and T2 tumors, resection of the chest wall muscles and the overlying skin, as performed in the radical mastectomy, is not necessary for improved survival. This trial also showed that the routine use of postoperative chest XRT after complete breast removal is not necessary for survival. Based on these results, the standard of care changed to a "total" (or "simple") mastectomy, which includes the removal of the breast bounded by the superficial fascia and the deep fascia, as well as the overlying nipple and areola complex, with the resection of any additional skin determined by the technical considerations necessary for the best cosmetic results and whether an immediate reconstruction procedure is to be done.

While the NSABP B-04 trial was ongoing, other investigators in Europe and in the United States were conducting studies on removing only the area of the breast involved with cancer. These procedures were called quadrantectomies and tylectomies. To test the role of whole-breast irradiation after local excision of the tumor (i.e., is irradiation necessary), and to compare these results with the total mastectomy procedure, was the study design of the NSABP B-06 trial. Long-term results of this trial as well as other studies that validated these results continue to uphold breast-conservative surgery, known as "lumpectomy," with whole-breast XRT of 50 cGy as an alternative to a total mastectomy as the standard of care. The surgery and irradiation performed in this trial were quite specific: the cancer was completely excised, and all resection margins were pathologically free from involvement with cancer cells; an acceptable cosmetic result was achieved, taking into consideration the size of the breast and the size of the tumor; only one cancer was present; the maximum tumor dimension was 4 cm or less; and with tangential fields, whole-breast XRT was delivered to a total dose of 50 cGy. Pathologically, the cancers were either invasive ductal or invasive lobular cancers. This trial did not include patients with multicentric cancers. Therefore patients with multicentric cancers are now best treated with a total mastectomy.

In addition to the primary breast surgery, which was either a mastectomy or lumpectomy, surgical removal of level I and level II ipsilateral axillary lymph nodes was performed. (Note: A total mastectomy plus an ALND also is known as a modified radical mastectomy). During the course of the dissection, the long thoracic nerve, supplying the serratus anterior muscle, should be identified and preserved. An injury to this nerve will cause a "winged" scapula. In addition, the thoracodorsal nerve, artery, and vein, supplying the latissimus dorsi muscle, should be identified and preserved. These vessels may be used by plastic surgeons to increase blood flow to a tissue-transfer flap during reconstructive surgery. Efforts should be made to preserve at least one of the intercostal brachial nerves, which supply skin sensation to the axilla and undersurface of the arm. For technical reasons, however, this nerve may sometimes be unable to be saved, and this should be discussed with the patient as part of the informed consent for surgery.

The removal of approximately 10 lymph nodes is considered adequate to determine the need for and type of adjuvant systemic therapy; to stratify patients, and to perform subset analysis of patients in adjuvant therapy trials; to provide regional control of cancer in the axilla; and to stage the lymph nodes according to the current AJCC system.

Sentinel Lymph Node Surgery

Prospective randomized controlled clinical trials are under way by the NSABP and by the American College of Surgeons Oncology Group (ACOSOG) to assess the role of sentinel lymph node surgery for patients with invasive T1 and T2 breast cancers. By definition, the sentinel lymph node or nodes are the first nodes in a regional lymphatic drainage area to receive lymph draining from the tumor. The sentinel lymph node is identified by injecting a radio-isotope, technetium sulfur colloid or a blue dye, isosulfan blue, or both, into the walls of the tumor cavity, the tissue on the outer edge of the tumor, or perhaps the overlying skin or subareolar area, and finding the node, nodes, or lymphatic channels in which one or both of these agents accumulate. If the sentinel lymph node is negative for metastases, it will be important to determine how accurately this predicts that the remaining level I and II axillary lymph nodes are all negative for metastases. The type of pathologic assessment of these nodes also is under clinical investigation. The role of IHC staining for breast cancer cells not identified on routine H&E staining is an important research question in terms of both staging and therapeutic management. Included in the sentinel node identification is an abnormal node identified by the surgeon during exploration of the axilla. Any lymph node replaced by cancer usually does not pick up the blue dye or radioisotope, but the surgeon should be able to feel this node.

In the NSABP B32 trial, patients with negative sentinel nodes are randomized to either no further surgery or to a completion ALND; patients with a positive sentinel node all undergo a completion ALND. This trial has achieved its accrual goal of more than 5200 patients. In the ACOSOG Z0011 trial, patients with negative sentinel nodes do not undergo an ALND; patients with a positive sentinel node are randomized to either no further surgery or a completion ALND.

Important issues under clinical investigation in these trials include the accuracy of sentinel lymph node surgery, which is dependent on surgical and pathologic expertise; the impact of this surgical procedure on the patient's distant disease-free and overall survival; the efficacy of maintaining regional control of cancer in the axilla; the occurrence of injury to the intercostal brachial nerve; and the occurrence of lymphedema after this procedure, especially if nodal irradiation is administered.

Reconstructive Surgery

In patients who will be treated with a total mastectomy, considerations concerning reconstructive procedures should be included as part of the preoperative discussion. Reconstruction can be performed immediately, at the time of the mastectomy, or as a delayed procedure. The main types are saline-filled implants, autologous tissue-transfer flaps, or a combination of both methods.

Implants are placed in a pocket beneath the pectoralis major muscle. A tissue expander is often placed first, and saline is injected through a small subcutaneous valve periodically over a period of several weeks or a few months until the desired volume and size is achieved. At a second operation, the expander is removed, and the permanent implant is placed.

The most common type of tissue-flap surgery involves transferring a section of skin, fat, and muscle with its own attached blood supply to the chest-wall defect and creating a shaped "breast." Tissue may be taken from the abdomen, using the rectus muscles, or from the back, using the latissimus dorsi muscle.

The nipple and areola also can be reconstructed by using several different techniques. In addition, contralateral breast reduction or augmentation may be appropriate for some patients to achieve a more symmetrical result. Today, many insurance companies will cover the costs of postmastectomy reconstruction. For patients not undergoing reconstruction, breast prostheses and bras fitted with pockets are available, although not all insurance carriers cover these costs.

The type of reconstructive procedure and whether it is performed at the same time the breast is removed or at a later date is dependent on many factors, including: body habitus, previous abdominal surgical procedures, age, history of cigarette smoking, diabetes, and hypertension. If XRT is planned, most patients are strongly advised to wait until the acute radiation changes have subsided before undergoing a reconstruction procedure.

Surgical Treatment Complications

A small hematoma or seroma may fill in the breast defect in patients treated with conservation surgery. This often provides a nice cosmetic result and, in the absence of an infection, no treatment is necessary. A large or expanding hematoma usually requires surgical evaluation. Obtaining careful hemostasis, placing drains in wounds that are large or deep or both, and having the patient wear supportive bras, perhaps reinforced with a compressive wrap, may all be helpful in reducing the occurrence of this complication.

Ischemia of wound edges occurring with breast-conservation surgery or mastectomy with or without a reconstruction procedure is a consequence of dissecting the skin flaps too thinly. This may occur with increased frequency in patients who smoke cigarettes or have small-vessel peripheral vascular disease, especially patients with diabetes. Close follow-up wound care, including débridement of necrotic tissue and antibiotics for secondary infections, is a mainstay of treatment.

Axillary seroma formation occurs as a result of disruption of lymphatic and vascular channels during the course of performing the lymph node dissection. Placement of closed suction-drainage catheters intraoperatively is helpful in minimizing this occurrence. Strict attention to sterile technique and to postoperative wound care to avoid the introduction of bacteria, resulting in an infected seroma, is important. Small seromas may resorb without intervention. Seromas that increase daily must be aspirated with sterile technique every 1 or 2 days; replacement of a closed suction-drainage catheter may be necessary if the seroma fails to resolve, although this is rarely needed.

The two most common long-term complications of ALND are paresthesias or pain of the undersurface or the posterior aspect of the arm and axilla and lymphedema. Injury to the intercostal brachial nerve is possible because anatomically it courses through the axillary fat pad. Although many surgeons will attempt to dissect the tissue away from this nerve, preservation may not always be technically possible. Discussing this with the patient as part of the preoperative informed consent process is important. Lymphedema was a well-known and frequent complication of the Halsted radical mastectomy. With the surgical procedures performed today, this complication occurs less frequently; unfortunately, however, the occurrence is still frequent, ranging from 5% to 36%. For women in whom lymphedema develops, this becomes an important issue in their quality of life. Research is needed to determine the contributing etiologic factors, to assess the degree of functional impairment and the best treatment modalities, and, perhaps most important, how to minimize the occurrence of this morbidity. Retrospective studies provide only potential hypotheses and anecdotal information. The NSABP B32 trial will obtain some prospective data on lymphedema. The hypothesis being tested is whether sentinel lymph node surgery is associated with a lower incidence of lymphedema, as compared with an ALND. Treatment of lymphedema usually includes physical therapy, lymphatic massage, and compressive wraps. Prevention, however, is the ultimate goal.

Stage IIB and Stage IIIA Breast Cancer

Historically, the majority of patients in Halsted's clinical series were patients first seen with large or locally advanced breast cancers. In consideration of the fact that neither chemotherapy nor XRT was available, the design of his operation and his 5-year results were quite good; however, his hypotheses on the biology of cancer spread, which formulated the scientific basis for the design of his operation, were not correct. Although today patients with operable stage III disease may be treated with a total mastectomy and ALND, followed by systemic chemotherapy and, often, chest-wall irradiation, this sequence of treatment modalities is now changing. During the last 10 years, clinical research has been performed in which patients with stage IIB and stage IIIA cancers have received "induction," or neoadjuvant chemotherapy, meaning that chemotherapy is given preoperatively. An unanticipated result of this treatment is that a large number of tumors have regressed sufficiently so that the patients could then choose breast-conservation surgery with XRT as an alternative to mastectomy. (Note: With either procedure, the patients also undergo an axillary lymph node assessment). The hypotheses under study in these trials, however, centered on learning more about the biologic behavior of the primary tumor in relation to the behavior of the metastases in the axillary lymph nodes and in distant "systemic" organs, rather than on breast preservation. No overall survival advantage has occurred as a result of induction chemotherapy; however, longer follow-up data from these completed trials are needed. A preliminary analysis of a subset of patients who had a complete pathologic response to the chemotherapy does show a survival benefit, but the number of patients in this group is small. Trials are now under way to access the role of additional systemic chemotherapy given sequentially preoperatively or postoperatively in patients who receive induction chemotherapy. These trials also are assessing the roles of different chemotherapy agents, sentinel lymph node surgery before or after induction cheomotherapy (or both), and identifying molecular targets for treatment.

Stage IIIB Breast Cancer

For patients with stage IIIB disease involving the overlying skin or the underlying chest wall, or in patients with fixed or matted axillary lymph nodes, preoperative chemotherapy is standard care. Most patients then undergo a total mastectomy and ALND. Postoperative treatment usually includes XRT as well as additional systemic therapy.

Inflammatory Breast Cancer (Stage III B)

One of the most rapidly progressive presentations of breast cancer, inflammatory carcinoma, is often confused with a breast infection. Clinically, women are first seen with breast pain, swelling, erythema, and edema; they are usually premenopausal, in their late 30s or 40s, and may or may not be breast feeding. Mammographic findings may include thickening of the dermis; an underlying mass is not always present. Expeditious diagnosis and treatment is important. Pathologically, the cell line is a poorly differentiated high-grade adenocarcinoma of ductal origin, extensively and diffusely involving the breast tissue. A biopsy of the overlying skin often shows tumor cells filling the lymphatic ducts of the dermis, thereby causing the erythema and edema, the "inflammatory" appearance of the skin.

If the presumptive diagnosis is a breast infection, the patient must be monitored closely for response to antibiotic therapy covering for gram-positive, gram-negative, and anaerobic organisms. If clinical improvement does not occur, a tissue diagnosis should be obtained. First-line therapy is combination chemotherapy. After a clinical response with near-resolution of the erythema, edema, and swelling, a total mastectomy and ALND are performed. Pathologic complete responses are seen on occasion; however, microscopic residual disease commonly occurs even in patients with an apparent complete clinical response. Postoperatively, patients are usually treated with additional systemic therapy and XRT. With this aggressive approach, significant improvements in 5-year survival rates have occurred.

Paget's Disease of the Breast

Clinically, Paget's disease of the breast initially is seen as an area of erythema and scaling, similar to eczema; with progression, erosion and ulceration develop. A biopsy demonstrating Paget's cells is diagnostic. This intraepithelial tumor begins in the skin of the nipple and areola and then extends into multiple ducts in the subareolar tissue. With progression, an invasive ductal cancer will develop and extend into the breast. Treatment is based on the extent of disease. Excision of the nipple and areola complex as well as the subareolar tissue will determine the tumor size and the presence or absence of invasion. If no evidence of invasive disease is found, the patient can be treated with lumpectomy and XRT or a total mastectomy. Patients with invasive disease are treated according to the same guidelines as for invasive ductal or lobular breast cancer, including an axillary lymph node assessment and adjuvant systemic therapy recommendations.

Breast Cancer in Males

Approximately 2% of all breast cancers occur in men. The presence of mutations in the *BRCA2* gene are associated with an increased risk of about 15% for male breast cancer; the risk factors for the majority of cases either are family history of breast cancer or are unknown. Clinical presentations include a hard mass, with or without fixation to the overlying skin or underlying chest muscle. Ulceration, bleeding, pain, and axillary lymphadenopathy occur with progressive disease. Nipple discharge, which may be serous or bloody, should be considered suggestive of an underlying breast malignancy.

Pathologically, these are almost always ductal in origin, because male breast tissue, unstimulated by estrogen, does not contain lobular elements. Mammography is performed. Diagnosis is made by biopsy. Hormone-receptor studies should be done; more than 50% of breast cancers in men are estrogen-receptor positive. Because of the small amount of tissue present, primary surgical treatment is a total mastectomy with an axillary lymph node assessment for T1 and T2 tumors. Recommendations for the treatment of stage III disease in men are the same as those for women. Although too few men with breast cancer exist to conduct clinical trials to assess the various adjuvant therapy programs, most oncologists follow the same recommendations as for women, including the use of tamoxifen if the hormone receptors are positive. Postmastectomy XRT may be recommended for some patients thought to be at high risk for local or regional recurrence. This is described in the next section.

Breast Cancer Radiotherapy

Radiation Therapy with Breast-conservation Surgery

XRT, delivered in small doses daily for several weeks, is effective in killing cancer cells while allowing surrounding normal tissue cells a chance for recovery. With the advent of supervoltage irradiation, the breast target volume can be treated to maximum tumor-cell kill while sparing the skin and thereby reducing the less than desirable cosmetic outcomes of breast edema, fibrosis, retraction, and skin telangiectasia. Whole-breast irradiation to a total dose of 50 Gy over a 5-week period is the usual course of treatment after breast-conservation surgery. Patients are usually treated daily, Monday through Friday, with fractions of 1.8 to 2.0 Gy each day. An additional boost dose of 10 to 20 Gy to the primary tumor site over another 1- to 2-week period is often recommended, especially in patients with an extensive intraductal component. In patients who will also receive systemic chemotherapy, the XRT is often given after the chemotherapy is completed.

Partial breast irradiation is under clinical investigation. Because only the tumor bed and surrounding tissue are treated, the research questions to answer include the ipsilateral local breast cancer recurrence rate and the overall cosmetic results as compared with whole-breast external-beam XRT. The NSABP and the RTOG are conducting large-scale prospective randomized trials to answer these questions.

Postmastectomy Radiation

After mastectomy for early-stage breast cancer, chest-wall XRT is currently not routinely recommended. Recent data, however, suggested a survival benefit when postmastectomy XRT is given to patients with four or more positive axillary lymph nodes or when the lymph nodes are found to have extracapsular spread of tumor. In terms of disease-free survival, an improvement has been seen with reduction in local and regional tumor recurrence. Trials are currently under way to test further the hypothesis that postmastectomy regional XRT improves overall survival and distant disease-free survival in patients who also receive aggressive chemotherapy and who have one to three positive axillary nodes.

Draining nodal basins in the axillary, supraclavicular, and internal mammary areas also are sometimes included in the treatment fields in these high-risk patients. As a result of this treatment, an increased risk of lymphedema occurs, as high as 25% when an ALND has been performed. Changes are observed on chest radiographs, including pulmonary fibrosis and pleural thickening; patients are usually clinically asymptomatic. Radiation pneumonitis, cardiomyopathy, and brachial plexus injury occur rarely when supervoltage therapy is administered with carefully planned fields.

Patients who undergo an immediate reconstruction procedure and postoperatively are treated with XRT have a less-than-desirable cosmetic outcome. Implants become hardened, with the development of capsular contractures; fat necrosis may occur in the transferred autologous tissue flaps. Delaying the reconstruction until after all treatment is completed is the best recommendation for these patients with more locally advanced cancers.

Palliative Radiation Therapy

Radiation also is recommended as palliative treatment for brain metastases and for some presentations of skeletal metastases. It also is recommended for patients with chest-wall or nodal recurrence of breast cancer. Unfortunately, in a patient in whom breast cancer develops in the same breast previously treated for cancer with breast-conservation surgery and XRT, another course of XRT cannot be recommended. In this situation, either a wide local excision or a mastectomy is the recommended treatment.

PEARLS FOR THE OR

Long thoracic nerve injury causes a "winged scapula."

Intercostalbrachial nerve injury causes pain or paresthesias of the axilla or arm or both.

Injection sites for sentinel node surgery include the subareolar area, the skin overlying the tumor site, and the walls of the tumor cavity or tissue immediately surrounding the tumor.

Proper handling of the lumpectomy or excisional biopsy specimen includes anatomic orientation, specimen mammography if the lesion is not palpable and was radiographically localized preoperatively, and request for appropriate tumor markers.

Removal of hard or enlarged nodes or both is part of sentinel node surgery, even with no tracer uptake.

Breast Cancer Systemic Therapy

Adjuvant Systemic Therapy

The treatment of presumed micrometastatic disease is known as *adjuvant* therapy. Endocrine-based therapy and combination chemotherapy are the current systemic adjuvant therapies available. Tamoxifen is the first-line endocrine therapy for both pre- and postmenopausal women with estrogen-receptor–positive tumors. Anastrozole instead of tamoxifen may be recommended in some postmenopausal women; the decision as to which drug is better awaits further long-term studies. The duration of treatment is usually 5 years; however, new information is emerging on using different hormonal agents sequentially for 3 to 5 years each. Potential toxicities as well as benefits must be assessed and explained to the patient. Some of these include exemestane, letrozole, toremifene, and faslodex.

In addition to endocrine agents, chemotherapy drugs used most often include doxorubicin, cyclophosphamide, fluorouracil, methotrexate, paclitaxel, or docetaxel in varying combinations and sequences. The duration of treatment is between four and eight cycles administered over a 4- to 6-month period. Recent preliminary data from the various cooperative groups suggest that improvement in survival is seen with the sequential administration of four cycles of two different non–cross-resistant chemotherapy programs in patients with positive axillary lymph nodes. Chemotherapy programs may be recommended for patients with negative axillary lymph nodes who are considered to be at high risk for metastatic disease. Newer trials will also include the use of targeted molecular agents and other endocrine agents.

Recent developments from clinical trials performed with trastuzumab, a monoclonal antibody to the Her-2/neu receptor, have shown significant benefit when given in the adjuvant setting in combination with chemotherapy when the gene is amplified.

Other targeted molecular therapies under investigation include epidermal growth factor inhibitors and anti-angiogenesis agents. The role of bisphosphonates in reducing the incidence of skeletal metastases has been under investigation for the past few years.

It is important to understand that, as new information becomes available through large-scale clinical trials, and the results are considered valid, changes in treatment recommendations will occur. Because so many studies in breast cancer are ongoing, and in many instances, benefits may be seen only in certain subsets of patients, it is a challenge to keep up with this new knowledge. It also is important to differentiate between proven treatments and those that are currently under clinical investigation. Providing patients with information from which they will make an informed-consent decision relies on explaining carefully the difference between the proven treatments and treatments that are still part of clinical research trials or have been extrapolated from other studies.

Dose intensity or *escalation* refers to increasing the total dose of a drug within a period of time; dose density refers to shortening the period of time between dosages. To date, most studies have shown no benefit for dose escalation; data are emerging on the potential benefit of dose density, but further studies are needed.

Toxicities of endocrine agents, chemotherapy agents, targeted molecular agents, and supportive therapies must be presented before the administration of any of these drugs. This includes both the short-term and long-term toxicities; these not only are specific for each agent but also vary when agents are used in certain combinations. Updated lists including their estimated severities and frequencies are available through the FDA and the National Cancer Institute.

Stage IV Breast Cancer (Metastatic Therapy)

Treatment approaches in patients with metastatic breast cancer are determined by the age of the patient; the hormone-receptor status of the original tumor; the Her-2/neu receptor assay on the primary tumor or, if amenable to biopsy, on the metastatic tumor; the extent of disease; and the previous treatment programs. Treatment is palliative, and the overall goal is to maintain the patient's quality of life and alleviate the symptoms associated with the metastatic disease. Surgery or XRT or both may be helpful in relieving spinal cord and central nervous system compression. Orthopedic procedures for stabilizing weight-bearing bones and avoiding painful pathologic fractures should always be considered but are needed infrequently.

Significant research activity continues in the development of new agents to treat these patients. This list changes frequently and includes liposomal doxorubicin, vinorelbine, capecitabine, epidermal growth factor inhibitors (e.g., gefitinib), and bisphosphonates such as pamidronate to stabilize lytic bone lesions, alleviate bone pain, and reduce the chance of pathologic fractures. In premenopausal women, hormone ablation continues to be used and studied.

Neoadjuvant or Induction Chemotherapy

Anthracycline-based regimens (doxorubicin) are preferred as first-line therapy for patients with large primary breast cancers or who have inoperable breast cancer to reduce the tumor so that surgery can be performed. The use of a taxane as a first-line therapy option or as a sequential agent before or after definitive surgical therapy also is under clinical trial investigation. In patients who receive induction chemotherapy followed by surgery, additional chemotherapy, especially if positive lymph nodes are identified pathologically, remains a research question. Tamoxifen or sometimes anastrozole is recommended in addition to the chemotherapy in patients with estrogen-receptor–positive tumors. The role of endocrine therapy instead of chemotherapy as an induction agent is under investigation by ACOSOG.

Patient Follow-up Care

Once therapy is completed, all of the treating oncologists must determine an appropriate follow-up schedule. For the first 2 to 3 years, the patient is seen every 3 to 4 months; for years 3 through 5, patients are usually seen every 6 months.

Mammography is usually performed 6 months after the completion of XRT in patients treated with breast-conservation surgery; thereafter, mammography is performed annually. Many oncologists obtain liver-function tests and alkaline phosphatase levels at least once a year. Bone scans and chest radiographs, which were once routinely performed annually, are now performed only if the patient is symptomatic. More frequent evaluations and organ-specific tests are performed based on the patient's symptoms and findings on clinical examinations. As part of good medical practice, patients with an intact uterus or ovaries should have an annual gynecologic examination. Pelvic ultrasounds and endometrial biopsies are not indicated in asymptomatic patients receiving tamoxifen therapy. ACS guidelines on colon cancer screening are part of good medical practice for these patients.

Recurrence of breast cancer may occur beyond 5 years from the day of diagnosis; therefore follow-up at least annually is important. These patients are at increased risk for a new contralateral breast cancer, a new primary colon or gynecologic malignancy, and as a consequence of some of the breast cancer treatments, acute myelogenous leukemia or angiosarcoma of the chest wall.

Complementary Therapies

Some patients are interested in trying other therapies because of their potential benefits. Herbs, vitamins, nutritional supplements, acupuncture, meditation, Reiki, and relaxation are just a few of these therapies.

These therapies are not alternatives to the standard-of-care treatments. For individual patients, however, potential benefits may be derived. Therefore consideration can certainly be given to those of particular interest, provided they are used as complementary to standard treatments.

The most important issue is that the patient keeps her oncologist informed of which therapies she is using to monitor for any potential side effects.

Patient Support

Throughout the past 10 to 20 years, a heightened awareness has existed of the emotional needs of the woman newly diagnosed with breast cancer. Recognizing and meeting these needs right at the start of her treatment planning is just as important as the recommended multimodality therapies. The patient should be encouraged to choose a companion—a spouse, a family member, or a close friend—to be present during consultations and discussions. Listening, taking notes, reminding the patient of certain questions she had wanted to ask, and facilitating arrangements for doctor visits, tests, and treatments are all immensely helpful.

During and after treatment, participation in a support group has been helpful for some patients. For other patients, meeting another patient who has already completed a similar treatment program and developing a "one-on-one" or "buddy" system of support has worked well.

Many local, regional, and national organizations are very generous in terms of their outreach activities: emotional support for the patients and their families; educational books, pamphlets and videos; and, in some instances, limited funding for special research projects. Included among these organizations are the following:

American Cancer Society, tel. 1-800-ACS-2345

Avon Breast Cancer Research and Care Programs, tel. 1-800-FOR-AVON

Y-ME 1-800-221-2141

Susan G. Komen Foundation, tel. 1-800-I'm-AWARE

National Alliance of Breast Cancer Organizations (NABCO), tel. 1-888-80NABCO

National Cancer Institute Cancer Information Service (CIS), tel. 1-800-422-6237

In addition, the Breast Cancer Research Guide of Massachusetts lists many more state and national organizations and resources that are available to breast cancer patients. Similar resource compendiums may be available in other states.

Physician Support

It is very challenging for physicians to be up to date on breast cancer. Numerous research studies are under way, and even more are being developed. As data mature, new information becomes available. Beliefs are either supported or negated by outcome data derived from large-scale prospective studies. This is truly a continuing educational experience for physicians who choose to take care of patients with breast cancer.

Physicians interested in participating in clinical trials can contact the various cooperative groups directly for referral to the nearest local site. If a site is not available, they can contact the Clinical Trials Support Unit. Resources for the latest information on cancer treatment, available trials, and educational materials are provided through the National Cancer Institute main home page:

www.nci.nih.gov

www.cancernet.nci.nih.gov

www.cancertrials.nci.nih.gov

Suggested Reading

Bear HD, Anderson S, Brown A, et al: The effect on tumor response of adding sequential preoperative docetaxel to preoperative doxorubicin and cyclophosphamide: Preliminary results from National Surgical Adjuvant Breast and Bowel Project protocol B-27. J Clin Oncol 21:4165–4174, 2003.

Fisher B, Constantino JP, Wickerham DL, et al: Tamoxifen for prevention of breast cancer: Current status of the National Surgical Adjuvant Breast and Bowel Project P-1 study. J Natl Cancer Inst 2005. In press.

Fisher B, Dignam J, Wolmark N, et al: Tamoxifen in treatment of intraductal breast cancer: National Surgical Adjuvant Breast and Bowel Project B-24 randomized controlled trial. Lancet 353:1993–2000, 1998.

Hortobagyi GN: Treatment of breast cancer. N Engl J Med 339: 974–984, 1998.

NIH Consensus Statement on Adjuvant Therapy for Breast Cancer, November 1–3, 2000 @ **http://consensus.nih.gov**

Ward E, Jemal A, Cokkinides V, et al: Cancer disparities by race/ethnicity and socioeconomic status. CA J Clin 54(2):78–93, 2004.

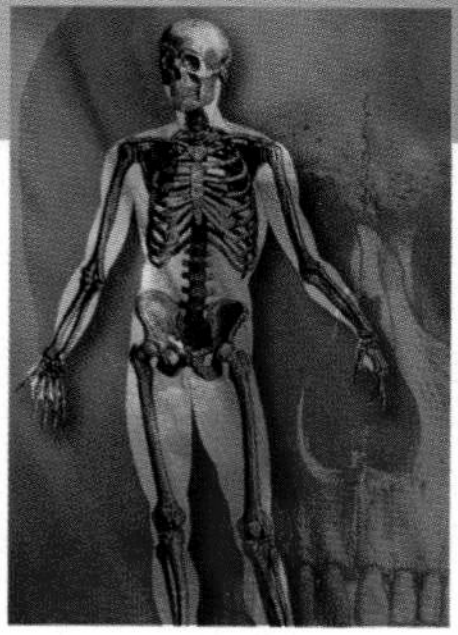

Chapter 41

Principles of Surgical Oncology

HAROLD J. WANEBO, MD, R. JAMES KONESS, MD, and MICHAEL P. VEZERIDIS, MD

Perhaps no other branch of surgery embraces as many aspects of medicine as does the discipline of surgical oncology. Working knowledge of pharmacology (chemotherapy), physics (radiation therapy), immunology, endocrinology, and pathology, as well as broad-based and intricate knowledge of surgical anatomy, are all required in the practice of a surgical oncologist. As the treatment of cancer is a major worldwide health issue, the history of surgical advances is intimately tied to advances in the treatment of cancer and benign neoplasms.

Although cancer care has become multidisciplinary and multispecialty, the surgeon nevertheless remains the primary caregiver in the treatment of resectable solid malignant neoplasms and the coordinator of treatment. Surgical oncology is a specialized-interest discipline within the realm of general surgery that focuses on the diagnosis and management of the cancer patient. The surgical oncologist brings a body of knowledge that extends to all facets of cancer, including prevention, diagnosis, treatment, rehabilitation, and surveillance. The salient feature of differentiation is that surgical oncology is both a technical and a cognitive specialty involving a chronic disease process that encompasses all organ systems and involves multiple physiologic and biologic processes.

The most common solid neoplasms in the United States arise in the lung, breast, colorectum, and prostate, and they are all covered extensively in site-specific chapters. Herein, we elucidate the principles of surgical oncology in four important areas: (1) the role of the surgeon in diagnosis and treatment of solid tumors; (2) urgent and special conditions or maladies unique to the cancer patient; (3) research and clinical investigation, development of new therapies, participating in clinical trials (adjuvant therapy); and (4) recruitment and fostering of education in surgical oncology.

The Surgical Role in Oncology: "The Team Leader"

The surgeon has a major role in oncology and commonly assumes the position of the team captain in patient management, as he or she is usually the first called to see the patient with suspicion of a tumor. The surgeon is frequently involved in screening programs for breast cancer and, to a lesser degree, for colorectal cancer. From that perspective, he or she is usually the first interventionalist involved in care of the patient and has the opportunity and responsibility to direct the effort to diagnose and provide therapy in the best possible way. This commonly means providing the entrée to a multidisciplinary care approach to the problem. The surgeon also has an obligation to promote the interdisciplinary approach to cancer diagnosis and care and to enroll patients in clinical trials wherever possible to advance the field in conjunction with other nonsurgical colleagues.

The Surgical Role in the Diagnosis

A new patient may be referred to a surgeon because of suspicion of cancer based on the presence of a mass in the breast or the recent demonstration of a mammographic abnormality; a finding of a large polyp in the rectum that may not be amenable to endoscopic removal, or, more commonly, a cancerous growth in the bowel. The finding of early changes suggestive of gastric mucosal migration into the esophagus with or without dysplasia (Barrett's esophagus) also causes problems to be sent to the surgeon for subsequent management.

Although gastric cancer is less commonly seen now, patients still have it and need surgical care. The surgeon is frequently asked to see the patient with a suggestive mole that is subsequently sampled and demonstrated to be melanoma, and he will determine the need for lymphoscintigraphy and sentinel node biopsy, based on the lesion microstage. Frequently consulted by the primary care physician regarding the patient with weight loss, early satiety, and a suspicion of malignancy, the surgeon may organize the patient's workup and subsequent management. A gastroenterologist may be involved and requested to perform an endoscopic retrograde cholangiopancreatography (ERCP) to exclude early cancer of the pancreas along with imaging studies to exclude a mass in the pancreas or biliary tree and, perhaps, to complement this with endoscopic ultrasound to facilitate earlier diagnosis.

Once the patient is enrolled in this progression, the surgeon has an obligation to be relentless in obtaining a diagnosis of cancer or to confirm a benign process. Thus in pursuing the diagnosis of a breast lesion, the surgeon must select the most direct and simple approach to the diagnosis from an array of approaches. A fine-needle aspiration of a palpable mass may yield serous fluid suggesting a simple cyst or may indicate a solid tumor that requires diagnosis by cytology. Complementary use of breast ultrasound or mammography to guide a core needle biopsy may indicate a suggestive lesion (or even a malignancy), for which an excisional biopsy may be required. In the event of having made the diagnosis of breast cancer, a melanoma, squamous cancer of the skin, or a combination of these, the current standard is to perform a sentinel node biopsy to determine the presence of nodal metastases.

Other, less common, problems seen by the surgeon may be a musculoskeletal mass or a radiographic retroperitoneal or extremity abnormality that may require a biopsy of the soft tissue or a bone biopsy to exclude a primary sarcoma of bone or soft tissue. The latter might be performed in conjunction with an orthopedic colleague.

Surgeons with specialized interest (i.e., head and neck oncology, thoracic oncology, or other colleagues in orthopedics [musculoskeletal oncology], urologic oncology) may be involved in the process to evaluate the patient completely and to expedite the diagnosis so that treatment can be initiated. In the event of demonstration of a chest lesion, a patient should be referred rapidly for a bronchoscopy. It should be considered whether to perform a needle biopsy or, perhaps, even a thoracoscopic removal or a biopsy of the nodule that, if cancerous, may require a subsequent staging maneuver by mediastinoscopy in addition to proper imaging studies. In head and neck cancers, the surgeon with head and neck experience must indeed be competent in the clinical examination of the oropharynx and larynx and be capable of conducting an endoscopic examination of the posterior pharynx and larynx to exclude a visible lesion. Based on the findings, the patient may need to be subjected to microlaryngoscopy to obtain tissue confirmation of any visualized abnormalities. In such cases, the presence of a squamous cancer of the larynx may prompt a careful examination of the lung by bronchoscopy and the esophagus by an esophagoscopy, as well, to exclude other areas that share the same aerodigestive pathway to carcinogenesis. The basics of the major diagnostic maneuvers are reviewed in the next section.

Surgical Objectives

Contemporary Imaging

The exploratory laparotomy in surgery and, particularly, in surgical oncology is a rare circumstance today. Computed tomography (CT) and magnetic resonance imaging (MRI), the workhorses of internal imaging, are highly indicative of the diagnosis before definitive histologic evaluation. CT uses advanced mathematical techniques to create two-dimensional images of the cross-sectional volume being scanned and uses basic radiologic principles to demonstrate differential blocking of x-ray transmission by dense structures in the body as the x-ray beam is moved around the body. The transmitted beam is detected and integrated into cross-sectional images. Spiral (helical) CT represents a further advancement, as the x-ray table moves rapidly through the gantry during a single breath-hold. This helix in space is interpreted by computer software as a three-dimensional data set that creates more precise and continuous images. MRI places the body in a superconducting magnet wherein pulses are created by brief applications of electric current. Hydrogen nuclei in protons within the body then resonate to varying degrees, generating electromagnetic waves or signals. A detecting coil notes these signals, and sophisticated data processing generates an image. With variation of the time between radiofrequency pulses (TR or time to repeat) and the time between applying the pulse and listening for the signal (TE or time to echo), different tissues in the body (including neoplastic growths) will generate different signals. T_1 and T_2 refer to physical properties of body tissue after exposure to a series of pulses at predetermined time intervals, afterward expressed as signal intensity (or brightness). For example, solid neoplasms are often bright on T_2-weighted images.

Whereas CT relies on intravascular and intraluminal contrast agents, MRI has the potential to image specific cells or tissues that might take up certain paramagnetic contrast agents that contain a paramagnetic label, such as gadolinium, iron, and manganese. The emerging field of MR spectroscopy relies on measurements made on the spectra of hydrogen nuclei (^{1}H, or proton). Nuclei with an odd number of protons or neutrons generate a net magnetic moment, behaving as a small bar magnet. The surrounding chemical environment affects a proton's position in an applied external magnetic field and is shifted accordingly (chemical shift). Thus spectral analysis can provide detailed information about types of molecules and their concentrations in a tissue sample.

Nuclear medicine is another imaging technique that provides functional information rather than structural or anatomic data. The presence of somatostatin receptors on some neoplasms (neuroendocrine tumors) allows diagnostic imaging with indium-111 [^{111}In]-pentetreotide, and [^{99m}Tc]-sestamibi has been found to be an excellent agent for abnormal parathyroid localization that currently is being explored for breast cancer imaging. Positron emission tomography (PET) uses cyclotron-produced positron emitters and a special camera to detect them by virtue of the concurrent production of a pair of photons traveling away from each other at 180 degrees after each positron undergoes an annihilation reaction. Because it produces isotopes of basic elements in the body and can follow key molecules in many metabolic processes, it can be used to evaluate data such as blood flow, blood volume, glucose metabolism, protein metabolism, oxygen concentration, and distribution of drugs. Although many radiopharmaceuticals have been labeled with positron emitters, fluorine-18-fluorodeoxyglucose ([^{18}F]FDG) has been the most widely used to date in oncology patients. It is taken into cells by the same membrane transport system as glucose and, like glucose, it is phosphorylated intracellularly. However, it cannot undergo further metabolism in the glycolytic pathway or rapidly diffuse back out of most cells. Trapped ^{18}F activity thus gives a measure of the intracellular accumulation of FDG. Because malignant cells often have an enhanced rate of glycolysis and because FDG competes with glucose for intracellular transport and phosphorylation, accumulation of FDG on whole-body images may indicate malignant disease. Most important, these data may help with response to therapy and in long-term follow-up in oncology patients.

Invasive ultrasound techniques are increasingly useful in the care of surgical oncology patients. Endoluminal transrectal ultrasound is the most accurate method for staging of early rectal cancers. It allows the surgeon to made decisions regarding local excision versus neoadjuvant radiotherapy, thus delivering the most effective treatment with the least morbidity. Endoluminal ultrasound via a flexible endoscope is increasingly important in staging, visualizing, and performing biopsies of lymph nodes, and it aids the surgeon with decisions regarding resectability of esophageal, gastric, pancreatic, biliary, upper gastrointestinal, and colorectal neuroendocrine neoplasms. Intraoperative ultrasound and laparoscopic ultrasound are frequently used to determine the stage and resectability of tumors, to screen for liver metastases, to localize nonpalpable tumors (i.e. insulinoma), and to confirm the completion of a procedure.

Serum Biochemical Markers

Appropriate Biopsy Techniques

A major role for the surgeon in the diagnosis of cancer lies in the acquisition of tissue to allow the pathologist to make the exact histologic diagnosis. To that end, several principles must be kept in mind:

1. Accurate pathologic diagnosis depends on obtaining a sample of viable, representative tumor. Some tumors may have areas of necrosis or desmoplastic reactions around them, and such tissue would be nondiagnostic. A frozen section may be needed to ensure that sampling is adequate, especially if an anesthetic has been required to do the biopsy.
2. The biopsy and its results should be obtained as rapidly as possible while inducing the least amount of pain and inconvenience to the patient.
3. Care should be taken so that the tissue to be examined is not contaminated during the biopsy. Hematomas after biopsy could lead to tumor spread along tissue planes and should be avoided. Instruments that come in contact with tumors should be discarded before further surgery on uncontaminated areas.
4. The surgeon must be familiar with fixatives and other transport media, and communication with the pathologist is vital to ensure that the tissue is handled properly so that pertinent questions can be answered and further testing can be performed if needed.
5. The importance of orientation of the biopsy cannot be overstated. This is essential in biopsies of a breast tumor where proper orientation by sutures is necessary to ensure that a follow-up excision can be appropriately done to remove a close or involved margin.

Further testing might include immunohistochemistry, electron microscopy, receptor analysis, and molecular biologic studies. Biopsy techniques available to the surgeon/clinician include fine-needle aspiration (FNA), core needle biopsy, incisional biopsy, excisional biopsy, punch biopsy, shave biopsy, and curettage.

Fine-needle aspiration yields specimens for cytologic rather than histologic diagnosis. It was first introduced in 1930 but became widespread in the 1970s, when the Papanicolaou stain and the field of cytologic diagnosis were popularized. Its advantages of minimal patient discomfort, minimal disturbance of tissue planes, and the ability to sample multiple areas of the tumor make it the procedure of choice to diagnose many solid neoplasms. Seeding of tumor along the needle tract is extremely rare, and the specificity of FNA approaches 100%, as false positives are unusual. Radiographic techniques such as CT and ultrasound may allow FNA of internal organs. Tru-cut and other core-needle–producing biopsies yield larger amounts of tissue used for histologic information, such as grade, and immunohistochemical staining that often provides subtype information. Commercially available needle biopsy "guns" allow for CT, ultrasound, and stereotactic-guided breast sampling of previously inaccessible tissue.

Tumors in which microscopic architectural organization is important for diagnosis, such as soft tissue sarcoma and lymphoma, often require an incisional biopsy to allow treatment planning. In these "open" procedures, attention to placement of the incision is often essential to future treatment. For example, if a core needle biopsy is not adequate, extremity sarcomas should be incised in a longitudinal direction to allow excision of the biopsy site at definitive resection. Internal biopsy sites such as the larynx, gastrointestinal tract, bladder, and cervix are preferably sampled with an instrument that provides a cupped biopsy, an extension of the incisional biopsy. Still more inaccessible areas of the body, such as the common bile duct and segmental bronchial tumors, are best diagnosed with brush cytology. Excisional biopsies are reserved for presumptively benign tumors and sufficiently small malignancies that can be completely excised without compromising cosmesis or function.

Curettage refers to the method whereby tissue is removed by using a curette in a repeated scraping motion, yielding crushed tissue for analysis. An example of this technique includes endocervical and endometrial sampling to evaluate postmenopausal bleeding and to evaluate and treat dysfunctional bleeding. Endometrial aspiration biopsies are easily accomplished and can rapidly provide satisfactory tissue for analysis in an office setting.

Lesions of the skin are ideally suited for biopsy via a conventional local excision under local anesthesia or by using a commercially available disposable dermal punch biopsy kit. Melanoma, in which the depth of invasion determines local and regional treatment, can be diagnosed and removed with a circular drill-type punch obtaining a full thickness of skin into the superficial fat. This is helpful for large lesions, whereas a standard excisional biopsy is usually accepted for smaller lesions. For nonpigmented skin lesions, the biopsy technique depends on size, location, and concern for malignancy. Many are amenable to definitive excisional removal. If clinical suspicion of cancer exists, then a core punch might be the best first step. Shave biopsies are not appropriate, as they provide no information as to depth, and they compromise subsequent treatment.

Improper handling of a tissue sample diminishes the diagnostic value of an otherwise adequate biopsy. Until the biopsy sample is delivered to the pathologist, the surgeon is responsible for the handling of the specimen, and he or she must be aware of certain principles. Neutral buffered 10% formalin provides prompt fixation, and most samples are best transported in this medium. Certain types of specimens, however, require preservation in other ways to maximize their diagnostic value. For example, tissue suggestive of lymphoma should be delivered fresh. The pathologist will fix part for morphologic analysis and immunologic marker studies. The rest may be sent for flow cytometry surface-marker analysis or frozen for molecular genetic studies. FNA cytology specimens must be fixed on glass slides or transported in red blood cell–lysing medium (i.e., Cytolyte). Inking or orienting the specimen is often of value to the surgeon in assessing adequacy of treatment or in helping to plan future local treatment and is best communicated directly to the pathologist. If a pathologist is not immediately available, a drawing is fashioned to orient the pathologist. Last, frozen sections are a source of stress to the pathologist and surgeon alike and should not be relied on as an initial biopsy, except to determine whether the specimen contains viable tissue for diagnosis. Frozen sections are best reserved for margin analysis at the time of major cancer extirpations. There are exceptions, of course (i.e., cancer of the pancreas or possible cancer of the lung in an excised pulmonary nodule).

Pathology

Standard histologic evaluation involves formaldehyde fixation, paraffin embedding, and staining with hematoxylin and eosin, followed by light microscopy. Oncologic pathologic evaluation involves a variety of evolving techniques that complement and accentuate conventional assessment. Electron microscopy, available for more than 40 years, helps to subcategorize certain types of tumors based on subcellular structural features. More recently, cytogenetics, immunohistochemistry, analysis of DNA content by flow cytometry, and molecular genetics have assumed an important role in the diagnosis of cancer.

Cytologic analysis is based on the morphologic examination of individual cells in the absence of their supporting stroma or parenchyma. Cells are obtained by FNA biopsy, brushing of visceral surfaces, or scraping epithelial surfaces (i.e., Papanicolaou cervical smear). If necessary, cells transported in suspension are centrifuged and the suspension smeared on glass slides, where they are subsequently fixed and stained. The primary goal of cytologic analysis is to differentiate tumors as benign or malignant, not to subclassify malignancies. Stains can be applied for more in-depth analysis; however, the surgeon should obtain a larger amount of tissue if this information is necessary. Further, although a laboratory with adequate expertise may have false-positive rates of less than 1%, false-negative and negative predictive rates are considerably higher.

Immunohistochemistry involves the use of antibodies to specific antigens, mostly proteins deposited on the microscope slide by an indirect procedure using antibodies tagged with fluorescent molecules, or with enzymes such as peroxidase or alkaline phosphatase that can catalyze in situ conversion of substrate to a colored reaction product. Some antigens recognized by diagnostically useful antibodies include some with known functions, such as surface receptors, hormones, or proteins controlling the cellular differentiation and proliferation, and some whose function is yet to be determined. Further, the production of monoclonal antibodies provides reagents that bind very specific portions of an antigen (epitope), can be produced in large quantities, and are highly reproducible. Occasionally, immunohistochemistry contributes to the distinction between benign and malignant tissue. Among non-Hodgkin's lymphomas and leukemias, the lymphocytes may demonstrate monoclonality, an important criterion for malignancy in these tumors. For instance, in B-cell lymphomas and leukemias, immunohistochemistry may detect cells bearing exclusively *kappa* or *lambda* light chains rather than the normal 2:1 kappa and lambda mixture. More frequently, immunohistochemistry is used to classify malignancies. Applying a battery of antibodies recognizing intermediate filaments and cell-surface antigens is highly effective in separating undifferentiated carcinomas from anaplastic lymphomas, melanomas, and sarcomas. The difficult task of classifying of lymphomas also is highly facilitated by the use of immunohistochemistry.

DNA content can be analyzed by either flow cytometry or image analysis microscopy applied to blood, body fluids, or solid tumors. Flow cytometry is performed on cells or their nuclei stained with fluorescent dyes that bind quantitatively to DNA. The stained cells in suspension are then exposed to a laser beam, and a photomultiplier tube, viewing cells passing one at a time, measures the fluorescence emitted. Image analysis uses microscopes to measure the amount of nonfluorescent dye bound to individual cells. Chromosome number (or ploidy) is measured, with malignant tissue often exhibiting an increased chromosome number (aneuploid). The S-phase fraction, or the proportion of cells in which the DNA content of the cell has doubled, also can be measured. This information can provide valuable prognostic information, but, in practice, results have been mixed, with some benign neoplasms demonstrating aneuploid populations and results being affected by the fixatives used and the conditions of fixation.

Molecular biologic techniques in cancer diagnosis involve the analysis of nucleotide sequences to detect the presence of malignant cells. Molecular genetic tests tend to be more objective than are those of light microscopy and require less experience to interpret. Further, molecular genetic tests are generally much more sensitive than either light microscopy or immunohistochemistry. To date, however, most molecular genetic tests require significant amounts of time and labor and are relatively expensive.

Fluorescence in situ hybridization (FISH) allows the detection of chromosomal abnormalities visible in the light microscope. Karyotypes, or portraits, are constructed from condensed chromosomes released from metaphase cells and banded by staining with Giemsa dye. Specific regions of interest are hybridized with DNA probes recognized by antibodies directed against the molecular tag and coupled to a fluorochrome. In situ hybridization, as distinct from FISH, is used to detect RNA and gene expression. This technique can be performed on formalin-fixed, paraffin-embedded tissues. Its chief diagnostic application is for the characterization of the tissue origin of a neoplasm, especially in genes that are encoded by neuroendocrine tumors.

Southern blot hybridization provides a means for detecting changes or differences in DNA nucleotide sequence, particularly large stretches of DNA, as in translations, large deletions, or amplifications. Foreign DNA, such as viral integration, also may be detected. The blot or transfer method also allows the detection of RNA (Northern blotting) or proteins (Western blotting).

A more recently developed and far more powerful technique is the polymerase chain reaction, a procedure in which regions of DNA can be enormously amplified in vitro, provided the nucleotide sequences immediately next to regions are known. A pair of oligonucleotides, or primers, is constructed in DNA synthesizers to be complementary to specific sequences in opposite strands of the template on either side of the region to be amplified. DNA polymerases then copy the DNA of the template by adding nucleotides to the 3-prime end of preexisting strands of DNA annealed to the template DNA. The procedure also may be applied to RNA by the initial transcription of RNA into a single-stranded complementary DNA (cDNA) under the direction of the RNA-dependent DNA polymerase reverse transcriptase.

Specific chromosomal abnormalities have most often been described in leukemias and lymphomas, although characteristic abnormalities are increasing, being described for solid tumors. The most common structural changes are balanced translations, deletions, and gene amplifications. The Philadelphia chromosome (Ph), present in approximately 99% of patients with chronic myeloid leukemia, was one of the first chromosome abnormalities described for malignant disease. The Ph chromosome was shown with banding to involve chromosome 22 and was later defined as a balanced translocation involving chromosomes 9 and 22. Similarly, osseous and nonosseous Ewing sarcomas consistently have the t(11;22) translocation.

Staging

The desire of clinicians to stage cancer has been evident for decades and is based on multiple important considerations. Cancer staging is based on the premise that tumors that are of the same histologic type and extent have similar natural histories. The TNM is now the established staging method. T stands for tumor size. For example, in breast cancer, it is simply categorized as T1, smaller than 2 cm; T2, 2 to 5 cm; T3, larger than 5 cm; and T4, a tumor of any size with extension to chest wall (T4a) or skin (T4b) or both (T4c) or represents inflammatory cancer (T4d). The N refers to regional nodes: N0, no nodal metastases; N1, metastases to ipsilateral nodes; N2, ipsilateral nodes fixed to each other, N3, metastasis to internal mammary nodes. M refers to the presence of distant metastases. M0, no distant metastases; M, presence of distant metastases; this can be followed by a number indicating the number of distant sites. The TNM classification system is applicable to all cancers, and the details for individual cancers are specified in the manual by the American Joint Committee for Cancer Staging.

Surgical Role: Triage Officer

Staging the Cancer: Introducing the Multidisciplinary Team

The surgeon may find him- or herself as a triage officer in a management of some oncologic problems (i.e., the patient with a lump in the neck, the patient with a breast mass, and the patient with suggestive lymphadenopathy may all ultimately require care by the medical oncologist or the radiation therapist). He or she is really the patient's entrée into their therapeutic world. In such cases, the surgeon can rapidly facilitate a biopsy, for example, frequently using FNA cytology to determine that a neck mass is indeed a squamous cancer versus an adenocarcinoma that requires divergent diagnostic and therapeutic approaches. Even a soft tissue tumor may be rapidly confirmed with an initial FNA biopsy (determining that the lesion is a suspected sarcoma vs. some other histogenesis). In any case, this moves the patient into the right potential treatment modality quickly. Depending on findings, an FNA biopsy may indicate the need for additional tissue confirmation. Although an FNA biopsy may suggest a breast cancer, and indeed may be the entrée into a treatment program for the breast, it is wise to have a tissue confirmation. If the lesion is small, this is usually obtained by a local excision (lumpectomy), with attention to detail regarding the margins of the excision and with an effort to have complete excision. This not only facilitates the obvious pathologic review, but also sets the stage for subsequent therapy. In such a patient, if the margins are clear from the initial excision, subsequent excision may not be needed. A sentinel node biopsy is done to indicate the stage of disease and, if positive, may indicate the need for axillary dissection. Completion radiation to the breast may be all of the additional treatment needed besides the sentinel node and axillary dissection as indicated.

Similarly, an FNA biopsy of a neck mass confirming a squamous cancer, and ruling out an adenocarcinoma or lymphoma or other lesion, would definitely set the stage for this patient to have a careful head and neck endoscopic examination to detect the primary source and to initiate a treatment program for the patient. In such patients, the early demonstration of a small cancer in the posterior pharynx or larynx may permit an early radiation attack on that site, usually in conjunction with chemotherapy, as suggested by protocols. This may permit the patient to have total local control of this primary site and subsequent control of the neck cancer through more conservative surgery. Of course, this greatly enhances the patient's quality of life. This is far better than the unwise approach of the "slash in the neck biopsy" as the first diagnostic approach when the disease is truly originating at a primary mucosal site such as the oropharynx or larynx. In these cases, the tumor can be adequately managed by combined surgical and chemoradiation therapy and treating the entire disease process rather than focusing merely on the neck problem.

One of the common disease sites seen by the general surgeon with an interest in cancer is the breast. Currently, the surgeon's role is heavily directed toward initiating the diagnosis, obtaining adequate excision of a primary lesion, and confirming the presence or absence of nodal metastases by sentinel node biopsy and with or without an axillary dissection. Evaluating the patient with the medical oncologist and radiation therapist by case discussion in the Tumor Board, and perhaps with a protocol nurse, generally leads to the best possible treatment for the patient, according to the stage of disease.

In patients with suspected colorectal cancer, which is second to lung cancer or the most common neoplasm in both sexes, the surgeon has an important role. Early rectal cancer demonstrated by the gastroenterologist or suspected by a primary care physician will require careful endoscopy and a clearing colonoscopy to exclude other sites in the colon. Subsequently, the patient will require scheduling for primary staging and therapy. In such patients, rectal ultrasound greatly enhances the endoscopic diagnosis and permits a decision regarding the potential value of local excision (for a UT-1 or UT-2 lesion with or without radiation) in conjunction with local radiation. In such cases, the local excision and the staging ultrasound may confirm the possibility of this being an acceptable primary treatment for early-stage rectal cancer. Controversy exists here as to the long-term value of local excision, especially in patients with UT-2 and certainly in those with UT-3 lesions in which increased risk of nodal disease is present.

It is here that enrollment of patients into clinical trial protocols is important, as it may permit a more conservative treatment of the patient under the aegis of a carefully monitored treatment program for lesions in the midrectum. Although low anterior resection with reconstruction may have the better outcome data versus local excision, it is obviously more intrusive and has higher morbidity and mortality than does a local excision. The consideration of preoperative chemoradiation versus postoperative therapy is under study by different groups, including National Surgical Adjuvant Breast and Bowel Project (NSABP), and should be considered and discussed with the patient. Patients with larger lesions (T3 to T4)

PEARLS FOR ROUNDS

Surgical oncology is a specialized interest discipline within the realm of general surgery that focuses on the diagnosis and management of the cancer patient.

Major areas of interest included diagnosis and treatment of solid tumors, management of acute and chronic problems related to malignancy, and guidance of patients through the obstacle course of specialists and special procedures to reach the optimum treatment.

The surgeon functions as the captain of the ship and aggressively pursues early diagnosis using all of the currently available techniques and assists the patient in the decision-making process about the optimum surgical and adjuvant therapy.

The surgeon frequently is involved in the screening process for common tumors such as breast and colorectal cancer.

The surgeon facilitates the multimodal treatment provided to the patient by inserting vascular access devices for chemotherapy and "PEG" tubes for management of nutrition (operative bypass may be needed).

The surgeon conducts the long-term post-op surveillance of cancer patients to facilitate early diagnosis and treatment of recurrence or palliation.

may be candidates for preoperative chemoradiation and subsequent resection. With careful attention to details, the accompaniment of preoperative radiation can be properly addressed in managing such patients also to permit sphincter-saving reconstruction to be done. The decision to use a temporary ileostomy or colostomy will be dictated by the findings and judgment of the surgeon. This important judgment can prevent anastomotic problems. One should not forget that an adequately performed resection (total mesorectal excision, as described by Heald) has perhaps the best outcome in the rectal cancer patient. Preoperative radiation therapy has recently been shown to improve survival significantly, and postoperative therapy is well documented to improve survival as well.

The patient with rectal cancer is generally a candidate for adjuvant therapy, and certainly such a patient should be enrolled in clinical trial protocols. Commonly, this can be done pending the discussion of the patient at the Tumor Board once the pathology and staging details are known.

In the patient with head and neck cancer, triple endoscopy and careful biopsy and staging of the primary lesion definitely augment subsequent therapy and influence the outcome. Early-stage disease may be managed with surgical resection with or without radiation or surgery alone, whereas patients with advanced disease, stage III and stage IV, are commonly treated by chemoradiation therapy. Such patients are usually entered into a study protocol that tends to optimize the therapeutic approach by the medical oncologist and the radiation therapist and ensures an adjustment of therapy according to toxicity levels. It is important to reflect on the quality of life and take all the steps necessary to maximize this in these patients with complex disease. Although the combined therapy programs are associated with improvements in disease outcomes, they also engender complicated toxicity and quality-of-life problems that must be addressed.

Similarly, evaluation of the patient with esophageal cancer requires a careful staging endoscopy (now supplemented with endoscopic ultrasound) to determine the depth of penetration, as well as either an endoscopic assessment or radiologic assessment of the length of lesion, the size of the lesion, and whether the mediastinum is involved. In such patients, numerous studies involve either neoadjuvant or combined therapy or postoperative chemoradiation therapy. The optimal treatment program is still under study. Commonly, these patients require a total esophagectomy either through a right thoracoabdominal approach (Ivor-Lewis) or the transhiatal approach (Bolton). Patients with more distal esophageal lesions may be managed through a left thoracoabdominal approach. Patients with gastroesophageal junction cancer or proximal gastric cancer will require complete resection of the distal esophagus and proximal stomach with regional node dissection commonly done through an abdominal or abdominal thoracic approach. In such cases, the utilization of neoadjuvant therapy appears promising but still is best done in a clinical trial. The interdisciplinary involvement of the gastroenterologist (especially someone who is facile with endoscopic ultrasound) and the radiologist, giving careful attention to involvement of mediastinal nodes, is essential for accurate staging.

In managing patients with head and neck cancer, esophageal cancer, and stomach or pancreatic cancer, nutritional considerations also are very important. Frequently, such patients have had major weight loss, approaching 10% or more, and may require a definitive program for supplementation (i.e., a jejunostomy feeding tube, or a G-tube in some cases, depending on the primary site). Alimentation through the gastrointestinal (GI) tract is still the optimal way to augment nutrition in such patients, rather than the use of intravenous hyperalimentation.

Hepatobiliary and pancreatic cancers are major diseases that confront the surgeon and can test the mettle of any treatment group. These patients truly require a multidisciplinary and interdisciplinary approach, involving not only the surgeons and his gastroenterology and radiology colleagues, but also the medical oncologist and radiation therapist. Cancer of the pancreas is still probably the most ominous of the diseases being frequently diagnosed very late and being underappreciated, unrecognized, and probably undertreated. Patients with apparent early lesions, as suggested by the ERCP and radiologic evaluation, may be candidates for a neoadjuvant protocol (i.e., laparoscopic staging, placement of jejunostomy or gastrostomy feeding tube, and subsequent chemotherapy and radiation as preludes to subsequent resection). This is with the understanding that the patient is in a clinical study, as no confirmed benefit of neoadjuvant therapy exists for this disease. However, this one option benefits patients with more advanced disease. In the patient with earlier disease, a resection and postoperative therapy by protocol is optimal and may carry an improved outcome. In some institutions with extensive experience, survival rates in the 18% to 20% range or higher have been reported, whereas the more commonly reported rate is approximately in the 5% range. Although staging probably has an impact here, the experience of the treating group and facility (the surgeon and his multidisciplinary team) likely improves the outcome.

Although hepatocellular cancer is rare in the United States (<10,000 cases), it is one of the major neoplasms worldwide. A commonly associated condition is cirrhosis secondary to hepatitis B or C. Hepatitis C is becoming an increasingly prevalent finding, as is hepatitis B, in this country. Treatment considerations are based on patient stage and the degree of cirrhosis. Small lesions in a patient with high-risk Child C cirrhosis may be managed with ethanol injection, saving such a patient the need for resection. Resection in the favorably staged patient is the optimal treatment with the best long-term outcome, however. Some centers offer liver transplants for patients that are carefully staged with marked cirrhosis and a relatively small lesion (3- to 4-cm lesion). The use of indocyanin green may help establish the functional reserve for such patients, in addition to other imaging studies, albumin, and liver-function measurements.

In the United States, hepatic neoplasms are more commonly secondary to metastases from colorectal cancer. The surgical role is well established here, and survival in the 25% to 30% range can be expected in well-selected patients. The addition of hepatic artery infusion to augment these results has recently been documented. A surgeon with an interest in this disease is best allied with an active hepatologist or medical oncologist or both to facilitate optimal management of these patients. The utilization of hepatic artery infusion devices is still experimental, in spite of the publications suggesting benefit to resection even in an adjuvant setting. In such cases, involvement of an interactive group of medical oncologist, surgeons, and radiologists will ensure optimal care of such patients.

The management of lung cancer, including diagnosis, staging, and treatment, is highly in the purview of the thoracic oncologist. Utilization of bronchoscopy, mediastinoscopy, and endoscopic or thoracoscopic approaches is important in the armamentarium of the thoracic surgeon. The medical and radiation oncologists are commonly involved in protocol management of these patients in an effort to ensure optimal care. Although the patient with true stage I cancer has an excellent prognosis, more commonly seen are patients with stage IIIA or B cancers, who should be considered candidates for protocol therapy in clinical trial settings.

Adjuvant Therapy

The surgeon serves as the patient's advocate in the interaction with other cancer-treating disciplines. Indeed, in the common malignancies, a well-established role exists for adjuvant therapy, especially in breast cancer management. Numerous well-designed protocols and studies document the benefit of chemotherapy with or without tamoxifen in patients at different stages of primary breast cancer. A role for neoadjuvant therapy also is found in patients with locally advanced disease. Although recently challenged, there may be a role for more aggressive care, up to even using stem cell support in very high risk patients. This has been under study but is controversial and still considered experimental. The surgeon may have various roles in such patients, ranging from being the primary therapist to being a coordinator of therapy by other specialists. For example, in patients with early-stage disease, especially the elderly, tamoxifen may be the only addition to local excision plus radiation for a small invasive cancer, or perhaps it may be the only therapeutic modality used after adequate resection of a favorably staged noninvasive breast cancer. In some cases, the surgeon may be the facilitator for more aggressive care, such as the placement of infusion ports for aggressive chemotherapy in high-stage patients. It also is the surgeon's role to participate in the active monitoring of such patients after therapy and to maintain a close involvement with these patients throughout the therapy and after therapy.

The surgical role in colorectal cancer, as well as in other cancers of the upper GI tract, will necessitate the surgeon's pursuing additional therapies by either chemotherapy or radiation or both. A plethora of protocols now exists to provide adjuvant care for all such patients. The surgeon has an important role in confirming that these patients are seen and discussed by members of the multidisciplinary team to ensure that adequate planning exists for adjuvant therapy. Again, the surgeon has an important role in monitoring of patients after therapy.

PEARLS FOR THE OR

Early diagnosis of solid tumors is facilitated by use of fine needle aspiration cytology or core needle biopsy of palpable masses.

Ultrasound can aid the surgeon in diagnosis of palpable breast thickening or lumps. Cysts or solid masses have distinctive ultrasound characteristics, and ultrasound directed FNA or core biopsy can provide histologic confirmation.

Excisional biopsies of suspicious tumors in the breast, head and neck, and soft tissue should be fully oriented by marking sutures prior to exam by the pathologist.

For melanoma or SCC of skin, proper biopsy techniques will ensure adequate histology. Full-thickness biopsy into subcutaneous tissue by core, punch, or incisional technique is needed. For sarcoma, initial FNA followed by core biopsy or proper oriented incisional biopsy may be done. Mucosal tumors require cup biopsy via endoscope and breast requires FNA, core stereotactic, or open biopsy.

Proper management of biopsied tissue is important:tissue for lymphoma assessment or for electron microscopy, or special antibody or molecular tests should be examined fresh.

Sentinel node biopsy optimizes lymphatic staging for melanoma, breast cancer, skin cancers, and certain GI tumors and commonly involves lymphscintigraphy to pinpoint the nodal site.

Role of Surgical Oncologist

Post-treatment Surveillance

The classic surveillance of patients with breast cancer may require a schedule of careful clinical examinations in breast cancer. This includes a yearly mammography of the contralateral (unaffected) breast and, perhaps, a 6-month mammography for at least 2 years of the ipsilateral (affected) breast. Periodic chest radiograph, CT scan of the abdomen, measurement of tumor marker CA27-29, and selective liver-function test (i.e., carcinoembryonic antigen [CEA] 27, 29) would be required, depending on the initial stage of disease and the prognosis.

Patients with GI cancer, especially colorectal cancer, are monitored at a frequency ranging from 3 to 6 months, depending on stage. This should include clinical examination, periodic endoscopy, a baseline and follow-up CT of the pelvis (in the patient with previous rectal cancer resection), and CEA measurements on a frequent basis, 2 to 3 months during the first 2 to 3 years and then at least at the time of the follow-up visit. Although the role of intensive monitoring of these patients is somewhat controversial, with lack of confirmation of benefit by random trial, the potential benefit to the patient with early diagnosis of recurrence provides an opportunity for treatment (e.g., liver metastases may be resected in the hope for cure in one third of such patients with metastatic colorectal cancer). A local recurrence in the rectum, if not previously treated with radiation, may be amenable to repeated resection plus radiation therapy, with a chance for long-term cure in approximately one third of the patients. In patients with other GI malignancies, careful follow-up is dictated by the site (i.e., endoscopy for esophageal and gastric cancer patients), is important, and is supplemented by radiologic studies and tumor markers, such as CEA or CA19-9, on periodic follow-up visits. Table 41-1 shows a suggested follow-up schedule after primary cancer resection.

TABLE 41–1 Monitoring Program after Primary Cancer Resection

	Colorectal	Gastric Esophageal Pancreatic	Breast	Melanoma Sarcoma	Head and Neck
Clinical visits for all of these cancers*			q 3 mo for the first 3 yr q 4 mo for the 4th yr q 6 mo for the 5th yr for all cancers		
Selected Tests					
Fecal occult blood	q 6–12 mo		—	—	—
Endoscopy	Clearing colonoscopy q 6–12 mo After 4 yr, q 3 yr	Each visit	—	—	Each visit
Imaging, baseline and follow-up	**For all GI cancers:** Baseline CT: abdomen and pelvis then q 12 mo–3 yr q 18 mo–4–5 yr Chest radiograph q 6 mo–3 yr then q 12 mo		**High risk:** CT abdomen and chest q 6 mo for up to 3 yr q 12 mo yr 4 and 5 **Low risk:** CT abdomen and chest q 6 mo for up to 18 mo q 12 mo yr 2 and 5	**High risk:** CT abdomen and chest q 6 mo for 2 yr then q 12 mo for 3–5 yr	Selected CT, head neck, and chest **High risk:** q 6 mo for 2 yr then q 12 mo for 3–5 yr
Bone scan	—		Baseline and with symptoms	If symptomatic	If symptomatic
Laboratory	**For all GI cancers:**				
CBC/Diff	q 12 mo or symptomatic		If symptomatic	If symptomatic	If symptomatic
CEA	q 3 mo for 1–3 yr q 4 mo for the 4th yr q 6 mo for the 5th yr				
CA 19-9	q 3 mo for 1–3 yr q 4 mo for the 4th yr q 6 mo for the 5th yr		q 2 mo for 3 yr		
CA 27-29			q 4 mo for 3–5 yr		
LDH, alk phosphatase				q 3 mo for 3 yr q 4 mo for 3–5 yr	

*Timing of visits may be adjusted according to risk of recurrence.
CBC, complete blood count; CEA, carcinoembryonic antigen; CT, computed tomography; LDH, lactate dehydrogenase.

Clinical Trialist

The surgeon with an interest in cancer care has additional obligations. He has an important responsibility to participate in some of the multidisciplinary clinical trial groups. Several organizations are well established. Surgeons have directed the NSABP for many years, led by clinical trial pioneer Dr. Bernard Fisher and his successors. The NSABP has been setting standards in breast cancer management and, to a large degree, also has contributed to management of colorectal cancer. Other such groups that have made important contributions include the regional cooperative groups Cancer and Leukemia Group B (CALGB), Eastern Cooperative Oncology Group (ECOG), Northern California Oncology Group (NCOG), and Southwest Oncology Group (SWOG), along with the recently developed American College of Surgeons Cooperative Study Group. Surgical participation in these groups permits the surgeon to be at the cutting edge of clinical trials, actually involved and able to take leadership roles in these organizations and "to spread the gospel" in his or her own institution to enroll patients in the clinical trials. The participation of American patients in clinical trials is still very low (probably 2% to 4% nationally), and thus it should be the goal of all surgeons to increase these numbers. It provides optimal care for patients in carefully designed and monitored treatment programs that also provide answers and advances to the malignancy under therapy.

New Therapies

Surgeons also have an opportunity to participate in some of the newer modalities that are continuing to evolve. In the past, the role of immunotherapy was quite limited to studies with **Bacille Calmette-Guérin** (BCG) and nonspecific immune stimulation using such agents as lavamisole and *Cryptosporidium parvum*. Now a more sophisticated armamentarium includes designer drugs such as numerous cytokines that can augment cellular and humoral immunity and colony-stimulating factors that can restore the depressed granulocyte count or platelet count and also can augment the red cell mass in the compromised cancer patient. Now promising monoclonal antibodies such as humanized monoclonal antibody to the Her-2/neu receptor (Herceptin) provide a great boost in breast cancer therapy. Recent studies show benefit of treatment with monoclonal antibodies or thymidine kinase inhibitors of tumor growth factors or their receptors such as epidermal growth factors types I and II or vascular endothelial growth factor. Numerous tumor vaccines are under study, and the suggestion is that these will be the important modalities in the future. The role of gene therapy is under study. The use of the adenovirus vector delivery systems, the use of vaccinia virus, and the use of viral oncolysates in the formation of vaccines also are under study. The surgeon may be involved with associates who have a primary role in these new treatment modalities and may assist patients for whom conventional therapy is no longer warranted.

Surgical Education

The surgical oncologist who is formally trained as such or the surgeon who is an oncologist by virtue of his or her self-training, interest, and discipline also has an obligation to participate in the education of younger colleagues in training residents and fellows with an interest in cancer care. Well-established fellowship programs in surgical oncology provide specialized training to surgeons with an interest in cancer, organized under the umbrella of the Society of Surgical Oncology. These are 2-year fellowship training programs with a strong focus on providing a multidisciplinary education to the surgeon, not only in the advancement in surgical skills, but also in the training in the use of the other disciplines to facilitate care of the patient with malignancy. The surgeon also has an obligation to participate in public education to improve cancer care within regions. The American Cancer Society (ACS) provides an excellent opportunity for the surgeon to work through an umbrella organization, involving the public in supporting cancer care and cancer research. The ACS has long involved volunteers from the community who have an interest in cancer and has had a position in creating education of the medical profession as well as that of the public so that the overall cancer care has really been greatly improved.

The surgeon has a great opportunity to provide a disciplined treatment approach to his or her patients and to collaborate with colleagues in collecting data and publishing important results, in this way advancing the field. The field of surgical oncology is expanding rapidly and offers a variety of opportunities to the surgeon in training.

Suggested Reading

American Joint Committee on Cancer: Staging Manual, 6th ed. Springer, New York, 2002.

Balch C, Bland K, Brennan M, et al: What is a surgical oncologist? Ann Surg Oncol 1(1): 2, 1994.

Ellis FH: Transthoracic resection for carcinoma of the thoracic esophagus and cardia. In Wanebo HJ (ed): Surgery for Gastrointestinal Cancer. New York, Lippincott-Raven, 1996, pp 217–229.

Ferrand SF, Chen CC, Dilsizian V, et al: What is new in nuclear medicine imaging? Surg Oncol Clin North Am 8(1):185, 1999.

Rosenberg S. Surgical oncology. In DeVita V, Hellman S, Rosenberg S (eds): Cancer Principles and Practice of Oncology. Philadelphia, Lippincott-Raven, 1997, pp 295–306.

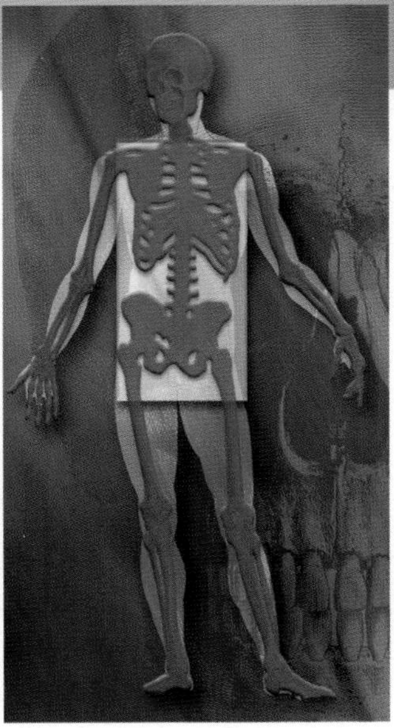

SECTION XI

ORTHOPEDIC SURGERY

Chapter 42

Diseases of the Bones and Joints

DONNA M. PACICCA, MD, RYAN R. SNYDER, MD, PETER DEWIRE, MD, and ANDREW B. STEIN, MD

Osteomyelitis

Infections of the bone may be acute or chronic, and the bone may be infected by organisms from a hematogenous or an exogenous source.

Acute hematogenous osteomyelitis is a blood-borne infection that occurs most commonly in children and involves the metaphyseal portion of the long bone. The metaphysis has an abundant blood flow with terminal capillary loops, and this predisposes it to infection. In immature bone, the physeal plate acts as a barrier to the spread of infection to the epiphysis. Acute hematogenous osteomyelitis is uncommon in adults and usually involves subperiosteal cortical bone and vertebral bodies. Risk factors include human immunodeficiency virus (HIV) infection, diabetes mellitus, sickle cell anemia, and intravenous drug abuse.

In some cases of **exogenous osteomyelitis,** organisms enter the bone directly after open fractures, missile wounds, or surgery. In **contiguous osteomyelitis,** the organisms spread to the bone from chronic tissue infections, such as decubitus ulcers.

Etiology

The most common bacteria associated with hematogenous osteomyelitis in children are the gram-positive cocci, *Staphylococcus aureus*, and streptococci (Table 42-1), whereas in adults, they are gram-negative bacteria, such as *Escherichia coli, Pseudomonas,* and *Salmonella.* In adults, gram-positive bacteria are the most frequent cause of exogenous osteomyelitis. Although any bacterium can be isolated from contaminated open fractures, the most common bacteria associated with osteomyelitis after an open fracture are *S. aureus, Staphylococcus epidermidis,* and nonenterococcal streptococci. Osteomyelitis caused by *Mycobacterium tuberculosis* is most commonly seen in patients from developing countries and frequently infects the vertebral bodies.

Mycotic infections of the skeleton occur by hematogenous spread or direct invasion and are most commonly caused by *Candida, Coccidioides, Sporothrix,* and *Actinomyces.*

Pathogenesis

The inflammatory process in acute osteomyelitis leads to an increase in intraosseous pressure. A focal area of necrotic bone (sequestrum) develops within the infected area, and the proliferation of bacteria within the sequestrum may result in chronic osteomyelitis. The normal host response is an attempt to isolate the infected bone by forming an envelope of new bone (involucrum). Depending on the status of the host's immune system and the virulence of the infecting bacteria, recurring draining sinuses may develop as a means of decompressing the contained infection. Patients with chronically draining sinuses may develop squamous cell carcinoma within the sinus tracts.

Evaluation

History and Physical Examination

In patients with osteomyelitis, a thorough physical examination and a complete review of systems and past medical history are essential, because systemic illnesses and previous medical or surgical treatment may alter the current treatment options.

Patients with acute hematogenous osteomyelitis are first seen with localized pain and tenderness. In children, pain may be elicited by palpation of the metaphyseal portion of the bone or by percussion of the spinous process at the involved level. Fever, localized swelling, and erythema are

TABLE 42–1 Causes of Osteomyelitis

Disease and Characteristics of Patients	Most Common Causes
Hematogenous Osteomyelitis	
Patients <4 mo old	*Staphylococcus aureus*, group B streptococci, and gram-negative bacilli
Patients from 4 mo to 21 yr	*S. aureus* and group A streptococci; rarely, coliforms
Patients > 21 yr	*S. aureus* and a wide variety of other aerobic and anaerobic cocci and bacilli
Patients of any age:	
With sickle cell anemia	*Salmonella* species
Undergoing hemodialysis	*S. aureus* and *Pseudomonas aeruginosa*
With intravenous drug abuse	*S. aureus* and *P. aeruginosa*
Contiguous Osteomyelitis	
Patients with vascular insufficiency (e.g., diabetic patients with neuropathy, patients with neurologic deficits and decubitus ulcers, and patients with atherosclerotic peripheral vascular disease)	Polymicrobic: gram-positive cocci (aerobic and anaerobic) and gram-negative bacilli (aerobic and anaerobic)
Patients without vascular insufficiency:	
After injury caused by stepping on a nail that penetrates the shoe and foot	*P. aeruginosa*
After reduction and internal fixation of a fracture	Coliforms, *S. aureus*, and *P. aeruginosa*
After sternotomy	*S. aureus* and *Staphylococcus epidermidis*
Chronic Osteomyelitis	*S. aureus*, Enterobacteriaceae, and *P. aeruginosa*

Data from Sanford JP: Guide to Antimicrobial Therapy. Hyde Park, VT, Antimicrobial Therapy, Inc., 1999.

often present. If the infection involves the lower extremity, an antalgic gait is common. Brodie's abscess may develop in the metaphysis of a long bone and often is seen as subacute osteomyelitis.

Elderly and immunocompromised patients often are seen initially with chronic osteomyelitis that occurs after the inadequate treatment of acute osteomyelitis or as an extension of a soft tissue wound. In chronic osteomyelitis, an intermittent draining sinus may develop, and typical local and systemic evidence of an infection may be absent.

Laboratory Studies

Laboratory evaluation should include a complete blood count, erythrocyte sedimentation rate, and measurement of C-reactive protein. An elevated white blood cell (WBC) count and an increase in the percentage of bands and polymorphonuclear leukocytes are common. The sedimentation rate and C-reactive protein level are elevated, and serial measurements are used to follow up the response to treatment. A nutritional screen should be obtained to detect predisposing factors for osteomyelitis and to assess the need for nutritional support.

Imaging Studies

Osteomyelitis is first evident on plain radiographs 1 to 2 weeks after the onset of infection. Radiographic evidence of the disease includes local areas of bone resorption and reactive new-bone formation. The borders of the infected bone are indistinct and irregular. Multiple sequestra may be present, each appearing as a dense island of bone surrounded by a radiolucent cavity. Laminations of newly formed bone have an onion-skin appearance. Nuclear imaging studies show increased tracer uptake within 48 to 72 hours of the infection. Magnetic resonance imaging (MRI) is the most sensitive means of detecting osteomyelitis. Early marrow changes are evident as decreased signal intensity on T_1- and T_2-weighted images.

Treatment

Treatment of osteomyelitis is based on the accurate identification of a pathogen. Antibiotics are given either intravenously or orally, depending on the clinical response and condition of the patient. The standard duration of antibiotic treatment for pyogenic osteomyelitis is 4 to 6 weeks.

In children, hematogenous osteomyelitis is often successfully treated with antibiotics alone. Infection involving a joint requires immediate irrigation and decompression to prevent subsequent joint destruction and growth abnormalities.

In adults, surgical treatment is often needed to eradicate the infection. Indications for surgery include the presence of an abscess or necrosis of the bone and soft tissue and the need for drainage. Chronically infected sinus tracts should be excised and examined for malignant tissue. Vascularized flaps are necessary for coverage of soft tissue defects. Cortical or cancellous bone grafts may be needed to restore or maintain mechanical stability to the bone.

Arthritis

Arthritis is a common cause of disability and affects people of all ages and ethnic backgrounds. Based on clinical, radiographic, and laboratory results, arthritis can be subdivided into three broad categories: inflammatory, noninflammatory, and infectious arthritis. The optimal management of patients with arthritis involves a combined approach that includes medical, surgical, and rehabilitation specialists.

Inflammatory Arthritis

Etiology and Classification

Inflammatory arthritis is a disorder that affects the synovial joints and may occur secondary to autoimmune or metabolic disorders. The analysis of **synovial fluid** is the primary means by which inflammatory arthritis is differentiated from noninflammatory arthritis. The number of WBCs found in synovial fluid is more than 2000/μL in inflammatory arthritis and is less than 2000/μL in noninflammatory arthritis (Table 42-2). In patients with autoimmune disorders, arthritides can be further subclassified into seropositive and seronegative inflammatory arthritis, based on the presence or absence of **rheumatoid factor** in the serum.

Seropositive Inflammatory Arthropathies. These arthritic conditions include not only rheumatoid arthritis but also several other rheumatic and nonrheumatic conditions, such as chronic infections, juvenile chronic arthritis, cryoglobulinemia, and Sjögren's syndrome.

Rheumatoid arthritis is a chronic, progressive, inflammatory disease of unknown etiology. It most commonly affects young women and results in a symmetric, destructive arthritis. The proximal joints of the hands and feet are most frequently involved, but any peripheral joint can be affected. Involvement of the atlantoaxial and subaxial joints may lead to instability and myelopathy. Diagnostic criteria for rheumatoid arthritis include morning stiffness of more than 1-hour duration, arthritis of three or more hand joints, symmetrical arthritis, rheumatoid nodules, and a positive test for rheumatoid factor. Periarticular erosions on radiographs of the hands and wrists are used to support the diagnosis.

Juvenile chronic arthritis (JCA) is a chronic, noninfectious inflammatory disease of childhood and is classified into three subgroups: pauciarticular, polyarticular, and systemic at onset. In **pauciarticular JCA,** fewer than five joints are involved at presentation, and patients may have iridocyclitis, which sometimes leads to irreversible blindness. Results of serum testing for antinuclear antibodies are frequently positive. In **polyarticular JCA,** which is the most common subtype of JCA, five or more joints are involved at presentation. Polyarticular JCA is encountered more often in girls than in boys and is most likely to progress to the adult form of rheumatoid arthritis. Results of serum testing for antinuclear antibodies are positive in 40% to 60% of patients with polyarticular JCA. Patients with **systemic JCA** have intermittent daily fevers and may have a rheumatoid rash. About 50% of patients with JCA have no long-term sequelae, and the remainder develop progressive, crippling arthritis.

TABLE 42–2 Classification of Synovial Effusions

Measure*	Findings			
	Normal	**Noninflammatory**	**Inflammatory**	**Septic**
Volume (knee)	<1 mL	Often >1 mL	Often >1 mL	Often >1 mL
Viscosity	High	High	Low	Variable
Color	Colorless to straw	Straw to yellow	Yellow	Variable
Clarity	Transparent	Transparent	Transparent	Opaque
White blood cells	<200/μL	200–2000/μL	2000–75,000/μL	Often >100,000/μL
Polymorphonuclear leukocytes	<25%	>25%	Often >50%	>85%
Culture	Negative	Negative	Negative	Often positive
Mucin clot	Firm	Firm	Friable	Friable
Glucose (morning testing) results	Nearly equal to blood results	Nearly equal to blood results	<50 mg/dL lower than blood results	>50 mg/dL lower than blood results

* Counts of white blood cells and percentages of polymorphonuclear leukocytes are lower if the organism is less virulent or if the disease is partially treated.

Data from Schumacher HR Jr: Synovial fluid analysis and synovial biopsy. In Kelly WN, Harris ED, et al (eds): Textbook of Rheumatology. Philadelphia, WB Saunders, 1993.

Seronegative Inflammatory Arthropathies. These arthritic conditions are associated with spondylitis and include ankylosing spondylitis, psoriatic arthritis, Reiter's syndrome, and enteropathic arthritis. The presence of human leukocyte antigen B27 (HLA-B27) is strongly associated with this group of disorders, which are inherited and characteristically involve the axial skeleton and the sacroiliac joints. Frequent findings in affected patients include enthesopathy, asymmetrical peripheral arthritis, and extra-articular involvement of the skin, eyes, and urogenital and gastrointestinal tracts.

Ankylosing spondylitis, the most common form of seronegative spondyloarthropathy, affects men more often than women. About 90% of patients are positive for HLA-B27. As the disease progresses, a rigid, stooped posture may develop. Pulmonary function is compromised by progressive ankylosis of the thoracic spine and costovertebral articulations.

Crystalline Deposition Diseases. These inflammatory arthritides are caused by a metabolic disorder and are characterized by recurrent attacks of acute arthritis. Gout and chondrocalcinosis are the most common types.

Gout occurs when monosodium urate, a by-product of purine metabolism, is overproduced or underexcreted. This leads to hyperuricemia and the formation of negatively birefringent crystals. The crystals are deposited in and around joints, and tophi then form in periarticular soft tissues. Recurrent attacks of severe arthritis lead to joint erosions and destruction and thereby cause crippling deformities. Although any joint can be involved, gout characteristically involves the metatarsophalangeal joint of the great toe, the knee joint, and the distal small joints of the hand. Gout is associated with obesity, diabetes mellitus, hyperlipidemia, hypertension, and excessive alcohol consumption.

Chondrocalcinosis, which is also called **calcium pyrophosphate deposition disease** or **pseudogout,** is a recurrent acute, subacute, or chronic form of arthritis that is caused by the deposition of calcium pyrophosphate dihydrate (CPPD) crystals in hyaline cartilage and fibrocartilage. The crystals are most commonly deposited in the knees, wrists, shoulders, and elbows, where they elicit an inflammatory response. The deposits are responsible for the characteristic radiographic finding of chondrocalcinosis. Under a polarizing microscope, the deposits appear as irregularly shaped and positively birefringent crystals. Chondrocalcinosis may be a heritable disorder and also occurs in association with several other conditions, including hyperparathyroidism, hemochromatosis, osteoarthritis, and hypomagnesemia.

Evaluation and Treatment

The effective treatment of inflammatory arthritides depends on an accurate diagnosis of the disorder. Clinical manifestations and laboratory findings are discussed earlier and in Table 42-2.

Rheumatoid Arthritis

Medical management of rheumatoid arthritis requires combination treatment with nonsteroidal anti-inflammatory drugs (NSAIDs), corticosteroids, and disease-modifying antirheumatic drugs (DMARDs). The DMARDs include methotrexate, sulfasalazine, hydroxychloroquine, and gold salts. Several new biologic agents have been developed to target specifically components of the inflammatory mechanism. Cyclosporine inhibits T-cell lymphocytes and is used in combination with methotrexate in severe rheumatoid arthritis. Other biologic agents include anti-cytokine and anti–T-cell monoclonal antibodies. Inhibitors of interleukin-1 (IL-1) and tumor necrosis factor α (TNF-α) have been identified and are being investigated for the management of patients with rheumatoid arthritis.

IL-1 blocker (anakinra) significantly reduced clinical symptoms of rheumatoid arthritis when used alone or in combination with weekly methotrexate. TNF inhibitors (etanercept, infliximib, and adalimumab) show similar effects, with higher response rates for clinical and radiographic parameters with the TNF inhibitors. Both show reduced radiographic disease progression at 6 and 12 months. Long-term effects are still unknown.

Surgical management of rheumatoid arthritis is indicated if medical management has proved ineffective after 6 months. The choice of surgical technique depends on the joint involved and the degree to which it is affected. Synovectomy may be beneficial early in the course of the disease, before joint destruction has occurred, because it may provide symptomatic relief and delay disease progression. Either resection arthroplasty or replacement arthroplasty is indicated if the disease is more advanced. In cases of rheumatoid arthritis involving the cervical spine, the disease is nonoperative in the absence of neurologic deficits. Decompression and fusion are indicated in the presence of progressive neurologic deficits or a mechanically unstable cervical spine segment.

Juvenile Chronic Arthritis

Treatment of JCA is best when using a multidisciplinary team approach. Medical management often includes combination therapy to achieve disease control. Initiation of medical treatment is usually with an NSAID. Naproxen is the most commonly used NSAID. In those with fevers and serositis associated with systemic arthritis, indomethacin is most effective. For those that continue to be symptomatic, combination therapy is initiated. Intra-articular corticosteroid injections have been efficacious in controlling the synovitis in JCA. Oral corticosteroids can also be used for rapid control of severe arthritis, but long-term use should be limited. Methotrexate and sulfasalazine have both been shown to be safe and effective in treating oligoarthritic and polyarthritic JCA but should not be used in those with systemic arthritis because of serious side effects. Physical and occupational therapists should initiate a teaching and treatment program which includes active-assisted range of motion (AROM) and passive range of motion (PROM) with gradual strengthening. The orthopedic surgeon has a limited role in the treatment of JCA, with no universal agreement about the procedures that are indicated. Surgical procedures are used to provide symptomatic relief and increase the functionality of the patient. Synovectomy and soft tissue releases were previously thought to have a more beneficial outcome; however, long-term studies have shown that ultimate outcome is not altered. Arthrodesis is most often indicated for severe joint destruction of the ankle or the atlantoaxial instability that is associated with JCA. Epiphysiodesis has a role for leg-length discrepancies with satisfactory results. Total joint replacement has a limited role, but newer technologies and techniques have led to improved long-term results. This has previously been limited to the hip and knee, but the shoulder and elbow studies have data that show encouraging results.

Ankylosing Spondylitis

Conventional medical therapy consists of NSAIDs and intra-articular corticosteroids. Methotrexate and sulfasalazine are used in cases of chronic synovitis. These forms of therapy have been shown to have limited efficacy. Recent advances in the biologic treatment of JCA with infliximab and etenercept (TNF inhibitors) led to their use in the treatment of refractory juvenile ankylosing spondylitis (JAS). There have only been case reports, but short-term results have been promising.

Crystalline Deposition Diseases

Treatment of crystalline arthritis most often involves the use of NSAIDs. Colchicine also may be used to treat acute episodes of gout. Corticosteroids and adrenocorticotropic hormone (ACTH) may be used if colchicine or NSAIDs are ineffective or contraindicated. To prevent attacks of gout, a uricosuric agent such as probenecid may be used in patients who underexcrete urate, whereas allopurinol, a xanthine oxidase inhibitor, can be used in patients who overproduce urate.

Noninflammatory Arthritis

Noninflammatory arthritis occurs in association with a wide variety of idiopathic, metabolic, and systemic disorders. Noninflammatory arthritis is characterized by joint effusions with WBC counts less than 2000/μL, and the arthritic component may or may not dominate the clinical picture.

Etiology and Classification

Disorders associated with noninflammatory arthritis include primary and secondary osteoarthritis, avascular necrosis (Fig. 42-1), osteochondritis dissecans, neurovascular disorders, Paget's disease, hemoglobinopathies, and endocrine disorders, such as acromegaly and hemochromatosis. Some hemoglobinopathies, such as sickle cell disease, may lead to osteonecrosis and secondary osteoarthritis. Patients with hemophilia have recurrent intra-articular bleeding that results in joint destruction. Inborn errors of metabolism, such as Gaucher's disease and ochronosis, also result in destructive arthropathy. Bone dysplasias, including osteogenesis imperfecta, dystrophic dysplasia, multiple epiphyseal dysplasia, and spondyloepiphyseal dysplasia, are uncommon disorders that affect bone growth and may result in symptomatic arthritis. Post-traumatic arthritis and sequelae of childhood hip disorders are common causes of hip pain in the young adult. Slipped capital femoral epiphysis, developmental dislocation of the hip, and Legg-Calvé-Perthe disease (all of which are discussed later in this chapter) are the most common childhood disorders that lead to early degenerative arthritis of the hip in the adult.

Osteoarthritis is the most common noninflammatory arthritic condition and is associated with significant disability, work loss, and hospitalizations. The disease is

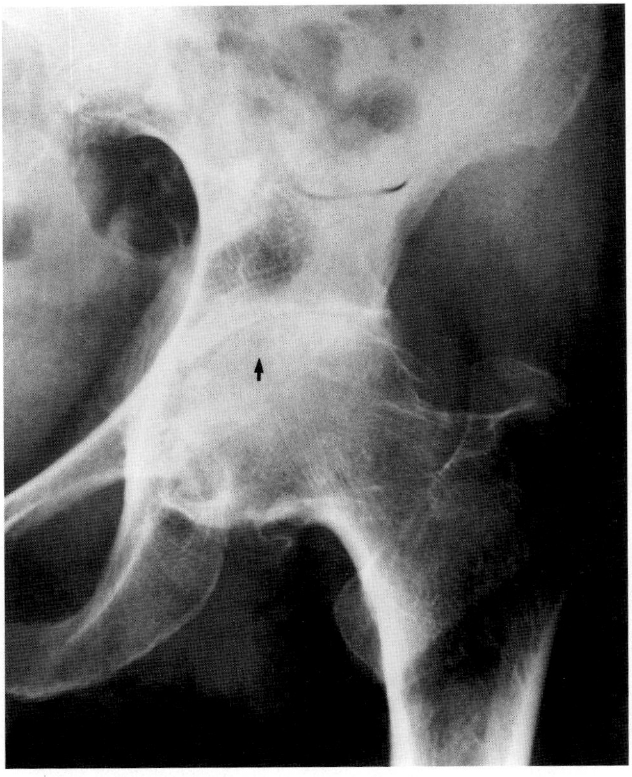

FIGURE 42–1 Avascular necrosis of the femoral head with associated osteoarthritis. Note area of collapse (*arrow*).

classified into two groups: **primary (idiopathic) osteoarthritis** and **secondary osteoarthritis.** Risk factors include advancing age, female sex, repetitive stress, and trauma. Causes of secondary osteoarthritis are listed in Box 42-1. Osteoarthritis is characterized by a progressive loss of articular cartilage and the formation of peripheral osteophytes and subchondral cysts. The pathologic changes in joints affected by osteoarthritis occur primarily in the articular cartilage. Initially, an increase in water content and in proteoglycan production is noted. Progressive damage to the articular cartilage results in areas of fibrillation and fissuring and in the eventual replacement of normal hyaline cartilage with fibrocartilage.

Evaluation

History and Physical Examination

Patients with osteoarthritis typically have activity-related pain that is relieved with rest. Stiffness occurs with prolonged rest, and intermittent flares of the disease are common. Loss of normal joint motion may occur and be followed by muscular atrophy and functional loss. Painful motion is often accompanied by crepitus. Joint enlargement may develop in association with structural changes in the cartilage and periarticular bone.

Laboratory Studies

The sedimentation rate and C-reactive protein level are typically normal. Results of synovial fluid analysis are shown in Table 42-2.

Imaging Studies

Radiographs are useful in cases of moderate to severe osteoarthritis but are unable to detect early cartilage changes associated with the disease. Radiographic findings characteristic of osteoarthritis include joint-space narrowing, subchondral sclerosis, subchondral cysts, and osteophyte formation.

Treatment

Nonoperative management of patients with osteoarthritis should begin with an alteration in activities and with the use of physical therapy and NSAIDs. Obese patients may slow the progression of their disease by weight reduction. Surgical options depend on the joint involved and include resection or replacement arthroplasty and arthrodesis.

BOX 42-1 Classification of Osteoarthritis

I. Primary (idiopathic) osteoarthritis
  A. Localized
    1. Hands (e.g., Heberden's nodes, Bouchard's nodes, and erosive osteoarthritis)
    2. Feet (e.g., hallux valgus and hallux rigidus)
    3. Knee (patellofemoral, medial or lateral compartment)
    4. Hip (e.g., eccentric, concentric, and diffuse)
    5. Spine (e.g., apophyseal disease, intervertebral joints, spondylosis, and diffuse idiopathic skeletal hyperostosis [DISH])
    6. Other single sites
  B. Generalized
II. Secondary osteoarthritis
  A. Trauma (acute or chronic)
  B. Congenital
    1. Localized disease (e.g., Perthes' disease, congenital dislocation of the hip [CDH], and slipped capital femoral epiphysis [SCFE])
    2. Mechanical factors
    3. Bone dysplasia (e.g., dysplasia epiphysealis multiplex and spondyloepiphyseal dysplasia)
  C. Metabolic (e.g., ochronosis, hemochromatosis, calcium pyrophosphate dihydrate [CPPD] disease, and gout)
  D. Endocrine (e.g., acromegaly, obesity, and diabetes)
  E. Other bone and joint disease (e.g., osteonecrosis, infection, Charcot's arthropathy, and rheumatoid arthritis)
  F. Disease of obscure etiology (e.g., Kaschin-Beck disease and Mseleni disease)

Data from Mankin HJ: Clinical features of osteoarthritis. In Sledge CB, Rubby S, et al (eds): Arthritis Surgery. Philadelphia, WB Saunders, 1994.

Infectious Arthritis

Etiology

Infectious arthritis most commonly affects infants and children. It often results from an intracapsular extension of metaphyseal osteomyelitis, and *S. aureus* is the usual pathogen (Table 42-3). The hips, shoulders, elbows, and ankles are involved most frequently.

In sexually active adults with acute monoarticular arthritis, an infection with *Neisseria gonorrhoeae* must be considered. However, intravenous drug abusers have an increased incidence of nongonococcal arthritis. In this group, the sternoclavicular and sacroiliac joints are commonly involved, and *Pseudomonas* and other gram-negative bacteria are the most likely pathogens.

Evaluation

History and Physical Examination

Patients with septic arthritis may present with complaints of pain (which is often severe), swelling, fever, chills, and limited mobility of the affected joint. Examination of the joint reveals pain with active and passive motion. Joint effusion, warmth, and erythema are usually present. A limp is often present when the infection involves a lower extremity joint.

TABLE 42–3 Causes of Infectious Arthritis

Characteristics of Patients	Most Common Causes
Patients <3 mo old	*Staphylococcus aureus*, Enterobacteriaceae, group B streptococci, and *Neisseria gonorrhoeae*
Patients from 3 mo to 14 years old	*S. aureus* (27%), *Streptococcus pyogenes* and *Streptococcus pneumoniae* (14%), *Neisseria* species (14%), gram-negative bacilli (6%), *Haemophilus influenzae* (3%), and unknown (36%)
Patients 15–40 years old with acute monoarticular arthritis	*N. gonorrhoeae, S. aureus,* and streptococci; rarely, aerobic gram-negative bacilli
Patients >40 years old with chronic monoarticular arthritis	*Brucella*, *Nocardia*, and *Mycobacterium* species and fungi
With polyarticular arthritis, usually acute	*N. gonorrhoeae*, *Borrelia burgdorferi*, acute rheumatic fever, viruses (e.g., hepatitis B virus and parvovirus B19), and rubella vaccine
With rheumatoid arthritis	*S. aureus*, streptococci, and gram-negative bacilli
Without rheumatoid arthritis	*N. gonorrhoeae* and *S. aureus*
With septic bursitis	*S. aureus*; rarely, *Mycobacterium tuberculosis* and *Mycobacterium marinum*
Patients after joint replacement or intra-articular administration of antibiotics in the infected joint	Methicillin-resistant or methicillin-sensitive *Staphylococcus epidermidis* (40%), methicillin-resistant or methicillin-sensitive *S. aureus* (20%), Enterobacteriaceae, and *Pseudomonas* species

Data from Sanford JP: Guide to Antimicrobial Therapy. Hyde Park, VT, Antimicrobial Therapy, Inc., 1999.

Laboratory Studies

Joint aspiration should be carried out in any joint in which infection is suspected. The synovial fluid should be cultured and a quantitative WBC count obtained. A complete blood count with differential and an erythrocyte sedimentation rate also should be obtained. A leukocyte count exceeding 50,000/μL with more than 80% polymorphonuclear leukocytes strongly supports the diagnosis of bacterial arthritis. A WBC count exceeding 100,000/μL in synovial fluid is considered diagnostic of septic arthritis. In patients with septic arthritis, synovial fluid viscosity is often diminished, and a poor mucin clot is found (see Table 42-2). Cultures are positive in nearly 100% of patients with nongonococcal bacterial arthritis but in only about 25% to 50% of those with gonococcal infections.

Imaging Studies

Plain radiographs of the joint should be evaluated for evidence of concurrent osteomyelitis. MRI, computed tomography (CT), and radionuclide scanning may be used to confirm the presence of a bone abscess and to evaluate soft tissue extension and the possibility of multifocal joint involvement.

Treatment

Empiric antibiotic treatment of patients with infectious arthritis should begin as soon as specimens for culture have been obtained. Intravenous antibiotics should be administered for at least the initial 2 weeks or until the patient demonstrates a clinical response. The antibiotic may be changed when culture results become available and should be continued for at least 4 weeks.

Prompt drainage of the infected joint is indicated. However, the optimal method of drainage is debated. Surgical drainage is always indicated in septic joint infections associated with osteomyelitis or abscess collection, in pediatric joint infections of the hip, and in cases in which needle aspiration is not feasible. Any joint that cannot be drained completely by needle aspiration should be drained surgically. Whether an arthroscopic or open drainage technique is used will depend on the joint involved. Needle aspiration may be used as the initial treatment in cases involving the knee, wrist, ankle, and other small joints of the hands and feet. If a rapid improvement in the clinical course is not seen with needle aspiration, then surgery is required.

Appropriate splinting of the joint should begin immediately to prevent contractures. Range-of-motion exercises and strengthening should be initiated to preserve motion and prevent periarticular muscular atrophy.

Complications

The amount of morbidity related to septic arthritis depends on several factors, including the infectious agent that is responsible, the length of time between the onset of infection and the initiation of treatment, and the presence or absence of coexisting diseases. Patients with rheumatoid arthritis have a greater risk of developing septic arthritis and an overall worse outcome than do those without an underlying inflammatory condition.

Arthritic and Other Disorders of the Hip

Symptomatic arthritis of the hip joint is a common reason for orthopedic referral. Patients with intra-articular and extra-articular involvement and referred pain all present with pain in and around the hip joint.

Intra-articular causes of hip pain include arthritis, osteonecrosis, injuries of the labrum, and loose bodies.

Extra-articular causes of hip pain include trochanteric bursitis, musculotendinous strains, and coxa saltans (snapping hip). Coxa saltans occurs when the iliotibial band, the gluteus maximus tendon, or the iliopsoas tendon snaps over the prominent greater or lesser trochanter or the femoral head.

Referred hip pain may be radicular in origin and secondary to lumbar disk herniation. It may also occur in association with low back pain, pelvic pain, genitourinary disorders, and gastrointestinal disorders.

Evaluation

History and Physical Examination

Patients with hip disorders require a thorough evaluation of the spine, pelvis, and lower extremities. Hip joint pain is most commonly felt in the groin, posterior thigh, or buttock, but it also may be felt in the knee. Walking, tying a shoe, and getting in and out of a car typically exacerbate pain that originates in the hip joint. Loose bodies and injuries of the labrum may cause acute, intermittent hip pain. Trochanteric bursitis produces pain along the lateral thigh and is easily reproduced by palpation. Lumbar disk disease may produce radicular symptoms in the hip with involvement of the upper lumbar roots.

Examination of the hip should include an assessment of the stance and swing phases of the patient's gait. An antalgic gait characteristically shortens the stance phase on the affected side. The gluteus medius gait is characterized by an abnormal pelvic tilt during the swing phase, with the unaffected side dropping because of the weakness of the contralateral gluteus medius. The Trendelenburg test is a test of hip-abductor strength of the contralateral hip. In single-leg stance, the unaffected hip tilts downward owing to weakness of the abductor muscle. An assessment of hip range of motion includes internal and external rotation, flexion, extension, adduction, and abduction. Decreased internal rotation and painful abduction are the earliest signs of hip arthritis. The Thomas test should be performed to check for hip-flexion contractures. Examination of the back and knee and evaluation of leg lengths are important aspects of a thorough hip examination.

Imaging Studies

Anteroposterior and lateral radiographs of the hip and an anterior view of the pelvis are necessary for the proper evaluation of hip disorders. In addition, patients whose symptoms suggest involvement of the back should have radiographs of the lumbosacral spine. MRI is indicated in the evaluation of avascular necrosis of the hip and is the most sensitive test of early disease. In some cases, MRI can detect labrum injuries, loose bodies, and synovial diseases. However, labrum defects are not always evident on MRI.

Treatment

Nonsurgical Treatment

Nonsurgical treatment of hip disorders may include the use of a cane or crutch, because these external supporting devices reduce the joint-loading forces. To maximize its mechanical benefit, a cane should be held in the hand opposite the involved joint. Lofstrand crutches have a platform on which to rest the forearm and are indicated when arthritis involves the upper extremity.

Physical therapy may be beneficial in improving flexibility and restoring strength and range of motion. Exercise should be individualized, and modified programs with low stress loads across the joints should be emphasized. Protection from hip overuse should be stressed, and weight reduction is important.

Medical therapies include the use of analgesic medications, such as acetaminophen and NSAIDs. The cyclo-oxygenase-2 (COX-2) inhibitors and nonacetylated salicylates may reduce the incidence of gastrointestinal side effects associated with the use of NSAIDs.

Surgical Treatment

Indications for Surgery. Surgical options for the management of hip disorders include arthroscopy, arthrodesis, osteotomy, and arthroplasty.

Arthroscopy is limited to the management of labrum tears, loose bodies, and chondral defects.

Arthrodesis is indicated in young patients with advanced unilateral hip arthritis. Ipsilateral knee involvement, spine disorders, and bilateral hip disease are relative contraindications to hip fusion.

Pelvic and femoral osteotomies are indicated for the treatment of several hip disorders. Developmental dysplasia of the hip in young patients is most successfully treated with a pelvic osteotomy. A young, active patient who has hip pain secondary to acetabular dysplasia but does not have degenerative hip arthritis is the ideal candidate for a pelvic osteotomy. The goal of the osteotomy is to reorient the acetabulum to a more mechanically favorable position to improve coverage of the femoral head. Femoral side osteotomies can be used to treat coxa valga, femoral neck nonunion, and osteonecrosis of the femoral head and to treat some cases of hip dysplasia. In patients with osteoarthritis, the use of femoral intertrochanteric osteotomies has largely been replaced by the use of resurfacing procedures, such as total hip arthroplasty.

Total hip arthroplasty (THA) is indicated if hip arthritis causes debilitating pain that is refractory to nonsurgical treatment. The procedure is ideally suited for patients older than 65 years, and it is recommended for younger patients who have ipsilateral knee and back disease but are not candidates for a hip arthrodesis. THA also is indicated for patients who require reconstructive surgery after tumor resection, osteonecrosis, developmental dysplasia of the hip, or JCA. In THA, the femoral component stem may be uncemented or cemented, with the uncemented stems indicated primarily for younger patients and for patients undergoing revision arthroplasty. The acetabular component is most commonly composed of an inner liner and outer shell. The liner is made of ultra–high-molecular-weight polyethylene, and the shell is a porous coated alloy that is press-fitted into the acetabulum.

Surgical Anatomy. An orientation to the surgical approaches to the hip joint begins with knowledge of the superficial landmarks of the pelvis and femur. The anterior superior iliac crest is easily palpated and is the site of attachment of the sartorius muscle and the inguinal ligament. The greater trochanter of the femur is palpable along the lateral thigh and is the insertion of the gluteus medius and minimus located proximally. The vastus lateralis originates along the inferior greater trochanter at the trochanteric ridge.

Surgical Approaches. Several surgical approaches to the hip joint are commonly used.

The **anterior** or **iliofemoral approach (Smith-Petersen approach)** gives access to the anterior hip joint and limited access to the anterior column of the pelvis and medial pelvic structures. This internerve approach uses the muscular interval between the following: (1) the sartorius and rectus femoris innervated by the femoral nerve and (2) the tensor fascia and gluteus medius innervated by the superior gluteal nerve. Care must be taken not to damage the lateral femoral cutaneous nerve of the thigh, the femoral nerve, and the ascending branch of the lateral femoral circumflex artery.

The **anterolateral approach (Watson-Jones approach)** is used in fracture reduction, anterior hip arthrotomy, and biopsies of the hip joint. This approach uses the plane between the tensor fascia and the gluteus medius. The femoral nerve, artery, and vein can be damaged if the retractor is inadvertently placed over the anterior column.

The **direct lateral approach** is used primarily during arthroplasty and provides an extensive exposure of the hip and proximal femur. The gluteus medius and vastus lateralis are split during this approach. The approach preserves the posterior external rotators and reduces the risk of posterior dislocation of the hip. However, abductor muscle strength may be compromised and result in an abductor limp. A modification of the approach is the trochanteric slide, which involves an osteotomy and mobilization of the greater trochanter.

The **posterolateral approach** is commonly used in hip arthroplasty procedures. It also may be used for drainage procedures, for management of fractures of the posterior acetabulum, and for pelvic reconstruction. The tensor fascia and gluteus maximus are split. The short external rotators from the piriformis proximally to the quadratus femoris distally are released, exposing the posterior hip capsule. The medial circumflex femoral artery is found beneath the quadratus femoris. The sciatic nerve coursing behind the piriformis is at risk during this approach.

Complications

Complications associated with hip arthroscopy include neurapraxias of the femoral and pudendal nerves. Long-term follow-up studies of patients undergoing hip arthrodesis have demonstrated a high rate of satisfaction and significant pain relief with good function after successful arthrodesis of the hip; however, studies also have shown an increase in the incidence of symptomatic back pain and ipsilateral knee pain after hip arthrodesis. THA is one of the most commonly performed orthopedic procedures and one of the most successful. Studies of patients after THA have documented significant alleviation of pain and improvement in mobility and quality of life. However, several potential complications after THA may occur and include persistent pain, prosthetic loosening, osteolysis, dislocation, infection, and periprosthetic fractures.

Arthritic and Other Disorders of the Knee

Disorders in and around the knee joint are common and may be secondary to both intra-articular and extra-articular involvement. Osseous disorders of the knee may be isolated to the femur, patella, or tibia.

Intra-articular causes of knee pain include arthritis, osteochondritis dissecans, and patellofemoral disorders. **Arthritis** is discussed in detail earlier in this chapter.

Osteochondritis dissecans is a disorder of unknown etiology and is characterized by an area of avascular subchondral bone. It most often affects the medial femoral condyle, and the overlying articular cartilage becomes secondarily affected. Intra-articular loose bodies are often the result of osteochondritis dissecans that fails to heal despite treatment.

Patellofemoral disorders (Box 42-2) are a common cause of knee pain and may be associated with acute trauma, a repetitive injury, patellofemoral malalignment, an abnormal patellar tilt or subluxation, synovitis, recurrent hemarthrosis, prolonged immobilization, patellar instability, bipartite patella, synovial plicae, and chondral defects.

BOX 42–2 Classification of Patellofemoral Disorders

I. Conditions caused by trauma in the otherwise normal knee
- A. Acute trauma
  - 1. Contusion
  - 2. Fracture
    - a. Patella
    - b. Femoral trochlea
    - c. Proximal tibial epiphysis (tubercle)
  - 3. Dislocation (rare in the normal knee)
  - 4. Rupture
    - a. Quadriceps tendon
    - b. Patellar tendon
- B. Repetitive trauma (overuse syndromes)
  - 1. Patellar tendinitis (jumper's knee)
  - 2. Quadriceps tendinitis
  - 3. Peripatellar tendinitis (e.g., anterior knee pain due to hamstring contracture in adolescents)
  - 4. Prepatellar bursitis (housemaid's knee)
  - 5. Apophysitis
  - 6. Osgood-Schlatter disease
  - 7. Sinding-Larsen-Johansson disease
- C. Late effects of trauma
  - 1. Post-traumatic chondromalacia patellae
  - 2. Post-traumatic patellofemoral arthritis
  - 3. Anterior fat pad syndrome (post-traumatic fibrosis)
  - 4. Reflex sympathetic dystrophy of the patella
  - 5. Patellar osseous dystrophy
  - 6. Acquired patella infra (patella baja)
  - 7. Acquired quadriceps fibrosis

II. Patellofemoral dysplasia
- A. Lateral patellar compression syndrome (LPCS)
  - 1. Secondary chondromalacia patellae
  - 2. Secondary patellofemoral arthritis
- B. Chronic subluxation of the patella (CSP)
  - 1. Secondary chondromalacia patellae
  - 2. Secondary patellofemoral arthritis
- C. Recurrent dislocation of the patella (RDP)
  - 1. Associated fractures
    - a. Osteochondral (intra-articular)
    - b. Avulsion (extra-articular)
  - 2. Secondary chondromalacia patellae
  - 3. Secondary patellofemoral arthritis
- D. Chronic dislocation of the patella
  - 1. Congenital
  - 2. Acquired

III. Idiopathic chondromalacia patellae

IV. Osteochondritis dissecans
- A. Patella
- B. Femoral trochlea

V. Synovial plicae*
- A. Medial patella (shelf)
- B. Suprapatella
- C. Lateral patella

*Anatomic variant made symptomatic by acute or repetitive trauma.
Data from Merchant AC: Classification of patellofemoral disorders. Arthroscopy 4:235, 1998.

Tendinitis of the proximal patellar tendon, or Sinding-Larsen-Johansson disease, is one example of a disorder caused by overuse. Traction apophysitis of the tibial tubercle, or Osgood-Schlatter disease, is another example of an overuse disorder and is typically seen in children and jumping athletes.

Extra-articular causes of knee pain include angular deformities of the tibia and femur, which result in abnormal loading of the medial or lateral tibiofemoral compartment and premature joint deterioration; inflammation of bursae, which is often caused by localized trauma, arthritis, gout, tendinitis, or sepsis; hip and back disorders; and degenerative arthritis of the lumbosacral spine, which may cause radicular symptoms referred to the knee.

Injuries to the knee are discussed in detail in Chapters 44 and 45.

Evaluation

In assessing a patient with disorders of the knee, it is necessary to have a systematic approach that includes a focused and thorough history and physical examination. Further workup may include laboratory and imaging studies necessary to support the diagnosis and to assist in the formation of a treatment plan.

Standard screening radiographs obtained to evaluate complaints about the knee include anteroposterior and lateral images. Preoperative planning for total knee arthroplasty requires full-length standing radiographs that allow determination of the mechanical and anatomic axes of the limb and assist in preoperative templating. Any prior injury or limb deformity requires a radiograph.

Treatment

Nonsurgical Treatment

Initial treatment of most nontraumatic disorders of the knee is nonsurgical and may include the following: activity modification; weight reduction in overweight patients; a supervised therapy program incorporating stretching, strengthening, and low-impact exercises; use of an external support, such as a cane or walker, to reduce activity-associated pain; use of braces or shoe inserts to lessen the load on the involved knee; use of anti-inflammatory and analgesic agents, such as NSAIDs, acetaminophen, corticosteroids, and synthetic hyaluronic agents; and use of nutritional supplements, such as chondroitin sulfate and glucosamine.

NSAIDs are generally well tolerated and provide symptomatic relief, but they should be used with caution in patients who have a history of an NSAID allergy, peptic ulcer disease, impaired renal or hepatic function, congestive heart failure, or hypertension. NSAID use should be carefully monitored in patients concurrently taking an anticoagulant, oral hypoglycemic agent, or other drug that may alter NSAID metabolism. The traditional NSAIDs act by inhibiting both COX-1 and COX-2, whereas the newer NSAIDs selectively inhibit COX-2. Selective COX-2 inhibitors and acetaminophen are pain-relieving agents that avoid the gastrointestinal side effects commonly seen with traditional NSAIDs.

Corticosteroids can be used for the management of patients with arthritic conditions of the knee. These drugs are administered by intra-articular injection, and they act by reducing the inflammatory response of the synovium.

Synthetic hyaluronic acid preparations are synovial fluid supplements that are primarily indicated for use in younger patients who have arthritic conditions of the knee and wish to delay undergoing total knee arthroplasty. The preparations may augment the viscoelastic effects of synovial fluid and are thought to have anti-inflammatory properties, but their precise mechanism of action is unclear. They must be administered two or three times a week by intra-articular injection, and their high cost makes them prohibitive for general use. Studies evaluating their efficacy in the management of osteoarthritis of the knee have shown beneficial effects lasting an average of 6 months.

Chondroitin sulfate and glucosamine are nutritional supplements available as over-the-counter medications. In patients with osteoarthritis, these agents may stimulate production of proteoglycans by chondrocytes and thereby contribute to articular cartilage regeneration. In addition, they may have anti-inflammatory properties.

Surgical Treatment

Indications for Surgery

Surgical options for the management of arthritic and other disorders of the knee include arthroscopy, chondrocyte transplantation, osteochondral grafting, osteotomy, unicompartmental knee arthroplasty, and total knee arthroplasty.

Knee arthroscopy is minimally invasive surgery performed on an outpatient basis. Arthroscopic débridement of the arthritic knee involves joint lavage and resection of torn meniscal fragments and is beneficial in many patients. However, in those who have advanced degenerative changes of the articular cartilage, arthroscopic lavage and débridement tend to be less beneficial. Abrasion chondroplasty may be helpful in patients with unstable chondral lesions.

Osteochondritis dissecans may be treated arthroscopically when the lesion remains attached to the underlying cancellous bone. Internal fixation of the lesion to its cancellous bed allows healing.

In unrepairable lesions of osteochondritis dissecans and in some osteochondral defects after fractures, arthroscopic drilling of subchondral bone may allow filling of the defect with fibrocartilage. **Autologous chondrocyte transplantation** can be used in the repair of isolated chondral defects of the tibiofemoral articular cartilage if they measure from 2 to 7 cm^2. Before transplantation takes place, articular cartilage must be harvested from a non–weight-bearing surface of the knee. The harvested chondrocytes are then cultured and reimplanted into the chondral defect. Early results are promising and suggest that improvement in function occurs in the majority of patients, but long-term clinical results and prospective randomized trials are needed. **Autologous osteochondral grafting** also has been used for the treatment of focal osteochondral defects in the weight-bearing portion of the knee, but few clinical reports on the results are available. In the procedure, small plugs from non–weight-bearing portions of the joint are harvested and implanted into the defect. After surgery, early motion is recommended, and weight bearing is delayed to allow adequate healing.

Osteotomy of the proximal tibia or distal femur is indicated in some cases of unicompartmental degenerative arthritis of the knee. Osteotomy transfers the weight-bearing forces to the uninvolved compartment and may delay the need for total knee arthroplasty. Patients with medial compartment osteoarthritis caused by a varus deformity may be candidates for a proximal tibial valgus osteotomy. This procedure is ideally suited for active patients who are younger than 60 years, have a varus deformity that is less than 15 degrees, and do not have lateral compartment arthritic changes. The procedure is contraindicated in patients who have inflammatory arthritis, lateral compartment disease, tibial subluxation, or a fixed flexion contracture greater than 15 degrees. Patients with lateral compartment osteoarthritis caused by a valgus deformity may be candidates for a varus osteotomy. If the valgus deformity is greater than 12 degrees and shows superolateral deviation of the joint line, distal femoral varus osteotomy is preferred. If the valgus deformity is less than 12 degrees, it may be managed with a proximal tibial varus osteotomy. Five-year follow-up studies of distal femoral and proximal tibial osteotomies show a high success rate. Success depends on the ability to obtain an adequate correction of the deformity at the time of surgery and on the ability to regain adequate postoperative range of motion.

Unicompartmental knee arthroplasty is another option for the management of patients with unicompartmental osteoarthritis. Advocates of this procedure cite the reduced cost of the prosthesis and successful long-term results. Sedentary patients who are older than 60 years, have greater than 90 degrees of flexion, and have a flexion contracture less than 15 degrees are the ideal candidates for the treatment. A functional anterior cruciate ligament (ACL) is necessary for long-term success of a unicompartmental arthroplasty. Difficult surgical technique and poor component design limit the use of unicompartmental arthroplasty. In addition, a total knee arthroplasty is more difficult after failure of unicompartmental implants.

PEARLS FOR ROUNDS

The most common bacteria associated with hematogenous osteomyelitis in children are the gram-positive cocci *Staphylococcus aureus* and streptococci, whereas in adults they are gram-negative bacteria, such as *Escherichia coli, Pseudomonas*, and *Salmonella*.

Magnetic resonance imaging is the most sensitive means of detecting osteomyelitis.

Inflammatory arthritis is a disorder that affects the synovial joints and may occur secondary to autoimmune or metabolic disorders. Analysis of synovial fluid is the primary means by which inflammatory arthritis is differentiated from noninflammatory arthritis.

Osteoarthritis is classified into two groups, primary (idiopathic) osteoarthritis and secondary osteoarthritis, and is the most common noninflammatory arthritic condition associated with significant disability, work loss, and hospitalizations.

Anteroposterior and lateral radiographs of the hip and an anterior view of the pelvis are necessary for the proper evaluation of hip disorders.

In patients with diabetes mellitus, damage to the peripheral nerves is the primary effect on the foot.

Total knee arthroplasty (TKA) is indicated in patients who have radiographic evidence of advanced intra-articular disease and have disabling knee pain and other symptoms that cannot be managed successfully with nonoperative treatment. Contraindications to TKA include joint infection, extensor mechanism failure, Charcot's joint and other advanced neuromuscular disorders, and prior knee arthrodesis or ankylosis. The overall clinical success rate of current total condylar knee designs is extremely high, with excellent pain relief and improvement in function. Survival of the original prosthetic components is greater than 90% at 10- to 15-year follow-up in most published series. Patients who are immunocompromised or have rheumatoid arthritis, systemic lupus erythematosus, diabetes mellitus, or previous prosthetic joint infections have a higher failure rate owing to prosthetic infection.

Surgical Anatomy

The knee is a complex joint composed of the tibiofemoral and patellofemoral articulations. Medial and lateral menisci are interposed between the tibia and femur and play an important functional role in load transmission, joint stability, and cartilage nutrition. The medial meniscus is more constrained than the lateral meniscus by its soft tissue attachments, and this predisposes it to more frequent injury. The peripheral one third of each meniscus is vascularized and is called the red zone, whereas the inner two thirds is avascular and is referred to as the white zone.

Several ligaments provide static stability to the tibiofemoral articulation. The medial collateral ligament (MCL) is composed of superficial and deep components. It attaches on the medial femoral condyle and inserts on the medial tibia. The primary function of the MCL is to prevent valgus instability. The lateral collateral ligament (LCL) originates on the lateral femoral condyle and inserts on the fibular head. It prevents varus instability and provides rotational stability. The ACL originates on the lateral intercondylar notch and inserts just anterior to the tibial spine (Fig. 42-2). The primary function of the ACL is to prevent anterior translation of the tibia on the femur. The posterior cruciate ligament (PCL) originates from the medial intercondylar notch and inserts in a broad band along the posterior tibia. Its primary function is to prevent posterior translation of the tibia on the femur. Both the ACL and the PCL contribute to rotational stability. In addition to the knee ligaments, several muscles and tendons traverse the joint and provide dynamic stability.

Surgical Approaches

The surgical approach to arthroscopic knee surgery requires the establishment of arthroscopic and working portals. The **standard arthroscopic portal** is the anterolateral portal, which is adjacent to the patellar tendon and just above the joint line. The **standard working portal** is the anteromedial portal, which is medial to the patellar tendon and just above the joint line. Several **auxiliary portals** may be used

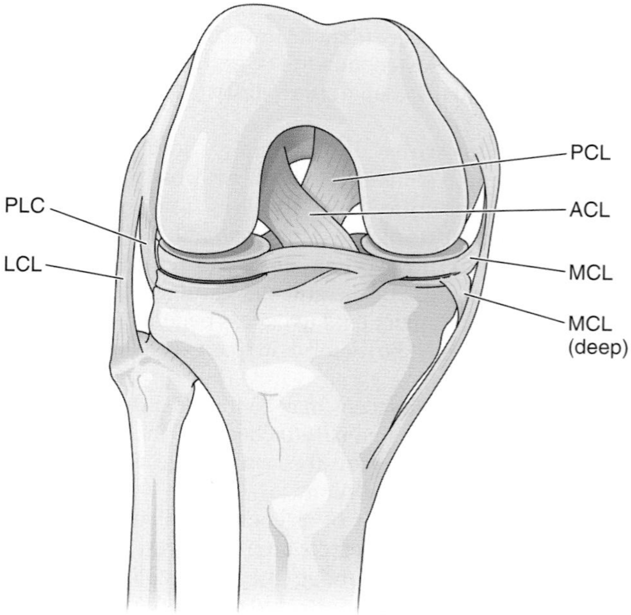

FIGURE 42–2 Anatomy of the knee.

and include superolateral, posteromedial, posterolateral, and medial and lateral parapatellar portals. A separate **inflow portal** may be established through the suprapatellar pouch.

The usual approach for a routine primary TKA is via an **anterior medial parapatellar incision.** Alternative approaches include a subvastus approach and a midvastus approach, which allow preservation of the quadriceps tendon.

Complications

Although arthroscopy is one of the most commonly performed orthopedic procedures, complications do occur. Complications include infection, deep venous thrombosis, pulmonary embolism, reflex sympathetic dystrophy, and neurovascular injury. Creation of the posteromedial portal may result in an injury to branches of the saphenous nerve. Creation of the posterolateral portal may result in an injury of the peroneal nerve.

Complications associated with osteotomies around the knee include overcorrection, undercorrection, nonunion, infection, avascular necrosis, intra-articular fracture, deep venous thrombosis, vascular injuries, and loss of correction. Additional complications associated with high tibial valgus osteotomies include peroneal nerve injuries and patella baja.

Complications associated with TKA include infection, venous thrombosis, thromboembolism, fat embolism, neurovascular injuries, and periprosthetic fractures.

The infection rate in patients who have undergone TKA is low, ranging from 0% to 14% in most series. Infection after TKA may occur at any time and may be low-grade, without classic symptoms and signs of septic arthritis. If infection is suspected, laboratory evaluation should include a WBC count, erythrocyte sedimentation rate, and measurement of C-reactive protein. Culture and Gram staining of material aspirated from the joint are indicated, although the rate of false-negative results may be as high as 25%. Leukocyte-labeled nuclear scans are more sensitive and specific than are technetium- and gallium-labeled scans in determining whether the joint is infected. In intraoperative frozen sections examined microscopically, the finding of more than five WBCs per high-power field is strongly suggestive of an infected joint.

Management of an infected TKA requires surgical drainage and débridement. In some cases, the TKA components are left intact, and intravenous antibiotic treatment (usually with tobramycin or vancomycin) is given for 6 weeks. This procedure may be successful if the infection occurs early in the postoperative period or if symptoms have been present for only a few days. In other cases, the TKA components are removed and then reinserted after a cement spacer containing antibiotics is placed between them. With this two-stage exchange procedure, successful reimplantation occurs in 90% to 95% of patients.

The risk of thromboembolism and deep venous thrombosis can be reduced with the use of prophylactic drugs (usually, warfarin or low-molecular-weight heparin), compressive stockings, foot and calf compression devices, and continuous passive motion.

Nondisplaced fractures associated with a stable, well-fixed prosthesis can often be managed nonoperatively. If the fracture pattern is unstable, surgical options may include plate-and-screw or cable fixation, intramedullary nailing, and revision arthroplasty with a stemmed prosthesis. If the prosthesis is loose or poorly functional, revision arthroplasty is the treatment of choice.

Disorders of the Foot and Toes

Heel Pain

Heel pain is possibly the most common and least understood complaint concerning the foot and ankle.

The skin under the heel is a complex structure composed of fat compartmentalized by fibrous septa. Compression of the heel pressurizes the fat, creating hydrostatic forces that resist further deformation of the heel pad and protect the calcaneus and the underlying soft tissues of the heel. The plantar fascia (plantar aponeurosis) is a ligament that originates on the inferior portion of the calcaneal tuberosity and inserts into the bases of the proximal phalanges of the toes (Fig. 42-3). When the toes are brought into dorsiflexion, the tension on the plantar fascia inverts the heel and raises the longitudinal arch of the foot. This helps stabilize the joints in the middle of the foot, allowing the gastrocnemius and soleus muscles to plantar-flex the rigid foot by exerting force on the heel.

Evaluation

Heel pain is typically of insidious, nontraumatic onset. Patients often describe the pain as worse in the morning when they take the first few steps out of bed. The pain is localized to the plantar heel and is usually exacerbated by activity. Plantar fasciitis may be present if pain and tenderness are worse when the toes are in dorsiflexion. Heel pain also may be caused by tarsal tunnel syndrome, a stress fracture of the calcaneus, or systemic rheumatoid disease. Radiographs should be obtained to eliminate stress fractures and unusual causes of heel pain, such as neoplasms.

Treatment

Nonsurgical Treatment. The use of NSAIDs may help relieve symptoms. The injection of steroids into the plantar fascia has been tried; however, this procedure is not recommended because several reports have associated it with atrophy of the fatty cushion and acute rupture of the plantar fascia. The use of soft heel cups will cushion the heel, help distribute the weight across the heel, and

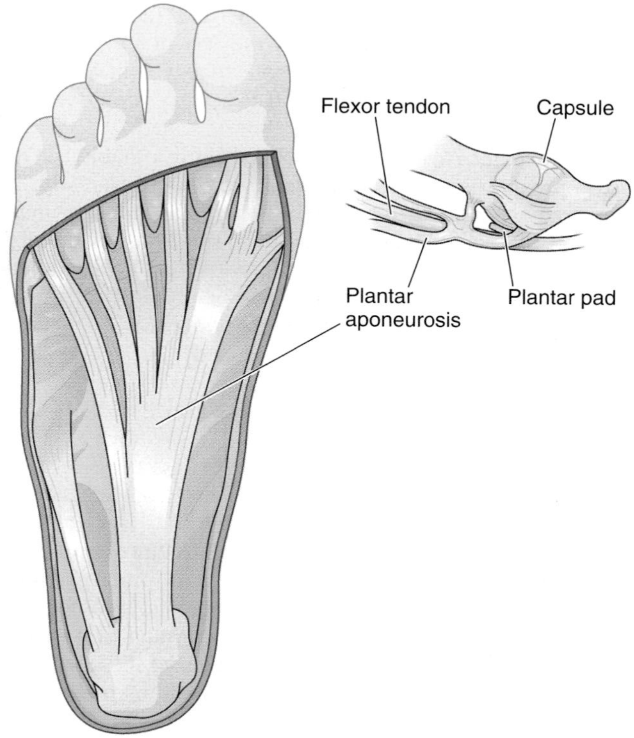

FIGURE 42–3 Plantar fascia.

decrease the tenderness. Bracing the foot into a neutral position at night effectively reduces the morning pain of plantar fasciitis and often reduces or eliminates overall symptoms. Prosthetic modification of the shoes to stiffen them to the toe helps by reducing repetitive traction on the plantar fascia during gait. Although nonoperative treatment may be protracted, it is generally quite effective.

Surgical Treatment. In patients with plantar fasciitis, surgery is occasionally indicated, but the results of plantar fascia release are unpredictable.

Complications

Plantar fascia release may cause worsening of the heel pain and sometimes causes neuromas of the medial calcaneal branch of the posterior tibial nerve.

Hallux Valgus

Hallux valgus is usually caused by wearing shoes that are too small or are improperly designed.

Evaluation

Hallux valgus characteristically causes pain along the medial aspect of the prominent first metatarsal head (Fig. 42-4). If pain is not present, another diagnosis such as sesamoiditis or hallux rigidus should be considered. Adequate vascularity is critical to the success of surgical reconstruction, so pulses and capillary refill should be assessed. Sensory testing often reveals numbness that extends to the dorsomedial hallux and is sometimes caused by irritation of the nerve crossing the medial eminence. Radiographs should be obtained to reveal whether degenerative changes are present, to help determine the amount of subluxation at the metatarsophalangeal joint,

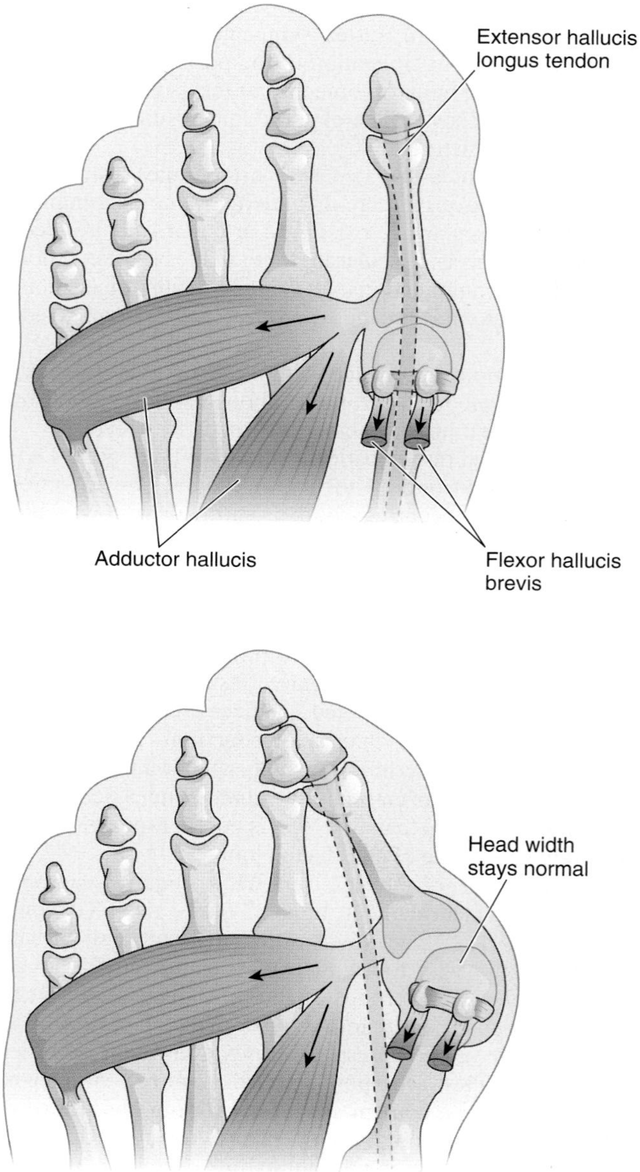

FIGURE 42–4 Pathophysiology of hallux valgus.

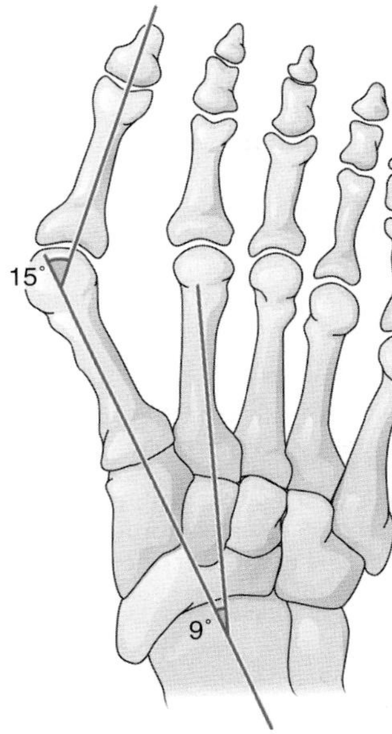

FIGURE 42–5 Hallux valgus radiographic measurements that should be obtained to reveal whether degenerative changes are present, to help determine the amount of subluxation at the metatarsophalangeal joint, and to determine the intermetatarsal and hallux valgus angles.

and to determine the intermetatarsal and hallux valgus angles (Fig. 42-5).

Treatment

Nonsurgical Treatment. Patients should be encouraged to wear comfortable shoes, preferably with laces. They should avoid wearing shoes with elevated heels or narrow toes and shoes made of unyielding synthetic fabrics. Stitching across the medial aspect of the shoe, as is commonly seen in sports shoes, can aggravate bunion pain.

Surgical Treatment. Surgery undertaken for cosmetic reasons is not appropriate. However, if pain persists despite the use of proper shoes, surgical reconstruction should be considered. In patients with a mild to moderate deformity, a distal metatarsal osteotomy with a plication of the medial soft tissues is a common and effective approach. In those with a severe or recurrent deformity, an arthrodesis of the metatarsophalangeal joint is effective and reliable.

Complications

Common complications of hallux valgus repairs include stiffness, neuromas (especially of the dorsomedial cutaneous branch of the hallux), nonunion, malposition of the first metatarsal, and recurrence of the deformity. Avascular necrosis has been reported after distal osteotomy, especially with significant soft tissue release.

Foot Problems Associated with Diabetes Mellitus

In patients with diabetes mellitus, damage to the peripheral nerves is the primary effect on the foot. The exact causes of nerve damage are unclear, but mechanisms are thought to include the nonenzymatic glycosylation of proteins, which impedes protein actions that are critical to nerve function; the intraneural accumulation of sorbitol, which may interfere with neural metabolism; and damage to the vascular nerves, which leads to localized ischemia and impairs nerve function. The extent of nerve damage is related to the duration of the diabetes, the degree of disease control, and the length of the nerve. The nerves to the feet are long and are therefore affected first. Damage occurs to sensory, autonomic, and motor fibers. The lack of sensory feedback allows prolonged and repetitive trauma to the foot to go unnoticed. Damage to the skin and joints causes neuropathic ulcers and arthropathy, which predispose the patient to infection and foot deformity.

Evaluation

Examination should begin by assessing the pulses of the foot and checking for other indications of vascular compromise, such as alopecia and decreased warmth. Proprioception and light touch are simple but crude indications of sensation. Sharp/dull discrimination should be assessed, with care to avoid excessively injuring the skin. Testing with Semmes-Weinstein monofilaments is a reliable and quantifiable means for evaluating the sensory threshold.

In patients with diabetic foot ulcers, a thorough assessment of vascularity is critical. Diabetics have an increased incidence of atherosclerotic disease, and if vascularity is insufficient, healing is unlikely to occur.

Radiographs should be obtained if osteomyelitis (Fig. 42-6) or neuropathic arthropathy (Charcot's arthropathy) is suspected. Diffuse calcification of the arteries and distal osteolysis are characteristic of diabetes. Further vascular evaluation, including arterial Doppler studies, may be necessary. MRI and bone scanning are useful for evaluating osteomyelitis or deep infection.

Treatment

Every patient with diabetes should be instructed about meticulous foot care before evidence of neuropathy is apparent, and instructions should be reinforced frequently. Patients should be advised to inspect their feet regularly and to seek immediate attention if changes are noted or problems occur. Because foot damage is not painful in these patients, they sometimes show an inappropriate nonchalance toward it.

Diabetic foot ulcers should be débrided and their depth determined. Some superficial ulcers can be managed by using a cushion insole to ease the load. Others are treated

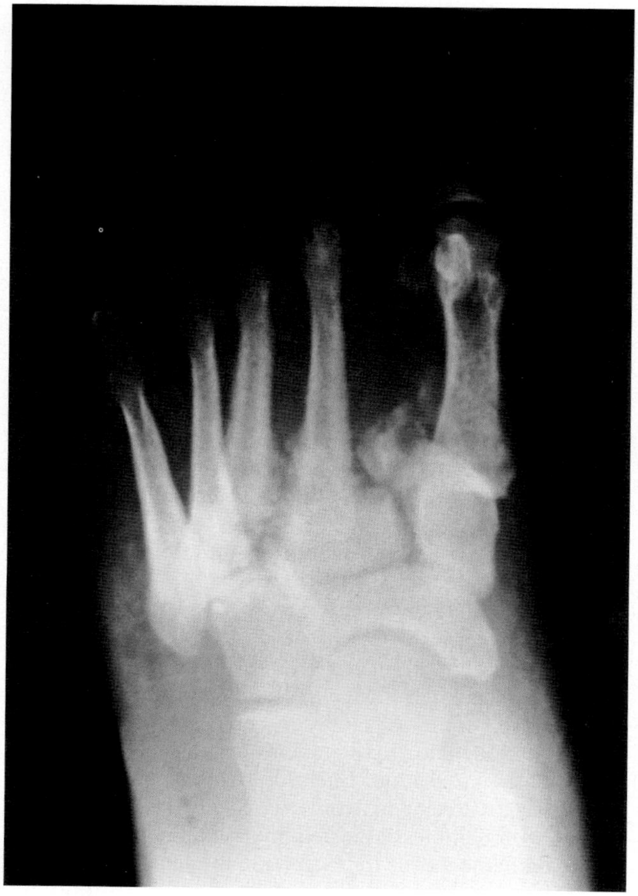

FIGURE 42–6 Radiograph of Charcot foot.

with total contact casting, which promotes healing by decreasing the motion of the foot within the cast and by decreasing plantar contact pressure on the skin. For ulcers that go beneath the dermis, surgical débridement is necessary. If infection is present, appropriate antibiotic treatment is begun. Use of topically applied growth factors shows promise as adjunct therapy. If a plantar ulcer occurs beneath a bony prominence, surgical removal of the prominence is often required. A common example of this is the excision of a metatarsal head when a plantar forefoot ulcer is found under it.

In patients with diabetes, the management of lower extremity fractures and soft tissue injuries is prolonged. Early return to unprotected ambulation carries a risk of collapse of the foot. The trauma associated with the onset of neuropathic arthropathy may be minimal, and the symptoms are often mild, but some degree of pain is often present. Immobilization and the avoidance of weight bearing are the initial treatment of choice, with the goal of achieving a braceable plantigrade foot. Surgical reconstruction is indicated for intractable ulcers associated with the deformed foot.

PEARLS FOR THE OR

Indications for surgery for osteomyelitis include the presence of an abscess or necrosis of the bone and soft tissue and the need for drainage.

In the surgical management of rheumatoid arthritis, synovectomy may be beneficial early in the course of the disease, before joint destruction has occurred, because it may provide symptomatic relief and delay disease progression. Either resection arthroplasty or replacement arthroplasty is indicated if the disease is more advanced.

Surgical options for the management of hip disorders include arthroscopy, arthrodesis, osteotomy, and arthroplasty.

Total knee arthroplasty is indicated in patients who have radiographic evidence of advanced intra-articular disease and have disabling knee pain and other symptoms that cannot be managed successfully with nonoperative treatment.

Foot Problems Associated with Rheumatoid Arthritis

Rheumatoid arthritis is an inflammatory disease of the joint synovium that affects 2% to 3% of people older than 55 years. The disease is autoimmune. Cartilage destruction is due to proteolytic enzymes released into the synovial fluid by the inflammatory process. Attenuation of the capsular ligaments around the joints leads to the deformities seen in the affected joints, especially in the hands and feet.

In the feet, attenuation of the plantar plate and collateral ligaments of the metatarsophalangeal joints leads to hyperextension and eventual dislocation of the toes (Fig. 42-7). The fat pad beneath the metatarsal heads migrates distally and dorsally with the toes. This causes the metatarsal heads to bear weight on plantar skin without the normal fatty cushion. With the dislocation of the lesser toes and pressure from the medial shoe, the hallux often drifts into valgus. Involvement of ankle tendons and ankle and hindfoot joints may subsequently cause hindfoot valgus and pes planus deformities.

Evaluation

After the painful portion of the foot is carefully inspected, examination should focus on detecting associated deformities and evaluating the relative flexibility of joints. If surgical treatment is necessary and will require endotracheal intubation, a lateral radiograph of the cervical spine in flexion should be obtained to determine whether atlantoaxial subluxation is present.

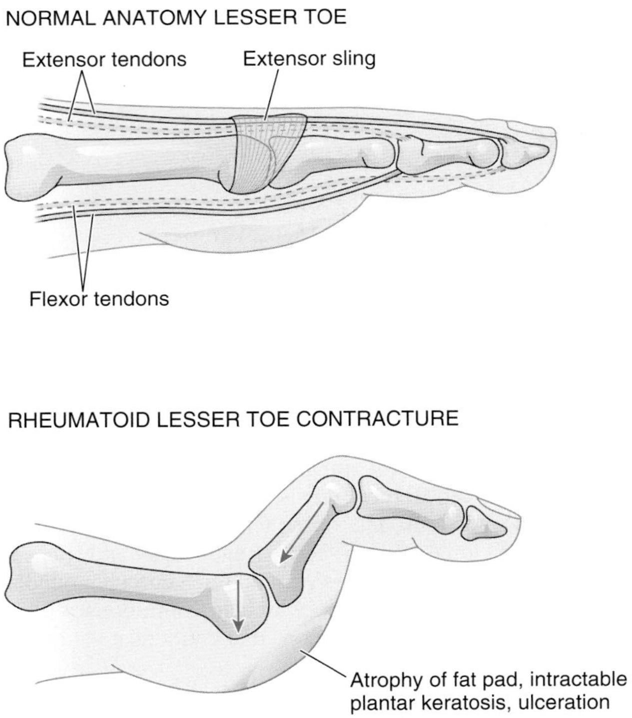

FIGURE 42–7 Pathophysiology of rheumatoid foot disease. In the feet, attenuation of the plantar plate and collateral ligaments of the metatarsophalangeal joints leads to hyperextension and eventual dislocation of the toes.

Treatment

Nonsurgical Treatment

In patients with rheumatoid arthritis, foot problems should first be managed nonsurgically. NSAIDs may provide symptomatic relief but have little effect on arresting the progression of disease. Other medications, such as gold salts, penicillamine, methotrexate, and glucocorticoids, can slow the progression of joint destruction. Extra-depth shoes and cushion inserts are helpful in accommodating forefoot deformities.

Surgical Treatment

Commonly performed soft tissue procedures that are successful in nonrheumatoid patients often fail in rheumatoid patients because their tissues are severely compromised by the progression of disease. Resection of the lesser metatarsal heads is effective in repositioning the plantar fat pad and reducing dislocations of metatarsal joints. A resection arthroplasty of either the proximal or the distal interphalangeal joint may be added if the patient has a toe deformity that will interfere with shoes. Fusion of the first metatarsophalangeal joint reduces the hallux valgus, adducts the metatarsal, and provides a solid weight-bearing support on the medial aspect of the foot.

Hindfoot reconstruction can be considered if brace management fails. Although synovectomy alone may be helpful early in the disease, fusion of the affected joints (commonly, the ankle, subtalar, or Chopart joints) is often necessary.

Complications

Because of the immunosuppressive effects of rheumatoid arthritis and the drugs that are often prescribed to treat it, patients with this disease are subject to a higher incidence of infection, slow healing, and skin breakdown. Osteopenia often precludes obtaining rigid fixation of the bone.

Suggested Reading

Broy SB, Schmid FR: A comparison of medical drainage (needle aspiration) and surgical drainage (arthrotomy or arthroscopy) in the initial treatment of infected joints. Clin Rheum Dis 12:501–522, 1986.

Goldenberg DL: Infectious arthritis complicating rheumatoid arthritis and other chronic rheumatic disorders. Arthritis Rheum 32:496–502, 1989.

Goldenberg DL: Bacterial arthritis. In Sledge CB, Ruddy S (eds): Arthritis Surgery. Philadelphia, WB Saunders, 1994, pp 495–509.

Goldenberg DL, Brandt KD, Cohen AS, et al: Treatment of septic arthritis. Arthritis Rheum 18:83–90, 1975.

Kelley WN, Schumacher R: Crystal-associated synovitis. In Kelley WN, Harris ED, Ruddy S, Sledge CB (eds): Textbook of Rheumatology. Philadelphia, WB Saunders, 1993, pp 1291–1354.

Tetsworth KD: Infection. Rosemont, IL, Academy of Orthopedic Surgeons, 1999.

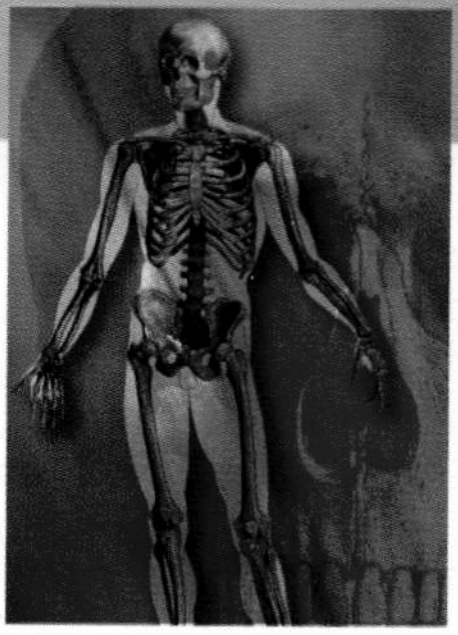

Chapter 43
Hand Surgery

ANDREW B. STEIN, MD, RYAN R. SNYDER, MD, and
DONNA M. PACICCA, MD

Injuries of the Wrist and Hand

Anatomy

Wrist

The distal radius has a biconcave articular surface, and the scaphoid and lunate facets are separated by a small ridge. The metaphysis of the distal radius is composed of mostly cancellous bone with thin cortices, especially on the dorsal and radial aspects. Extrinsic ligaments link the distal radius to the proximal carpal row, with the volar ligaments intrinsically stronger and more essential than the dorsal ones. In the normal adult, the average radial length (relative ulnar variance) is 11 mm, whereas the average radial inclination is 23 degrees and the average palmar inclination is 11 degrees (Fig. 43-1). About 80% of the axial load across the wrist is normally borne by the radius and 20% by the ulna, but changes in the radial length or angulation can significantly alter this relation.

Hand

Extrinsic and intrinsic muscles are necessary for normal function of the hand. The extrinsic muscles originate in the forearm and insert in the hand, whereas the intrinsic muscles have both their origins and insertions in the hand. The extrinsic flexors of the fingers include the flexor digitorum profundus (FDP) and the flexor digitorum superficialis (FDS). The FDP inserts at the base of the distal phalanx and can flex both the proximal interphalangeal (PIP) and distal interphalangeal (DIP) joints. The FDS inserts at the base of the middle phalanx and can flex only the PIP joint. Active DIP flexion confirms the integrity of the FDP tendon. The integrity of the FDS tendon can be tested by demonstrating PIP flexion with all but the examined finger held in extension, because the profundus tendons of the three fingers near the ulna share a common muscle belly. By restricting FDP excursion, PIP flexion can be initiated only by an intact FDS tendon, which itself is independent.

The intrinsic muscles of the hand include the thenar and hypothenar muscles; four dorsal interosseous muscles, which are abductors of the fingers; three palmar interosseous muscles, which are adductors of the fingers; and four lumbrical muscles, which arise from the FDP tendons and are the only muscles that directly relax their own antagonist. The interosseous and lumbrical muscles act together to flex the metacarpophalangeal (MP) joints and extend the interphalangeal (IP) joints through their insertion into the complex dorsal extensor apparatus (Fig. 43-2).

Considerable differences exist between flexor tendons and extensor tendons. The flexor tendons are composed of fascicles of long tendon cells (tenocytes) and dense, predominantly type I collagen fibers. Each collagen bundle is covered by an endotenon, which is continuous with a fine fibrous outer layer (epitenon) that contains most of the blood supply to the tendon.

The tendons are enclosed in synovial sheaths that start in the distal palm and extend into the fingers. The sheaths are important for hand function and for tendon nutrition. Segmental thickenings of the sheath form a series of five strong annular pulleys. Interposed between these pulleys are thin synovial cruciate sections that collapse during flexion (Fig. 43-3). The A2 and A4 pulleys are the most important biomechanically, and their damage will cause bow-stringing of the tendons and a loss of digital motion and power.

Tendon nutrition is derived not only from an extrinsic blood supply through the vinculum circulation but also from synovial fluid diffusion within the tendon sheath. Tendon healing is thought to occur through intrinsic and extrinsic mechanisms, the relative contributions of which depend on such factors as the type of injury, the method of repair, and the type of postsurgical rehabilitation program.

Surgical Techniques and Approaches

The skin of the hand is highly specialized. The glabrous skin on the palm is thick, irregular, and extensively tethered, allowing traction and durability. In contrast, the skin on the back of the hand is thin and mobile, allowing motion of the joints. Sensibility is of paramount importance for volar skin but is easily sacrificed for dorsal skin. These differences are reflected in commonly used operative exposures. **Longitudinal incisions** are commonly used through dorsal skin because they allow extensile approaches and because the resultant scar is easily tolerated in this loose, redundant skin. Incisions through volar skin, however, should never be longitudinal, because the ensuing scar formation will

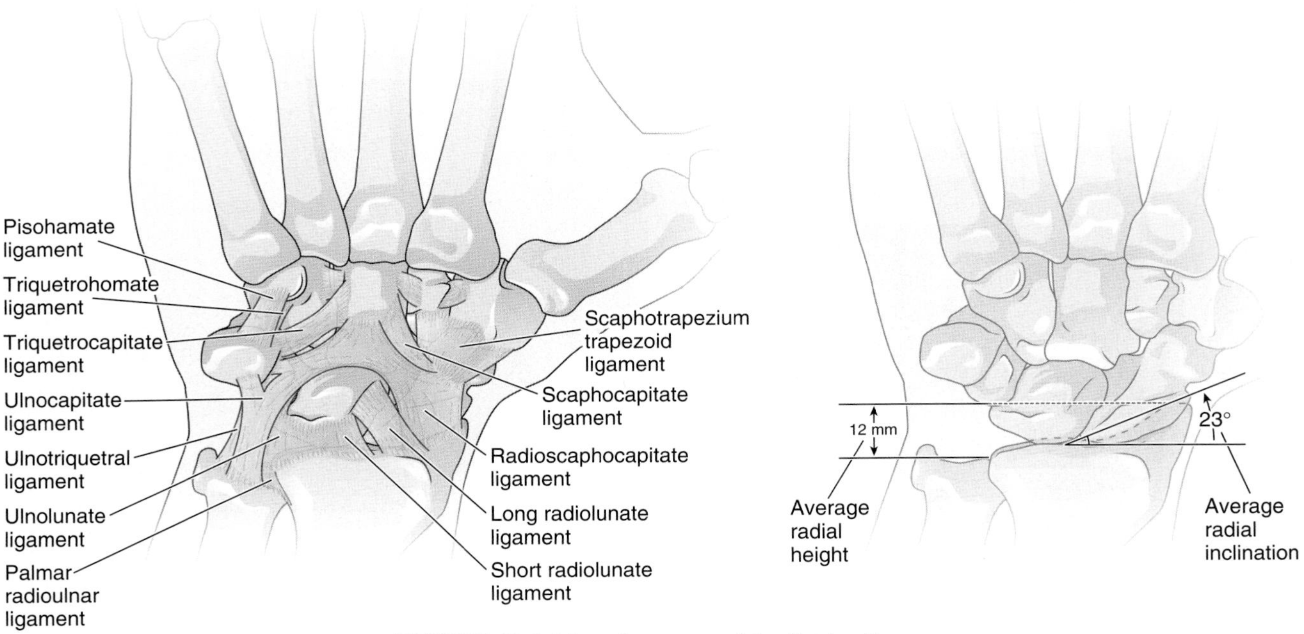

FIGURE 43–1 Normal anatomy of the distal radius.

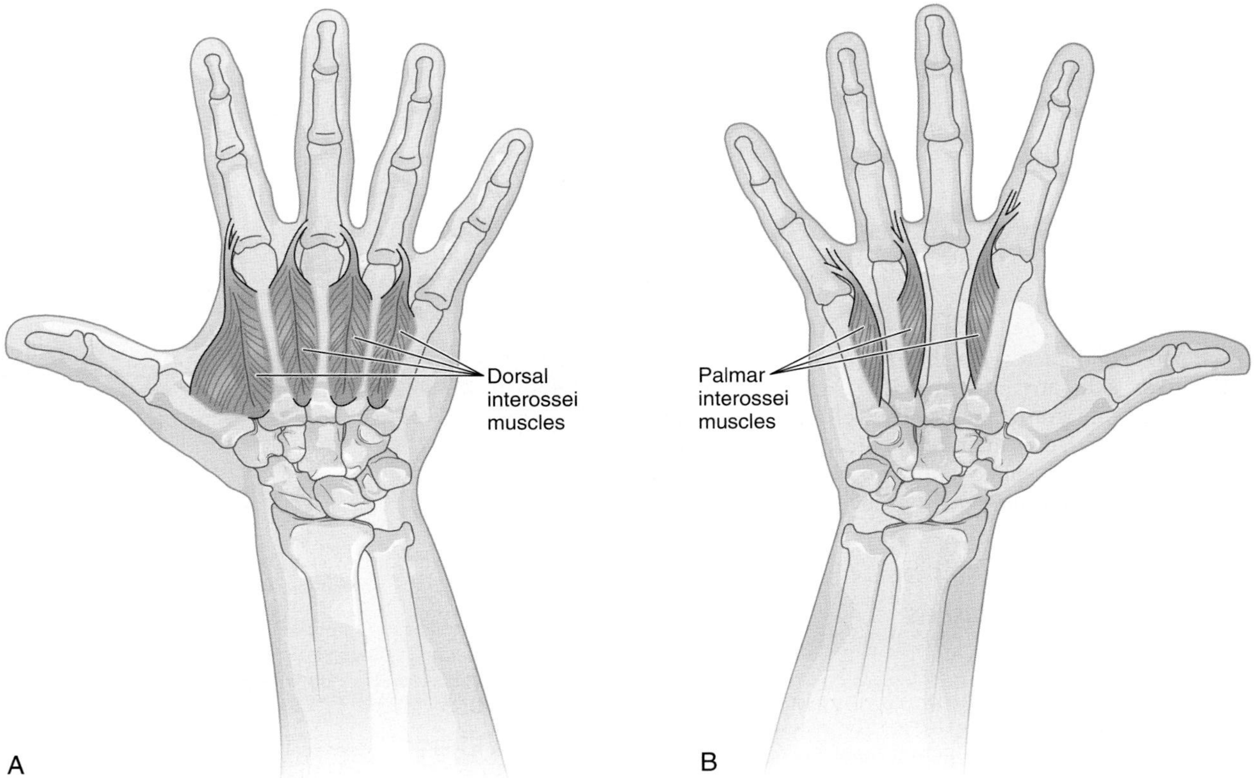

FIGURE 43-2 Lateral *(A)* and dorsal *(B)* views of the complex dorsal extensor apparatus of the finger. The interosseous and lumbrical muscles act together to flex the metacarpophalangeal (MP) joint and extend the proximal interphalangeal (PIP) and distal interphalangeal (DIP) joints through their insertion into the complex dorsal extensor apparatus.

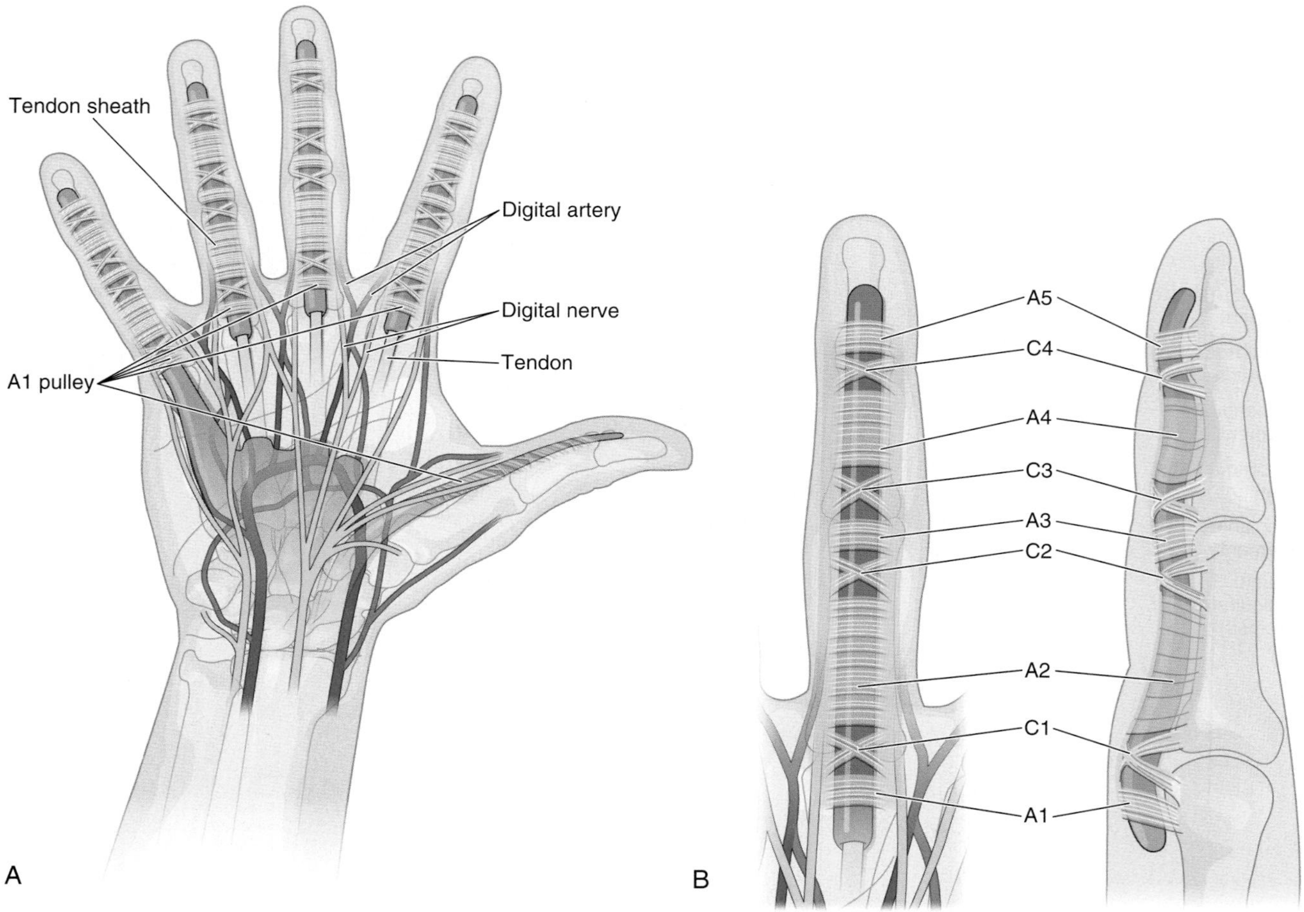

FIGURE 43–3 *A*, Palmar view of the flexor tendon sheath of the finger. *B*, Lateral view. The sheath is composed of annular pulleys (A1, A2, A3, A4, and A5), cruciate pulleys (C1, C2, and C3), and the palmar aponeurosis pulley (PA).

cause flexion contractures. For this reason, **zigzag incisions** of the volar skin are preferred (Fig. 43-4). Similarly, although free skin grafts are usually well accepted on the dorsum of the hand, they are rarely indicated on the palmar aspect, because they cannot supply the requisite sensation and cannot withstand the repetitive shear forces imparted during grip.

Distal Radius Fractures

Etiology and Classification

Fractures of the distal radius are quite common and account for up to 15% of all fractures. The peak incidence is in patients age 60 to 70 years. In this age group, the usual mechanism of injury is a fall onto the outstretched hand. In young patients, the usual mechanism is a high-energy trauma, and associated injuries are frequently found.

PEARLS FOR ROUNDS

The peak incidence of distal radius fractures is in patients age 60 to 70 years. In this age group, the usual mechanism of injury is a fall onto the outstretched hand. In young patients, the usual mechanism is a high-energy trauma, and associated injuries are frequently found.

Carpal tunnel syndrome is characterized by pain, paresthesia, and numbness in the palmar radial aspect of the hand.

Zone I extensor tendon injuries, such as mallet finger and swan-neck deformity, involve the terminal insertion of the conjoined lateral bands at the level of the distal interphalangeal joint.

From 30% to 50% of phalangeal fractures are open, and more than half of these open fractures occur in the workplace.

After phalangeal fracture, early mobilization of the fingers is important to prevent finger stiffness.

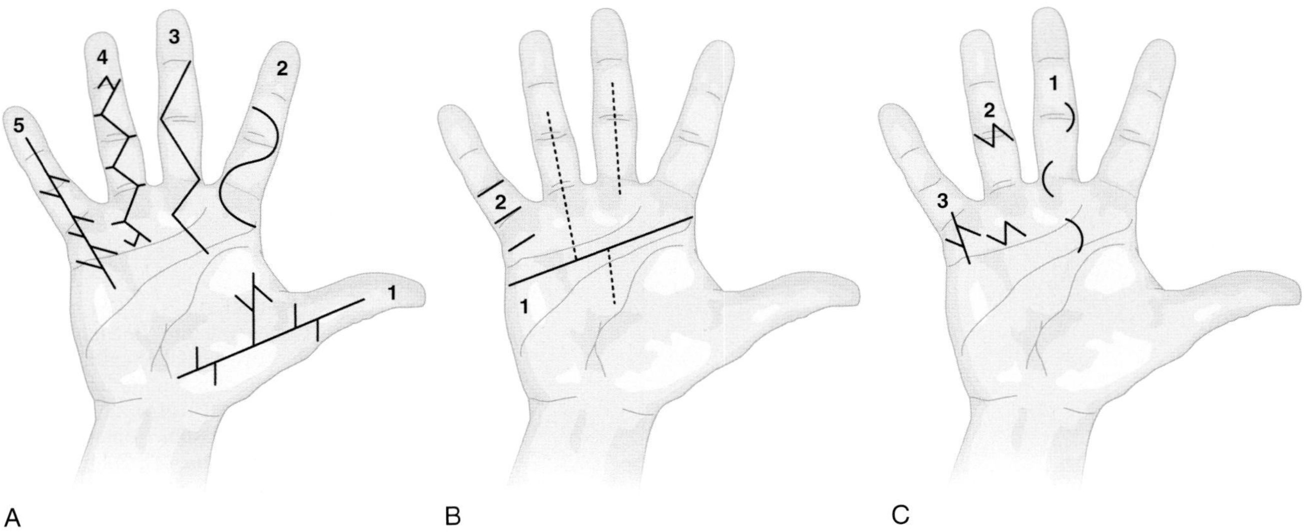

FIGURE 43–4 Basic incisions. *A*, Longitudinal incisions. (1) A T-shaped incision exposes all three cords that contract the thumb and first web space. The incisions are closed with Z-plasties. (2) A lazy-S incision is not recommended in the palm or the finger because it becomes straight and contracts. (3) The Bruner incision is preferred to the lazy-S because sharp angles remain and prevent scar contracture. (4) A multiple Y-V incision with a Z-plasty at either end provides good exposure and corrects relative skin shortage. (5) A midline longitudinal incision, closed with Z-plasties. *B*, Transverse incisions. (1) Most of the palmar aponeurosis can be removed through an incision that begins in the distal palmar crease on the ulnar side and ends in the proximal crease on the radial side of the hand. A proximal extension is unnecessary but is used by many surgeons. A variety of distal incisions, separate or in continuity, can be added to remove digital disease. (2) Multiple, short, transverse incisions. The transverse incision can be sutured, skin grafted, or left open. *C*, Minimal exposure. (1) Moermans' short, curved incisions used for segmental fasciectomy. The incisions for fasciotomy (2) and limited fasciectomy (3). (Adapted from Green D, Hotchkiss R, Pederson W (eds): Green's Operative Hand Surgery, 4th ed. Philadelphia, Churchill Livingstone, 1999, p 572.)

A fall onto the hand with the wrist in extension and the forearm in pronation results in a bending force at the metaphysis. The metaphysis fails in tension volarly and in compression dorsally. This is the most common pattern of injury, and the resulting dorsally displaced fracture is referred to as **Colles' fracture** (Fig. 43-5). A fall onto the hand with the wrist in flexion and the forearm in supination results in a volarly displaced fracture that is referred to as **Smith's fracture.** When shearing forces result in an articular fragment and either dorsal or volar displacement of the carpus, the fracture is called a **dorsal** or **volar Barton fracture.** Axial loading of the carpus can cause intra-articular fractures, the most common of which is called the **lunate-load fracture** or **die-punch fracture** and is characterized by depression of the lunate facet. A number of classification systems have been proposed as alternatives to these sometimes confusing terms, but no system has been universally accepted.

Evaluation

The diagnosis of distal radius fracture is suggested by pain, swelling, and tenderness at the wrist after a traumatic event and is often associated with a gross deformity. High-quality plain radiographs are usually the only imaging studies needed for diagnosis and treatment, although tomography or CT scanning can be quite helpful in understanding the anatomy of fractures with complex intra-articular patterns.

Treatment

The choice of treatment depends on various factors, including the fracture pattern, the associated soft tissue injuries, and the age and health of the patient.

If the fracture is stable and no significant soft tissue injuries are found, treatment usually consists of closed reduction and plaster immobilization in a well-molded cast. The intact periarticular ligaments and soft tissues will apply traction on the distal osseous structures and thereby reduce the fracture fragments. Immobilization is required for 4 to 8 weeks, during which time weekly radiographs should be taken.

If significant comminution is seen at the fracture site, treatment with closed reduction and the application of an external fixation device will prevent unacceptable settling over time. The device has rigid bars and uses ligamentotaxis to maintain reduction (Fig. 43-6). A major pitfall to be avoided is overdistraction or prolonged immobilization, because this can lead to wrist stiffness and loss of finger motion.

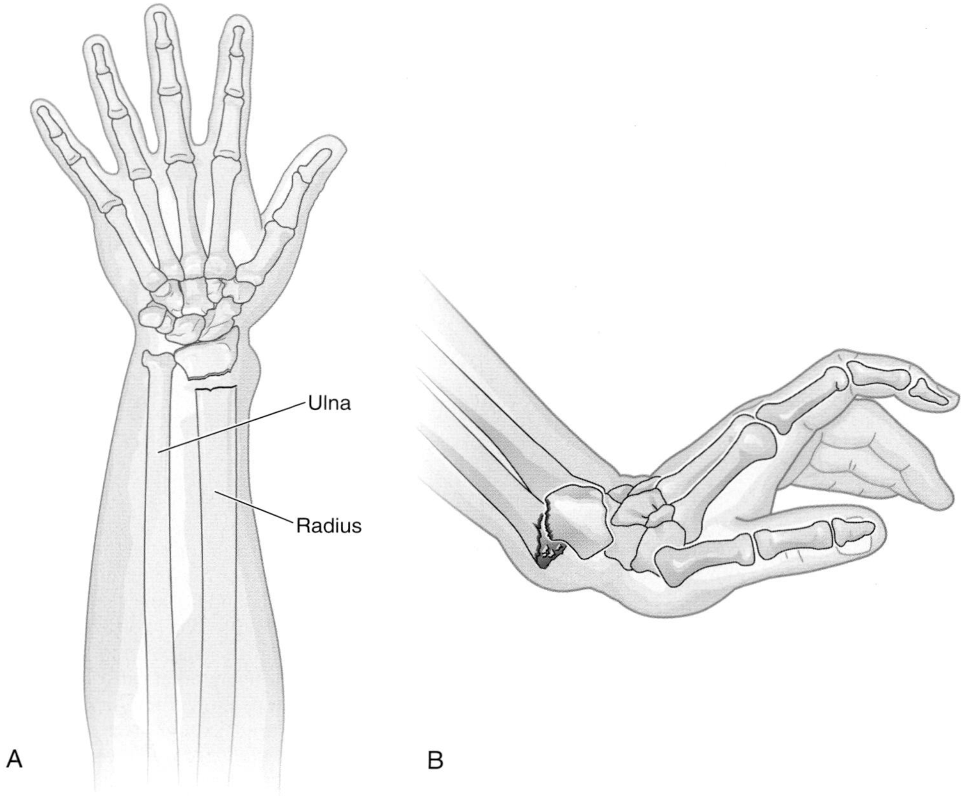

FIGURE 43–5 *A*, Classic Colles' fracture showing a dorsally displaced extra-articular fracture of the distal radius. *B*, This fracture typically results from an attempt to break a fall by using the hands and arms.

External fixation is often combined with percutaneous pinning or limited open reduction of displaced articular fragments with or without bone grafting. The combined treatment may allow earlier removal of the external frame. Arthroscope-assisted reduction of intra-articular fractures is another minimally invasive technique that has been gaining in popularity. For unstable periarticular fracture patterns, such as dorsal or volar Barton fractures, formal open reduction and internal fixation are indicated.

Complications

Residual articular step-offs that exceed 1 mm after reduction will predispose the patient to post-traumatic arthritis. Radial shortening and angulation alter the wrist mechanics and load transmission and will also predispose the patient to degenerative arthritis and distal radioulnar joint problems. The exact amount of malunion that is acceptable remains unknown, although it is clear that younger patients can tolerate less anatomic disruption than can older patients, so every effort should be made to achieve and maintain an anatomic reduction in the younger group.

Post-traumatic arthritis and median nerve dysfunction are relatively frequent complications and may require operative decompression. Rupture of the extensor pollicis longus (EPL) tendon is a delayed complication that occurs 6 to 8 weeks after a distal radius fracture and is thought to represent a vascular insult to the tendon at the level of Lister's tubercle. Reflex sympathetic dystrophy occurs in some patients, and pin-tract or deep infections may arise after surgical intervention.

Carpal Tunnel Syndrome

Carpal tunnel syndrome is the most common compressive neuropathy of the upper extremity. The syndrome is characterized by pain, paresthesia, and numbness in the palmar radial aspect of the hand.

Etiology and Pathogenesis

Carpal tunnel syndrome is caused by compression and dysfunction of the median nerve at the level of the carpal tunnel in the wrist. Compression initially reduces the epineurial blood flow and causes ischemia. With compression for extended periods, axonal transport becomes impaired. In patients with long-standing disease, endoneurial fibrosis occurs and causes mechanical symptoms that are less likely to improve after decompression.

Factors implicated in the development of carpal tunnel syndrome include displaced distal radius fractures, lipomas

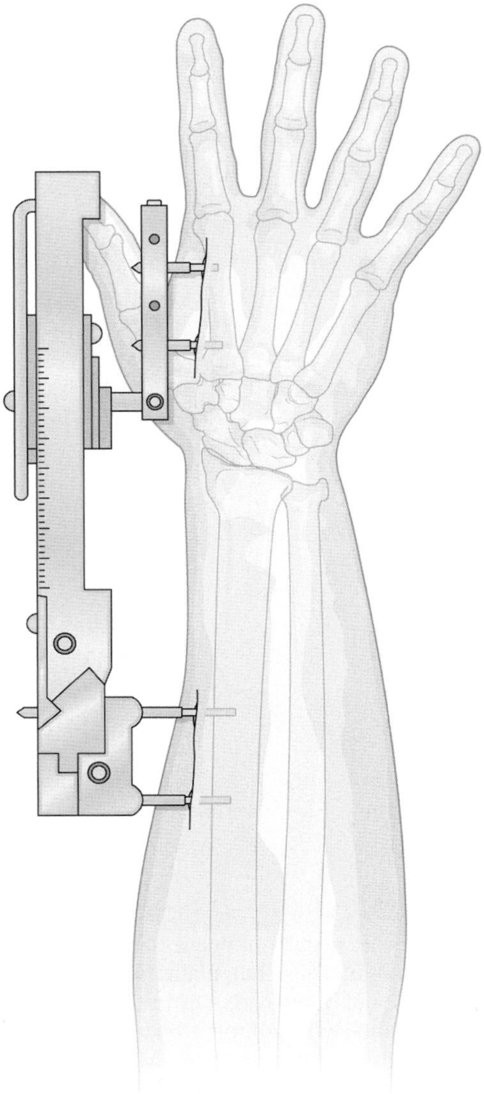

FIGURE 43–6 An external fixation device uses ligamentotaxis to maintain reduction of a distal radius fracture.

arising within the carpal tunnel, and repetitive mechanical stress. Indeed, classic carpal tunnel syndrome, which was once considered to be primary (idiopathic), is now believed to be secondary to fibrous hypertrophy of the flexor tendon synovium as a result of repetitive mechanical stress that induces local necrosis and collagen fragmentation. These pathologic changes increase the contents of the carpal tunnel and thereby decrease the space available for the nerve. As a result, the nerve is compressed.

Studies indicate that conditions such as diabetes mellitus, hypothyroidism, alcoholism, and aging can cause global depression of peripheral nerve function and thereby lower the threshold for developing a compressive neuropathy. In addition, a compressive lesion at one point on a nerve lowers the threshold for developing a compressive lesion at another level of the same nerve because of a disturbance in axonal transport mechanisms. This is termed the *double-crush phenomenon* and is often seen in patients who have a cervical root lesion in addition to median nerve compression at the carpal tunnel. Failure to recognize the cervical root compression may result in the persistence of symptoms of carpal tunnel syndrome despite an adequate surgical release.

PEARLS FOR THE OR

Longitudinal incisions are commonly used through dorsal skin because they allow extensile approaches and because the resultant scar is easily tolerated in this loose, redundant skin. Incisions through volar skin, however, should never be longitudinal, because the ensuing scar formation will cause flexion contractures. For this reason, zigzag incisions of the volar skin are preferred.

Although free skin grafts are usually well accepted on the dorsum of the hand, they are rarely indicated on the palmar aspect, because they cannot supply the requisite sensation and cannot withstand the repetitive shear forces imparted during grip.

If conservative management of carpal tunnel syndrome is ineffective, surgical release of the transverse carpal ligament is indicated.

Zone II injuries of the flexor tendon are generally considered the most challenging to treat, given the difficulty of repairing both tendons in close opposition within the tendon sheath.

Evaluation

Patients commonly feel pain and tingling or numbness in the thumb, index, and long finger and in the radial half of the ring finger. They complain that these symptoms often awaken them from sleep and are exacerbated by repetitive use of the hand. Physical examination may reveal dry skin on the affected fingers. Thenar atrophy may be present in advanced stages of nerve compression.

Numerous tests should be performed, because no single test is entirely conclusive. In Phalen's maneuver, passive wrist flexion reproduces symptoms within 60 seconds. In the carpal compression test (Durkin's maneuver), direct pressure over the carpal tunnel reproduces symptoms within 30 seconds. In Tinel's test, percussion over the nerve may cause paresthesia at the carpal tunnel or in the fingers.

Sensibility testing is an important part of the examination and should include vibrometry and Semmes-Weinstein monofilament testing. Both of these are threshold tests that reflect the function of a single nerve fiber and are therefore likely to detect a gradual decline in nerve function. Static and moving two-point discrimination tests are used to measure innervation density and will reflect complex cortical integration of overlapping sensory units. However, these discrimination tests are better for assessing nerve regeneration after repair than they are for diagnosis.

Electrodiagnostic testing remains the diagnostic gold standard. Although its results are highly operator dependent and its use entails an added cost, it is valuable because it provides the only objective measure of nerve function.

Treatment

Nonsurgical Treatment

Conservative management of carpal tunnel syndrome includes nighttime splinting of the wrist in a neutral position to reduce carpal tunnel pressures; use of oral anti-inflammatory drugs to reduce synovitis; use of diuretics to reduce edema; and good management of any underlying systemic conditions. Corticosteroid injections also are of value, because they provide transient relief in about 80% of patients and relief for up to a year in about 20%.

Surgical Treatment

If conservative management is ineffective, surgical release of the transverse carpal ligament is indicated. An open procedure is generally recommended because it is safe and reliable. Endoscopic devices have been developed; but aside from reducing the size of the scar, they seem to offer no significant advantages over an open technique, and they are associated with an increase in the risk of iatrogenic nerve injury and an attendant increase in cost. Although neurolysis was previously combined with release of the transverse carpal ligament, numerous studies have failed to demonstrate any added benefit, so it is no longer routinely recommended.

Flexor Tendon Injuries

Flexor tendon injuries have been divided into five zones, based on anatomic considerations (Fig. 43-7). They are zone I, distal to the superficialis insertion; zone II, the fibro-osseous tunnel (A1 pulley to zone I); zone III, the carpal tunnel to the A1 pulley; zone IV, the carpal tunnel; and zone V, proximal to the carpal tunnel.

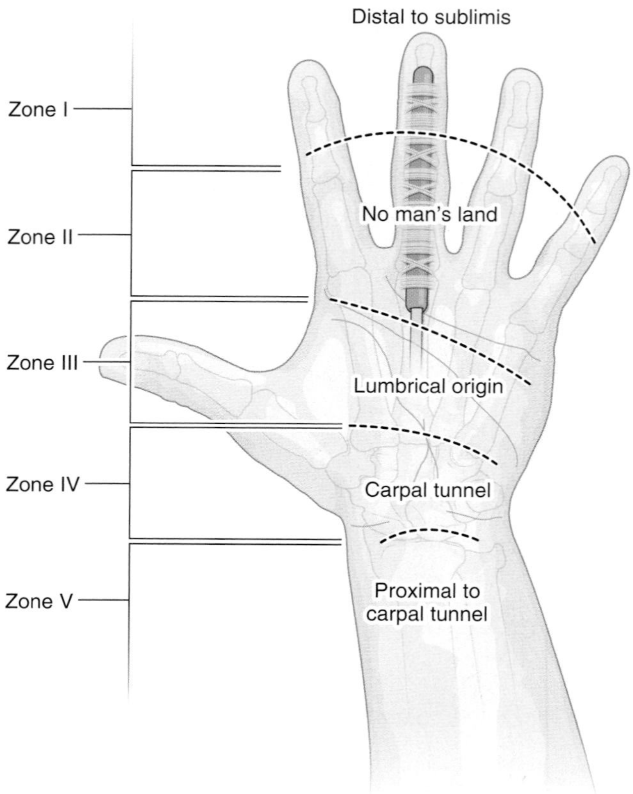

FIGURE 43–7 Five zones of flexor tendon injury.

Evaluation

History and Physical Examination

An alteration in the normal resting posture and cascade of the fingers (Fig. 43-8) is highly suggestive of tendon discontinuity. The alteration can be amplified by passively flexing and extending the wrist. Functional testing of each tendon is easily performed and is always indicated. In children or unresponsive patients, squeezing the flexor muscle bellies in the forearm will passively initiate tendon excursion. Pain with flexion is suggestive of a partial tendon laceration.

Imaging Studies

Imaging studies are usually not necessary for the diagnosis of flexor tendon injuries, but plain radiographs may be indicated to rule out bony avulsions in patients with closed injuries or patients with complex open injuries in which associated fractures are suspected. MRI and ultrasound studies also may be used if the diagnosis remains in question.

Treatment

Although partial tendon lacerations involving less than 60% of the flexor tendon need not be repaired, treatment is indicated for more severe injuries.

Zone II injuries are generally considered the most challenging to treat, given the difficulty of repairing both tendons in close opposition within the tendon sheath. However, both tendons should be repaired in severe injuries involving any zone. Unless associated vascular compromise is found, treatment should be done on a semi-elective basis when a skilled surgeon is available. A primary repair can be delayed for up to 3 or 4 weeks in an adult and perhaps up to 6 weeks in a child. With a longer delay, myostatic contracture will occur and will prevent the tendon from

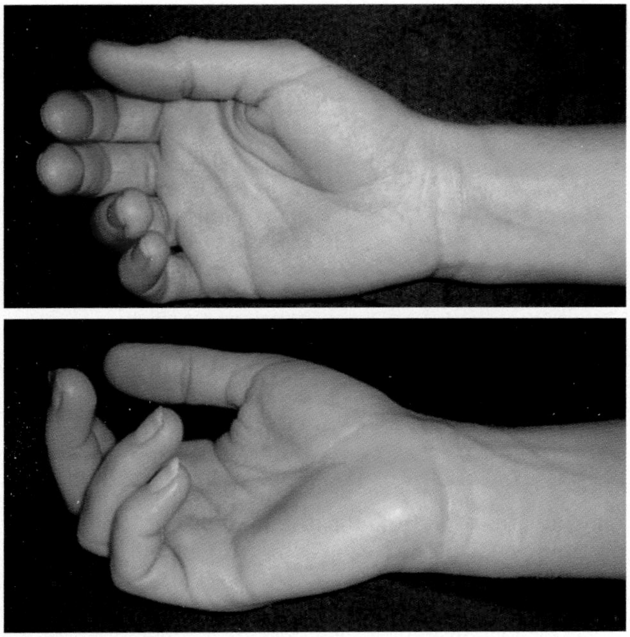

FIGURE 43–8 Normal resting posture and cascade of the fingers.

being brought out to length. In this case, free tendon grafting or staged reconstruction will be necessary.

Although much debate exists regarding the ideal repair technique, general agreement indicates that the A2 and A4 pulleys must be preserved to prevent bow-stringing, that the tendons must be handled carefully to minimize the risk of adhesion formation, and that appropriate suture materials and techniques must be used to prevent gaps at the tendon-repair juncture. In most cases, 3-0 or 4-0 braided polyester sutures are used because of their strength, minimal reactivity, and ease of placement. Suture techniques for tendon repair all involve grasping the tendon with multiple passes. The number of suture strands that cross the repair site appears to be the most important factor in preventing breakdown. A four-stranded core repair is most often used, because it provides significantly more strength than a two-stranded repair and is easily applied to tendons of almost all dimensions.

Rehabilitation involves the use of an extension block splint and passive motion or controlled active-motion exercises. The goal is controlled early movement, because it will help prevent adhesion formation and will improve the tensile strength of the repaired tendon.

Complications

Clean sharp injuries herald a better outcome than crushing injuries or injuries associated with fractures, neurovascular damage, and skin loss. Zone II injuries have the worst prognosis. The prognosis for a successful repair and the avoidance of adhesion formation is better in younger patients than in the elderly, although children may pose problems if they are unable to cooperate with postoperative instructions.

Extensor Tendon Injuries

Etiology and Classification

Extensor tendon injuries have been divided into nine zones (Fig. 43-9). Zone I and zone III injuries affect the fingers and are among the most common types.

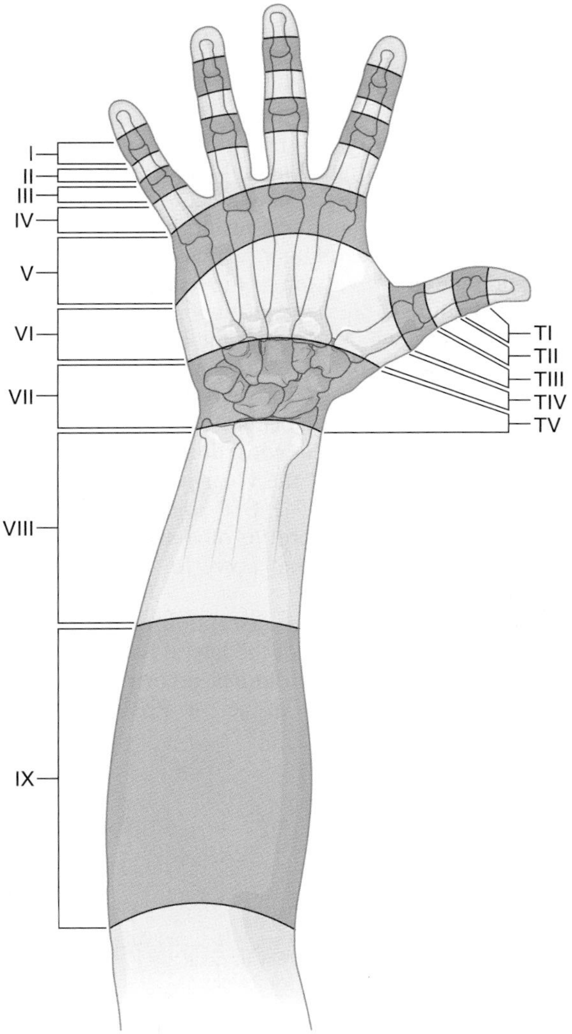

FIGURE 43–9 Nine zones of extensor tendon injury: I, distal interphalangeal joint; III, proximal interphalangeal joint; V, metacarpophalangeal joint; VII, wrist; and II, IV, VI, VIII, the sections in between; IX, distal forearm.

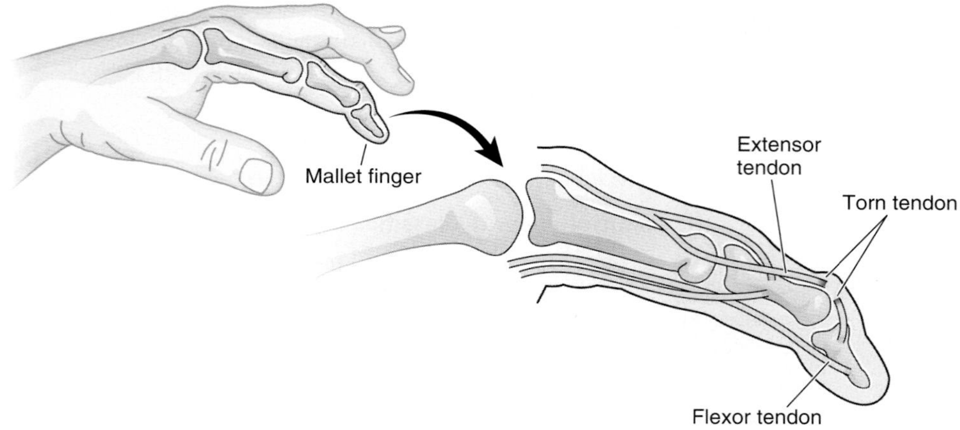

FIGURE 43–10 The mallet finger deformity causes a droop of the fingertip. The relative size of the flexor tendon compared with the smaller size of the extensor tendon shows the need to have a strongly healed extensor tendon before removing the splint.

Zone I injuries, such as **mallet finger** (Fig. 43-10) and **swan-neck deformity** (Fig. 43-11), involve the terminal insertion of the conjoined lateral bands at the level of the DIP joint. Mallet finger may occur from a laceration; however, it more commonly results from sudden forced flexion of the extended finger, which causes rupture of the terminal tendon or avulsion of the tendon with a fragment of bone. Failure to treat mallet finger may result in swan-neck deformity, which is one of the classic manifestations of an imbalance between the intrinsic and extrinsic extensor mechanisms. With disruption of the terminal tendon, relative overpull occurs at the level of the PIP joint, and this increases with dorsal migration of the lateral bands. If laxity of the volar plate coexists, the PIP joint will hyperextend. The DIP joint assumes a flexed position (similar to the profile of a swan) as a result of unopposed pull from the powerful flexor digitorum profundus.

Zone III injuries involve disruption of the central slip and allow volar migration of the lateral bands. If a zone III injury is not corrected, **boutonnière deformity** (Fig. 43-12), may occur, with a loss of active PIP extension, and unopposed flexion from the displaced lateral bands causes overpull and hyperextension at the DIP joint.

Evaluation

Extensor tendon injuries can usually be diagnosed on the basis of clinical findings alone. Finger extension is actually more complex than finger flexion, because extension is dependent both on the extrinsic extensors innervated by the radial nerve and on the intrinsic extensors innervated by the ulnar and median nerves. During evaluation, remember that the juncturae tendinum join the communis tendons at the level of the MP joints and that they may allow active MP extension despite the presence of a complete tendon laceration proximal to the fibrous interconnections (Fig. 43-13). In addition, remember that the intrinsic muscles provide for MP joint flexion and IP joint extension, which can occur even with complete disruption of the extensor digitorum communis (EDC) tendon. Simultaneous extension of the MP and IP joints requires both an extrinsic and intrinsic contribution. Thus a careful physical examination and a high index of suspicion are often needed to make an accurate diagnosis.

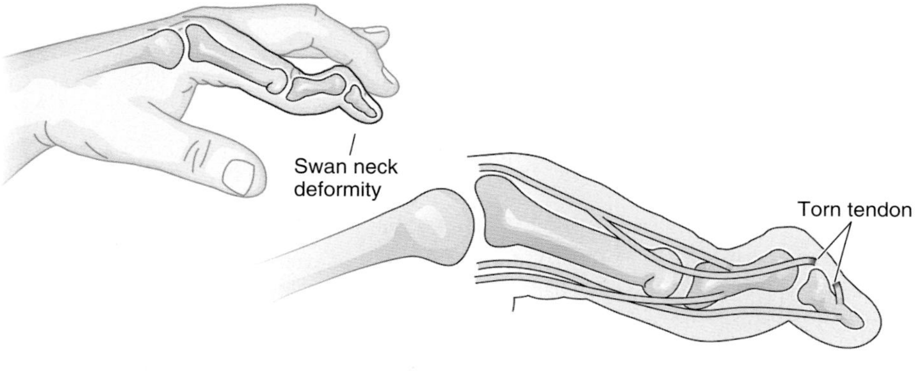

FIGURE 43–11 Swan-neck deformity.

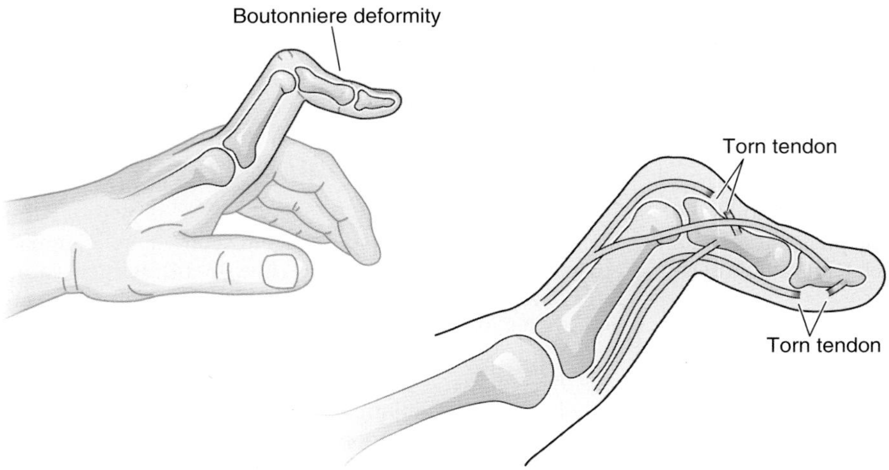

FIGURE 43–12 Boutonnière deformity.

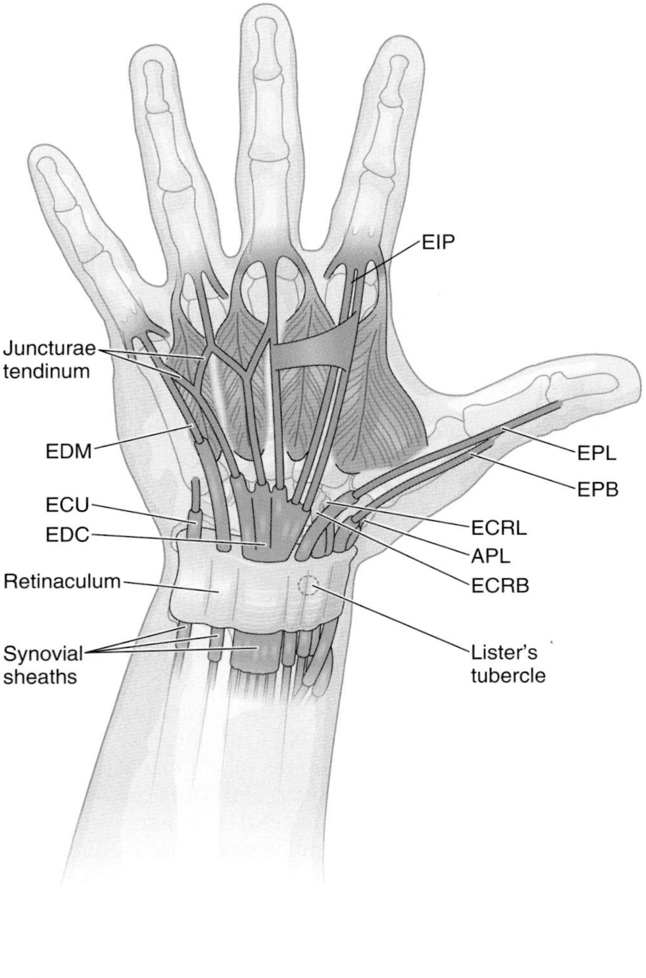

FIGURE 43–13 Extensor tendons of the hand. The extensor tendons gain entrance to the hand from the forearm through a series of six canals. Note that the juncturae tendinum may provide full extension even if the EDC tendon is completely cut. APL, abductor pollicis longus; ECRB, extensor carpi radialis brevis; ECRL, extensor carpi radialis longus; ECU, extensor carpi ulnaris; EDC, extensor digitorum communis; EDM, extensor digiti minimi; EIP, extensor indicis proprius; EPB, extensor pollicis brevis; EPL, extensor pollicis longus.

Although lacerations are a frequent cause of extensor tendon injuries, closed injuries are more common and are often missed initially because of an inadequate physical examination and the fact that it usually takes from 2 to 3 weeks for the classic imbalance between the intrinsic and extrinsic extensor mechanisms to develop. Forceful flexion of the extended PIP joint is the usual initial injury, and patients typically are first seen with a swollen PIP joint and tenderness at the dorsal base of the middle phalanx. A small avulsion fracture is sometimes seen on a lateral radiograph.

Treatment

For soft tissue mallet injuries or bony injuries involving a small fragment of bone, treatment consists of continuous extension splinting of the DIP joint for 6 to 8 weeks. Direct repair of the tendon is not recommended, because the tendon is quite thin in zone I and has a tenuous blood supply. Swan-neck deformity is easily prevented by correction of the underlying mallet deformity. Once the deformity is present, correcting it may require a DIP fusion or more involved soft tissue reconstruction.

If a small avulsion fracture is present, treatment should initially consist of maintaining the PIP joint in extension either with an external splint or with transarticular pinning. If more than a third of the articular surface has been avulsed, some surgeons recommend open reduction and internal fixation. However, the complication rate has been reported to be greater than 50%, and some studies suggest that remodeling of the articular surface always occurs with extension splinting, despite the original loss of joint congruity. For this reason, many surgeons recommend closed reduction and transarticular pinning of the DIP joint in extension if volar subluxation of the joint is found or if the patient cannot tolerate external splinting for a prolonged period.

Treatment of boutonnière deformity most often entails dynamic extension splinting of the PIP joint, combined with DIP flexion exercises. If this fails to overcome a fixed PIP flexion deformity and to allow dorsal migration of the lateral bands, surgical intervention may be necessary. Numerous procedures have been described and involve either soft tissue release or tendon reconstruction. The outcome of these procedures is unpredictable, so they should be tried only if prolonged closed treatment has failed.

Complications

In the past, extensor tendons were repaired in the emergency department and then splinted for 3 or 4 weeks with the wrist in extension and the fingers in slight flexion. This often resulted in adhesions between the repaired tendon and the surrounding soft tissues, especially if the primary injury was associated with a crushing force or concomitant fracture. For this reason, an increased push occurred to treat tendon injuries in a controlled operating room setting, with the attention to detail and improved suture techniques described earlier for flexor tendon injuries. In the postoperative period, controlled motion has been shown to give better results than prolonged immobilization. Dynamic extension splinting is often used immediately with cooperative patients.

Metacarpal and Phalangeal Fractures

Metacarpal and phalangeal fractures are quite common, comprising 10% of all fractures (Fig. 43-14). In most cases, the border digits are involved. Mechanisms of injury are varied and include simple torsional and bending injuries, which often occur during sporting competitions, and severe crushing injuries, which are frequently associated with complex soft tissue injuries. From 30% to 50% of phalangeal fractures are open, and more than half of these open fractures occur in the workplace.

Evaluation

History and Physical Examination

The history should include the patient's occupation, hand dominance, and presence of preexisting systemic illnesses. The physical examination begins with an assessment of the extent and severity of any associated soft tissue injuries, because these often take precedence over bony injuries or dictate the treatment of the fractures. The three essential anatomic requirements of the digits that allow normal finger function are normal length, rotation, and angular alignment. After a fracture, length and angulation may be appreciated on radiographs, but rotational alignment can be determined only by physical examination. This is most easily accomplished by checking that the digital nailplates remain parallel to one another in full extension as well as in full flexion. If uncorrected, rotational deformities will cause digital scissoring.

Imaging Studies

The only imaging studies needed are high-quality plain radiographs in three planes. To avoid misdiagnosis of finger injuries, the radiographic views should be of the involved digit, rather than of the hand.

Treatment

Early mobilization of the fingers is important to prevent finger stiffness. In this regard, three general principles should be kept in mind. First, if immobilization is necessary, it should rarely be allowed to exceed 3 weeks. Second, immobilization should always be with the fingers in the intrinsic plus position (safe position), with the MP joints in maximal flexion and the IP joints in full extension. Third, if open reduction is needed, internal fixation must be stable enough to allow immediate range-of-motion exercises.

Operative intervention is indicated if closed reduction of the fracture fails to maintain adequate length, rotation, or

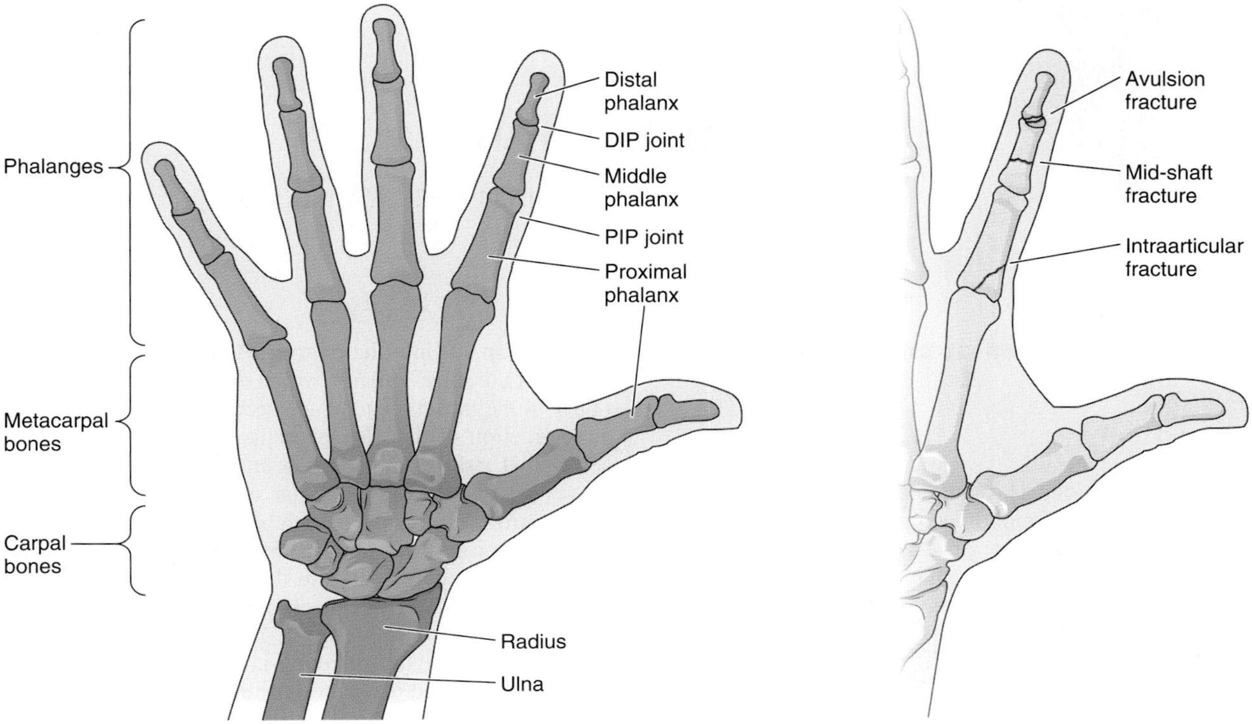

FIGURE 43–14 Metacarpal and phalangeal finger fractures.

angular alignment of the finger. Operative intervention also is indicated if patients have intra-articular fractures with loss of joint congruity or if they have potentially unstable fracture patterns associated with soft tissue injuries whose treatment is facilitated by early motion (such as a flexor tendon laceration that occurs in zone II and is associated with a fracture of the proximal phalanx). Various types of fixation can be used. These include percutaneous pinning, static and dynamic external fixation, and formal open reduction with internal fixation using interosseous wiring or miniplates and screws.

Although antibiotic prophylaxis helps reduce the infection rate associated with open fractures in many parts of the body, it has not proved efficacious in reducing the infection rate associated with open fractures of the fingers. For this reason, it is crucial to remove all nonviable or marginally viable tissue during the initial débridement of the wound.

Complications

The incidence of loss of motion of the injured finger is increased in patients with fractures accompanied by extensive soft tissue injuries and in those with periarticular and articular fractures. Nonunions and infections are seen most often after open fractures.

Suggested Reading

Gellman H, ed: Fractures of the Distal Radius. Rosemont, IL, American Academy of Orthopaedic Surgeons, 1998.

Green DP (ed): Operative Hand Surgery, 5th ed. Philadelphia, Churchill Livingstone, 2005.

Hoppenfeld S, de Boer P, eds: Surgical Exposures in Orthopaedics: The Anatomic Approach. Philadelphia, Lippincott, 1984.

Manske PR, ed: Hand Surgery Update, Vol 1. Rosemont, IL, American Society for Surgery of the Hand, 1994.

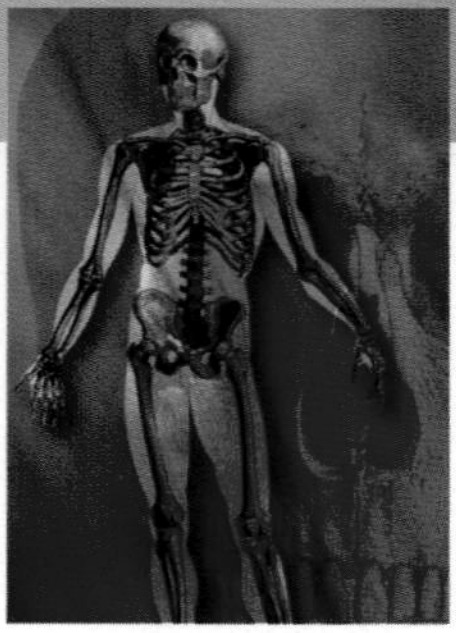

Chapter 44
Soft Tissue Injuries

RYAN R. SNYDER, MD, DONNA M. PACICCA, MD, and
PETER DEWIRE, MD

Soft Tissue Injuries of the Shoulder

Anatomy

Shoulder

The glenohumeral joint is a ball-and-socket–type joint that permits a wide range of motion, with stability conferred by a number of structures that provide static and dynamic restraints to excessive motion. Static constraints to glenohumeral motion include the humeral head and glenoid, joint capsule, glenohumeral ligaments, glenoid labrum, and negative intra-articular pressure. The rotator-cuff muscles and the deltoid and accessory muscles of the shoulder provide dynamic restraints to shoulder instability.

Rotator Cuff

The rotator cuff is composed of the tendons of the supraspinatus, infraspinatus, teres minor, and subscapularis muscles. The primary function of the rotator-cuff muscles is to center the humeral head in the glenoid during shoulder motion. Abduction of the shoulder is caused by the deltoid and supraspinatus muscles. The subscapularis is the primary internal rotator of the shoulder, and the teres minor and infraspinatus externally rotate the arm.

The blood supply to the rotator cuff is derived from branches of the circumflex humeral, subscapular, and thoracoacromial arteries. About 1 cm from the insertion of the supraspinatus tendon is a hypovascular zone. This is the most common location of rotator-cuff tears. The supraspinatus is thought to be more susceptible to injury and subsequent tearing because of the relatively decreased vascularity.

Surgical Techniques and Approaches

Shoulder and Proximal Humerus

Several surgical approaches are used for access to the shoulder joint and proximal humerus. The **anterior approach (deltopectoral approach)** is used to access the glenohumeral joint for reconstruction, arthroplasty, drainage procedures, and biceps tendon repairs. This approach begins at the coracoid process and continues in the deltopectoral groove. The muscle interval is developed between the pectoralis major and the deltoid. Beneath this layer is the tendon of the subscapularis, which overlies the joint capsule. Injury to the musculocutaneous nerve can occur with vigorous retraction of the coracobrachialis tendon. The axillary nerve is at risk of damage beneath the subscapularis as it passes through the quadrangular space.

The **anterolateral approach** is used primarily for repair of the rotator cuff and subacromial decompressions. It can be extended to gain access to the acromioclavicular joint. This approach requires detachment of the deltoid muscle from the anterior acromion.

The **direct lateral approach** is also useful for repair of the rotator cuff and insertion of intramedullary rods. It can be extended for access to the proximal humerus for open reduction and internal fixation of greater tuberosity fractures and fractures of the neck of the humerus. The axillary nerve is at risk of damage in the distal part of the incision as it wraps around the humerus approximately 5 to 7 cm from the acromion.

The **posterior approach** to the shoulder is useful in posterior instability procedures, glenoid osteotomies, and drainage procedures. The deltoid is lifted from its origin, and the interval between the teres minor and the infraspinatus muscles is developed. Both the axillary and the suprascapular nerves are at risk in this approach.

Middle and Distal Humerus

Surgical exposure of the humerus is primarily used for biopsies, osteotomies, and the open reduction and internal fixation of fractures. The commonly used surgical approaches are anterior, anterolateral, and posterior.

The **anterior approach** develops proximally from the deltopectoral groove. Distally, the interval divides the medial and lateral fibers of the brachialis muscle. The musculocutaneous and radial nerves are encountered in the exposure of the middle and distal humerus and must be protected.

The **anterolateral approach** is extensile, allowing for more distal exposure of the humerus and elbow. The lateral cutaneous and radial nerves are at risk with this approach. The interval is between the brachialis and brachioradialis muscles. The radial nerve can be identified between these muscles at the elbow joint. The brachialis muscle is elevated on its lateral border to expose the humerus.

The **posterior approach** divides the fasciae between the lateral and long heads of the triceps muscle and then splits the medial head fibers to reach the posterior humerus. The radial nerve is at risk as it travels in the spiral groove. The ulnar nerve is deep to the medial head of the triceps muscle and is at risk during elevation of these fibers. Subperiosteal dissection is necessary to protect these structures.

Shoulder Instability

Etiology and Classification

Symptoms of shoulder instability are more frequently seen in athletes involved in overhead sports activities than in the general population. Shoulder instability can result from an acute traumatic event or from excessive joint laxity and volume. Acute shoulder instability can be classified into three groups, based on the direction of the humeral head dislocation: anterior (the most common), posterior, and inferior. In those with unidirectional instability after a traumatic dislocation, the risk of recurrent instability is related primarily to the age at which the initial dislocation occurred. The risk approaches 100% when the initial dislocation occurs before the patient is 17 years old. In some cases, shoulder instability is unidirectional. In other cases, it is multidirectional.

Anterior shoulder instability usually occurs when the arm is forced into external rotation, abduction, and extension. Patients with anterior dislocations have been divided into three groups. Type I patients are stable on examination under anesthesia (EUA) and have inferior capsular hemorrhage. Type II patients show anterior subluxation on EUA and may have a Hill-Sachs lesion of the humeral head. Type III patients show dislocation on EUA and have a complete glenoid labrum avulsion called the Bankart lesion. This injury results in recurrent anterior instability and often requires surgical repair.

Posterior shoulder instability is much less common than anterior instability. On physical and radiographic examination, signs of posterior instability are subtle and are frequently overlooked. Posterior dislocations most often occur in association with a seizure or electric shock and are caused when the internal rotators of the shoulder, including the subscapularis, pectoralis major, and latissimus dorsi muscles, overpower the external rotators. A direct blow to the anterior shoulder or a fall on the outstretched arm also may lead to a posterior dislocation.

Inferior shoulder instability and anterior shoulder instability are the two types that most often contribute to multidirectional instability (MDI). In patients with MDI, recurrent shoulder instability is common.

MDI occurs as a result of excess laxity of the capsular and ligamentous supporting structures of the shoulder. In MDI, the glenoid labrum is typically intact. The distended joint capsule is unable to restrain excessive humeral head translation during extremes of motion. Muscle weakness often accompanies this condition.

Evaluation

History and Physical Examination

Evaluation of a patient with complaints of shoulder pain and instability requires a thorough history. Patients should be asked questions about their age and the position that their arm was in at the time of the first dislocation. Symptoms of anterior instability are exacerbated with abduction and external rotation of the shoulder (apprehension test), whereas symptoms of posterior instability occur with adduction and internal rotation. Patients with voluntary or habitual subluxation often have MDI. A sulcus sign may be present, which indicates inferior instability. MDI is often associated with generalized ligamentous laxity and can be checked by apposition of the thumb to the volar surface of the forearm, or elbow hyperextension.

In all cases of acute dislocation of the shoulder, a thorough assessment of the neurovascular status of the limb must be done before attempts at reduction. Vascular injuries occur more frequently in older patients after an acute dislocation and may result in ischemia of the extremity.

Imaging Studies

Diagnostic workup of the patient with acute unilateral shoulder instability should include anteroposterior, lateral (scapular Y), and axillary radiographs to help assess the location of the humeral head and any associated fractures. Repeated radiographs should be obtained after reduction of a dislocated shoulder. Magnetic resonance imaging (MRI) or computed tomography (CT) scanning is indicated in recurrent dislocations to determine whether a Bankart lesion or any bony injuries are present. CT scanning also may demonstrate abnormalities of glenoid morphology, such as excessive retroversion or hypoplasia. MRI may detect tears of the inferior glenohumeral ligament.

EUA and diagnostic arthroscopy may be indicated in cases in which the cause of the symptoms remains unclear. Diagnostic arthroscopy may help guide surgical treatment and identify associated conditions. Lesions of the superior labrum and biceps anchor, undersurface rotator cuff tears, and posterior labrum tears may be diagnosed during diagnostic arthroscopy and are often difficult to diagnose clinically.

Treatment

Nonsurgical Treatment

Acute anterior or posterior dislocations of the shoulder require closed reduction. Before reduction of an anterior dislocation is performed, the patient may require analgesics, muscle relaxants, or tranquilizers to overcome the pain, muscle spasms, and anxiety. Intra-articular lidocaine also may provide adequate pain relief to allow reduction. In general, traction on the flexed and abducted arm will effect the reduction. Adequate countertraction is usually necessary. The hippocratic method of placing the foot in the axilla and applying traction is associated with a high complication rate and therefore should be avoided.

After the reduction of an anterior or posterior dislocation, it is necessary to assess the stability of the shoulder and to reassess the neurovascular status of the extremity. Repeated radiographs should be obtained to determine the adequacy of the reduction and to recheck for fractures.

The duration of treatment after reduction of an acute shoulder dislocation is controversial and depends on age and other factors. In patients who are 30 years old or younger, the shoulder should be placed into a shoulder immobilizer for 2 to 5 weeks to prevent recurrence. A supervised therapy program directed at isometric exercises is then begun and is followed by progressive exercises for rotator cuff strengthening and motion. In patients who are older than 30 years, shoulder motion is begun earlier to prevent stiffness. Modification of activities is encouraged.

Recurrent instability of the shoulder and symptomatic MDI are managed with a brief period of rest. Early motion and rehabilitation of the rotator-cuff and shoulder-girdle muscles should be instituted. Failed nonoperative treatment may be an indication for reconstructive surgery. Patients with MDI have a better response to therapy than do those with traumatic causes of shoulder instability.

Surgical Treatment

Indications for Surgery

If a shoulder dislocation occurs in association with avulsion of the rotator cuff, early surgery is indicated to remove interposed bone fragments and soft tissues. If greater tuberosity fractures remain displaced after reduction, surgery and internal fixation are indicated. If large glenoid rim fractures are displaced or compromise the stability of the joint, fixation is indicated.

Surgical stabilization is an option for patients whose occupations require absolute shoulder stability. In addition, surgical stabilization may be indicated for elite young athletes because of the high incidence of recurrent dislocation in these patients.

Surgical Techniques

The choice of technique depends on whether the shoulder instability is anterior, posterior, inferior, or multidirectional.

For recurrent anterior instability caused by a detachment of the labrum and capsule from the glenoid rim, anatomic repair is indicated. Bankart and capsular-shift procedures can be done either arthroscopically or with open techniques that use the deltopectoral approach to the anterior shoulder. In the Bankart procedure, the avulsed tissue is reattached to the glenoid rim. The labrum and capsule are repaired by using either suture anchors or drill holes in the glenoid, through which sutures are passed. The subscapularis is not reefed but is repaired anatomically. The open Bankart procedure is the gold standard for management of the Bankart lesion and is successful in eliminating redislocation in more than 90% of patients in whom it is performed. Arthroscopic capsular-shift procedures and Bankart repairs using bioabsorbable tacks and suture anchors are gaining greater acceptance and popularity. Procedures with laser thermal capsular shrinkage have been developed, but long-term data on these procedures are still lacking.

Several nonanatomic procedures reduce anterior instability by limiting external rotation. These include soft tissue transfers and bony blocks. The subscapularis transfer to the greater tuberosity (Magnuson-Stack method), subscapularis and capsular advancement procedure (Putti-Platt method), and the coracoid transfer (Bristow procedure) are examples. These procedures do not correct excessive capsular laxity, so they have been replaced largely by the more anatomic reconstructive procedures.

For recurrent posterior instability, a posterior inferior capsular-shift procedure is indicated. If excessive glenoid retroversion is the cause of the instability, glenoid neck osteotomy will restore stability by increasing glenoid anteversion.

In patients with recurrent MDI, it is necessary to determine preoperatively what directions are most unstable or symptomatic. The inferior capsular-shift procedure is used to decrease the capsular volume and reinforce incompetent capsular tissue. This can be done arthroscopically or with open techniques that use the anterior or posterior approach. Results after capsular-shift procedures have generally been good. Capsular shrinkage can be accomplished either by arthroscopic techniques or by laser capsulorrhaphy.

Complications

Complications associated with reconstructive surgery for shoulder instability include recurrent instability, loss of motion, and weakness. Patients who undergo Bankart and capsular-shift reconstruction may experience loss of shoulder motion and loss of strength resulting from excessive capsular shift or subscapularis plication. Athletes in throwing sports often complain of a loss of strength after anatomic or nonanatomic stabilization procedures. Synovitis has been reported when bioabsorbable tacks are used in surgery.

Rotator Cuff Disorders

Etiology and Classification

Intrinsic causes of rotator-cuff damage include age-related degeneration, hypovascularity, and repetitive microtrauma. Extrinsic causes of rotator-cuff damage include congenital subacromial stenosis, recurrent instability, overuse, trauma, and mechanical impingement.

Disorders of the rotator cuff include impingement syndrome, rotator-cuff tears, tendinitis, bursitis, and rotator-cuff arthropathy.

In impingement syndrome, encroachment of the rotator cuff can be caused by proximal migration of the humeral head or by components of the coracoacromial arch. In the Neer classification system, impingement syndrome is classified into three stages. In stage I, patients are younger than 25 years, and the rotator cuff is edematous and hemorrhagic. In stage II, patients are 25 to 40 years old, and tendinitis and degenerative fibrosis of the rotator cuff are found. In stage III, patients are older than 40 years, and acromial spurs and rotator-cuff tears are usually present.

The anterior acromion may be flat (type I), curved (type II), or hooked (type III). Rotator-cuff impingement and tearing are strongly associated with the type III acromion. Subacromial spurring also may contribute to the impingement syndrome.

Trauma is frequently responsible for damage to the rotator cuff. Microtrauma associated with repetitive overuse can lead to tendinitis and rotator-cuff failure. Acute macrotrauma also can result in partial or complete rotator-cuff tears (Fig. 44-1). Cuff tears sometimes occur in association with anterior dislocations, particularly in older patients during their first dislocation. Acute cuff tears can result from trauma without dislocation, but this is uncommon. Hemorrhagic bursitis can mimic a rotator-cuff tear in young athletes with an acute traumatic injury to the shoulder.

Rotator-cuff arthropathy occurs in association with chronic, massive cuff tears. The humeral head moves proximally, and this leads to chronic impingement. Destruction of the glenoid, humeral head, and arch can follow. Varying degrees of functional loss and pain result.

Evaluation

History and Physical Examination

Patients with rotator-cuff damage most often complain of pain over the anterolateral shoulder and along the deltoid muscle to its insertion. Symptoms typically are worse with activity, particularly with overhead activity. Pain often occurs at night, hindering the ability to sleep on the affected side. The pain may be acute or gradual in onset. The patient should be questioned concerning previous symptoms of instability or dislocation. Patients often complain of shoulder weakness and stiffness and should be questioned about neck pain and radicular symptoms. Cardiac, gastrointestinal, and pulmonary disorders may be responsible for pain referred to the shoulder.

Examination of the shoulder should begin with inspection of the shoulder-girdle muscles to detect signs of asymmetry and atrophy. The shoulder should be palpated and any local pain noted. Tenderness under the posterior and lateral acromion suggests rotator-cuff damage or bursa inflammation.

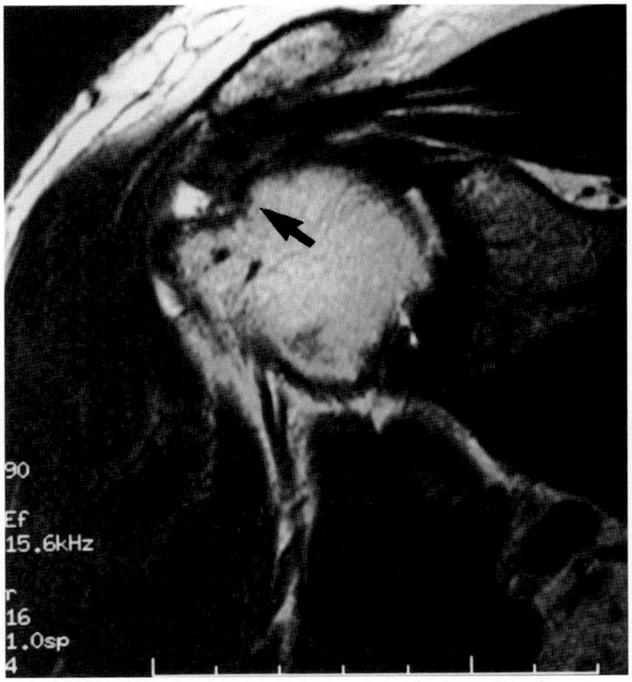

FIGURE 44–1 Magnetic resonance imaging of shoulder with rotator-cuff tear.

The range of motion should be measured. Normal active elevation is 180 degrees. Internal rotation is typically assessed by having the patient put the hand on the back and determining to what spinal level the hand can reach. External rotation should be measured with the elbow flexed to 90 degrees from the resting arm position. Normal external rotation is 90 degrees.

Shoulder strength should be assessed with particular attention to the rotator-cuff muscles. Pain or weakness with resisted motion may indicate a rotator-cuff tear or tendinitis. Pain with resisted external rotation at 0 and 90 degrees of shoulder abduction suggests damage to the infraspinatus and teres minor muscles. In the subscapularis test (lift-off test), the shoulder is fully internally rotated with the hand behind the back. The strength of the hand push-off is a measure of subscapularis muscle function. In the supraspinatus test, the arm is abducted 90 degrees, forward flexed 30 degrees, and internally rotated. In the drop-arm test, the patient is asked to lower the arm slowly from full elevation. With a full-thickness cuff tear, the arm may drop.

Patients should be tested for the Hawkins and Neer signs of impingement. In the Hawkins test, forceful internal rotation of the 90-degree abducted and forward flexed arm forces the greater tuberosity and supraspinatus tendon into the coracoacromial arch. Painful symptoms reproducing the patient's complaints are consistent with the diagnosis of impingement syndrome. In the Neer test, the scapula is stabilized, and the arm is internally rotated and forward flexed in the plane of the scapula. This forces the greater tuberosity into the anterior acromion and coracoacromial arch. Resulting pain suggests impingement. The relief of impingement symptoms by an injection of lidocaine into the subacromial space is helpful in making the diagnosis of impingement syndrome and distinguishing it from instability and rotator-cuff tears.

Imaging Studies

Anteroposterior radiographs in internal rotation are useful for identifying proximal migration of the humerus. The finding of less than 7 mm between the acromion and humeral head is suggestive of chronic rotator-cuff insufficiency. Subchondral sclerosis and cysts are seen in chronic rotator-cuff disease. Calcium deposits in the rotator-cuff tendon are seen in calcific tendinitis. The anteroposterior, axillary, and scapular Y radiographs are all evaluated for arthritic changes, subluxation or dislocation, and for acromion morphology.

MRI is the most sensitive and specific study for diagnosing full-thickness and partial-thickness rotator-cuff tears, cuff degeneration, and tendinopathy. MRI also can be useful in the diagnosis of impingement secondary to acromial spurring or a hooked acromion. If an MRI cannot be obtained, arthrography is a reliable method for detecting full-thickness tears. Ultrasonography may be reliable in detecting large full-thickness tears but is less reliable in small full-thickness tears and partial-thickness tears.

Treatment

Nonsurgical Treatment

Patients with rotator-cuff damage and impingement syndrome are initially treated with nonoperative techniques. The only exceptions are young patients first seen with an acute traumatic tear of the cuff. The goal of nonoperative treatment is to restore rotator-cuff function and eliminate pain. At least 3 months of conservative treatment is indicated before any surgical intervention is warranted.

Activity modification should be instituted so that painful motion is avoided. Ice massage is recommended after activity and shoulder rehabilitation exercises. Nonsteriodal anti-inflammatory drugs (NSAIDs) and occasional cortisone injections into the subacromial space may be given to reduce the inflammatory response of the tendon and subacromial bursa. Cortisone injections should be used judiciously and only after 6 to 8 weeks of conservative treatment. Careful avoidance of intratendinous injections is necessary to minimize the risk of tendon rupture. Excessive use of injections will compromise the integrity of the tendon and make repair more difficult. No definitive evidence indicates that cortisone injections alter or improve the outcome in rotator-cuff disorders and impingement syndrome.

The cornerstone of treatment of rotator-cuff damage and impingement is a focused shoulder-rehabilitation program designed to strengthen the rotator cuff and periscapular muscles and maximize their function. This will bring the humeral head back down into its functional position in the glenoid and will thereby reduce the amount of rotator-cuff impingement. The program begins with pendulum exercises and passive range-of-motion exercises. Once motion is restored, rotator-cuff and periscapular strengthening is begun.

In elderly, less active patients with partial-thickness rotator-cuff tears, nonoperative treatment will often result in good function. In patients with stage I rotator-cuff impingement, nonoperative techniques are usually successful; however, if pain and disability persist after an appropriate interval of nonoperative treatment, further workup is indicated to determine whether surgical intervention is needed.

Surgical Treatment

Surgical management of impingement syndrome consists of subacromial decompression and release of the coracohumeral ligament. Decompression can be performed with open surgery or arthroscopy. Arthroscopic decompression is associated with a lower morbidity rate and a quicker rehabilitation and return of motion. In addition, arthroscopy allows the evaluation of the glenohumeral joint. Most studies have shown good to excellent results with open surgery or arthroscopy.

In patients with symptomatic acromioclavicular arthrosis, distal clavicle excision may be indicated. This also can be performed with open surgery or arthroscopy. Undersurface acromioclavicular osteophytes may be debrided during arthroscopic subacromial decompression.

In patients with massive rotator cuffs (cuffs that exceed 5 cm in size), direct surgical repair of cuff tears may not be possible. Options for management include subacromial decompression and cuff débridement, autograft and allograft reconstruction, and tendon transfer.

In patients with normal-sized rotator cuffs and partial-thickness cuff tears, treatment may consist of subacromial decompression and cuff débridement or may consist of acromioplasty and cuff débridement. Successful results have been reported with both techniques.

In patients with normal-sized rotator cuffs and full-thickness cuff tears, subacromial decompression is routinely performed. Open surgical repair is the standard treatment if the tear is large and complex or if evidence exists of cuff retraction. A "mini" open repair, which combines arthroscopic subacromial decompression with a small incision for the cuff repair, can be used if the tear is small and is not retracted. Arthroscopic repair also has been used for small tears. After subacromial decompression and cuff repair have been performed, pendulum exercises and assisted motion are begun immediately. Active motion should be delayed for 4 to 6 weeks after repair.

Complications

Poor results after repair of torn rotator cuffs have been associated with inadequate decompression and continued cuff impingement. Repair of repeated cuff tears is associated with a worse outcome than is repair of initial cuff tears.

Acromioclavicular Joint Injuries

Etiology and Classification

Injuries to the acromioclavicular joint range from simple sprains to complete dislocations. They may result from direct force to the joint caused by a fall onto the shoulder or from indirect force caused by a fall onto the outstretched hand.

In the most common classification system, acromioclavicular joint injuries are divided into six types. **Type I injuries** are acromioclavicular sprains. **Type II injuries** are acromioclavicular ligament tears with coracoclavicular ligament sprains. **Type III injuries** are tears of both the acromioclavicular and coracoclavicular ligaments. **Type IV injuries** are type III injuries with the coracoclavicular ligament avulsed and the distal clavicle displaced posteriorly into or through the trapezius. **Type V injuries** are type III injuries with the clavicle severely displaced superiorly. **Type VI injuries** are type III injuries with the clavicle displaced inferiorly and laterally beneath the acromion and with the deltoid and trapezius muscles detached from the distal clavicle.

Evaluation

In type I injuries, findings on physical examination include local tenderness and swelling of the acromioclavicular joint, with no palpable deformity. Anteroposterior radiographs of the acromioclavicular joint show normal results.

In type II injuries, examination reveals the presence of subluxation of the acromioclavicular joint. The clavicle is mobile and tender on palpation at the acromioclavicular joint and in the coracoclavicular space. Motion of the shoulder causes localized acromioclavicular joint pain. Anteroposterior radiographs show the clavicle to be slightly higher than the acromion and the acromioclavicular joint space to be slightly wider. Stress films yield normal results.

In type III injuries, pain is felt in the acromioclavicular joint and coracoclavicular space and is exacerbated with any shoulder motion. Anteroposterior radiographs demonstrate that the clavicle is superior to the acromion, and stress views demonstrate an increased coracoclavicular space.

In type IV injuries, patients have all the physical findings seen in type III injuries. In addition, the clavicle is displaced posteriorly, and it may tent the skin if it buttonholes through the trapezius. Axillary radiographs or CT scans demonstrate posterior displacement.

In type V injuries, findings are an exaggeration of type III findings. The clavicle is grossly displaced, and tenting of the skin is present. The extremity is displaced downward, and occasional traction brachial plexopathies can result. Radiographs demonstrate an increase in the coracoclavicular space to be 100% to 300% as compared with that of the normal shoulder.

In type VI injuries, the shoulder appears flat, and the acromion is prominent. Brachial plexus injuries, rib fractures, and clavicle fractures may be present. Imaging studies show the clavicle to be in either a subacromial or subcoracoid position.

Treatment

Nonsurgical Treatment

In patients with a type I, II, or III injury, symptoms are treated with analgesics, ice, and a sling. Range of motion may be instituted after 1 or 2 weeks, when the patient feels comfortable moving the arm. Although some recommend surgical treatment for type III injuries, long-term results in those treated nonoperatively are satisfactory and do not justify surgical intervention.

Surgical Treatment

In patients with a type IV, V, or VI injury, surgery is indicated. It usually consists of open reduction of the clavicle and repair of the coracoclavicular ligament to restore vertical stability to the clavicle. Coracoclavicular fixation is provided by a Dacron suture, wire loop, screw, or ligament transfer.

Soft Tissue Injuries of the Knee

Meniscal Tears

Etiology and Classification

Meniscal tears are rare in children younger than 10 years, but they are one of the most common knee injuries in adolescents and adults. Most meniscal tears result from twisting or rotational forces during weight-bearing or sporting activities. Knee instability secondary to an anterior cruciate ligament (ACL) tear will frequently lead to a meniscal tear.

Several systems exist for classifying meniscal tears. Based on their orientation, meniscal tears are classified as **bucket-handle, radial, horizontal,** and **longitudinal tears.** Based on their placement, they are classified as **displaced** and **nondisplaced tears.** Based on their location, they can be classified as **red-zone, white-zone,** and **red-and-white zone tears.** The red zone of the meniscus is peripheral and has a blood supply, so tears in this zone have the best healing potential. The white zone is avascular, so tears in this zone do not heal. The decision about whether to attempt repair of a meniscal tear should take the zone into account.

Evaluation

History and Physical Examination. Symptoms of a meniscal tear may be intermittent and vague. Swelling typically occurs 2 or 3 days after a tear, and the patient may complain of tenderness localized to the joint line. A clicking sensation may be reported. Complaints of buckling, giving way, or locking of the knee suggest a mobile fragment or bucket-handle tear. An inability to extend the knee fully also suggests a bucket-handle tear.

Whenever a meniscal tear is suspected, the knee joint, knee ligaments, and patellofemoral mechanism should be evaluated. Knee examination may reveal an effusion. Palpation along the medial or lateral joint line commonly elicits pain, and pain may be exacerbated by fully flexing the knee or squatting. In the McMurray test for meniscal tears, a rotational force and valgus or varus stress are applied while the knee is extended. If the meniscus is torn, it will be trapped under the femoral condyle, and this will cause an audible click or snap. In the Apley grind test, the patient is prone, and the knee is flexed to 90 degrees. The tibia is rotated while a compression force is applied across the knee joint. This may reproduce the painful sensation of a torn meniscus. Neither the McMurray test nor the Apley grind test is specific to meniscal tears.

Imaging Studies. Plain radiographs in anteroposterior, lateral, and merchant views should be obtained but usually yield normal results. MRI is the best noninvasive test for demonstrating a torn meniscus (Fig. 44-2).

Treatment

In patients with asymptomatic degenerative tears, non-operative treatment may be appropriate. In other patients with meniscal tears, surgery is usually indicated and is most often performed arthroscopically.

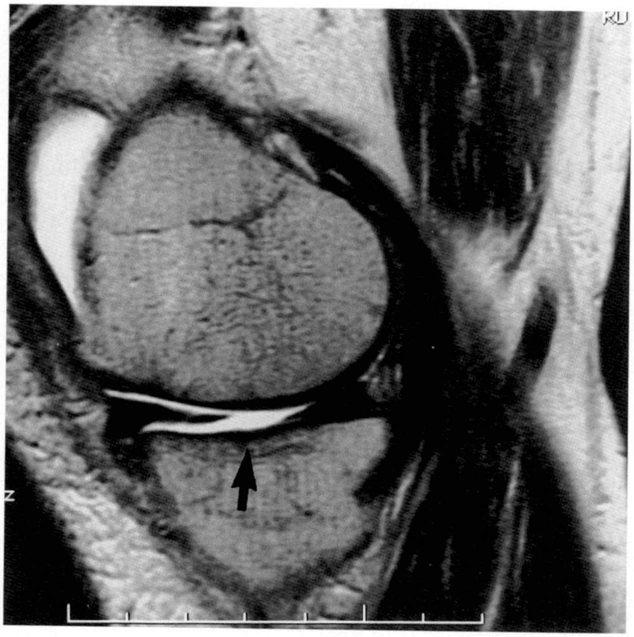

FIGURE 44–2 Magnetic resonance imaging of knee with meniscus tear.

For meniscal tears that are peripheral longitudinal tears in the red zone, surgical repair is appropriate. Meniscal tears heal more reliably in those with ACL tears if they are repaired simultaneously with ACL reconstruction. Suturing techniques include inside-out, all-inside, and outside-in suturing. Nonabsorbable sutures are the most reliable. The newer absorbable darts, anchors, and arrows may be used to augment suture repairs. In cases of an isolated repair of a torn meniscus, the knee is immobilized in flexion, and the patient is generally advised to avoid weight bearing for 3 to 6 weeks.

Tears that occur in the white zone do not reliably heal. These are often treated arthroscopically by partial meniscectomy. Minimizing the amount of excised meniscus may diminish the risk of later developing osteoarthritis. After resection of a meniscal tear, patients should be encouraged to undertake range-of-motion exercises and weight bearing as tolerated.

Complications

During repair of a lateral meniscal tear, the peroneal nerve may be injured while the sutures are passed or the knots are tied. During repair of a medial meniscal tear, the saphenous nerve is at risk of injury. Implanted devices may break or become loose within the knee.

Anterior Cruciate Ligament Tears

Etiology

Tears of the ACL most often result from a noncontact injury with a pivoting, decelerating, or cutting maneuver. ACL tears are frequently accompanied by other ligament or soft tissue injuries about the knee.

Evaluation

History and Physical Examination. Patients often report feeling a popping sensation when the ACL is torn. Hemarthrosis causes immediate swelling of the knee, and pain and guarding of the knee may make it difficult to examine the knee and check for associated injuries, including neurovascular injuries and dislocations. Several tests can be used to detect a torn ACL. The Lachman test, which is the most sensitive, examines forward translation of the tibia when the femur is stabilized and the knee is flexed 20 degrees. The pivot shift test detects anterior subluxation of the tibia when the knee is extended and reduction when the knee is flexed. Abduction and external rotation during leg extension may increase tibial subluxation. The anterior drawer test examines how far forward the tibia can be drawn when the knee is flexed 90 degrees.

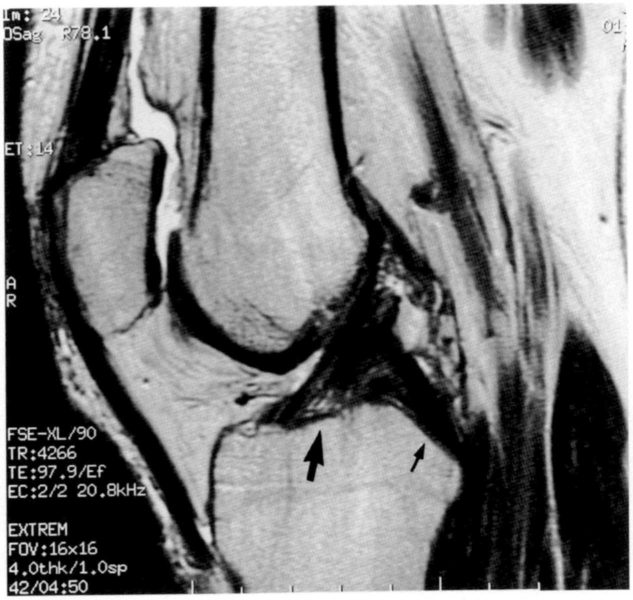

FIGURE 44–3 Magnetic resonance imaging of normal knee with intact anterior cruciate ligament and posterior cruciate ligament.

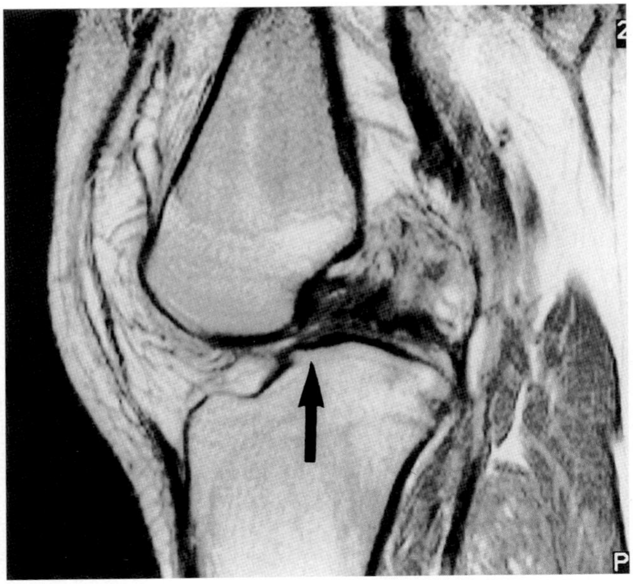

FIGURE 44–4 Magnetic resonance imaging of knee with anterior cruciate ligament tear.

Imaging Studies. In patients with an acute knee injury, initial imaging studies include plain radiographs with anteroposterior, lateral, and oblique views. An ACL injury is suggested by the radiographic finding of an avulsion fracture of the lateral tibial margin (Segond fracture) or an avulsion fracture of the tibial spine. MRI should be performed to evaluate the ACL and to assess further any associated injuries (Figs. 44-3 and 44-4). MRI is able to detect about 98% of ACL tears but is less frequently able to distinguish complete tears from partial tears.

Treatment

Whether a torn ACL is treated surgically or nonsurgically depends on the patient's activity level and age, the degree of knee instability caused by the tear, and the presence of associated injuries.

Nonsurgical Treatment. For patients who are willing to avoid high-demand activities that involve jumping, pivoting, or heavy manual labor, nonoperative treatment may be appropriate. The goal is to eliminate recurrent knee instability. The hamstring muscles are agonists of the ACL, and strengthening the thigh muscles and gastrocnemius complex through a physical therapy program may reduce the instability of the knee. Proprioceptive training may help restore function of the knee. Functional bracing may offer support and may also provide resistance to tibial translation at low loads. However, bracing may diminish normal reaction times, and buckling episodes often continue.

PEARLS FOR ROUNDS

The rotator cuff is composed of the tendons of the supraspinatus, infraspinatus, teres minor, and subscapularis muscles.

Symptoms of shoulder instability are more frequently seen in athletes involved in overhead sports activities than in the general population.

In all cases of acute dislocation of the shoulder, a thorough assessment of the neurovascular status of the limb must be done before attempts at reduction. Vascular injuries occur more frequently in older patients after an acute dislocation and may result in ischemia of the extremity.

Magnetic resonance imaging is the most sensitive and specific study for diagnosing full-thickness and partial-thickness rotator-cuff tears, cuff degeneration, and tendinopathy.

Most meniscal tears of the knee result from twisting or rotational forces during weight-bearing or sporting activities. Knee instability secondary to an anterior cruciate ligament (ACL) tear will frequently lead to a meniscal tear.

Tears of the ACL most often result from a noncontact injury in which a pivoting, decelerating, or cutting maneuver takes place. ACL tears are frequently accompanied by other ligament or soft tissue injuries about the knee.

Ankle sprains are the most common athletic injury. An inversion of the ankle typically causes damage to ligaments in the lateral ligament complex.

Surgical Treatment. ACL reconstruction reliably restores ACL function. After the acute injury, reconstruction is delayed until inflammation subsides and the normal range of motion is restored. A delay of at least 3 weeks has been shown to reduce the postoperative risk of arthrofibrosis.

Arthroscope-assisted surgery is currently the standard technique used for ACL reconstruction. An autologous bone-patella-bone (BPB) graft or an autologous or allogeneic tendon graft can be used. Tendons that are commonly grafted include the achilles, semitendinous, and gracilis tendons. When an autologous BPB graft is used, the central 10 mm of the patellar tendon is harvested, along with the bony attachments to the tibial tubercle and patella. Autologous tendons are harvested from the ipsilateral knee and are double-looped.

Tibial and femoral tunnels are made through the native ACL origin and insertion sites, and the grafts are then fixed within these tunnels. Joint laxity can be decreased by tensioning the graft before the tibial side of the graft is fixed.

Postoperative rehabilitation focuses on exercises to prevent stiffness and restore the full range of motion and quadriceps strength. A brace is used, and the patient is encouraged to begin weight bearing as tolerated. It generally takes 6 to 9 months before the patient can return to sports activities. The likelihood that patients will return to their preinjury sports level is high. Over time, progressive laxity may ensue, resulting in increased instability.

Complications

Stiffness often develops in patients who undergo immediate surgery, rather than waiting for the return of full motion of the knee. Complications after ACL reconstruction include failure of graft incorporation, pain associated with the presence of hardware, and problems related to malpositioned tunnels. Most often, the femoral tunnel is placed too far forward, and this results in loss of knee extension. The incidence of postoperative anterior knee pain and patellar fractures is higher in patients who undergo BPB reconstruction than in those who undergo other types of reconstruction. Few complaints are made regarding the donor site in patients with hamstring grafts.

Posterior Cruciate Ligament Tears

Injuries of the posterior cruciate ligament (PCL) are much less common than are those of the ACL. PCL injuries can result from hyperextension of the foot or from hyperflexion when the foot is planted. They also can result from a direct injury to the anterior tibia, as occurs with automobile accidents in which a passenger's leg strikes the dashboard or a pedestrian's leg is struck by the bumper of a car. Tears of the posterolateral ligament complex of the knee are the most common associated injury. In patients with a knee dislocation, a combination of tears of the PCL, ACL, and medial collateral ligament may be found.

Evaluation

PCL injuries usually do not cause knee instability, and high levels of activity may be possible with an isolated PCL tear. However, because PCL tears subject the medial compartment of the knee to higher loading pressures, these tears are associated with an increased incidence of patellofemoral pain and degenerative changes.

If the PCL is torn, a posterior sag of the tibia is seen when the knee is flexed 90 degrees. The sag is due to posterior subluxation of the tibia. The most sensitive test for detecting a torn PCL is the posterior drawer test, which examines how far back the tibia can be drawn when the knee is flexed 90 degrees. The quadriceps active drawer test will demonstrate anterior tibial translation when the knee is flexed 90 degrees and the quadriceps muscle is activated. If the posterolateral complex also is torn, increased external rotation of the foot will be present when checked from a prone position.

Treatment

Nonsurgical Treatment. In most cases, an isolated PCL injury is treated nonsurgically, with management focusing on strengthening the quadriceps muscle.

Surgical Treatment. PCL reconstruction may be indicated in high-level athletes if more than 10 mm of posterior tibial translation exists, and this causes knee pain. PCL reconstruction also may be indicated in patients with combined injuries of the PCL and other ligamentous structures. Grafts for PCL reconstruction include BPB and hamstring autografts and allografts. With a combined injury of the PCL and the posterolateral complex, repair of both is generally necessary. With a combined injury of the PCL and medial collateral ligament (MCL), repair of both is indicated.

Medial Collateral Ligament Tears

Injuries of the MCL result from a valgus strain on the knee. The origin of the MCL on the medial femoral condyle is the most common site of the injury.

Evaluation

If an MCL injury is present, the application of valgus stress on the knee when it is flexed 30 degrees will reproduce medial pain. The injury is classified on the basis of the amount of medial joint opening observed during this maneuver. In **grade I injuries,** the opening is less than 5 mm. In **grade II injuries,** it is 6 to 10 mm. In **grade III injuries (complete tears),** it is more than 10 mm.

Treatment

In all cases of isolated MCL injuries, nonoperative treatment with NSAIDs and support devices is indicated. Patients with grade I injuries are advised to use crutches until they are comfortable without them. Patients with grade II injuries should use a hinged knee brace with crutches for

PEARLS FOR THE OR

After the reduction of an anterior or posterior dislocation, it is necessary to assess the stability of the shoulder and to reassess the neurovascular status of the extremity.

If a shoulder dislocation occurs in association with avulsion of the rotator cuff, early surgery is indicated to remove interposed bone fragments and soft tissues.

Anterior cruciate ligament (ACL) reconstruction reliably restores ACL function, and arthroscopy-assisted surgery is currently the standard technique used for ACL reconstruction.

several weeks, whereas those with grade III injuries should use these devices for 3 to 4 weeks. Patients should begin weight bearing as tolerated, and rehabilitation of the thigh muscles should be stressed. On average, it takes 6 weeks for a torn MCL to heal.

Posterolateral Complex Injuries

The posterolateral complex of the knee consists of the lateral collateral ligament (LCL), the popliteus tendon and its attachments, the arcuate ligament, the biceps tendon, and the lateral head of the gastrocnemius muscle. The LCL is the primary restraint against varus instability.

Injuries to the posterolateral complex are uncommon. When they do occur, they are usually the result of direct trauma to the medial knee or anteromedial tibia when the foot is planted. They also may be seen after knee dislocations in which both the ACL and PCL are torn.

Evaluation

Patients with posterolateral complex injuries complain of knee instability, which may be aggravated when they descend the stairs. Examination of the knee reveals increased external rotation of the tibia at 30 and 90 degrees of knee flexion. A reverse pivot shift may be present. Posterior drawer recurvatum and varus instability also may be found. In about 10% of cases, a peroneal nerve is injured and causes ankle- and foot-extensor weakness.

Treatment

In patients with acute injuries of the posterolateral complex, surgical repair of each of the injured structures is indicated. This should be done within several weeks of the injury. In patients with chronic injuries and symptoms of knee instability, reconstructive surgery with autograft or allograft is indicated.

Ankle Sprains

Ankle sprains are the most common athletic injury. An inversion of the ankle typically causes damage to ligaments in the lateral ligament complex (Fig. 44-5). This complex

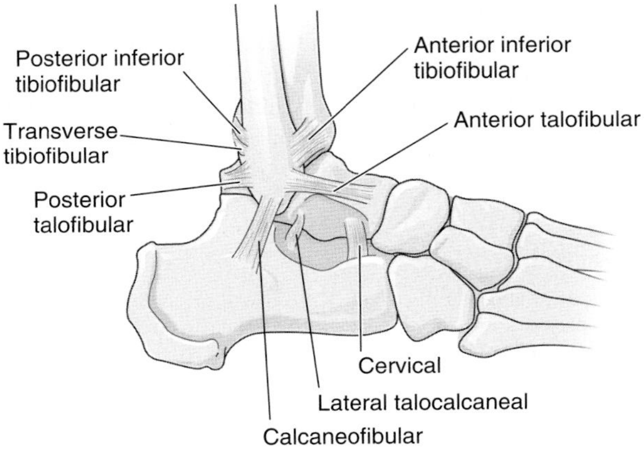

FIGURE 44–5 Diagram of lateral ankle ligaments.

includes the anterior talofibular ligament (which is most frequently injured), the calcaneofibular ligament, and the posterior talofibular ligament.

Evaluation

Physical examination is directed toward localizing the pain. Because of initial pain and inflammation, ligament laxity may be difficult to assess. Careful evaluation of the ankle should rule out other soft tissue injuries, such as Achilles tendon ruptures, injuries to the ankle syndesmoses, and peroneal tendon dislocations or tears. Evaluation also should include a search for fractures that can mimic ankle sprains. Radiographs are necessary in nearly every case. If the ankle injury does not heal as expected, further radiographic evaluation, possibly with the addition of MRI, CT scanning, or bone scanning, will be necessary to rule out an occult injury. Among the injuries that are not always obvious with standard ankle radiographs are osteochondral fractures of the talus and fractures of the lateral process of the talus, the anterior process of the calcaneus, the proximal fifth metatarsal, and the proximal fibula.

Treatment

Nonsurgical Treatment

Rest, ice, compression, and elevation (RICE) should be initiated as soon as the injury occurs. Cast immobilization may be necessary, with the length of treatment time depending on the degree of injury. Often functional bracing is implemented while the ligament(s) heal. Gradually, the leg should be used for weight bearing as tolerated. If peroneal muscle strength does not return to normal in the first few weeks, strengthening exercises should be instituted.

Surgical Treatment

Surgical repair is indicated if the ligaments heal in an elongated position, causing recurrent instability. Although surgical repair usually brings good results, reconstruction with other tissue is sometimes necessary. Some reconstructive operations use a portion of the peroneus brevis muscle and place it through bony tunnels in the fibula, talus, or calcaneus. This routing is meant to simulate the normal ligamentous architecture, but postoperative stiffness is sometimes a problem.

Suggested Reading

Albright JC, Carpenter JE, et al: Knee and Leg: Soft-Tissue Trauma. Orthopaedic Knowledge Update 6. Rosemont IL, American Academy of Orthopaedic Surgeons, 1999.

Andrew JG, Herrick AL, Marsh DR: Musculoskeletal Medicine and Surgery. Philadelphia, Churchill Livingstone, 2000.

Barnes CL, Barrack RL, et al: Knee Reconstruction. Orthopaedic Knowledge Update 6. Rosemont IL, American Academy of Orthopaedic Surgeons, 1999.

Enneking WF, Rathe R, et al: Clinical Musculoskeletal Pathology. Gainesville, FL, Office of Medical Informatics at the University of Florida, 1998.

Evans RP, Nelson CL, et al: Surgery of the Musculoskeletal System. New York, Churchill Livingstone, 1990.

Richards RR: Soft Tissue Reconstruction in the Upper Extremity. New York, Churchill Livingstone, 1995.

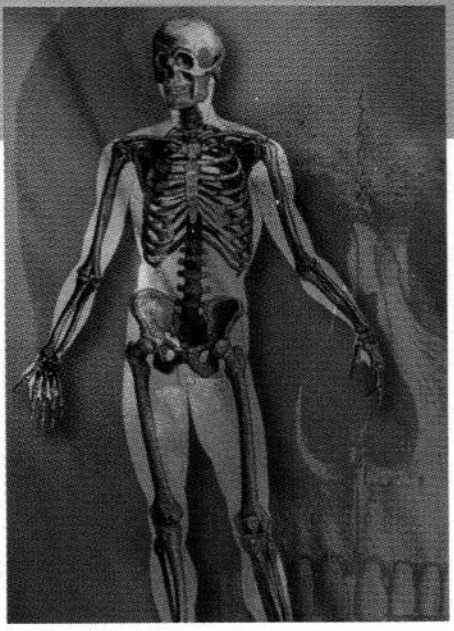

Chapter 45
Fractures

DONNA M. PACICCA, MD, RYAN R. SNYDER, MD, and
PETER DEWIRE, MD

Systems for Classifying Fractures

Numerous systems exist for classifying fractures. Common systems are based on etiology, fracture pattern, location, alignment, and associated injuries. Fractures classified on the basis of etiology include pathologic, traumatic, and stress fractures. **Pathologic fractures** are found in an area of bone that has been weakened by a disease process. These fractures commonly occur after some trivial injury and may occur spontaneously. **Traumatic fractures** result from a substantial impact on the bone. **Stress fractures** result from repeated low-level stress that exceeds the strength of the bone.

Fractures classified according to common patterns often reflect the mechanism of injury. Common fracture patterns include **spiral, oblique, transverse, compression, avulsion, segmental** (two separate fractures), **comminuted** (three or more fragments)**,** and **greenstick** (incomplete) **fractures.** Transverse and greenstick fractures result from a bending force, whereas spiral fractures follow a twisting injury. Greenstick fractures occur only in children.

Fractures are described according to their location as proximal-, middle-, or distal-third fractures. They also are described as intra-articular or extra-articular fractures.

Fractures are described by their alignment, displacement, and angular deformity in terms of the relation of the distal fragment to the proximal fragment. The amount of displacement is commonly expressed as a percentage of apposition of the fracture fragments. Associated characteristics, such as open fractures and fracture dislocation, are included in descriptions of fractures.

The Comprehensive Classification of Fractures of Long Bones applies to all long-bone fractures and is based on the work of the AO Foundation, a Swiss orthopedic group whose initial system of osteosynthesis has been the basis for current fracture treatment throughout the world. In this system, the three primary types are type A, extra-articular fractures; type B, partial articular fractures; and type C, complete articular fractures. Type A fractures are more easily treated than are types B and C. Type C fractures generally have a worse prognosis because of the amount of intra-articular damage.

Fractures associated with soft tissue injuries frequently are the result of high-energy injuries. Open fractures are often associated with other major trauma. The Gustilo classification of open fractures is the most widely used classification system and is described in Table 45-1.

Assessment of the **mangled extremity severity score (MESS) variables** listed in Table 45-2 can be used to predict whether a patient who has a serious injury of an extremity is likely to benefit most from limb amputation or a limb-salvage operation. Variables include the types of skeletal and soft tissue injuries, the limb ischemia time, the presence of shock, and the age of the patient. Patients with MESS scores of 7 or more are likely to require limb amputation, whereas those with scores lower than 7 are likely to have a functional limb after a limb-salvage operation.

Injuries of the Spine

Anatomy

The spine is composed of 33 vertebrae: 7 cervical, 12 thoracic, 5 lumbar, 5 sacral, and 4 coccygeal. Several

TABLE 45–1 Classification of Open Fractures

Type	Description
Type I	Skin opening of ≤ 1cm, quite clean. Most likely from inside to outside. Minimal muscle contusion. Simple transverse or short oblique fractures
Type II	Laceration >1 cm long, with extensive soft tissue damage, flaps, or avulsion. Minimal to moderate crushing component. Simple transverse or short oblique fractures with minimal comminution
Type III	Extensive damage to soft tissue, including muscles, skin and neurovascular structures. Often, a high-velocity injury with a severe crushing component
Type IIIA	Extensive soft tissue laceration with adequate bone coverage. Segmental fractures and gunshot injuries
Type IIIB	Extensive soft tissue injury with periosteal stripping and bone exposure. Usually associated with massive contamination
Type IIIC	Vascular injury requiring repair

Data from Gustilo RB, Mendoza RM, et al: Problems in the management of type III (severe) open fractures: A new classification of type III open fractures. J Trauma 24:742–746, 1984.

TABLE 45–2 Mangled Extremity Severity Score (MESS) Variables

Component	Points*
A. Skeletal and Soft Tissue Injury	
Low-energy injury (stab, simple fracture, or civilian gunshot wound)	1
Medium-energy injury (an open or multiple fractures or a dislocation)	2
High-energy injury (a close-range shotgun or military gunshot wound or a crush injury)	3
Very high energy injury (same as high-energy injury, plus gross contamination or soft tissue avulsion)	4
B. Limb Ischemia (Score Is Doubled if Ischemia Lasts Longer than 6 Hours)	
Pulse reduced or absent but perfusion normal	1
Pulseless, with paresthesia or diminished capillary refill	2
Cool, paralyzed, insensate, or numb	3
C. Shock	
Systolic blood pressure always >90 mmHg	0
Transient hypotension	1
Persistent hypotension	2
D. Age	
<30 yr	0
30–50 yr	1
>50 yr	2

*Patients with MESS scores of ≥7 are likely to require limb amputation, whereas those with scores <7 are likely to have a functional limb after a limb-salvage operation.

Data from Johansen K, Daines M, Howey T, et al: Objective criteria accurately predict amputation following lower extremity trauma. J Trauma 30:568–573, 1990.

landmarks are used to determine the spinal level and are helpful in determining the surgical approach. The C2–C3 interspace is at the level of the mandible; the hyoid cartilage is at C3; the thyroid cartilage at C4–C5; the cervical prominence at C7; the tip of the scapula at T7; and the iliac crest at L4–L5.

In the cervical spine, neural foramina are found within the transverse processes. The atlas (C1) does not have a body or spinous process but has two lateral masses that articulate with the superior facets of the axis (C2) and the occiput. The odontoid process of C2 projects superiorly and articulates with the atlas. The primary stabilizer of the atlantoaxial joint is the transverse ligament. Apical and alar ligaments are specialized ligaments that contribute to the stability of the atlanto-occipital joint.

The lumbar vertebrae are the largest in the spine. They have articular facets and short, stout laminae and pedicles. Each lumbar vertebra has a pair of transverse processes. Strong iliolumbar ligaments attach these transverse processes to the ilium. Fractures through the processes are seen in pelvic fractures.

Superior and inferior articular facets are present on each vertebra, and their orientation determines spinal mobility. The orientation of the spinal facets changes at each spinal level. Because the thoracic spine also has costal facets that articulate with the ribs, the thoracic spine is less mobile than either the cervical or the lumbar spine. Most pathologic changes are seen in the more mobile cervical and lumbar segments of the axial spine.

Anterior and posterior longitudinal ligaments run the length of the spinal column and the vertebral bodies and are responsible primarily for interspinous stability. The ligamenta flava (yellow ligaments) are short interspinous ligaments connecting each lamina. They contribute to nerve root impingement in degenerative diseases of the spine. Intervertebral disks are fibrocartilaginous structures between each pair of vertebrae. Each disk is composed of an anulus fibrosus and a nucleus pulposus.

The spinal cord runs from the brainstem to L1. The terminal portion of the spinal cord is the conus medullaris, which becomes the cauda equina at about the L2 level and is entirely enclosed within the spinal canal. The spinal nerves are formed from dorsal and ventral roots within the subarachnoid space. The nerve roots exit through the intervertebral foramen. In the cervical spine, the numbered root exits above the corresponding vertebral level (for example, the C4 root exits at C3–C4). In the lumbar spine, the nerve root exits beneath the pedicle of the same vertebra.

Surgical Techniques and Approaches

The surgical approach to the spine can be either posterior or anterior. The pathologic changes often determine which approach is chosen.

The **midline posterior approach to the cervical spine** is the most common approach and can be used for posterior fusions, diskectomies, reductions of facet dislocations, and nerve root explorations. In the posterior approach to the C1–C2 interspace, care must be taken to avoid injuring the greater occipital and the third occipital nerves as they cross the surgical field and to avoid damaging the vertebral artery that exits the transverse foramen to enter the occiput.

The **anterior approach to the cervical spine** exposes the spine from C3 to T1. This approach is used for disk excisions, interbody fusions, biopsies, and drainage procedures. The recurrent laryngeal nerve is at risk during this approach, particularly on the right side as it nears the trachea. Many surgeons therefore favor the left side for the anterior approach to the cervical spine.

The **midline posterior approach to the lumbar spine** allows access to all of the spinal elements. From this approach, diskectomies, spinal fusions, and nerve root explorations are possible.

The **anterior transperitoneal approach to the lumbar spine** allows access to the lower lumbar segments, whereas the anterolateral retroperitoneal approach allows access to the entire lumbar spine. These approaches are used for spinal decompressions, fusions, resections, and biopsies of the spine, in combination with either axial compression or distraction. The injury pattern often results from a combination of these forces.

Cervical Spine Fractures and Dislocations

Etiology and Classification

Injuries to the adult cervical spine occur at all levels. They most often result from a fall or motor vehicle accident in which a direct injury to the head causes flexion, extension, lateral bending, or rotation of the cervical spine.

Occiput-C1 dislocations result from distraction, hyperextension, or translation forces. The main stabilizer of the articulation between the occiput and C1 is the tectorial membrane, which is disrupted as a result of the injury. The dislocation is classified as either anterior or posterior, based on the relation of the occiput to C1. Anterior dislocations are the most common type. Associated injuries include lacerations of the chin and posterior pharynx and fractures of the mandible. Cranial nerve injuries, vertebral artery lacerations, and injuries to the first three cervical roots also are commonly seen and are frequently fatal.

Occipital condyle fractures may be seen simultaneously with C1 fractures. The mechanism of injury is compression or lateral bending, which fractures the condyle or causes an avulsion of the alar ligament. Cranial nerve palsies are often seen in association with occipital condyle fractures.

C1 fractures result from an axial load across the atlas in combination with a flexion or extension force. C1 fractures are classified as anterior arch, posterior arch, or combined anterior and posterior arch (Jefferson or burst) fractures. Although C1 fractures are generally not associated with neurologic damage, about 50% of them are associated with fractures in other parts of the cervical spine. The most common association is an odontoid fracture occurring with a posterior arch fracture. Fractures of the transverse process and inferior tubercle of C1 result from avulsion injuries.

C1–C2 traumatic instability is uncommon but can occur in association with a forced flexion injury. Disruption of the transverse ligament leads to subluxation of C1–C2. The normal interval between the atlas and dens (atlanto-dens interval, or ADI) is less than 3 mm. When the ADI is 3 to 5 mm, the transverse ligament is disrupted. When the ADI is greater than 5 mm, the alar ligament also is disrupted. Although dislocations are often fatal, a complete spectrum of neurologic injuries can be seen. Rotary subluxation and dislocation of the atlantoaxial joint occur when a flexion or extension force combines with rotation. In this case, torticollis and neck pain are frequently the presenting complaints, and neurologic injury is uncommon.

C2 fractures may involve the odontoid process, vertebral body, lateral mass, or isthmus. **Fractures of the odontoid process of C2** result from flexion, extension, and rotation forces and are grouped into three types, based on the Anderson and D'Alonzo classification system. In type 1 fractures (the least common type), the tip of the odontoid is avulsed. In type 2 fractures (the most common type), damage occurs to the base of the odontoid at the junction with the body of C2, and the rate of fracture nonunion is high if more than 5 mm of displacement or 11 degrees of angular deformity is found. In type 3 fractures, injury occurs through the body of C2. **Fractures of the lateral mass of C2** result from a compression injury, and neurologic deficits are uncommon. **Fractures through the isthmus of C2,** or **hangman's fractures,** lead to traumatic spondylolisthesis of the axis. These fractures may result from flexion or extension and an axial load or from hyperextension and distraction. They are usually seen in association with motor vehicle accidents, falls, or hanging. Accompanying injuries include fractures at another cervical spine level, rupture of the C2–C3 disk, unilateral or bilateral C2–C3 facet dislocation, and damage to the vertebral arteries and cranial nerves. Spinal cord injury is uncommon in nondisplaced injuries.

Fractures of C3–C7 are seen most frequently in association with blunt trauma, motor vehicle accidents, diving accidents, and falls. In the Allen and Ferguson classification system, the fractures are grouped according to mechanism of injury. The most common mechanism consists of compression and flexion.

Compression flexion injuries of the subaxial cervical spine cause progressive failure of the posterior structures in distraction and failure of the anterior structures in compression. These injuries progress from vertebral end plate fractures to complete displacement and comminution of the vertebral body and failure of the posterior ligament complex. **Compression extension injuries** can cause progressive injury from the posterior arch to the anterior vertebral body and ligamentous structures. **Vertical compression injuries** can burst the end plates of the vertebral bodies. In less severe injuries, no significant displacement occurs. However, with increasing forces, displacement of bone fragments into the neural canal may occur and result in neurologic injury. The most common injury level is the C6–C7 level (Fig. 45-1).

Distraction injuries of the subaxial cervical spine occur with flexion or extension. Distraction and flexion can cause failure of the posterior ligamentous structures. As a result, unilateral or bilateral facet dislocations or perched facets may be seen. With progressive anterior translation of the cephalad vertebral body, spinal canal narrowing occurs, leading to neurologic injury. A spinal cord injury is strongly associated with a sagittal canal diameter of less than 13 mm. Distraction and extension can cause failure of the anterior ligamentous structures or fracture of the anterior vertebral body. Widening of the anterior disk space results. As the

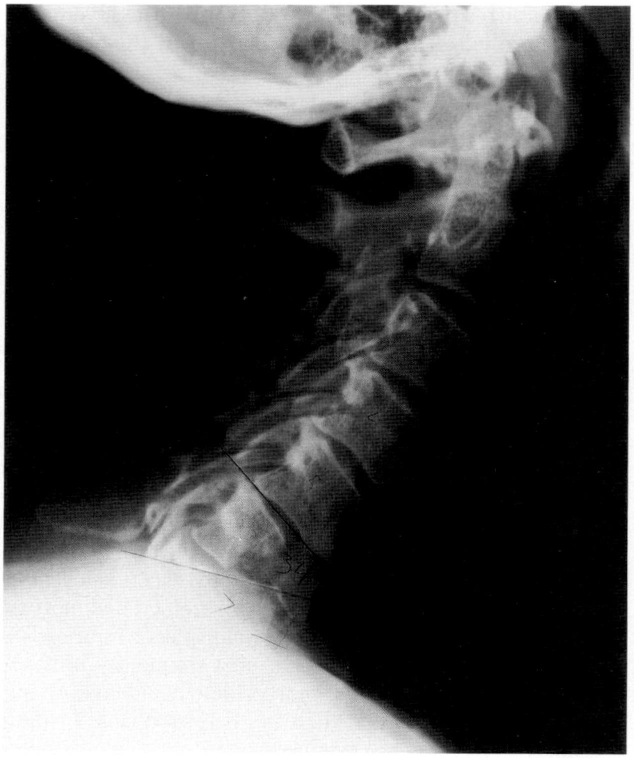

A

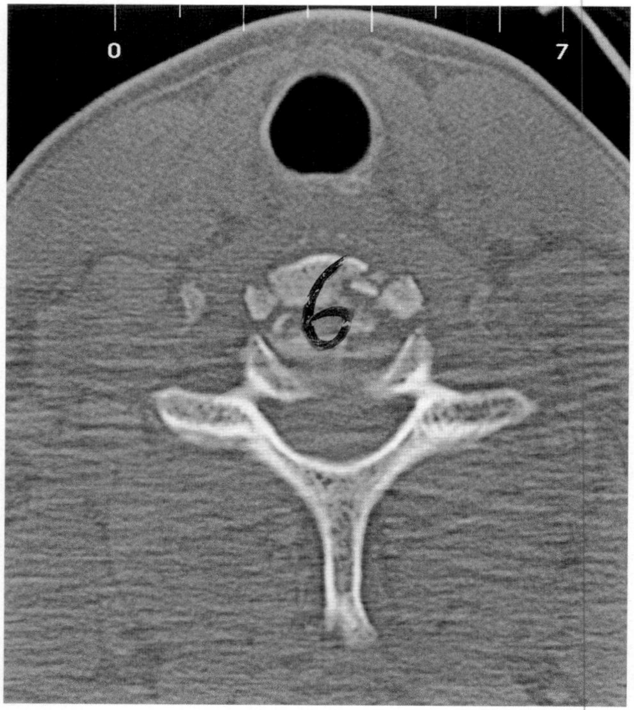

B

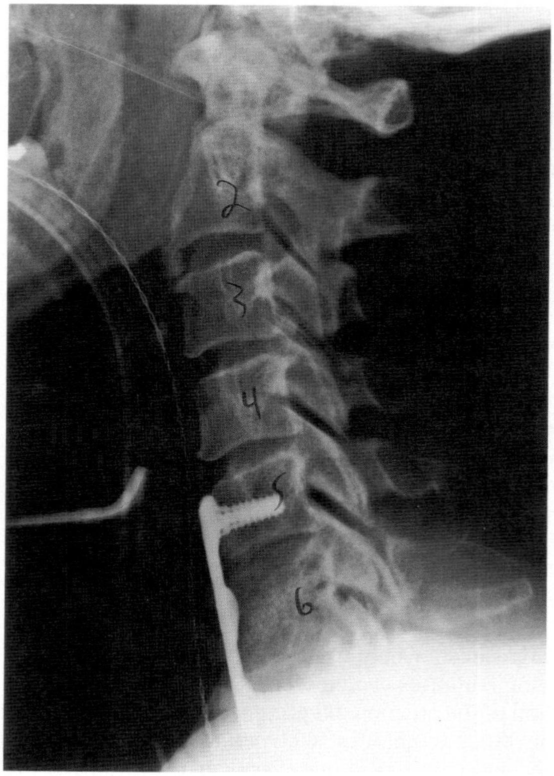

C

FIGURE 45–1 Radiographs of C6 burst fracture. *A*, Lateral C-spine. *B*, Computed tomography scan. *C*, After anterior corpectomy and fusion with instrumentation.

injury progresses, the posterior structures are injured, and posterior displacement of the superior vertebral body occurs.

Lateral flexion injuries of the subaxial cervical spine result from an asymmetrical injury to the side of the head. Ipsilateral arch and contralateral ligament injuries are seen. Displacement of either the arch or the articular facets on the side of the ligament injury may occur.

Avulsion fractures of the spinous process, or **clay shovelers' fractures,** result from flexion and are seen from C3 to T1. The most common site is C7, but C6 and T1 are also frequently affected.

Evaluation

Spinal injury should be suspected in any patient involved in a fall, an automobile accident, or other traumatic incident. Management begins at the site of the accident, where emergency medical technicians immobilize the spine for transport of the patient to a trauma center. Resuscitation and stabilization should follow the advanced trauma life support (ATLS) guidelines of the American College of Surgeons.

History and Physical Examination. After ATLS, a complete history and physical examination should be performed. Injuries to the face, head, neck, and abdomen should raise the suspicion of a concomitant spinal injury. Spinal examination requires that each level of the spine be palpated for tenderness, asymmetry, or step-off of the spinous processes. A thorough neurologic examination includes evaluation of sensation, motor strength, and reflexes (Box 45-1). Evaluations of rectal tone and perirectal sensation are required to assess for spinal shock. The presence of a bulbospongiosus (bulbocavernosus) reflex at the time of initial examination indicates that spinal shock is absent and that any neurologic deficit is due to spinal cord injury. The absence of the reflex indicates that spinal shock is present. Once the bulbospongiosus reflex returns, usually after 24 to 48 hours, spinal shock has ended, and neurologic deficits are attributable to structural cord damage.

Spinal cord injuries may cause complete or incomplete neurologic deficits. A **complete neurologic deficit** is characterized by the lack of sensory and motor function below the level of the injury. An **incomplete neurologic deficit** is characterized by the preservation of some spinal cord function below the level of the injury. Four recognized types of incomplete deficit are found:

1. The **central cord lesion,** which is the most common type, causes quadriplegia with sparing of the bowel and bladder function. Return of function is greater in the lower extremities than in the upper extremities.
2. The **anterior cord syndrome** preserves deep sensation and proprioception but causes loss of motor function and sensation. Motor function recovery is poor.
3. The **posterior cord syndrome** preserves motor function and sensation but causes loss of proprioception and deep pressure and pain sensation.
4. **Brown-Séquard's syndrome** is a unilateral cord injury that results in ipsilateral motor loss and contralateral sensory and temperature loss.

BOX 45–1 Patient Assessment in Spinal Injury

Major Sensory Levels (Nerve Root and Region of Innervation)

C4	Clavicle
C5	Deltoid region
C6	Radial forearm and thumb
C7	Middle finger
C8	Fifth finger
T1	Medial and proximal arm
T5	Nipples
T7	Costal margins
T10	Umbilicus
T12	Inguinal ligament
L3	Anterior thigh
L4	Medial aspect of knee
S1	Lateral foot and fifth toe
S2	Posterior thighs
S3–4	Buttocks and perianal regional

Major Motor Levels (Level, Muscle Group, and Action)

C5	Deltoid and shoulder rotators	Abduction of shoulder and external rotation of arm
C6	Biceps, brachial, and wrist extensors	Flexion of elbow
C7	Triceps and wrist flexors	Extension of elbow and wrist
C8	Intrinsic hand muscle	Abduction and adduction of fingers
L2–3	Iliopsoas	Hip flexion
L4	Quadriceps	Extension of knee
L5	Tibialis anterior and posterior and extensor hallucis longus	Dorsiflexion of foot and great toe
S1	Gastrocnemius	Plantar flexion of foot
S4–5	Anal sphincter	Voluntary contraction of anal sphincter

Segmental Reflexes (Level and Reflex)

C5	Biceps
C6	Brachioradialis
C7	Triceps
T7–10	Upper abdominal
T10–12	Lower abdominal
L1	Cremasteric
L4	Knee jerk
L5	Posterior tibial jerk
S1	Ankle jerk
S1–4	Bulbospongiosus (bulbocavernosus)
S4–5	Anocutaneous

Imaging Studies. In the emergency department, a lateral radiograph of the cervical spine should be obtained and must also include the C7–T1 level. Once the patient is stabilized, a complete set of cervical radiographs should be obtained, including an anteroposterior (AP) view and an odontoid view. Radiographic evaluation should focus on bone or soft tissue abnormalities and vertebral alignment. The normal distance between the basion and dens in an adult is 4 to 5 mm. Any increase in this distance suggests an occipitoatlantal dislocation. C1–C2 instability should be suspected if the lateral cervical spine radiograph shows an increase in the ADI. Rotary subluxations of C1–C2 should be suspected if an open-mouth view shows asymmetry of the lateral masses.

Other imaging studies to detect and evaluate soft tissue and spinal cord injuries include magnetic resonance imaging (MRI) and computed tomography (CT) scanning. Because some patients with cervical dislocations are unable to report neurologic symptoms during reduction of the dislocation, an MRI should be obtained before reduction. Occult fractures of the cervical spine are best detected by CT scanning.

Treatment

Injuries of C1 and C2. Occiput-C1 dislocations can be treated with halo immobilization or with fusion of the occiput to C2. It is critical to avoid overdistraction when using halo immobilization. Occipital condyle fractures are treated with a collar if they are stable or with a halo if they are unstable. C1 anterior arch and burst fractures are usually treated with halo immobilization, although chronic instability and pain are indications for a C1–C2 fusion. C1 posterior arch fractures are usually stable and can be treated with an orthosis. C1–C2 traumatic instability often requires treatment with a posterior fusion. C1–C2 dislocation and rotary subluxation require reduction with traction, followed by fusion or halo immobilization.

Management of C2 fractures depends not only on the type of fracture but also on whether any associated displacement or deformity is present. In type 1 fractures of the odontoid process, a cervical orthosis is indicated. In nondisplaced type 2 and type 3 fractures, halo immobilization for 12 weeks is indicated. In displaced type 2 fractures, reduction is required. If residual C1–C2 displacement larger than 5 mm, an angular deformity, or a nonunion is found, then a posterior spinal fusion should be performed. In nondisplaced fractures of the isthmus of C2, halo immobilization is indicated. In displaced and angulated fractures of the isthmus of C2, reduction and halo immobilization are necessary. If progressive neurologic deficits and an associated disk herniation are noted, anterior C2–C3 decompression and fusion are indicated. If severe angulation and facet dislocations are present, posterior C1–C2 fusion is indicated.

Injuries of C3–C7. In flexion compression injuries of the subaxial cervical spine, when the middle and posterior columns remain intact, the cervical spine remains stable and therefore can be treated with a halo for 8 to 12 weeks. However, when the middle and posterior columns are disrupted, surgical treatment may be necessary to prevent late deformity. Surgical treatment includes an anterior corpectomy and interbody fusion. A posterior fusion also may be necessary if posterior dislocation or instability is present.

In vertical compression injuries of the subaxial cervical spine, patients without neurologic deficits can usually be treated adequately with halo immobilization. Patients with neurologic deficits usually require anterior decompression and fusion.

In distraction injuries of the subaxial cervical spine, treatment depends on whether the injury occurs with flexion or extension. Distraction flexion injuries are unstable and are often associated with disk herniation. They should be treated with closed reduction and posterior fusion. MRI should be performed before reduction in the presence of an incomplete neurologic deficit and unilateral or bilateral facet dislocations. In distraction extension injuries with an intact posterior longitudinal ligament, halo immobilization is adequate. Anterior decompression and fusion with a cervical plate are necessary when the posterior longitudinal ligament also is injured.

Lateral flexion injuries of the subaxial cervical spine require open stabilization procedures when ligament injuries result in instability or when displacement of the arch is found.

Thoracolumbar Injuries

Because the thoracolumbar junction is the most mobile segment, the majority of spinal injuries occur at this level. Associated injuries to the chest, head, abdomen, pelvis, and lower extremities are common. Neurologic injuries caused by trauma to the thoracic spine are usually complete. Injuries at the thoracolumbar junction affect the conus, and injuries to the lumbar spine affect the cauda equina and nerve root.

Injuries of the spinal column may be stable or unstable. If left untreated, an unstable spine can cause pain, neurologic deterioration, and progressive spinal deformity. The model most commonly used in the clinical and biomechanical assessment of spinal stability is the Denis three-column model of the spine. According to this model, spine instability results from an injury that affects at least two of the following three columns: (1) the anterior column, which consists of the anterior longitudinal ligament, anterior vertebral body, and anterior annulus; (2) the middle column, which consists of the posterior longitudinal ligament, posterior vertebral body, and posterior annulus; and (3) the posterior column, which consists of the pedicles, laminae, and spinous and transverse processes.

Etiology and Classification

Injuries to the thoracolumbar spine are most often associated with falls and motor vehicle accidents. The injuries may result from flexion, rotation, compression, distraction, shear forces, or a combination of these mechanisms. The most frequent combinations are flexion-rotation and flexion-distraction. The basic fracture patterns include compression fractures, burst fractures, seat-belt injuries, and fracture dislocations. Isolated minor fractures of the lamina, pars interarticularis, or spinous process also may occur.

Compression fractures damage the anterior column and may cause a distraction injury of the posterior column, particularly if significant flexion occurs at the time of injury. Compression fractures involve the superior end plate, inferior end plate, or both. They are generally not associated with spinal cord injuries or neurologic deficits.

Burst fractures occur if an axial load is applied when the spine is relatively straight. The anterior and middle columns are generally damaged. With severe burst fractures, the posterior column also may be injured, leading to fractures of the facet, lamina, or spinous process. Fracture fragments may compromise the spinal canal, resulting in variable neurologic compromise. Spinal instability may eventually lead to a kyphotic deformity.

In **flexion-distraction injuries**, or **seat-belt injuries,** the axis of rotation is anterior to the spine. The anterior column acts as a hinge, and tension causes the posterior column to fail. The force disrupts either the disk or the vertebral body (Chance fracture). This results in failure of the middle column and an unstable fracture pattern.

Flexion-rotation injuries cause fracture dislocations and failure of all three columns. This is the most unstable pattern of injuries to the thoracolumbar spine. The anterior column fails under compression, with tearing of the anterior longitudinal ligament or annulus. The posterior column fails as a result of a facet fracture, dislocation, or disruption of posterior ligamentous supports. Shear stress contributes to the degree of injury. Flexion-rotation injuries are frequently associated with significant neurologic deficits.

Evaluation

The initial management of patients with thoracolumbar injuries is the same as that for patients with cervical spine injuries (see earlier) and includes immobilization, resuscitation, and stabilization. Careful attention should be paid to the abdominal examination, as patients often have associated hollow viscus injury.

History and Physical Examination. Patients must have a complete neurologic examination. They should be gently rolled over ("log-rolled") to inspect the back for deformity and ecchymoses, to palpate the spine for pain, and to palpate for step-off of the spinous processes.

Imaging Studies. Radiographs of the thoracic spine, thoracolumbar junction, and lumbosacral spine should be obtained and should include lateral cross-table radiographs of the thoracolumbar spine. MRI and CT scanning of the involved area of the spine should be performed to evaluate fully the spinal canal, spinal cord, and associated bone and soft tissue injuries.

Treatment

Management of thoracolumbar injuries depends on the nature of the injury, associated neurologic deficits, and stability of the spine.

Nonsurgical Treatment. A stable injury without neurologic deficits or with a stable neurologic deficit can be treated nonoperatively. Orthotics may be prescribed to decrease the mobility of the spine and are indicated in some compression fractures, flexion-distraction injuries, and extension-distraction injuries. A variety of braces are available and include the thoracolumbosacral orthosis (TLSO), hyperextension, Jewett, and corset types. The Jewett brace does not immobilize the spine below the thoracolumbar junction. Custom-molded braces can immobilize the lower lumbar spine if a leg extension is added. Hyperextension bracing is used to treat flexion-distraction injuries in which the anterior longitudinal ligament is intact. It is also used to treat compression fractures with more than 50% loss of anterior vertebral height or more than 30 degrees of kyphosis. When multiple consecutive compression fractures exist, bracing may reduce the development of a progressive kyphotic deformity.

Surgical Treatment. Surgical management of thoracolumbar injuries is indicated if the patient has an unstable spine or has progressive or complete neurologic deficit. In patients with incomplete neurologic deficit, decompression and stabilization of the spine may prevent further neurologic loss and allow some recovery of function. In patients with complete neurologic deficit, decompression of the spinal cord at the level of the injury does not significantly alter the outcome of the neurologic loss, but it does allow early mobilization.

Although some burst fractures can be treated nonoperatively with a customized TLSO, surgical management of burst fractures is indicated if deformity of more than 20 degrees, a loss of 40% or more of the vertebral body height, or a neurologic injury is found. It also is indicated if retropulsion of fracture fragments into the spinal canal reduces the canal size by more than 50%.

Fracture dislocations of the thoracolumbar spine are treated surgically, and this allows early mobilization. Either an anterior or a posterior approach may be used for decompression and fusion, but the most common approach is the posterior one. A posterior lateral fusion instrumented with hooks and rods across the level of injury will stabilize the spine and prevent further injury. The canal may be decompressed indirectly through the use of distraction instrumentation or directly by the posterolateral or transpedicle approach. It is important to assess the disk and check for bony fragments to ensure that distraction does not lead to disk herniation and further neurologic insult. Direct decompression is used in injuries below the conus at L1. Segmental fixation with pedicle screws also may be used to fuse the spine. Bone grafting is necessary in addition to the instrumentation, and autologous iliac crest bone grafting is preferred.

Failure to obtain adequate posterior stabilization or decompression is an indication for an anterior decompression and fusion. The anterior approach also may be used in the management of unstable thoracolumbar injuries. Because large central fragments are not easily removed by posterior decompression, anterior decompression is preferred. Cages and screw-and-plate devices may be safely used for anterior stabilization.

Clavicle Fractures

Etiology and Classification

Fractures of the clavicle most commonly result from a direct fall onto the shoulder. These fractures involve the middle third in most of the cases. The fractures are stable and tend to heal well, with a low risk of nonunion. High-energy injuries and open fractures of the clavicle are more commonly associated with neurovascular injury and nonunion.

Evaluation

History and Physical Examination

The patient with a clavicle fracture is seen after a fall onto the shoulder or outstretched hand. Examination reveals localized tenderness of the affected area. Deformity is often present, and tenting of the skin may occur. Crepitus at the fracture can be elicited with palpation. Examination of distal pulses and a neurologic examination of the affected extremity should be performed routinely in any patient with a clavicle fracture.

Imaging Studies

AP radiographs of the clavicle will demonstrate most fractures.

Treatment

Nonsurgical Treatment

Treatment with a sling or figure-of-eight brace will result in fracture healing in more than 95% of patients.

Surgical Treatment

Indications for open treatment include open fractures and injuries to the subclavian vessels. Clavicle fractures associated with scapulothoracic dissociation should be treated with internal fixation. Surgical treatment may be indicated in patients who show skin tenting but lack normal pain mechanisms. Painful nonunions of clavicle fractures are uncommon, but when they do occur, internal fixation is necessary. Plate fixation with a 3.5-mm compression plate gives the optimal results. Intramedullary wires are no longer used because of their high complication rate.

Proximal Humerus Fractures

Etiology and Classification

Fractures of the proximal humerus are common injuries. The most frequent cause is a fall in an elderly patient with osteoporosis. In younger patients, high-energy injuries account for most fractures of the proximal humerus. Dislocations of the humeral head may accompany these injuries.

Fractures may involve the humeral head, greater tuberosity, lesser tuberosity, and humeral shaft. The Neer classification of fracture patterns is based on the number of parts of the proximal humerus that are displaced more than 1 cm or angulated more than 45 degrees. Fractures through the anatomic neck are associated with a high incidence of avascular necrosis because these fractures disrupt the blood supply to the humeral head from the anterior circumflex arteries.

Evaluation

History and Physical Examination

Patients with a fracture or fracture dislocation of the proximal humerus are initially seen after a fall onto the outstretched arm or after a direct blow to the shoulder. Examination of the shoulder reveals pain, swelling, and possible deformity. A neurologic examination of the extremity is necessary to assess the brachial plexus. Vascular injury is suggested by the presence of an expanding axillary hematoma or diminished wrist pulses.

Imaging Studies

AP, scapular Y, and axillary radiographs should be taken. The axillary radiograph is the optimal view for assessing dislocations and checking the glenoid articular rim for fractures. CT scanning may be useful for evaluating articular fragments and for preoperative planning.

Treatment

Impacted, nondisplaced fractures that occur through the surgical neck are stable and are treated with a sling and early mobilization. When pain subsides, progressive range-of-motion and isometric exercises are begun.

Two-part Fractures

Treatment of two-part fractures of the proximal humerus will depend on a variety of factors, including the configuration and stability of the fracture and the age of the patient.

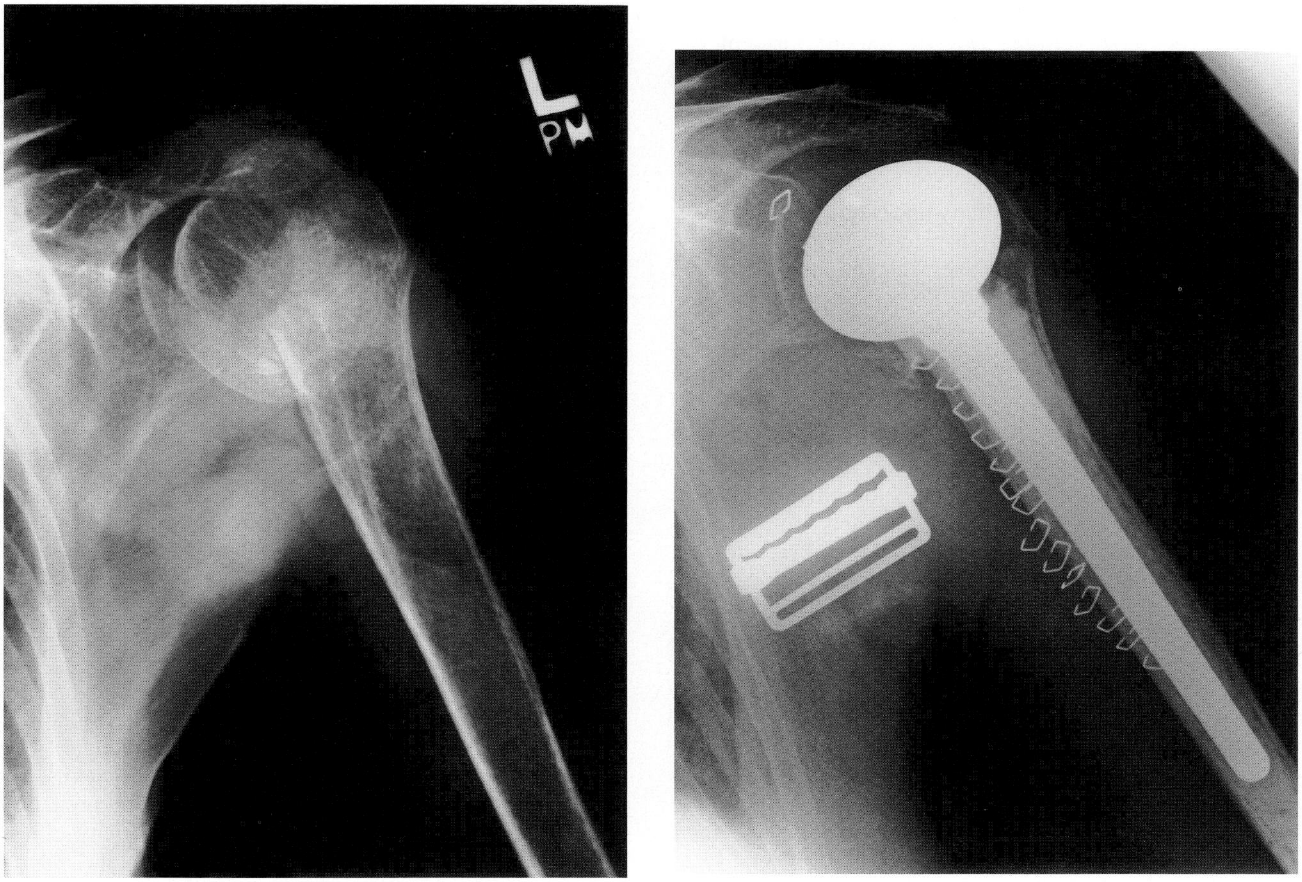

A B

FIGURE 45–2 Radiographs of a two-part anatomic neck proximal humerus fracture. *A*, After injury. *B*, After proximal humeral hemiarthroplasty.

In two-part fractures of the anatomic neck, the fracture occurs above the greater and lesser tuberosities (Fig. 45-2). Because the humeral head is split and its vascular supply is disrupted, a high risk is present of developing avascular necrosis of the humeral head. Prosthetic replacement is the treatment of choice in elderly patients, but open reduction and internal fixation are indicated in younger patients. In two-part fractures of the surgical neck, treatment depends on angulation and stability. If the parts are initially angulated more than 45 degrees, closed reduction should be performed. If the fracture is unstable after attempted reduction or is accompanied by multiple traumatic injuries, percutaneous pinning with 2.5-mm Schanz pins is indicated.

Two-part fractures of the greater tuberosity are accompanied by tears of the rotator cuff and require open reduction with internal fixation and cuff repair. If the greater tuberosity fracture is associated with anterior dislocation of the humeral head, a reduction of the anterior dislocation may reduce the greater tuberosity fragment. Two-part fractures of the lesser tuberosity are associated with posterior glenohumeral dislocations. Large fragments require open reduction and internal fixation.

Three-part Fractures

Most three-part fractures are unstable, with the head and greater tuberosity displaced from the shaft. These fractures require open reduction and either percutaneous or internal fixation. Percutaneous fixation is difficult in osteoporotic bone, so hemiarthroplasty may be preferable in elderly patients. Internal fixation is indicated for irreducible and unstable fractures. A plate with screws or a tension band is used in younger patients with good bone quality.

Four-part Fractures

In elderly patients with osteoporosis, four-part fractures are treated with a prosthetic replacement. In younger patients with good bone quality, open reduction and internal fixation is attempted; however, the risk of osteonecrosis of the humeral head is high.

Complications

Complications associated with the treatment of fractures of the proximal humerus include shoulder stiffness, loss of motion, and injuries to the axillary artery and to the brachial plexus and nerve. Malunion of displaced tuberosity fractures frequently results in pain, impingement, and limited motion. Repeated closed reductions are associated with the late development of myositis ossificans.

Humeral Shaft Fractures

Etiology and Classification

Fractures of the humeral shaft most commonly result from direct trauma, a fall onto the outstretched arm, a penetrating wound, or a motor vehicle accident. Fractures are classified by their location, fracture pattern, and degree of comminution.

Evaluation

History and Physical Examination

Fractures of the humeral shaft usually do not present a diagnostic dilemma. Clinical manifestations include pain, deformity, crepitus, and swelling at the level of the injury. Because a change in the neurovascular status of the extremity may occur during reduction maneuvers, it is imperative to perform a neurologic and vascular examination before reduction is attempted. In up to 20% of patients with humeral shaft fractures, radial nerve injuries are seen in association with the injury or as a result of fracture manipulation. Radial nerve palsies most frequently occur in fractures at the metaphyseal-diaphyseal junction (Holstein-Lewis fractures) and in middle-third fractures. Compartment syndrome also may be seen in association with fractures of the humeral shaft.

Imaging Studies

AP and lateral radiographs of the entire humerus should be obtained. The humeral head and elbow should be visible. If intra-articular extension is present, radiographs of the involved joint also should be obtained. Pathologic lesions must be imaged further with bone and CT scans or with MRI.

Treatment

Nonsurgical Treatment

Most fractures of the humeral shaft are treated nonoperatively. The wide range of motion of the glenohumeral joint compensates for deformities of the humeral shaft. About 20 degrees of anterior angulation, 30 degrees of varus or valgus angulation, and 3 cm of shortening are acceptable and do not compromise function. Treatment begins with an initial period of immobilization in a coaptation splint, hanging arm cast, or functional brace. Hanging casts may cause distraction of the fracture and produce an angular deformity. Functional bracing uses the soft tissue envelope to compress the fracture and maintain alignment.

Surgical Treatment

Surgery is indicated for treatment of open fractures; segmental fractures; pathologic fractures; fractures associated with floating elbows, vascular injuries, or brachial plexus injuries; and fractures that fail to respond to nonoperative treatment. Surgery also is indicated for patients with bilateral humeral shaft fractures and multiple trauma injuries.

Surgery usually consists of open reduction and internal fixation with plates, screws, or intramedullary nails. External fixation is indicated in patients with significant bone loss, comminuted fractures, associated burns, and open fractures with significant soft tissue injury.

Fractures about the Elbow

Anatomy

The elbow is a modified hinge joint, consisting of the articulation between the distal humerus and the radius and ulna. This allows flexion and extension as well as pronation and supination of the forearm. The bony anatomy of the distal humerus consists of diverging medial and lateral columns, bridged by the trochlea and capitellum. This construct allows the distal humerus to have two functionally independent joints. The lateral column terminates with the capitellum, which articulates with the radius and allows rotation. The medial column ends with the trochlea, which articulates with the olecranon process of the ulna and allows flexion and extension.

Distal Humerus Fractures

Etiology and Classification

The mechanism of injury is most commonly a fall on an outstretched hand or secondary to direct impact to the elbow. This can occur with the elbow in various degrees of flexion or extension and varus or valgus load, all of which contribute to the injury pattern. Classification is based on anatomic location and, to a certain extent, mechanism of injury.

Distal humerus fractures are divided into supracondylar, transcondylar (with and without intercondylar extension), and condylar fractures.

Supracondylar fractures are extra-articular by definition and occur through the metaphysis of the distal humerus. They are rare in adults and, when diagnosed, radiographs

PEARLS FOR ROUNDS

Pathologic fractures are found in an area of bone that has been weakened by a disease process. These fractures commonly occur after some trivial injury and may occur spontaneously. Traumatic fractures result from a substantial impact on the bone. Stress fractures result from repeated low-level stress that exceeds the strength of the bone.

Common fracture patterns include spiral, oblique, transverse, compression, avulsion, segmental (two separate fractures), comminuted (three or more fragments), and greenstick (incomplete) fractures.

Fractures are described according to their location as proximal-, middle-, or distal-third fractures. They also are described as intra-articular or extra-articular fractures.

Fractures are described by their alignment, displacement, and angular deformity in terms of the relation of the distal fragment to the proximal fragment.

Because the thoracolumbar junction is the most mobile segment, the majority of spinal injuries occur at this level.

Fractures of the clavicle most commonly result from a direct fall onto the shoulder. These fractures involve the middle third in most of the cases.

Fractures of the proximal humerus are common injuries. The most frequent cause is a fall in an elderly patient with osteoporosis. In younger patients, high-energy injuries account for most fractures of the proximal humerus.

Fractures of the pelvis can result directly from blunt trauma or indirectly from forces transmitted through the lower extremity. The fractures can be classified on the basis of their anatomic location, mechanism of injury, or stability.

The incidence of hip fractures is highest in elderly white women. Risk factors include smoking, inactivity, osteoporosis, dementia, and the use of psychotropic medications.

Tibial plateau fractures most often result from a fall, a motor vehicle collision, or an accident in which a pedestrian is struck by the bumper of a car.

should be scrutinized for possible intercondylar extension. They can be subdivided by mechanism (flexion or extension). Extension supracondylar fractures account for more than 80% of supracondylar fractures in adults.

Transcondylar fractures occur primarily in the elderly with osteopenic bone and may or may not have intercondylar extension. This is the most common distal humerus fracture in the adult. Fragments are often displaced and rotated because of muscle pull at the medial and lateral epicondyles.

Condylar fractures are very rare in the adult population. Lateral condylar fractures are more common than medial. Lateral condyle fractures involve the capitellum, and medial condyle fractures involve the trochlea.

Evaluation

History and Physical Examination

As is true with all fractures about the elbow, a careful neurovascular examination should be obtained. Marked swelling usually occurs, and compartment pressures should be monitored if a question occurs about compartment syndrome.

Imaging Studies

Standard AP and lateral views of the elbow are obtained. Oblique views are often helpful in complicated fracture patterns. Radiographs of the wrist and elbow should be obtained if any question exists about the possibility of another injury. Traction radiographs may sometimes be useful for preoperative planning.

Treatment

Nonsurgical treatment is indicated for nondisplaced and severely comminuted fractures in the elderly with limited functional capacity.

Surgical treatment is indicated for displaced fractures, vascular injury, and open fractures. Open reduction and internal fixation with a plate and screws on each column is required. Interfragmentary screws are often used in addition to plates in the transcondylar-type fracture with intercondylar extension. Percutaneous pinning is not biomechanically sound enough to hold these fractures rigidly in an adult. Total elbow arthroplasty may be considered in severely comminuted fracture patterns and in osteoporotic bone.

Complications

The most common complications related to the treatment of these fractures include loss of elbow motion, malunion, and nonunion. Malunion can lead to cubitus valgus, which increases the risk of developing a tardy ulnar nerve palsy.

Proximal Radius and Ulna Fractures

Etiology and Classification

These fractures are divided into olecranon and radial head fractures. Olecranon fractures occur by either direct trauma to the olecranon, or a fall onto an outstretched hand with a strong contraction of the triceps. Radial head fractures occur by direct trauma, or by a fall with impaction of the radial head into the capitellum.

Evaluation

History and physical examination should rule out any possible neurovascular deficits. Tenderness will be elicited with direct palpation of the fracture site. In radial head fractures, hemarthrosis should be aspirated, and intra-articular lidocaine injected to better assess for a possible bony block to pronation and supination. Competence of the ulnar collateral ligament also should be assessed to rule out valgus instability. A good wrist and shoulder examination should be performed to rule out any other possible injuries.

Imaging studies should include the standard AP and lateral of the elbow. Anterior and posterior fat pad signs are indications of a hemarthrosis and are highly suggestive of a fracture if present. The radial head should point to the capitellum on all radiographs, and a dislocation should be suspected if it does not.

Treatment

Nonsurgical treatment of olecranon fractures in a long-arm cast is indicated for nondisplaced fractures. Follow-up radiographs should be taken at 1 week to rule out displacement. Protected range of motion may be started at 3 weeks if the fracture remains stable. Indications for nonoperative treatment of radial head fractures include those that are nondisplaced or that involve less than 25% of the head. Fractures that are displaced more than 2 mm may be treated nonoperatively if no bony block to motion exists. Patients are placed into a sling, and early range of motion is encouraged.

Surgical treatment for the olecranon is indicated for comminuted or displaced fractures or both. Treatment usually consists of a K-wire and tension-band construct. Specially contoured plates and screws are used in comminuted fracture patterns. Surgical treatment for radial head fractures include those that are displaced more than 2 mm, involve more than 25% of the head, have significant comminution, or are associated with a bony block to motion. Open reduction and internal fixation is usually performed with K-wires or an articular screw. In those fractures that are severely comminuted, radial head excision is sometimes indicated.

Complications

Complications of the treatment of olecranon fractures include malunion, nonunion, loss of motion, and tardy ulnar nerve palsy. Those associated with radial head fracture treatment include loss of motion, nonunion, malunion, reflex sympathetic dystrophy, and proximal radial migration when radial head excision is used.

Fractures of the Forearm

Anatomy

The forearm is composed of the radius and ulna, with the ulna acting like an axis around which the radius rotates, allowing pronation and supination. The radius has a bow associated with it that allows this rotation. Loss of the radial bow due to an inadequately treated fracture will result in loss of rotation. The radius and ulna articulate with each other at both the proximal and distal ends, and any fracture that creates shortening will result in fracture or dislocation at the proximal or distal radioulnar joint.

Etiology and Classification

Fractures of one or both bones of the forearm are usually due to a high-energy mechanism. This may be from a motor vehicle accident, gunshot wound, or fall from a height. They are classified into radial and ulnar diaphyseal fractures, Monteggia fractures, and Galeazzi fractures. Radial and ulnar diaphyseal fractures usually occur together but may occur in isolation. A Monteggia fracture is a fracture of the ulnar diaphysis, with an associated radial head dislocation. A Galeazzi fracture is a fracture of the radial diaphysis with an associated disruption of the distal radial ulnar joint.

Evaluation

Radial and ulnar diaphyseal fractures often occur together and have an obvious forearm deformity. A careful physical examination is performed, and the presence or absence of specific examination findings should be noted for the median nerve, anterior interosseous nerve, posterior interosseus nerve, radial nerve, ulnar nerve, and radial and ulnar pulses. Any suspicion for an impending compartment syndrome should be evaluated by checking compartment pressures.

Imaging studies should be obtained, with a good AP and lateral view of the elbow, forearm, and wrist.

Treatment

Nonsurgical treatment is rarely indicated. This should be used only in the nondisplaced fracture of the radius or ulnar diaphysis or both.

Surgical treatment should be used for any displaced fracture of the radius or ulnar diaphysis or both. Monteggia and Galeazzi fractures are considered "fractures of necessity," and surgical treatment is almost universally used. Fixation is usually accomplished with a dynamic compression plate. Approach to the distal radius is through a volar incision, whereas the ulna and proximal radius are approached through a dorsal incision. Intramedullary fixation for the radius and ulna has been developed and may be used in certain situations.

Complications

Complications of treatment include malunion or nonunion, synostosis, and nerve injury. As stated previously, if malunion results in loss of the radial bow, pronation and supination may be lost. The risk of synostosis between the radius and ulna may be lessened if two incisions are used, rather than plating each bone through the same incision. Anterior interosseus and posterior interosseus nerve injury may occur and are often due to overtraction rather than direct laceration.

Fractures of the Pelvis and Acetabulum

Anatomy

Pelvis

The pelvis is a ring composed of two innominate bones. The bones articulate posteriorly with the sacrum and articulate anteriorly at the symphysis pubis. Each innominate bone is formed by the fusion of the ilium, pubis, and ischium. Ligaments connect the innominate bones to the sacrum, lumbar spine, and each other. These ligaments provide vertical and rotational stability to the pelvis.

Acetabulum

The acetabulum is contained within the anterior and posterior columns of the pelvis, and it articulates with the femoral head to form the hip joint. The labrum surrounds the margin of the acetabulum.

Surgical Techniques and Approaches

Pelvis

Surgical approaches to the pelvis are used to obtain bone grafts and perform open reduction and internal fixation of pelvic fractures.

Anterior and posterior approaches to the ilium can be used for cortical and cancellous bone grafts. In the anterior approach, care must be taken to avoid injury to the lateral femoral cutaneous nerve of the thigh as it passes the anterior superior iliac spine. In the posterior approach, the cluneal nerve is at risk of injury.

A **midline anterior approach to the symphysis pubis** is used for open reduction and internal fixation of widely displaced symphyseal disruptions associated with pelvic injuries. The pubic tubercle and symphysis are palpable subcutaneous structures. The rectus abdominal muscle and rectus sheath must be released from their attachment on the pubis. The superficial epigastric artery and vein must be ligated. The bladder can be gently released from the back of the pubis to gain access to the posterior symphysis.

Acetabulum

Surgical approaches to the acetabulum are used for fracture treatment and reconstructive procedures.

The **anterior approach** is used in the treatment of anterior wall fractures, anterior column fractures, transverse fractures, and fractures involving both the anterior and posterior columns of the acetabulum. The anterior approach uses the interval between the sartorius muscle and the tensor fasciae latae. The gluteus medius and minimus are elevated from the outer table of the pelvis. The internervus plane is between the femoral and superior gluteal nerves.

The **posterior approach** is used in the treatment of posterior wall fractures and posterior column fractures. To gain access to the posterior wall, the short external rotators are released. Further exposure of the posterior column may require a trochanteric osteotomy and elevation of the gluteus medius and minimus from the outer table of the ilium. The superior gluteal artery, sciatic nerve, and inferior gluteal artery are at risk during this approach and must be protected. The superior gluteal artery is often injured in pelvic fractures that involve the greater sciatic notch, and this may result in significant blood loss.

Pelvic Fractures

Etiology and Classification

Fractures of the pelvis can result directly from blunt trauma or indirectly from forces transmitted through the lower extremity. The fractures can be classified on the basis of their anatomic location, mechanism of injury, or stability.

Stable pelvic fractures are often low-energy injuries that do not disrupt the pelvic ring and can withstand physiologic loading. Stable fractures are often isolated injuries and may affect any part of the pelvis. The most common type affects the pubic ramus or ischial ramus (or both) and results from a fall in an elderly patient with osteoporosis. Isolated iliac wing fractures are usually stable and result from a fall or blunt trauma. Avulsion fractures are seen in young athletes and result from forceful contractions of the rectus femoris or hamstring muscles.

Unstable pelvic fractures are rotationally unstable, vertically unstable, or both. The vector that leads to unstable pelvic fractures may be an anterior-posterior force, lateral compression, external rotation-abduction, or shear force. Unstable and high-energy pelvic disruptions are associated with life-threatening injuries and require prompt recognition and management.

Evaluation

History and Physical Examination. The patient is initially assessed for hemodynamic stability and associated life-threatening injuries to the head, chest, and abdomen. The neurologic and vascular status of the lower extremities and perianal area is then evaluated.

In patients with high-energy pelvic trauma, massive hemorrhage and hemodynamic instability are usually the result of a venous plexus injury. Arterial injuries, particularly of the iliac vessels or superior gluteal artery, may result in loss of arterial pulses to the extremity. ATLS protocol should be started and resuscitation begun as soon as possible. Medical antishock trousers (MAST), pelvic external fixation, and angiographic embolization may be necessary to control bleeding secondary to pelvic injury. Indications for arteriography and arterial embolization include ongoing hemodynamic instability that is not attributable to associated injuries to the chest, abdomen, or retroperitoneum.

Neurologic injuries to the lumbosacral plexus occur in approximately 50% of patients with unstable pelvic injuries or fractures involving the sacrum. Deformity of the lower extremity in the absence of an extremity fracture is common with unstable pelvic fractures. Asymmetrical rotation or shortening of the limb may be found. Palpation of the posterior pelvis, sacrum, and lumbar spine may reveal a hematoma, fracture, or dislocation. A single examiner should assess for pelvic instability by looking for abnormal motion caused by anterior, posterior, or lateral compression.

Associated injuries occur commonly with high-energy pelvic trauma. A search must be made for open wounds, including perineal, genital, and rectal wounds. Flank swelling and ecchymoses are suggestive of massive bleeding. Rectal and vaginal examinations should be performed to search for urethral injuries, which occur in about 20% of patients with pelvic trauma, are more common in male than in female patients, and are most frequently associated with fractures that involve the pubic rami. A urethral injury is suggested by the presence of blood at the urethral meatus and the finding of a high-riding prostate. Before a catheter is placed, a retrograde urethrogram should be performed in hemodynamically unstable male patients suspected of a urethral injury.

Imaging Studies. Imaging studies should include the following: an AP radiograph of the pelvis, which can detect injuries to the anterior pelvis, sacroiliac joint, sacrum, and ilium; a pelvic inlet view, which is useful in evaluating posterior displacement of the sacrum, sacroiliac joint, iliac wing, and pubic ramus and in identifying rotational deformities of the hemipelvis; a pelvic outlet view, which is useful in evaluating the sacrum and sacral foramina and in detecting vertical displacement of the hemipelvis; and radiographs of the lumbar sacral spine, which may reveal fractures of the transverse processes. CT scanning is useful for assessing injuries to the pelvic ring and detecting posterior displacement and instability. Signs of pelvic instability include the presence of more than 5 mm of posterior sacroiliac displacement, posterior fracture gaps, and transverse process avulsion fractures.

Treatment

Treatment of pelvic fractures is based on the fracture pattern and the types of associated injuries.

Stable Fractures. Pelvic fractures that are stable include pubic ramus fractures, sacral impaction fractures, avulsion fractures, and most isolated iliac wing fractures. Stable pelvic fractures that do not involve the pelvic ring can be treated nonoperatively, with early mobilization and ambulation.

Unstable Fractures. Pelvic fractures that are rotationally unstable but are vertically and posteriorly stable include open-book and lateral compression fractures. Treatment consists of pelvic stabilization with internal fixation or an external frame or both. The frame generally requires the placement of two or three pins in each anterior iliac crest.

Pelvic fractures that are rotationally unstable and are also vertically or posteriorly unstable require open reduction and internal fixation with plates, screws, or bars.

Acetabular Fractures

Etiology and Classification

Fractures of the acetabulum are high-energy injuries that may result from either direct or indirect blunt trauma. Most commonly, acetabular fractures are caused by forces transmitted through the femoral head when the knee strikes the dashboard during an automobile accident. The position of the femur at the time of the impact determines what part of the acetabulum is injured. If the femur is externally rotated, the anterior column will be fractured. If the hip is flexed, the posterior column or posterior wall will be injured. The femoral head also may be fractured or dislocated.

Acetabular fractures have been classified on the basis of the columns and walls involved. According to the classification system of Judet and Letournel, five elementary and five associated fracture patterns exist. The five elementary patterns are the **anterior wall fracture, posterior wall fracture, anterior column fracture, posterior column fracture,** and **transverse fracture.** Associated fracture patterns involve more than one elementary type of fracture. The classification of acetabular fractures is useful in planning treatment and predicting outcome.

Evaluation

History and Physical Examination. Because many fractures of the acetabulum are associated with life-threatening injuries, the patient should be initially resuscitated and stabilized in accordance with the ATLS guidelines of the American College of Surgeons. The neurologic function of the involved extremity should be evaluated. In light of the high incidence of injury to the sciatic nerve, particularly its peroneal branch, a thorough examination of sensory and motor function should be performed. The position of the involved extremity also should be noted. Shortening of the leg suggests either dislocation or ipsilateral long-bone fracture. Soft tissue injuries to the lateral thigh may cause degloving of the superficial tissues.

Imaging Studies. An AP radiograph of the pelvis will show the position of the femoral head in relation to the acetabulum and will help visualize the anterior and posterior lips of the acetabulum. The iliopectineal and ilioischial lines delineate the anterior and posterior columns. Oblique views taken in internal and external rotation (Judet views) will better define the acetabular injury. An iliac oblique view will outline the posterior column and anterior wall of the acetabulum, whereas an obturator oblique view will outline the anterior column and the posterior wall. A CT scan will help detect intra-articular fragments, femoral head fractures, and dislocations.

Treatment

Dislocations of the femoral head must be reduced immediately to minimize the risk of avascular necrosis. Skeletal traction should be applied to maintain reduction, stabilize soft tissues, and maintain limb length.

Nonsurgical Treatment. Nonoperative management of acetabular fractures may be appropriate if imaging studies show that the femoral head remains congruent within the acetabulum, the weight-bearing superior acetabulum is intact, and the 45-degree roof arcs are intact and unaffected by the fracture. Although some posterior wall fractures are unstable and require open reduction and internal fixation, nonoperative management may be appropriate if the fracture is stable and involves less than 50% of the posterior wall. Impaction fractures with a step-off that is 2 mm or less can be treated nonoperatively. Fractures that involve both the anterior and posterior columns and have secondary congruence also can be successfully treated by nonoperative measures.

Surgical Treatment. The goals of surgical treatment are to restore joint congruity and stability, minimize the risk of post-traumatic arthritis, and allow early mobilization. Fracture dislocations are treated as an emergency and require open reduction and internal fixation. Loose fragments within the joint must be excised to prevent post-traumatic arthritis. Fracture fragments that result in incongruous joints with a step-off that is more than 2 mm should be surgically reduced and stabilized.

Complications

Complications associated with surgical treatment of acetabular fractures include infections, femoral and sciatic nerve palsies, and heterotopic bone formation.

Fractures of the Hip, Femur, and Tibia

Hip Fractures

The incidence of hip fractures is highest in elderly white women. Risk factors include smoking, inactivity, osteoporosis, dementia, and the use of psychotropic medications. The 1-year mortality rate after a hip fracture in an elderly patient ranges from 12% to 36%.

The anatomy of the hip and surgical approaches to the hip joint are discussed in Chapter 42. See the section entitled Arthritic and Other Disorders of the Hip.

Etiology and Classification

Hip fractures can be broadly classified into two groups: femoral neck fractures and intertrochanteric hip fractures.

PEARLS FOR THE OR

Surgical management of thoracolumbar injuries is indicated if the patient has an unstable spine or has progressive or complete neurologic deficit.

Indications for open treatment of clavicle fractures include open fractures and injuries to the subclavian vessels.

The goal of surgical treatment of hip fractures is to provide stability for appropriate healing and early mobilization, because early full weight bearing will limit loss of function and reduce postoperative complications.

Femoral shaft fractures are best treated with intramedullary nails, because their use results in union in more than 95% of cases.

Femoral neck fractures are intracapsular. The primary blood supply of the femoral head is from the lateral epiphyseal arteries, which are branches of the cervical arteries. These vessels traverse the capsule of the posterior femoral neck before supplying the femoral head. In cases of femoral neck fracture, disruption of these vessels may lead to avascular necrosis or fracture nonunion. Some femoral neck fractures are displaced, whereas others are impacted but nondisplaced. Fractures that are displaced have a poorer prognosis when treated with internal fixation rather than hemiarthroplasty.

Most hip fractures result from a low-energy fall directly onto the greater trochanter or from a twisting injury to the lower extremity. However, femoral neck fractures also result from repetitive stress. Femoral neck stress fractures may be of the tension type or the compression type. **Tension-type stress fractures** occur along the superior femoral neck and are seen most often in young athletes and military recruits. These fractures require surgical treatment. **Compression-type stress fractures** occur along the inferior femoral neck. They are seen in elderly patients with osteoporosis and can be successfully managed nonoperatively with protected weight bearing. Metastatic cancer and other pathologic bone lesions frequently are found in the proximal femur and may eventually cause a hip fracture. To prevent this, lesions that are longer than 2.5 cm or occupy more than 50% of the cortical bone should be repaired.

Intertrochanteric hip fractures are extracapsular fractures. Because they occur in cancellous bone, where numerous muscle attachments contribute to an ample blood supply, they are rarely associated with avascular necrosis and fracture nonunion.

Intertrochanteric fractures are subclassified on the basis of the fracture pattern and secondary fracture stability. The posteromedial cortex provides stability to the fracture after open reduction and internal fixation. Intertrochanteric fractures with separate posteromedial fragments are unstable and may collapse into varus. Fractures with reverse obliquity occur at the level of the lesser trochanter medially and extend into the subtrochanteric region laterally. Because of the deforming effects of the muscle attachments, intertrochanteric fractures tend to shorten and externally rotate the extremity.

Evaluation

History and Physical Examination. In younger patients, a hip fracture is usually the result of a high-energy injury and must be treated as a surgical emergency. In elderly patients, comorbid conditions should be evaluated and managed before hip surgery or other hip treatment is undertaken.

In patients with a stress fracture of the femoral neck, hip pain has an insidious onset and is relieved with rest. In patients with a displaced femoral neck or intertrochanteric hip fracture, shortening and external rotation of the affected limb can be noted. Patients with a nondisplaced fracture or a stress fracture usually do not have associated deformity of the limb, but movement of the leg will result in pain. Pain may be localized to the hip or knee region in femoral neck fractures and may radiate laterally in intertrochanteric fractures.

Imaging Studies. If a hip fracture is suspected, radiographs of the hip and pelvis should be obtained. AP and cross-table lateral views of the hip will help determine the fracture pattern and amount of displacement. If a femoral neck fracture is suspected but is not apparent on plain radiographs, MRI should be performed. Bone scanning also may be helpful but may not yield positive results for up to 48 hours after the injury.

Treatment

Nonsurgical Treatment. Although most patients with hip fractures are treated surgically, the exceptions are patients who are nonambulatory and have advanced dementia and patients in whom the surgical risks outweigh the benefits.

Surgical Treatment. The goal of surgical treatment of hip fractures is to provide stability for appropriate healing and early mobilization, because early full weight bearing will limit loss of function and reduce postoperative complications. The surgical technique to be used will depend on the type of fracture, the age of the patient, and the presence or absence of associated medical conditions.

In patients with hip fractures and associated conditions such as rheumatoid arthritis, Paget's disease, advanced osteoarthritis, chronic renal failure, hyperparathyroidism, and some types of metabolic bone disorders, surgical fixation with screws or nails is usually inappropriate. Depending on the extent of the joint-space loss that is associated with the fracture, either total arthroplasty or hemiarthroplasty may be indicated. Unipolar and bipolar hemiarthroplasties are available, and the benefits of each design are debated. Bipolar designs tend to be more expensive than unipolar designs, but they may reduce acetabular erosion. Other indications for arthroplasty include pathologic fractures, irreducible fractures in the elderly, fractures in nonambulatory patients, and fractures in patients with a neurologic condition such as Parkinson's disease or stroke. Long-term studies show that the results with cemented prostheses are superior to those with uncemented prostheses.

In patients who do not have associated medical conditions, an impacted and nondisplaced fracture of the femoral neck may be treated by placing three cancellous lag screws across the fracture and screwing them into the subchondral bone of the femoral head (Fig. 45-3). In patients with a displaced fracture of the femoral neck, treatment will depend on factors such as the patient's age and activity level. In an older, relatively inactive patient, prosthetic replacement is indicated. In a young, active patient, closed reduction and stabilization with cannulated screws are indicated.

In most cases of intertrochanteric hip fracture, the internal fixation apparatus used is the sliding hip screw. This apparatus has a large lag screw, which is placed into the femoral head and slides to allow fracture impaction, and has a side plate with angles fixed between 130 and 150 degrees (Fig. 45-4). With impaction of the fracture, greater stability is achieved. Reverse obliquity and some unstable intertrochanteric fractures may be treated with intramedullary hip screws or gamma nails. These devices provide a more biomechanically sound construct for healing the unstable fractures.

Complications

In femoral neck fractures treated with internal fixation, healing should occur in 6 to 12 months. Complications associated with treatment of these fractures include nonunion and avascular necrosis. Nonunion is more frequent in displaced than in nondisplaced fractures and occurs in as many as 25% of cases. Avascular necrosis occurs in as many as 33% of cases. A delay in the reduction of displaced femoral neck fractures increases the risk of avascular necrosis. Femoral neck nonunion causes pain and disability and usually requires additional surgery. Avascular necrosis can be treated nonoperatively, but about 33% of patients will require additional surgery. Failure of fixation in femoral neck fractures is uncommon but sometimes occurs in patients with osteoporosis.

In intertrochanteric fractures, complications of treatment include loss of fixation, acetabular penetration of the screws, thromboembolism, infection, and malunion. Loss of fixation is the most frequent complication and is usually due to improper positioning of the lag screw. Placement of the screw in an anterior and superior position is the most common error and leads to screw dislodgement or plate breakage.

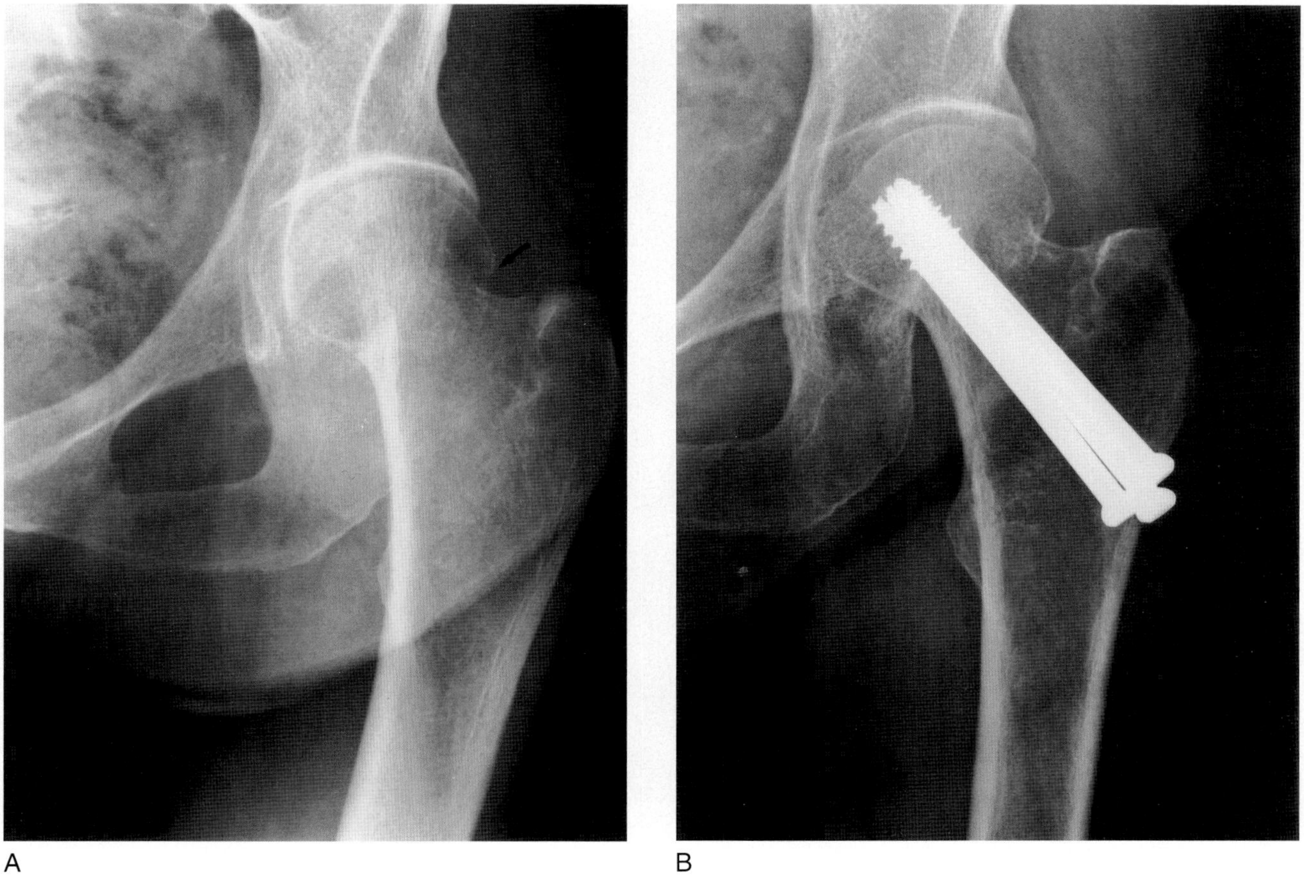

FIGURE 45–3 Radiographs of a valgus-impacted femoral neck fracture. *A*, After injury. *B*, After open reduction internal fixation.

Femoral Diaphyseal Fractures

Etiology and Classification

Fractures of the femoral diaphysis are usually the result of a low-energy twisting injury in elderly osteoporotic patients or the result of a high-energy injury in younger patients. However, they also may occur in association with metastatic lesions. Femoral shaft fractures can be classified by their location as subtrochanteric, shaft, or distal fractures.

Subtrochanteric femoral fractures begin below the lesser trochanter, but they may extend proximally to involve the piriform fossa or intertrochanteric region (Fig. 45-5). The subtrochanteric region of the femur is subjected to high bending moments and axial loads. Tensile forces are greatest laterally, whereas compressive forces are greatest on the medial cortex. Because the subtrochanteric region has a high proportion of cortical bone, vascularity to the region is relatively decreased. This can lead to slower fracture healing and a greater failure rate of internal fixation.

Femoral shaft fractures may be spiral, oblique, or transverse. The fracture pattern, amount of comminution, and associated injuries guide the method of treatment. In fractures caused by a motor vehicle accident, fall, or gunshot wound, associated injuries are common and may include vascular damage, compartment syndrome, ipsilateral knee injuries, and axial fractures. An ipsilateral femoral neck fracture occurs in about 5% of patients with femoral shaft fractures.

Distal femoral fractures occur within 9 cm of the articular surface. Because of the deforming forces of the gastrocnemius muscle, the distal fragment is often flexed and posteriorly displaced. Some distal fractures are extra-articular, whereas others are intra-articular. Intra-articular fractures may be unicondylar or bicondylar.

Evaluation

History and Physical Examination. Fractures of the femoral diaphysis are usually obvious and cause pain,

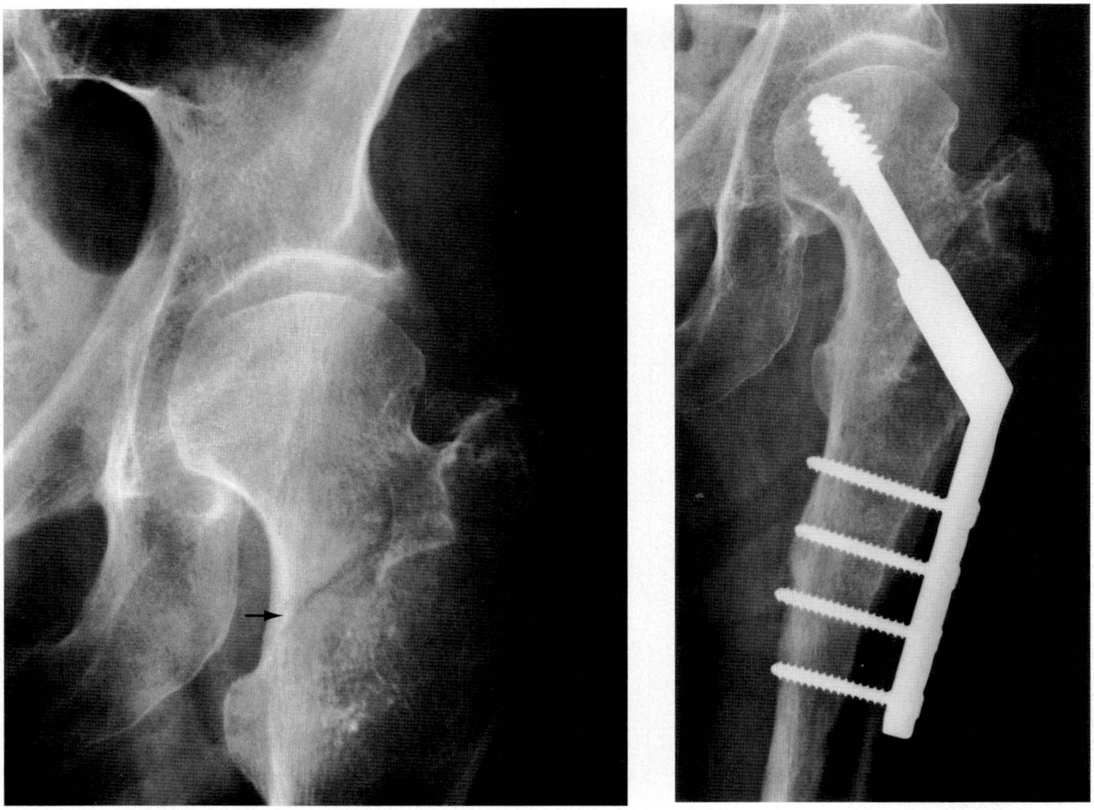

A B

FIGURE 45–4 Radiographs of an intertrochanteric hip fracture. *A*, After injury. *B*, After open reduction internal fixation.

deformity, and crepitus at the fracture site. The patient should be checked for associated injuries, especially in cases involving high-energy trauma. Particular attention must be given to the neurovascular examination of the leg. Lack of a pulse, decreased capillary refill, and pallor suggest a vascular injury that requires immediate intervention. Significant swelling of the thigh may lead to compartment syndrome, so compartment pressures should be assessed.

Imaging Studies. Radiographs should include an AP and cross-table lateral view of the femur, an AP and lateral view of the hip to rule out a hip fracture, and radiographs of the knee to assess for an associated fracture or ligament avulsion. CT scanning of distal femoral fractures may help evaluate intra-articular and coronal plane fractures.

Treatment

Nonsurgical Treatment. Nonoperative management is reserved for patients in whom the risks of surgery outweigh the benefits.

Surgical Treatment. Femoral diaphyseal fractures in adults are generally treated surgically, because this allows early stabilization and reduces the rate of complications.

In the surgical treatment of subtrochanteric femoral fractures, the type of fixation to be used depends on the fracture pattern. If the fracture does not extend proximally and the lesser trochanter is intact, standard interlocked anterograde nails are used. If the fracture is unstable owing to the loss of the medial buttress, then a second-generation intramedullary nail or gamma nail with fixation into the femoral head is indicated. If the fracture involves both the piriform fossa and the lesser trochanter, a sliding hip screw, gamma nail, or 95-degree fixed-angle plate may be used.

Femoral shaft fractures are best treated with intramedullary nails, because their use results in union in more than 95% of cases. Proximal and distal interlocking of these nails will allow rotational control of the fracture. The nails can be placed anterograde through the piriform fossa or retrograde through the intercondylar notch. Retrograde nailing is preferred in the treatment of ipsilateral tibial shaft

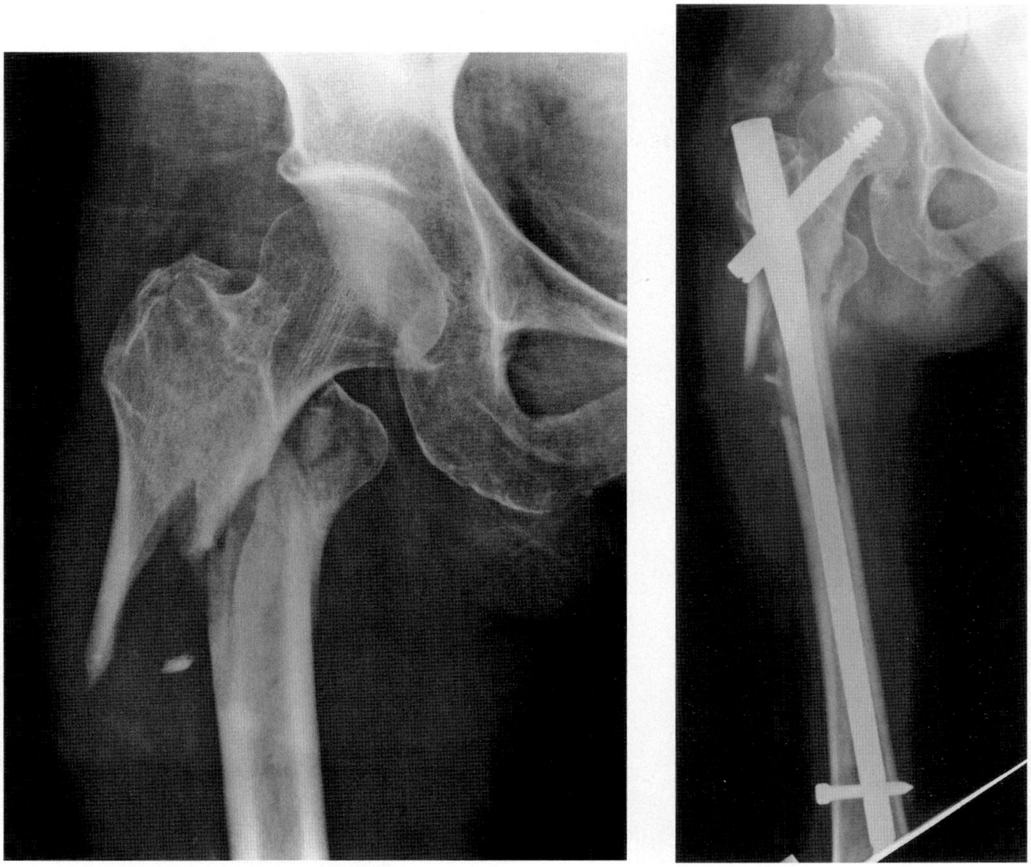

FIGURE 45–5 Radiographs of a subtrochanteric hip fracture. *A*, After injury. *B*, After open reduction internal fixation.

fractures, periprosthetic fractures, and ipsilateral femoral neck fractures.

Other options for the management of femoral shaft fractures include plate fixation and external fixation. Plate fixation may be indicated for ipsilateral femoral neck fractures or fractures with vascular injury. External fixation is used in the management of most type IIIC open fractures and some type IIIB open fractures, as well as in some shaft fractures associated with severe burns or vascular compromise. In patients too unstable for immediate surgery, skeletal traction may be applied until surgery can be performed.

Distal femoral fractures are generally treated surgically. In extra-articular supracondylar fractures, intramedullary nails may be used. In T-type intercondylar fractures that can be anatomically reduced, management may include lag-screw fixation of the intercondylar component and a retrograde intramedullary nail. Open reduction and internal fixation with fixed-angle blade plates, a dynamic condylar screw, or buttress plates have also been used with success in the management of supracondylar femur fractures with or without an intercondylar extension (Fig. 45-6). Buttress plates are indicated in the management of severely comminuted fractures that cannot be treated with a fixed-angle device. Supplemental medial plate fixation may be necessary when the medial cortex is deficient. Spanning external fixation may be used until surgery can be performed in patients with multiple fractures, vascular injuries, or open fractures.

Complications

Nonoperative treatment with skeletal traction, bracing, and casting is associated with a high rate of complications, including prolonged immobility, pin-tract infection, malunion, and nonunion.

Complications associated with surgical treatment of femoral diaphyseal fractures include nonunion, delayed union, malunion, loss of fixation, and failure of fixation. Distraction and lengthening can occur at the fracture site. Infection and nerve injuries are rare. External fixation is associated with stiffness, pin-tract infections, and osteomyelitis. The use of anterograde femoral nails is associated

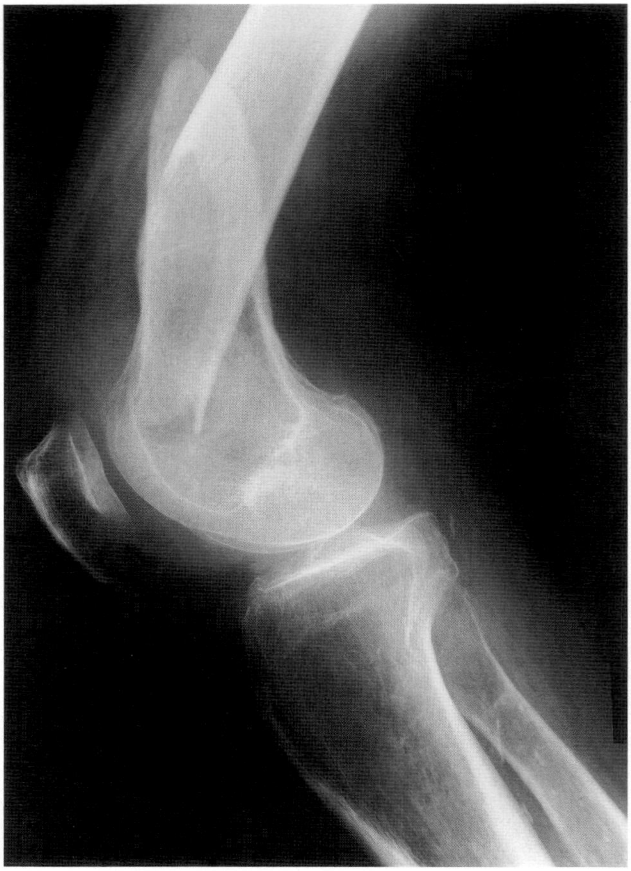

A

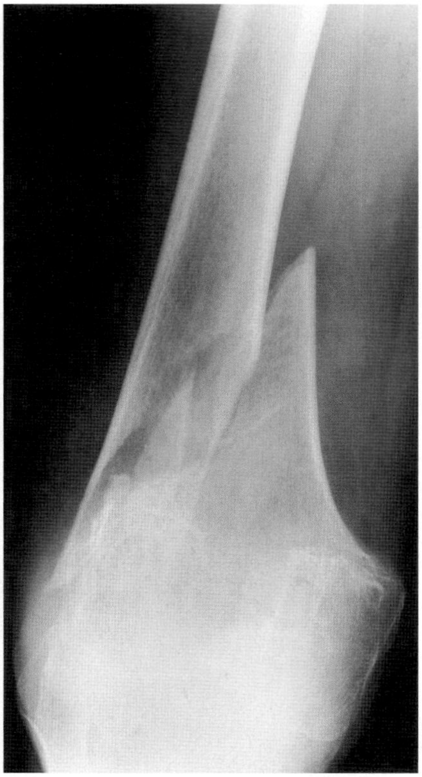

B

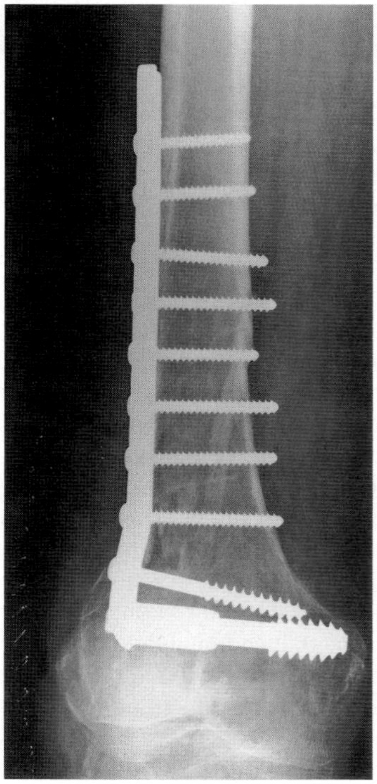

C

FIGURE 45–6 Radiographs of a supracondylar femur fracture. *A* and *B*, After injury. *C*, After open reduction internal fixation.

with iatrogenic femoral neck fractures and heterotopic ossification.

Fractures about the Knee and Lower Leg

The anatomy of the knee and surgical approaches to the knee joint are discussed in earlier chapters. See the section in Chapter 42 entitled Arthritic and Other Disorders of the Knee.

Patellar Fractures

The patella is the largest of the sesamoid bones. It is attached at its proximal pole to the quadriceps tendon and at its distal pole to the patellar tendon. Its primary function is to improve the mechanical advantage of the quadriceps muscle by increasing the moment arm from the axis of knee rotation. The patella moves within the intercondylar groove of the femur and slides up to 7 cm between full flexion and extension. The medial and lateral retinacula attach along the margins of the patella and into the proximal tibia and contribute to the knee-extensor mechanism and patellar stability.

Etiology and Classification

Patellar fractures most commonly result from a direct blow, such as that associated with a fall on the knee or with an automobile accident in which the knee hits the dashboard. Patellar fractures less frequently result from indirect forces, such as eccentric quadriceps contraction with the knee in a flexed position.

Patellar fractures may be either nondisplaced or displaced, with **displaced fractures** having more than a 2-mm step-off. On the basis of the fracture pattern, patellar fractures can be classified as **comminuted fractures, transverse fractures, vertical fractures, osteochondral fractures,** and **fractures involving the apical or inferior pole.**

Evaluation

History and Physical Examination. Knee examination reveals localized pain and swelling. Active knee extension must be assessed to determine the competence of the extensor mechanism. Dashboard injuries are frequently associated with ipsilateral femur fractures, posterior cruciate ligament tears, and hip dislocations, so a search should be made for these types of injuries.

Imaging Studies. AP, lateral, and axial radiographs of the knee should be obtained. A bipartite patella is evident by its superolateral position and its sclerotic smooth margins. This condition is bilateral in 50% of patients.

Treatment

Nonsurgical Treatment. A patellar fracture that is displaced 2 mm or less and has an intact extensor mechanism can be treated with a knee immobilizer or cylinder cast, with the knee kept in full extension for 4 to 6 weeks. Patients may begin weight bearing as tolerated.

Surgical Treatment. Indications for open reduction and internal fixation include open fractures, comminuted fractures, and fractures that show more than 2 mm of articular incongruity or displacement. Transverse fractures can be fixed with a tension band and either Kirschner wires or screws. Comminuted fractures may require additional lag screws or Kirschner wires. Inferior pole fractures may require reattachment of the patellar tendon and excision of the fragment if it is too small to be stabilized. Partial or total patellectomy is indicated only in severely comminuted fractures that cannot be reduced and stabilized. If the retinaculum is disrupted, it must be repaired.

Complications

Complications of patellar fractures include loss of motion and extensor strength. Nonunion, malunion, infection, and post-traumatic arthritis may occur after internal fixation.

Tibial Plateau Fractures

The proximal tibia is composed of the medial and lateral plateaus and the nonarticulating intercondylar eminence. The anterior and posterior tibial spines onto which the cruciate ligaments attach are found along the intercondylar eminence. The medial tibial plateau has a concave contour and is larger than the lateral plateau, which has a convex contour. In the sagittal plane, the proximal tibia has a 10-degree inferior slope from anterior to posterior. Fibrocartilaginous menisci cover the peripheral medial and lateral tibial plateaus and function to dissipate forces transmitted through the proximal tibia during weight bearing.

Etiology and Classification

Tibial plateau fractures most often result from a fall, a motor vehicle collision, or an accident in which a pedestrian is struck by the bumper of a car. Lateral plateau fractures are more common than medial plateau fractures and generally result from low-energy trauma in elderly patients with osteoporosis. Ligament injuries, peroneal nerve injuries, and popliteal vessel injuries occur more frequently with medial plateau fractures caused by high-energy trauma.

According to the Schatzker classification system, six types of tibial plateau fractures occur. **Type I** is a split fracture of the lateral plateau; **type II** is a split depression fracture of the lateral plateau**; type III** is a depressed fracture of the lateral plateau; **type IV** is a medial plateau fracture**; type V** is a bicondylar fracture; and **type VI** is a bicondylar fracture with extension into the diaphysis.

Evaluation

History and Physical Examination. In patients with a tibial plateau fracture, a thorough assessment of the knee, soft tissues, and neurovascular condition of the involved extremity will guide the timing of surgery and the extent of the surgical exposure. Knee examination will reveal effusion. If the fracture is not clearly apparent on radiographs, aspiration of the knee may yield marrow fat and blood. Acute compartment syndrome may develop in patients who have a Schatzker type V or VI fracture or a vascular injury. Most nerve injuries associated with tibial plateau fractures are neurapraxias. Other associated injuries include meniscal tears and collateral or cruciate ligament sprains and tears.

Imaging Studies. Plain radiographic images of the knee should be obtained if tibial plateau fracture is suspected. AP, lateral, and internal and external rotation views are necessary to characterize the fracture and the amount of articular incongruity. Stress views may demonstrate collateral ligament disruption. Traction radiographs to assess reduction by ligamentotaxis may aid in preoperative planning. CT scanning also may be beneficial in preoperative planning. In cases of suspected arterial injury, arteriography is necessary. MRI may be used to assess meniscal injuries and damage to the collateral and cruciate ligaments.

Treatment

Nonsurgical Treatment. Nonoperative treatment is indicated for nondisplaced or minimally displaced tibial plateau fractures. The knee is immobilized with a hinged brace, and the patient is instructed to avoid weight bearing for 4 weeks. Early motion may be instituted to prevent stiffness and encourage cartilage healing.

Surgical Treatment. Surgical treatment is indicated for the following: displaced fractures; fractures with an articular depression exceeding 4 mm; fractures that show more than 10 degrees of varus or valgus instability when the knee is in full extension; fractures associated with compartment syndrome or vascular injury; open fractures; and ipsilateral femoral shaft fractures.

In displaced or depressed fractures, the goal of surgery is to restore the articular surface. Depressed fragments are elevated, and metaphyseal defects are filled with grafted bone. Tibial buttress plates are used to stabilize the condyles. Arthroscopy may be useful to assess articular congruity after reduction. Menisci should be preserved and repaired when possible.

In nondisplaced split fractures, if open reduction is limited by the extent of soft tissue injury, internal fixation with percutaneous lag screws can be used. Supplemental fixation with a hybrid external ring device may be necessary for type V comminuted bicondylar fractures, type VI fractures, and fractures with extensive soft tissue injuries. Spanning external fixation is indicated if extensive comminution of the fracture is seen. Balanced suspension and skeletal traction may be used until soft tissue swelling diminishes and surgery can be performed, or it may be the definitive treatment if associated medical conditions preclude surgery.

Associated injuries to the menisci or collateral ligaments should be repaired at the time of surgery. If the anterior cruciate ligament has been avulsed with a fragment of the tibial spine, the tibial spine should be reattached. If the midsubstance of the anterior cruciate ligament has been torn, reconstruction should be delayed until the fracture has healed.

Complications

Complications associated with tibial plateau fractures include malunion, nonunion, compartment syndrome, and nerve injury. Complications of nonsurgical treatment include post-traumatic arthrosis, whereas those of surgical treatment include post-traumatic arthrosis, wound infection, and failure of fixation. Pin-tract infections sometimes occur with the use of hybrid external fixation.

Tibial Shaft Fractures

The tibia is a long tubular bone that is subcutaneous throughout its length. In cross section, the tibia has a triangular shape. The blood supply is relatively poor. The nutrient artery is derived from the posterior tibial artery and gives rise to the intramedullary blood supply. The periosteal blood supply is derived primarily from the anterior tibial artery.

Etiology and Classification

Tibial shaft fractures can result from direct or indirect trauma and are the most common of the long bone fractures. These fractures can be classified according to location as proximal-third, middle-third, or distal-third fractures. They also can be classified according to their fracture patterns. The most common fracture patterns are simple, comminuted, and butterfly. Tibial stress fractures also are seen.

Simple fractures are subclassified as transverse, spiral, and oblique. **Transverse** and **oblique fractures** result from high-energy injuries, such as falls and motor vehicle accidents, or from three-point bending. **Spiral fractures** result from low-energy twisting injuries. **Comminuted fractures** may be segmental and may result from high-energy torsion, four-point bending, or crush injuries. **Butterfly fractures** result from a twisting and bending force. **Tibial stress fractures** are repetitive overuse injuries and are most often seen in military recruits and dancers.

Evaluation

History and Physical Examination. Evaluation begins with a complete neurovascular assessment of the involved extremity. Soft tissues must be assessed for open wounds or tenting of the skin. Malaligned fractures must be reduced immediately and splinted to minimize further soft tissue injury. Open fractures must be treated as a surgical emergency. An initial assessment for an acute compartment syndrome should be followed by serial examinations for signs of an impending compartment syndrome. The earliest signs are sensory loss and intense pain. Pulses are present until late in the course of a compartment syndrome. Compartment pressures should be measured. A four-compartment fasciotomy must be done if clinical evidence of compartment syndrome exists.

Imaging Studies. Plain AP and lateral radiographs that include the knee and ankle should be obtained. If a vascular injury is suspected, an angiogram is necessary. A radiograph of the contralateral tibia is useful for preoperative templating of segmental and comminuted fractures.

Treatment

Nonsurgical Treatment. Nonoperative treatment is most successful in patients whose tibial shaft fractures are caused by low-energy injuries and show minimal displacement. If the fracture pattern is stable, with less than 1 cm of shortening and less than 5 degrees of varus or valgus angulation, it can be treated nonsurgically. If the fracture is associated with less than 10 degrees of rotational deformity, it also can be treated nonsurgically. After the fracture is reduced, a long-leg cast is used for stabilization, and radiographs are taken on a weekly basis. Bracing and early weight bearing may begin about 4 weeks after the injury, when pain and swelling will have diminished. The average time to healing is 4 to 5 months.

Surgical Treatment. Indications for surgical treatment of tibial shaft fractures include open fractures, unstable fracture patterns, and fractures with unacceptable alignment. Surgical options for stabilization include the use of intramedullary nails, external fixation, and plate and screws.

Intramedullary nails are indicated for the treatment of most tibial shaft fractures, including type I, II, and IIIA open fractures. Interlocking screws proximally and distally provide rotational control and maintain length. Unreamed (solid) and reamed nails are available. In open fractures, unreamed nails are used. In closed fractures, intramedullary reaming allows the use of larger nails, but the reaming may compromise the endosteal blood supply.

External fixation of tibial shaft fractures is indicated for patients with type IIIB and IIIC open fractures; patients who have multiple traumatic injuries and require urgent stabilization; and patients who have periarticular fractures associated with significant soft tissue injuries that preclude open reduction and internal fixation. External fixation also is indicated for some patients who have closed fractures.

Few indications are found for fixation of tibial fractures with plate and screws. Shaft fractures that extend proximally into the knee or distally into the tibial plafond may be treated with plate osteosynthesis.

Complications

Complications associated with tibial fractures include deep venous thrombosis, reflex sympathetic dystrophy, compartment syndrome, malunion, and nonunion. The rate of nonunion in fractures treated nonoperatively is about 5%. Ankle and hindfoot stiffness caused by prolonged immobilization may be seen after cast treatment. Up to 20% of patients initially treated with a cast will require subsequent surgical treatment. Nonunion or delayed union after intramedullary nailing may be treated with dynamization of the proximal locking screw to allow fracture impaction. When the proximal surgical approach is used for placement of tibial nails, knee pain sometimes develops.

Fracture of the Foot and Ankle

Ankle Fractures

Fractures of the ankle are among the most common major joint injuries. Recognizing the concurrent ligamentous component of these injuries is critical to treatment. The proximal portion of the ankle joint consists of the tibia and fibula. These bones are held tightly together by the syndesmotic ligaments, which encompass the talus on three sides. The lateral collateral and deltoid ligaments securely bind the structures together. After injury, the stability of the ankle is directly related to the integrity of these structures.

Evaluation

Examination begins with an assessment of the neurovascular status of the extremity and with palpation of the fibula up to the knee. The specific points of tenderness and swelling should be identified, because they correspond with damaged structures. The standard radiographic views of the ankle should be supplemented by views of the foot or the entire tibia if the tenderness extends to these areas. The ankle mortise should be scrutinized for evidence of widening as a result of injury to the syndesmoses.

Treatment

Anatomic restoration of the articular surface is necessary for acceptable results. Joint surface incongruity leads to stress within the joint and predisposes the ankle to early arthritis. If the mortise is not displaced, cast immobilization of the fracture is sufficient. To decrease the rotation of the cast around the leg, it may be necessary to extend the cast above the knee. Fractures with any degree of articular displacement require internal fixation. If the fracture is accompanied by severe damage to the soft tissues, internal fixation may need to be delayed until satisfactory healing has occurred.

Suggested Reading

An HS, Jenis LG, Vaccaro AR, et al: Adult Spine Trauma: Orthopaedic Knowledge Update 6. Rosemont, IL, American Academy of Orthopaedic Surgeons, 1999, pp 653–672.

Berry DJ, Garvin KL, Lee SH: Hip and Pelvis Reconstruction: Orthopaedic Knowledge Update 6. Rosemont, IL, American Academy of Orthopaedic Surgeons, 1999, pp 455–504.

Browner BD, Jupiter JB (eds): Skeletal Trauma: Fractures, Dislocations, and Ligamentous Injuries. Philadelphia, WB Saunders, 1998.

Bucholz RW, Heckman JD (eds): Rockwood and Green's Fractures in Adults, 5th ed. Philadelphia, Lippincott, 2002.

Canale ST (ed): Campbell's Operative Orthopaedics, 10th ed. Philadelphia, Mosby, 2003.

McCarthy JC, Busconi B: The role of hip arthroscopy in the diagnosis and treatment of hip disease. Can J Surg 38(suppl 1):S13–S17, 1995.

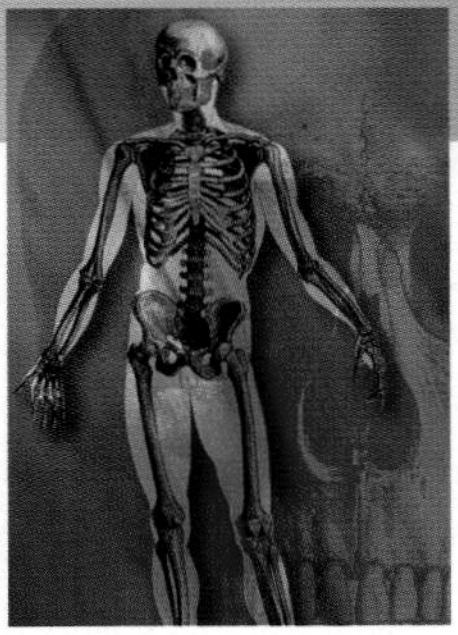

Chapter 46
Pediatric Orthopedics

DONNA M. PACICCA, MD, RYAN R. SNYDER, MD, and
PETER DEWIRE, MD

Orthopedic surgeons treat a wide variety of disorders that involve the growing skeleton in children. Because of the limitations of space, only the most common disorders are discussed here. For additional information, readers are referred to the list of selected readings at the end of the chapter.

Pediatric Infections of the Bones and Joints

Osteomyelitis

Osteomyelitis is one of the more devastating diseases that can affect a child, especially if left untreated. Worldwide, it remains one of the leading causes of death and dysfunction. In the United States, the morbidity and mortality rates associated with osteomyelitis in children have decreased as a result of early diagnosis and treatment.

Etiology and Pathogenesis

As discussed in Chapter 42, **acute hematogenous osteomyelitis** in children is most commonly caused by *Staphylococcus aureus* or *Streptococcus*. The infection is presumed to arise from sluggish blood flow in the metaphyseal sinusoids and may be incited by local trauma (bone contusion). White blood cells are unable to access the sinusoid area and clear pathogens from it, so the pathogens multiply.

Chronic osteomyelitis may occur despite adequate drainage and antibiotic treatment for acute infection, or it can develop in association with an inciting event, such as an open fracture. In patients with acute osteomyelitis caused by *S. aureus*, chronic osteomyelitis is more likely to develop.

Evaluation

Physical Examination and Laboratory Studies. Children with osteomyelitis complain of pain and refuse to use the affected limb. The erythrocyte sedimentation rate is elevated in more than 90% of patients, but the white blood cell count varies and is a less reliable indication of infection. Aspiration of the affected area is essential to determine the infecting organism, because blood cultures yield positive results in only 40% to 50% of cases.

Imaging Studies. Radiographs do not show bony involvement for 7 to 14 days. Bone scanning can be performed in the setting of aspiration, as long as it is done within 48 hours. Magnetic resonance imaging (MRI) is quite sensitive for osteomyelitis but is not specific for it. In the early stages of disease, ultrasonography may be useful for detecting localized soft tissue changes and periosteal abscess.

Differential Diagnosis. Acute hematogenous osteomyelitis can be confused with rheumatic fever, septic arthritis, bone cancer, sickle cell crisis, and Gaucher's disease.

Treatment

In children with acute infection, the use of antibiotics alone may be effective if antibiotic treatment is begun within 72 hours of the onset of symptoms. If a periosteal abscess is present or if the patient has not responded to antibiotic treatment, surgical treatment should be performed to decompress and débride the bone.

In children with chronic osteomyelitis, surgical intervention is required to débride necrotic infected bone, and adjuvant antibiotic therapy is necessary to effect remission. Patients may require multiple surgeries, and antibiotic cement bead placement may be useful to assist in the eradication of infection.

Septic Arthritis

As discussed in Chapter 42, septic arthritis in infants and young children is usually caused by *S. aureus*. It most commonly affects the knees, hips, ankles, and elbows. Because the sequelae of the disease can be devastating in pediatric patients, rapid diagnosis and treatment are required.

Evaluation

History and Physical Examination. Septic arthritis is most commonly seen in infants and children younger than 2 years. These patients usually are first seen with an elevated temperature, restricted joint motion, effusion, warmth, and tenderness. However, they may have irritability and slight asymmetry in motion. A careful history is important for establishing any possible antecedent traumas.

Laboratory and Imaging Studies. The white blood cell count is elevated in 30% to 60% of patients. The erythrocyte sedimentation rate is more sensitive and is usually high, except in neonates, patients with sickle cell anemia, and patients treated with corticosteroids. Blood cultures yield positive results in only 40% to 50% of cases. Plain radiographs may show subtle joint-space widening or obliteration of fat planes. Needle aspiration of the affected joint is the definitive test and should be performed expeditiously. If infection of the hip joint is suspected, aspiration should be performed in the operating room with the patient under anesthesia, so no delay in surgical incision and drainage will occur if infection is present.

Differential Diagnosis. The differential diagnosis includes juvenile arthritis, Schönlein-Henoch purpura, Lyme disease, sickle cell crisis, and transient synovitis.

Treatment

As soon as blood, synovial fluid, and other pertinent specimens are obtained, appropriate antibiotics should be started. An organism identifiable on Gram stain is the best guide for antibiotic therapy. In the absence of an organism, the choice of antibiotic depends on the child's age, immune status, and local epidemiologic data. Neonates are more susceptible to group B streptococcal infection, whereas adolescents may have a gonococcal infection. Surgical intervention is required to remove the microorganisms and associated debris from the joint and thereby prevent cartilage destruction.

Pediatric Fractures

Long-Bone Fractures

In children, fractures have the remarkable ability to remodel because of concurrent longitudinal growth. Treatment generally involves closed reduction and casting to maintain alignment while the bones heal. However, if the fracture is displaced, surgical intervention may be necessary to restore articular congruity. Although closed treatment is still considered the standard of care for long-bone fractures, some fractures may require operative intervention because of concomitant traumatic injuries. For example, if a femur fracture occurs in a patient with a closed head injury, operative stabilization of the fracture may be required to control alignment and facilitate early mobilization of the patient (Fig. 46-1).

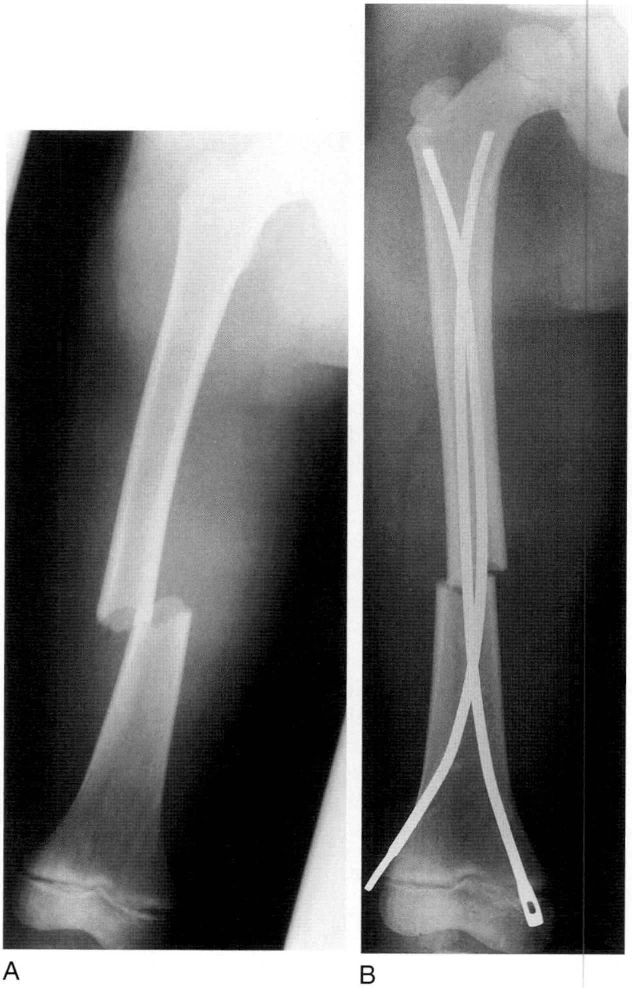

FIGURE 46–1 Radiographs of a femoral shaft fracture. *A*, After injury. *B*, After flexible nails.

Growth Plate Fractures

Growth plate fractures, or **physeal fractures**, involve the portion of the bone where endochondral ossification is occurring. Because this portion is primarily cartilaginous, it is often the site of injury and a site for deformity after fracture.

Classification

The Salter-Harris classification system is most commonly used to classify physeal fractures (Fig. 46-2). This system delineates five types, based primarily on radiographic findings. In **type I**, which generally occurs in younger children, the epiphysis is completely separated from the metaphysis and may be displaced or nondisplaced, but no evidence of metaphyseal fracture is found. In **type II**, which is the most common type, the fracture occurs transversely through the physis before exiting through the metaphysis. The metaphyseal fragment is often referred to as a *Thurston-Holland fragment*. In **type III**, the fracture begins at the articular surface and propagates peripherally to exit through the physis. This fracture pattern occurs commonly in the ankle during physeal closure (juvenile Tillaux

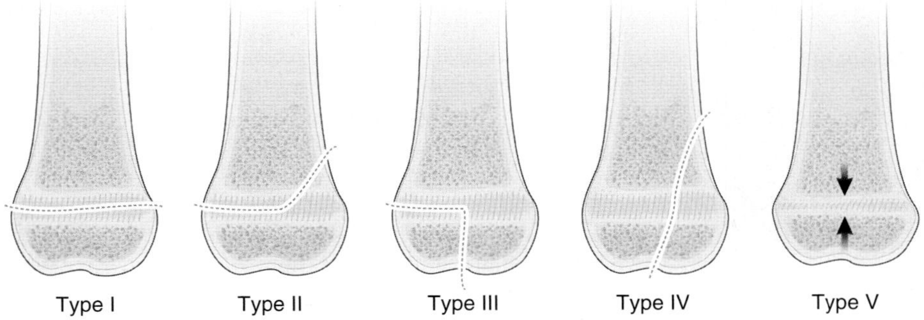

FIGURE 46–2 Salter-Harris classification for physeal fractures. (Adapted from Bora FW: The Pediatric Upper Extremity. Philadelphia, WB Saunders, 1986.)

fracture). In **type IV**, the fracture is a vertical split that begins at the epiphysis, moves across the physis, and exits through the metaphysis. This fracture pattern is associated with a higher incidence of partial growth arrest. In **type V**, the fracture is one that cannot be diagnosed at the time of initial injury. It is caused by a severe crush to the physis and leads to cessation of growth in the affected area.

Treatment

In type I physeal fractures, closed reduction with casting is usually sufficient. Smooth pins may be inserted across the physis if reduction is not thought to be stable. In type II, closed reduction with casting is performed by using the intact hinge of periosteum for stability. Occasionally, a screw is inserted parallel to the physis to help hold the metaphyseal fragment in place. Type III fractures require anatomic reduction, and usually screws or pins are used parallel to the physis to hold the fragment into place. Type IV also requires anatomic reduction, with the assistance of pins or screws to help hold alignment. Type V fractures are usually recognized only after the growth plate has shut down, and management is directed at correcting the residual deformity.

Buckle Fractures

Buckle fractures, or **torus fractures**, are unique to childhood. They affect the metaphysis and result from a compressive load. They are usually found in the distal radius but are occasionally found in other bones. Rather than completely fracturing, the bone buckles, creating a stable injury pattern.

Because buckle fractures are stable, surgical intervention is unnecessary. However, immobilization for a short period is recommended to protect the healing bone from further injury.

Greenstick Fractures Associated with Plastic Deformation

In children, the haversian canals in the bones are large. This makes the bones more porous and therefore more susceptible to deformation. A longitudinal compressive force directed against a curved immature bone will increase the curvature. If the compression is continued beyond the bone's ability for elastic recoil, plastic or permanent deformation will occur.

Plastic deformation often occurs in conjunction with a greenstick fracture, which is an incomplete fracture with intact periosteum. This type of fracture is commonly seen in the ulna and fibula.

Treatment is usually nonsurgical. Closed reduction under anesthesia is performed. Occasionally in a two-bone forearm fracture, the greenstick fracture must be completed to achieve an adequate reduction. In greenstick fractures, the deformity is first increased, which unlocks the periosteum. Reduction is then able to be performed by using the intact periosteum to stabilize the fragments. A well-molded cast is then placed. If closed reduction results in unsatisfactory results, open reduction may be performed with flexible intramedullary nailing, percutaneous pinning, or internal fixation with plates and screws to stabilize the fracture.

Plastic deformation is almost always treated closed. Reduction is performed under anesthesia by placing the apex of the deformity over a wedge and applying a constant force at points proximal and distal to the apex of the bow over a period of 2 to 3 minutes. A well-molded cast is then applied.

Fractures Associated with Osteogenesis Imperfecta

Osteogenesis imperfecta is a genetic disorder caused by qualitative or quantitative defects in the formation of type I collagen. Affected children have brittle bones and are susceptible to multiple fractures (Fig. 46-3) even with minimal trauma. It is important to distinguish fractures caused by child abuse (see below) from fractures associated with osteogenesis imperfecta, since the clinical and radiographic presentation may be similar.

Evaluation

The clinical features of osteogenesis imperfecta can be quite variable and will depend on the specific collagen abnormality that is responsible. Patients may have blue sclerae, hearing loss, dentinogenesis imperfecta, short

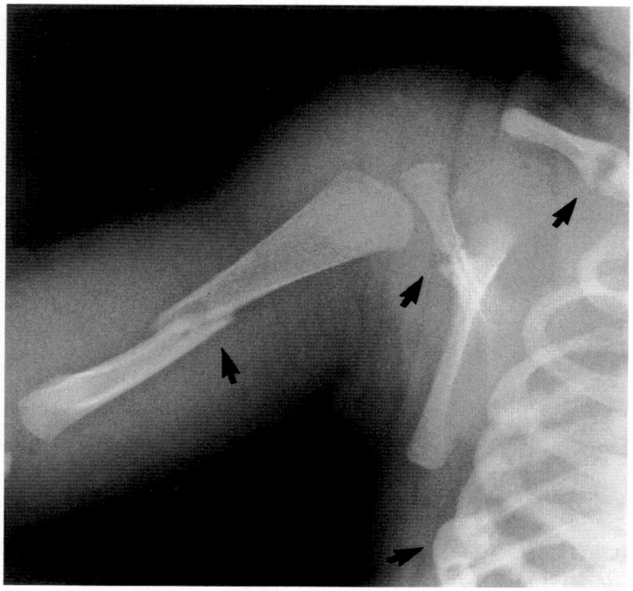

FIGURE 46–3 Radiograph of a 5-day-old patient with osteogenesis imperfecta and multiple fractures in different stages of healing.

stature, and skin fragility. Patients with more severe forms of disease are seen at birth with multiple fractures and resultant deformity. Spinal deformity occurs in 40% to 80% of patients. One of the radiographic hallmarks of osteogenesis imperfecta is osteopenia.

Treatment

Nonsurgical Treatment. To prevent fractures and deformities in infants with osteogenesis imperfecta, parents and caregivers should be instructed about appropriate positioning and handling of the infant and about the techniques of physical therapy. Therapy designed to improve muscle strength will increase bone strength by placing increased stress on the bones.

Orthotics and casts may be used to treat fractures and prevent deformities caused by bowing of long bones. A short period of casting and functional bracing is optimal, because prolonged immobilization will lead to disuse osteopenia and repeated fractures.

Surgical Treatment. Some patients will require surgical correction of long-bone deformities and scoliosis. Management of anesthesia can be challenging in these patients because they often have restricted motion of the neck and jaw, pulmonary-function abnormalities associated with thoracic distortion, and valvular heart disease. In addition, anesthesia-induced hyperthermia, with acidosis, hypoxia, tachycardia, fever, and elevated levels of creatine phosphokinase may develop. This hypermetabolic state is not true malignant hyperthermia but mimics it. The use of succinylcholine and anticholinergic drugs should be avoided.

Fractures Associated with Child Abuse

If fractures are found in an infant who is not yet walking, child abuse should be considered.

Evaluation

The most common long-bone fractures seen in abused children are fractures of the humerus, tibia, and femur. Although spiral fractures are sometimes associated with child abuse, transverse diaphyseal long-bone fractures are the ones that are most commonly associated and should raise suspicion. Metaphyseal "corner" fractures are considered suggestive of abuse.

Other evidence of abuse is frequently present and may include bruises, burns, skin marks, signs of neglect, and radiographic evidence of multiple fractures that are in various stages of healing. For children younger than 5 years, a skeletal survey is helpful for diagnosing additional bony injuries. Bone scans also can be helpful, especially if the child has head trauma or is younger than 2 years.

Treatment

Treatment of child abuse requires a team approach, with involvement of pediatricians, social workers, and other specialists.

Pediatric Disorders of the Spine and Hip

Scoliosis

Scoliosis is characterized by lateral deviation and rotation of the spinal column (Fig. 46-4).

Etiology and Classification

Although a familial predilection appears to be present in scoliosis, in most cases the cause is unknown.

Idiopathic scoliosis is generally divided into three types, based on age. **Infantile scoliosis** appears before patients reach the age of 3 years and is extremely rare in North America. **Juvenile scoliosis** appears between ages 3 and 10 years, and **adolescent scoliosis** appears after age 10 years. Juvenile scoliosis and adolescent scoliosis are seen more frequently in girls than in boys. Adolescent scoliosis is the most common type, with radiographic studies showing that from 1.3% to 3% of patients have a spinal curvature of 10 degrees or greater.

Congenital scoliosis is the result of abnormal vertebral development. Affected patients often have associated visceral abnormalities, particularly involving the cardiac and renal systems. Associated skeletal deformities include Klippel-Feil syndrome (congenital cervical spine fusion), Sprengel's deformity, and radial club hand.

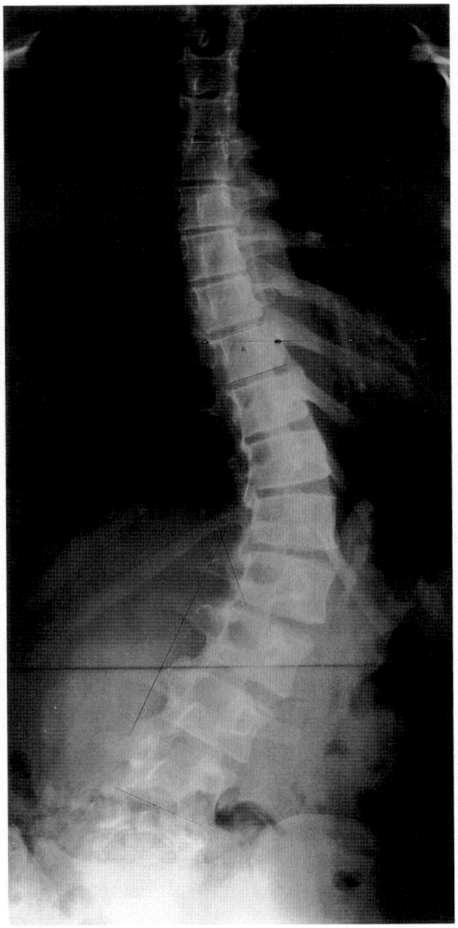

FIGURE 46–4 Radiograph of an adolescent patient with scoliosis.

In some cases, scoliosis occurs secondary to neuromuscular conditions, such as cerebral palsy, muscular dystrophy, meningomyelocele, and poliomyelitis (see Neuromuscular Disorders in Children, later). Progressive scoliosis develops in virtually all patients with Duchenne's muscular dystrophy and coincides with the loss of ambulation and confinement to a wheelchair. Patients with meningomyelocele have a high incidence of scoliosis secondary to muscle paralyses or to vertebral anomalies.

Evaluation

School screening programs are recommended for girls 11 to 13 years old and boys 13 to 14 years old. Adolescents are examined for trunk asymmetry, generally on a forward-bending test. A scoliosometer is used to quantify truncal rotation, and children with angles measuring 7 degrees or greater are referred for a complete physical examination and neurologic evaluation.

Physical examination may reveal lateral trunk shift, flank crease asymmetry, leg-length discrepancy, asymmetrical rib hump, and shoulder asymmetry. In patients with scoliosis, curves are described by their apex. The types of curves, listed from the most frequent to the least frequent, are as follows: right thoracic curves; double major (right thoracic and left lumbar) curves; left lumbar curves; right lumbar curves; and left thoracic curves. This last type of curve is associated with a high rate of intrathecal abnormalities, and evaluation by MRI is recommended. Curve progression is related to the magnitude of the curve, the age of the patient, and skeletal maturity. Severe thoracic curves may be associated with cardiopulmonary dysfunction. Severe lumbar curves may be associated with pain.

Standing anteroposterior and lateral radiographs are used to quantify the curve. In the case of a leg-length discrepancy, sitting films or leg-length–corrected standing films (i.e., films taken with the patient standing on blocks) should be obtained. A film that includes the pelvis will allow Risser staging, which is based on ossification of the iliac crest apophysis and ranges from grade 0 to grade 5.

Treatment

Physical therapy, electrostimulation, and manipulation have not been found to influence the natural history of scoliosis. All patients should be observed for curve progression. Bracing is used to treat patients in whom curve progression is documented and to treat skeletally immature patients who have a curve that is 30 to 40 degrees and is categorized as grade 0, 1, or 2. Surgery is indicated if curve progression continues despite bracing or if the curve exceeds 40 degrees.

Developmental Dislocation of the Hip

Developmental dislocation of the hip is the most common hip disorder that affects children. Most patients show dislocation at birth (the incidence ranges from 2.7 to 17 per 1000 live births), but some are first seen with late subluxation and acetabular dysplasia. The cause of the disorder is multifactorial. Ligament laxity, mechanical factors, breech presentation, and family history have all been implicated.

Evaluation

In neonates and infants up to age 3 months, the Ortolani maneuver and Barlow test may reveal hip instability and dislocation. The Ortolani maneuver reduces the dislocated hip via gentle abduction and forward translation of the femoral head. The Barlow test dislocates or subluxates the unstable hip via adduction of the flexed hip and gentle pressure directed posteriorly and applied through the knee. In older infants, hip instability and dislocation are characterized by a loss of abduction secondary to shortening of hip musculature or by apparent shortening of the thigh (Galeazzi sign).

Treatment

Treatment focuses on obtaining and maintaining reduction of the femoral head while allowing development of the acetabulum. The Pavlik harness allows hip motion within a stable arc. Most older children are treated with closed reduction and casting, but a small percentage require open reduction.

Legg-Calvé-Perthes Disease

Legg-Calvé-Perthes disease is an unusual condition that causes varying degrees of femoral head fragmentation and repair. The disease is seen in children age 2 to 12 years, with a peak incidence in those who are age 4 to 8 years. Boys are affected 4 to 5 times more commonly than girls, and the disease is bilateral in about 10% of cases. Although Legg-Calvé-Perthes disease is generally considered to be a sequela of idiopathic osteonecrosis, it may represent a more generalized disorder of the epiphyseal cartilage. No evidence yet exists that it is a genetic or coagulation disorder.

Evaluation

Patients may be seen initially with a limp and occasional pain in the groin, thigh, or knee. Laboratory results are normal. Plain radiographs may reveal fragmentation or flattening of the femoral ossific nucleus, but they occasionally yield normal results. MRI can show the extent of involvement.

Treatment

Treatment focuses on reduction of pain, improvement of function, and minimization of femoral head deformity. Bed rest, traction, and bracing have all been used, with varying degrees of efficacy. Some patients require surgery to achieve containment of the hip. The prognosis is better for children younger than 6 years than for older children.

Slipped Capital Femoral Epiphysis

Slipped capital femoral epiphysis is a disorder in which the proximal femoral epiphysis becomes displaced on the femoral neck. The disorder affects boys twice as often as girls, and it is more common in black children than in white and Asian children. The prevalence of symptomatic bilateral slips is reported to be 37%. The cause of the disorder is unknown. Patients with endocrine abnormalities (most commonly, hypothyroidism) appear to have a predilection for the femoral disorder. Mechanical factors, such as obesity and rapid growth spurts, also may play a role. Trauma does not appear to be a significant cause.

Evaluation

The clinical presentation is quite variable. Some patients complain of the sudden onset of groin, thigh, or knee pain, whereas others note an insidious onset of pain over several weeks or months. Patients are often able to bear weight, but they may have a limp and walk with the affected leg in external rotation. Attempts at internally rotating the hip will duplicate the pain, and hip flexion may cause obligate external rotation.

Anteroposterior and lateral radiographs are essential for making the diagnosis. The earliest radiographic sign is slight widening and irregularity of the physis seen on the anteroposterior view. In a mild slip, the height of the epiphysis on the affected side may be slightly decreased in comparison with that on the unaffected side. Klein's line (tangential to the superior femoral neck) will not intersect the lateral aspect of the femoral head. The lateral view will show the femoral head displaced posterior to the neck, and it may show remodeling of the femoral neck on the affected side, making it appear bowed in comparison with the unaffected side. The severity of the slip is judged by the amount of displacement seen on the lateral view.

Treatment

Treatment focuses primarily on preventing progression of the slip. A corrective osteotomy to redirect the femoral head into a more normal weight-bearing position can be considered. However, the current recommendation is for in situ screw fixation of the slip, by using fluoroscopic control. A single screw is appropriate for a stable slip, defined as a slip that with motion does not fluoroscopically demonstrate independent movement of the epiphysis. Two screws may be needed to fix an unstable slip. Most patients will experience some improvement in hip motion after fixation. Screw fixation also will induce premature physeal closure, but this may take up to 14 months to occur.

Complications

Realignment osteotomies may improve the range of motion, but they are associated with a higher rate of complications such as osteoarthritis. Osteonecrosis and chondrolysis are complications that can occur with or without treatment. The incidence of osteonecrosis is increased in unstable slips, in stable slips undergoing aggressive reduction, and in slips treated with multiple screw fixation into the anterolateral or posterolateral femoral head. Chondrolysis in patients with untreated slips may be a result of an immune-mediated process. In treated slips, it is associated with mechanical damage caused by permanent pin or screw placement into the joint.

Pediatric Disorders of the Lower Extremities

One of the more common reasons for orthopedic consultation is the evaluation of a child's walking pattern. An abnormal pattern is usually benign and self-limited, but evaluation will help rule out the presence of a pathologic condition.

Pigeon Toe

Pigeon toe, or **in-toeing**, may be the result of a rotational disorder of the lower extremities. Physical examination is important to rule out a disorder or delineate the cause of the disorder.

In infants younger than 1 year, a common problem is **metatarsus adductus** (Fig. 46-5), or adduction of the forefoot at the level of the tarsometatarsal joints. This problem usually resolves spontaneously. Passive stretching exercises are generally recommended for feet that can be passively but not actively corrected to the neutral position.

In toddlers, the most common cause of in-toeing is **tibial torsion** (Fig. 46-6). The thigh-foot axis (which normally shows 0 to 15 degrees of external rotation) is internally rotated in this condition. The condition is usually bilateral, but it can be unilateral and is generally worse on the left side. In most children, tibial torsion resolves spontaneously. Although a Denis Browne splint is sometimes used, the efficacy of this device is uncertain. Operative correction through a supramalleolar osteotomy is generally reserved for severe cases.

In children who are age 3 to 6 years old**, femoral anteversion** (Fig. 46-7) is the most common cause of in-toeing. These children have increased internal rotation of the hip and decreased external rotation. They will often sit with their legs in a W position. The disorder generally resolves by the time the child reaches age 10 years. If it is severe and continues to be symptomatic after this age, surgical correction may be indicated, because in older children with persistent femoral anteversion and compensatory external tibial torsion, patellofemoral problems may develop.

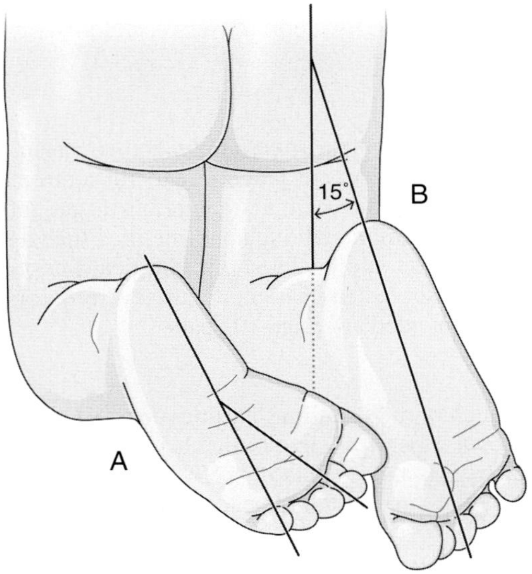

FIGURE 46–5 Common measurements for torsional disorders. *A*, Metatarsus adductus. *B*, Normal thigh-foot angle. Negative thigh-foot angles (<10 degrees) are seen in tibial torsion.

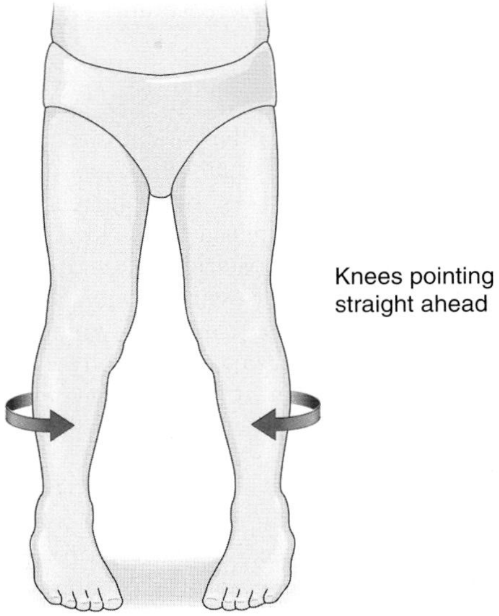

FIGURE 46–6 Tibial torsion.

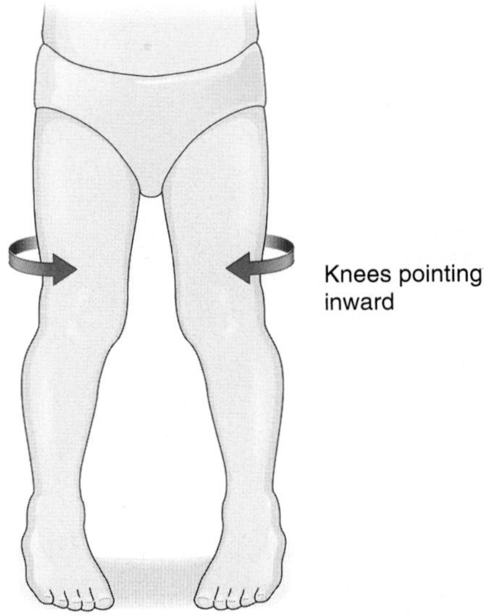

FIGURE 46–7 Femoral anteversion.

Genu Varum

Genu varum, or **bowleg,** is physiologic in newborns and young infants. At birth, the tibiofemoral angle is about 10 to 15 degrees of varus. In most cases, this gradually corrects to neutral alignment by age 2 years. However, in children who are early walkers or have an above-average weight, this bowing may increase up to about 18 months before it begins to correct.

Evaluation

If the bowing persists after the patient reaches age 2 years, it is important to rule out pathologic conditions such as vitamin D–dependent rickets, hypophosphatemic rickets, metaphyseal chondrodysplasia, and tibia vara (Blount disease). Standing anteroposterior radiographs of the lower extremities are helpful in assessing for tibia vara (Fig. 46-8), a condition that may be seen in young children or adolescents. The finding of a metaphyseal diaphyseal angle that is greater than 16 degrees in a young child is considered predictive of Blount disease.

Treatment

Bracing may be helpful in children younger than 3 years but is controversial. Surgery is reserved for patients who have not improved by age 4 years. The goal is to overcorrect, because recurrence of the deformity is common.

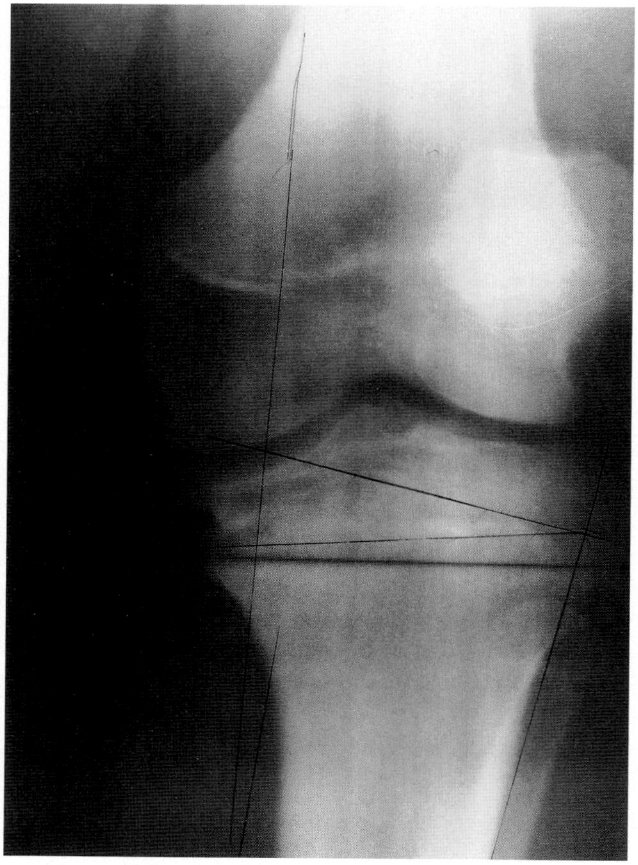

FIGURE 46–8 Radiograph of a patient with adolescent Blount disease.

PEARLS FOR ROUNDS

In children, fractures have the remarkable ability to remodel because of concurrent longitudinal growth. Treatment generally involves closed reduction and casting to maintain alignment while the bones heal. However, if the fracture is displaced, surgical intervention may be necessary to restore articular congruity.

If fractures are found in an infant who is not yet walking, child abuse should be considered. The most common long-bone fractures seen in abused children are fractures of the humerus, tibia, and femur.

Scoliosis is characterized by lateral deviation and rotation of the spinal column.

Developmental dislocation of the hip is the most common hip disorder affecting children.

Slipped capital femoral epiphysis is a disorder in which the proximal femoral epiphysis becomes displaced on the femoral neck.

Pigeon toe, or in-toeing, may be the result of a rotational disorder of the lower extremities. Physical examination is important to rule out a disorder or delineate the cause of the disorder.

In infants younger than 1 year, a common problem is metatarsus adductus, or adduction of the forefoot at the level of the tarsometatarsal joints.

Clubfoot consists of ankle equinus, heel varus (inversion), forefoot adduction, and forefoot equinus.

Adolescents with tibia vara are generally obese and do not respond to bracing. Surgical management, either by hemiepiphysiodesis or corrective osteotomy, is the treatment of choice.

Genu Valgum

Genu valgum, or **knock knee**, is physiologic from age 2 years and peaks on average at age 3 years. In some cases, it results from a proximal tibia fracture. In a patient with severe genu valgum, metabolic abnormalities such as renal osteodystrophy should be ruled out. Surgical intervention is generally reserved for patients with severe deformities and is recommended after age 10 years.

Clubfoot

Congenital clubfoot, or **talipes equinovarus,** is a deformity seen in about 1 per 1000 live births. It is more common in boys than in girls and is bilateral in 30% to 40% of patients.

Evaluation

Clubfoot consists of ankle equinus, heel varus (inversion), forefoot adduction, and forefoot equinus. The affected leg and foot are smaller and shorter than normal. The cause of clubfoot is multifactorial and is not well understood;

however, the deformity is sometimes seen in association with disorders such as myelomeningocele, diastrophic dwarfism, and Larsen's syndrome. It also is seen in patients with vertebral, anal, cardiac, tracheal, esophageal, renal, and limb (VACTERL) anomalies.

Treatment

During the first 3 months of life, patients with congenital clubfoot are treated with gentle manipulation and serial casting of the foot. When they reach age 3 months, radiographs are obtained to determine whether nonsurgical treatment should be continued. Lateral views with forced dorsiflexion and anteroposterior views with simulated weight bearing are taken, and the talocalcaneal angle is evaluated. If the goal of convergence has not been met or is unlikely to be met with nonsurgical treatment, surgery is indicated. Surgery is undertaken when the patient is between ages 6 and 12 months and is designed to address all aspects of the deformity, so that additional operative interventions are not required in the future. The goal is a plantigrade foot that is pain free, functional, and stable.

Tarsal Coalition

In patients with tarsal coalition, a congenital failure of differentiation and segmentation of the tarsal bones results in a fibrous, cartilaginous, or osseous connection. The most common types of coalition are calcaneonavicular and talocalcaneal. Tarsal coalition may occur in isolation or may be associated with another disorder, such as Apert's syndrome or fibular hemimelia. Because tarsal coalition is usually asymptomatic, its true prevalence is unknown.

Evaluation

Symptoms occur in about 25% of cases. Patients are first seen with activity-related pain that localizes to the area of the sinus tarsi and may be described as an ankle sprain. Progressive valgus of the hindfoot, flattening of the longitudinal arch, and limitation of subtalar motion may develop. Standard anteroposterior and lateral radiographs may not show the abnormality. The calcaneonavicular coalition is best seen on an oblique view, whereas the talocalcaneal coalition may be demonstrated by an axial (Harris) view. Computed tomography (CT) scanning will best demonstrate a subtalar coalition. MRI may be necessary to diagnose a fibrous coalition.

Treatment

Treatment is indicated only for symptomatic patients. Immobilization and orthotics are used initially to try to alleviate the symptoms. Surgical intervention is reserved for patients in whom symptoms persist.

Flexible Flatfoot

The average normal arch height is lower in children than in adults. The arch height increases during the first decade of life, and the range of normal arch heights in all ages is quite wide. Large-scale population studies show that most young children have "flat" feet that fall in the "normal" range. Recent studies of the effect of shoe modifications and inserts on arch height show no benefit, because spontaneous improvement of the longitudinal arch will occur with or without intervention.

Flexible flatfoot is a variant of normal. In patients with this condition, a loss of the longitudinal arch occurs during weight bearing, with reconstitution of an arch on toe standing. The length of the Achilles tendon is normal, and good subtalar mobility is present. Although flexible flatfoot rarely causes disability, some children may complain of activity-related foot pain. Shoe inserts may alleviate this discomfort, as well as extend the life of the shoe. However, the inserts will not improve the appearance of the foot.

Neuromuscular Disorders in Children

Cerebral Palsy

Cerebral palsy is a static encephalopathy, or nonprogressive motor disorder of the central nervous system. The disorder may occur in association with prematurity, anoxic injuries, head trauma, meningitis, or perinatal infections such as toxoplasmosis, rubella, cytomegalovirus, and herpes simplex (TORCH infections).

Evaluation and Classification

Patients with cerebral palsy usually are first seen with motor milestone delays. In infants as young as 4 months, predictive signs of cerebral palsy can be identified by evaluating the extension tone of the neck, head control in the sitting position, and weight bearing through the arms in the prone position.

Cerebral palsy can be classified physiologically, according to the type of movement disorder that is present. **Spasticity** is the most common and is characterized by increased tone and hyperreflexia. **Athetosis** is more frequently seen in patients with kernicterus and is characterized by writhing movements and lack of muscle control. **Ataxia**, or **extrapyramidal cerebral palsy,** is characterized by decreased coordination, lack of balance, and a wide-based gait. In some cases, patients have a mixed picture, with spasticity and athetosis involving the entire body.

Cerebral palsy also can be classified topographically, according to the area of involvement. **Hemiplegia** involves the upper and lower extremity on the same side; **diplegia** involves lower extremities more than upper extremities; and **quadriplegia** involves the entire body. Hemiplegic patients have early hand dominance, and a leg-length discrepancy may develop. All hemiplegics and most diplegics have the ability to walk. Quadriplegics are less likely to walk.

Treatment

The mainstay of treatment is physical therapy. Muscle-stretching and -strengthening exercises are indicated to minimize contractures and maximize muscle function. Therapy also is important for improving function in patients who undergo surgery.

In ambulatory patients, surgical management requires careful planning and an understanding of the primary deformities, which require treatment, as well as the compensatory deformities, which do not. Common problems include windswept hip deformity and hip subluxation, crouched gait, equinovarus deformity of the ankle, and scoliosis.

In patients with spasticity, several treatment options exist to diminish spasticity and thereby improve integrated muscle function and muscle strength. The first option is medical treatment with baclofen, a γ-aminobutyric acid (GABA) agonist that acts by inhibiting the release of excitatory neurotransmitters. Baclofen can be given orally or via continuous intrathecal pump infusion. Clinical studies have shown that treatment via pump infusion causes a significant reduction of spasticity without systemic side effects but with a high rate of complications. The second option is selective dorsal rhizotomy. Results of rhizotomy are promising, but concerns exist about post-operative weakness, spinal deformity, and rapid hip subluxation. The third and newest option is injection of botulinum A toxin, which acts at the level of the motor end plate to "paralyze" the spastic muscles. The effects of the toxin generally last from 2 to 4 months. In patients with significant spasticity at an early age, the use of botulinum toxin may delay the need for surgical intervention and help identify the muscles that require intervention.

Myelomeningocele

Myelomeningocele, or **spina bifida cystica**, is a neural tube defect that results from failure of the neural tube to close during early embryonic development. Hereditary factors and environmental factors, including folate deficiency, are implicated. In the United States, the incidence of neural tube defects has decreased over the last few decades and is expected to decrease further, partly because of early screening and partly because of periconceptual administration of folic acid.

Evaluation

Hydrocephalus that requires shunting is found in 70% to 85% of patients, and syringomyelia is seen in up to 54% of patients. About 90% of patients have a type II Arnold-Chiari malformation with displacement of the brainstem into the foramen magnum. Patients with myelomeningocele have varying degrees of spinal cord dysfunction, ranging from complete paraplegia to only bowel and bladder dysfunction. Children with myelomeningocele are prone to develop symptomatic tethering of the spinal cord, which can alter the bowel and bladder function; cause progressive scoliosis, spasticity, and weakness; and lead to worsening of foot deformities. According to recent studies in adults with sacrum-level lesions, up to 30% of patients lose their ability to ambulate independently by age 30 years. This implies that myelomeningocele causes a slow deterioration of function over time.

Orthopedic problems are related to the level of neurologic function and can include such problems as hip dislocation, clubfoot, and congenital vertical talus. Patients with myelomeningocele are susceptible to pathologic fractures. The affected limb may become hot and swollen, with the appearance of a septic process.

Latex allergy is seen in 18% to 40% of children with myelomeningocele and is thought to be due to multiple exposures to latex catheters early in life. For this reason, latex-free environments are generally recommended for patients with myelomeningocele.

PEARLS FOR THE OR

If a periosteal abscess is present or if the patient has not responded to antibiotic treatment, surgical treatment should be performed to decompress and débride the bone.

In children with chronic osteomyelitis, surgical intervention is required to débride necrotic infected bone, and adjuvant antibiotic therapy is necessary to effect remission.

Severe cases of in-toeing caused by tibial torsion can be corrected surgically with a supramalleolar osteotomy.

Treatment

A multidisciplinary approach is used in the treatment of myelomeningocele. The neurosurgery, orthopedic, and rehabilitation services must work together to help children maintain functional mobility by ambulation or by a wheelchair and to prevent neurologic deterioration. The mainstays of treatment are bracing and assist devices. Specific surgical intervention is determined on an individual basis as the need arises. This is most often related to detethering of the cord, contracture releases, or spinal deformity correction.

Muscular Dystrophies

The muscular dystrophies are a group of hereditary disorders characterized by progressive muscle weakness that is unrelated to an inflammatory condition.

Duchenne's muscular dystrophy is a sex-linked recessive disorder in which dystrophin is absent and levels of creatine phosphokinase become markedly elevated. Affected patients will demonstrate normal developmental milestones in the early years but will begin to show signs of weakness around age 4 years. At this time, because of significant weakness in the gluteus maximus and quadriceps muscles, patients will be unable to rise from a seated position on the floor without rolling over, kneeling, and pushing their hands against their shins, knees, and thighs (Gowers sign). As a compensation for proximal motor weakness, they will walk on their toes and demonstrate lumbar lordosis.

Children with Duchenne's muscular dystrophy lose their ability to ambulate independently by age 10 years. Once they are wheelchair-bound, scoliosis progresses rapidly, because no muscular support exists for the growing spine. Spinal instrumentation and fusion to the pelvis can prevent patients from becoming bedridden and can help their pulmonary function. Death of cardiopulmonary complications usually occurs by the third decade.

Facioscapulohumeral muscular dystrophy is an autosomal dominant disorder that is seen in older children and adolescents and is characterized by muscle abnormalities of the face, scapula, and arm. The creatine phosphokinase levels are normal. Treatment is aimed at restoring the mechanical advantage of the deltoid and rotator-cuff muscles (which are usually spared). The technique of scapulothoracic fusion has been shown to increase shoulder flexion and abduction and allows patients to raise their arms above their heads.

Myotonic myopathies are autosomal dominant disorders that are characterized by the inability of muscles to relax after contraction. Congenital myotonic myopathy is also called floppy-infant syndrome. Aggressive orthopedic management improves quality of life. Treatment is primarily orthotic, with contracture release when necessary. Scoliosis also is common and may require surgical stabilization as life expectancy is until the adult years.

Poliomyelitis

Poliomyelitis is caused by poliovirus, an enterovirus that attacks the anterior horn cells in the brain and spinal cord. Because of wide-scale vaccination, the disease has been eradicated in the United States but is still found in many other parts of the world.

Poliomyelitis is characterized by muscle weakness with normal sensation. Affected patients can demonstrate a wide range of deformities, depending on the extent of involvement. Bracing is used to prevent deformity and maximize function. Surgical intervention may be indicated to balance muscle forces and to correct deformity in ambulatory patients.

Suggested Reading

Benson MKD, Fixsen JA, MacNicol MF (eds): Children's Orthopaedics and Fractures, 2nd ed. Philadelphia, Churchill Livingstone, 2002.

Weinstein S: The Pediatric Spine: Principles and Practice. New York, Raven Press, 1994.

Wenger D, Rang M: The Art and Practice of Children's Orthopaedics. New York, Raven Press, 1993.

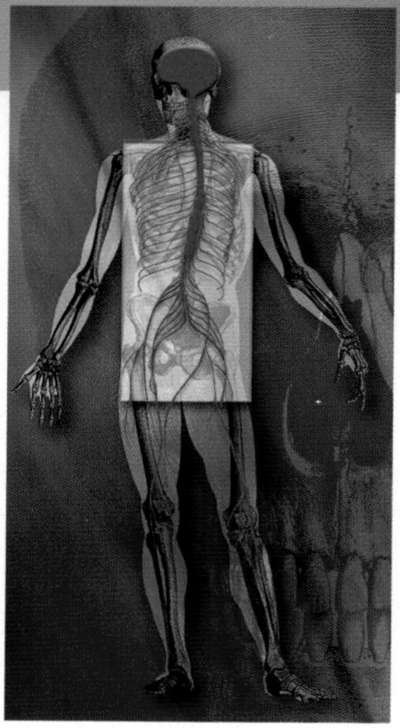

SECTION XII

NEUROSURGERY

Chapter 47

Management of Patients with Neurosurgical Diseases

ROGER HARTL, MD, and PHILIP E. STIEG, MD, PhD

Trauma

Traumatic Brain Injury

Traumatic brain injury (TBI) is a leading cause of death and disability in children and in adults in their most productive years. Overall, each year there are approximately 52,000 deaths from TBI and an estimated 70,000 to 90,000 are left with permanent neurologic disabilities. Thus neurotrauma is a serious public health problem mandating continuing efforts in the areas of prevention and treatment. During the past two decades, understanding of the pathophysiology of TBI has increased remarkably. One central concept is that not all neurologic damage occurs immediately at the moment of impact (primary injury), but evolves over the ensuing minutes, hours, and days. This theoretically preventable secondary brain injury can increase mortality and worsen disability.

In this chapter, we refer to recently published, evidence-based documents containing guidelines for the medical and surgical management of patients with TBI (see J Neurotrauma 17:449–554, 2000). These documents have been accepted by the American Association of Neurological Surgeons and the World Health Organization and can be accessed via the Internet at *www.braintrauma.org*.

TBI is graded as mild, moderate, and severe on the basis of the Glasgow Coma Scale (GCS) after resuscitation. Mild TBI (GCS, 13–15) in most cases results from a concussion, and full recovery ensues. In moderate head injury, the patient is lethargic or stuporous (GCS, 9–13), and in severe head injury, the patient is comatose and unable to open the eyes (GCS, 3–8).

Glasgow Coma Scale

The GCS scoring system is routinely used as part of the neurologic examination in severe head injury. Note that the GCS represents the best response elicited from the patient. This is particularly relevant to the motor score, which represents the response of the best responding limb. The GCS should be recorded with the patient off paralytics and sedatives. Motor and verbal responses are assessed (Table 47-1).

The best response of any limb is recorded. If the patient is paralyzed or heavily sedated, score the best response that you actually observe. If the score cannot be assessed, assign a value of 1. Standard painful stimulus is an axillary pinch to elicit a localization response. For all other responses, use nail-bed pressure. If both eyes cannot be assessed or if the patient underwent tracheostomy or intubation, assign a value of 1.

Motor function

- Localizes pain: The patient crosses the midline, reaches toward and attempts to remove the painful/noxious stimuli.
- Flexion withdrawal: The patient pulls the extremity or body part away from the painful/noxious stimuli.

TABLE 47–1 Glasgow Coma Scale

Score	Eyes	Verbal	Motor
6	—	—	Obeys commands
5	—	Oriented and converses	Localizes painful stimuli
4	Spontaneously	Disoriented and converses	Flexion withdrawal
3	To verbal command	Inappropriate words	Flexion abnormal
2	To painful stimuli	Incomprehensible sounds	Extension
1	No response	No response	No response

* Total score is between 3 and 15. GCS score <9 indicates coma.

- Flexion abnormal (decorticate): The arms are tightly flexed over the chest. The elbows, wrists, and fingers are flexed, and the legs are rigidly extended and internally rotated.
- Extension (decerebration): The arms are rigidly extended and close to the body. The legs are rigidly extended, and the feet are plantar flexed.

The verbal assessment entails asking the patient for the month and year.

Initial Assessment and Clinical Examination of Patients with Severe Traumatic Brain Injury

Prehospital evaluation and management of patients with TBI is similar to the protocol in other trauma patients (Table 47-2 *A* and *B*). The cornerstones of the resuscitation of severely head-injured patient are as follows:

- Primary survey with cervical spine control and brief neurologic assessment
- Resuscitation (airway, breathing, circulation)
- Secondary survey with complete neurologic examination and determination of the GCS score

General principles of the TBI workup are the following:

- Unless signs of cerebral herniation (pupillary asymmetry, dilated/fixed pupils, extensor posturing or flaccidity to noxious stimuli, or a combination of these) are noted, patients should not be hyper-

TABLE 47–2A Outline of the Initial Assessment of a Comatose Patient or a Patient Who Has Been Intubated and Sedated

	Critical Findings	Intervention
Oxygenation/ventilation	Apnea, cyanosis, Sa_{O_2} <90%	Intubation if hypoxemic despite supplemental O_2, keep Pa_{CO_2} at 35 mmHg
Blood pressure	SBP <90 mmHg	Isotonic fluid resuscitation, MAP >90 mmHg, consider arterial line
Spinal stability	Pain, mechanism, radiography, severe TBI	Immobilization, imaging
Postresuscitation GCS <9	Herniation syndrome, posturing	Consider sedation ± pharmacologic paralysis for transport and intubation Short-term hyperventilation ± mannitol, head CT
Pupillary diameter, light reflex	Dilated pupil: diameter ≥ 4mm Asymmetry: ≥ 1 mm difference between pupils Fixed pupil: constricts, < 1mm to light	If herniation suspected: short-term hyperventilation ± mannitol

CT computed tomography; MAP, mean arterial pressure, TBI, traumatic brain injury.

TABLE 47–2B Outline of a Detailed Neurologic Examination*

	Critical Findings	Intervention
Visual inspection, external signs of cranial trauma	Raccoon's eyes, Battle sign, CSF leak from ears and/or nose, hematotympanon, facial fractures, proptosis, direct orbital trauma, skull-base fractures	Prophylactic antibiotics controversial
Mental status	Decreased level of consciousness	If herniation suspected: Short-term hyperventilation ± mannitol
Cranial nerves	Visual fields/acuity changes, pupillary abnormalities, nystagmus, absent oculocephalic response ("doll's eyes," do not test in patients with possible cervical spine injury), abnormal oculovestibular response ("cold calories"), nerve III, VI, and VII palsy	Consider head CT Monitoring in ICU
Motor examination	Abnormal flexion, abnormal extension, or flaccid to noxious stimuli	
Sensory examination	Abnormal finding with pin-prick and light touch, position sense, vibration. No withdrawal from noxious stimuli	
Reflexes and muscle tone	Abnormal deep-tendon reflexes Babinski sign (upgoing toe) Abnormal rectal tone and/or bulbocavernosus reflex	

*Some tests may not be possible in comatose patients.
CSF cerebrospinal fluid; CT, computed tomography; ICU, intensive care unit, MAP, mean arterial pressure.

ventilated and the arterial P_{CO_2} should be maintained around 35 mmHg, the lower limit of normocapnia.

- Isotonic fluids should be used for resuscitation to avoid free-water overload.
- Computed tomography (CT) is the imaging study of choice to detect skull fractures or intracranial injury with hemorrhage and to assess the necessity of surgical evacuation of a mass lesion. A head CT scan also can demonstrate pathology that is closely associated with intracranial hypertension, such as obliterated basal cisterns, compressed cerebral ventricles, and midline shift. Magnetic resonance imaging (MRI) scanning is usually not indicated in the acute phase after TBI. A cerebral angiography or magnetic resonance angiography (MRA) is helpful if a traumatic dissection of the carotid artery is suspected. This should be considered if unilateral neurologic deficits cannot be explained by the head CT.
- All comatose patients with an abnormal CT scan and a GCS score of 8 or less should undergo intracranial pressure (ICP) monitoring.
- Obtain plain radiographs of the cervical spine as soon as possible and a CT scan of suggestive areas.
- Once the patient has been stabilized, a careful physical examination should be conducted.
- Scalp wounds should be thoroughly inspected and sutured to prevent blood loss.

Surgical Indications in Traumatic Brain Injury

The decision to operate on a patient with an intracranial traumatic mass lesion has sometimes to be made within a few minutes and is influenced by many factors (Fig. 47-1). Some general comments can be made. Consider surgery for the following:

- Open, depressed skull fractures
- Any symptomatic extra-axial lesion, such as a subdural hematoma (SDH) or epidural hematoma (EDH)
- Intracranial hematoma causing more than 5-mm midline shift
- Brain contusion causing more than 5-mm midline shift, unless it is found in an "eloquent" area of the brain, such as the speech cortex, the motor or sensory areas, thalamus, or basal ganglia
- Lesions in the posterior fossa should be considered for operation even if they appear small and do not cause neurologic problems, because of the risk of rapid expansion

A large question mark–shaped incision for the trauma craniotomy has classically been used for the evacuation of most supratentorial traumatic mass lesions. If high ICP is suspected or expected to develop postoperatively, the bone flap can be stored in the bone bank for later reimplantation. This is called a *decompressive craniectomy*.

Specific Lesions

Acute and Chronic Subdural Hematoma. An SDH is a collection of blood between the dura and the brain surface, usually due to injury to cortical blood vessels or bridging veins (Fig. 47-2). Frequently, subdural hematomas are associated with underlying injury to the brain, such as contusions, lacerations, and hematomas, so SDHs sometimes show a complicated postoperative course with secondary brain swelling and increases in ICP. Other neurotoxic factors and the presence of blood also have been implicated in secondary ischemia after SDH, even if the hematoma was evacuated in a timely fashion. Treatment recommendations for patients with acute SDH are summarized in Figure 47-3.

One of the most feared complications during surgery is the development of malignant brain swelling, which can result in massive herniation of the brain through the craniotomy defect. If this cannot be controlled with hyperventilation and mannitol, a new contralateral mass lesion should be suspected. This can be ruled out with intraoperative ultrasound.

Chronic SDHs are more frequent in infants and in the elderly after minor head trauma. They arise from tears in the bridging veins; the blood liquefies over time and becomes encased by fibrous membranes and slowly increases in size. Patients can sometimes be completely asymptomatic or can have focal deficits, hemiparesis, and papilledema. Surgical treatment includes craniotomy or burr-hole drainage in the operating room (OR). If the CT scan demonstrates that the SDH is homogeneous and not septated, twist-drill craniostomies can be attempted in the intensive care unit (ICU) or in the OR. The fluid drained typically has a "motor oil" appearance.

Epidural Hematoma. In these lesions, the blood is located usually in the temporal region between the dura and the inner table of the skull (Fig. 47-4). It is usually attributed to an injury to the middle meningeal artery. EDHs are more frequently seen in younger patients between ages 20 and 40 years. The classic presentation of EDHs has been described as a patient who loses consciousness immediately after injury, followed by a lucid interval shortly after trauma, and then a secondary loss of consciousness. Only up to one third of patients appear like that; the majority remain unresponsive after trauma. Prompt evacuation of an EDH can result in an excellent outcome, even though the patient may have been in a deep coma preoperatively. Any symptomatic EDH, an acute asymptomatic EDH with greater than 15-mm thickness, and any posterior fossa EDH should be considered for surgery. Treatment recommendations for acute EDH are presented in Figure 47-5.

Intraparenchymal Lesions. Contusions occur in up to 90% of patients who die of a severe TBI. Most

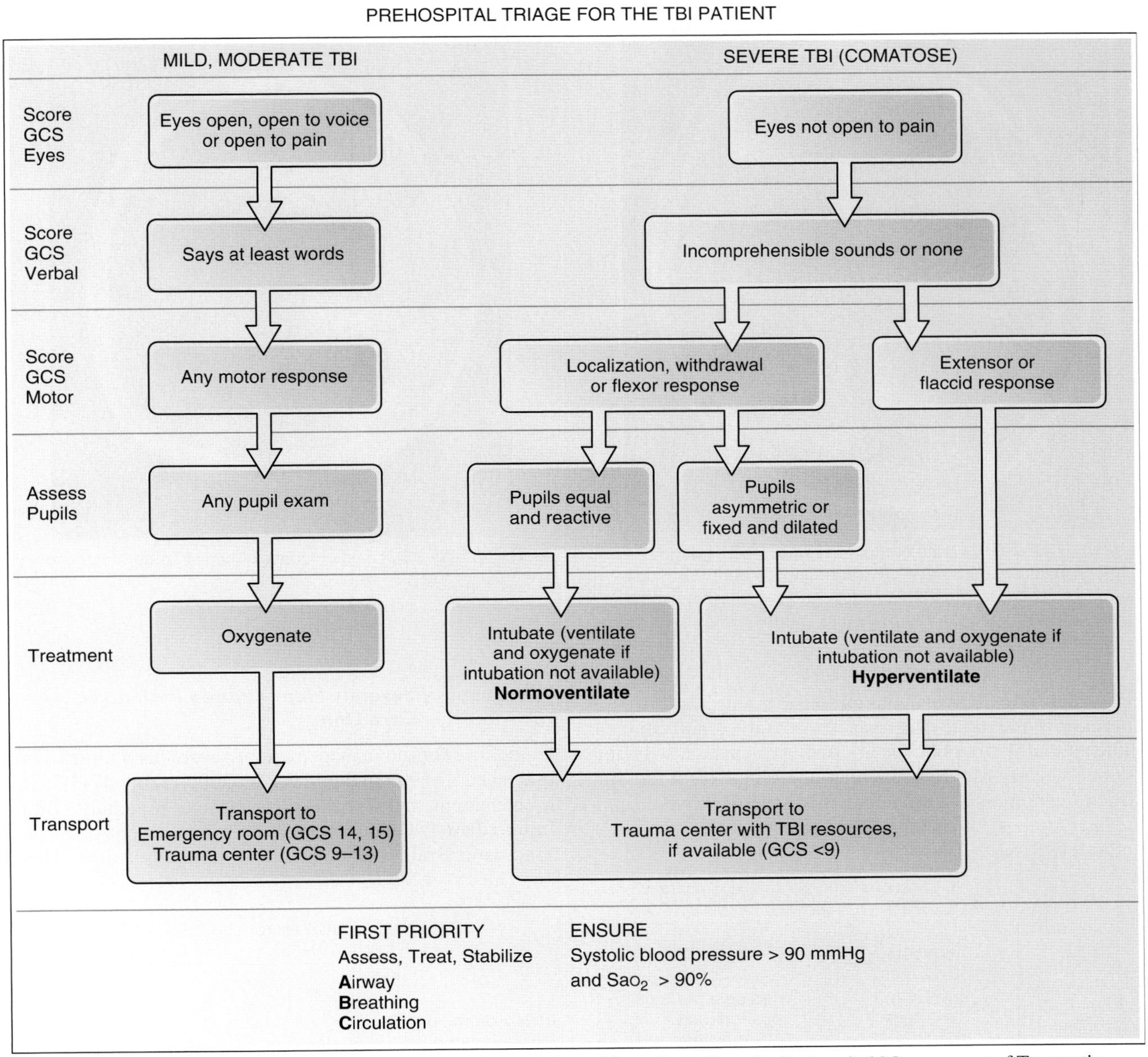

FIGURE 47–1 Algorithm for neurotrauma treatment triage. (Adapted from Guidelines for Prehospital Management of Traumatic Injury. Brain Trauma Foundation, Inc. New York, New York, 2000, with permission.)

contusions are located in the frontal and temporal lobes. They tend to increase over time and may contribute significantly to the development of intracranial hypertension. Temporal lobe contusions are especially dangerous because they may compress the brainstem without causing high ICPs. A patient's brain may therefore herniate, even though the ICP readings were relatively low. Temporal lobe lesions and large contusions should undergo surgical removal.

Decompressive Craniectomy. Decompressive craniectomy has been proposed for the treatment of established severe intracranial hypertension or if the development of high ICP is anticipated while operating on a traumatic

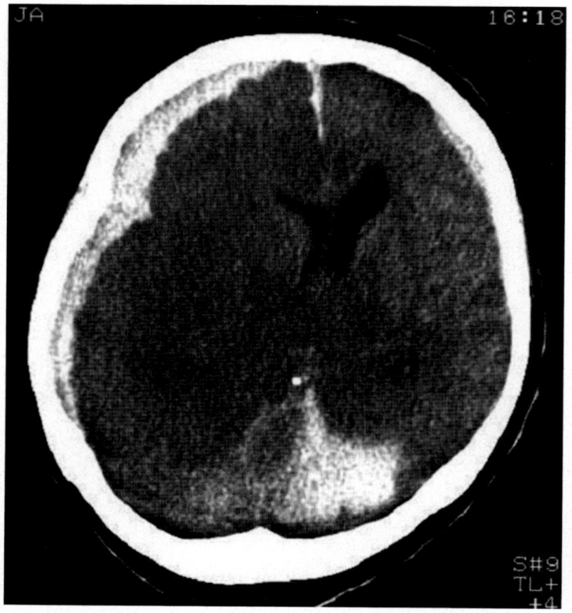

FIGURE 47–2 This axial computed tomography image depicts an acute right-sided crescent-shaped subdural hematoma (SDH). The SDH extends into the interhemispheric space anteriorly. A tentorial SDH and significant midline shift are noted.

cerebral lesion. For a decompressive craniectomy to be successful, the bone flap has to be large, and studies indicate that it works better in young patients and when it is done as early as possible. Other neurologic disorders for which decompressive craniectomies have been advocated are large strokes, intracerebral hemorrhages, Reye syndrome, and rarely SAH.

	GCS score 9–15	GCS score < 9
Clot thickness > 10 mm *or* MLS > 5 mm	Early surgery	Surgery as soon as possible with post-operative ICP monitoring
Clot thickness < 10 mm *and* MLS < 5 mm	Non-operative management	Surgery if: •GCS decrease by 2 or more points prior to admission •ICP > 20 mmHg or abnormal pupillary exam •ICP monitoring required

FIGURE 47–3 Treatment options for patients with acute subdural hematoma.

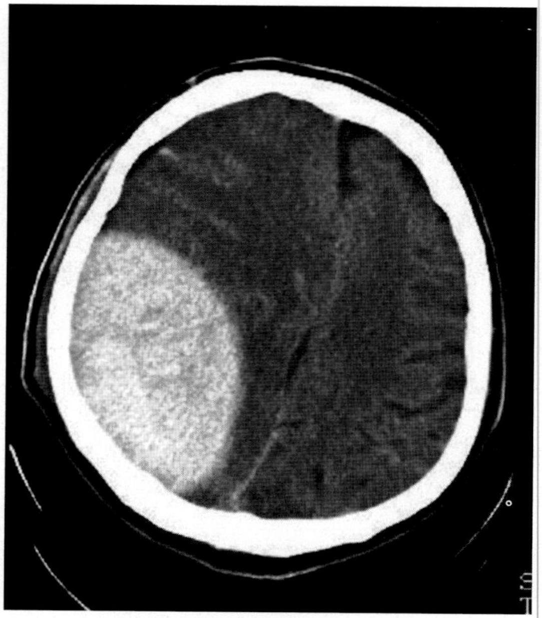

FIGURE 47–4 A classic biconvex-shaped epidural hematoma.

Treatment of Severely Head-Injured Patients in the Intensive Care Unit

Guidelines for the management of severe head injury were published in 1995 and updated in 2000 (Table 47-3). (See Management and Prognosis of Severe Traumatic Brain Injury: Part I, Guidelines for the Management of Severe Traumatic Brain Injury, at www.braintrauma.org). These

	GCS score 9–15	GCS score < 9
EDH > 30 mL *or* MLS > 5 mm *or* Clot thickness > 15 mm	Consider surgery	Surgery as soon as possible
EDH < 30 mL *and* MLS < 5 mm *and* Clot thickness < 15 mm	Non-operative management	Consider surgery

FIGURE 47–5 Treatment plan for patients with acute epidural hematoma.

TABLE 47–3 Summary of the Guidelines for Management of Severe Traumatic Brain Injury

Topic	Standard Recommendations	Guideline Recommendations	Options
Trauma systems		All regions in the United States should have an organized trauma care system	Neurosurgeons should initiate neurotrauma care, planning to include prehospital management and triage, maintenance of appropriate call schedules, quality improvement measures for trauma care, and participation in trauma-education programs.
Integration of brain-specific treatment into the initial resuscitation			The first priority for the head-injury patient is rapid and complete physiologic resuscitation. No specific treatment should be directed at intracranial hypertension in the absence of signs of transtentorial herniation or progressive neurologic deterioration not attributable to extracranial explanations.
Resuscitation of blood pressure and oxygenation		Hypotension (systolic blood pressure <90 mmHg) or hypoxia (apnea or cyanosis in the field or a $Paco_2$ <60 mmHg) must be scrupulously avoided, if possible, or corrected immediately.	The mean arterial pressure should be maintained above 90 mmHg throughout the patient's course in an attempt to maintain cerebral perfusion pressure (CCP) >70 mmHg.
Indications for intracranial pressure (ICP) monitoring		ICP monitoring is appropriate in severe head injury patients (GCS 3–8) with an abnormal CT scan, or a normal CT scan if two or more of the following are noted on admission: SBP <90 mmHg, age >40 yr, unilateral or bilateral motor posturing.	
ICP treatment threshold		ICP treatment should be initiated at an upper threshold of 20–25 mmHg.	
Cerebral perfusion pressure			Cerebral perfusion pressure should be maintained at a minimum of 60 mmHg.
Hyperventilation	In the absence of increased intracranial pressure, prolonged hyperventilation therapy ($Paco_2$ ≤25 mmHg) should be avoided after severe TBI.	The use of prophylactic hyperventilation ($Paco_2$ ≤35 mmHg) therapy during the first 24 hr after severe TBI should be avoided because it can compromise cerebral perfusion.	Hyperventilation therapy may be necessary for brief periods with acute neurologic deterioration, or for longer periods if intracranial hypertension is refractory to sedation, paralysis, CSF drainage, and osmotic diuretics.
Mannitol administration		Mannitol is effective for control of raised ICP after severe head injury. Intermittent bolus doses may be more effective than continuous infusions. Effective doses	The indications for the use of mannitol before ICP monitoring are signs of transtentorial herniation or progressive neurologic deterioration not attributable to systemic pathology. Serum osmolarity should be kept

Continued

TABLE 47–3 Summary of the Guidelines for Management of Severe Traumatic Brain Injury (*cont'd*)

Topic	Standard Recommendations	Guideline Recommendations	Options
		are 0.25 g–1 g/kg body weight.	<320 mOsm. Euvolemia should be maintained by adequate fluid replacement. A Foley catheter is essential in these patients.
Barbiturate administration		High-dose barbiturate therapy may be considered in hemodynamically stable, salvageable patients with severe head injury, with intracranial hypertension refractory to maximal medical and surgical therapy aimed at lowering increased ICP.	
Glucocorticoid administration	The use of glucocorticoids is not recommended for improving outcome or reducing intracranial pressure in patients with severe head injury.		
Nutritional support		Replace 140% of resting metabolism expenditure in nonparalyzed patients and 100% resting metabolism expenditure in paralyzed patients by using enteral or parenteral formulas containing ≥15% of calories as protein by the seventh day after injury.	
Antiseizure prophylaxis	Prophylactic use of phenytoin, carbamazepine, or phenobarbital is not recommended for preventing late post-traumatic seizures.		Use anticonvulsants to prevent early post-traumatic seizures in patients at high risk for seizures after head injury. Phenytoin and carbamazepine have been demonstrated to be effective in preventing early post-traumatic seizures.

guidelines were based on three levels of clinical certainty, supported by clinical research.

- Standards: Represent accepted principles of patient management that reflect a high degree of clinical certainty
- Guidelines: Represent a particular strategy or range of management strategies that reflect a moderate degree of clinical certainty
- Options: Are there remaining strategies for patient management for which unclear clinical certainty is present?

These guidelines cover 14 topics critical for the medical treatment of patients with severe TBI.

Treatment of Patients with Increased Intracranial Pressure

Increased ICP is a frequent complication of severe TBI and many other neurologic disorders, and it is directly related to morbidity and mortality after trauma. The ICP should be monitored in all patients with severe TBI (GCS <9) and abnormal head CT. Studies have shown that it also should be monitored in severe TBI patients with normal head CT, provided that they fulfill at least two of the following three criteria: age over 40 years, unilateral or bilateral motor posturing, SBP less than 90 mmHg. ICP treatment should be initiated at an upper threshold of 20 to 25 mmHg.

PEARLS FOR ROUNDS

Signs of increased intracranial pressure (ICP) on head computed tomography (CT) scans are midline shift, compression or enlargement of the cerebral ventricles, and effacement of basal cisterns.

Cerebral vasospasm after subarachnoid hematoma occurs between days 3 and 20; it peaks on day 7. Angiographic spasm occurs in 50% to 70% of patients; symptomatic spasm, in 30%. The mortality rate is 7%.

ICP monitoring is appropriate in severe head injury patients (Glasgow Coma Scale, 3–8) with an abnormal CT scan, or a normal CT scan if two or more of the following are noted on admission:
SBP, <90 mmHg
Age older than 40 years
Unilateral or bilateral motor posturing

Immediate and complete physiologic resuscitation with avoidance of arterial hypotension or hypoxia in patients with severe head injury is the single most important factor improving outcome in this patient group.

Treatment of patients with severe traumatic brain injury with steroids is not indicated. A recent prospective, randomized multicenter trial showed that the mortality of patients with traumatic brain injury who received high-dose dexamethasone infusion was increased compared with that of a control group.

General measures that should be taken to prevent ICP increases:

- Make sure that no venous outflow obstruction is present: check for tight tracheostomy collar or C-collar. An abnormal head position also may cause venous outflow obstruction.
- Make sure that the patient does not receive unnecessary free water, which may worsen brain edema and increase ICP. IV medication should, if possible, be dissolved in normal saline.

A critical pathway for the treatment of ICH is presented in Figure 47-6. In this algorithm for established ICH, the treatment steps are determined by the risk/benefit ratio of individual treatment maneuvers.

Traumatic Brain Injury in Children: Child Abuse

Traumatic brain injury is the most common cause of death and disability in children. Mechanisms of trauma frequently differ from those seen in the adult. Child abuse is the second most frequent cause of death in childhood after motor vehicle accidents, with approximately 1500 pediatric deaths per year in the United States. The "shaking impact syndrome" should be suspected in children younger than 3 years who are first seen with one of the following:

- Retinal hemorrhages
- SDH, shearing injury, or localized ICH
- Multiple skull fractures, fractures of the ribs and long bones, and bruises in various stages of healing
- History of trauma that does not account for the severity of actual injury

No relation is obvious to race, gender, socioeconomic status, or education among victims of shaking impact syndrome. Overall, up to one third of affected children die, one third to half remain severely disabled, and only one third have a chance of a meaningful recovery.

Spine Trauma

Acute spinal cord injury should always be assumed in trauma patients, especially if they are unconscious with significant trauma, or complain of neck and spine tenderness and pain, tingling in their extremities, weakness, or with a history of these symptoms.

Patients who are completely alert, oriented, not intoxicated, and do not complain of spine tenderness, pain, or neurologic deficits may be cleared clinically without obtaining cervical radiographs.

Initial Assessment and Treatment

The following points are cornerstones in the early treatment of patients with suspected spine injury:

- Assure proper immobilization on backboard with cervical collar or sandbags or both. After radiologic studies are done, the backboard should be removed to avoid unnecessary discomfort and decubitus ulcers. The patient should always be log-rolled.
- Monitor and maintain SBP at less than 90 mmHg. Use dopamine as a pressor to maintain blood pressure, if needed. IV fluids are used to replace fluid loss.
- Maintain adequate oxygenation.

A quick neurologic examination should be performed as soon as possible:

- Obtain a focused history: Mechanism of injury, time of injury, transient weakness, tingling in extremities
- Palpation of spine, detection of soft tissue trauma, bone deformities ("step-off")
- Motor examination
- Sensory examination: sensation to pinprick to localize dermatomes and to test the spinothalamic tract, light/crude touch to test the anterior spinothalamic tract, and proprioception/joint position to test the posterior columns
- Rectal examination: test voluntary anal sphincter contraction. Anal sphincter reflex: Contraction of anal sphincter in response to scratching the perianal skin. Bulbocavernosus reflex: rectal contraction in response to squeezing the glans penis. The bulbocavernosus reflex also can be elicited in patients with a Foley catheter by a tug on the catheter.
- Muscle-stretch reflexes, abdominal cutaneous reflexes. Reflexes are frequently absent immediately after SCI.

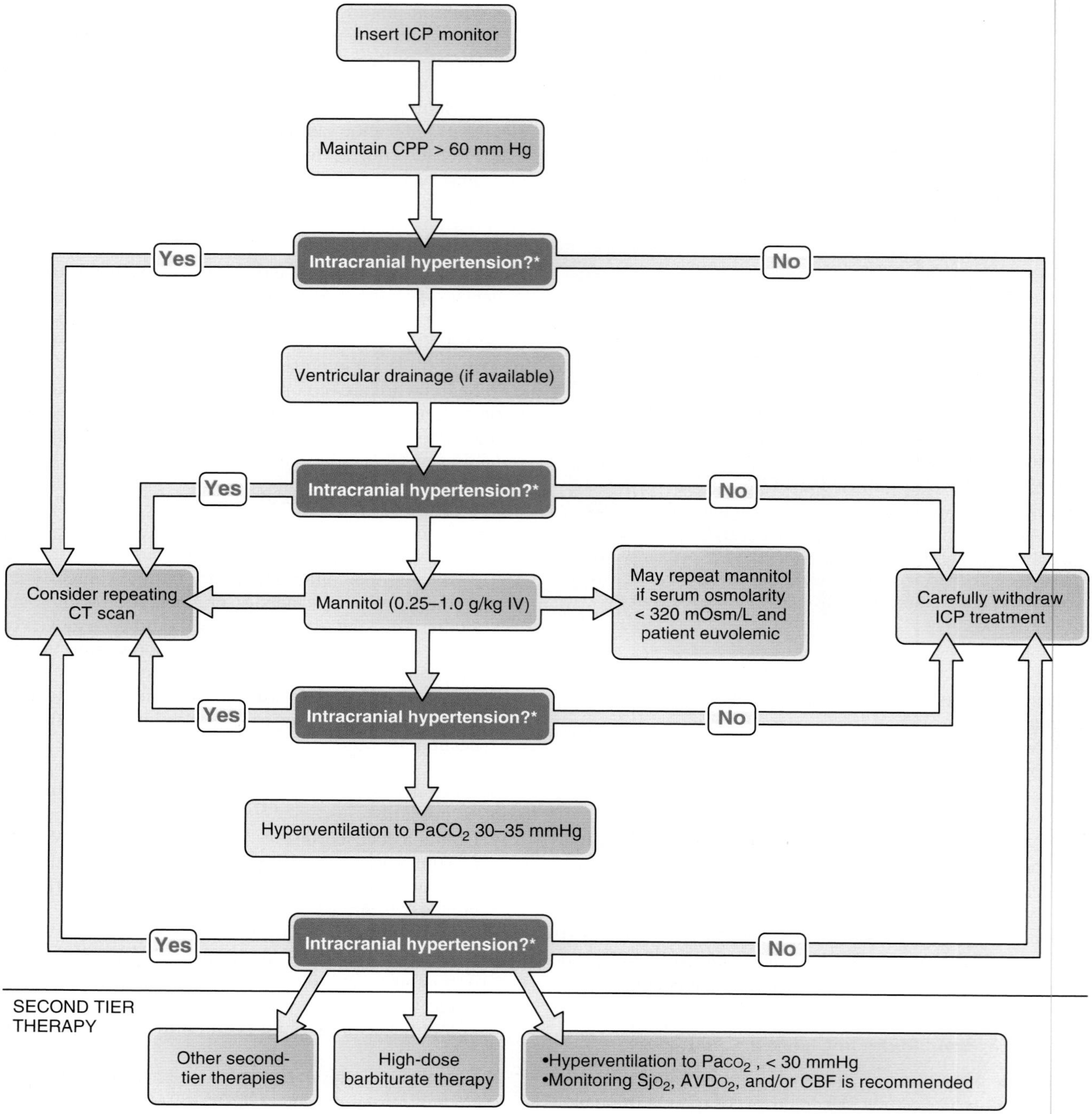

*Threshold of 20–25 mmHg may be used. Other values may be substituted in individual conditions.

FIGURE 47–6 Critical pathway for the treatment of intracranial hypertension in patients with traumatic brain injury according to Guidelines for the Surgical Management of Traumatic Brain Injury (see www.braintrauma.org). Second-tier therapies include decompressive craniectomy and intravenous hypertonic saline infusion.

BOX 47-1 Radiographic Signs of Cervical Spine Trauma

Retropharyngeal space >6 mm at C2 or retrotracheal space >22 mm at C6
Tracheal deviation
>3.5 mm subluxation on any level on cross-table lateral C-spine
Acute kyphotic angulation
Loss of lordosis
Widened interspinous space
Narrowed or widened disk space
Distance between atlas and dens on lateral C-spine, >4 mm

Treatment of acute SCI with methylprednisolone is not recommended because its negative side effects outweigh its benefits.

The basic radiographic evaluation comprises the following examinations (Box 47-1):

- Cervical spine radiographs consisting of at least a lateral cervical spine radiograph demonstrating all seven cervical vertebral bodies down to the C7/T1 junction, anteroposterior cervical spine radiograph and open-mouth odontoid view to evaluate the C1/C2 junction and the dens. A "swimmer's view" may be necessary to visualize the cervicothoracic junction. If all studies fail to demonstrate the C1/C2 region or the cervicothoracic junction or both, a CT scan through those areas should be obtained.
- AP and lateral views of thoracic or lumbar spine or both if abnormalities are suspected.

A fine-cut CT scan should be obtained from one to two levels above to one to two levels below the level demonstrating radiographic abnormalities. The purpose of the CT scan is to assess bony abnormalities and to aid in preoperative planning.

An MRI or, rarely, a myelogram is performed if the patient has a neurologic deficit, especially if deficits are not explained by other radiographic findings or if a neurologic deterioration developed after admission or after treatment. MRI scanning detects soft tissue injuries, intraspinal hematomas, and spinal cord edema and hemorrhage.

Flexion/extension (F/E) cervical spine films are obtained if a patient complains of neck pain, has negative spine radiographs, and the physician wants to rule out injury to the ligaments. The patient has to be neurologically intact, completely awake, cooperative, and alert. During flexion and extension, the alignment of the cervical spine on the lateral films should be maintained. Sometimes F/E films have to be obtained 2 to 3 weeks after injury because of post-traumatic muscle spasms that make it impossible to the patient to move the neck adequately.

Spine Fractures

Atlanto-occipital Dislocation. This fracture results from disruption of the ligaments connecting C1 (atlas) to the skull. Patients may be neurologically intact or demonstrate bulbar-cervical dislocation resulting in respiratory arrest and quadriplegia. Treatment requires either operative fusion or prolonged immobilization in a halo. Craniocervical traction may worsen the injury.

Atlas (C1) Fractures. The most common C1 fracture is the Jefferson fracture, which results from axial loading and leads to fracture of the arch of C1. Jefferson fractures make up for up to 13% of all cervical spine fractures and are usually benign. Treatment is with a collar or, in severe cases, with immobilization in a halo vest.

C2 Fractures. Fractures of the axis account for approximately 20% of all cervical spine fractures. The "hangman fracture" results from hyperextension plus axial loading during injury. Most patients are neurologically intact. The great majority of fractures heal with immobilization alone, and operative fusion is rarely needed.

Fractures through the odontoid process, or dens, are more frequent and can result in significant neurologic deficits. They result from flexion and are easily missed on plain films. Depending on the anatomic site of the fracture line, they have been divided into three different types. Treatment of these fractures is sometimes controversial. Surgery is usually advocated for severely displaced fractures and after failure of external immobilization.

Fractures from C3 to C7. The "clay shoveler's fracture" results from an avulsion of the spinous process due to sudden forced neck hyperflexion. The fracture is stable and is treated with a cervical collar, mainly for pain control. The majority of fractures between C3 and C7 are compression/flexion fractures. Classic presentation is after diving accidents. If the fractures are mild and stable, they can be treated with external immobilization. Teardrop fractures are more extensive, involve the disk space, and frequently show retropulsed bone fragments in the spinal canal. Patients may be quadriplegic. Most of these fractures require surgical stabilization.

Locked Facets. Very extensive flexion can lead to bilaterally "locked," "sprung," or "jumped" facets. In the normal situation, facets overlap, meaning that the inferior surface of the superior facet rests on the superior surface of the inferior facet. Flexion injury can lead to distraction of neighboring facets to the degree that this relation is reversed. "Perched" facets refers to a milder degree of dislocation. Hyperflexion plus rotation leads to unilaterally jumped facets. These injuries are frequently associated with neurologic deficits. Treatment can be complicated. Closed reduction of locked facets involves the application of so-called Gardner-Wells tongs or a halo ring to the head. A special headboard is required that allows the attachment of a rope and weight to the head ring. Traction is applied by adding weight in 5- to 10-pound increments until control radiographs demonstrate satisfactory alignment. Sometimes, locked facets have to be aligned under visual control in the OR.

It is important to remember that cervical facet dislocation can be associated with disk herniation that is not appreciated on plain radiographs and CT scans. During cervical traction and realignment, the herniated disk can extrude further and lead to additional neurologic injury. Therefore some authors recommend a pretreatment MRI to rule out disk herniation.

Thoracolumbar Spine Fractures. A three-column model has been devised to evaluate the stability of thoracolumbar spine fractures.

- The anterior column is composed of the anterior half of the disk and the vertebral body and the anterior longitudinal ligament.
- The middle column consists of the remaining part of the disk and the vertebral body plus the posterior longitudinal ligament.
- The posterior column comprises the posterior bony elements, ligaments, the ligamentum flavum, and the facet joints.

Injuries to the anterior or posterior column alone are usually considered stable. Injuries involving the middle column are frequently unstable. Typical injuries can be divided into

- Compression fractures, involving only the anterior column
- Burst fractures, affecting the anterior and middle column
- Seat-belt or chance fractures: these are fractures parallel to the disk space, in a horizontal plane, that result from flexion injuries and affect all three columns
- Fracture-dislocation fractures involve all three columns and are highly unstable.

General Principles of Surgical Management of Spine Trauma

Surgical management of spine fractures is frequently discussed controversially. Some basic principles are as follows:

- Bone or other material in the spinal canal compressing the cord should be removed operatively if the patient does not improve with conservative treatment or deteriorates neurologically.
- Operating on patients who have complete spinal cord lesions has not been shown to improve their function.

PEARLS FOR THE OR

In patients with incomplete spinal cord injury, bone or other material in the spinal canal compressing the spinal cord should be removed operatively if the patient does not improve with conservative treatment or deteriorates neurologically.

Operating on patients who have complete spinal cord lesions has not been shown to improve their function. Therefore indications for spine-stabilization surgery in this patient group are to improve their capacity to participate in rehabilitation and pain control.

Stable thoracolumbar spine fractures are treated with an orthosis, such as a molded thoracolumbar sacral orthosis (TLSO). Unstable thoracolumbar spine fractures with neurologic deficit frequently should undergo surgical stabilization. Posterior approaches are usually preferred, but surgical decompression and vertebral body resection sometimes require access via an anterior, transthoracic, or transabdominal approach.

Antibiotic-coated ventriculostomy catheters have been shown to reduce the rate of infections associated with intracranial (ICP) monitoring.

A ventricular catheter connected to an external strain-gauge device is the most accurate and cost-effective way of measuring ICP. It also allows therapeutic drainage of cerebrospinal fluid (CSF). Parenchymal monitors for fiberoptic monitoring of brain-tissue pressure are also accurate but more expensive, and they do not allow CSF drainage. Recently introduced combined catheters allow CSF drainage as well as continuous uninterrupted monitoring of ICP via fiberoptic or strain-gauge technology.

- Stable thoracolumbar spine fractures are treated with an orthosis, such as a molded thoracolumbar sacral orthosis (TLSO). Unstable thoracolumbar spine fractures with neurologic deficit frequently should undergo surgical stabilization. Posterior approaches are usually preferred, but surgical decompression and vertebral body resection sometimes require access via a transthoracic or transabdominal approach.

Cerebrovascular Disease

Types of Strokes

Cerebrovascular diseases affect the vascular system of the brain or the spine and can lead to stroke. A typical stroke is characterized by a sudden onset of neurologic deficits that are frequently focal. Strokes can be divided into the following:

- Cerebrovascular accident (CVA) or completed strokes in which the neurologic deficit is permanent
- Reversible ischemic neurologic deficit (RIND) in which the deficit disappears after 24 hours
- Transient ischemic attack (TIA), in which the deficit completely resolves within 24 hours

Strokes also can be divided based on the underlying pathology into

- Embolic or thrombotic ischemic strokes
- Hemorrhagic strokes including ICH and SAH

Treatment depends on the nature of the underlying disease (Box 47-2).

During the initial evaluation, the physician should attempt to determine whether the stroke is ischemic or hemorrhagic (Fig. 47-7). This is crucial, because ischemic stroke may require immediate treatment with thrombolytics, which would have catastrophic consequences if administered in patients with blood in their heads.

Hemorrhagic Stroke

Subarachnoid Hemorrhage due to Aneurysms

SAH is defined as bleeding between the brain and the arachnoid membrane, a thin layer of cells that surrounds the brain parenchyma and the main blood vessels. An SAH typically causes severe headaches, photophobia, and neck stiffness, but many patients can actually be initially seen in stupor or coma. The most common cause of SAH is trauma. Spontaneous (i.e., nontraumatic) SAH is caused by rupture of a cerebral aneurysm in approximately 80% of cases. We discuss aneurysmal SAH in detail.

Pathophysiology and General Management. Most aneurysms are congenital, and in autopsy studies, up to 5% of the population were found to have cerebral aneurysms. Cigarette smoking, hypertension, and certain drugs like ethyl alcohol (ETOH) and cocaine also have been associated with aneurysms and SAH. Fully 20% of all SAHs occurs in the age group between 20 and 45 years. Aneurysmal SAH carries a grave prognosis. Approximately 10% of patients die before reaching the hospital, and the overall mortality is about 45%. Aneurysmal SAH is frequently associated with a complicated and protracted clinical course. The key points concerning pathophysiology and general management are the following:

The biggest risk immediately after the initial hemorrhage is rerupturing of the aneurysm. Early surgical intervention

BOX 47–2 Most Common Etiologies of Stroke

Hemorrhagic Stroke

1. ***Vascular Disorders***
   Arteriovenous malformation
   Aneurysm
   Cavernous malformations
   Venous malformations
   Capillary telangiectasias
   Moya-Moya disease (children)
   Sturge-Weber syndrome (children)
2. ***Vasculopathy***
   Amyloid angiopathy
3. ***Coagulation Disorders***
   After thrombolytic treatment for ischemic stroke or MI
   Use of anticoagulants
   Leukemia, thrombocytopenia
4. ***Hemorrhagic Transformation of Ischemic Stroke***
5. ***Hypertension***
6. ***Drugs: ETOH, Cocaine***
7. ***Brain Tumor (Primary or Metastatic)***
8. ***Post-traumatic***
9. ***Postoperative: after Carotid Endarterectomy***

Ischemic Stroke

1. ***Arterial Vascular Occlusion***
   Trauma: Arterial dissection
   Atherosclerosis: Carotid artery stenosis
   Fibromuscular dysplasia
   Infection: Meningitis, systemic
   Moya-Moya
   Vasculitis: SLE, polyarteritis
   Vasospasm from migraine or subarachnoid hemorrhage
2. ***Dural Sinus or Venous Thrombosis***
3. ***Hematologic: Antiphospholipid Antibodies, Antithrombin III Deficiency, etc.***
4. ***Drugs: Oral Contraceptives, Cocaine, Amphetamines***
5. ***Embolic: Arrhythmia, Congenital Heart Defect, Endocarditis, Prosthetic Valves***

ETOH, ethyl alcohol; MI, myocardial infarction; SLE, systemic lupus erythematosus.

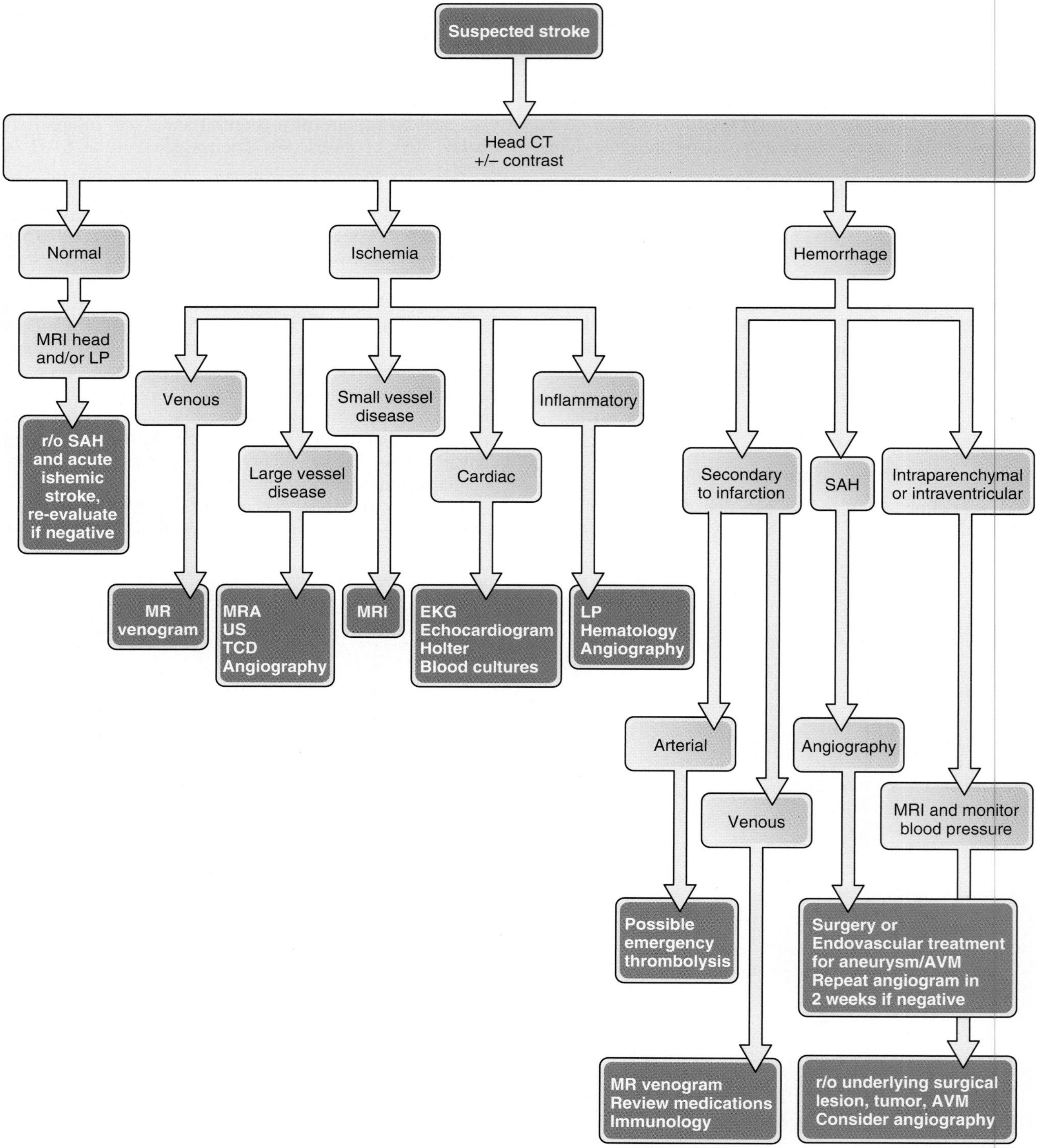

FIGURE 47–7 Algorithm for the evaluation of stroke patients.

to eliminate this risk has become a well-accepted standard, except in patients in very poor clinical condition.

Cerebral vasospasm, critical narrowing of cerebral arteries that can lead to strokes, brain edema, and herniation, threatens the patient between days 4 and 21 after initial hemorrhage. Clinically significant vasospasm occurs in 20% to 30% of patients and is the most important cause of morbidity and mortality in patients who survive the hemorrhage. Vasospasm is diagnosed clinically by detecting a sudden neurologic worsening of the patient and is confirmed with cerebral angiography. Transcranial Doppler examination of the intracerebral vasculature can be used as a daily screening test in the ICU. A sudden increase in flow velocities indicates vasospasm. Treatment of cerebral vasospasm includes pharmacologically induced hypertension, hypervolemia, and hemodilution (hyperdynamic therapy, HHH therapy) in the ICU. Another treatment option is cerebral angiography with angioplasty intra-arterial injection of potent vasodilators by interventional neuroradiologists. Effective HHH therapy requires the aneurysm to be surgically or endovascularly secured. Vasospasm is caused by breakdown products of the subarachnoid blood.

The vast majority (80% to 90%) of cerebral aneurysms are located in the "anterior" part of the cerebral circulation (i.e., the internal carotid artery [ICA] and the middle and anterior cerebral arteries [MCA and ACA], the posterior communicating artery [p-com], and the anterior communicating artery [a-com]). The remaining aneurysms are found in the "posterior" circulation (i.e., the basilar artery, the vertebral arteries and the posterior cerebral artery [PCA]). Location of the aneurysm, age of the patient, and clinical grade determine the type of treatment.

Differential Diagnosis. SAH not caused by an aneurysm can be seen in the presence of an arteriovenous malformation (AVM; see later), and sometimes it is seen in patients who have been taking cocaine.

Workup and Evaluation. SAH is first seen with

- Severe headaches, often referred to as "the worst headache of my life"
- Neck stiffness
- Decreased mental status

The Hunt and Hess classification is used to characterize the clinical severity of SAH (Table 47-4).

A CT scan without contrast is the imaging study of choice to detect blood in patients with suspected SAH. The Fisher Scale (Table 47-5) is used to characterize CT scan findings after SAH. A CT angiogram should be considered in a patient without history of trauma who needs to go to the OR urgently for evacuation of an intracranial blood clot associated with SAH. Occasionally, a cerebral aneurysm can be detected. Ventriculomegaly is frequently seen in patients with SAH and is treated with a ventriculostomy. If the initial CT scan is negative for SAH, a lumbar puncture to look for red blood cells or xanthochromia should be considered. If an SAH is confirmed, the patient must undergo cerebral angiography of both carotid and vertebral arteries. Cerebral angiography will detect cerebral aneurysms in 80% to 85% of cases. If a cerebral angiogram is negative, it should be repeated in 1 to 2 weeks. Patients with SAH should be admitted to the ICU. Blood pressure must be controlled tightly to reduce the risk of aneurysm rerupture. If a ventriculostomy catheter is in place, overdrainage of CSF should be avoided, because this could theoretically increase the rerupture risk. Antiseizure prophylaxis should be initiated. The calcium channel–blocker nimodipine has been shown to improve outcome from aneurysmal SAH by reducing the incidence of vasospasm. Hyponatremia is a common problem in patients with SAH, and serum sodium should be monitored.

TABLE 47–4 Hunt and Hess Classification for Assessing Subarachnoid Hemorrhage

Grade	Description
0	Asymptomatic
1	Mild headache with neck stiffness
2	Cranial nerve palsy, moderate to severe headache, neck stiffness
3	Mild focal deficit, lethargy, confusion
4	Stupor, moderate to severe hemiparesis
5	Deep coma, decerebrate rigidity

*Based on a 70-kg adult.

Treatment Alternatives. The goals of early treatment of ruptured aneurysms are the following.

- To prevent potentially fatal rebleeding, the risk of which is highest immediately after the initial hemorrhage (20% in the first 14 days after the initial hemorrhage)
- To avoid operating during cerebral vasospasm with neurologic deterioration

TABLE 47–5 Fisher Scale for Vasospasm

Grade	CT Findings
1	No SAH
2	Diffuse or vertical layers <1 mm thick
3	Localized blood clot or vertical layers 1 mm
4	Intracerebral or intraventricular blood with diffuse or no SAH

CT, computed tomography; SAH, subarachnoid hemorrhage.

- To allow treatment of vasospasm with HHH therapy or angioplasty, once an aneurysm has been secured

The main treatment options include

- Surgical exposure of the aneurysm with placement of a clip across the neck of the aneurysm to exclude it from the circulation
- Endovascular placement of small platinum coils into the aneurysm to promote thrombosis
- Vascular bypass procedures with trapping of the aneurysm

Surgery for the clipping of most anterior circulation aneurysms is typically done with the patient in the supine position, the head immobilized in a Mayfield headholder and turned to one side. The craniotomy exposes the sylvian fissure and part of the temporal and frontal lobes. By using the operating microscope and microsurgical techniques, the surgeon carefully exposes the aneurysm and places a clip across the aneurysm neck. Patency of surrounding blood vessels can be checked with intraoperative angiography or micro-Doppler. Postoperatively, the patient is kept in the ICU.

Endovascular treatment of cerebral aneurysms has evolved over the past 10 to 15 years into a viable alternative to surgery in many situations. The interventional neuroradiologist advances a microcatheter into the aneurysm and electrolytically detaches platinum coils into the aneurysmal sac. Long-term outcome results are not available, and a direct comparison between surgery and endovascular treatment has not been conducted. The decision to coil versus clip an aneurysm depends on the

- Neurologic grade (surgery is currently preferred for better-grade patients)
- Patient age (older patients are more likely to receive coils)
- Comorbidities and life expectancy (coiling is preferred in patients who are sicker)
- Aneurysm location and anatomy

Treatment of Unruptured Cerebral Aneurysms

Recent recommendations for the treatment of unruptured cerebral aneurysms stated that asymptomatic aneurysms with a diameter greater than 10 mm should be considered for treatment. Aneurysms smaller than 10 mm have a lower risk of hemorrhage, and the decision to treat them has to be made in conjunction with other factors, such as patient age, existing medical and neurologic conditions, and the relative risks of repair. Re-evaluation of the aneurysm should be done periodically with cerebral angiography, MRA, or CT angiography (Fig. 47-8).

Arteriovenous Malformations

Intracranial AVMs are relatively uncommon, but increasingly recognized congenital lesions that can cause serious neurologic symptoms. Although AVMs can be first seen with hemorrhage or seizure, an increasing number are detected before rupture since the advent of contemporary brain-imaging techniques. Over the last decade, significant developments have been made in the management of intracranial AVMs, with an evolution of microsurgical as well as endovascular and radiosurgical techniques to treat these lesions.

Pathophysiology. Among the four different types of cerebral vascular malformations, AVMs are the most frequent. Morphologically, AVMs consist of dilated arteries and veins without a capillary bed. They are less common than intracranial aneurysms but can be associated with them in 7% to 18% of the cases. Patients first seen with a hemorrhage or seizures caused by AVMs are generally younger than are aneurysm patients. On cerebral angiography, AVMs appear as "tangles" of vessels. Morbidity and mortality of AVM rupture are 30% to 35% and 10%, respectively. The risk of treatment must be weighed against a hemorrhage risk of approximately 2% to 4% per year.

Workup and Evaluation. CT without contrast has a low sensitivity, but calcification and hypointensity may be noted; enhancement is seen after contrast administration. CT angiography is sometimes an alternative to cerebral four-vessel angiography. MRI is very sensitive, showing an inhomogeneous signal void on T_1- and T_2-weighted sequences, commonly with hemosiderin suggesting prior hemorrhage. MRI also can provide critical information detailing the localization and topography of an AVM, as intervention is being considered. Arteriography is the "gold standard" for defining the arterial and venous anatomy. In addition, superselective angiography can provide functional and physiological data important to clinical decision analysis. Patients with hemorrhage due to AVMs must be monitored in the ICU.

Treatment Alternatives. At present, four major treatment options are available for patients with an AVM. The lesion can be followed up expectantly with the understanding that the patient has some risk of hemorrhage or other neurologic symptoms. Alternatively, intervention can be undertaken with the goal of complete AVM obliteration, because subtotal therapy does not confer protection from hemorrhage. Management strategies include single or combined therapy by applying microsurgery, endovascular techniques, or radiosurgery (focused radiation).

Each treatment option has associated risks and benefits. Surgery is still the treatment of choice for AVMs. The risk of surgery is determined by the location of the AVM and the size and the pattern of venous drainage. The main advantage of surgery is that it eliminates the risk of

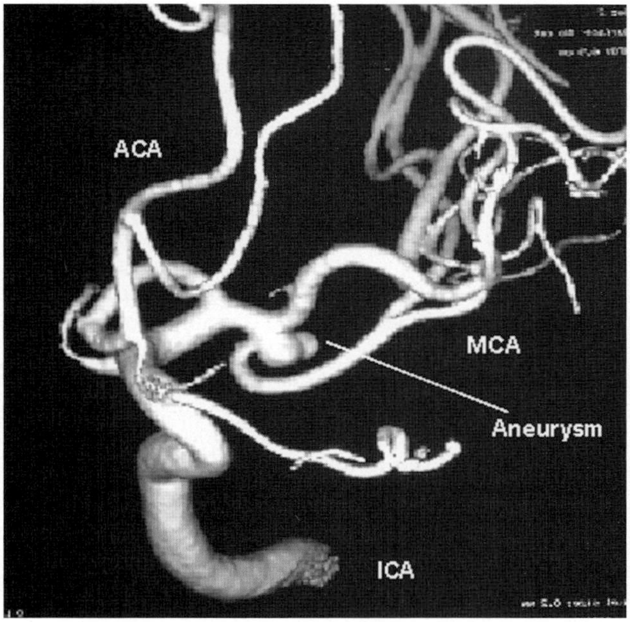

A

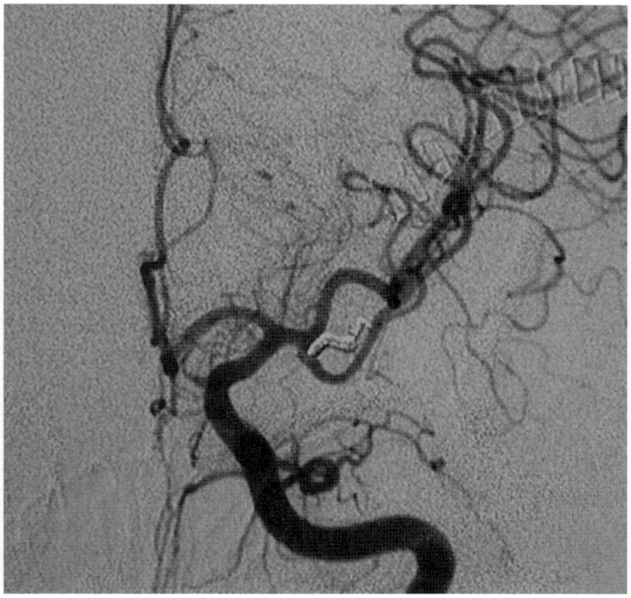

B

FIGURE 47–8 Three-dimensional cerebral angiography demonstrating a bilobulated left middle cerebral artery aneurysm. *A*, Before surgical treatment. *B*, After clipping on conventional angiography. ACA, anterior cerebral artery; ICA, internal cerebral artery; MCA, middle cerebral artery.

bleeding immediately. Stereotactic radiosurgery can be considered for small AVMs (less than 10-cc volume), but it can take up to 3 years before obliteration of the AVM is observed. Endovascular techniques can be used as an adjunct to surgery or sometimes as the main treatment modality. During endovascular procedures, glue is injected into the AVM under fluoroscopic control. If an AVM is associated with an aneurysm, the aneurysm is usually treated first, because of its higher risk of hemorrhage. At many centers, AVMs are treated in collaboration between neurointerventionalists and neurosurgeons.

Spinal Arteriovenous Malformations

Spinal vascular malformations are relatively rare and are seen with a progressive myelopathy. Treatment options include embolization, surgical resection, and a combination of surgical and endovascular treatments.

Cavernous Malformations

Cavernous malformations (CMs) comprise 5% to 13% of all vascular malformations in the brain and spinal cord. They are increasingly recognized with improved imaging techniques such as MRI in patients with negative CT scan and angiography. Autopsy series have revealed CMs in approximately 0.5% of the population.

Pathophysiology. CMs are well-defined, lobulated lesions that occur in the parenchyma of brain or spinal cord and gradually enlarge because of recurrent hemorrhages. Patients frequently have multiple lesions, and the presentation depends on the anatomic location. Supratentorial CMs are located in and around the cortex and occur with seizures, hemorrhage, and progressive neurologic deficit. Brainstem lesions will likely be seen with cranial nerve palsies. Depending on the location, the annual bleeding rate is between 0.25% and 2.7%.

Workup and Evaluation. A patient with suspected CM should undergo MRI imaging, which will disclose the well-circumscribed and mixed-signal-intensity lesion with high accuracy. Characteristically, CMs do not show up on CT imaging or on cerebral angiography.

Treatment Alternatives. Asymptomatic or minimally symptomatic CMs can be observed initially, because they may remain quiescent, and recurrent hemorrhage is usually not catastrophic. Observation also should be considered for multiple lesions and lesions in critical areas of the brain that are not amenable to surgical excision. Stereotactic radiosurgery has been used to treat CMs in critical brain lesions, but long-term results are not available. Indications for surgical excision are recurrent hemorrhage, progressive neurologic deficit, and intractable epilepsy when the risk/benefit ratio is acceptable. By using microsurgical technique, the successful resection of even certain brainstem CMs can be accomplished.

Spontaneous Intracerebral Hemorrhage

Pathophysiology. ICH refers to bleeding within the brain parenchyma. It accounts for approximately 10% of all strokes. Many cases are associated with arterial hypertension, but a strict causality has not been established. It also can occur in areas of previous ischemic stroke, after aneurysm or AVM surgery, after carotid endarterectomy, or because of vascular abnormalities. In young adults, it is more likely to be associated with vascular abnormalities or abuse of ETOH, cocaine, or amphetamine. In elderly patients, it can be due to amyloid angiopathy, but this can be confirmed only by pathological examination of tissue. ICH occurs as a catastrophic complication of anticoagulation with warfarin in patients with cardiovascular disease. Brain tumors associated with ICH are glioblastoma multiforme and some metastatic tumors. The most common locations of ICH are the basal ganglia, followed by thalamus, brainstem, and cerebral white matter. Lobar hemorrhages may be more likely to require surgical intervention because of mass effect. After the initial bleed, patients can deteriorate because of rebleeding, the development of brain edema and mass effect, hydrocephalus, or seizures.

Workup and Evaluation. Patients are first seen with headaches, nausea/vomiting, and with progressive neurologic deterioration over minutes or hours. Deficits are frequently focal and indicate the site of the lesion. Initial evaluation includes a head CT scan without contrast. Contrast can be given if an underlying abnormality is suspected, such as an AVM, large aneurysm, or brain tumor, and an MRI is not readily available or feasible. Further workup should include an MRI to determine the age of the hemorrhage and underlying pathology. Cerebral angiography is conducted at a later point if an underlying vascular abnormality is suspected. Key points in managing these patients are the following:

- As soon as the diagnosis of ICH is made, it is important to stop and reverse all anticoagulation. Studies have shown that patients taking warfarin for cardiac problems can be safely taken off their anticoagulants for days and up to weeks if managed and monitored properly. Coagulation parameters should be checked in every patient.
- Blood pressure should be monitored but not aggressively reduced by more than 30% or below premorbid levels.
- A ventriculostomy may have to be placed to monitor ICP and drain CSF. If the patient demonstrates signs of herniation, mannitol should be given, and the patient should be hyperventilated. Surgery should be considered in these patients.

Treatment Alternatives. Considerable controversy exists regarding the indications for surgery in these patients. The decision whether to operate must take into consideration the location of the hematoma, time frame of deterioration, patient age, life expectancy, medical comorbidities, and neurologic function at the time of presentation. Surgery should be considered in patients who demonstrate

- Signs of significant mass effect on the head CT scan, such as midline shift and compression of basal cisterns
- Neurologic deficits that can be clearly attributed to a surgical lesion
- Progressive neurologic deterioration in the face of an intracranial mass lesion
- Lesions that are located in parts of the brain that can be operated on without causing additional neurologic deficits

If the ICH is located in the posterior fossa, the decision to operate is made more liberally, because expansion of the mass or development of brain edema may quickly lead to hydrocephalus, herniation, or both, even if the patient appears in good neurologic condition at the time of the bleed. Evacuation of some deep ICHs by using endoscopic techniques is a promising alternative to open craniotomy and may be associated with less surgical morbidity. Overall mortality from ICH has been reported to be about 44% at 1 month after the bleed. Patients with ICHs located in deep structures tend to do worse.

Occlusive Cerebrovascular Disease

Ischemic strokes are characterized by an abrupt onset of neurologic symptoms. They can be classified as arterial thrombosis and embolic strokes. Carotid artery atherosclerosis is frequently one of the underlying problems and is treated by neurosurgeons and vascular surgeons with carotid artery endarterectomy.

Arterial Thrombosis and Embolic Strokes

Pathophysiology. Risk factors for cerebrovascular disease include

- Arterial hypertension
- Cardiac diseases
- Diabetes
- Oral contraception
- Elevated cholesterol levels
- Smoking
- Obesity
- Family history

Approximately 50% of all strokes are due to thrombotic occlusion of cerebral arteries or occlusion caused by vasculitis, rheumatoid arthritis, or traumatic vessel dissection. One fourth of strokes are due to embolic occlusion from atheromatous plaques in the aortic arch, arrhythmias or valvular heart disease, or fat and air emboli. Coagulopathies and venous thrombosis account for approximately 5% of all strokes.

Once the cerebral blood flow decreases below an ischemic threshold, neurologic symptoms will develop. The progression from reversible to permanent infarction depends on the severity and duration of blood-flow compromise. Based on the arterial vessel occluded, different clinical syndromes can be differentiated.

Differential Diagnosis. Occlusion of small, deep, penetrating arteries in the basal ganglia can result from long-standing hypertension and is characterized by small areas of infarct called "lacunar strokes." Clinically, this leads to distinctive syndromes with very localized deficits, such as pure motor hemiplegia, pure sensory deficits of certain limbs, or brainstem syndromes described earlier (Table 47-6).

Other than thromboembolic stroke, the differential diagnosis also should include hemorrhagic stroke, seizure, and brain tumors. Carotid artery stenosis is an important cause of stroke, and it is discussed later. Stroke-like symptoms even after mild trauma or external manipulation of the neck should bring up the possibility of carotid or vertebral artery dissection.

Workup and Evaluation. All patients should initially have a head CT scan. Infarction will be visible as a low-density lesion after approximately 12 hours to 2 days on CT. Blood will be seen as a hyperdense lesion. MRI is more sensitive than CT for the detection of ischemia, especially if the lesion is located in the posterior fossa or brainstem. An angiogram is indicated if other vascular malformations must be excluded, or a vessel dissection or large-vessel stenosis is suspected. Treatment of thromboembolic strokes is usually the domain of neurologists and endovascular neuroradiologists.

Treatment Alternatives. Intravenous thrombolytic therapy with tissue plasminogen activators may be a treatment option if the patient can be worked up within a few hours after onset of symptoms. Medical treatment relies mainly on the control of underlying comorbidities and long-term anticoagulation with warfarin, aspirin, and other drugs. The neurosurgeon becomes involved if a cerebral angiography, an MRA, or carotid artery ultrasound demonstrates high-grade carotid artery stenosis or carotid artery dissection after trauma.

Carotid Endarterectomy

Carotid endarterectomy can be considered in asymptomatic and symptomatic patients with more than 60% or 70% narrowing of the carotid artery, respectively. During the procedure, neurologic function is monitored either by EEG or by measuring flow velocities in intracranial arteries with transcranial Doppler technique. Some surgeons prefer clinical monitoring of the patients under local anesthesia. In surgery, the carotid bifurcation is identified. The common, external, and internal carotid arteries are cross-clamped, opened, and the atherosclerotic plaque is removed. Surgeons have controversial opinions as to whether to use a shunt during the cross-clamping to maintain carotid flow. In experienced hands, morbidity and mortality of the procedure are approximately 5%.

TABLE 47–6 Clinical Syndromes Associated with Occlusion of Major Cerebral Arteries*

Artery Occluded	Clinical Syndrome
Internal cerebral artery	Decreased mental status Homonymous hemianopsia of the contralateral side Contralateral hemiparesis and sensory disturbance (numbness, tingling, etc.) Gaze palsy to the opposite side Global aphasia if the dominant hemisphere is affected Amaurosis fugax with carotid artery stenosis
Anterior cerebral artery	Contralateral lower extremity weakness and sensory deficit Incontinence Bilateral occlusion may cause akinetic mutism
Middle cerebral artery	Contralateral weakness and sensory deficits arm > legs Aphasia if dominant side affected
Posterior cerebral artery	Contralateral homonymous hemianopsia
Basilar artery	Mental status changes, coma Bilateral motor and sensory deficits Cranial nerve deficits Cerebellar deficits

*The degree of deficits may vary, and some patients may be asymptomatic. This will depend on the degree and localization of occlusion.

Suggested Reading

Bederson J, Awad I, Wiebers D, et al: Recommendations for the management of patients with unruptured intracranial aneurysms: A statement for healthcare professionals from the Stroke Council of the American Heart Association. Stroke 31:2742–2750, 2000.

Brain Trauma Foundation and the American Association of Neurological Surgeons, Joint Section on Neurotrauma and Critical Care: Guidelines for the management of severe traumatic brain injury. J Neurotrauma 17:449–554, 2000.

Brilstra E, Rinkel G, van der Graaf Y, et al: Treatment of intracranial aneurysms by embolization with coils: A systematic review. Stroke 30:470–476, 1999.

Brott T, Bogousslavsky J: Treatment of acute ischemic stroke. N Engl J Med 343:710–722, 2000.

Fernandes H, Gregson B, Siddique S, et al: Surgery in intracerebral hemorrhage: The uncertainty continues. Stroke 31:2511–2516, 2000.

Ghajar J: Traumatic brain injury. Lancet 356:923–929, 2000.

McLone D: Pediatric neurosurgery: Surgery of the developing nervous system. Philadelphia, WB Saunders, 2001.

Ogilvy C, Stieg P, Awad I, et al: Recommendations for the management of intracranial arteriovenous malformations. Stroke 32:1458–1471, 2001

Rinkel G, Djibuti M, Algra A, van Gijn J: Prevalence and risk of rupture of intracranial aneurysms: A systematic review. Stroke 29:251–256, 1998.

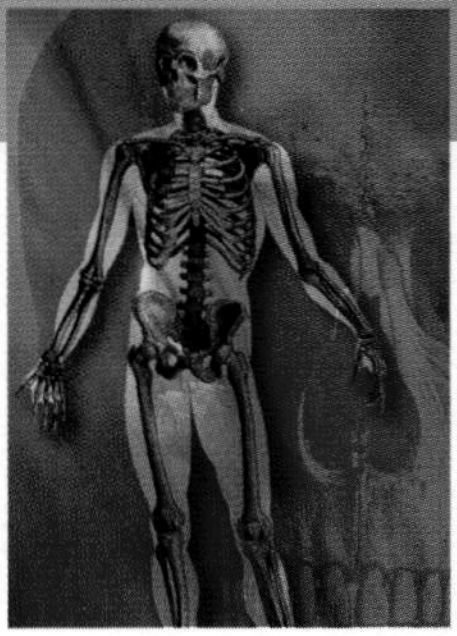

Chapter 48

Central Nervous System and Spinal Degenerative Diseases and Infections

ROGER HARTL, MD, and PHILIP E. STIEG, MD, PhD

Low Back Pain

Low back pain is a common complaint among patients, and, in the majority of cases, no specific diagnosis can be made. Some of the pathologies that can cause lower back pain and may require neurosurgical intervention are

- Metastatic and primary cancer to the spine or the spinal cord or cauda equina or both
- Infection, spinal osteomyelitis
- Trauma to the spine, fractures
- Spinal stenosis
- Lumbar disk herniation

Some of the most frequent operations in neurosurgery are lumbar diskectomies for lower back pain or sciatica and laminectomies for lumbar stenosis.

Lumbar Disk Herniation

Pathophysiology

Lumbar disk herniation (LDH) can be regarded as the acute exacerbation of a chronic problem. Over time, increased mechanical stress leads to loss of hydration, degeneration, and tearing of the lumbar disk. Protrusion of the disk into the spinal canal compresses the nerve root and causes acute pain. It is important to remember that most lumbar disk herniations, in contrast to cervical disk herniations, will lead to compression of the nerve root exiting one level below (i.e., a right L4–L5 disk will cause a right L5 radiculopathy (Fig. 48-1). The vast majority of LDHs occur at the L4–L5 and L5–LS1 levels. Herniated lumbar disk can further be divided depending on the degree of protrusion into "bulging" disks, "free fragments," and, depending on the orientation, into central, lateral, and far lateral disk herniations. Several clinical syndromes can be attributed to lumbar disk or leg herniation (Table 48-1).

Most patients are first seen with recurrent low back pain, frequently bilateral, that is associated with muscle spasms and made worse by sitting or walking or both. Treatment is usually conservative.

An acute monoradiculopathy is the most frequent indication for surgery. A herniated disk compresses one particular nerve root, and the patient experiences pain and weakness along the course of the sciatic nerve and in the distribution of the affected nerve root. This is what is usually referred to as sciatica.

The most severe neurologic compromise is associated with the cauda equina syndrome. In this syndrome, a central disk herniation will compress the cauda equina and cause acute onset of urinary retention, loss of anal sphincter tone, saddle anesthesia, and progressive bilateral lower extremity weakness. Patients are at high risk for permanent neurologic deficits and should undergo surgery as soon as possible.

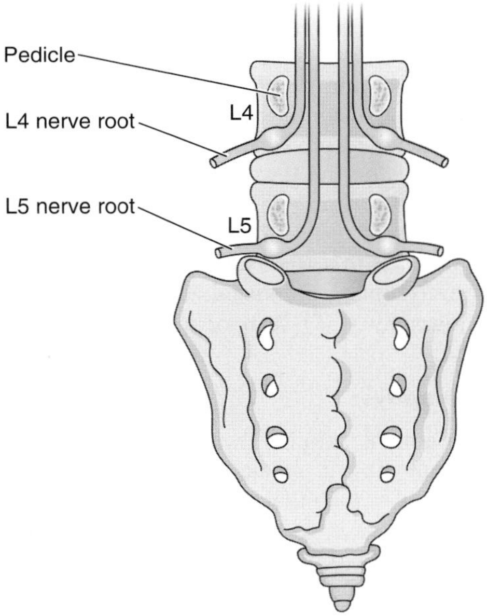

FIGURE 48–1 In the lumbar spine, the nerve root exits below its like-numbered vertebral body. For example, the L4 nerve root exits between L4 and L5. With an L4–L5 disk herniation, the affected nerve root is the L5 root. In contrast, in the cervical region, nerve roots exit above their like-numbered vertebral bodies. For example, the C6 nerve root exits between the C5 and C6 vertebrae. A C5–C6 disk herniation leads to a C6 radiculopathy.

TABLE 48–1 Neurologic Deficits Expected with Lumbar Disk Herniation

Deficit	Locations		
Herniation	L3–L4	L4–L5	L5–S1
Radiculopathy	L4	L5	S1
Motor weakness	Foot dorsiflexion	Extension great toe	Foot plantarflexion
Sensory deficit	Medial foot	Dorsum foot	Lateral foot
Reflex	Knee jerk	—	Ankle jerk

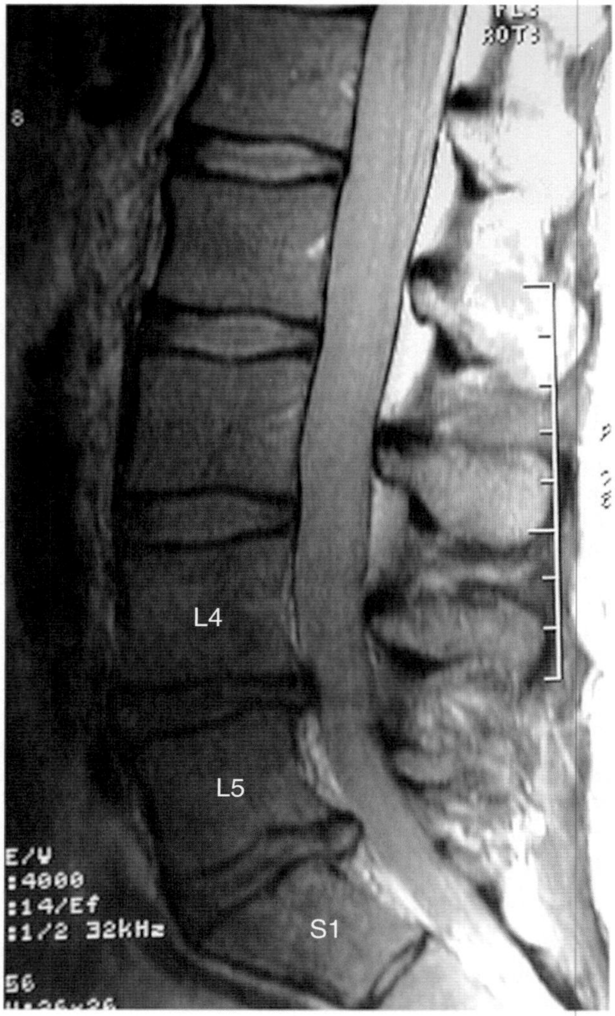

FIGURE 48–2 Sagittal magnetic resonance image of the lumbar and sacral spine demonstrating two disk herniations at L4–L5 and L5–S1.

The failed-back syndrome describes a situation in which the patient complains of persisting pain after one or more back surgeries that interferes significantly with daily activities. When all other conservative therapies and repeated surgeries have been exhausted, spinal fusion is frequently the only option left for these patients.

Workup and Evaluation

Initial evaluation of a patient with low back pain and suspected lumbar disk herniation starts with a detailed history. The physician should document previous malignancies, medication, IV drug abuse, steroid use, infection and fevers, weight loss, history of previous surgeries, and trauma, etc. The goal of the initial workup is to exclude the possibility of a serious underlying problem other than LDH. A cauda equina syndrome should be excluded by asking about urinary retention, incontinence, saddle anesthesia, and leg weakness. A detailed physical examination should be done next with focus on the lower extremities. A positive straight leg–raising test (Lasegue's sign) supports an LDH.

The imaging study of choice for LDH is an MRI without contrast (Fig. 48-2). If this study cannot be obtained or if the bony anatomy must be visualized, a lumbosacral computed tomography (CT) scan or a CT myelography should be done.

Treatment Alternatives

Conservative treatment should always be the first step, unless the patient has a cauda equina syndrome or significant weakness or pain that cannot be controlled with medication, in which case, an emergency diskectomy may be indicated. Keep in mind more than 90% of patients with low back pain will improve within 1 month, even without treatment. Bed rest, analgesics, muscle relaxants, and anti-inflammatory drugs should be considered initially, but the period of immobilization should not extend beyond the first 2 to 4 days, and the patient should be encouraged to pick up activities of daily living as possible. Physical therapy with physical exercise may be a helpful addition to therapy. No good evidence exists that epidural injection of steroids or analgesics or both improves long-term symptoms.

Surgery should be considered if the symptoms persist for longer than 1 to 2 months despite conservative treatment. One of the most widely accepted procedures for LDH is **microdiskectomy**. In the prone position, the patient undergoes a microsurgical excision of the herniated disk fragment and partial laminectomy, conducted under the microscope. For larger disk fragments or cauda equina syndrome, it may be necessary to do a complete laminectomy with diskectomy. Instrumentation or fusion is rarely necessary. These procedures are successful in more than 90% of cases. Postoperative complications include wound infection, persisting pain or weakness or both, injury to the dura with cerebrospinal fluid (CSF) leak, and recurrence of disk herniation at the same level. After a microdiskectomy, the patient typically returns home the next morning or on the same day.

Lumbar Stenosis

Pathophysiology

Congenital or degenerative narrowing of the spinal canal in the lumbar region leads to a syndrome called *neurogenic claudication*. The patients have problems standing straight and walking downhill. They find relief when sitting and bending forward, because that increases the spinal canal diameter. Riding the bicycle, for example, is much better tolerated than other exercise.

Differential Diagnosis

In contrast to vascular claudication, the pain and sensory deficits associated with neurogenic claudication follow dermatomes. In contrast to LDH, the pain with spinal stenosis is frequently bilateral in the hips, thighs, and legs.

Workup and Evaluation

Initial evaluation is similar to that for LDH and focuses on the exclusion of more serious underlying pathology. Plain lumbosacral spine radiographs usually demonstrate degenerative bone disease, a mixed picture of bone hypertrophy and erosion and narrowing of the spinal canal. Myelograms have an important role in the workup for this disease, because they allow functional imaging of the degree of spinal and root canal stenosis. Magnetic resonance imaging (MRI) is poor in visualizing bone, but it depicts compression of nerve roots, narrowing of the spinal canal, and thickening of the ligaments. MRI is the imaging study of choice.

Treatment Alternatives

As with LDH, conservative treatment is attempted first. If this fails, a lumbar laminectomy can be considered. During this procedure, the patient is in the prone position, and the spinous process, the lamina, and the ligamentum flavum are resected, which decompresses the nerve roots in the spinal canal. If necessary, the decompression should be extended laterally to relieve pressure from the nerve roots as they exit the spinal canal. Fusion or instrumentation or both are not mandatory after a routine laminectomy and should be reserved for demonstrated instability and failure to relieve symptoms (failed back syndrome).

Cervical Disk Herniation

Pathophysiology

The cervical segments that are most commonly affected by intervertebral disk herniation are C5, C6, and C7. In younger patients, cervical disk herniation (CDH) is usually an acute event with sudden onset of pain and sometimes neurologic deficits in the shoulder and arm. The important difference between lumbar and cervical disk herniations is that in the cervical region, a herniated disk can lead to myelopathy with neurologic symptoms in all segments below the herniation. The affected nerve root is the one that exits the spinal canal at the same level. The nerve roots exit above their like-numbered vertebral bodies, so that a C5–C6 disk causes a C6 radiculopathy. In older patients, chronic degenerative changes are more frequently the cause of CDH. These degenerative changes with bony osteophytes are caused by cervical spondylosis. Characteristic features of CDH are neck pain, paresthesias, and weakness along the nerve root distribution. Neck extension frequently worsens the symptoms. Central disk herniation with myelopathy results in increased muscle tone and reflexes, incontinence, unsteadiness, and clumsiness in the hands (Table 48-2).

PEARL FOR ROUNDS

The role of neurosurgery in the workup of patients with HIV infection is very limited. An invasive biopsy can usually be avoided with appropriate diagnostic workup including imaging studies such as contrast MRI.

Differential Diagnosis

As with LDH, other processes such as cancer, trauma, and infection must be ruled out. A left C6 radiculopathy can sometimes demonstrate pain similar to that with myocardial infarction. Moreover, consider brachial plexus lesions including Pancoast tumors, as well as ulnar and median nerve entrapment syndromes.

Workup and Evaluation

MRI is the imaging study of choice for evaluation of CDH. A myelogram has similar benefits but is invasive. A careful neurologic examination may reveal motor and sensory deficits in the distribution of affected nerve roots. Sometimes the Spurling sign can be positive; in patients with foraminal stenosis and compression of a cervical nerve root, lateral head movements or pressure on the top of the head can elicit pain and paresthesias in the distribution of the nerve root.

TABLE 48–2 Neurologic Deficits Expected with Cervical Disk Herniation

Deficit	Locations			
Herniation	C4–C5	C5–C6	C6–C7	C7–T1
Radiculopathy	C5	C6	C7	C8
Motor weakness	Deltoid	Forearm flexion	Forearm extension	Hand intrisics
Sensory deficit	Shoulder	Thumb	Fingers 2 and 3	Fingers 4 and 5
Reflex	—	Biceps	Triceps	—

PEARL FOR THE OR

Artificial cervical and lumbar disks have been introduced for the treatment of patients with cervical radiculopathy, myelopathy, or chronic disabling lower back pain. These procedures have the potential to replace fusion surgery, which has been considered the standard of care for some of these disorders. The advantage of artificial disks is that they preserve motion at the affected segment and may prevent degenerative disk disease at adjacent levels.

Treatment Alternatives

As in LDH, the majority of patients with CDH will improve with conservative treatment alone. Surgery should be considered for patients with severe or progressive neurologic deficits, myelopathy, or those for whom conservative treatment fails. The surgical options include

- Cervical laminotomy (posterior decompression) and diskectomy
- Anterior cervical diskectomy
- Anterior cervical diskectomy with fusion (ACDF)
- Anterior cervical diskectomy with fusion and plating.

A cervical laminotomy is probably the least invasive procedure and can provide good results if the disk herniation is lateral and focal without diffuse degenerative disease. Anterior approaches provide the advantage of much better removal of osteophytes and larger disk herniations but carry the risk of injury to the esophagus, the laryngeal nerves, and the development of postoperative hematomas. Controversy exists over the indication of bone graft fusion and instrumentation in anterior approaches, and no well-accepted guidelines have been formulated.

Infection of the Central Nervous System and Its Coverings

Bacterial, fungal and other infections may occur in every part of the brain, spinal cord, and its coverings. Treatment and prognosis depend on the patient's condition (immune defense) and the virulence of the infecting organism. The most commonly seen infections are meningitis and ventriculitis due to ventriculostomies in trauma patients and after subarachnoid hemorrhage (SAH), shunt systems in pediatric patients, and CSF fistulas after craniotomies or after trauma. The normal laboratory values of human CSF should be known (Box 48-1).

Meningitis and Ventriculitis

Cerebrospinal Fluid Sampling and Ventriculostomy Management in the Intensive Care Unit

In the intensive care unit (ICU), ventriculostomies are used mainly in patients with head injury or SAH for monitoring of intracranial pressure (ICP) or treatment of hydrocephalus.

BOX 48–1 Normal Laboratory Values of Human CSF

Normal CSF

- Clear and colorless
- 0 polymorphonuclear leukocytes (PMNs), 0 red blood cells, and 0 to five monocytes
- Protein, 15 to 45 mg/dL
- Glucose, 50% of serum glucose

Bacterial meningitis

- CSF glucose, less than 35 mg/dL
- CSF protein, more than 220 mg/dL
- Up to 2000 and more white blood cells/mL, mostly PMNs

- The average rate of bacterial colonization of catheters is between 4% and 14%. Clinically significant intracranial infections are uncommon.
- Neurosurgical technique significantly affects infection rate. Tunneling of the ventricular catheter decreases infection rate.
- Irrigation of fluid-coupled ICP devices and frequent sampling of CSF significantly increase bacterial colonization.
- CSF should not be sent routinely and only for a new-onset fever.
- Prophylactic antibiotics have not been shown to decrease infection rate.
- Ventriculostomy catheters should be removed as quickly as possible, as the risk of infection increases with length of monitoring.
- Whether and when to change a ventricular catheter in the absence of infection has been discussed controversially.

Once a catheter is infected (positive CSF culture or high clinical suspicion), it should be removed and replaced on the contralateral side if clinically indicated. Ventriculitis is treated with systemic and sometimes intrathecal antibiotics.

Cerebrospinal Fluid Fistulas

CSF fistulas can occur spontaneously, or as the result of traumatic skull-base fractures or dural defects after craniotomy. Infection resulting from a CSF fistula can occur weeks and months after the initial event. Most common CSF pathways are through the middle ear into the nose or nasopharynx (rhinorrhea) or through the ruptured tympanic membrane into the external auditory canal (otorrhea). The incidence of meningitis after traumatic CSF leak is up to 10%. Uncertainty may exist as to whether clear fluid observed in the nose or ear actually is CSF. β-Transferrin is a marker for CSF, and its presence would support the diagnosis of CSF fistula. Air may be seen on imaging studies in the intracranial compartment. Intrathecal injection of tracer material can sometimes be helpful in the determination of the pathway of a CSF fistula. Prophylactic antibiotics have not proven helpful. Initial treatment includes bed rest, keeping the head elevated and sometimes lumbar drainage to decrease the CSF pressure. Direct surgical repair of the leak may require a complicated skull-base approach and is frequently not successful. In these cases, placement of a ventriculoperitoneal shunt may be the only alternative.

Bacterial Meningitis

Meningitis is an infection of the coverings of the brain and it is clinically characterized by headaches, nuchal rigidity, fevers, and sometimes decreased mental status. It occurs most commonly as a complication of craniospinal surgery or after trauma. Seizures and cranial nerve palsies can occur, and coma develops in up to 10% of patients. CSF sampling usually reveals the offending organism.

Brain Abscess

A brain abscess is usually secondary to a focal infection elsewhere and develops most frequently in the white matter of the frontal or temporal lobe. An underlying bacterial endocarditis, a pulmonary infection, or a traumatic brain injury is the most likely source. Symptoms are frequently focal (paresis, seizures) and sometimes due to mass effect and surrounding brain edema. Signs of infection may be absent, with low white blood cell counts, negative blood cultures, and no fevers. CT and MRI imaging with and without contrast will reveal a ring-enhancing mass, which may be difficult to differentiate from a brain tumor. Medical treatment for small or multiple lesions includes systemic antibiotics. Steroids are controversial and reserved for patients with progressive deterioration secondary to edema and mass effect. Surgical excision via stereotactic aspiration or open craniotomy for accurate diagnosis and decompression is frequently indicated.

Human Immunodeficiency Virus and Brain Lesions

Multiple ring-enhancing lesions in a middle-aged patient should raise the suspicion of acquired immunodeficiency syndrome (AIDS)–related infections such as toxoplasmosis. Empiric treatment with pyrimethamine is the initial step in therapy. Other lesions with AIDS are primary CNS lymphoma, progressive multifocal leukoencephalopathy, and cryptococcal abscess. Stereotactic biopsies are occasionally required for diagnosis in these patients.

Osteomyelitis

Osteomyelitis can occur with result of an infection around the spine, the mastoids, or the sinuses, from contamination during surgery or trauma, or, rarely, from hematogenous spread from another infection. Presenting symptoms may be limited to pain, muscle spasms, and fever. Neurologic symptoms develop if the infection spreads into the epidural space and compresses the brain or spinal cord. Frequently a biopsy is required for diagnosis. Treatment includes systemic antibiotics, drainage, and débridement of infected bone.

Diskitis

Disk-space infections are seen after lumbar puncture, laminectomy, diskectomy, or spontaneously. Presenting symptoms are severe lower back tenderness, pain, and muscle spasm. Although the white blood cell count may be normal, the erythrocyte sedimentation rate is always elevated. Treatment requires a CT-guided or open biopsy for cultures and systemic antibiotics.

Suggested Reading

Benzel E (ed): Spine Surgery: Techniques, Complication Avoidance, and Management. Oxford, UK, Churchill Livingstone, 1999.

Management of acute central cervical spinal cord injuries. Neurosurgery 50(3 suppl):S166–S172, 2002.

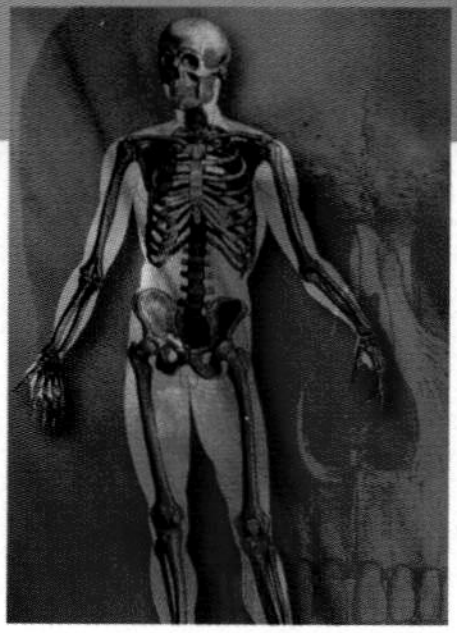

Chapter 49
Neoplasms

ROGER HARTL, MD, and PHILIP E. STIEG, MD, PhD

Intracranial Neoplasms

Incidence, Location, and Pathophysiology

With better availability of imaging techniques, intracranial neoplasms are diagnosed more frequently and earlier during their course. Primary brain tumors are the cause of death in approximately 13,000 patients per year in the United States and more than 100,000 patients each year die with symptomatic intracranial metastases. In adults, the most common tumors are gliomas, metastases, and meningiomas. Up to 85% of these tumors are located in the supratentorial compartment. In children, the most frequent tumors are medulloblastoma and cerebellar astrocytomas, and 60% of childhood tumors are located in the infratentorial compartment. Ionizing radiation is the only risk factor that has been identified for glial and meningeal neoplasms. A current classification is shown in Box 49-1.

Clinical Presentation

Symptoms develop either secondary to mass effect and increased intracranial pressure or because of focal damage. Consequently, brain tumors can cause either generalized symptoms, such as headache, nausea, vomiting, sixth nerve palsy, and decreased mental status, or they cause local symptoms such as hemiparesis, aphasia, ataxia, and seizures.

Workup and Evaluation

The best imaging technology available is magnetic resonance imaging (MRI), with and without gadolinium enhancement. Computed tomography (CT) can miss structural abnormalities, especially lesions in the brainstem and posterior fossa. A normal MRI virtually excludes the possibility of a brain tumor. Cerebral angiography can be helpful for preoperative embolization of very vascular brain tumors, such as meningiomas. Positron emission tomography (PET) scanning is sometimes done to differentiate between hypometabolic low-grade astrocytomas and hypermetabolic high-grade astrocytomas.

Treatment Alternatives

Treatment depends on many factors, including the type of tumor, the location, and the degree of disease progression. Treatment of many tumors combines surgery, radiotherapy, and chemotherapy.

Surgery

Surgical treatment usually involves a craniotomy and microsurgical resection of the brain tumor, sometimes assisted by an image-guided system. Before surgery, it is sometimes helpful with large tumors to treat with steroids. This minimizes intra- and postoperative brain swelling. Preoperative angiographic embolization may decrease bleeding from vascular brain tumors. A lumbar drain is sometimes inserted in the operating room to drain cerebrospinal fluid (CSF) during surgery. This reduces the amount of brain retraction needed to reach deep parts of the brain and minimizes brain injury. During surgery, frameless stereotactic devices, ultrasound, and an intraoperative MRI are sometimes used to identify deep lesions, or tumors that are not distinct from surrounding brain tissue. Antiseizure prophylaxis is not routinely used after craniotomy for tumors. The type of procedure—biopsy, partial tumor removal/decompression, or complete removal—depends on the nature of the tumor and its size.

The main surgical approaches used are

- a simple burr hole for a stereotactic biopsy,
- frontal, temporal, parietal, or occipital craniotomy; these are the standard approaches for most brain tumors located in the supratentorial compartment,
- trans-sphenoidal route for pituitary tumors, through the nose and sphenoid sinus into the pituitary fossa,
- transoral route for tumors located around the clivus and atlas, and
- suboccipital craniectomy; for lesions in the cerebellum and posterior fossa. *Craniectomy* means that the bone is not reinserted after surgery.

Radiotherapy

Radiotherapy uses ionizing radiation such as x-rays or gamma rays to cause cell death or to stop cell replication in tumors. The effect of radiotherapy depends on the total dose of radiation delivered, usually up to 60 Gy (Gray), and treatment duration. This must be balanced with the adverse effect on normal tissue. One disadvantage of radiotherapy is

BOX 49-1 Classification of CNS Tumors

Tumors of Neuroepithelial Tissue

Astrocytic tumors

- Astrocytoma
- Anaplastic astrocytoma
- Glioblastoma multiforme
- Pilocystic astrocytoma
- Pleomorphic xanthoastrocytoma
- Subependymal giant-cell astrocytoma

Oligodendroglial tumors

- Oligodendroglioma
- Anaplastic oligodendroglioma

Ependymal tumors

- Ependymoma
- Anaplastic ependymoma
- Myxopapillary ependymoma
- Subependymoma

Choroid plexus tumors

- Choroid plexus papilloma
- Choroid plexus carcinoma

Neuronal and mixed neuronal-glial tumors

- Gangliocytoma
- Dysembryoplastic neuroepithelial tumor
- Ganglioglioma
- Anaplastic ganglioglioma
- Central neurocytoma

Pineal parenchymal tumors

- Pineocytoma
- Pineoblastoma
- Embryonal tumor
- Medulloblastoma
- Primitive neuroectodermal tumor

Meningeal Tumors

- Meningioma
- Hemangiopericytoma
- Melanocytic tumor
- Hemangioblastoma

Primary Central Nervous System Lymphoma

Germ Cell Tumors

- Germinoma
- Embryonal carcinoma
- Yolk-sac tumor (endodermal sinus tumor)
- Choriocarcinoma
- Teratoma
- Mixed germ-cell tumor

Tumors of the Sellar Region

- Pituitary adenoma
- Pituitary carcinoma
- Craniopharyngioma

Metastatic Tumors

the delayed treatment effect. Three types of radiotherapy are used:

- Conventional external-beam radiation. Standard x-ray radiotherapy is administered, but the beams are shaped with collimators to protect normal brain. Treatment is typically fractionated over a period of several weeks. The usual dose for malignant gliomas, for example, is 50 to 60 Gy, spread out over a 6-week period.
- Stereotactic radiosurgery. Multiple converging beams deliver high doses of γ-rays or electrons from a linear accelerator in a single treatment session to the lesion. The gamma knife and Linac are examples.
- Interstitial treatment with radiation, called *brachytherapy.* The tumor is treated by the implantation of radioactive material.

Complications of radiotherapy include

- Increased brain edema immediately after treatment,
- Demyelination after weeks and months, which may be partially reversible
- Radionecrosis after years, which is nonreversible.

Chemotherapy

Chemotherapeutic agents have been used for many years in the management of brain tumors. Carmustine (BCNU) is an alkylating agent that is used for malignant gliomas in combination with surgery and radiotherapy. Oligodendrogliomas respond well to chemotherapy, and central nervous system (CNS) lymphomas are treated primarily with methotrexate.

Treatment of Selected Brain Tumors

Gliomas (Neuroepithelial Tissue Tumors)

Gliomas can be divided into astrocytomas and oligodendrogliomas. The degree of malignancy depends on histologic features such as the presence of nuclear atypia, mitotic rate, vascular proliferation, and necrosis. Prognosis after treatment depends on patient age, preoperative condition, and tumor pathology. Median survival for low-grade lesions is 8 to 10 years, and for high-grade tumors, less than 2 years.

Low-grade astrocytomas are first seen in younger patients (peak in the third to fourth decade), frequently with seizures. MRI typically demonstrates a nonenhancing mass in one of the cerebral hemispheres. Patients in good neurologic condition are initially monitored, and seizures are controlled pharmacologically. Radiographic studies should be performed at regular intervals. When clear clinical and radiologic evidence of tumor progression appears, surgery combined with radiotherapy should be considered. Unfortunately, most low-grade astrocytomas will eventually progress to malignancy.

Malignant astrocytomas (anaplastic astrocytoma and glioblastoma multiforme) affect patients in their 40s and 50s and are the most common glial tumors (Fig. 49-1).

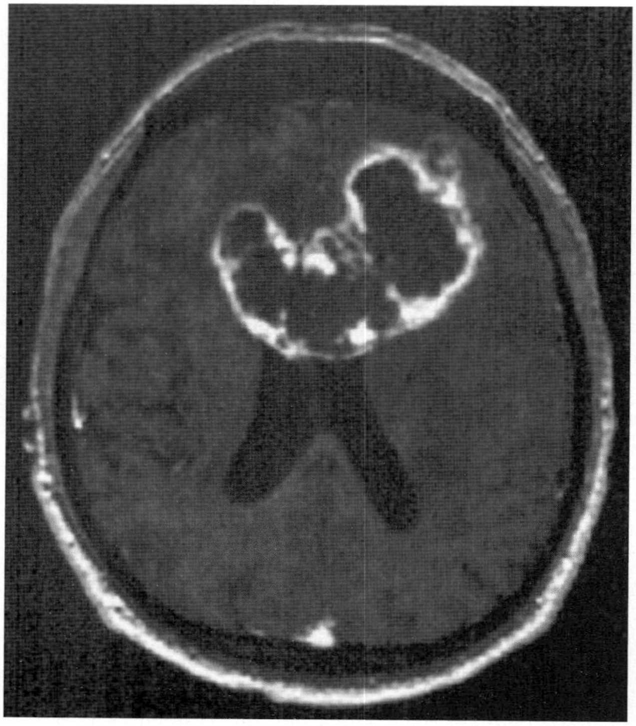

FIGURE 49–1 This axial magnetic resonance image with contrast shows a ring-enhancing, cystic glioblastoma that crosses the midline (*butterfly glioma*).

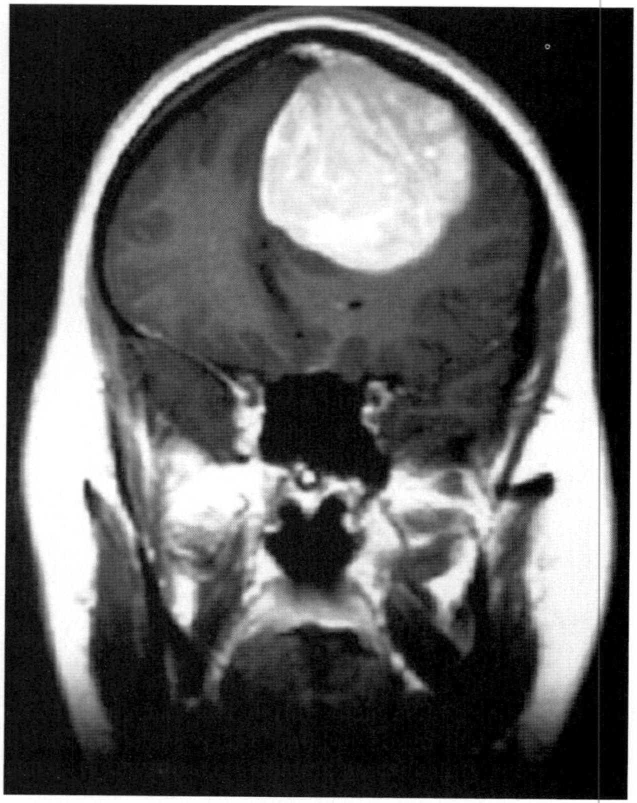

FIGURE 49–2 This coronal magnetic resonance image with contrast demonstrates a homogeneously enhancing, parasagittal, large meningioma with characteristic *dural tail sign*.

Typically on MRI, a ring-enhancing mass is seen, and the lesion can spread across the midline. Treatment consists of gross total resection, conventional conformal radiotherapy up to a total dose of 60 Gy, and sometimes chemotherapy with BCNU. If the lesion recurs, a second resection should be attempted.

Oligodendroglial tumors also can be divided into low-grade and high-grade lesions. These tumors show sensitivity to chemotherapy. Treatment consists of surgery and focal radiation followed by chemotherapy. Median survival with optimal treatment for low-grade lesions may be up to 16 years.

Meningiomas

Meningiomas arise from arachnoid cells in the meninges and constitute approximately 20% of all intracranial neoplasms. On MRI scanning, they typically appear as a homogeneously enhancing, well-circumscibed mass (Fig. 49-2). The vast majority of these are slow growing, benign lesions, but over time, they can cause neurologic deficits such as hemiparesis, cranial nerve dysfunction, and epilepsy. Surgery can be curative and is indicated for symptomatic lesions. Resection followed by radiotherapy can be considered for recurrent meningiomas.

Metastasis

Metastases are the most commonly seen intracranial supratentorial tumors in adults. Common primary sites include the lungs, breasts, and kidneys; in 25% of all patients with

PEARLS FOR ROUNDS

Treatment of brain tumors depends particularly on the type of tumor, the location, and the degree of progression of disease. Treatment often combines surgery, radiotherapy, and chemotherapy.

The most common presentation of brain tumors overall is slow progressive neurologic deficit, usually motor weakness. This is followed by headaches in approximately 50% of patients and seizures in 25%. Headaches and nausea/vomiting are the most common presenting symptoms in posterior fossa tumors.

Magnetic resonance imaging with and without gadolinium is the imaging study of choice for brain tumors, especially for tumors in the posterior fossa.

PEARLS FOR THE OR

The role of conventional, open surgery for certain brain tumors has been challenged by advances made with radiosurgery. Today, radiosurgery—with either gamma knife or cyberknife technology—is an accepted first-line treatment for solitary cerebral metastases or acoustic neuromas smaller than 3 cm. More frequently, radiosurgery can be used as an adjunct to open surgery after partial resection of a brain tumor.

In patients who are medically stable and with a reasonable life expectancy, spinal epidural metastases should be surgically resected. If signs and symptoms of spinal instability are noted, such as radiographic evidence of spinal cord compression, progressive neurologic deficit, pain, or deformity, resection should be followed by instrumentation. In the absence of these findings, radiosensitive tumors can be radiated as a first-line treatment, but the patients must be monitored closely.

lung or breast cancer, cerebral metastases develop. Among primary cancers, melanoma most commonly spreads to the brain (40%). Patients frequently are first seen with epilepsy or other focal neurologic deficits. Treatment depends on location and number of lesions. Corticosteroids are very effective in controlling associated brain edema. A solitary metastasis is removed surgically, followed by whole-brain radiation or stereotactic radiotherapy or both. If multiple lesions are present, radiotherapy will be the mainstay of treatment, even though sometimes surgery may be performed to remove large lesions that are in an amenable location.

Spinal Neoplasms

Approximately 20% of all CNS tumors are located in the spine. Spinal neoplasms are classified as either intradural or extradural. Of all intradural tumors, only 16% are located within the spinal cord (intramedullary). Most intradural tumors are primary CNS tumors. Metastases are found in the extradural compartment. The best study for diagnosing spinal tumors is MRI, with and without gadolinium.

The most common intramedullary spinal cord tumors are nonmalignant astrocytoma and ependymoma. Astrocytoma is more common in children, and ependymomas, in adults. Intramedullary tumors usually appear with pain, motor weakness, and gait disturbances. Treatment for ependymoma is surgical. Astrocytomas are more diffuse, cannot always be removed, and may require radiotherapy.

Neurofibromas are the most common spinal cord tumors located intradurally but outside the spinal cord (extramedullary). They frequently involve the nerve roots and may occur with a radiculopathy. Treatment is surgical removal.

Metastases to the spinal column are the most frequently seen forms of spine tumors. Common primary sites include breast, lung, and prostate. Surgical excision is the treatment of choice in the presence of spinal cord compression. Radiosensitive tumors include lymphoma, multiple myeloma, and renal cell metastases. Bony destruction by the metastatic tumor may render the spine unstable and require extensive surgery with stabilization and instrumentation.

Suggested Reading

DeAngelis LM: Brain tumors. N Engl J Med 344:114–123, 2001.
Gutin P, Posner J: Neuro-oncology: Diagnosis and management of cerebral gliomas, past, present, and future. Neurosurgery 47:1–8, 2000.

SECTION XIII

OTORHINOLARYNGOLOGY

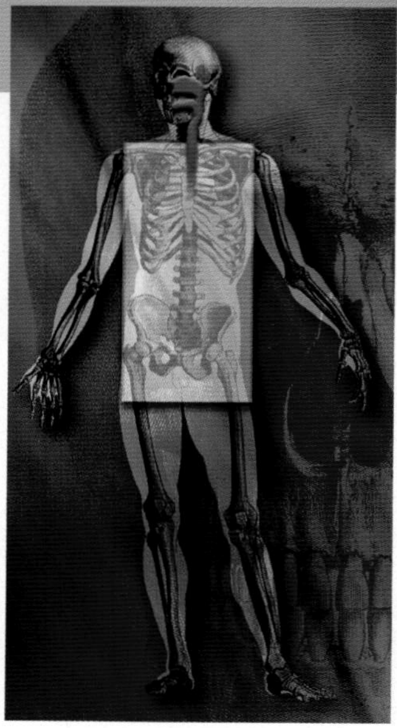

Chapter 50

Otologic and Neuro-otologic Diseases

ANAND K. DEVAIAH, MD, NEIL E. BROWN, MD, DANIEL K. SMITH, MD, and KENNETH M. GRUNDFAST, MD

A wide variety of diseases affect the ear and the temporal bone. Collectively, they are categorized as otologic/neuro-otologic disorders. Otologic diseases are those that affect any portion of the ear, including external and internal structures. Neuro-otologic disorders generally affect the lateral skull base, at the interface between the structures of the ear and the brain. Both groups of disorders are found in a portion of the skull base with a complex anatomy encased in a labyrinth of bone, which can make this area challenging to treat with medical and surgical means. This chapter serves as a surgeon's introduction to the anatomy and associated disorders.

Anatomy

The anatomy of the ear and the lateral skull base is complex, with several key components that are important to understanding the pathophysiology of diseases and disorders of that area.

Auricle

The auricle, or pinna, comprises several anatomic subunits (Fig. 50-1). The helix and antihelix define much of the overall shape of the ear. The configuration of the ear not only lends familiar aesthetic definition to the face but also is useful in the amplification of selected frequencies. The ear's neural supply is from a variety of sources, including the vagus, facial, trigeminal, and third cervical (greater auricular branch) nerves. The vascular supply is derived from the posterior auricular and superficial temporal arteries.

External Auditory Canal and Tympanic Membrane

The lateral two thirds of the external canal is a soft-tissue structure comprising primarily cartilage and skin. Cerumen is formed within the lateral portion of the external canal. The medial third of this structure is an osseous canal covered with soft tissue. A continuous slough of epidermis and cerumen occurs in the healthy ear. Its neural supply is based on the same nerves that supply the auricle.

The tympanic membrane serves as the dividing structure between the external and middle ear (Fig. 50-2). It consists of inner and outer epithelial layers surrounding middle fibrous layers. This structure is designed to begin the translation of sound from the external ear into the middle ear. It is attached to the malleus, which serves as the beginning of the ossicular chain.

Middle Ear and Ossicular Chain

The middle-ear space is bounded laterally by the tympanic membrane and medially by the mucosa-lined temporal bone. This space is normally a real space, clear of fluid or debris. The eustachian tube begins in this space. One opening to the eustachian tube is in the anteromedial aspect of the middle ear, and the other opening is in the nasopharynx. This tube helps to equalize pressure and serves as a drainage conduit for the middle ear.

The facial nerve is a bone-covered structure that courses through the entire temporal bone (Fig. 50-3). In about 50% of people, this nerve is dehiscent within the middle-ear space. This structure has several functions, with most of its fibers responsible for ipsilateral volitional movement of the muscles for facial expression. A branch of this nerve, the chorda tympani, also courses through the space to join the facial nerve. This nerve carries special sensory fibers from the anterior two thirds of the tongue.

Another component of the middle ear is the ossicular chain, comprising the malleus, incus, and stapes (Fig. 50-4). These three ossicles serve as a complex lever arm to

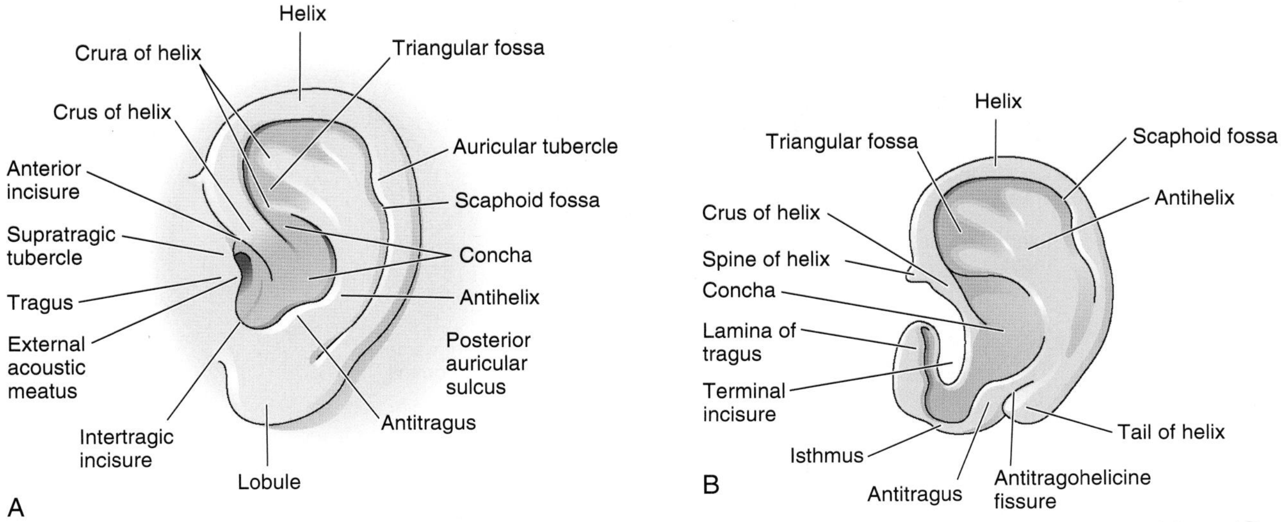

FIGURE 50–1 Anatomic subunits of the ear. *A*, The structural subunits of the auricle. *B*, The cartilaginous framework of the auricle, which underlies the corresponding subunits. (Adapted from Cummings C, Frederickson J, Harker L, et al (eds): Otolaryngology, 3rd ed: Head and Neck Surgery. Philadelphia, Mosby, 1998, p 2539.)

conduct vibrations from the tympanic membrane into the cochlea.

Cochlea and Semicircular Canals

The cochlea and semicircular canals (SCCs) are complex translational sensory units housed in an osseous labyrinth within the temporal bone (Fig. 50-5). The cochlea turns sound vibrations into neural signals. Sound is conducted into the inner ear by the stapes at the oval window and is then transmitted through the cochlea. This in turn causes stimulation of specific hair cells on the basis of sound frequency. Stimulation of the hair cells results in the creation of neural impulses, which are carried by the cochlear portion of the eighth cranial nerve (the vestibulocochlear nerve).

The semicircular canals comprise a significant portion of the peripheral vestibular system (see Fig. 50-5). Each of the three canals is oriented to respond in different planes of movement. Motion causes displacement of specially arranged hair cells, which translate the motion into neural signals carried by the vestibular portion of the vestibulocochlear nerve.

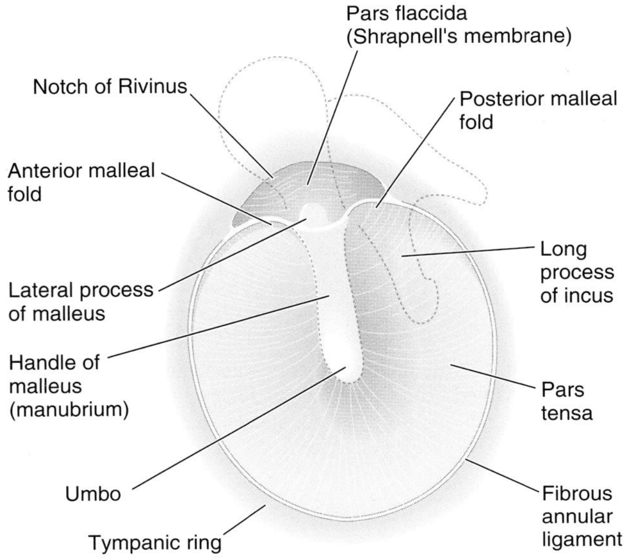

FIGURE 50–2 The tympanic membrane viewed through the external canal.

Internal Auditory Canal and Medial Temporal Bone

The internal auditory canal contains the fibers of the vestibulocochlear nerve (both the superior and inferior vestibular nerves as well as the cochlear nerve), facial nerve, and labyrinthine artery. It is the conduit for these structures between the brainstem and the medial aspect of the temporal bone. A lesion of one structure within this canal may affect the function of the other structures within the canal, given their close proximity.

Special Considerations in Temporal Bone Anatomy

The temporal bone has complex relations with structures in addition to the auditory and vestibular apparati (Fig. 50-6). These relations must be taken into account when addressing temporal bone diseases. One such structure is the temporal lobe of the brain, which is in close proximity to the temporal bone. The caudal temporal lobe is supported

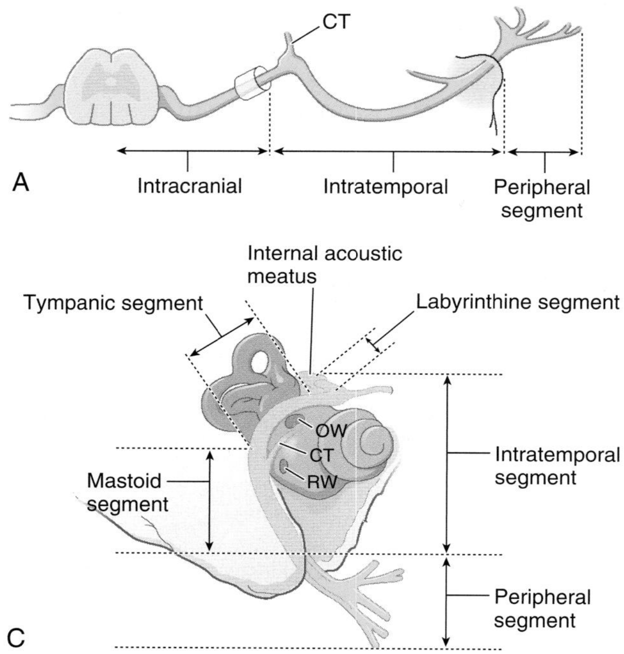

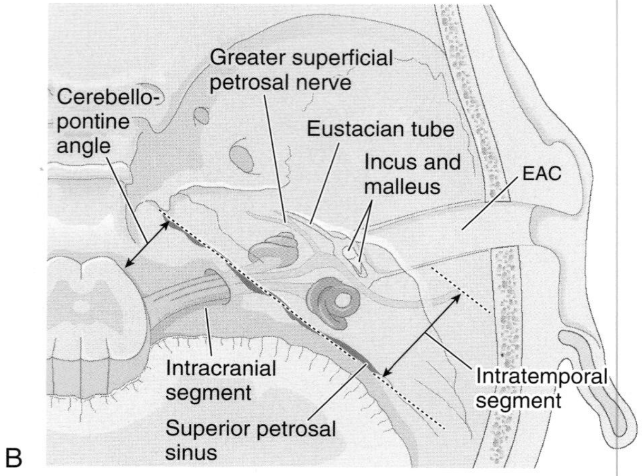

FIGURE 50–3 The facial nerve. *A*, From the brainstem root to the peripheral segment. *B*, An axial view as the nerve courses from the brainstem through the temporal bone. *C*, The segments of the facial nerve as they drape over the labyrinth on lateral view. CT, chorda tympani; EAC, external auditory canal; OW, oval window; RW, round window. (Adapted from Brackmann D, Arriaga M (eds): Otologic Surgery, 2nd ed. Philadelphia, Saunders, 2001, p 319.)

by the temporal bone and separated from it by an osseous plate called the tegmen.

Another important structure is the sigmoid sinus, which accepts venous drainage from the cerebral vasculature and courses through the mastoid portion of the temporal bone. It intersects with a portion of the tegmen designated as the sindural angle, which is another important surgical landmark. Adjacent to the sigmoid sinus are the posterior fossa and the cerebellum. As the sigmoid sinus exits the temporal bone, it may be seen in the middle ear; it also may be dehiscent in this area. It exits through the jugular foramen as the internal jugular vein.

The internal carotid artery also passes through the temporal bone (Fig. 50-7). A portion of its outline, covered in bone, can be seen in the middle ear as it courses rostral. Rarely, it may be dehiscent in the middle ear.

As mentioned earlier, the facial nerve also courses through the temporal bone. The nerve makes two turns (each

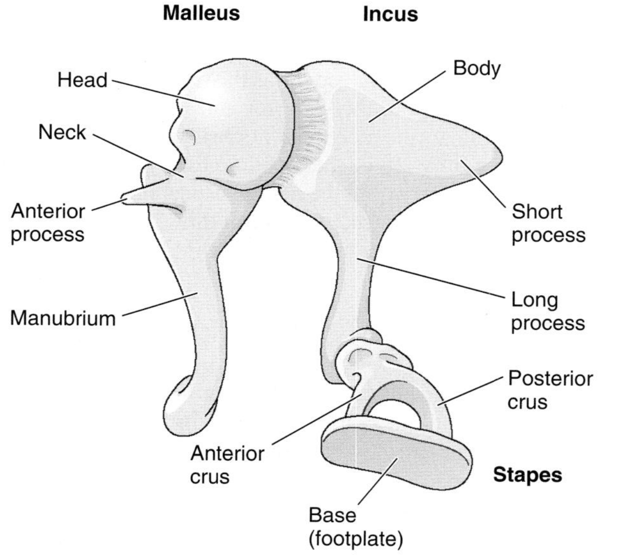

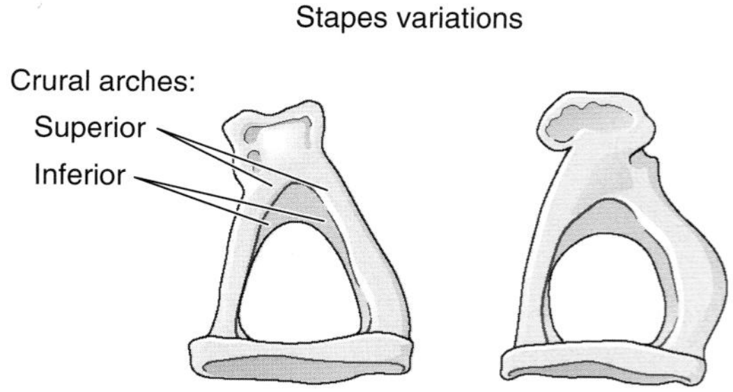

FIGURE 50–4 Articulation and anatomic subunits of the ossicles. (Adapted from Cummings C, Frederickson J, Harker L, et al (eds): Otolaryngology, 3rd ed: Head and Neck Surgery. Philadelphia, Mosby, 1998, p 2545.)

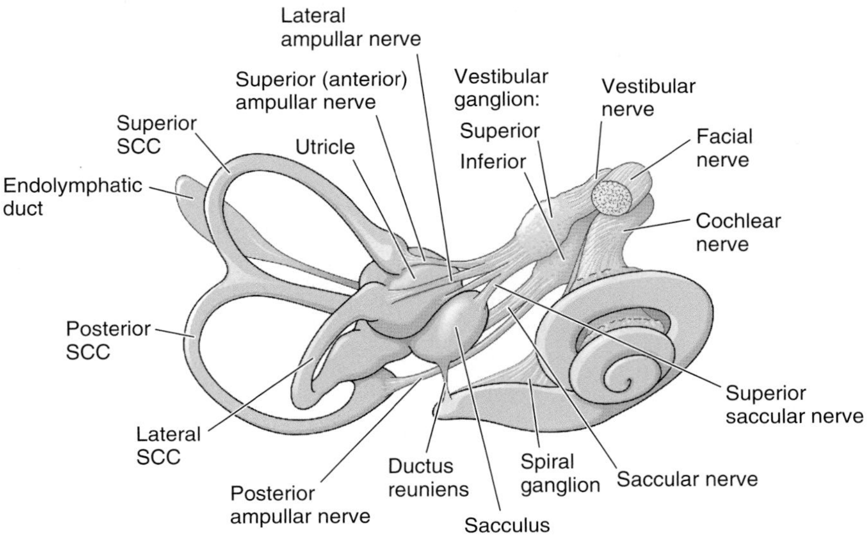

FIGURE 50–5 The membranous labyrinth, showing the relation between the auditory and vestibular portions with innervation. (Adapted from Cummings C, Frederickson J, Harker L, et al (eds): Otolaryngology, 3rd ed, Head and Neck Surgery. Philadelphia, Mosby, 1998, p 2564.)

of which is called a genu) before exiting the stylomastoid foramen (see Fig. 50-3). This nerve has a complex relation to the cochlea, labyrinth, and ossicles as it passes through the temporal bone. It is another important surgical landmark and is monitored during surgery to avoid injury.

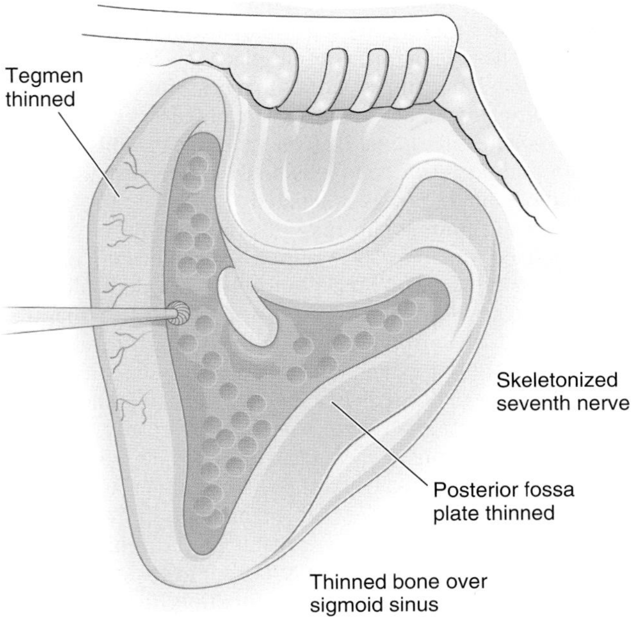

FIGURE 50–6 Relations among temporal bone structures in the mastoid portion. In this mastoidectomy cavity, note the thin plate of the tegmen, posterior fossa plate, sigmoid sinus, and facial nerve. (Adapted from Brackmann D, Arriaga M (eds): Otologic Surgery, 2nd ed. Philadelphia, Saunders, 2001, p 160.)

Disorders of the External Ear

Infectious and Inflammatory Disorders

Impetigo involves the epidermis of the auricle and is usually caused by *Staphylococcus aureus* or *Staphylococcus epidermidis*. Clinically, it manifests as red papules, which can progress into vesicles. These vesicles can further coalesce and develop into open, crusting sores. Systemic symptoms such as fever are not characteristic. Treatment consists of antibiotics (typically penicillin) and local wound care for areas of skin in which debris has collected. Lesions that do not respond should be examined carefully for resistant organisms or a different type of infectious process.

Erysipelas involves the dermis of the ear and is most commonly caused by group-A hemolytic streptococcus. The patient has pain, erythema, and edema of the auricle. The affected area is usually well demarcated from surrounding

PEARLS FOR ROUNDS

Sensation for the external ear is from the facial, vagus, trigeminal, and third cervical root nerves.

The most frequent organisms in acute otitis media are *Streptococcus pneumoniae, Haemophilus influenzae,* and *Moraxella catarrhalis.*

Acquired cholesteatoma most often begins in the pars flaccida.

Transverse temporal bone fractures are less common than longitudinal or oblique fractures, but are associated with a higher risk of facial nerve injury.

The most common tumor of the cerebellopontine angle is acoustic neuroma.

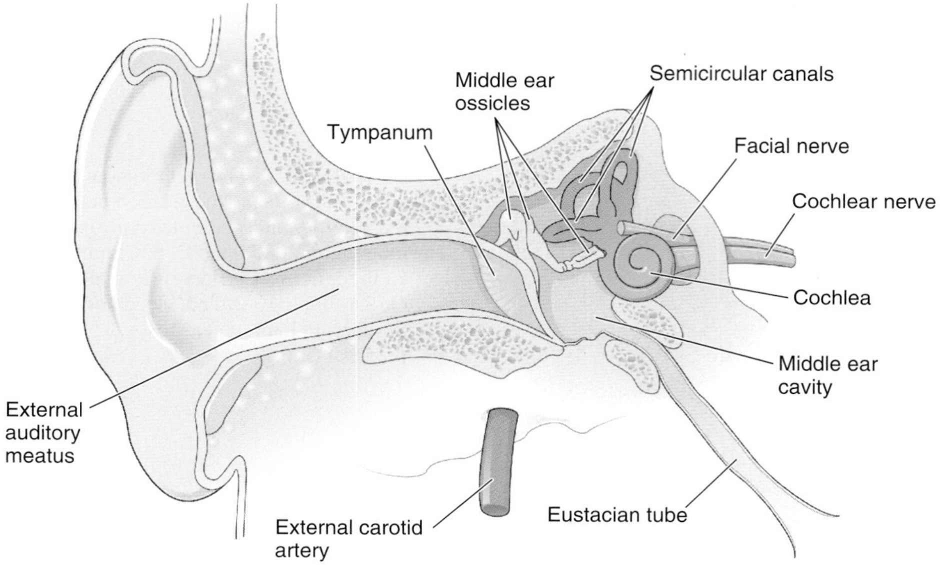

FIGURE 50–7 Structures of the inferior temporal bone. Note the relations between the carotid artery, jugular foramen structures, and facial nerve at the skull base. This area is richly supplied in vasculature and innervation.

uninvolved skin. Systemic symptoms of fever, nausea, and malaise also may be present. Initial treatment with orally administered antimicrobials is acceptable, but if prompt diminution of the erythema and edema is not observed within 48 hours, use of intravenous antibiotics is indicated. If left untreated or inadequately treated, the infection may progress to involve the perichondrium and the cartilage.

Other disorders can mimic these infections. One example is relapsing perichondritis, an autoimmune disorder in which the patient may initially have edema and erythema suggestive of erysipelas. However, erysipelas causes the entire auricle, including the lobule, to become red and swollen, whereas relapsing perichondritis typically involves only the skin adherent to the cartilage, with the lobule remaining normal in appearance.

Trauma

Trauma to the pinna is classified as either blunt or penetrating. Blunt trauma can result from a variety of activities, including wrestling, boxing, and self-mutilation. This can lead to an auricular hematoma or seroma with separation of the perichondrium and underlying cartilage. When this occurs, it deprives the cartilage of its nutritional support. If not corrected, this process can lead to destruction and remodeling of the cartilage (e.g., formation of a so-called cauliflower ear).

To prevent such adverse sequelae, these fluid collections should be treated promptly with incision and drainage. To prevent reaccumulation of the fluid, bolsters are sutured in place to close the space and keep the soft tissue reapproximated to the underlying cartilage (Fig. 50-8). This procedure is usually performed with use of a dental roll, gauze packing, or cotton secured with nylon sutures. First, a local anesthetic is injected to anesthetize the auricle; use of a preauricular and postauricular injection will typically provide an adequate regional block for the ear. The fluid collection is incised and completely drained in relation to the natural contours of the ear. Next, a dental roll or packing coated with an antibiotic ointment is placed anteriorly into the concha so as to contour the normal shape of the cartilage. Posteriorly, a roll of cotton is placed to apply pressure from a posterior direction. The rolls are secured in place, and to each other, with use of nylon mattress sutures that pass through each roll and the auricle. As many sutures as are necessary are used to reapproximate all drained areas of the ear. This allows anterior and posterior compression of the dead space from which the hematoma was evacuated.

Penetrating trauma can range from a simple laceration to complete avulsion of the auricle. With lacerations, the edges are approximated in one to three layers, depending on whether the cartilage is involved (two layers) or whether the anterior and posterior aspects of the pinna are affected (three layers). Loupe magnification is of benefit for precise approximation of the edges. Exposed cartilage should be covered with soft tissue, or excised if cosmetically feasible, to prevent chondritis. Once the edges are approximated, small stab incisions can be made in the pinna to prevent accumulation of a seroma or hematoma, if substantial potential space is present as a result of the injury. If the auricle is avulsed, cartilage may be found exposed at the site where it was severed. In this situation, the remaining viable cartilage can be buried in a postauricular pocket for later use in a delayed reconstruction of the pinna.

If the auricle is completely avulsed, options include reattachment with or without microvascular anastomosis, or burying the cartilage framework in a postauricular pocket

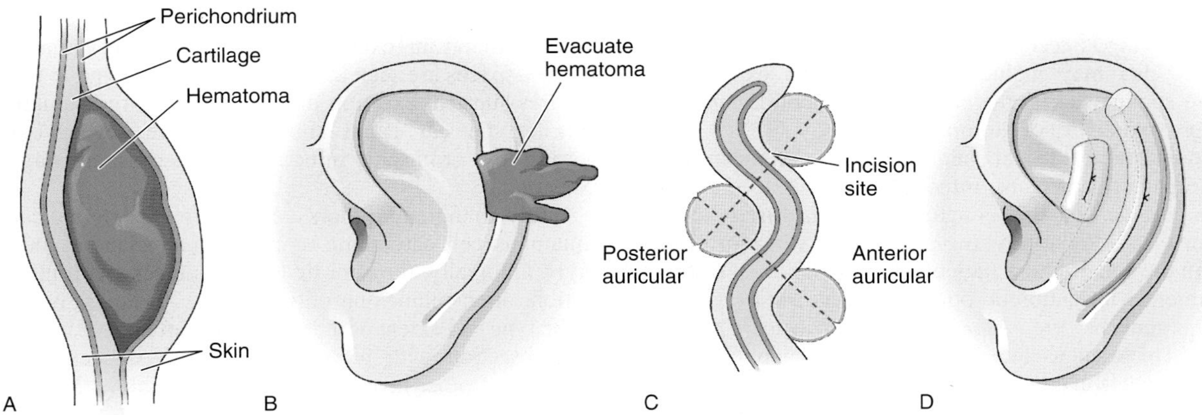

FIGURE 50–8 Treatment of an auricular hematoma. *A*, Hematoma is noted under the perichondrium. *B*, A cosmetic incision is performed to evacuate the collection. *C*, Bolsters are placed to hold the skin and perichondrium to the underlying cartilage. *D*, A side view of the bolsters in place. (Adapted from Cummings C, Frederickson J, Harker L, et al (eds): Otolaryngology, 3rd ed: Head and Neck Surgery. Philadelphia, Mosby, 1998, p 2988.)

for delayed reconstruction. When the auricle is reattached, close follow-up is required to monitor for signs of avascular necrosis or venous congestion. Antibiotics should be used to prevent infection; the utility of antithrombotics such as aspirin and heparin has been suggested in animal studies as a benefit to microvasculature patency but has not been proven in prospective randomized human trials for auricular avulsion.

Tumors

Basal cell carcinoma is the most common skin cancer of the auricle and shares the same histopathologic subtypes as cancer found in other areas of the skin. Treatment generally consists of local excision. A Mohs excision may be necessary, depending on factors such as whether the lesion is recurrent and its histologic subtype.

Squamous cell carcinoma of the auricle is less common and may be more difficult to treat than basal cell carcinoma. Small lesions may be treated with local excision, ensuring clear margins. If the lesion is sizable and involves underlying structures, then complete excision may require resection of the auricle with underlying portions of the temporal bone, parotidectomy, and neck dissection. Postoperative irradiation is typically used for extensive lesions.

Malignant melanoma also may involve the auricle. The accepted methods of treatment include wide local excision and Mohs excision; again, clear margins must be established. Further treatment for extensive lesions can include parotidectomy and regional neck dissection. The use of sentinel node mapping to guide the need for nodal dissection in high-risk patients is under investigation and appears to have utility.

PEARLS FOR THE OR

Tympanostomy tubes are placed in the anteroinferior aspect of the tympanic membrane.

The chorda tympani arises from the facial nerve and traverses the middle ear, passing between the malleus and the incus.

In the middle ear, the facial nerve is dehiscent in about 50% of people.

The internal auditory canal transmits the superior and inferior vestibular nerves, the cochlear nerve, and the labyrinthine artery.

Acoustic neuromas typically arise from the intracanalicular vestibular portion of the eighth cranial nerve but have no predilection for either the superior or the inferior branch.

Disorders of the External Ear Canal

Infectious and Inflammatory Disorders

Otitis externa is an inflammatory process of the external auditory canal that most commonly is caused by *Pseudomonas aeruginosa*. Repeated trauma to the external canal (e.g., use of cotton swabs in the ears) can contribute to the development of otitis externa. Simple cases can be treated with ototopical agents that have activity against this organism, such as fluoroquinolones. In addition, keeping water out of the ear canal helps to promote aural hygiene and to resolve the infectious process. Most acute external ear infections, including those caused by *P. aeruginosa,* resolve with this regimen. Little need to obtain cultures of liquid or debris from the external canal exists, except in the case of infections refractory to medication. In such cases, or in those involving considerable debris in the external canal, careful cleaning is needed to improve aural hygiene. Local treatment also may include insertion of an expandable cellulose spongewick in the canal to help débride material and improve delivery of ototopicals.

Although most external canal infections are bacterial, a fungal organism can cause infection as well, especially in patients who are diabetic. Fungal infection is differentiated from bacterial infection by the presence of white or black spores in the canal. These patients often will have a history of treatment with antibiotic otic drops. The most common fungal organisms are *Aspergillus niger* and *Candida albicans*. Treatment usually consists of topical application of antifungal agents in combination with serial débridements.

Malignant, or necrotizing, otitis externa is the term used to describe an unusually invasive infection. The responsible organism is usually *P. aeruginosa*. The host most often has an element of immunocompromise, such as diabetes. On examination, granulation tissue is seen on the floor of the external canal near the cartilaginous-osseous junction. The infection can invade and destroy soft tissue, cartilage, and bone. If it progresses, it can involve multiple cranial nerves as it tracks along the skull base. This is potentially life threatening. Treatment consists of topical and systemic antibiotics and local care, including serial débridements. Computed tomographic imaging is useful to determine the extent of the destructive infection. A technetium scan also can be used in the initial diagnosis to evaluate the extent of disease. Gallium scanning can help in monitoring the progress of therapy and in charting the resolution of the disease.

Rarely, viral organisms also cause external otitis. For example, Ramsay Hunt syndrome is a herpes zoster infection of the ear. Examination reveals painful vesicles involving the epithelium of the external canal. Vesicles may be present on the auricle or the face as well. Hearing loss, vertigo, and facial nerve paralysis can be associated with this infection. Corneal involvement also is common and should be assessed. In addition to local care, antivirals (acyclovir, valacyclovir) are used.

Trauma

Trauma to the external canal is generally self-inflicted, commonly through the patient's attempts to clean the ears with a variety of objects. The canal is designed to be a self-cleaning entity, and traumatic manipulation can result in cerumen impactions, otitis externa, or abrasions. Abrasions typically respond to a short course of ototopical medications and avoidance of canal irritation.

Tumors

Benign tumors of the external canal include exostoses and osteomas. A propensity exists for exostoses to develop because of repeated cold-water exposure, whereas osteomas develop independent of such exposure. Exostoses also exhibit a different histologic pattern than osteomas; layered bone is found in exostoses, whereas mature bone and marrow spaces are seen in osteomas. Neither type of tumor requires surgical excision unless it grows large enough to obstruct the ear canal substantially; in severe cases, hearing loss or chronic infection may necessitate surgical excision.

Rarely, malignant tumors can involve the external canal. Squamous cell carcinoma or malignant melanoma occurs rarely. Clinically, they are first seen as ulcers with inflammation, often mimicking otitis externa. Treatment is based on the type and extent of the tumor and can include temporal bone resection with parotidectomy, neck dissection, and resection of other involved soft tissue and bone. Radiation therapy is often used.

Disorders of the Middle Ear and Tympanic Membrane

Infectious and Inflammatory Disorders

Otitis media is more common in children than in adults. The organisms that most commonly cause it are *Streptococcus pneumoniae, Haemophilus influenzae*, and *Moraxella catarrhalis*.

In most cases, otitis media resolves spontaneously or with medical therapy. However, when children or adults have frequently recurring acute otitis media or middle-ear effusion that persists for a considerable time after an acute episode, then surgical intervention may be warranted. Surgical procedures that are helpful in the management of otitis media, along with their indications, are summarized later.

Tympanocentesis

In this procedure, an opening is made in the eardrum with a needle, usually to obtain a sample of middle-ear fluid for culture. Indications are acute otitis media in a neonate younger than 6 weeks old, in a patient of any age who is immunocompromised, or in a patient who has not had diminution of fever and relief of pain within 24 hours after initiation of appropriate medical therapy.

Myringotomy

This procedure involves making an incision in the eardrum, usually to initially drain pus from the middle ear or to create an opening into which a tympanostomy (ventilating) tube can be inserted. Indications include a suspicion of impending complications from acute otitis media (e.g., facial paralysis ipsilateral to acute otitis media, or vertigo secondary to acute otitis media labyrinthitis). A myringotomy incision without insertion of a ventilating tube will typically close within several days; this is not ideal in clinical scenarios that require a more persistent drainage path, such as for management of chronic otitis media or for complications from otitis media.

Insertion of a Tympanostomy Tube

Because inadequate ventilation of the middle ear is believed to be an important factor predisposing patients to otitis media, insertion of a tympanostomy tube helps to diminish the frequency of ear infections by providing a more consistent path for middle-ear ventilation. These tubes are generally placed in the anteroinferior aspect of the tympanic membrane. Indications include frequently recurring acute otitis media (three or more infections over a 6-month period, or four or more infections over a 12-month period), persistent middle-ear effusion accompanied by conductive hearing loss in the affected ear, or complications from otitis media (e.g., coalescent mastoiditis, facial nerve paralysis, or sigmoid sinus thrombosis). Most tympanostomy tubes will extrude on their own and do not require removal by a physician.

Adenoidectomy

This procedure consists of removal of the adenoids. Numerous reports suggest that adenoidectomy helps to diminish the frequency and duration of otitis media. Indications include recurrent otitis media and persistent middle-ear effusion after extrusion of a tube.

Common Sequelae of Otitis Media

If left untreated, or as a consequence of refractory disease, otitis media can result in problems such as eardrum perforation, eardrum atrophy with retraction, middle-ear adhesions, erosion of the ossicles, sclerotic plaques (known as tympanosclerosis), and acquired cholesteatoma (which is discussed later). Many of these disorders respond to medical or surgical treatment, but others may progress despite treatment. The primary goal of treatment is the establishment of a "safe" ear that is free of infection; this reduces the risk of continued inflammation and progression to a complication. The improvement of hearing also is a goal of treatment but is considered secondary to preventing the complications of disease.

A destructive process seen commonly in the middle ear is cholesteatoma. Cholesteatoma may be either congenital (from a developmental source) or acquired (as a result of chronic infection and more common); in the following, we discuss acquired cholesteatoma. Acquired cholesteatoma (referred to hereafter as cholesteatoma) occurs when an eardrum becomes markedly retracted, usually in the posterosuperior area (the pars flaccida). Desquamating keratin debris becomes trapped in the developing retraction pocket and forms an expanding mass, which can invade the middle ear and mastoid. If left to progress, it can result in more infections, destruction of the middle-ear and temporal bone structures, intracranial erosion with abscess formation, or thrombosis of the intracranial sinuses. Initial evaluation with a computed tomography (CT) scan of the temporal bone can be useful in delineating disease (Fig. 50-9).

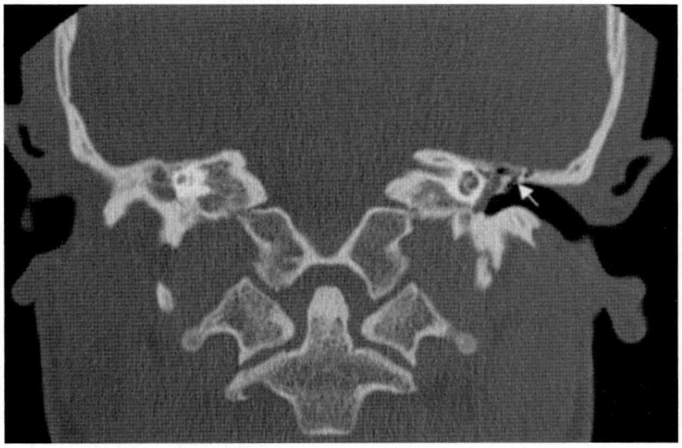

FIGURE 50–9 Appearance of cholesteatoma on coronal computed tomography scan. Note the left-sided soft tissue density (*arrow*), consistent with cholesteatoma matrix within the middle ear space, eroding a portion of the bony canal (the scutum).

Surgery on the eardrum, middle ear, and mastoid may be required to treat the sequelae of otitis media.

Tympanoplasty

Tympanoplasty is the repair of a defect in the tympanic membrane, such as a persistent perforation. Graft material, such as temporalis fascia, is placed either medial or lateral to the drum remnant to reestablish continuity of the tympanic membrane.

Ossicular Reconstruction

Ossicular reconstruction is restoration of continuity of the middle-ear ossicular chain to maintain or improve hearing. The patient's own ossicles can be repositioned, or prosthetic ossicles can be inserted to recreate the mechanical advantage provided by the natural ossicular chain.

Mastoidectomy

Mastoidectomy is drilling into and opening the mastoid to remove cholesteatoma or trapped, chronically infected granulation tissue. The mastoid may be opened to improve middle-ear aeration. In some cases, sequestered tissue is exteriorized by creating a large common cavity between the middle ear and the mastoid.

Less Common Complications of Otitis Media

Coalescent mastoiditis can occur with otitis media. In this disease, the infection causes destruction of the mastoid bone. This also can manifest as a subperiosteal abscess with anterior displacement of the auricle. Inflammatory material also can be trapped in the mastoid tip, resulting in a tip abscess (Bezold abscess). Treatment of these disorders involves opening the mastoid and affected areas to allow adequate drainage. In most cases of acute mastoiditis, placement of a tympanostomy tube also is required to improve aural hygiene.

Sigmoid sinus thrombosis can result from middle-ear and mastoid infection. In this disorder, the close proximity of the sigmoid sinus and associated communicating venous channels allows inflammatory material to promote thrombus formation. The thrombus can propagate proximally and distally, involving more intracranial venous sinuses as well as descending into the cervical portions of the jugular system. Treatment consists of surgery to remove trapped infectious material in the mastoid and middle ear, as well as antibiotics. Thrombectomy or ligation of involved thrombosed sinuses and veins is controversial, as is the use of anticoagulants.

Brain abscess also can occur as a result of invasive infection from otitis media or mastoiditis. The adjacent temporal lobe or cerebellum can be involved. In the case of a small abscess, the pocket may be drained across the mastoid. In a larger or more mature encapsulated abscess, a more extensive craniotomy may be needed for adequate drainage. The nidus of disease in the ear also should be treated.

Noninfectious Disorders of the Middle Ear

Disorders of the ossicular chain, independent of otitis media, may occur. Trauma can result in disruption of the ossicular chain. This can be corrected with use of ossicular chain reconstruction, as noted earlier. Leakage of perilymphatic fluid from around the oval or round window also may occur, causing hearing loss and dizziness. This is treated by exploring the middle ear, investigating for a leak, and patching leaking areas using a variety of materials.

Other disorders of the middle ear can result from autoimmune processes such as Wegener's granulomatosis or sarcoidosis. These may be initially seen as hearing loss or with otorrhea. Other systemic signs should be investigated to evaluate for such disorders.

Tumors of the middle ear are uncommon. One type of tumor that may be found is a glomus tumor, or paraganglioma. Glomus tympanicum often appears as a red mass behind the tympanic membrane. Patients frequently report hearing loss with pulsatile tinnitus. Some forms of glomus tumors may secrete catecholamines, although this is exceedingly rare in glomus tympanicum. If left to grow, these become locally destructive. Glomus tumors in other areas of the skull base (e.g., the glomus jugulare) may grow to large sizes and also impinge on temporal bone structures. This can cause multiple cranial neuropathies.

Disorders of the Lateral Skull Base and Temporal Bone

Temporal Bone Trauma

Approximately 30% of patients who sustain major trauma also have a fracture of the base of the skull, and 18% have a fracture of the temporal bone. A small subset of patients with temporal bone fracture also have injuries of the cervical spine or the internal carotid artery, facial trauma, or other intracranial injuries necessitating further evaluation.

Fractures due to temporal bone trauma have been classically described as longitudinal, transverse, or oblique, on the basis of their location relative to the petrous apex. These fracture patterns were determined according to impact studies on human skulls. Longitudinal fractures are the most common and are associated with facial nerve injury in approximately 10% of patients. Ossicular dislocation also can occur, with the incudostapedial joint most commonly affected. Transverse temporal bone fractures are less common, occurring in approximately 20% of patients with temporal bone trauma. Facial nerve injury occurs more often in association with transverse fractures, in about 50% of cases.

A patient who has major head trauma and is suspected to have, or has been diagnosed with, a temporal bone fracture, should be examined for the following:

- External auditory canal skin lacerations, bleeding, or osseous irregularity
- Leakage of clear (possibly cerebrospinal) fluid
- Gray or white debris in the external canal, which could be herniated brain material from the temporal lobe
- Blood within the middle ear (hemotympanum)
- Facial tone and volitional movement, to look for asymmetry. Asymmetry may indicate injury to the facial nerve. Immediate versus delayed paralysis should be documented, as they often require different types of treatment
- Nystagmus, which could indicate a fracture through the labyrinth with associated cochleovestibular damage

At the bedside of a patient with a suspected temporal bone fracture, two complementary tuning-fork tests can be used to assess hearing. The Weber test is done by placing the shaft of the tuning fork (preferably one with a 512-Hz frequency) firmly on the midline of the forehead or on the front teeth. The patient is then asked if the sound generated by the vibrating fork is heard better in one ear as compared with the other. The Weber test lateralizes *either* toward the ear with a conductive hearing loss or away from the ear with a sensorineural hearing loss. The same instrument can then be used to do a Rinne test, which involves placing the tines of the vibrating fork close to the ear. First, the tines are struck and held about one inch (2.54 cm) away from the external auditory meatus; the shaft is then pressed against the skin overlying the mastoid bone behind the same ear. The patient should always hear the sound next to the ear (air conduction) louder than that behind the ear (bone conduction). If bone conduction is louder than air conduction, then the patient has a conductive hearing loss in the ear being tested.

Once the patient has been stabilized and other injuries have been properly managed, a fine-cut CT scan (1.5-mm cuts through the temporal bone) and audiogram can be obtained. These tests give insight into the radiographically documented and functional injuries of the temporal bone. If facial nerve injuries are seen on physical examination, stimulatory testing can be performed to determine objective measures of function, which can give clues to recovery.

Most temporal bone fractures do not require surgical management. However, surgery may be necessary to treat facial nerve injury, cerebrospinal fluid otorrhea, perilymphatic fistula, and ossicular disruption.

Tumors of the Temporal Bone and the Lateral Skull Base

The most common tumor of the cerebellopontine angle is vestibular schwannoma, also known as acoustic neuroma. This benign tumor generally arises from the intracanalicular vestibular portion of the eighth cranial nerve. No predilection exists for either the superior or inferior branch of the nerve. The lesion grows within the internal auditory canal and can extend into the cerebellopontine angle. If it continues to grow, it may compress the brainstem. The early signs of acoustic tumor include unilateral hearing loss, ipsilateral tinnitus, and a poor word-discrimination score on audiologic testing of the involved ear. Although unilateral symptoms may suggest the rare acoustic neuroma, even rarer are bilateral acoustic neuromas; finding these should alert the clinician to the possibility of a form of neurofibromatosis. Auditory brainstem response (ABR) testing can be helpful in confirming the presence of an acoustic tumor. However, magnetic resonance imaging with gadolinium contrast medium is more sensitive and can detect small tumors that may be missed by using ABR (Fig. 50-10). These lesions may be observed or surgically removed, depending on their characteristics and those of the patient. The removal of such lesions requires a team approach; the team should include an otolaryngologist trained in neuro-otologic techniques and a neurosurgeon. The surgical approach varies according to the tumor size and location as well as the hearing status of the ipsilateral ear. Removal can be performed by drilling through the mastoid and the labyrinth, through a craniotomy to expose the middle cranial fossa, or through a suboccipital craniotomy.

Another common lesion of the lateral skull base is meningioma, a benign meningeal neoplasm that may be found in locations similar to schwannoma within the temporal bone. It can be distinguished from schwannoma on magnetic resonance imaging by the presence of a dural tail. Removal can be accomplished with use of the same approaches as those for schwannoma.

A petrous apex granuloma, also known as a cholesterol granuloma or cholesterol cyst, is a lesion of the medial portion of the petrous bone. The cells of the petrous apex can become infected and bleed, and the debris can become sequestered to form an expanding inflammatory lesion. If expansion is allowed to continue, it can result in erosion of the petrous bone (Fig. 50-11). Evacuation, exteriorization, or excision of the cyst is curative. Treatment may consist of drilling beneath the cochlea, below the inferior semicircular canal, through the sphenoid paranasal sinus, or through a middle-fossa craniotomy.

In summary, the ear and temporal bone can be a challenging anatomic area for the surgeon. A basic understanding of the anatomy and pathophysiology can lead to improved recognition of dangerous conditions. This can help in coordinating the team effort that may be required to care for patients who have associated disorders.

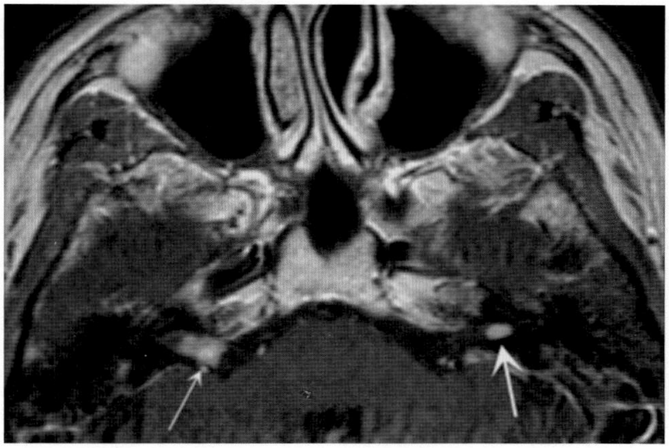

FIGURE 50–10 Appearance of schwannoma on axial T1-weighted magnetic resonance imaging with contrast. A right-sided schwannoma is seen in the internal auditory canal (*small arrow*). A smaller schwannoma is seen on the contralateral side (*large arrow*). This patient was diagnosed with neurofibromatosis type 2.

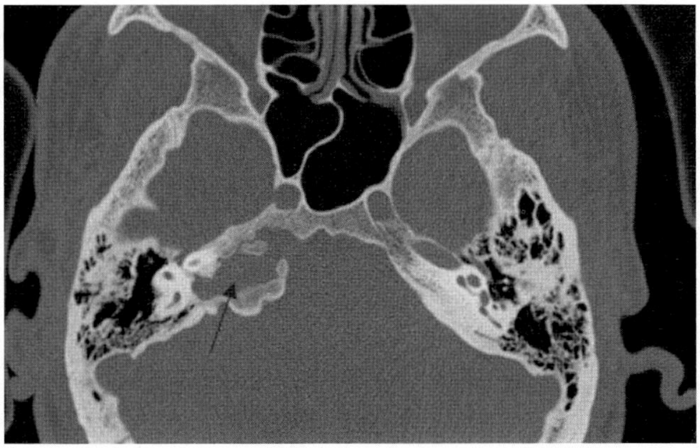

FIGURE 50–11 Computed tomography appearance of petrous apex granuloma. The petrous portion of the temporal bone has been eroded away (*arrow*) because of chronic infection.

Suggested Reading

Canalis RF, Lambert PR: Anatomy and embryology of the auditory and vestibular systems. In Canalis RF, Lambert PR (eds): The Ear: Comprehensive Otology. New York, Lippincott, 2000, pp 17–65.

Friedman RA, Kesser BW: Surgery of ventilation and mucosal disease. In Brackmann DE, Shelton C, Arriaga MA (eds): Otologic Surgery, 2nd ed. New York, WB Saunders, 2001, pp 68–81.

Hirsch BE: Infections of the external ear. Am J Otolaryngol 13:145–155, 1992.

Janfaza P, Nadol JB Jr: Temporal bone and ear. In Janfaza P, Nadol JB Jr, Galla RJ, et al. (eds): Surgical Anatomy of the Head and Neck. New York, Lippincott, 2001, pp 420–479.

Nadol JB Jr: Cerebellopontine angle tumors. In Nadol JB Jr, Schuknecht HF (eds): Surgery of the Ear and Temporal Bone. New York, Raven Press, 1993, pp 391–413.

Nosan DK, Benecke JE Jr, Murr AH: Current perspective on temporal bone trauma. Otolaryngol Head Neck Surg 117:67–71, 1997.

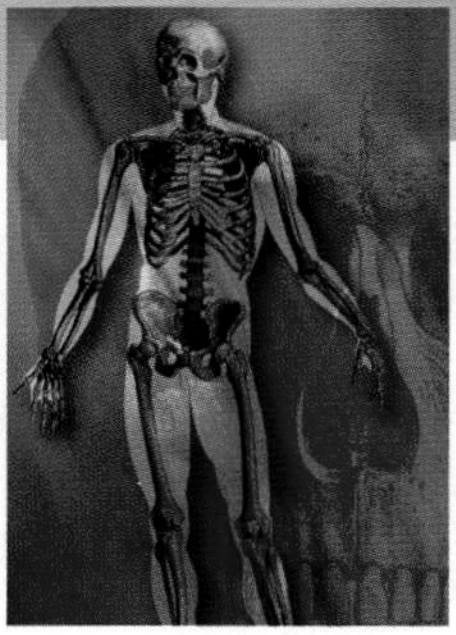

Chapter 51

Head and Neck Oncologic Surgery

SCHARUKH JALISI, MD, NEIL E. BROWN, MD, and
DANIEL K. SMITH, MD

Epidemiology

Carcinoma of the oral cavity, pharynx, and larynx accounts for about 5% of mortality in all cancers. Of these three types, about 75% are oral cavity and pharyngeal cancers, and the rest are laryngeal cancer. In the United States, the rates of head and neck cancer have declined over the last 20 years for both men and women. The risk of oral and pharyngeal cancer is higher in African Americans than in whites. This has been attributed to the higher prevalence of alcohol and tobacco consumption in the former group.

Etiology

The most important risk factor for head and neck cancer is tobacco and alcohol consumption. Smoking cessation causes the risk of oral dysplasia to decrease to the levels of nonsmokers after 15 years. Smoking has a strong predilection to cause laryngeal cancer, whereas alcohol consumption is associated with pharyngeal cancer. Other risk factors include the consumption of betel nuts (in parts of South Asia) and chronic denture use. Occupational exposure to wood, leather, textiles, and nickel increases the risk of oral, pharyngeal, laryngeal, and paranasal sinus carcinomas.

Infectious etiologies have been implicated, including the human papilloma virus, human immunodeficiency virus, herpes simplex virus, and Epstein-Barr virus. Gastroesophageal reflux disease has been suggested to increase the risk of laryngeal and hypopharyngeal cancer. An increased prevalence also is noted in immunosuppressed patients and in those with a genetic history of head and neck cancer.

Evaluation

Any patient in whom head and neck cancer is suspected requires a careful evaluation, starting with a comprehensive medical history and physical examination. Any history of cancer, surgery, or radiation therapy is noted. A history of smoking or alcohol intake also must be recorded. Comorbidities, particularly those of the pulmonary and cardiovascular systems, should be documented. Physical examination comprises assessment of the head and neck, with thorough palpation of the neck for any nodal disease. Mirror or flexible fiberoptic examination is performed to evaluate the upper aerodigestive tract mucosa.

A number of radiographic and laboratory studies should be performed, including computed tomographic scanning (CT), magnetic resonance imaging (MRI), chest radiograph, complete blood count (especially when lymphoma is suspected), liver enzyme tests (to assess for metastasis), thyroid-function tests, and electrolytes and Epstein-Barr-virus titers (if nasopharyngeal cancer is suspected).

Histopathologic diagnosis based on tissue samples is very important, and most patients with oral cavity, pharyngeal, and laryngeal malignancies will need laryngoscopy, esophagoscopy, bronchoscopy, and biopsy of the lesion. The most important point to remember is that a chronic neck mass may be a sign of mucosal malignancy of the upper aerodigestive tract and hence must be evaluated by a head and neck surgeon. Most patients with head and neck cancer need a multidisciplinary approach to therapy, with evaluation by specialists in otolaryngology–head and neck surgery, radiation oncology, medical oncology, speech pathology, and radiology.

Classification of Neck Dissection

A neck dissection refers to the removal of lymph nodes from the neck, with or without nonlymphatic structures, including the sternocleidomastoid muscle, spinal accessory nerve, and internal jugular vein.

In 1988, the Committee for Head and Neck Surgery and Oncology of the American Academy of Otolaryngology–Head and Neck Surgery (AAO-HNS) developed a standard classification system for neck dissections. This was later revised (Table 51-1), along with the classification of lymph-node levels in the neck (Table 51-2), which correspond to the six levels and sublevels of the neck (Fig. 51-1).

Site-specific Malignancies

Cutaneous

Basal cell carcinoma accounts for 90% of all cutaneous neoplasms in the head and neck, followed by squamous

TABLE 51–1 Classification of Neck Dissections

Type	Description
Radical neck dissection	Removal of all lymph nodes and nonlymphatic structures from neck
Modified radical neck dissection	Type I: all lymph nodes + sparing of SAN Type II: all lymph nodes + sparing of SAN + IJV Type III: all lymph nodes + sparing of SAN + IJV + SCM
Selective neck dissection	Preservation of ≥1 lymph-node groups and *all* nonlymphatic structures
Extended neck dissection	Removal of ≥1 additional lymph-node groups or nonlymphatic structures not encompassed by radical neck dissection (e.g., parapharyngeal nodes, carotid artery)

SAN, spinal accessory nerve; IJV, internal jugular vein; SCM, sternocleidomastoid muscle.
Modified from Robbins KT, Clayman G, Levine PA, et al: Neck dissection classification update: Revisions proposed by the American Head and Neck Society and the American Academy of Otolaryngology–Head and Neck Surgery. Arch Otolaryngol Head Neck Surg 128:751–758, 2001.

cell carcinoma. The least common form is melanoma. Risk factors for basal cell carcinoma and squamous cell carcinoma include an age of older than 60 years, exposure to ultraviolet-B light, white complexion and features, and a history of multiple severe sunburns. The symptoms of cutaneous malignancy include incidental findings of a suggestive enlarging lesion, pruritis, bleeding, and neck mass. Basal cell carcinoma commonly is first seen as a discrete lesion with an ulcerative center and rolled edges; squamous cell carcinoma usually has an erythematous, crusted, ulcerated appearance. Melanoma classically is initially seen as a pigmented lesion that is Asymmetrical, with Border variations, Color variations, and Diameter increases (ABCD) over time. Staging is performed with CT and MRI. Tissue diagnosis is very important. Treatment is mainly surgical, with or without neck dissection, depending on the stage of the disease. Disease with distant metastases is managed with chemotherapy and radiation therapy.

Paranasal Sinuses and Nasal Cavity

Symptoms of tumors in this region usually include nasal obstruction, epistaxis, nasal discharge, anosmia/dysosmia, and pain. On physical examination, numbness may occur in the distribution of the trigeminal nerve. Ocular findings such as proptosis, diplopia, extraocular muscle involvement, and fullness of the cheek or gingivobuccal sulcus may be noted. CT and MRI are important in delineating the anatomic extent of these tumors.

Benign lesions are far more common than malignant lesions. The most common benign lesions of the nasal cavity and paranasal sinuses are sinonasal polyps. The exact etiology of polyps is not clearly understood. They cause symptoms because of mechanical obstruction to airflow and natural drainage of sinuses, which in turn cause rhinosinusitis. Medical management in the form of antihistamines, nasal steroids, and immunotherapy is the key in providing relief. If medical treatment is unsuccessful, endoscopic surgery may be performed to improve ventilation and aeration of the sinuses.

Other benign lesions include papilloma, inverting papilloma (which has a tendency to turn into squamous cell carcinoma), hemangioma, and teratoma.

Only 3% of malignancies of the upper respiratory tract are in the sinonasal region. Squamous cell carcinoma is the most common malignant lesion in this area; others include adenocarcinoma, adenoid cystic carcinoma (which has a predilection for early neurovascular spread), melanoma, sarcoma, olfactory neuroblastoma, and sinonasal undifferentiated carcinoma. These lesions are usually managed with a combination of surgery, radiation therapy, and chemotherapy. Staging is very important in determining therapy and prognosis.

Pharynx

The pharynx is divided into the oropharynx, nasopharynx, and hypopharynx. The oropharynx involves the soft palate superiorly, the anterior tonsillar pillars anteriorly, and the pharyngeal walls laterally, and it extends to the floor of the vallecula. The anatomic boundaries of the nasopharynx are the skull base superiorly, the walls of the superior constrictor laterally and posteriorly, the choanae anteriorly, and the soft palate inferiorly. The hypopharynx begins at the vallecula and extends to the inferior margin of the cricoid cartilage.

Nasopharynx

Symptoms of nasopharyngeal tumors include nasal obstruction, bleeding, and unilateral otitis media (due to obstruction of the eustachian tube); neurologic symptoms are due to cranial invasion. The differential diagnosis of lesions in this location includes nasopharyngeal carcinoma, lymphoma, rhabdomyosarcoma, neuroblastoma, and juvenile nasopharyngeal angiofibroma.

Of the various head and neck cancers, nasopharyngeal carcinoma has one of the poorest prognoses because of its proximity to the skull base and cranial structures. According to the World Health Organization, nasopharyngeal carcinoma has three types: squamous cell carcinoma (type I), nonkeratinizing carcinoma (type II), and undifferentiated carcinoma (type III). Treatment includes radiation and

TABLE 51–2 Lymph Node Groups Found Within the Six Levels and the Six Sublevels

Lymph Node Group	Description
Submental (sublevel IA)	Lymph nodes within the triangular boundary of the anterior belly of the digastric muscles and the hyoid bone. These nodes are at greatest risk for having metastases from cancers arising from the floor of mouth, anterior oral tongue, anterior mandibular alveolar ridge, and lower lip
Submandibular (sublevel IB)	Lymph nodes within the boundaries of the anterior belly of the digastric muscle, the stylohyoid muscle, and the body of the mandible. It includes the preglandular and the postglandular nodes and the prevascular and postvascular nodes. The submandibular gland is included in the specimen when the lymph nodes within the triangle are removed. These nodes are at greatest risk for having metastases from cancers arising from the oral cavity, anterior nasal cavity, soft tissue structures of the midface, and submandibular gland
Upper jugular (includes sublevels IIA and IIB)	Lymph nodes located around the upper third of the internal jugular vein and adjacent spinal accessory nerve extending from the level of the skull base (above) to the level of the inferior border of the hyoid bone (below). The anterior (medial) boundary is the stylohyoid muscle (the radiologic correlate is the vertical plane defined by the posterior surface of the submandibular gland) and the posterior (lateral) boundary is the posterior border of the sternocleidomastoid muscle. Sublevel IIA nodes are located anterior (medial) to the vertical plane defined by the spinal accessory nerve. Sublevel IIB nodes are located posterior (lateral) to the vertical plane defined by the spinal accessory nerve. The upper jugular nodes are at greatest risk for having metastases from cancers arising from the oral cavity, nasal cavity, nasopharynx, oropharynx, hypopharynx, larynx and parotid gland
Middle jugular (level III)	Lymph nodes located around the middle third of the internal jugular vein extending from the inferior border of the hyoid bone (above) to the inferior border of the cricoid cartilage (below). The anterior (medial) boundary is the lateral border of the sternohyoid muscle, and the posterior (lateral) boundary is the posterior border of the sternocleidomastoid muscle. These nodes are at greatest risk for having metastases from cancers arising from the oral cavity, nasopharynx, oropharynx, hypopharynx, and larynx
Lower jugular (level IV)	Lymph nodes located around the lower third of the internal jugular vein extending form the inferior border of the cricoid cartilage (above) to the clavicle below. The anterior (medial) boundary is the lateral border of the sternohyoid muscle and the posterior (lateral) boundary is the posterior border of the sternocleidomastoid muscle. These nodes are at greatest risk for having metastases from cancers arising from the hypopharynx, thyroid, cervical esophagus, and larynx
Posterior triangle group (includes sublevels VA and VB)	This group is composed predominantly of the lymph nodes located along the lower half of the spinal accessory nerve and the transverse cervical artery. The supraclavicular nodes are also included in posterior triangle group. The superior boundary is the apex formed by convergence of the sternocleidomastoid and trapezius muscles; the inferior boundary is the clavicle, the anterior (medial) boundary is the posterior border of the sternocleidomastoid muscle, and the posterior (lateral) boundary is the anterior border of the trapezius muscle. Sublevel VA is separated from sublevel VB by a horizontal plane marking the interior border of the anterior cricoid arch. Thus, sublevel VA includes the spinal accessory nodes, whereas sublevel VB includes the nodes following the transverse cervical vessels and the supraclavicular nodes with the exception of the Virchow node, which is located in level IV. The posterior triangle nodes are at greatest risk for having metastases from cancers arising from the nasopharynx, oropharynx, and cutaneous structures of the posterior scalp and neck
Anterior compartment group (level VI)	Lymph nodes in this compartment include the pretracheal and paratracheal nodes. precricoid (delphian) node, and the perithyroidal nodes including the lymph nodes along the recurrent laryngeal nerves. The superior boundary is the hyoid bone, the inferior boundary is the suprasternal notch, and the lateral boundaries are the common carotid arteries. These nodes are at greatest risk for having metastases from cancers arising from the thyroid gland, glottic and subglottic larynx, apex of the piriform sinus, and cervical esophagus

From Robbins KT, Clayman G, Levine PA, et al: Neck dissection classification update: Revisions proposed by the American Head and Neck Society and the American Academy of Otolaryngology—Head and Neck Surgery. Arch Otolaryngol Head Neck Surg 128:751–758, 2002, with permission.

chemotherapy, with surgery reserved for patients who have residual or recurrent disease.

Oral Cavity, Oropharynx, and Hypopharynx

Symptoms in this region typically include dysphagia, odynophagia, weight loss, voice change, neck mass, and bleeding. The most common type of tumor is squamous cell carcinoma; others include lymphoma, sarcoma, and tumors of the minor salivary gland.

Most nodal metastases arise from the base of the tongue and the tonsils (both of which form part of the oropharynx). Treatment depends on stage and includes surgery with or without radiation and chemotherapy. Lymph-node metastasis is treated with neck dissection or chemoradiotherapy.

Tumor resection may result in large soft-tissue and osseous defects. These defects can be reconstructed by the otolaryngologist in various ways, including regional flaps such as pectoralis major flaps and free flaps. Free flaps

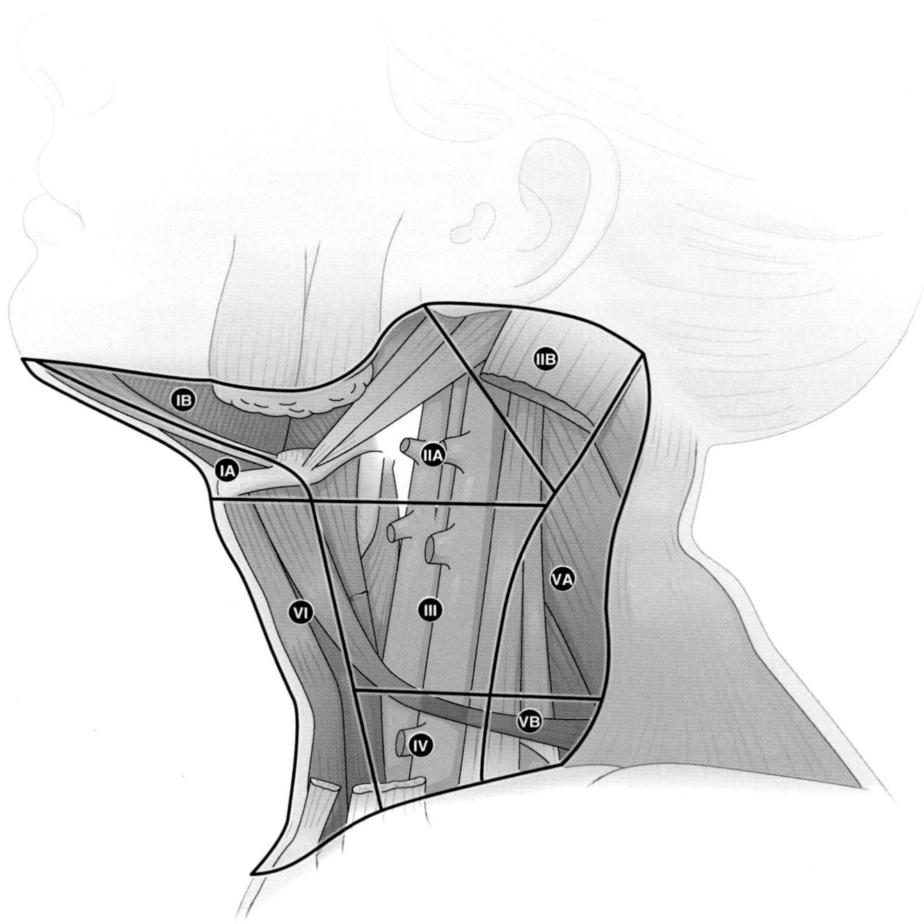

FIGURE 51–1 Six levels of the neck, with sublevels. See also Table 51-2. (Adapted from Robbins KT, Clayman G, Levine PA, et al: Neck dissection classification update: Revisions proposed by the American Head and Neck Society and the American Academy of Otolaryngology–Head and Neck Surgery. Arch Otolaryngol Head Neck Surg 128:751–758, 2002, with permission.)

are transferred tissue segments with their own independent blood supply; using them allows a healthy reconstruction in a poorly vascularized tissue bed. Examples of free flaps include fibular or scapular osteocutaneous flaps, radial forearm fasciocutaneous flaps, and jejunal flaps. The osseous portion of these flaps can be used to reconstruct the mandible or maxilla as needed. Free flaps have the best functionality and flexibility of any reconstructive option.

Larynx

The most common benign lesions of the larynx are vocal cord polyps and nodules. Other benign masses include papilloma, cysts, granuloma, granular cell tumor, chordoma, and neurogenic tumor. Most of these lesions are treated with microsurgical techniques.

PEARLS FOR ROUNDS

Pleomorphic adenoma is the most common tumor of the parotid.

Inverting papilloma is a benign tumor of the paranasal sinuses that has the potential to become malignant.

The stage of the cancer is the most important factor in predicting survival.

Encapsulation distinguishes schwannoma from neurofibroma.

Nasopharyngeal cancer has been associated with Epstein-Barr virus.

PEARLS FOR THE OR

Removal of all lymph nodes and sparing of the spinal accessory nerve only is referred to as type I modified radical neck dissection.

A glottic carcinoma with vocal cord fixation is considered a T3 lesion.

A neck mass in a patient without infectious symptoms should be evaluated with endoscopy to rule out a primary mucosal malignancy of the upper aerodigestive tract.

Surgery for adenoid cystic carcinoma of the parotid requires sacrifice of the facial nerve because of the tendency of this cancer to invade neurovascular structures.

Healthy vascularized tissue in the form of a free flap may be needed to reconstruct a large defect in a previously irradiated tissue bed.

According to the National Cancer Data Base, the larynx is the most common site of head and neck cancer and accounts for 20% of all cases. Squamous cell carcinoma is the most common form of laryngeal cancer and accounts for 90% of all cases; survival ranges from 42% to 77%. The most common subsite of laryngeal cancer is the glottis (56%), followed by the supraglottis (41%) and the subglottis (1% to 3%). Symptoms include hoarseness, stridor, voice change, cough, odynophagia, dysphagia, hemoptysis, and neck mass.

Tumors in each of these three subsites behave differently. Supraglottic cancer tends to be identified in advanced stages because it does not cause symptoms until late in the disease process. These lesions tend to metastasize to regional lymph nodes in the neck. Glottic carcinoma is generally detected early because even small lesions can cause at least a voice change, so these patients can be referred for otolaryngologic evaluation. Because this region has poor lymphatic drainage, the chance of nodal metastasis is low. Subglottic tumors are first seen late and usually with respiratory distress and biphasic stridor. Advanced laryngeal cancers are classified as stage III or IV.

Treatment can be surgical or nonsurgical. Surgical treatment involves either total laryngectomy or, in selected patients, partial laryngectomy. Early-stage cancers can be treated equally well with partial laryngectomy or radiation therapy. Advanced-stage cancers require total laryngectomy; however, the Veterans Affairs Laryngeal Study Group has demonstrated that a combination of radiation and chemotherapy is an alternative to surgery when organ preservation is desired. Neck disease must be addressed with lymph-node dissection, particularly in patients with supraglottic carcinoma.

The most important issue after total laryngectomy is voice rehabilitation. Many ways exist to restore the voice after total laryngectomy, including use of an electrolarynx, esophageal speech, and tracheoesophageal puncture with insertion of a speech prosthesis. The latter method is the one most commonly used in the United States.

Salivary Glands

The major salivary glands are the parotid, submandibular, and sublingual glands. In addition, thousands of minor salivary glands are found in the upper aerodigestive tract. Approximately 75% of tumors in large salivary glands are benign, and 75% in small salivary glands are malignant; 75% of parotid tumors, 50% of submandibular tumors, and only 20% of sublingual gland tumors are benign. The most common benign neoplasm of the parotid is pleomorphic adenoma, accounting for about 75% of these tumors. The next most common is Warthin's tumor, which is bilateral in 10% of cases. Other benign parotid tumors are oncocytoma and monomorphic adenoma. Mucoepidermoid carcinoma is the most common malignant tumor of the parotid and the second most common malignant tumor of the submandibular gland, after adenoid cystic carcinoma. Mucoepidermoid carcinoma can be high grade or low grade, depending on the amount of epidermoid cells present. High-grade tumors are more aggressive. Other malignant tumors of salivary glands are adenoid cystic carcinoma (which can appear with facial paralysis), acinic cell carcinoma (which is bilateral in 3% of cases), adenocarcinoma, and carcinoma ex pleomorphic adenoma.

The most common symptom in these patients is an asymptomatic, slowly enlarging mass. The presence of pain and facial nerve paralysis indicates a malignant tumor. A thorough physical examination, followed by appropriate imaging, must be performed. Fine-needle aspiration may be done to obtain a diagnosis. If it is nondiagnostic, then a biopsy of the parotid gland, which is equivalent to removal of the superficial lobe of the parotid gland, must be performed. Incisional biopsy is to be avoided because it can seed the overlying skin and surrounding tissues with tumor cells.

The treatment of choice for salivary neoplasms is surgical excision. Most of these tumors are superficial to the facial nerve, so a superficial parotidectomy may be performed. For deep-lobe parotid tumors, a total parotidectomy may be needed. The facial nerve is preserved unless it is involved with cancer cells, in which case, it is resected to a tumor-free margin. It can then be repaired with a nerve graft with the aim of obtaining a better facial mimetic movement than total facial paralysis.

Vascular Tumors

The most common benign vascular lesion of the head and neck is hemangioma, which must be distinguished from vascular malformation. Hemangioma is not present at birth; it proliferates in the first year of life and involutes by 5 to 8 years in most cases. Vascular malformation is present at birth; it grows with the child and does not involute. Hemangiomas are noncompressible and firm, whereas vascular malformations are compressible and soft. Treatment for hemangioma involves observation, unless it affects vital structures, in which case, it is treated with surgical excision, carbon dioxide laser excision, sclerosing agents, and steroid therapy. Vascular malformations can be treated in a similar fashion, except that the Nd:YAG laser is beneficial in these lesions.

Other vascular tumors include paragangliomas, carotid body tumors, peripheral nerve neoplasm, and lipoma. Paraganglioma derives from neural crest cells and is multicentric. The paraganglia can be found in the larynx, aortic arch, carotid and vagal bodies, and jugulotympanic region. These lesions are routinely identified on head and neck examination. Workup includes CT and MRI with magnetic resonance angiography; angiography with embolization may be done preoperatively to reduce intraoperative bleeding. Carotid body tumors are characteristically pulsatile masses in the neck, which are mobile in the lateral but not in the superior-to-inferior direction. The classic finding on an arteriogram is widening of the carotid bifurcation with a tumor blush. These lesions are treated surgically.

Peripheral nerve neoplasms include schwannoma and neurofibroma. Schwannomas are slow-growing, encapsulated tumors arising from Schwann cells; they are characterized by spindle cells. Tumors with thick concentrations of these cells are classified as Antoni type A, and those with sparser concentrations, as Antoni type B. Neurofibromas are unencapsulated and hence more difficult to dissect from the nerves. They may occur as isolated or multiple lesions associated with type 1 neurofibromatosis. The treatment of choice for patients who are symptomatic is surgical excision.

Staging

Head and neck cancers are primarily staged clinically. All head and neck sites, with the exception of thyroid, use the same classification system for regional lymph nodes. The American Joint Committee on Cancer (AJCC) cancer staging manual (6th edition) provides detailed descriptions of the components and other staging guidelines. Brief summaries of the staging guidelines for head and neck cancers are shown in Boxes 51-1 through 51-6.

Complications

The most common complications of head and neck oncologic surgery are generally due to the wound and include hematoma, infection, seroma, wound breakdown, fistula (aberrant connection between two cavities), dysphagia, aspiration, voice and speech changes, and multiple nerve paralysis/pareses with resulting functional deficit.

BOX 51-1 Thyroid Gland Cancer Staging

T1, ≤2 cm limited to thyroid
T2, >2 cm but <4 cm limited to thyroid
T3, >4 cm limited to thyroid or any tumor with minimal extrathyroid extension
T4a, Extending beyond thyroid capsule to invade subcutaneous soft tissue, larynx, trachea, esophagus, or recurrent laryngeal nerve
T4b, Invades prevertebral fascia or encases carotid artery or mediastinal vessels

From American Joint Committee on Cancer (AJCC): AJCC Cancer Staging Manual, 6th ed. New York, Springer-Verlag, 2002, with permission.

BOX 51-2 Paranasal Sinuses Cancer Staging

TX, Primary tumor cannot be assessed
T0, No evidence of primary tumor
Tis, Carcinoma in situ

Maxillary Sinus

T1, Limited to maxillary sinus mucosa with no erosion or destruction of bone
T2, Causing bone erosion or destruction including extension into hard palate and/or middle nasal meatus, except extension to posterior wall of maxillary sinus and pterygoid plates
T3, Tumor invades any of the following: bone of the posterior wall of maxillary sinus, subcutaneous tissues, floor or medial wall of orbit, pterygoid fossa, ethmoid sinuses
T4, Invades anterior orbital contents, skin of cheek, pterygoid plates, infratemporal fossa, cribriform plate, sphenoid, or frontal sinuses
T4b, Invades any of the following: orbital apex, dura, brain, middle cranial fossa, cranial nerves other than maxillary division of trigeminal nerve (V2), nasopharynx, or clivus

Nasal Cavity and Ethmoid Sinus

T1, Confined to ethmoid with or without bone erosion
T2, Invading two subsites in single region or extending to involve adjacent region within nasoethmoidal complex, with or without bony invasion
T3, Extends to invade medial wall or floor of orbit, maxillary sinus, palate, or cribriform plate
T4a, Invades any of the following: anterior orbital contents, skin of nose or cheek, minimal extension to anterior cranial fossa, pterygoid plates, sphenoid, or frontal sinuses
T4b, Invades any of the following: orbital apex, dura, brain, middle cranial fossa, cranial nerves other than (V2), nasopharynx, or clivus

From American Joint Committee on Cancer (AJCC): AJCC Cancer Staging Manual, 6th ed. New York, Springer-Verlag, 2002, with permission.

BOX 51–3 Pharynx Cancer Staging

TX, Primary tumor cannot be assessed
T0, No evidence of primary tumor
Tis, Carcinoma in situ

Oropharynx

T1, 2 cm or less
T2, >2 but <4 cm
T3, >4 cm
T4, Invades adjacent structures
T4a, Invades larynx, deep/extrinsic muscle of tongue, medial pterygoid, hard palate, or mandible
T4b, Invades lateral pterygoid muscle, pterygoid plates, lateral nasopharynx, or skull base, or encases carotid artery

Hypopharynx

T1, Limited to one subsite of hypopharynx and 2cm or <
T2, >2 but <4 cm without fixation or more than one subsite or adjacent site
T3, >4 cm or with hemilarynx fixation
T4a, Invades thyroid/cricoid cartilage, hyoid bone, thyroid gland, esophagus, or central compartment soft tissue
T4b, Invades prevertebral fascia, encases carotid artery, or involves mediastinal structures

Nasopharynx

T1, Confined to nasopharynx
T2, Extends to soft tissue of oropharynx and/or nasal fossa
T2a, Without parapharyngeal extension
T2b, With parapharyngeal extension
T3, Invades bony structures and/or paranasal sinuses
T4, Intracranial extension, and/or involvement of cranial nerves, infratemporal fossa, hypopharynx, or orbit

From American Joint Committee on Cancer (AJCC): AJCC Cancer Staging Manual, 6th ed. New York, Springer-Verlag, 2002, with permission.

BOX 51–4 Lip and Oral Cavity Cancer Staging

T1, ≤ 2 cm
T2, >2 but <4 cm
T3, >4 cm
T4 (lip), Invades through cortical bone, inferior nerve, floor of mouth, or skin of face (i.e., chin or nose)
T4a, (oral cavity) Invades adjacent structures (e.g., through cortical bone, into deep [extrinsic] muscle of tongue [genioglossus, hypoglossus, palatoaglossus, and styloglossus], maxillary sinus, skin of face)
T4b, Invades masticator space, pterygoid plates, or skull base and/or encases internal carotid artery

Note: Superficial erosion alone of bone/tooth socket by gingival primary is not sufficient to classify as T4.
From American Joint Committee on Cancer (AJCC): AJCC Cancer Staging Manual, 6th ed. New York, Springer-Verlag, 2002, with permission.

BOX 51–5 Larynx Cancer Staging

TX, Primary tumor cannot be assessed
T0, No evidence of primary tumor
Tis, Carcinoma in situ

Supraglottis

T1, Limited to one subsite, with normal vocal cord mobility
T2, Invades mucosa of >1 adjacent subsite of supraglottis or glottis or region outside the supraglottis; without fixation of larynx
T3, Limited to larynx with vocal cord fixation and/or invades postcricoid area, pre-epiglottic tissues, paraglottic space, and/or minor thyroid cartilage erosion
T4a, Invades through thyroid cartilage and/or tissues beyond larynx
T4b, Invades prevertebral space, encases carotid artery, or invades mediastinal structures

Glottis

T1, Limited to vocal cord(s), with normal mobility
T1a, Limited to one vocal cord
T1b, Involves both vocal cords
T2, Extends to supraglottis, and/or subglottis, and/or with impaired cord mobility
T3, Limited to larynx with vocal cord fixation
T4, Invades through thyroid cartilage and/or other tissues beyond larynx
T4a, Invades through thyroid cartilage and/or tissues beyond larynx
T4b, Invades prevertebral space, encases carotid artery, or invades mediastinal structures

Subglottis

T1, Limited to subglottis
T2, Extends to vocal cord(s) with normal/impaired mobility
T3, Limited to larynx with vocal cord fixation
T4a, Invades cricoid or thyroid cartilage and/or tissues beyond larynx
T4b, Invades prevertebral space, encases carotid artery, or invades mediastinal structures

From American Joint Committee On Cancer (AJCC): AJCC Cancer Staging Manual, 6th ed. New York, Springer-Verlag, 2002, with permission.

BOX 51–6 Salivary Glands Cancer Staging

T1, ≤2 cm without extraparenchymal extension
T2, >2 cm but <4 cm without extraparenchymal extension
T3, >4 cm and/or extraparenchymal extension
T4a, Invades skin, mandible, ear canal, and/or facial nerve
T4b, Invades skull base and/or pterygoid plates and/or encases carotid artery

From American Joint Committee on Cancer (AJCC): AJCC Cancer Staging Manual, 6th ed. New York, Springer-Verlag, 2002, with permission.

TABLE 51–3 Five-Year Survival by Cancer Location and Stage

	Percentage by Stage			
Location of Tumor	**Stage I**	**Stage II**	**Stage III**	**Stage IV**
Oral cavity	70%–90%		50%–60%	
Oropharynx–base of tongue	50%–100%	44%–77%	45%–76%	11%–59%
Oropharynx–tonsils	83%–100%	57%–77%	23%–56%	15%–29%
Oropharynx–soft palate	80%–90%		30%–60%	
Nasopharynx (epithelial carcinoma only)	63%–78%	63%–70%	42%–55%	0%–42%
Larynx				
CIS	95%–100%			
Glottic	85%–97%		54%–91% (all three regions)	
Supraglottic	76%–95%			
Hypopharynx	74%	45%–63%	32%	0%–14%
Paranasal sinuses (squamous cell carcinoma only)	90%	80%	30%	20%
Salivary gland (all histological types)	75%	53%–63%	41%–51%	24%–32%

Data from Shah JP, Patel SG (eds): American Cancer Society Atlas of Clinical Oncology, Cancer of the Head and Neck. Hamilton, Ontario, Canada; BC Decker, 2001; Greene FL, Page DL, Fleming ID, et al: AJCC Cancer Staging Manual, 6th ed. New York, Springer-Verlag, 2002.

Prognosis

The five year survival by cancer location and stage is shown in Table 51-3.

Suggested Reading

Bailey BJ, Calhoun KH, Healy GB (eds): Atlas of Head and Neck Surgery–Otolaryngology, 3rd ed. Philadelphia, Lippincott Williams & Wilkins, 2001.

Carew JF: The larynx: Advanced stage disease. In Shah JP, Patel SG (eds): American Cancer Society Atlas of Clinical Oncology, Cancer of the Head and Neck. Hamilton, Ontario, Canada, BC Decker, 2001, pp 156–168.

Davidson BJ: Epidemiology and etiology. In Shah JP, Patel SG (eds): American Cancer Society Atlas of Clinical Oncology, Cancer of the Head and Neck. Hamilton, Ontario, Canada, BC Decker, 2001, pp 1–18.

Morse DE, Katz RV, Pendrys DG, et al: Smoking and drinking in relation to oral epithelial dysplasia. Cancer Epidemiol Biomarkers Prev 5:769–777, 1996.

Mulliken JB, Glowacki J: Hemangiomas and vascular malformations in infants and children: A classification based on endothelial characteristics. Plast Reconstr Surg 69:412–420, 1982.

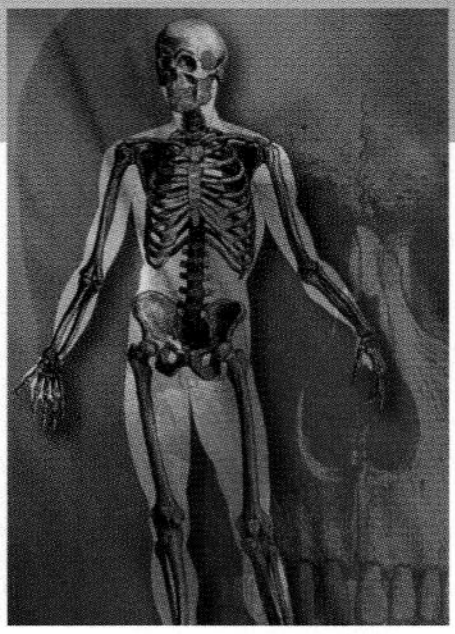

Chapter 52
Pediatric Otolaryngology

NEIL E. BROWN, MD, ELIZABETH J. MAHONEY, MD, and KENNETH M. GRUNDFAST, MD

Purview of Pediatric Otolaryngology

Although pediatric otolaryngology has become a recognized subspecialty within otolaryngology-head and neck surgery, many community-based practicing otolaryngologists care for children with otolaryngic disorders. Most otolaryngic surgery in children is done to help manage such common disorders as otitis media, tonsillitis, pharyngitis, and snoring. In addition, children born with congenital anomalies of the head and neck may require reconstructive surgery, those with tumors need extirpative surgery, and those with congenital or acquired airway abnormalities may require surgery to create or restore an adequate upper airway.

Surgery of the Ear

Ear: Preauricular Pits and Cysts

A preauricular pit is an indentation in the skin just anterior to the root of the helix of the pinna. Preauricular pits, more common in African Americans than in whites, can be unilateral or bilateral but do not always need surgical removal. The key to knowing if and when surgery is needed to remove preauricular pits is infection. If unilateral or bilateral preauricular pits are noted on routine physical examination, with no history of redness, swelling, or drainage of purulent liquid from the pit, then no need exists to recommend surgery. However, if a child has had signs of infection of a preauricular pit, surgical excision is indicated. When a child has bilateral preauricular pits and only one side has been infected, surgical excision of the preauricular pit on the side that has not previously manifested signs of infection is optional and considered elective. To avoid the need for a second general anesthesia, parents often opt to have both pits excised, although only one is infected.

Achieving successful outcome with excision of a preauricular pit can be difficult. Surgical excision of a preauricular pit is deceptive, seeming to be merely a quick and simple procedure, but complete excision requires adequate exposure with meticulous dissection. Without *complete* excision of the pit and the underlying sinus tract, recurrence can easily occur with need for multiple surgical excisions. When a child initially is seen with an infected preauricular pit, it is best to treat with orally administered antimicrobial agents rather than incising and draining the red swollen mass anterior to the pinna. Incising the infected preauricular pit/cyst/sinus will provide egress for the pathogens, but the incision creates scarring and multiple fibrous connections between the cyst wall and the surrounding subcutaneous skin, and this makes ultimate complete excision more difficult. Therefore treating the infected preauricular pit/cyst with antibiotics and warm compresses is preferable to incision and drainage, even if the infected cyst ruptures spontaneously. The steps to be used in excision of a preauricular pit are as follows:

1. Place an elliptical incision *only* through the dermal layer of skin surrounding the orifice of the pit; from the posterior aspect of the elliptical incision, extend an incision through the subcutaneous skin layer superior and posterior to the pinna.
2. Through the incision, expose the fascia of the temporalis muscle.
3. Use blunt dissection to create a plane separating the temporalis muscle deep from the skin and subcutaneous tissue that contains the pit/cyst/sinus.
4. Using a skin hook to retract the skin and fine forceps, fine hemostat, and sharp-end iris scissors, undermine the skin for 3 to 5 mm around the elliptical incision separating the skin from the soft tissue that contains the pit/cyst/sinus tract.
5. Grasp the soft tissue containing the pit/cyst/sinus, and dissect free from surrounding normal subcutaneous tissue.
6. The pit/cyst/sinus is likely to be adherent to the root of the cartilaginous helix of the pinna, so that complete excision of the epithelial lined pit will require excision of 2 to 3 mm of the root of the helix.
7. Primary closure with absorbable sutures is preferable if the entire pit/cyst/sinus has been excised cleanly; however, if doubt exists about the adequacy of the excision or if the defect is too big to close primarily, then partial primary closure combined with iodoform strip gauze packing, with healing by secondary intention, offers the best chance for reasonable cosmetic result and minimal chance for recurrence.

Otologic Procedures of the Ear

Tympanocentesis and **myringotomy** are two procedures done in the eardrums of children and are commonly confused with each other.

In tympanocentesis, an opening is made in the eardrum with a needle to remove a sample of the liquid contents of the middle ear, usually for culture and sensitivity testing so that organisms present can be identified precisely. Typical indications for tympanocentesis include concern that a middle-ear effusion in a neonate could be causing sepsis, acute otitis media in an immunocompromised child (e.g., one who has severe combined immunodeficiency disorder [SCID] or known infection with human immunodeficiency virus [HIV], or one who is having bone-marrow transplantation), and acute otitis media in an otherwise healthy child who has not had defervescence and relief of pain within 48 hours after initiation of appropriate medical therapy.

In myringotomy, an incision is made in the eardrum to gain access to the middle ear to evacuate fluid or a mass, or to create an opening for insertion of a tympanostomy tube. Myringotomy with insertion of a tympanostomy tube is the operation done most frequently in children in the United States.

Myringoplasty is surgery done on the eardrum, usually to repair a hole. Although traumatic eardrum perforations usually heal without surgery, a perforation that persists for more than 6 months after either a traumatic event or extrusion of a tympanostomy tube may require surgical repair. Repair is accomplished with use of a graft, either with adipose obtained from the earlobe or with fascia from the temporalis muscle.

Because inadequate ventilation of the middle ear is believed to be an important factor predisposing otitis media to develop in children, insertion of a **tympanostomy (ventilating) tube** helps to diminish the frequency of ear infections. Indications for this procedure include frequently recurring acute otitis media (occurring four or more times during a 3-month period) and persistent middle-ear effusion (present for more than 10 weeks and accompanied by conductive hearing loss in the affected ear). When a child has persistent otitis media and major conductive hearing loss in both ears, the indication for aspiration of fluid and insertion of tubes is stronger compared with when fluid is found in only one ear or minimal hearing loss occurs in both ears. Almost no risk is associated with insertion of a tympanostomy tube, except that the opening in the eardrum at the site of insertion may not heal after the tube has become extruded, so a minor surgical procedure may be needed to repair the eardrum.

Middle-ear Surgery

A **tympanoplasty** is any operation done within the middle ear, also known as the tympanum. This procedure may be done to provide exposure for repair of the eardrum or to gain access to the middle-ear ossicles. When an eardrum perforation is too large for a simple myringoplasty, involving surgery only on the eardrum, the eardrum remnant is elevated, and the middle ear is entered to provide better exposure for placement of a fascia graft. Because the fascia graft can be placed either medial or lateral to the fibrous annulus of the eardrum, tympanoplasty can be performed with use of either a medial or a lateral graft.

When a child has a conductive hearing loss, it can be assumed that the middle-ear bones either are not in continuity with each other or are fixed in some way. **Ossiculoplasty,** also known as ossicular reconstruction, can be done to restore ossicular continuity and normal transmission of vibration from the eardrum to the stapes footplate and oval window. This procedure can be performed by removing, reshaping, and then reinserting the patient's own ossicles or by using an allograft ossicular replacement prosthesis that is available commercially. Middle-ear prostheses that are commonly used are made of hydroxyapatite or titanium.

Middle-ear surgery is done with an otomicrosope. The risks of any middle-ear surgery include hearing loss, damage to the chorda tympani nerve with resulting loss of taste sensation on the ipsilateral side of the tongue, and damage to the facial nerve with ipsilateral facial paralysis that may be temporary or permanent, depending on the site and extent of the injury.

Mastoid Surgery

Mastoidotomy involves creating an opening in the mastoid, whereas **mastoidectomy** consists of exenteration of the mastoid air cells. Both procedures are done with use of a drill, to gain a view of the mastoid air cells to provide egress for infection, to allow better aeration and create an air reservoir for the middle ear through the aditus ad antrum (the connection between the middle ear and the mastoid), or to remove lesions such as cholesteatoma. Cholesteatoma is an ingrowth of keratin-producing epithelium that extends into the middle ear or the mastoid, or both. Decades ago, before the advent of antibiotics, the primary indication for mastoidectomy in children was for the treatment of mastoiditis. However, in recent years, this procedure has been done mainly to remove cholesteatoma or to improve aeration to the middle ear during a tympanoplasty performed to repair a chronic eardrum perforation. The risks of mastoid surgery include accidental injury of the dura with cerebrospinal fluid leak and damage to the facial nerve with resulting facial paralysis.

Surgery in the Nasopharynx

Adenoidectomy is the removal of adenoids from the nasopharynx. The adenoids are present at birth, tend to enlarge until the child is about 5 years old, and usually diminish in size by approximately 8 years. The two main reasons for removing the adenoids in a child are (1) to provide an improved nasal airway if they are so large that they block airflow through the choanae at the junction between the nose and the nasopharynx. This condition is manifest when a child snores loudly and breathes almost entirely through the mouth rather than through the mouth and nose; and (2) as adjunct treatment for children with frequent otitis media, the rationale for this being that the adenoids harbor pathogens that can predispose a child to develop middle-ear infections. Risks of adenoidectomy include postoperative bleeding and hypernasality resulting from inadequate closure of the soft palate against the posterior pharyngeal wall, where the adenoids might previously have added bulk necessary for adequate closure.

PEARLS FOR ROUNDS

The most significant risk of tonsillectomy in children is postoperative hemorrhage. The literature reports an occurrence of approximately 2% to 4%.

The two most common indications for tonsillectomy in children are recurrent infection and tonsillar hypertrophy.

The three organisms most frequently cultured from middle ear infections in children include *Streptococcus pneumoniae*, *Haemophilus influenzae*, and *Moraxella catarrhalis*.

Second branchial arch anomalies are the most common and represent 90% of branchial cleft cysts and associated sinuses.

The most common malignant tumor of the neck in children is lymphoma.

Surgery in the Oral Cavity and Oropharynx

Congenital cysts and solid lesions can be found in the tongue or on the floor of the mouth. Lesions in the tongue include lymphangioma, hemangioma, and lingual thyroid, and those on the floor of the mouth can be a ranula. Whereas a hemangioma tends to regress and involute before a child reaches puberty, a lymphangioma usually does not involute. A hemagioma can be treated with systemic steroids or sclerotic agents, or both. If a lymphangioma of the tongue is large enough to cause difficulty with feeding or eating, surgical excision may be necessary. Children with Beckwith-Wiedemann syndrome have macroglossia, an excessively large tongue that may protrude from the mouth and may require partial glossectomy.

When operating on a child's tongue, major postoperative edema can be anticipated. Sometimes the patient remains intubated for 1 or 2 days until the edema subsides and an adequate airway can be ensured.

The most common operation done in the oropharynx of children is tonsillectomy. Indications include frequent (chronic) tonsillitis and tonsillar hypertrophy. In general, a child who has had three or more episodes of tonsillitis a year for more than 2 years is considered to be a candidate for tonsillectomy. Another indication is sleep-disordered breathing in a child who has markedly enlarged tonsils on physical examination. Tonsillectomy and adenoidectomy are often performed together in a child. The main risk of tonsillectomy is bleeding that can occur within the first 10 hours or as late as 10 days after surgery. Before recommending tonsillectomy for a child, it is important to question the parents about nosebleeds, easy bruisability, or any other clue that might suggest a bleeding diathesis.

Surgery of the Nose and Sinuses

Except for repair of a nasal septal deformity or incision and drainage of a septal hematoma or abscess, surgery of the nose is not commonly done in children. Children who are born with a pit or dimple in the midline dorsum of the nose are likely to have a congenital dermoid cyst that needs excision. The presence of nasal polyps should raise the suspicion of cystic fibrosis, as these lesions rarely occur in children who do not have this disease. Nasal polyps are almost never detected in children who are younger than 18 months. Therefore when a lesion appearing to be a polyp is seen in the nose of an infant, this should raise the suspicion that the lesion may be an encephalocele rather than an ordinary allergic polyp, and appropriate imaging studies should be obtained to look for a defect in the skull base and specifically in the region of the cribriform plate.

In the past, sinus surgery was done in children only for the treatment of acute infection, but in recent years, children with symptoms and radiographic evidence of chronic sinusitis have been managed with endoscopic sinus surgery. This procedure is performed with telescopes and specially designed instruments, so incisions on the face are not required.

Surgery of the Larynx and Trachea

The most common cause of stridor in newborn infants is a condition known as laryngomalacia. The diagnosis can easily be made if the characteristic finding of a floppy epiglottis and aryepiglottic folds is noted with use of a flexible fiberoptic telescope during an office examination. Most children outgrow laryngomalacia without ever requiring surgical intervention. However, when a child with inspiratory stridor and laryngomalacia fails to gain weight, an **epiglottoplasty** can be done with a laser to recontour the epiglottis and aryepiglottic folds.

Lesions of the larynx include cysts, polyps, nodules, and hemangioma. Vocal cord nodules are usually the result of improper use of the voice and are generally treated with voice therapy rather than surgical excision. The most common laryngeal lesion requiring surgery in children is benign squamous papilloma, which is usually caused by infection with human papillomavirus type 6 or 11. Laryngeal papillomata in children tends to recur relentlessly after excision or removal with a laser; therefore the disorder is described as recurrent respiratory papillomatosis. Better treatments to prevent recurrence are continually being sought.

Paralysis of a vocal cord causing hoarseness and a raspy voice can be corrected with laryngeal surgery to medialize the vocal cord or to insert cartilage in it for added bulk. Paralysis of both vocal cords usually causes airway compromise sufficient to require a tracheotomy.

Tracheotomy

A **tracheotomy** is an opening made in the trachea through which a tracheotomy tube is inserted. Usually a tracheotomy is temporary and can be removed when the airway obstruction is alleviated. A **tracheostomy** is the creation of a stoma, with skin being sutured to the tracheal wall. A tracheostomy is more permanent than a tracheotomy. The two main indications for tracheotomy in children are an anticipated need for prolonged endotracheal intubation and a need to provide an alternate airway when a major obstruction of the upper airway is found at the base of tongue or at the oropharynx, larynx, or subglottic trachea.

Although children tend to tolerate prolonged endotracheal intubation better than adults, when a child has been intubated for 2 to 3 weeks and a need is anticipated for additional lengthy intubation, a tracheotomy is indicated. When a child has severe laryngeal papilloma, subglottic hemangioma, bilateral vocal cord paralysis, or any lesion or condition that substantially compromises airflow to the lungs, a tracheotomy also should be considered. If the airway compromise is severe enough to suggest that a tracheotomy may be necessary, it is best to perform the procedure immediately rather than to wait and see if the child can survive without it.

Although emergency cricothyrotomy can establish a secure airway for an adult, the cricothyroid space is small or nonexistent in infants. Therefore this procedure should not be considered as a potential life-saving maneuver in a child who has airway compromise. A planned tracheotomy is *always* preferable to an emergency cricothyrotomy.

Surgery of the Neck

Children frequently have cervical adenopathy. In addition, congenital cysts and other masses are relatively common in children. Malignant and benign neoplasms can be encountered. Taking an accurate history is important in the evaluation of a pediatric neck mass, specifically including the duration the mass has been present and any factors that might have preceded the appearance of the mass. Exposures to ticks and cats or a history of foreign travel should raise concern for a chronic cervical infection. A congenital mass is likely to be the result of an error in embryogenesis. Lesions that have grown rapidly in size can be malignant. Fever and night sweats may mean that a neck mass is an infected lymph node or an abscess. A neck mass that is enlarging without any signs of infection in the head may mean that the mass is malignant.

The consistency, mobility, tenderness, color and laterality of the mass also are important in the diagnostic evaluation. A unilateral solid mass is more likely to represent a neoplastic process, whereas any type of cystic mass is more suggestive of an inflammatory or congenital process. A purpuric mass at the angle of the mandible is suggestive of a mycobacterial infection and should be managed medically before surgical excision is attempted. Many practitioners find ultrasound useful for determining whether a mass is cystic or solid, and computed tomography (CT) is helpful for delineating relations of a mass to surrounding structures. Laboratory evaluation should include a complete blood count and purified protein derivative tests.

Initial management of a neck mass that could be an enlarged lymph node should be broad-spectrum antibiotics. In general, if a child's neck mass is thought to be an enlarged lymph node, incisional biopsy or excision of the node can be deferred until the child has had complete medical evaluation and treatment with antibiotic. However, open surgical biopsy is indicated if a neck mass is greater than 2 cm in diameter, unilateral, and persistent more than 4 weeks after antimicrobial therapy.

If a neck mass is cystic rather then solid, and signs of infection are present, then the surgeon must keep in mind that the localized infection that may be apparent on examination and confirmed with CT scan could be an infected branchial cleft cyst instead of an abscess from a necrotic lymph node with cystic degeneration. This being the case, the surgeon must be cautious in proceeding to incision and drainage of any localized infection in a child's neck. What appears to be a simple neck infection could be an infected branchial cleft cyst. Complete excision of a branchial cleft cyst with minimal chance for recurrence is far more difficult to

PEARLS FOR THE OR

The blood supply to the tonsil includes (1) facial artery (tonsillar branch), (2) dorsal lingual artery, (3) ascending palatine artery, (4) lesser palatine artery, and (5) ascending pharyngeal artery.

The chorda tympani nerve innervates the anterior two thirds of the tongue.

The facial nerve innervates the stapedius muscle, which is attached to the stapes.

The second branchial cleft sinus tract runs lateral to the carotid bifurcation; it passes between the internal and external carotid arteries.

The tensor veli palatini, innervated by the trigeminal nerve, opens the eustachian tube.

TABLE 52–1 Differences between Dermoid and Thyroglossal Duct Cysts

	Dermoid Cyst	Thyroglossal Duct Cyst
Embryology	Arises from mesodermal and ectodermal layers	Arises from the embryologic tract of the thyroid's descent from the foramen cecum into the lower anterior neck
Physical findings	Midline cystic mass present at birth or noticed after birth; can be located in the dorsum of the nose	Midline neck mass, usually at or near hyoid bone
Position of cyst in neck	Can present as midline masses that do not elevate with tongue protrusion; any midline cyst caudal to palpable thyroid isthmus is most likely a dermoid cyst	Most common at level of hyoid but can be anywhere along the tract of the thyroid gland's descent; *moves with tongue protrusion*
Treatment	Local excision	Sistrunk procedure: surgical excision of entire tract to the level of the tongue base including a central portion of the hyoid bone

achieve after the cyst has been incised and drained. When a branchial cleft cyst has become infected, the best treatment is antimicrobial therapy and excision after the infection has subsided.

The most common reason for neck surgery in children is to remove a congenital cyst. The position of the cyst within the neck helps to determine the embryologic origin of the cyst. The two most commonly encountered midline congenital cysts are thyroglossal duct cyst and dermoid cyst. Differentiating between them is important because complete removal of a thyroglossal duct cyst requires removal of the body of the hyoid bone, whereas removal of a dermoid cyst does not necessarily require removal of the mid-portion of the hyoid (Table 52-1). The most common cysts that are located lateral in the neck are branchial cleft cysts (Table 52-2). When a child has an infected cyst in either the midline or the lateral neck, it is preferable to treat the infection with parenteral antibiotics and to strive for total excision of the cyst (Figs. 52-1 and 52-2) after the infection has resolved rather than to incise and drain the cyst. Only when a concern exists for impending airway obstruction should an infected congenital cyst be drained. Incision and drainage tends to disrupt the cyst capsule, resulting in local scarring and adhesions that can obscure the dissection plane and interfere with precise surgical excision at a later time.

Suppurative infection of the retropharyngeal or parapharyngeal spaces typically occurs in younger children. After

TABLE 52–2 The Four Types of Branchial Cleft Cysts

Arch	Derivative: Nerve	Derivative: Artery	Tract
First	Trigeminal (V)	External maxillary (degenerates)	*Type I*: cyst or tract orifice is anteroinferior to lobule; tract parallels ear canal; runs lateral to facial nerve *Type II*: cyst or tract orifice is located below angle of mandible, and sinus tract runs superiorly to enter ear canal; may run superficial or deep to facial nerve
Second	Facial (VII)	Stapedial (degenerates)	Cyst or tract orifice is located at anterior margin of SCM at junction of middle and lower thirds tracking between internal and external carotid and inserting into the tonsillar fossa
Third	Glossopharyngeal (IX)	Common and internal carotids	Cyst is low in anterior neck and more commonly on the left side; tracks under the glossopharyngeal nerve and internal carotid artery but superficial to the vagus nerve; travels through the thyrohyoid membrane and inserts into the pyriform fossa
Fourth	Vagus (X)	Aortic arch and right proximal subclavian	Extremely rare; may present as cyst or abscess in thyroid gland or perithyroid space; tracks posterior to the common carotid artery to insert at the apex of the pyriform sinus Left: tract passes underneath the aorta Right: tract passes underneath the subclavian artery, superior to the recurrent laryngeal nerve and inferior to the superior laryngeal nerve

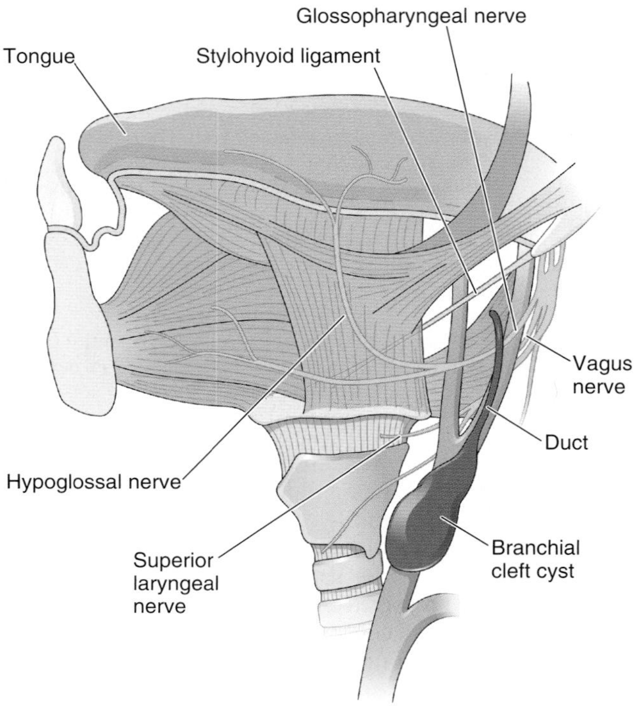

FIGURE 52–1 Excision of second branchial cleft sinus tract.

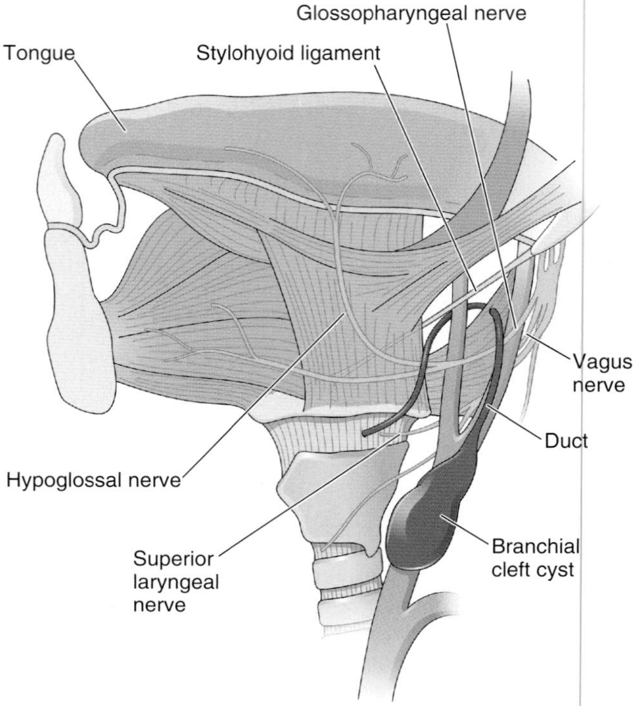

FIGURE 52–2 Excision of third branchial cleft sinus tract.

age 5 years, the lymph nodes in these regions begin to involute, and infections in these areas become less likely. Signs and symptoms suggestive of a deep-neck-space infection include fever, refusal to eat or drink, neck stiffness, drooling, and trismus. A lateral neck radiograph may show widening of the prevertebral soft tissues. If the clinical picture is suggestive or if the lateral neck radiograph raises concern, a contrast-enhanced CT of the neck should be obtained. If the CT shows a phlegmon, parenteral antibiotics are indicated for 2 to 3 days, and the patient's clinical progress is monitored. If the CT shows a frank abscess, surgical drainage is necessary. Infections of the retropharyngeal and parapharyngeal spaces should always be taken seriously because of their potential to spread rapidly along fascial planes. Infection can extend into the mediastinum. Complications of deep-neck-space infections include airway compromise, sepsis, septic venous thrombosis, and mediastinitis.

Congenital Hearing Impairment

Children can be born with sensorineural hearing loss or conductive hearing loss, or both (known as mixed hearing loss). About 1 of every 1000 children born in the United States is profoundly deaf. These children often have no traits that identify them as having hearing loss. Neonatal screening has been used to identify children with isolated hearing loss so that appropriate intervention can be begun early in life. Screening can be performed easily in the hospital nursery before discharge, either by otoacoustic emission testing or auditory brainstem-response testing.

Congenital hearing impairment can be caused by a maternal infection such as rubella or cytomegalovirus or by factors such as maternal alcohol consumption resulting in fetal alcohol syndrome. Alternatively, a newborn's hearing impairment can be inherited. More than 200 genes cause hereditary hearing impairment; about one third of affected children have associated findings that are recognizable as a syndrome, whereas two thirds have no associated findings and are considered to have the nonsyndromic type of this disorder.

Purely conductive hearing loss that is present at birth and caused by abnormally formed middle-ear bones in one or both ears may go undetected for several years, depending on its severity and whether it is bilateral. Congenitally fixed or abnormally formed middle-ear ossicles can be repositioned or replaced with prosthetic ossicles.

Suggested Reading

Albright JT, Topham AK, Reilly JS: Pediatric head and neck malignancies. Arch Otolaryngol Head Neck Surg 128:655–659, 2002.

Bodenstein L, Altman RP: Cervical lymphadenitis in infants and children. Semin Pediatr Surg. 3:134–141, 1994.

Brookhouser PE, Beauchaine KL, Osberger MJ: Management of the child with sensorineural hearing loss: Medical, surgical, hearing aids, cochlear implants. Pediatr Clin North Am 46:121–141, 1999.

Chandler JR, Mitchell B: Branchial cleft cysts, sinuses, and fistulas. Otolaryngol Clin North Am 14:175–186, 1981.

Palmer PM, Dutton JM, McCulloch TM, Smith RJ: Trends in the use of tracheotomy in the pediatric patient: The Iowa experience. Head Neck 17:328–333, 1995.

Windfuhr JP, Chen Y: Post-tonsillectomy and adenoidectomy hemorrhage in nonselected patients. Ann Otol Rhinol Laryngol 112:63–70, 2003.

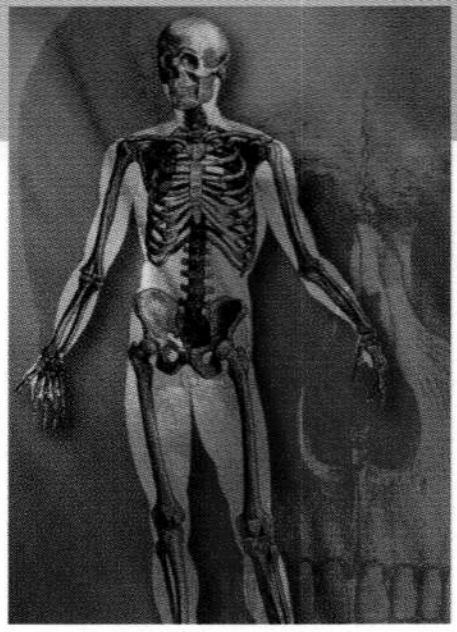

Chapter 53
Facial Plastic and Reconstructive Surgery

JEFFREY H. SPIEGEL, MD, and PUSHKAR MEHRA, BDS, DMD

The well-trained facial plastic surgeon needs a broad knowledge base. The anatomy of the head and neck is complicated, and the anatomy that the surgeon must deal with to obtain high-quality results is particularly challenging. This is partly due to the large number of important motor and sensory nerves in that area, but it also is because the anatomic relations between structures that the facial plastic surgeon must be familiar with are different from those that are typically learned. For most physicians, it would not be crucial to know the entire course of the temporal branch of the seventh cranial nerve, according to surface landmarks and tissue planes—from the temporal bone to the stylomastoid foramen, across the parotid, through the temporalis fascia, and across the temple—but for the facial plastic surgeon, this information is vital. Similarly, knowledge of the relative intermingling of fibers at the lateral edge of the orbicularis occuli muscle as it interacts with the zygomaticus major is important for some facial plastic surgery techniques.

Facial plastic surgeons must also know much general medicine to assess the impact of comorbid diseases on healing after surgical procedures, as well as much about the biocompatibility of medical materials. Because they must routinely insert expanded tetrafluoroethylene, gold, titanium, silicone, silicon, bovine cartilage, porcine intestinal submucosa, and many other materials into the face, they must know the appropriate indications for each.

An in-depth understanding of photographic principles also is required. This is necessary for photodocumentation of patients and their surgical results, and, importantly, it provides an understanding of the interplay between light and shadow, which can help the surgeon to understand where to place incisions and how to hide scars. A good grasp of psychology is another important skill, as the goals and motivations of patients desiring a change in their appearance must be assessed carefully to determine whether they are suitable candidates for surgery. Also useful is a good background in mathematics and physics. Many facial plastic surgical techniques require detailed knowledge of geometry, and the frequent use of lasers and similar equipment necessitates an understanding of physics beyond the basics.

The full extent of information pertaining to facial plastic and reconstructive surgery would require a large volume. For the purposes of this chapter, fundamental concepts and procedures are considered.

Rhinoplasty and Septorhinoplasty

Rhinoplasty refers to the group of surgical procedures that focus on changing the external shape and appearance of the nose. However, not all rhinoplasty is performed for that reason. An important aspect of this procedure is to improve the function of the nose as it relates to the passage and humidification of inspired air. The more complete set of procedures to change both the appearance and function of the nose is often referred to as septorhinoplasty.

From an anatomic standpoint, several critical components of the nose require consideration. Cephalically, the nasal structure is based on paired nasal bones. These bones should be symmetrical in appearance, with a smooth dorsum. Nasal trauma can result in asymmetry and the appearance that the nose is deviating to one side or the other. Similarly, the nasal bones can deviate laterally or into the nasal vault, resulting in a flattened nasal dorsum. The midportion of the nose has upper lateral cartilages, which ideally are symmetrical and which connect in the midline to the dorsal aspect of the nasal septum. The nasal septum is a cartilaginous, osseous structure that should extend in a straight sagittal plane from the nasal dorsum to the floor of the nose, where it rests in an osseous ridge in the midline of the nasal floor, known as the maxillary crest. When the septum is not straight, when it deviates to one side, or when its inferior aspect does not sit straight within the maxillary crest, nasal obstruction can develop. A nasal septoplasty is frequently performed to correct this problem. Typically, this procedure involves removal or modification of obstructing sections of bone and cartilage after elevation of the mucoperichondrium on both sides of the septum.

The most caudal aspect of the nose is the nasal tip. The tip is formed by paired lower lateral cartilages, each of which has a medial, a lateral, and an intermediate crura. The medial crus on each side meet in the midline to form the support of the columella (the central part of the nose as seen from the basal view). The cartilages are important with respect to the internal and external nasal valves. These anatomic regions form one of the greatest areas of resistance to airflow and

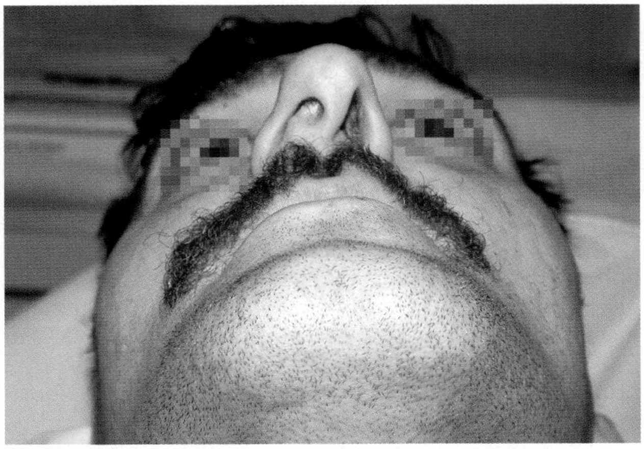

FIGURE 53–1 Patient with a major nasal obstruction and twisting of the columella due to malpositioning of the nasal septum.

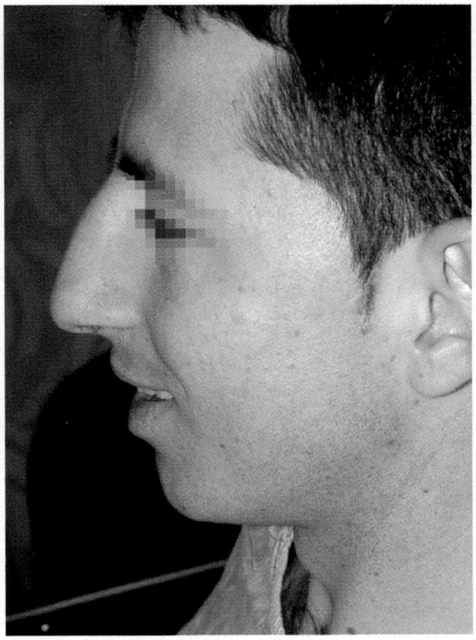

FIGURE 53–2 Patient with a prominent nasal dorsal hump.

perceived nasal obstruction (Fig. 53-1). Nasal tape strips are sometimes worn by athletes to open the nasal valve and improve airflow during competitions.

Much discussion over the years has concerned the ideal shape of the nose. Clearly, this is a question without one true answer. The criteria for physical attractiveness vary among social and ethnic groups, within those groups, and over time. However, in general, proportion and symmetry are valued highly. The nose should be straight, symmetrical, and neither too large nor too small for the person's face. You will find many mathematical formulae and anatomic benchmarks that surgeons have constructed to calculate ideal facial proportions (Fig. 53-2).

For the surgeon who is performing rhinoplasty, or any facial plastic surgery for that matter, it is paramount that the goals of the patient be understood. In a case of nasal fracture due to trauma, the patient usually wants only to restore his or her appearance to what it was before the injury. However, in elective aesthetic procedures, the surgeon should ask each patient to name the specific aspects of the nose or face that he or she desires to change. Patients with a large dorsal hump will often want only the tip changed. They may like the hump, or it may be a family trait, and the surgeon's suggestion that it should be changed can be offensive. Aspects of the nose that may be considered for change include the length, projection, nasolabial angle, width, bulbosity of the tip, presence of a hump, and straightness. Although the surgeon should not tell the patient what about the nose requires change, it is important to explain how the desired change can be achieved while maintaining overall balance.

Rhinoplasty can be done through a number of incisions and under general or local anesthesia. A patient seen within 7 to 10 days of a nasal fracture may require no incision at all. A straight elevator (e.g., a Boise elevator) can be placed under the nasal bones, which are then lifted back into anatomic position. Tape and a dorsal splint are used to hold the nose in the desired location while it heals. For patients requiring only a reduction in the dorsum, rasping of the nasal bones and excision of excess dorsal cartilage can be achieved through an intercartilaginous incision. This incision goes through the scroll area, which is the junction of the upper and lower cartilages on each side. The nasal skin can then be elevated superior to the tip, and the desired changes can be achieved. Sometimes, enough rasping and excision is done to create a wide or flat nasal dorsum. This is frequently called an *open roof deformity,* and it can be corrected by allowing the nasal bones to collapse into each other after releasing them laterally (through a lateral osteotomy). It also can be corrected by replacement with a soft-tissue or cartilage dorsal **onlay** graft. Excessive resection of the nasal dorsum can result in a **ski-slope nose,** which once was popular but today is considered unnatural and is thus an undesirable outcome. Destruction of the septum, as from cocaine use or Wegener's vasculitis, can lead to a **saddle-nose deformity** with collapse of the dorsum. Rib or calvarial bone grafts are often needed to reconstruct these more major defects.

Nasal tip surgery can be done through a delivery approach or a columellar incision. After appropriate exposure is obtained, the nasal tip is shaped by removing cartilage or by suturing the cartilage into the desired position. Excessive cartilage resection results in an "operated-on" or pinched appearance, which is undesirable. Cartilage grafts also may

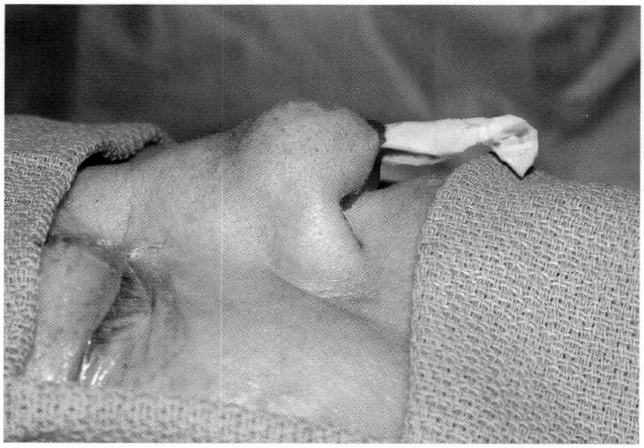

FIGURE 53–3 Patient with a synthetic implant used by a surgeon outside of the United States to augment the nasal dorsum. The implant became infected and extruded.

be used to support the nose, to help change the shape of the nasal valves to improve airflow, or to alter the shape of the nasal tip as desired.

Some physicians, particularly those outside of the United States, use synthetic materials as grafts to shape the nose. In some areas of Southeast Asia in particular, rhinoplasty surgeons will typically use a silicone or plastic insert for this purpose. However, this material is never fully integrated into the body, thereby posing a life-long risk of infection and extrusion to the patient (Fig. 53-3).

The patient will typically need to wear a nasal splint for 7 days after rhinoplasty. The application of ice to the face can help to reduce the discomfort and ecchymosis that can result after osteotomies of the nasal bones. Some postoperative nasal bleeding is to be expected, but it is rarely necessary to "pack" the nose. Overall discomfort is minimal, and most patients are ready to resume a less strenuous version of their normal routine after just over 1 week.

Rhinoplasty seems simple, but volumes have been written on the subject. With so many factors contributing to the final outcome, many facial plastic surgeons consider this to be the most challenging procedure that they perform.

Rhytidectomy/Facelift

Because of the interplay among genetics, exposures, experience, gravity, and the passage of time, the soft tissues of the face start to sag. This causes larger facial wrinkles and folds and can eliminate the smooth attractive contour of the mandible and the neck. A rhytidectomy (removal of rhytids, or wrinkles) is an attempt to restore the tissues to a position closer to the facial skeleton, with less redundancy. The position of the hyoid in the neck is important to consider before rhytidectomy, as a posteriorly positioned hyoid allows for a more acute cervicomental angle and a better potential outcome. An anterior hyoid, or a retrognathic chin, leads to a less acute cervicomental angle, and in this situation, even the best rhytidectomy surgeon may not be able to achieve the patient's desired goals. In some cases, additional procedures (e.g., mentoplasty or insertion of a chin implant) can reduce this problem.

Facelifts have evolved over time. Originally, an incision was made around the ears, and skin was elevated and then pulled back. This resulted in a good but short-lived improvement. Eventually, the anatomic concept of the superficial musculoaponeurotic system (SMAS) was incorporated. The SMAS is a fascial layer that is found deep to the facial skin. It incorporates many of the muscles of facial expression. Surgeons found that, by pulling back on the SMAS, a more natural and longer-lasting result could be obtained while minimizing the risk to the underlying motor branches of the facial nerve. More recently, the **deep-plane facelift** has become increasingly common. This technique is an attempt to further improve on the 5- to 10-year longevity of the result by lifting even deeper tissues. The plane of dissection varies, depending on which part of the face is being operated on in an attempt to minimize risk to the facial nerve. The most common complications after facelift surgery include hematoma (which may initially manifest as unusually severe postoperative pain), numbness (as from injury to the greater auricular nerve), and, less frequently, facial weakness. The skilled rhytidectomy surgeon knows not to pull the tissues to the extent that important facial landmarks (such as the position of the orbital or oral commissures) are changed. The position of the incision varies but should be as hidden as possible without substantially changing the patient's hairline (Fig. 53-4).

Innovative surgeons are continually trying variations on the standard rhytidectomy. These include the **neck lift,** which targets the neckline, and the **mini** or **weekend facelift,** in which a minimal amount of skin is elevated to provide a lesser degree of correction for patients with milder indications for facelift. Some surgeons offer a **two-stitch facelift,** in which a minimal incision is made in the temple, and the midface tissues are elevated by passing a long permanent suture. Each of these less extensive procedures requires a shorter time for recovery.

Brow Lift

The upper third of the face, comprising the forehead and the brow, is often overlooked when a patient seeks cosmetic surgery. The frontalis and corrugator muscles create transverse and vertical rhytids, respectively. Also important is that gravity can eventually pull the eyebrows from their position above the orbital rim. Sagging eyebrows can give a vibrant, well-rested person a tired or sad appearance. Sometimes a person will consult a facial plastic surgeon about a blepharoplasty when a brow lift would actually provide a better

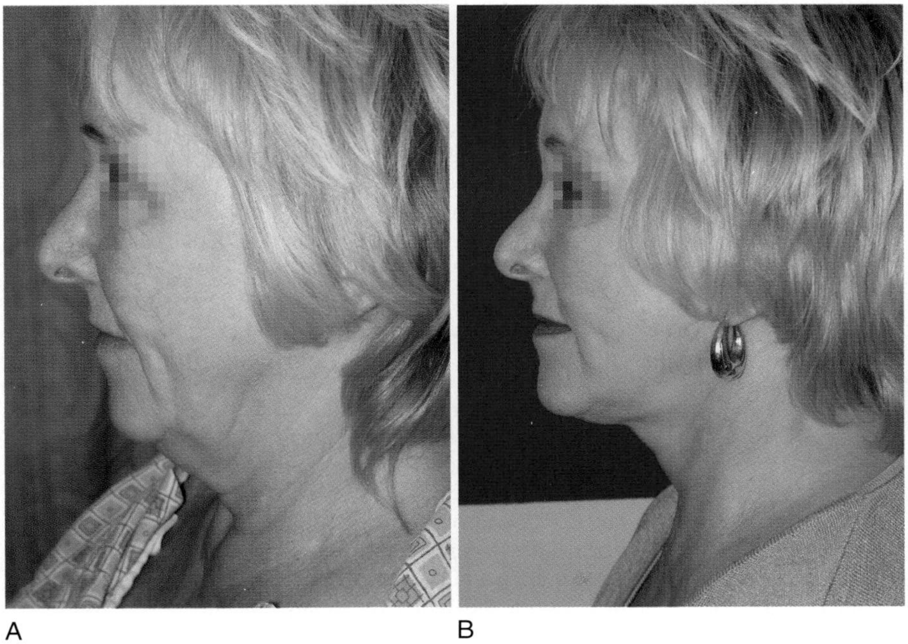

FIGURE 53–4 *A*, Lateral view before rhytidectomy. Note the sagging jowls and angulation of the neck skin. *B*, Two weeks after rhytidectomy, a natural-looking improvement is seen in the jowling and neck skin.

result. In this group of patients, blepharoplasty may lead to a worsened appearance, as the already sagging eyebrows are pulled inferiorly by removing upper eyelid skin.

A number of techniques are used to elevate the brow. In the traditional browlift, a somewhat long incision is made behind the hairline, almost from ear to ear. The tissues of the forehead are then elevated in the subperiosteal plane (laterally in the plane deep to the superficial fascia of the temporalis muscle, to avoid injury to the superior branches of the facial nerve). The forehead is then retracted posteriorly, and excess tissues are excised before closing the incision. In a now less commonly done version of this procedure, sections of forehead skin are removed superior to the eyebrows, both to elevate and to attempt to camouflage the incision in them. In an endoscopic browlift, a series of two to six small incisions are made behind the hairline. With use of an endoscope and long-handled, curved tissue elevators, the same elevation is done as in the traditional browlift; however, rather than removing any scalp, the elevated periosteum is simply pulled posteriorly and affixed to the skull through a screw, suture, or other method. Attaching the periosteum to the calvarial bone in this way holds the forehead in the appropriate position until the periosteum heals back to the frontal bone. Endoscopic browlift has a much shorter recovery period compared with traditional browlift.

Blepharoplasty (Eyelid Surgery)

Blepharoplasty is one of the most commonly performed surgical procedures involving the eyelids. It refers to the removal of excess skin or fat or both from under the eyelids. Although most often performed for cosmetic reasons, the procedure also can be used to treat functional problems, including superior visual eye-field loss due to overhanging skinfolds. As people age, dermatochalasis occurs because of skin laxity from breakdown of collagen and elastic fibers within the dermis. Sun damage and genetics also are predisposing factors for this condition. The epidermis becomes atrophic, accompanied by abnormal changes in melanocytes and keratinocytes, as well as by changes in dermal mucopolysaccharides and proteins. This leads to sagging of eyelid skin and herniation of orbital fat into the eyelids (Fig. 53-5).

A thorough preoperative general systemic and ocular examination is essential. Specific tests, such as the snap test and the lid-distraction test, also are helpful in diagnosis and treatment planning. Changing the position of the eyelid can modify a patient's refractive error, which can result in postoperative visual disturbance. The practitioner must be cognizant about conditions such as thyroid-function disorders, dry eyes, lid ptosis due to levator aponeurosis, and Müller's muscle problems. It is important that the patient demonstrate an adequate tear film and blink reflex, as well as good eyelid closure, before blepharoplasty.

As upper lid blepharoplasty almost always requires skin removal, a transcutaneous approach is used. In cases of lower lid blepharoplasty requiring only fat removal, a transconjunctival approach is preferred, as this procedure avoids the need for skin incisions. The procedure is commonly performed under local anesthesia with intra-

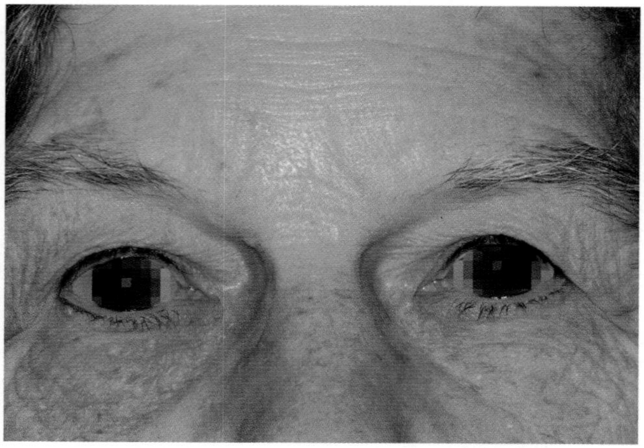

FIGURE 53–5 Frontal view of a patient showing age-related changes in the periorbital anatomy. Note drooping of upper eyelid skin and bulging of fat in the lower eyelid area.

venous sedation. After the patient has been prepped and draped, a surgical marker is used to outline areas for skin incision and the amount of skin to be removed (Fig. 53-6). After local anesthetic with epinephrine has been infiltrated, the skin incision is made with a number 15 scalpel blade; in the upper eyelid, the inferior border of the incision is usually made at the eyelid crease (approximately 10 mm above the upper eyelid margin). Medially, the incision stops at the level of the punctum; laterally, it generally extends to 1 to 2 mm beyond the lateral canthus, but this is variable depending on the amount of skin to be removed.

After the initial incision has been made, sharp scissors are used to excise excess skin with a superficial rim of orbicularis oculi muscle. Slight pressure is exerted on the globe to prolapse fat from underneath the orbital septum. The upper eyelid contains two discrete fat pads and the lacrimal gland, whereas the lower eyelid has three discrete fat-deposit pads. The orbital septum is incised across its medial two thirds, and the fat is allowed to herniate through the fat pads. The fat is teased gently from its attachments and excised with electrocautery or laser. Closure of the skin incision is completed with a subcuticular or running suture

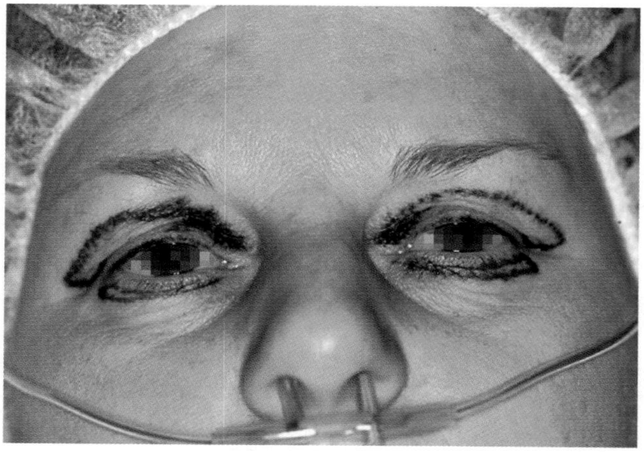

FIGURE 53–6 Frontal view of a patient planned for upper and lower lid transcutaneous blepharoplasty. Markings have been made for incisions and excess skin removal.

Liposuction

Aesthetically objectionable fat deposits are often seen in the central submental area and the region of the midjowl. Often the condition is hereditary and resistant to diet and exercise. Although the fat is usually distributed evenly throughout the central area, it extends bilaterally from the anterior border of the sternocleidomastoid on one side to the other side. A simple pinch test, in which the intervening dermal elements and subdermal fat are grasped and pinched in between the index finger and the thumb, is useful for evaluation of these fat deposits. Patients should be asked to tighten the platysma muscle so the surgeon can evaluate for platysmal banding. This condition occurs because of decussation of muscle fibers in the midline of the neck and requires platysmal plication for optimal correction.

The procedure is usually performed with the patient under intravenous sedation. Initially, surgical markings are made with the patient in an upright position. The planned site of the entry port and the location of the greatest fat deposits are marked at this time, as these areas often shift when the patient is placed in the supine position for the procedure. Identification of the inferior border of the mandible and the anterior border of the sternocleidomastoid muscles is essential, as these landmarks represent the superior and posterior boundaries for liposuction.

Once the patient is positioned comfortably in the supine position, the neck is prepped and draped in a sterile manner. A small 5-mm incision is made for the entry port. Tumescent infiltration of the neck area is achieved by local anesthetic deposition in a spokes-of-the-wheel advancement of the multiport infiltrator. It is not uncommon to infiltrate 75 to 100 mL of 0.1% lidocaine with 1:100,000 epinephrine into the neck region. Use of such volumes promotes a hydro-dissection plane, which facilitates fat removal and minimizes damage to deeper structures. A series of suction cannulas is then used to remove fat systematically (Fig. 53-7).

Laser Skin Resurfacing

Skin resurfacing has gained considerable popularity since the introduction of short-pulsed, high-energy, carbon dioxide (CO_2) lasers. Although other procedures such as chemical peels and dermabrasion are available for removal of facial

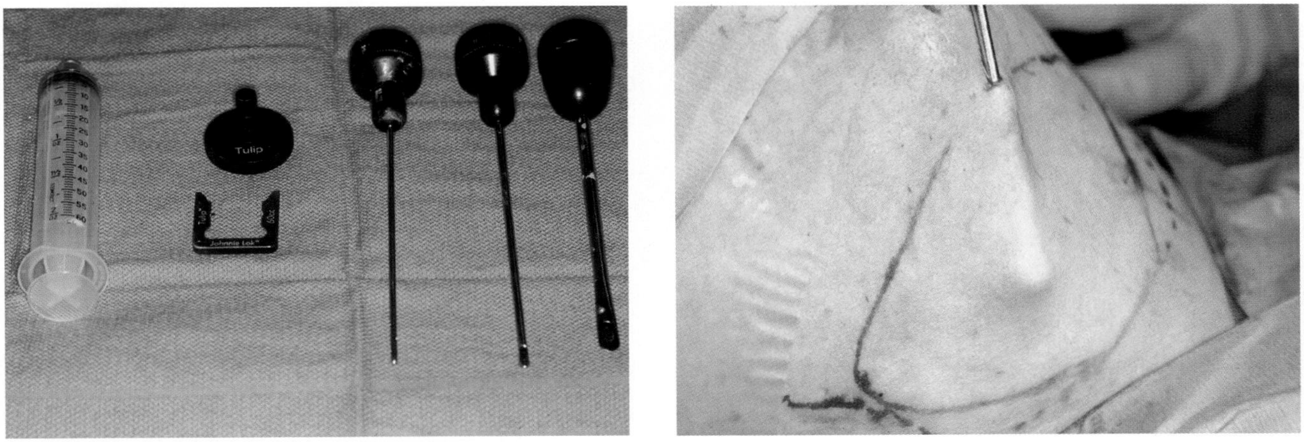

A B

FIGURE 53–7 *A*, Different-sized Tulip syringe and cannulas used for cervicomental liposuction. *B*, Intraoperative view of the liposuction technique.

lines and wrinkles, aesthetic cutaneous laser surgery remains the mainstay for facial rejuvenation in patients who are not candidates or who do not opt for facelift procedures. It is the action of the CO_2 laser on its chromophore, water, that makes it so useful clinically in the treatment of skin, as water constitutes 80% to 95% of the epidermis. As the laser is applied to the epidermis, the water component is heated rapidly to boiling temperature. This action effectively ablates the epidermis with thermal damage up to a depth of 100 μm. Subsequent passes to the skin repeat these effects and remove facial wrinkles. In addition to removal of the epidermis and the papillary layer of the dermis, a beneficial effect of laser thermal damage is to shorten the collagen fibers in the dermis by 20% to 30%; this is followed by substantial neocollagen formation. The combination of epidermal removal, dermal shrinkage, and neocollagen formation is tighter, fresher, more youthful-appearing skin with less-visible wrinkles

Unfortunately, cutaneous resurfacing with an ablative laser such as the CO_2 laser or with an ablative technique such as coblation results in a fairly long recovery period, during which time the patient will have a weepy, raw wound on the face. Other disadvantages include the possibility of hypopigmented or hyperpigmented skin in the area of the resurfacing. Newer laser techniques include treatment with intense pulsed light (IPL), in which energy passes through the epidermis and results in collagen remodeling in the deeper dermis. This remodeling can improve the appearance of fine facial rhytids. Although the effect is considerably less than that achieved with an ablative laser, virtually no recovery period occurs; IPL could easily be done during a person's lunch break, after which he or she could return to work with few visible signs of having had an aesthetic procedure.

Facial Augmentation

Hard-tissue and soft-tissue augmentations of the facial area have become popular in the last few years. These techniques are used to manage congenital and acquired defects and include augmentation of the lips, nasolabial grooves, and chin, temporal, zygomatic, and midface areas. Soft-tissue grafts commonly used in contemporary maxillofacial augmentation include homogenous grafts harvested from the patient's mucosa, skin, dermis, cartilage, and fat. Alternatively, soft-tissue augmentation can be performed with heterogenous grafts such as lyophilized dura and human dermis grafts. Commonly used hard-tissue replacement techniques include use of autogenous bone grafts harvested from the rib, cranium, or iliac crest, and use of freeze-dried cadaveric bone.

As biotechnology has advanced, newer materials have been introduced into the market. Although ceramics are still used with good results, hard-tissue polymers of various shapes and sizes are increasingly popular (Fig. 53-8). These materials include copolymers of polyethylene (Porex), polytetrafluoroethylene (Gore), polymethylmethacrylate (Biomet), and hydroxyapatite (Interpore). Advances in radiology and CAD/CAM technology have made it possible to obtain highly accurate three-dimensional stereolithographic models to order customized implants (Fig. 53-9), and to perform surgery with more predictable results.

Mentoplasty (Surgery of the Chin)

Hypoplasia, hyperplasia, and asymmetry of the genial are relatively common conditions. Before treatment, an accurate diagnosis must be established on the basis of clinical examination, photographic evaluation, and radiographic results. A

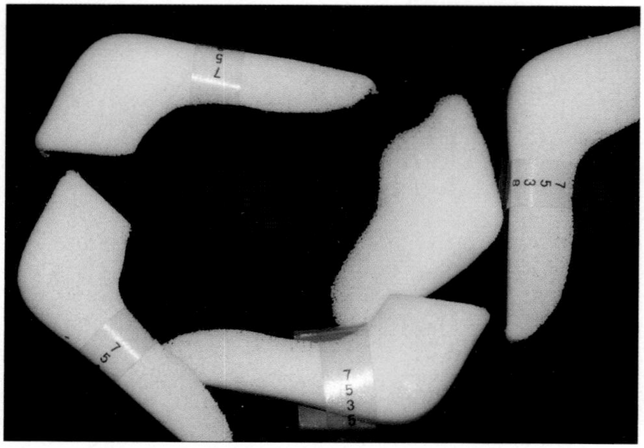

FIGURE 53–8 Alloplastic implants of varying sizes and shapes are available for cosmetic facial augmentation.

PEARLS FOR THE OR

The best tissue to use in replacing lost tissue is adjacent tissue. For a defect of the cheek skin, for example, rotating adjacent cheek skin into the defect will usually provide a better aesthetic outcome than repairing the area with a skin graft from the thigh. Many local skin flaps have been developed to facilitate the transfer of adjacent tissue. These include the note flap, the rhomboid flap, the rotation advancement flap, and the bilobed flap. The geometry of these flaps is fascinating, and their applications are quite varied.

Autologous tissues are preferable to synthetic or other implants. When cartilage is needed for a repair, it is better to borrow from the conchal bowl of the ear, the rib, or the septum than to use a synthetic material that will have a greater risk of infection and extrusion.

Straight lines occur rarely in the human body. Thus straight-line scars may be revised to be longer but to have a curved and broken course to help camouflage them.

cephalometric radiograph is ideal for evaluation of this area, as it gives detailed information about soft and hard tissues, as deficiency or excess of these tissues can contribute to the clinical picture. Most soft-tissue chin deformities can be corrected by procedures such as mentalis suspension or by camouflage with techniques such as hard-tissue augmentation of the bone in the region of the mentolabial folds. Osseous deficiencies are usually managed with sliding genioplasty (Fig. 53-10) or alloplastic augmentation (Fig. 53-11). A sliding genioplasty permits three-dimensional repositioning of the chin and involves an osteotomy of the anterior mandible with maintenance of the lingual and inferior soft-tissue pedicle for blood supply. The chin is placed in the optimal position and secured with bone plates or screws. All of these procedures are easily accomplished through an intraoral approach, thereby avoiding unnecessary scars.

Minimally Invasive Procedures

Increasingly, people desire procedures that provide a noticeable improvement in facial appearance but with a minimal recovery time. Such procedures that are now available include use of botulinum toxin and use of injectable fillers.

Botulinum toxin is used to treat facial rhytids caused by the dynamic action of the facial musculature. Originally

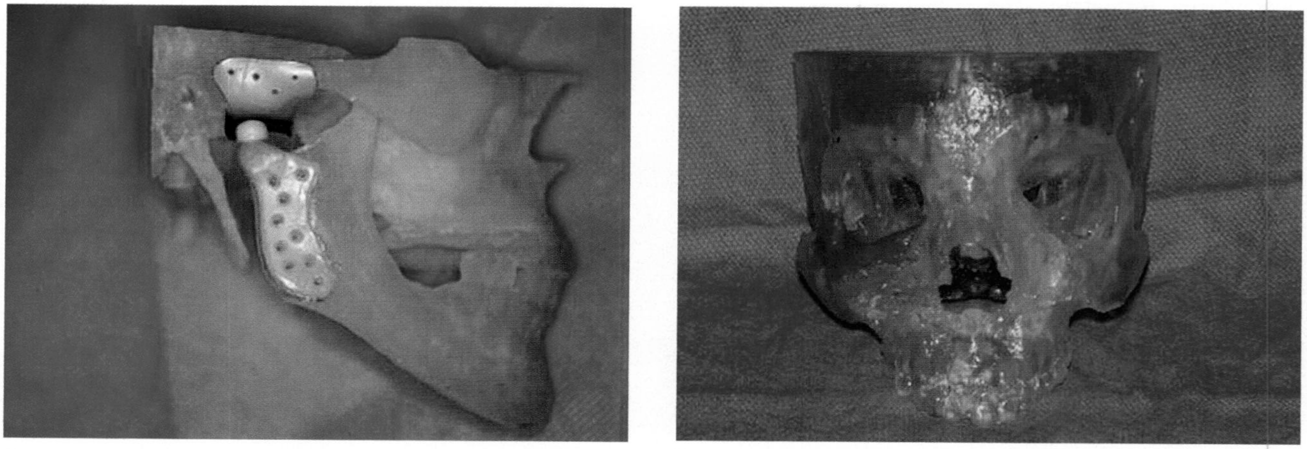

A B

FIGURE 53–9 *A*, A 3-D model manufactured before mandibular reconstruction. Wax-ups of the mandible and temporal fossa regions have been made for fabrication of customized implants by using CAD/CAM technology. *B*, A 3-D model manufactured before orbital reconstruction. Wax-up of the planned surgery has been performed for fabrication of surgical guides.

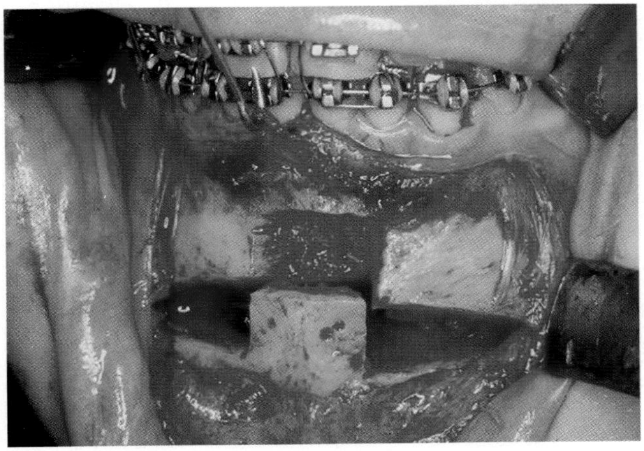

FIGURE 53–10 An intraoperative view of a bony sliding genioplasty for chin advancement. The osteotomized bone segment is secured with bone plates or screws or both.

approved by the Food and Drug Administration (FDA) to treat vertical glabellar furrows caused by the corrugator muscles, it is commonly used for transverse brow rhytids due to the frontalis muscles, for crow's feet due to the orbicular muscle of the eye, and for transverse glabellar and dorsal nasal rhytids due to the procerus muscle. Some surgeons even inject it to treat fine lines around the neck, mouth, and lower eyelids, although these uses are less common and have higher risk with reduced benefit. The toxin paralyzes the muscle for 3 to 4 months, after which time the muscle has healed and typically returns to its preinjection strength and function.

Injectable filler materials include bovine and human collagen, hyaluronic acid, medical-grade silicone, and hydroxyapatite. These materials are placed into or beneath the dermis to fill in facial rhytids. They range in duration from 3 months to 5 years, depending on the material. Each of these materials can be placed with just an injection through a needle that is 25 gauge or finer. Typical uses for filler materials include reduction in the nasolabial folds, treatment of fine perioral rhytids, enlargement of the lips, and filling in depressed facial scars.

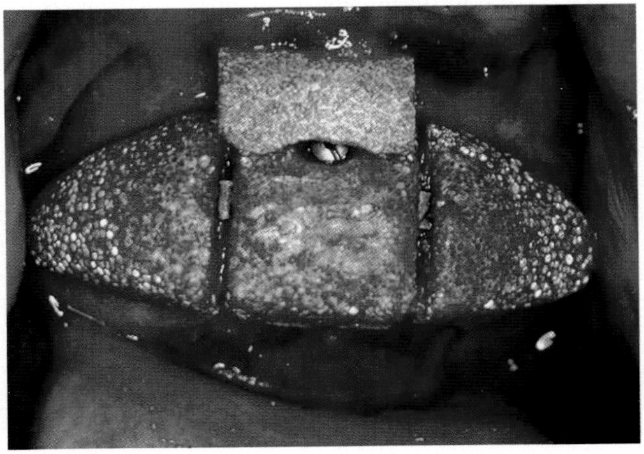

FIGURE 53–11 An intraoperative view of a chin implant being placed for chin augmentation.

Reconstructive Surgery

The need for reconstructive facial plastic surgery is unfortunately high. For the reasons mentioned at the beginning of this chapter, the face is perhaps the area of the body that generates the highest level of concern for a person. Consequently, when someone has a congenital, traumatic, or postablative defect of the head or neck, reconstructive surgery is of paramount importance.

The face can be divided into aesthetic subunits. These include, for example, the periorbital region and the perioral region; the latter can be divided further into the area between the nasolabial folds and area of the nasal tip. When a large portion of tissue in an aesthetic subunit must be replaced, it may be preferable to remove the remaining normal tissue and replace the entire area.

The repairing of defects typically involves bringing new tissue to an area of tissue loss. As mentioned earlier, this can sometimes be done by relocating adjacent tissue. Small areas can be repaired with random-pattern flaps, but larger tissue transfers require a defined blood supply for the tissue to survive. For example, axial flaps (which include nasolabial flaps and deltopectoral flaps) have a known blood vessel traveling the length of the tissue, which remains intact and provides nourishment to the transferred tissue.

Regional flaps can be composite tissues. For example, the pectoralis major is regularly transferred to the head and neck for reconstructive purposes. This muscle receives its blood supply through the pectoral branch of the thoracoacromial artery. Overlying skin is supplied by perforators from the underlying muscle. The artery comes down from above the clavicle toward the abdomen, on the undersurface of the muscle. An island of vascularized skin can be transferred by releasing three sides of the muscle and rotating it on its clavicular origin into the neck. The overlying skin island can be placed into the oral cavity or oropharynx for reconstruction of a defect after tumor extirpation. Other commonly used flaps for head and neck reconstruction include those obtained from the sternocleidomastoid muscle, the trapezius muscle, and the latissimus dorsi.

When a large amount of tissue or more pliable tissue or bone is needed, the reconstructive surgeon may elect to use a microvascular free tissue transfer, also known as a free flap. This form of reconstruction is essentially a transplant, except that the tissue donor and the recipient are the same person. Useful donor sites have an area of tissue that is predictably supplied by an artery and vein, and that can be removed without leaving a major functional or aesthetic defect.

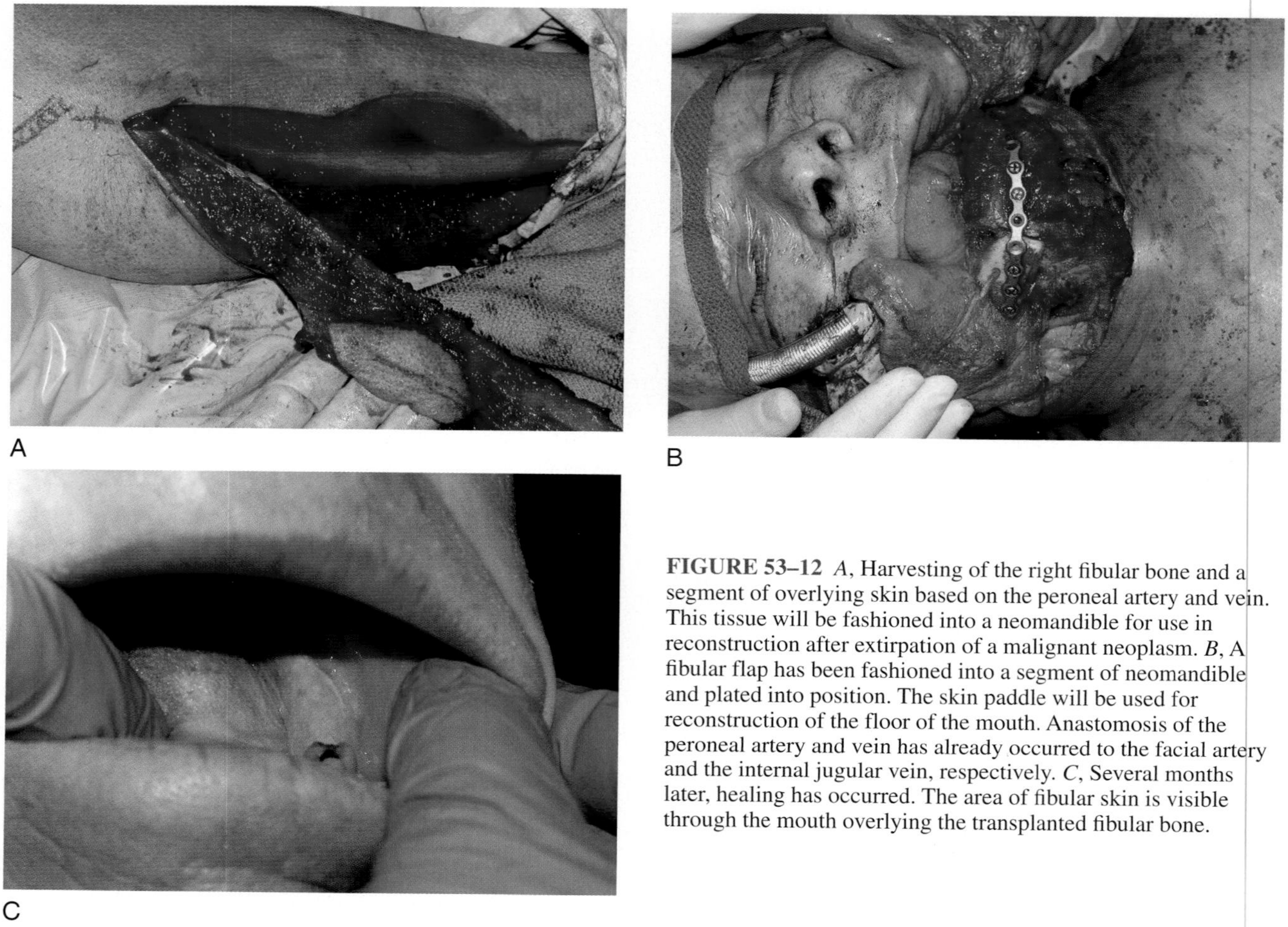

FIGURE 53–12 *A*, Harvesting of the right fibular bone and a segment of overlying skin based on the peroneal artery and vein. This tissue will be fashioned into a neomandible for use in reconstruction after extirpation of a malignant neoplasm. *B*, A fibular flap has been fashioned into a segment of neomandible and plated into position. The skin paddle will be used for reconstruction of the floor of the mouth. Anastomosis of the peroneal artery and vein has already occurred to the facial artery and the internal jugular vein, respectively. *C*, Several months later, healing has occurred. The area of fibular skin is visible through the mouth overlying the transplanted fibular bone.

PEARLS FOR ROUNDS

If a patient complains of significant pain or discomfort after rhytidectomy, it is neccessary to remove the dressing and check for a hematoma, as this will be the most common cause.

When a skin graft is placed, it receives nutrients and oxygen through three distinct stages: (1) imbibition (graft absorbs wound exudate); (2) inosculation (vascular buds in the wound connect to preexisting and new vascular channels in the skin graft); and (3) revascularization (new vessel growth).

In repair of mandible and midface fractures, wherever possible, make certain the patient's teeth are in proper occlusion at the outset of the case. This allows proper alignment of fractured fragments. When this is not possible, correct reduction can sometimes be accomplished by working down off of stable bone from the skull.

Mandibular reconstruction is often best accomplished with a free tissue transfer; flaps commonly used for the procedure include those from the fibula (Fig. 53-12), the iliac crest, and the scapula. These flaps transfer bone, muscle, and skin with an artery and vein, which are then reanastomosed to vessels in the neck. Other common free flaps include radial forearm flaps, lateral arm flaps, rectus abdominis muscle flaps, and gracilis muscle flaps.

Repair of Facial Fractures

Thanks to front and side airbags, laws mandating seat-belt and motorcycle-helmet use, and other safety innovations, people involved in even major motor vehicle collisions are more likely than ever to walk away with only minor injuries. However, facial fractures are still often sustained in these accidents, with nasal fractures being the most common.

These patients typically are first seen with epistaxis, nasal obstruction, and cosmetic deformity. In addition to determining if other fractures and injuries are present, the physician performing the initial assessment must evaluate the patient for hematoma of the nasal septum. If such a lesion is present, it must be drained rapidly. Blood accumulates between the septal cartilage and the perichondrium; however, the blood supply to the cartilage is delivered through the overlying perichondrium. The hematoma interferes with blood flow and can result in cartilage necrosis with resultant collapse of the nasal dorsum in what is known as a *saddle-nose deformity*. This type of deformity also can result from cartilage loss due to cocaine use or to Wegener's vasculitis.

Nasal fractures are diagnosed clinically. Except for medicolegal reasons, radiographic confirmation is required only rarely. The nose is tender, with a visible deformity, and typically feels mobile.

These fractures are treated with closed reduction, which involves replacing the nasal bones into position and then using an external cast or splint to hold them in anatomic position as they heal. The cast or splint is typically kept in place for 1 week. Because of swelling of the overlying nasal tissues, the closed reduction is best done either within the first hour after injury or after 7 to 10 days. After more than 2 weeks, closed reduction becomes difficult, as the bones begin to heal in their new position. Repair of the deformity after this time period is perhaps best accomplished by formal rhinoplasty several weeks later.

The zygomatic arch also is a common site of fracture, as the temporalis muscle passes beneath the arch en route to its insertion on the coronoid process of the mandible. Fractures of the zygomatic arch typically result in trismus and pain with movement of the mandible. Repair of the arch can be done through a small scalp incision over the temporalis muscle. An elevator is then passed deep to the superficial fascia of the temporalis muscle to prevent injury to the upper branches of the facial nerve. This elevator is then used to lift up the depressed fracture. A similar repair can be accomplished through a small intraoral incision.

The zygomaticomalar complex is commonly known as the cheekbone. The malar eminence has four primary osseous attachments: to the zygomatic arch, to the frontal bone at the zygomaticomaxillary suture line, along the inferior orbital rim, and to the maxilla in what is known as the lateral buttress. When the zygomaticomalar complex is fractured, the patient may have a flattened appearance to that side of the face. As the second branch of the trigeminal nerve passes through the infraorbital foramen in this region, numbness at the fracture site is common. A coexisting vision loss or orbital floor fracture must be sought. When the orbital floor is fractured, the globe can herniate inferiorly into the maxillary sinus. The entire globe does not usually fall, but some of the periorbital fat can pass down or the inferior rectus muscle can become entrapped in a fracture line along the floor, resulting in gaze restriction and diplopia. Inferior rectus entrapment can be detected by the forced duction test, in which the conjunctiva is anesthetized topically, and a forceps is used to grab its inferior fold in the midline, near the insertion of the inferior rectus. If the globe does not roll easily superiorly by pulling with forceps, inferior rectus entrapment is suspected.

Fractures of the zygomaticomalar complex that are minimal or not displaced can be watched, and the patient can be restricted to a soft diet. If the fracture is displaced or major, open reduction with internal fixation is performed. An intraoral incision is commonly used, although a brow, subciliary, or transconjunctival approach also may be required. After the fracture is exposed in the subperiosteal plane, it is reduced and held in position with small metal plates and titanium-alloy screws, which keep the bones in proper position while they heal. Although their necessity fades over subsequent weeks, they are typically never removed unless a problem such as infection or extrusion develops. Increasingly, absorbable plates and screws are being used. These provide strength for several weeks and then are absorbed gradually, leaving behind no foreign material.

Orbital floor fractures may require repair in which a segment of cartilage, gelatin film, bone, or a synthetic material is placed beneath the globe to prevent it or other orbital contents from herniating into the maxillary sinus through the fracture line. Care must be taken when shaping the implant so that it does not extend too far posteriorly and impinge on the important neurovascular structures of the orbit.

Mandibular fractures are another common facial fracture. These fractures generally occur in the subcondylar region, although any part of the mandible can become fractured. The most important aspect of the repair is to restore proper dental occlusion. Often, repair begins by placing the patient in maxillomandibular fixation, sometimes known as intermaxillary fixation, or, in common terms, as wiring the jaws shut. The fracture line can then be exposed through either an intraoral or a neck incision, and it can be held in proper reduction with metal plates and screws. Care must be taken not to place any screws into the tooth roots or the path of the mental nerve as it passes along the mandible toward the mental foramen on each side. If you have an interest in physics and geometry, you may be especially drawn to the study of proper plating techniques, as a detailed understanding of force vectors, physics, and mechanical properties greatly enhances the ability to repair mandibular fractures correctly.

The frontal sinus is another common site of facial fracture. This structure comprises two osseous "tables": an anterior table, which forms the visible external contour of the forehead, and an inner table, which forms the posterior wall of the sinus separating it from the cranial vault. Fractures that involve only the anterior table can be repaired by simple open reduction and internal fixation. However, fractures that pass through and disrupt the drainage passage of the frontal sinus, or those that substantially involve the posterior table, require a more elaborate repair. In these situations, it is likely that the frontal sinus will cease to function properly, resulting in chronic infections for the patient. Therefore the frontal sinus is eliminated when the repair is done. After removal of all mucosa from the sinus, the drainage passages are plugged, and either the sinus is filled (for example, with an abdominal fat graft to obliterate the space) or the posterior table is removed entirely. The latter process is known as sinus cranialization, as after being removed, the frontal sinus becomes part of the cranial vault. Dural tears are commonly encountered during repair of a posterior table fracture and must be repaired either primarily or with a fascia or other graft.

Maxillofacial Surgery

Maxillofacial osteotomies are considered routine procedures and are often performed for correction of congenital or acquired facial deformities. Indications for these procedures include craniofacial syndromes, dentoskeletal or traumatic facial deformities, and obstructive sleep apnea.

Although osteotomies of many facial bones are possible, the most common include those of the upper and lower jaws (orthognathic surgery). The Le Fort 1 osteotomy is the most frequently performed maxillary procedure; it involves separation of the maxilla from the nasal, maxillary sinus, and skull base areas (Fig. 53-13). The most commonly performed mandibular osteotomy is that of the sagittal split-ramus osteotomy, which involves splitting of the buccal and lingual cortices of the mandible (Fig. 53-14). Both procedures are performed with use of intraoral techniques

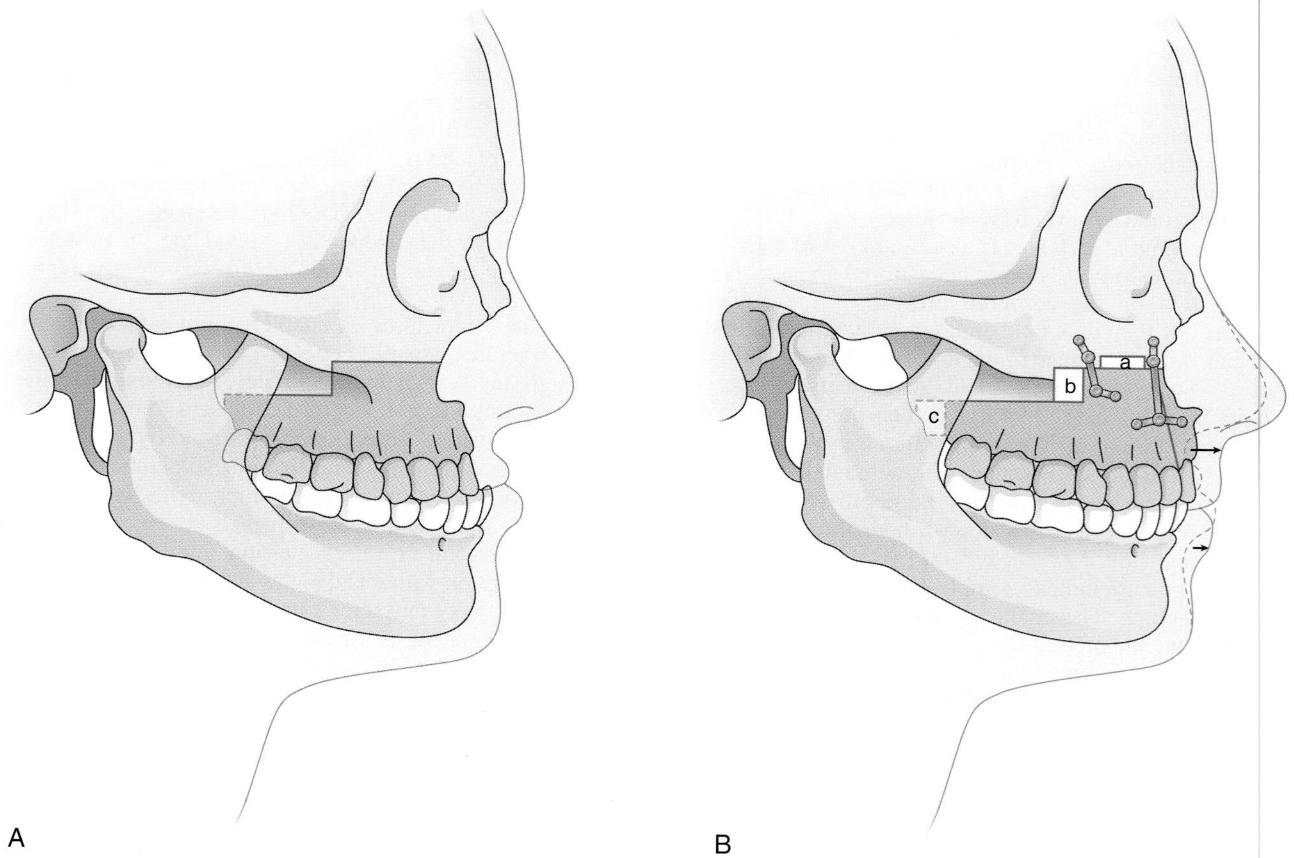

FIGURE 53–13 The Le Fort 1 osteotomy procedure. *A*, The maxilla is separated from the skull base at the level of the nasal pyriform rim (anteriorly) and the pterygomaxillary fossa (posteriorly). A vertical step is made at the level of the zygomatic buttress. *B*, The osteotomized maxilla is moved to its new position and stabilized with bone plates and screws in the lateral nasal wall and zygomatic buttress areas. Bone grafts (a, b, c) are often placed in the gaps to promote healing and maintain long-term stability.

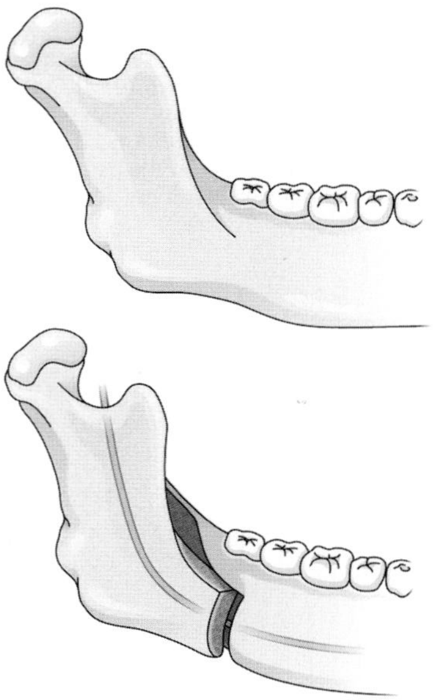

FIGURE 53–14 The sagittal-split osteotomy procedure. The mandible is split into buccal and lingual cortices, and the teeth-bearing segment can be advanced forward or backward, as desired.

and instrumentation and permit three-dimensional repositioning of the upper and lower jaws as required.

The surgery is initially planned on the basis of clinical and radiographic evaluations. The desired changes are mapped out on acetate tracings and then duplicated on dental-impression models to facilitate fabrication of surgical acrylic splints in the laboratory. The osteotomies are surgically completed in the operating room, and the prefabricated splints are used to position the jaws accurately.

In patients with extensive deformities, adjunctive procedures such as liposuction, rhinoplasty, facial augmentation, and genioplasty are often performed in combination with orthognathic surgery, either as a one-stage procedure or as secondary procedures at a later date (Fig. 53-15).

In conclusion, reading a single chapter on facial plastic surgery is analogous to seeing only the preview of an outstanding film. The most that could be accomplished in this chapter is to provide highlights of some of the many exciting and useful techniques that facial plastic surgeons have at their disposal to help improve or restore facial appearance and function. The future of this field is very bright, as new technologies continually inspire innovative surgeons to expand on and improve their offerings. As their armamentarium increases, so too do the benefits that patients can enjoy. The creative, clever student who

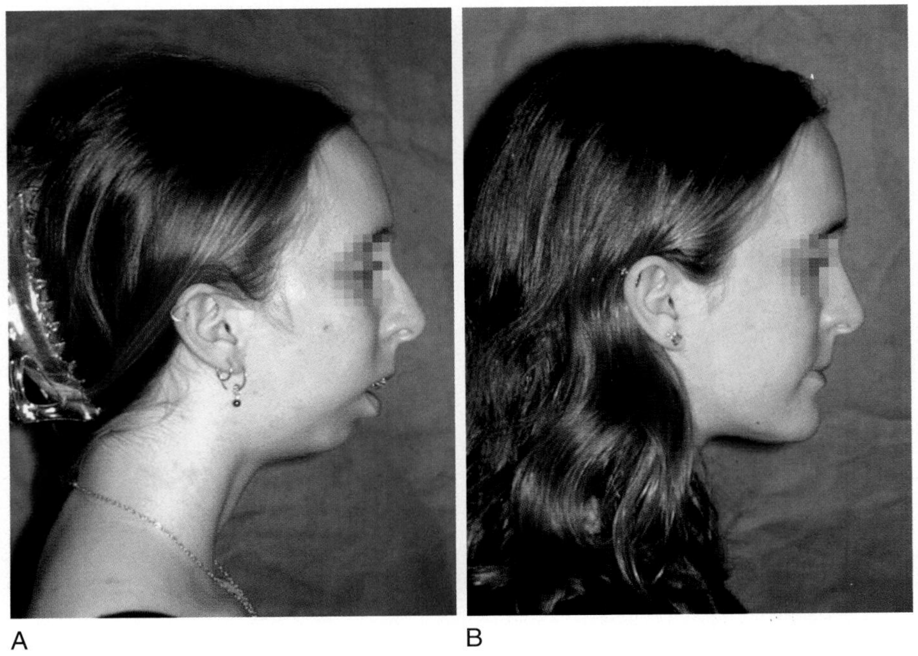

FIGURE 53–15 *A*, Preoperative view of the patient before complex facial reconstruction. *B*, Postoperative view of the patient after upper and lower jaw-advancement surgery.

chooses facial plastic surgery as a career is unlikely to be disappointed.

Acknowledgment

The authors thank Dr. Larry Wolford, Dallas, Texas, for photographs of patients from his practice.

Suggested Reading

Bradley DT, Park SS: Preoperative analysis and diagnosis for rhinoplasty. Facial Plast Surg Clin North Am 11(3):377–390, 2003.
Cheng ET, Perkins SW: Rhytidectomy analysis: Twenty years of experience. Facial Plast Surg Clin North Am 11(3):359–375, 2003.
Dayan SH, Bassichis BA: Evaluation of the patient for cosmetic Botox injections. Facial Plast Surg Clin North Am 11(3):349–358, 2003.

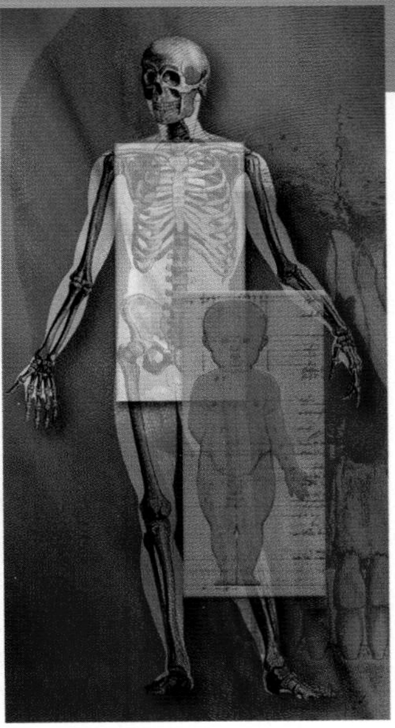

SECTION XIV

PEDIATRIC SURGERY

Chapter 54

Newborn and Pediatric Perioperative Care

ELIZABETH RENAUD, MD, HAROON I. PATEL, MD, and
STEVEN L. MOULTON, MD

Pediatric surgery is a broad-based subspecialty that encompasses a wide variety of procedures, including the correction of congenital malformations, the treatment of childhood cancers, transplantation, fetal surgery, and pediatric trauma. Management of pediatric surgical patients is based on a growing understanding of embryology, physiology, and pathology.

Terminology

Prematurity is defined as a gestational age of less than 37 weeks. Premature neonates can be further described as being **very low birth weight** (<1500 g) or **extremely low birth weight** (<1000 g). The smaller and more premature a newborn, the higher the likelihood of morbidity and mortality. Premature neonates are more likely to develop respiratory failure, circulatory problems, intracranial hemorrhage, sepsis, hyperbilirubinemia, and hypothermia than term neonates. The **neonatal period** begins at birth and extends through the first month of life. Newborns that are small for their gestational age have had **intrauterine growth retardation (IUGR)** due to maternal, placental, or fetal abnormalities. Newborns with IUGR are at increased risk for cardiopulmonary complications, hypoglycemia, dehydration, and problems related to congenital anomalies and infection. **Infants** are babies who are age 1 month to 1 year. **Congenital** refers to a condition present at birth and does not specify whether the problem is developmental or inherited. A **genetic** defect is an inherited condition that may or may not be apparent at birth.

Neonatal Physiology

Temperature Regulation

Neonates are at high risk for hypothermia because of their high surface area–to–body weight ratio. Persistent hypothermia can lead to metabolic acidosis because of a combination of decreased perfusion and increased metabolic demand. A vicious hypoxic cycle can develop when hypothermia induces pulmonary artery vasoconstriction, which increases right- to left-heart shunting via the ductus arteriosis. This, in turn, can lead to worsening hypoxemia and acidosis. To prevent heat loss, newborns should be bundled, and stressed neonates should be kept normothermic in temperature-controlled isolettes or radiant warmers. Surgical neonates are at added risk for hypothermia during transport and in the operating room, where the ambient temperature should increase and a warming blanket placed underneath the baby to maintain core body temperature as close to 37°C degrees as possible.

Cardiovascular Physiology

The fetal circulation is characterized by three shunts, all of which normally disappear after birth. These shunts, together with the high oxygen affinity of fetal hemoglobin, allow the fetus to cope with the relatively hypoxic environment of the womb. Oxygenated blood flows from the placenta through the umbilical vein and largely bypasses the liver via the ductus venosus (Fig. 54-1). It then flows into the inferior vena cava (IVC) and the right atrium. The two ventricles of the fetal heart work in parallel to supply blood to the systemic circulation.

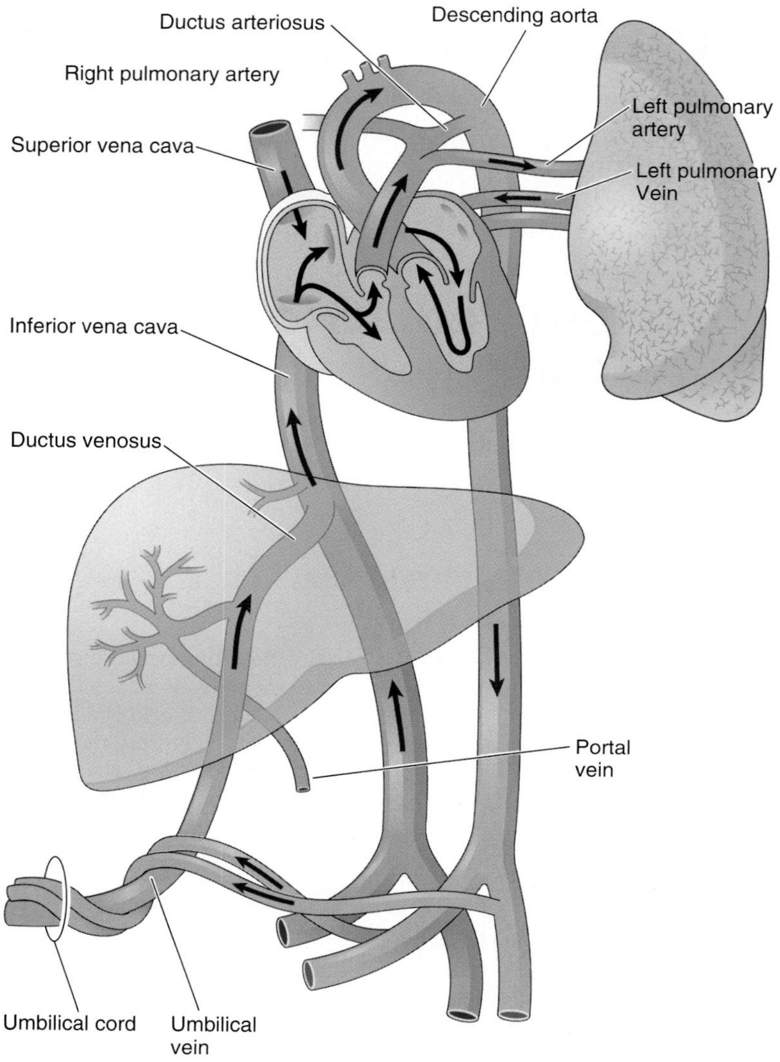

FIGURE 54–1 Fetal circulation.

A portion of the oxygenated blood entering from the IVC is shunted across the foramen ovale to the left side of the heart, where it is preferentially directed to the coronary circulation and the brain. The remainder enters the right ventricle, where it mixes with deoxygenated blood returning from the superior vena cava. Most of this mixed blood leaves the right ventricle and bypasses the remainder of the cardiac system and pulmonary vasculature by exiting through the ductus arteriosus, a communication between the pulmonary artery and the aorta. After exiting the ductus, blood circulates to the abdomen, lower extremities, and the placenta (see Fig. 54-1)

Multiple postnatal changes occur to transform the fetal circulation into the adult pattern (Fig. 54-2). At birth, the low-resistance placental circulation is removed; this event increases the overall resistance of the left ventricular outflow tract and the systemic circulation. Meanwhile, expansion of the lungs with the neonate's first breaths causes a marked reduction in the pulmonary vascular resistance. The change in the resistance patterns of the left and right ventricular outflow tracts functionally closes the foramen ovale. Although a degree of pulmonary hypertension still exists immediately after birth, pulmonary artery pressure is less than the aortic or systemic pressure. Any residual shunting across the ductus arteriosus is now from left to right, from the aortic to the pulmonary vasculature. Under normal circumstances, the increase in oxygen saturation of the blood that occurs at the time of birth both dilates the pulmonary vascular bed and closes the ductus arteriosus. These effects appear to be mediated by

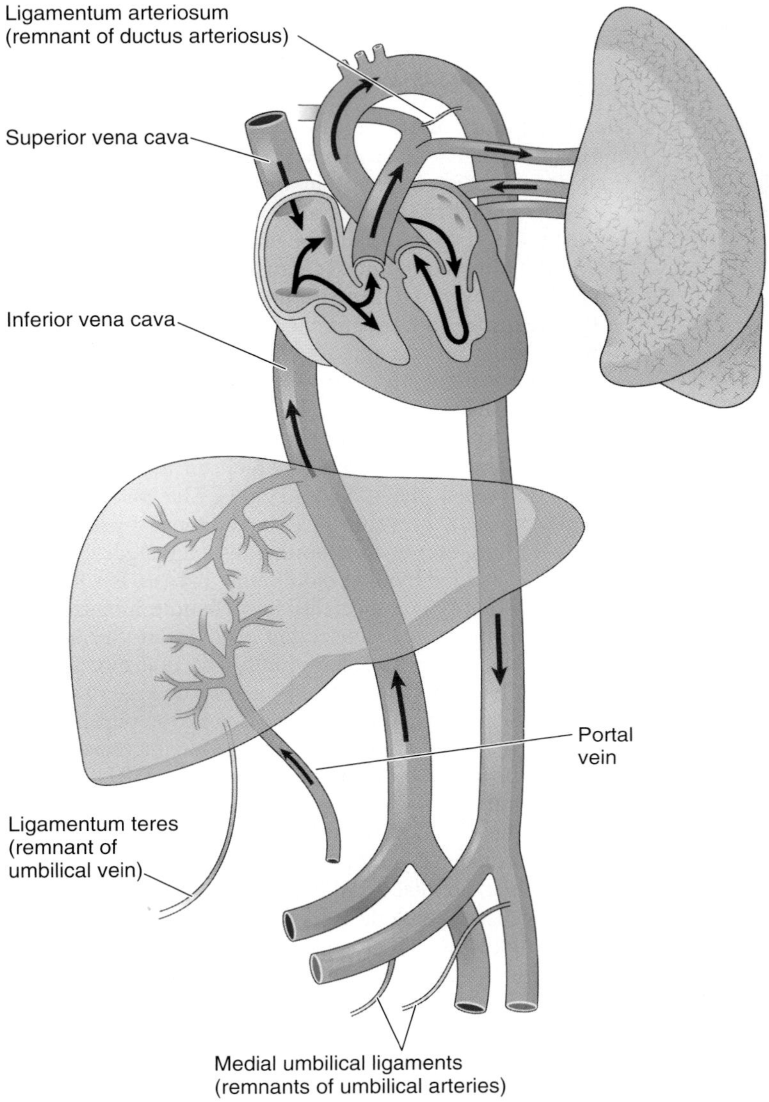

FIGURE 54–2 Adult circulation.

prostaglandins. Sometimes, however, the ductus arteriosus fails to close, particularly in premature neonates. These babies may have persistent shunting from left to right across the ductus; this shunting places them at risk for fluid overload and pulmonary edema. In contrast, neonates with persistent pulmonary hypertension due to prematurity, hypoxemia, or congenital cardiac anomalies may shunt from right to left and force already deoxygenated blood to bypass the pulmonary system and enter the systemic circulation, which can worsen hypoxemia. In either shunting situation, the patent ductus arteriosus may need to be closed pharmacologically with indomethacin or through surgical means.

The small ventricular size of the neonatal heart limits its capacity to respond to increases in diastolic volume (preload) with a commensurate increase in stoke volume. The primary mechanism for increasing cardiac output in neonates is therefore an increase in heart rate, rather than stroke volume. Neonates with congenital heart disease such as tetralogy of Fallot (TOF) and ventricular septal defect (VSD) are especially sensitive to physiologic stresses that tax cardiac reserve. A cardiac echocardiogram to rule out congenital cardiac anomalies is often included among the first preoperative tests for a neonate with a congenital anomaly that will require surgical correction, such as an omphalocele or a tracheoesophageal fistula.

PEARLS FOR ROUNDS

The fetal circulatory system uses the ductus venosus, the foramen ovale, and the ductus arteriosus to shunt oxygenated blood preferentially to the brain and upper body; these shunts close at or shortly after birth.

The oxyhemoglobin dissociation curve for fetal hemoglobin is shifted to the left, because of lower 2,3-DPG binding by fetal hemoglobin.

Total body water and extracellular fluid decrease between fetal life and adulthood, whereas intracellular water increases.

The functional immaturity of the newborn kidney predisposes the neonate to hypernatremia.

Associated congenital heart disease may complicate the timing of surgery and the administration of anesthesia.

Hemodynamic Monitoring and Support

Hemodynamic monitoring consists of readily measurable parameters such as heart rate and blood pressure, which vary by age (Table 54-1). An elevated heart rate is often the first indicator of volume depletion or blood loss. But unlike adults, in whom ongoing blood loss causes a steady decline in blood pressure, infants and children typically maintain their blood pressure until they experience blood loss greater than 40% of total blood volume. At this point, they may undergo rapid and irreversible decline. The management of hemodynamically unstable neonates includes optimization of volume status and, in some cases, various types of pharmacologic support. The latter may include the use of inotropes such as dopamine, dobutamine, and epinephrine. Conversely, critically ill neonates with pulmonary hypertension due to congenital diaphragmatic hernia or respiratory distress syndrome (RDS) may be treated with pulmonary vasodilators such as nitric oxide. Patients with cyanotic heart disease such as a hypoplastic left heart or transposition of the great vessels may benefit from continued patency of the ductus arteriosus to permit the delivery of oxygenated blood to the cerebral and systemic circulations. These neonates may be treated with prostaglandin E_1 to maintain ductus patency while they await more definitive surgical repair.

TABLE 54–1 Average Values for Normal Vital Signs

Age	Heart Rate	Respiratory Rate	Systolic BP (mmHg)
Premature infant	140	40	40–60
Term infant	120	40	80–100
1 yr	100	30	100
6 yr	80–100	20–30	100–120
12 yr	60–80	20	120

Respiratory Physiology

The respiratory tract begins as an outcropping of the embryonic gastrointestinal tract at 3 to 4 weeks of gestational age. As it elongates in front of the esophagus, it forms the trachea and bronchi. Complex interactions between the respiratory endoderm and the surrounding mesoderm direct continued branching of the secondary bronchi and eventual formation of the terminal alveoli. Both structural and functional components of the lung continue to grow and mature throughout pregnancy and well into postnatal life. The fetal lungs are incapable of adequate gas exchange before 23 to 24 weeks of gestational age, which is therefore the lower limit of extrauterine viability. This also is the point at which surfactant synthesis by type II alveolar pneumocytes begins. This phospholipid-rich glycoprotein prevents alveolar collapse by reducing surface tension, thereby promoting gas exchange.

RDS, also called hyaline membrane disease, is a leading cause of morbidity and mortality in premature infants. RDS results from inadequate surfactant production. Surfactant-deficient lungs are stiffer, less compliant, and more prone to microatelectasis than normal lungs. The risk of developing RDS is proportional to the degree of prematurity. Antenatal maternal steroid administration increases fetal surfactant production and reduces the risk of RDS. Early postnatal intratracheal administration of surfactant can further reduce RDS mortality. Additional therapeutic measures include oxygen and various types of ventilatory therapy, which are discussed later. Other causes of neonatal respiratory distress include aspiration of meconium, amniotic fluid, or blood; neonatal sepsis or pneumonia; asphyxia; pulmonary hypertension; pneumothorax; and anatomic pulmonary and cardiac malformations. Surgically treatable congenital anomalies such as tracheoesophageal fistula and small-bowel obstruction with polyhydramnios may be associated with respiratory distress and, depending on the underlying cause, respiratory compromise may affect the timing of surgery to correct a congenital malformation.

Signs of respiratory distress in the neonate include tachypnea, grunting respirations, flaring of the nasal alae, chest-wall retractions, and the use of accessory muscles or "abdominal breathing." Auscultation may reveal fine or coarse rales, rhonchi, and reduced air exchange. Asymmetrical breath sounds may indicate a pneumothorax, which can occur with aspiration syndromes because of a ball-valve effect of the aspirated material on the conducting airways. Infants in respiratory distress are placed on continuous cardiopulmonary monitors and pulse oximetry in a neonatal or pediatric intensive care unit. Initial clinical evaluation includes a careful history and physical examination followed by complete blood count (CBC) and blood culture, blood gas, and chest radiograph. The radiologic appearance of aspiration pneumonia is that of patchy or segmental pulmonary densities. Pneumonia also may be associated with the development of a pleural effusion.

Respiratory support can vary from simple oxygen therapy to complex forms of mechanical ventilation. Hood or nasal-cannula oxygen may be sufficient for mild to moderate respiratory distress. When these treatments prove inadequate, the next level of intervention is nasal or nasopharyngeal continuous positive airway pressure (CPAP) at 4 to 7 cm of water pressure. The failure of noninvasive respiratory support mandates endotracheal intubation and mechanical ventilation. Ventilation can be either volume or pressure limited. In general, alternative modes of ventilation should be sought when the peak inspiratory pressure approaches the patient's gestational age in weeks. More complex ventilatory options include high-frequency oscillatory and jet ventilation.

Antibiotic therapy is usually empirical. Additional pharmacologic agents may be added to increase lung compliance and thereby reduce barotrauma. Because meconium aspiration can cause inactivation of native surfactant, these patients may benefit from exogenous surfactant replacement. Nitric oxide (NO) can treat pulmonary hypertension by dilating the pulmonary vasculature and reducing lung inflammation. If NO fails for the patient, extracorporeal membrane oxygenation (ECMO) is an option for infants over 2 kg. Partial liquid ventilation is a novel technique that is currently undergoing clinical trials.

Renal Physiology

Total body water (TBW) is divided into intracellular and extracellular water compartments and accounts for about 80% of body weight at 32 weeks of gestation; it thereafter gradually decreases to about 70% at term. Neonates experience a relatively rapid 5% to 10% decrease in TBW during the first week of life. Preterm neonates, who have higher amounts of TBW than do those at term, are especially susceptible to the adverse effects of fluid overload during the first week of postnatal life, when they have not yet offloaded their excess water. Higher circulatory volumes can increase the likelihood of persistent patent ductus arteriosus, left ventricular failure, RDS, and necrotizing enterocolitis. TBW approaches adult levels (60% of body weight) by about age 1 year (Fig. 54-3).

The renal function of a neonate differs significantly from that of an adult. This is largely because the glomerular filtration rate (GFR) of a newborn is only one fourth that of an adult. Because renal potassium regulation is dependent on GFR, neonates and especially premature newborns are at risk for hyperkalemia. The neonatal kidney also has a lower tubular concentrating ability because of its decreased tubular sensitivity to antidiuretic hormone. Term infants can maximally concentrate their urine to approximately 600 mOsm/kg, whereas adults can concentrate their urine

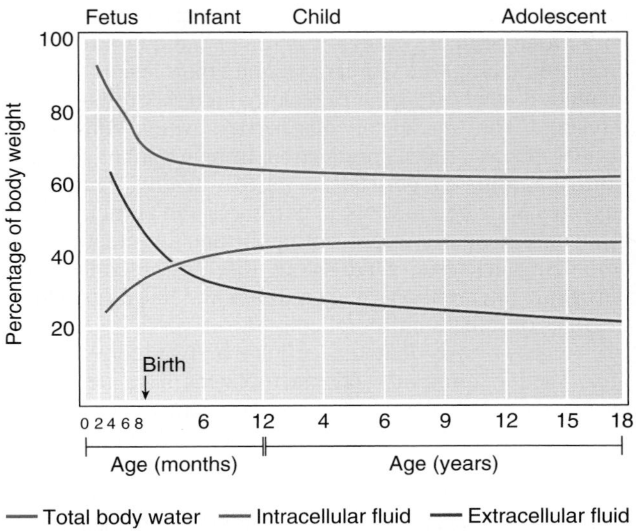

FIGURE 54–3 Distribution of extracellular and intracellular fluid by age.

to 1200 mOsm/kg. The neonatal kidney also can readily retain sodium, by excreting very dilute urine (as low as 30 mOsm/kg vs. 100 mOsm/kg in adults). These two features make the neonate prone to hypernatremia. Judicious fluid and electrolyte management is therefore an important consideration in any newborn who is not taking oral feeds. Five percent dextrose in water (D%W) is given in the first 24 hours, after which D5 0.25% normal saline with potassium should be started. Neonates should have an average urine output of 1 to 2 mL/kg/hr and a urine osmolality of approximately 250 mOsm/kg.

Hepatic Physiology

Newborns are susceptible to cholestasis and drug overdose because of their immature hepatic enzyme systems. For example, immaturity and thus deficiency of the glucuronyl transferase enzymes responsible for bilirubin conjugation and excretion can result in physiologic jaundice in the first weeks of life. Extreme cases of rapidly increasing unconjugated bilirubin levels may require phototherapy and, infrequently, exchange transfusion. The latter would be undertaken in an effort to prevent kernicterus, which is a type of central nervous system toxicity that is caused by the deposition of unbound bilirubin in the basal ganglia. Kernicterus can result in seizures, hearing loss, mental retardation, and cerebral palsy.

Immunology

Bacterial colonization begins at delivery. By age 3 days, the skin and upper respiratory tract are colonized with gram-positive organisms. By age 1 week, gram-negative and aerobic and anaerobic bacteria have colonized the gastrointestinal tract. Hospitalized infants are usually colonized with more virulent organisms and, depending on the flora present in their particular care unit and their level of instrumentation, they may be at especially high risk for systemic infection. The mucocutaneous barrier, which consists of normal mucosa, mucus production, immunoglobulins, local flora, coordinated peristalsis, gastric acidity, and other enzymes, may be too weak in newborns and particularly in premature neonates to prevent opportunistic infections by colonizing bacteria. Underlying disease processes and iatrogenic interventions, such as tubes and lines, can add to the risks of infectious complications.

Newborns have deficient cellular and humoral immunity. Their neutrophils and macrophages have decreased chemotactic and adhesive abilities; their complement system functions at 50% of adult capacity; and they exhibit diminished T-cell activity. Most neonates also have a relative immunoglobulin deficiency at birth, which increases their risk of infection by encapsulated organisms and viruses. In the first months of life, breast milk can compensate for many of these deficiencies. Breast milk contains polymorphonuclear white blood cells, macrophages, lymphocytes, complement, immunoglobulins, enzymes, lactoferrin, lysozyme, interferon, and many growth factors. Many of these factors contribute to passive protection of the infant, until its own immune system can mature.

Mortality rates due to infectious agents are moderately high, especially for preterm neonates and those with systemic infections (sepsis). The most common pathogens in the first weeks of life include group B *Streptococcus*, *Escherichia coli*, and *Listeria monocytogenes*. Infections occurring after this period in hospitalized newborns are usually nosocomial in origin and include coagulase-negative staphylococci, gram-negative enteric bacilli, and yeast. Clinical manifestations of sepsis in neonates include lethargy, irritability, oliguria, focal neurologic signs, jaundice, respiratory distress, apnea, feeding intolerance and abdominal distention, temperature instability, and cardiovascular collapse. The workup for sepsis in a newborn often requires a spinal tap, because approximately one third of neonates with sepsis have concomitant meningitis. The management of sepsis includes hemodynamic and respiratory support, empirical broad-spectrum antibiotic coverage, and later adjustment of antibiotic therapy based on microbiologic data.

Hematology

Premature neonates have an average blood volume of 100 mL/kg, whereas term newborns have an estimated blood volume of 80 to 85 mL/kg. Blood replacement is usually recommended if blood loss exceeds 10% of the estimated blood volume, although the threshold for transfusion will vary according to the initial hemoglobin concentration. Thus for a 3.2-kg neonate with a blood volume of 250 mL, an estimated blood loss of 25 mL at the time of surgery should trigger blood replacement. Blood loss is replaced with packed red blood cells in 10-mL/kg aliquots, each of which will increase the hematocrit by 3%.

Newborns are initially polycythemic with a hemoglobin of 15 to 20 g/dL. They subsequently develop a physiologic anemia between 3 and 5 months postpartum as they transition from fetal to adult hemoglobin. Platelet counts in neonates are similar to adult normal levels; however, if thrombocytopenia develops, one should be wary of an underlying systemic infection. Neonates may also have deficiencies of clotting factors V, XIII, and the vitamin K–dependent factors (II, VII, IX, and X). Vitamin K is routinely administered to all newborns to prevent hemorrhagic disease of the newborn. Neonates with persistent bleeding should be suspected of having an inherited coagulation disorder, vitamin K deficiency, a platelet disorder, or disseminated intravascular coagulation (DIC). Causes of bleeding abnormalities are evaluated through history, physical examination, and laboratory tests including prothrombin time (PT), partial thromboplastin time (PTT), fibrinogen, platelet count, and rarely, bleeding time.

PEARLS FOR THE OR

Metabolic alkalosis is caused by electrolyte loss and may occur with prolonged gastric suctioning or vomiting; metabolic acidosis is usually the result of poor tissue perfusion and lactic acidosis.

Parents are less troubled about the length of their child's incision than by its width and contour irregularities.

Parents will inspect the dressing you place on their child's wound and inevitably judge the skill and carefulness of the surgery that preceded it.

Pediatric Physiology

Pediatric Fluids and Electrolytes

Infants and young children experience greater insensible respiratory and transepithelial water loss than do their adult counterparts. Proper humidification of inspired air and maintenance of adequate ambient humidity can minimize these losses. Third-space losses represent the sequestration of fluid into extracellular tissue; they occur as the result of capillary leakage due to the inflammatory response caused by surgery and sepsis. These losses are associated with an overall decrease in circulatory volume despite a gain in weight. Patients with third-space losses require more fluid to replenish their intravascular volume depletion. Urine output (1 to 2 mL/kg/hr) and urine concentration are good indicators of overall fluid status and perfusion. Other methods of evaluating volume status include serial body weights, electrolyte panels, acid-base

TABLE 54–2 Approximate Composition of Body Fluids

Type of Fluid	Sodium	Potassium	Chloride	Bicarbonate	Replacement Fluid
Stomach	60	15	140	Minimal	0.45 NS
Pancreas	130	10	60	120	LR with HCO_3
Biliary	130	10	100	100	LR
Ileostomy	100	10	100	40	0.9 NS

measurements, and hemodynamic monitoring (pulse, blood pressure, and central venous pressure.) Intravenous fluid therapy is divided into three categories: resuscitation, maintenance, and replacement.

Resuscitation

The goal of fluid resuscitation is to correct existing deficits. These deficits can be estimated by obtaining a detailed patient history (volume of fluid lost through emesis or diarrhea, presence of fever) and performing a complete physical examination (evaluating hydration of mucous membranes, presence or absence of tears, heart rate, skin turgor, depression of anterior fontanel, changes in mental status, urine output, and concentration of urine). Resuscitation efforts should begin with a fluid bolus of isotonic normal saline (20 mL/kg). This can be repeated 2 or 3 times until the patient's vital signs or physical findings improve. Packed red blood cells (10 mL/kg) should be used in the setting of hypovolemia due to blood loss or anemia. Constant reevaluation of the patient's fluid status is essential to avoid overcorrection. Hypotonic fluids (D5W, 0.2%, 0.45%) should be avoided in the process of resuscitation to prevent iatrogenic hyponatremia. Dextrose-containing resuscitation fluids also should be avoided, as they can cause hyperglycemia and result in an osmotic diuresis, which can further exacerbate dehydration.

Maintenance

Maintenance fluid requirements can be estimated using the 4:2:1 rule, which is based on body weight:

Less than 10 kg: 4 mL/kg/hour
10 to 20 kg: add 2 mL/kg/hour to above value
More than 20 kg: add 1 mL/kg/hour to the above values

For example, a 22-kg child requires maintenance fluid of 62 mL/hour (40 mL for the first 10 kg, 20 mL for the next 10 kg, and 2 mL for the remaining 2 kg). The choice of maintenance fluid for the postoperative surgical patient varies depending on the patient's age and the clinical situation. Maintenance fluids are based on quarter (0.25) or half (0.45) normal saline with 5% dextrose; additional potassium and other electrolytes are added as needed. Normal saline (0.9%) should be avoided for protracted periods because it can result in a hyperchloremic acidosis if given in large volumes. Maintenance fluid rates may be increased in the postoperative period to account for unmeasured fluid losses, such as insensible and third-space losses.

Replacement

Replacement fluids are given for measured ongoing losses, including nasogastric tube losses, ileostomy output, and fluids from other tubes and drains (such as chest tubes and biliary drainage tubes). The composition of the output (Table 54-2) determines the character of the replacement fluid. These fluids are usually replaced milliliter per milliliter every 8 hours. Last, these recommendations for resuscitation, maintenance, and replacement serve only as guidelines. Frequent reevaluation of every child's fluid status is essential to avoid both under- and overhydration.

Nutrition

Pediatric nutritional requirements vary according to weight and age (Table 54-3). Planning must also consider the nutritional requirements of growth, especially in younger children. For example, the nongrowth nutritional needs of a preterm neonate are 50 to 60 kcal/kg/day; normal growth requires twice this amount. Stressed neonates and preterm neonates less than 1000 g will have even greater caloric

TABLE 54–3 Approximate Caloric Needs by Age

Age	Total Kilocalories (kcal/kg Body Weight)	Protein (g/kg Body Weight)	Fats (g/kg Body Weight)
Preterm infant	150	3.5	3.5
Term infant	120	3	3
1 yr	100	2.5	2.5
6 yr	70	2	2
12 yr	30	1.5	1

requirements. Carbohydrates (approximately 4 kcal/g) provide the majority of nonprotein calories; fats (9 kcal/g) provide the remainder. Essential fatty acids (linoleic acid and linolenic acid) should be supplemented at least twice weekly. Protein requirements are high during the first year of life to compensate for the infant's relative deficit in nitrogen content. Children require the same eight essential amino acids as adults (threonine, leucine, isoleucine, valine, methionine, lysine, tryptophan, phenylalanine), plus histidine. Newborn infants require these nine essential amino acids, plus cysteine and tyrosine; premature infants require all of these plus taurine.

Nutrition can be provided either enterally or parenterally. Enteral nutrition is the preferred method; however, some clinical situations, such as the inability to swallow or prolonged gastroparesis may limit the use of oral feeds. In these situations, enteral feeds may be given via a nasogastric, nasoduodenal, gastrostomy, or jejunostomy tube. If available, the best "formula" is breast milk; it is well tolerated and provides 20 kcal/ounce, which is about the same as most commercially available formulas. Infants and children who are unable to tolerate enteric feeds, for example, those with necrotizing enterocolitis, pancreatitis, or short-bowel syndrome, can be sustained with total parenteral nutrition (TPN) for prolonged periods. While receiving TPN, these patients require monitoring of catheter position with periodic radiographs and evaluation of electrolytes, trace elements, and vitamins with frequent laboratory testing.

Perioperative Care

Surgery is a stress-provoking event for children and their families. To alleviate this stress and make the experience more enjoyable, many institutions employ Child Life Specialists (CLSs) to provide preoperative counseling, visual preparation, play therapy, and accompaniment in the operating room. CLSs are well versed in childhood development and especially trained to recognize and address the emotional needs of children and their families. During visual preparation in the surgeon's office they use age-appropriate material to inform children about what will happen before, during, and after surgery. The children are encouraged to ask questions and express any fears they may have, so that misconceptions can be cleared up well before the day of surgery.

On the morning of surgery, the CLS meets each family member, gauges the level of anxiety, allays fear, and offers developmentally age-appropriate toys to the children. Toys divert attention and oftentimes lead to an activity that the children can share with their parents while waiting to enter the operating room. Minor dressing supplies, caps, and masks also may be offered. These items are provided well ahead of time to allow the children to touch, feel, and smell them in a safe, nonthreatening environment. Younger children whose anesthesia will be induced with an inhalation agent are asked to smell and choose a pleasing flavor, which is then used to coat the inside of their anesthetic mask.

For straightforward cases, parents may be invited into the operating room to comfort their child during the induction of anesthesia. This policy avoids separation of parent and child at the most stressful point during the entire operative process. To make this work, parents must be provided with information about what they might see, experience, and feel during their child's induction. Inhalational agents cause children to go through multiple stages of anesthesia, including an excitatory stage, during which they can appear quite agitated. This can be alarming and frightening to parents if they are not well prepared. All of this preparatory effort by the CLS lets the parents know that someone is looking out for them and their child, helping to facilitate the operative experience.

Infants may need to be premedicated with anticholinergic agents to prevent bradycardia, which can occur during induction. Induction of anesthesia is commonly performed by using inhalation anesthetics such as nitrous oxide and halothane. An intravenous peripheral line is placed after induction for delivery of other medications to maintain anesthesia. Regional anesthesia (spinal anesthesia, epidural, and caudal anesthesia) also may supplement general anesthesia or can be used exclusively in some children, with great benefit to the patient. For example, premature infants often undergo hernia repair under a spinal anesthetic; this permits a quicker recovery and less postoperative apnea. The combination of general and regional anesthesia can also provide a "lighter" general anesthesia and prolonged postoperative pain control.

Suggested Reading

Chesney RW, Zelikovic I: Pre- and postoperative fluid management in infancy. Pediatr Rev 11:153, 1989.

Gregory GA, ed: Pediatric anesthesia, 2nd ed. New York, Churchill Livingstone, 1990.

Lee H, Jain L: Physiology of infants with very low birth weight. Semin Pediatr Surg 9(2):50, 2000.

Mahaffey SM: Neonatal and pediatric physiology. In Greenfield LJ, Mulholland M, Oldham KT, et al (eds): Surgery: Scientific Principles and Practice, 2nd ed. Philadelphia, Lippincott-Raven, 1997.

Polin RA, Fox WW (eds): Fetal and Neonatal Physiology, 3rd ed. Vol. 1. Philadelphia, WB Saunders, 2003.

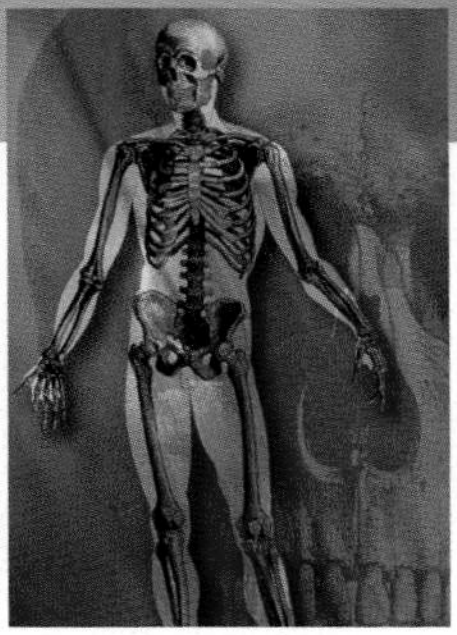

Chapter 55

Pediatric Trauma and Burns

STEVEN L. MOULTON, MD

Demographics

Trauma is the second leading cause of hospitalization for children and the number one cause of childhood death. Each year in the United States, more than 100,000 children are permanently disabled, and nearly 10,000 children die because of traumatic injury. Blunt trauma is the most common mechanism of childhood injury. Motor vehicle–related injuries are the leading cause of fatal trauma in childhood, with head injuries causing the majority of motor vehicle–related fatalities.

Patterns of and Response to Injury in Children

Clear differences exist between children and adults in the patterns of injury they sustain, as well as their physiologic and emotional responses to injury. The most prominent part of a young child's anatomy is the head, which is the point of initial impact in the majority of blunt pediatric injuries. A young child's head is supported by relatively underdeveloped musculature and ligaments of the neck. Young children are therefore at risk for upper (atlanto-occipital and C1-C3), lethal, cervical spine injuries, whereas older children and adults tend to have lower cervical spine injuries (C4-C8). As children become older and taller, their torsos reach the level of automobile fenders and bumpers, making torso injuries more common. Blunt impact on a child's torso can lead to significant injury with little evidence of external trauma, because of the resilient nature of the incompletely calcified skeleton. Deformation of the skeleton, along with diminished body fat and close proximity of a child's organs can therefore lead to severe, multiple organ injuries.

A child's physiologic response to injury is typically rapid and compensatory. The duration of compensation, however, is typically shorter in children than adults. This is partly due to the small size of the pediatric heart and its limited capacity to increase stroke volume. As a result, cardiac output (stroke volume × heart rate) in young children is almost entirely dependent on heart rate. Thus monitoring heart rate is a fairly accurate means of measuring the adequacy of volume replacement in a child. Hypotension is a late sign of shock in children and therefore an indication of extreme blood loss.

Adjusting and controlling the rate and quantity of resuscitation fluid in infants and children requires close monitoring to avoid under-resuscitation or fluid overload. Transfusion of large quantities of intravenous fluids or cold blood may cause hypothermia. The increased surface area/body weight ratio of children puts them at greater risk for heat loss and evaporative water loss. Young children have particularly thin skin and a relative absence of insulating fat. These conditions promote hypothermia and can lead to an increase in O_2 consumption, as the metabolic rate increases to maintain normal temperature. This can lead to lactic acidosis, a decrease in myocardial contractility, worsening acidosis, and coagulopathy. It is important, therefore, to keep children covered with warm blankets, to warm large transfusion volumes, and to keep the resuscitation suite and operating room temperatures above 75°F (24° C).

Resuscitation

Resuscitation of a pediatric trauma victim is best carried out at a facility committed to providing appropriately trained pediatric staff, equipment, and support services. In a pediatric setting, instrumentation and therapy are tailored in accordance with variable patient size, injury severity, and psychological makeup. The team leader focuses on establishing an adequate airway, while an associate confirms or establishes IV access. If the child is conscious, a calm, friendly approach provides comfort and emotional support in the setting of pain and unfamiliar surroundings. If the child is unconscious with a Glasgow Coma Score (GCS) of eight or less or has evidence of respiratory difficulty, preparations should be made for endotracheal intubation. This prevents airway obstruction, improves oxygenation and ventilation, and decreases the risk of aspiration.

The child's head should be kept in a neutral position during airway management. This is best accomplished by assigning an individual to hold the head and neck. Children younger than 2 years should be immobilized on a spine board with the torso on a folded blanket, to keep the head and cervical spine in alignment with the axial spine. Positioning in this manner compensates for occipital bossing, which causes neck flexion. The airway can be opened by positioning the child's head slightly forward in the "sniffing position." The mouth and pharynx are suctioned, and oxygen is provided in preparation for intubation. The use of rapid-sequence medications is preferred to minimize the risks of vomiting and intracranial hypertension.

As soon as a secure airway and ventilatory support have been established, the patient's circulation should be assessed. The presence of hypovolemic shock is usually clinically apparent. Infants and young children who are in shock tend to have mottling of the skin, cool and pale extremities, poor capillary refill, a rapid and thready pulse, poor heart sounds, and a diminished neurologic response in the absence of head injury. The neck veins are usually collapsed. If they are distended, an intrathoracic injury should be suspected, especially a tension pneumothorax. This may be difficult to diagnose clinically in a small child, as breath sounds are widely transmitted. If the situation is acute, needle decompression followed by tube thoracostomy on the suspected side is usually a safe course to follow. It is essential, however, to differentiate a pneumothorax from a right or left mainstem intubation. If pericardial tamponade is suspected as a cause for jugular venous distention, a pericardiocentesis is indicated.

Venous access is first attempted by using the veins on the back of the hands. If venous access cannot be achieved here, antecubital, femoral, and subclavian attempts should follow in that order. If venous access cannot be gained quickly, intraosseous access is a quick and reliable—but temporary—means to achieve rapid administration of resuscitation fluid and medications (Box 55-1). Fluid resuscitation in children is monitored by observing the heart rate and blood pressure, and periodically assessing perfusion (capillary refill, absence of skin mottling, urine output >1 mL/kg/hr, and central venous pressure 5 to 10 mmHg). The most common cause of persistent shock in children is acute blood loss from intracavitary bleeding, external bleeding, or an extremity injury. Neurogenic shock should be considered if hypovolemic shock can been ruled out and suspicion exists of a spinal cord injury.

BOX 55-1 Maintenance and Resuscitation Fluids for Children

Maintenance fluids

Infant 0–10 kg = 100 mL/kg D5 0.2NS with KCl 10 mEq/500 mL
Next 10 kg = 50 mL/kg D5 0.45NS with KCl 20 mEq/1000 mL
Adult = 30 mL/kg D5 0.45NS with KCl 20 mEq/1000 mL

Resuscitation fluids

Infants and children = 20 mL/kg LR × 2, then PRBCs 10 mL/kg prn
Adults = 1000 mL LR × 2, then PRBCs 10 mL/kg prn

Management

Pediatric Head Injuries

Central nervous system injury is the most devastating component of childhood trauma. It is the leading cause of death of the injured child and produces immeasurable suffering, in terms of both functional disability and diminished quality of life for the patient and family. It is generally accepted, however, that children have a lower risk of mortality from head injury than do their adult counterparts. One reason for this is the higher incidence of mass lesions such as subdural and epidural hematomas in adult patients, as opposed to children, who are more likely to have diffuse cerebral edema and contusions.

It is well accepted that brain injuries can be categorized as primary or secondary. Primary injuries are those inflicted immediately by the trauma and include skull fractures, contusions, or lacerations of the brain; subarachnoid hemorrhage; and hematomas. Secondary injuries are a result of ischemia, hypoxia, hypotension, infection, hydrocephalus, or increased intracranial pressure due to cerebral edema or intracerebral or extra-axial blood collections or both. Secondary injuries caused by hypoxia and hypotension are independently associated with significant increases in morbidity and mortality from head injury. Thus optimal management of severe closed head injury should be directed toward prevention of further secondary damage by providing adequate oxygenation, ventilation ($Paco_2$ = 34 ± 2 torr), and volume resuscitation in an appropriately monitored setting.

Shaking is a prevalent cause of intracranial injury in infants and young children. It is associated with intracranial hemorrhage, cervical spinal cord injury, and intraocular injuries. When an infant is shaken, the head moves in a complex oscillatory pattern. As oscillation proceeds, the brain may be moving in one direction while the skull is moving in the opposite. Impact of the brain against the skull, along with tearing of the bridging veins, causes cerebral contusions and intracranial bleeding. Shaking may be inflicted in combination with an impact injury, giving rise to the term "shake/slam syndrome." Accompanying fractures of the skeletal system are identified in up to 50% of cases of abusive head injury. Their presence, if properly documented, is powerful evidence of an abusive etiology of injury, as is the presence of retinal hemorrhages. Retinal hemorrhages can occasionally be seen after a prolonged increase in intracranial pressure and after cardiopulmonary resuscitation. For these reasons, it is imperative that an ophthalmologic examination be done as early as possible in the child's hospital course.

Pediatric Thoracic Trauma

A young child's ribs are extremely pliable. Compression of a child's chest may therefore cause major internal injury with little evidence of external injury and no fracture of the bony thorax. The greater mobility of a child's mediastinum may compound the degree of internal injury. This is particularly true of the infant, in whom wide shifts of the mediastinum can dislocate the heart or angulate and rupture the great vessels or major airways. The consequences of these pronounced cardiopulmonary derangements can be life threatening, owing to major blood loss or air leak into one or both hemithoraces.

Lung contusions are the most frequent intrathoracic injuries in children. They are often accompanied by lacerations of the lung parenchyma and are frequently associated with pneumothorax, hemothorax, or both. First-rib fractures and multiple rib fractures indicate more significant blunt chest trauma. Consider a computed tomography (CT) scan of the chest in a child with any one of the following conditions:

- Opacified hemithorax on initial chest radiograph
- Unexplained physiologic shunt (Po_2 <50 on 100% Fio_2)
- First or multiple rib fractures
- Unexpected pneumothorax on an abdominal CT for trauma
- Possible mediastinal widening on the initial chest radiograph in a stable patient.

Injuries to the great vessels are rarely seen in children. Most children with these injuries die in the field after ejection from a motor vehicle or a high-speed auto-versus-pedestrian accident. Tracheobronchial injuries also are rare. Most chest injuries in children occur concomitant with head or abdominal trauma. Thus all children with significant trauma to the chest require a thorough neurologic examination and appropriate studies to rule out intraabdominal injury.

Pediatric Abdominal Trauma

One of the principal differences between pediatric and adult abdominal trauma is the observation that children with solid-organ injuries are more likely to stop bleeding without operation than are their adult counterparts. CT evaluation provides an accurate assessment of the degree of solid-organ injury and the extent of hemoperitoneum or blood loss; however, for both liver and spleen injuries, the hemodynamic status of the child is the most accurate predictor of the need for operative intervention. Guidelines for nonoperative management of blunt abdominal trauma include accurate radiographic assessment, careful fluid management with transfusion of less than 40 mL/kg (one-half of the total blood volume) over the first 24-hour period, serial examinations and laboratory blood work, as well as a high index of suspicion for occult injury. Associated hollow viscus injuries tend to be first seen with early fever, abdominal distention, and subsequent peritonitis. Bile duct injuries, which occur in 3% to 4% of children with blunt liver injuries, can appear days or weeks after the initial injury with persistent abdominal pain, low-grade fever, ileus, biliary ascites, or jaundice.

The pancreas can be crushed or lacerated when a high-riding lap belt or handlebar compresses it against the underlying spinal column. Optimal CT scan evaluation of a suspected pancreatic injury should include oral contrast and fine cuts through the pancreas. Most children with pancreatic injuries can be managed nonoperatively; however, those with transection of the main pancreatic duct in the midbody or tail of the pancreas are probably best managed with a spleen-preserving distal pancreatectomy. Complications of both operative and nonoperative management include pseudocyst formation, pancreatic fistula, and diabetes. Pseudocysts that are larger than 10 cm can be treated with internal or percutaneous drainage; those smaller than 10 cm usually resolve spontaneously. Children with pancreatic duct injuries who are managed nonoperatively and who require long-term total parenteral nutrition are at risk for electrolyte disturbance, central venous catheter infection, and chronic pain syndromes.

Children with major renal injuries typically are first seen with flank pain and gross hematuria. Most can be managed nonoperatively, regardless of whether CT scan evidence of urinary extravasation is found. Operative management of a renal injury due to hemodynamic instability usually leads to loss of the kidney. All patients with renal injuries, especially those with high-grade injuries, require long-term follow-up with blood pressure monitoring and serial renal ultrasound evaluation of the collecting systems.

PEARLS FOR ROUNDS

The pediatric airway is more anterior, shorter, and more fragile than the adult airway.

Cardiac output in children is dependent primarily on heart rate. Corollary: Tachycardia usually indicates hypovolemia.

Optimal management of closed head injury includes prevention of secondary brain injury.

Prolonged arterial spasm is the most common presentation of pediatric vascular injury.

The duration of submersion in a near-drowning accident is the most important factor associated with intact survival; survival after prolonged submersion (>5 minutes) is closely related to water temperature.

Pediatric Orthopedic Trauma

The timing of fracture fixation for the multiply injured child is controversial, just as it is for the multiply injured adult trauma patient. Early fracture fixation in the adult population has been shown to decrease pulmonary complications and may limit the systemic inflammatory response to injury. However, in the setting of severe head injury or multiple blunt trauma, the risks of intraoperative hypotension and hypoxia during the orthopedic procedure may outweigh the benefits of early fracture stabilization. In many cases, the clinical judgment of the pediatric trauma and orthopedic surgeons must be relied on to decide the optimal timing for operative orthopedic intervention.

Pediatric Vascular Trauma

Prolonged arterial spasm is the most common presentation of vascular injury in childhood. It is important to remember, however, that spasm usually resolves within 3 hours. Vigilance and repeated examinations during this period may help to uncover a false sense of vessel integrity and avoid delay in the diagnosis and treatment of a surgically correctable lesion. Adults who experience sudden disruption of arterial flow usually have signs of limb hypoperfusion, followed by rapid onset of soft tissue ischemia. Children, in contrast, usually have adequate collateral flow to maintain tissue viability, but *insufficient* collateral flow for normal growth and development of the involved limb. Thus many infants and children are able to overcome an initial vascular insult only to demonstrate significant limb-length discrepancy months to years after the original injury.

Immediate surgical exploration is warranted if the patient has a penetrating vascular injury with obvious signs of vascular compromise, such as absent or diminished pulses, active bleeding, an expanding or pulsatile hematoma, a bruit or thrill, or evidence of distal ischemia. Fasciotomy should be considered whenever prolonged arterial inflow occlusion has occurred. Any child with blunt injury to a limb and clear-cut signs of vascular compromise should undergo arteriography because of the potential for widespread tissue damage. Children with soft signs of vascular injury, such as a stable hematoma, injury to an anatomically related nerve, unexplained hypotension, a history of hemorrhage, or injury in proximity to a major vessel, should be observed for 24 hours. In specific cases, such as in children younger than 2 years who do not have limb-threatening ischemia, as well as those who are especially ill but under close observation, it may be reasonable to observe some arterial lesions with the expectation that spontaneous resolution will occur.

Pediatric Drowning and Near-Drowning

Death from drowning is the second leading cause of traumatic death in children. Infants are most likely to drown in bathtubs, young children in swimming pools, and older children and adolescents in natural bodies of fresh water. Near-drowning implies submersion followed by survival, wherein the duration of submersion is the most important factor associated with intact survival. In general, survival after prolonged submersion (>5 minutes) is closely related to water temperature. Cold-water submersion promotes rapid brain cooling, a process that is facilitated by a young child's large surface area-to-mass ratio. Rapid cooling may be further enhanced by early aspiration of cold water with heat exchange via the pulmonary circulation. Outcome is further improved if mouth-to-mouth resuscitation is begun by on-site individuals. Children with mental-status changes who are arousable have a better than 90% survival rate without neurologic compromise, whereas those who arrive at a hospital comatose have a 70% survival rate, of which fewer than 50% will be neurologically intact.

PEARLS FOR THE OR

A child's trachea is soft and pliable; use care when handling or incising it.

Insertion of central venous catheters in children is the same as that for adults, except that the tolerance for error is less.

A child's chest wall is thin, and the chest cavity is small; use care when inserting chest tubes.

Hemodynamic status is the most accurate predictor of the need for transfusion or operative management or both of a pediatric solid-organ injury.

A child with a lap-belt mark and an abdominal computed tomography scan showing free fluid, but no solid organ injury, has a hollow viscous injury until proven otherwise.

Pediatric Burns

Burns are the third leading cause of traumatic death in children. The majority of pediatric burn deaths are caused by house fires. Scald burns are much more common in children and are generally more superficial. Burns are classified according to their depth:

First-degree burns involve the epidermis only and produce erythema, such as a sunburn.

Second-degree burns are partial-thickness burns that involve the dermis; they are generally described as superficial or deep. Second-degree burns usually blister and are extremely painful.

Third-degree burns penetrate the full thickness of the dermis to the subcutaneous tissue; the skin is typically leathery and insensate.

The "rule of nines" that is used to calculate the percentage of total body surface area (TBSA) burned does not accurately apply to children because of their proportionately larger head and smaller leg sizes. Instead, a Lund and Browder chart should be used, totaling all second- and third-degree burns to estimate the percentage burned (Fig. 55-1).

Fluid resuscitation during the first 24 to 48 hours after burn injury can prevent hypovolemia, reduce the incidence of renal failure, and decrease the mortality rate. The most widely used formula for estimating the amount of fluid required to resuscitate a burned child is the Galveston formula, which is based on the body surface area (BSA) of the child. For older children and adults, the Parkland formula—which is based on body weight—is more commonly used (Box 55-2). The amount of fluid given during the resuscitation phase is adjusted according to the patient's physiologic response, as measured by the vital signs, urine output (1 mL/kg/hr),

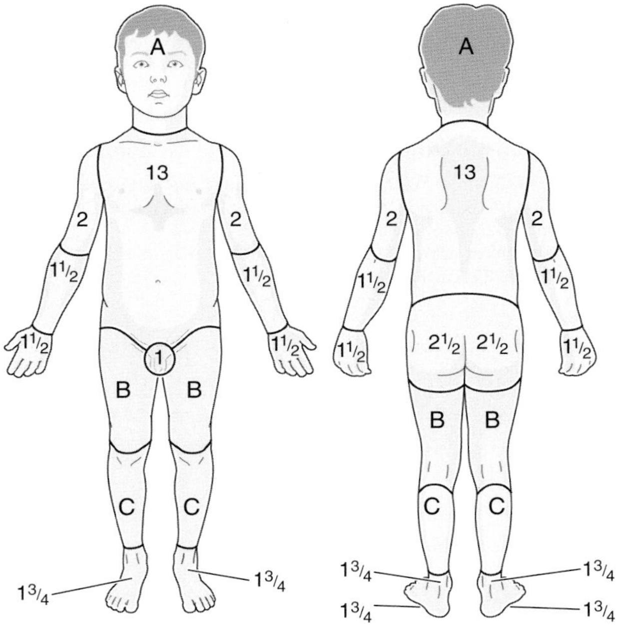

Age (yr)	<1	1	5	10	15	Adult
A half of head	$9\frac{1}{2}$	$8\frac{1}{2}$	$6\frac{1}{2}$	$5\frac{1}{2}$	$4\frac{1}{2}$	$3\frac{1}{2}$
B half of thigh	$2\frac{3}{4}$	$3\frac{1}{4}$	4	$4\frac{1}{4}$	$4\frac{1}{2}$	$4\frac{3}{4}$
C half of leg	$2\frac{1}{2}$	$2\frac{1}{2}$	$2\frac{3}{4}$	3	$3\frac{1}{4}$	$3\frac{1}{2}$

FIGURE 55–1 Lund Browder chart to estimate pediatric burn size.

central venous pressure (5 to 10 mmHg), and base deficit. Fluid requirements during the initial resuscitation may be higher or lower, depending on the depth of the burn and whether there are other, concomitant injuries.

An inhalation injury may be present with a history of exposure to smoke in a confined space, loss of consciousness, an impaired mental status, or head injury. Obvious clinical signs include flame burns to the face or soot about the nostrils. Other signs of an airway burn include hoarseness, stridor, wheezing, and carbonaceous sputum production. Oxygen should be given and an arterial blood gas obtained, including a carboxyhemoglobin (COHb) level. If the COHb is greater than 10%, an inhalation injury is suspected, and 100% oxygen should be given to wash out the carbon monoxide.

Superficial (first- and second-degree) burns are treated with topical agents until re-epithelialization occurs. These agents include synthetic materials (e.g., Biobrane, or hydrocolloid dressings for small burns), composite materials (e.g., TransCyte), and topical antimicrobials, such as mafenamide acetate (Sulfamylon) or silver sulfadiazine (Silvadene). The burn wound should be cleansed and dressed once or twice per day. Clean technique is used, and sterile dressings are applied to reduce the risks of burn-wound infection and the conversion of a partial-thickness burn into a full-thickness wound. Intact blisters are generally left alone. Third-degree burns and occasional deep second-degree burns mandate early burn-wound excision and grafting (24 to 48 hours after burn injury), not only for reasons of infection control, but also to reduce blood loss during the procedure when compared with that at a later time. The most favorable coverage for the excised wound is an autologous skin graft; however, temporary coverage with homograft or heterograft skin may be necessary until enough autologous skin can be cultured or regenerated. Intravenous antibiotics are used for perioperative prophylaxis, suspected pulmonary infection, or sepsis, but not for the burn wound in general, as this tissue is poorly perfused, and antibiotic delivery is unreliable.

BOX 55–2 Calculation of Resuscitation Fluid Requirements for Burns

Children

Galveston Lactated Ringer's 5000 mL/m^2 BSA burn + 2000 mL/m^2, 1/2 during the first 8 hr after burn, other 1/2 over next 16 hr period

Adults

Parkland Lactated Ringer's 4 mL/kg/% burn, 1/2 during the first 8 hr after burn, other 1/2 over next 16 hr period

Children with extensive burns require early nutritional supplementation to counteract the hypermetabolic burn response, which is marked by an increase in cardiac output and an increase in resting energy expenditure. Rehabilitation may be prolonged and often includes the use of compressive, elastic garments or silicon sheeting to limit hypertrophic scarring of the burn wound. Psychological problems are common after severe burn injury. Post-traumatic stress disorder (PTSD) in particular may arise from the injury or the dressing-change experience. Symptoms of this disorder include intrusive recollections and hyperarousal. Ultimately, PTSD can interfere with a child's social, educational, and biologic development.

Outcome

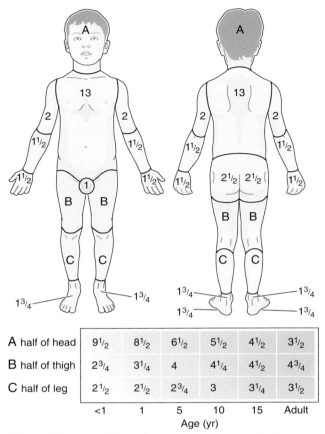

A major consideration in dealing with injured children is the effect that injury may have on subsequent growth and development. Recent evidence suggests that the majority of children who sustain severe multisystem trauma have residual personality changes at 1 year after hospital discharge, whereas half show cognitive and physical handicaps. Severely disabled children may require years of custodial or institutional care, and others have the misery of a life-long functional impairment. Childhood injuries have a significant impact on the family structure as well. Personality and emotional disturbances are seen in two thirds of uninjured siblings. A child's injuries also can strain a family's marital relationship, forcing financial and sometimes employment hardships. Thus how a family responds to a child's injuries may affect the structure and quality of family life for years to come.

Injury Prevention

Considering the devastating impact that childhood injuries may have on the child and his or her family, the physicians and nurses involved in the care of injured children have an obligation to be engaged in efforts directed toward injury prevention. This can take the form of local community support for injury prevention, involvement in community or state-wide violence prevention and conflict-resolution programs, or national participation in the debate over gun control.

Suggested Reading

Alexander RC, Smith WL (eds): Abusive Head Trauma: Proceedings of a Consensus Conference, Supported by the Brain Trauma Foundation. Ames, University of Iowa Press, 1991.

Gheen KM: Near-drowning and cold water submersion. Semin Pediatr Surg 10:26–27, 2001.

Herndon DN, Spies M: Modern burn care. Semin Pediatr Surg 10:28–31, 2001.

Ramenofsky ML, Moulton SL: The pediatric trauma center. Semin Pediatr Surg 4:128–134, 1995.

Tepas JJ, Mollitt D: Vascular injuries. In O'Neill JA, Rowe MI, Grosfeld JL, et al (eds): Pediatric Surgery, 5th ed. St. Louis, Mosby, 1998, pp 337–342.

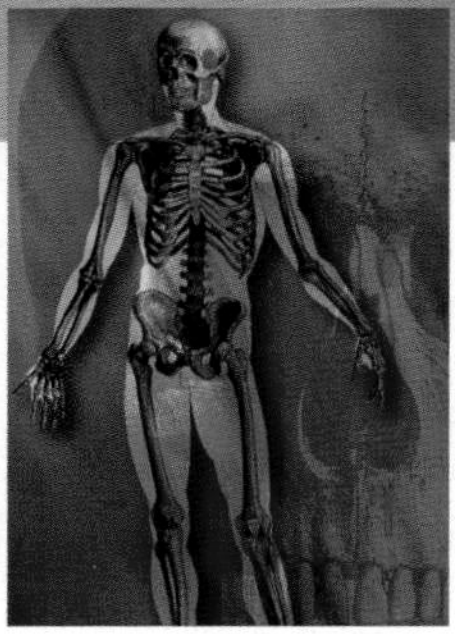

Chapter 56

Pediatric Head, Neck, and Thoracic Disorders

STEVEN L. MOULTON, MD

The Newborn Airway

Surgical Anatomy

The infant larynx is located higher and more anterior in the neck (C4) than the adult larynx (C7). This superior location places the upper tip of the epiglottis behind the soft palate, which explains the preferential nasal breathing of the newborn. The ability to breath through the mouth may take weeks or months to acquire. The infant airway also is narrow, easily traumatized, and highly prone to edema formation. Airway infection and endotracheal intubation can exacerbate airway edema and cause significant loss of lumen cross-sectional area, leading to stridor and laryngospasm. An uncuffed 3.5-mm endotracheal tube should easily pass through the larynx of a term newborn infant. When positive-pressure ventilation is provided, an air leak should be detectable at 15-cm of water pressure to assure that the endotracheal tube is not too large.

Physiology

The majority of newborns with cyanosis at birth have cardiopulmonary (congenital heart disease or pulmonary hypertension), gastrointestinal (tracheoesophageal fistula or gastroesophageal reflux), and central nervous system (CNS) disorders (maternal anesthesia, birth trauma with an intracranial bleed, or CNS malformation). Symptomatic obstruction may occur anywhere from the nasal cavities and nasopharynx, to the larynx, trachea, or the main-stem bronchi below. Initial management of the newborn with cyanosis and respiratory distress at birth includes immediate suctioning and pulling the tongue forward (this ensures a patent airway above the larynx). If the obstruction persists, a laryngoscope is inserted to lift the base of tongue and epiglottis to visualize the larynx. An appropriate-sized endotracheal tube is passed, and if respiratory distress continues, a chest radiograph should be obtained to assess for an intrinsic problem with the trachea, lungs, or pleural cavities. Once an adequate airway is established, a systematic evaluation should be carried out to determine the level of obstruction.

Congenital Anomalies

A variety of congenital anomalies are associated with obstruction of the newborn airway. Some occur in isolation, whereas others occur in association with one or more syndromes. **Choanal atresia** is complete obstruction of the posterior nares; it may be membranous or bony, unilateral or bilateral. The diagnosis is confirmed by the inability to pass a catheter through one or both nares into the nasopharynx. Emergency management consists of maintaining a nipple with the tip cut off in the infant's mouth to keep the tongue forward and open the oropharynx. A computed tomography (CT) scan of the nasopharynx is helpful in preparation for surgery, as it will define the type and level of obstruction.

Micrognathia, commonly seen in Pierre Robin syndrome, is associated with a retroposed tongue and is usually clinically obvious. The small lower jaw and strong sucking action of the infant allow the tongue to be sucked back and occlude the laryngeal airway. This can be life threatening. Infants with symptomatic micrognathia should be kept prone so that the tongue is positioned forward, and consideration should be given to insertion of a nasopharyngeal tube; symptoms usually self-resolve by age 3 months.

Laryngomalacia is the most common congenital laryngeal anomaly and the most frequent cause of *inspiratory* stridor in infants. It is manifested by inward collapse of supraglottic structures during inspiration. **Tracheomalacia** represents subglottic airway flaccidity and accounts for almost half of all congenital tracheal anomalies that occur with stridor. Intrathoracic tracheomalacia is first seen with *expiratory* stridor or wheezing, much like asthma. A diagnosis of laryngomalacia or tracheomalacia is best made by direct examination of the larynx or trachea during spontaneous breathing. Expectant observation is suitable in most cases except secondary tracheomalacia, in which removal of the cause of the extrinsic compression, such as a vascular ring or bronchogenic cyst, may improve airway dynamics.

Anomalies of the aortic arch and great vessels may form **vascular rings** that encircle and compress the trachea and esophagus, producing respiratory distress and symptoms of obstruction on swallowing. The most common yet least symptomatic vascular ring is an **aberrant right subclavian artery**. This vessel arises from the descending left-sided thoracic aorta and crosses the mediastinum behind the esophagus to supply the right arm. Diagnosis can be made on a barium-swallow study, which shows a midline esophagus with posterior indentation. Correction is by surgical division of the anomalous right subclavian artery at its origin. A **double aortic arch** forms when the distal portion of the right aortic arch persists in tandem with the left aortic arch. The persistent right arch is usually dominant and passes behind the esophagus. Operative repair entails complete division of the smallest arch. The least common and most severe vascular ring is a **pulmonary artery sling**. In this case, the left pulmonary artery arises from the right pulmonary artery and traverses the mediastinum between the trachea and the esophagus. A pulmonary artery sling is corrected by dividing the origin of the left pulmonary artery and anastomosing it to the main pulmonary artery anterior to the trachea. If complete tracheal rings, tracheal stenosis, or tracheomalacia accompanies any of these vascular anomalies, then a sleeve resection of the abnormal portion of the trachea or bronchus or both should be performed.

Surgical Disorders of the Head and Neck

Cysts and Sinuses of the Neck

Cervical Lymphadenopathy and Lymphadenitis

Cervical lymphadenopathy refers to all causes of lymph node enlargement, including tumor and infection. Cervical lymphadenitis denotes inflammatory enlargement of one or more lymph nodes of the head and neck. Most children with cervical lymphadenitis have an acute presentation and are treated as outpatients by their pediatrician. A surgical consultation may be requested if the presumptive infection does not respond to antibiotic therapy or if the lymph node enlargement becomes chronic and persists for weeks or months. In this situation, the question of malignancy often arises, but benign causes predominate.

Several groups of lymph nodes have been anatomically defined for ease of description. The lymph nodes of the anterior triangle include the submandibular and deep anterior cervical nodes. These nodes drain most of the face, nasopharynx, mouth, and oropharynx and are commonly affected in acute cervical lymphadenitis. The posterior triangle and supraclavicular nodes are less commonly affected in acute cervical lymphadenitis and, because of their different drainage pattern, are more likely to denote systemic disease, neoplasia, or both.

Cervical lymphadenitis in children is most commonly the result of a viral illness and is usually self-limited. The most common bacterial pathogens are **penicillin-resistant staphylococci** and **group A β-hemolytic streptococci**. Bacterial pathogens tend to cause suppuration (abscess formation) of the involved lymph nodes, and staphylococcal infections usually have less erythema of the overlying skin and follow a slower course to resolution. **Haemophilus influenzae type b,** another organism increasingly recognized as a pathogen in children, also may cause cervical lymphadenitis.

Clinical Presentation and Diagnosis. The history should be queried for duration, constitutional symptoms, exposure to tuberculosis, and possible exposure to a cat or kitten. The physical examination should note whether the child has unilateral or bilateral disease. Careful attention should be paid to the anterior and posterior cervical triangles, any overlying skin changes, the oropharynx, dentition, scalp, hands, and arms. Both axillae should be assessed and the chest examined. If the disease is thought to be infectious, a pharyngeal culture should be obtained and therapy started before species identification.

Treatment and Prognosis. A 10-day outpatient course of an oral, β-lactamase–resistant antibiotic is usually effective. Improvement should be noted within 2 or 3 days of initiating therapy, but complete resolution of the lymphadenopathy may take several weeks. If the patient appears ill, has significant associated cellulitis, or is a young infant, therapy should be initiated with an intravenous (IV) β-lactamase–resistant antibiotic. Children with cervical lymphadenitis who are managed in an outpatient setting should be re-evaluated in 2 to 3 days for evidence of clinical improvement. If no improvement is noted or the condition is worse, the therapy is inadequate or the diagnosis is wrong. If the child appears well, it may be prudent to change the antibiotic before continuing to monitor the child as an outpatient; otherwise, the child should be admitted for IV antibiotics. If the child does not improve with a change in antibiotic therapy or is admitted to the hospital for IV therapy, ultrasound examination of the infected node should be considered; if any evidence of abscess formation is found, this fluid should be drained with a needle or surgically. The fluid should be sent for aerobic and anaerobic bacterial culture, fungal culture, and acid-fast bacillus (AFB) culture and staining. A purified protein derivative (PPD) should be placed and, if exposure to tuberculosis is known or supraclavicular or posterior cervical lymphadenopathy is present, a chest radiograph should be obtained. If culture of the lymph node shows no growth or the patient has not improved in 2 weeks or both, antibiotics should be stopped and consideration given to an excisional lymph node biopsy. This is especially true if the involved lymph nodes are clustered, hard or matted, larger than 2 cm and have shown rapid growth, or are located in the posterior triangle.

Given the variety of infectious agents associated with cervical lymphadenitis in children, it is imperative to follow a systematic approach. If that approach does not yield improvement or a diagnosis, then one must consider other causes. Lymphadenopathy may be associated with certain underlying diseases (e.g., acquired immunodeficiency syndrome [AIDS]) or may herald the presentation of a systemic illness that will become more obvious as it evolves (e.g., Kawasaki disease).

Other Causes of Cervical Lymphadenopathy and Lymphadenitis. Tuberculosis that presents with cervical lymphadenitis has been described since ancient times. In underdeveloped countries, the causative agent is almost exclusively *Mycobacterium tuberculosis*. Tuberculous lymphadenitis is frequently seen in the supraclavicular region, as the mode of entry is through the respiratory tract, and the disease may be bilateral. A strongly positive PPD skin test result is indicative of tuberculosis, whereas a negative result essentially excludes the diagnosis; intermediate reactions are not definitive. An excisional lymph node biopsy may be necessary to confirm the diagnosis before initiating one of several drug regimens.

An atypical or **nontuberculous mycobacterial infection** should be considered when the lymphadenitis is chronic and indolent and has failed to respond to standard antibiotic therapy. *Mycobacterium avium-intracellulare*, *M. scrofulaceum*, and *M. kansasii* are the most common causes of nontuberculous mycobacterial lymphadenitis in young children. Atypical mycobacterial lymphadenitis usually occurs in young children between ages 1 and 5 years. The submandibular nodes are most often involved (due to an oropharyngeal reservoir), and unilateral disease is the rule. The lymphadenopathy is generally nontender and constitutional symptoms are mild or absent. The chest radiograph result is normal and the PPD result is variable (usually negative). Aspiration or simple incision and drainage of nontuberculous mycobacterial lymphadenitis is not usually curative and may produce a chronically draining sinus tract. The mainstay of therapy has therefore been surgical curettage or excision of the most involved "culprit" nodes. Either procedure is made difficult, however, by the inflammatory nature of the involved nodes and their often intimate association with the mandibular branch of the facial nerve. Alternatively, a 6-week course of clarithromycin may be offered.

Lymphadenitis secondary to **cat-scratch disease** is generally benign and self-limited. Contact with a cat, usually a kitten, can be documented in a majority of cases. The infectious agent is a gram-negative bacillus, *Bartonella henselae*. Inoculation occurs via a skin break such as an old wound, scratch, or bite. A characteristic papule at the site of infection appears after 3 to 5 days, and lymphadenopathy evolves over the next 1 to 2 weeks. Mild constitutional symptoms such as body aches, malaise, anorexia, or low-grade fever are common. Because contact usually involves the hand or arm, epitrochlear and axillary nodes are frequently involved; however, the cervical lymph nodes also may be involved. In the vast majority of cases, the lymphadenopathy resolves over a period of weeks to months without treatment, and no current therapy is known to be effective. Rarely, complications including encephalitis, retinitis, and osteomyelitis may be encountered.

Toxoplasmosis may initially be seen with cervical lymphadenopathy. Although the lymphoglandular form is more common in adults, the disease does occur in children. Multiple lymph nodes are usually involved, and signs of acute inflammation are absent. The infecting agent is *Toxoplasma gondii*, the definitive host is the cat, and human infection occurs through contact with cat feces or through consumption of contaminated meat or milk. Diagnosis is usually made by biopsy and supported with antitoxoplasma serum titers. Antibiotic therapy is effective.

Infectious mononucleosis is an Epstein-Barr virus infection. It may be associated with isolated cervical lymphadenopathy, although diffuse lymphadenopathy with systemic signs such as fever and hepatosplenomegaly are more common. Heterophile antibody and atypical lymphocytes are diagnostic.

Branchial Anomalies

Branchial anomalies are remnants of the branchial apparatus, which forms during the third embryonic week, reaches its maximum development in the fifth week, and disappears by the eighth week. The paired branchial arches are defined by the four external clefts and four pharyngeal pouches that develop on each side of the primitive neck. The mesoderm that separates the clefts and pouches gives rise to the facial cartilages and bones with their attached muscles. The muscular components of each arch are innervated by the corresponding nerve of that arch (Table 56-1). A branchial anomaly may be seen as a significant facial deformity or a minor skin tag or cartilaginous remnant. In some cases, a complete fistula exists between the pharynx and the anterior neck, or one end may be obliterated to form an internal or external sinus. A cyst may form if both ends resorb and an aggregate of cells persists within the mesoderm.

Clinical Presentation and Diagnosis

Anomalies of the first-arch complex include cleft lip and palate, as well as abnormalities of the external and middle ears. A fistula of the first branchial arch is rare. The external opening is found near the upper anterior border of the sternocleidomastoid muscle (Fig. 56-1). Excision of a first branchial cleft anomaly requires formal exploration of the parotid gland and use of a nerve stimulator, to avoid injury to the facial nerve. Second branchial cleft anomalies are the most common and typically appear as a sinus, fistula, or cyst along the lower third of the anterior border of the sternocleidomastoid muscle. A second branchial cleft fistula runs superomedially between the internal and external carotid arteries to the tonsillar fossa. Third branchial

TABLE 56–1 The Branchial Arches

Structure	Nerve	Bone and Muscle
First (mandibular) branchial arches		
Auditory canal	Mandidular branch of CN V	Mandible and maxilla
Tympanic membrane	Chorda tympani nerve	Zygoma
Upper part of pinna of ear		Malleus, incus
Parotid gland		Tensor tympani
		Tensor palati
		Anterior belly digastric
		Muscles of mastication
Second (hyoid) branchial arches		
Helix	CN VII, facial nerve	Muscles of facial expression
Antihelix		Platysma, occipitalis
Lobe of the pinna		Posterior belly digastric
Palatine tonsil		Stapedius and stylohyoid
Tonsillar fossa		Stapes and styloid process
		Upper body/low cornu hyoid
Third branchial arches		
Common carotid	Glossopharyngeal, CN IX	Lower body/ upper cornu hyoid
Inferior parathyroid		Superior pharyngeal m.
Thymus		Stylopharyngeus m.
Fourth branchial arches		
Thyroid cartilage		Intrinsic muscles of larynx
Cuneiform cartilage of larynx		Cricothyroid muscles
Lateral thyroid	Sup. laryngeal branch of CN X	Inf. pharyngeal constrictor
Ultimobranchial bodies (calcitonin)		
Rt: subclavian artery		
Lt: arch of aorta		
Superior parathyroid glands		

CN, cranial nerve.

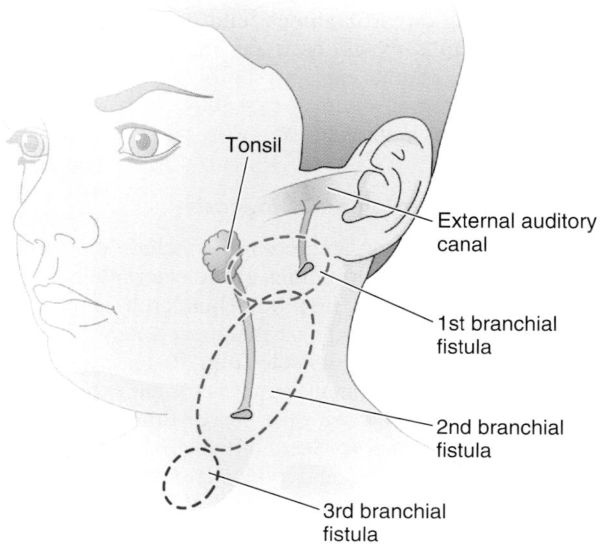

FIGURE 56–1 The typical internal and external openings of the first three branchial cleft fistulae.

cleft fistulae are located along the lower portion of the sternocleidomastoid muscle; they course behind the internal carotid artery to reach the pyriform fossa. Fourth branchial cleft anomalies are rare.

Treatment and Prognosis

All suspected branchial anomalies are managed with surgical excision, as cysts and sinuses are prone to recurrent infection. Fistulae must be completely excised to the level of the pharynx for cure. Very rarely, carcinoma may develop in a branchial cleft remnant.

Thyroglossal Duct Remnants

The thyroglossal duct begins as a midline pharyngeal diverticulum, which descends from the foramen cecum at the base of the tongue to the isthmus of the thyroid. The thyroglossal duct is joined in its descent by thyroid tissue arising from the fourth branchial arches. Normally, the thyroglossal duct becomes obliterated; failure of obliteration leads to formation of a thyroglossal duct cyst. The hyoid bone, originating from the second and third arches, fuses anteriorly and becomes intimately associated with the thyroglossal duct. As a result, the duct can be located anterior to, in the substance of, or behind the hyoid bone.

Clinical Presentation and Diagnosis

A thyroglossal duct cyst usually presents between ages 2 and 10 years as an asymptomatic, round, smooth, anterior midline neck mass overlying the hyoid bone. Occasionally it will be found just lateral to the midline or above the hyoid bone at the base of the tongue. Because of its association with the base of the tongue, the cyst may be noted to rise in the neck with tongue protrusion. The differential diagnosis includes an ectopic midline thyroid, a benign or malignant thyroid nodule, cervical lymphadenopathy, a hemangioma or vascular malformation, a lipoma, or a dermoid cyst.

A preoperative ultrasound of the neck should be obtained to avoid removal of an ectopic midline thyroid, which may be a patient's only functioning thyroid tissue. If the ultrasound indicates that the neck mass is cystic, one may safely proceed to surgical excision. If the mass is solid or thyroid tissue cannot be demonstrated in the normal location, a thyroid scan should be obtained along with thyroid-function tests. If the thyroid scan shows activity in the mass, treatment with exogenous thyroid hormone may result in reduction in the size of the ectopic gland. If the mass is found to be solid at the time of surgery, a frozen section should be obtained to confirm the diagnosis, after which the ectopic thyroid gland may then be divided and tucked behind the strap muscles or autotransplanted in the rectus abdominis muscle to fix the cosmetic defect. Adherence to this diagnostic algorithm should avoid iatrogenic hypothyroidism.

Treatment and Prognosis

Thyroglossal duct cysts are prone to infectious complications because of persistent communication with the base of the tongue (Fig. 56-2). An infected cyst should be treated with oral or IV antibiotics and, if necessary, needle aspiration. Once the infection has resolved, formal excision of the cyst in continuity with the central portion of the hyoid bone will ensure that all ductal remnants are removed. Carcinoma developing in a thyroglossal duct cyst is rare.

Dermoid Cysts

Dermoid cysts are congenital inclusions of skin and related appendages. They develop at sites of embryonic fusion, so are typically found in the subcutaneous tissues of the eyebrow, the midline of the neck, and in the nasal and frontal regions. Rarely, midline nasal and frontal dermoids may have intracranial extensions; midline facial lesions should therefore be evaluated with a preoperative CT scan. Infection commonly develops within dermoid cysts, and infants with an intracranial extension are at risk of meningitis and intracranial abscess formation. Treatment consists of complete surgical excision.

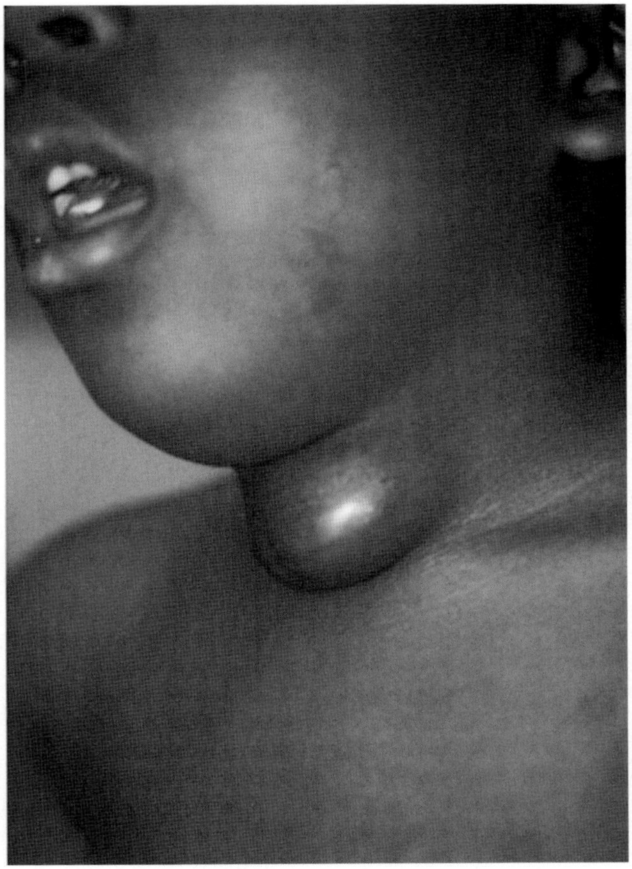

FIGURE 56–2 Thyroglossal duct abscess.

Preauricular Cysts and Sinuses

Preauricular cysts and sinuses are common and often bilateral. They are distinguished from first branchial cleft anomalies by their preauricular location. They are thought to arise from anomalous formation of the external ear. External sinuses that periodically drain should be excised, as they are prone to infection.

Muscular Torticollis

Torticollis is a congenital muscular disorder characterized by fibrosis and shortening of the sternocleidomastoid muscle. Shortening of the muscle leads to the development of a palpable swelling in all or part of the muscle, as well as rotation of the head toward the opposite side of the tumor. Torticollis may be related to abnormal in utero positioning, as the reported incidence of breech and complicated deliveries is much higher in affected infants.

Clinical Presentation and Diagnosis

Torticollis usually is first seen at 2 to 3 weeks of age as a hard, spindle-shaped, discrete mass 1 to 3 cm in diameter, in the midportion of one or both sternocleidomastoid muscles. The parents and pediatrician may initially be concerned about a neoplasm. With time, as the sternocleidomastoid muscle shortens, limitation occurs in turning the head toward the side of the tumor. Impaired rotation of the supine infant's head allows gravity to deform the posterior occiput and contralateral forehead. This asymmetrical skull deformity is called *plagiocephaly,* and it develops in the first few months of life. A progressive facial deformity will follow if there is no intervention. Significant facial deformity takes about 8 months to develop and is an indication for surgical division of the affected sternocleidomastoid muscle.

Treatment and Prognosis

Initial management is usually conservative. The parents are taught to stretch the involved sternocleidomastoid muscle several times a day by placing the infant supine (or prone in the parent's lap) and gently rotating the infant's head toward the involved muscle. The infant's head is held in this position for about 1 minute to stretch the sternocleidomastoid muscle. Initially, the baby will cry because this maneuver is painful. The process should be gently repeated 10 times to the right and left sides, 3 times per day. Over a period of several weeks, the involved muscle becomes supple, and the pain resolves. The goal is to turn the head so that the chin reaches the shoulder. Eventually, the infant's head should be able to rotate equally to the right and to the left. Physiotherapy will fail if the parents do not comply, in which case, it will be necessary to divide the sternocleidomastoid muscle at the sternal and clavicular heads.

Disorders of the Breast

Congenital Anomalies

Most neonates have palpable breast tissue because of the influence of maternal hormones late in gestation. In many instances, the breast bud will express a colostrum-like, milky substance, which will disappear in a few weeks and has no clinical significance. Abnormalities of breast development include **polymastia** (supernumerary breast tissue, with or without nipple or areola) and **polythelia** (nipple or areola only). These accessory breast elements may be ectopic or may develop anywhere along the line of the primitive mammary ridge, which extends from the lateral third of the clavicle to the symphysis pubis bilaterally. Supernumerary nipples should be excised for cosmetic reasons, as should supernumerary or ectopic breast tissue in view of its propensity to develop during puberty and even lactate during pregnancy. Absence of the breast (amastia) or the nipple (athelia) is uncommon and may be associated with an underlying abnormality of the chest wall, such as **Poland's syndrome** (absence or deformity of the cartilages and ribs at levels 2, 3, 4, and 5 in association with mammary and pectoralis muscle hypoplasia).

Breast infections in children are most common in the neonatal and adolescent periods. Induration, cellulitis, and breast tenderness are the presenting signs and symptoms. Abscess formation is common and *Staphylococcus aureus* is the most likely causative organism. Intravenous antibiotics along with prompt drainage through a circumareolar incision are indicated; however, one must avoid injury to the breast bud in neonates to prevent later breast deformity.

Breast Masses in Children

Discrete breast masses in male and postpubertal female patients are almost always benign. The most common finding in women is a **fibroadenoma**, which is a discrete, smooth, firm, and fairly mobile breast mass that is typically painless and slow growing. **Giant fibroadenomas** have a similar smooth, round surface, but they grow rapidly, displace normal tissue, and can significantly distort the normal breast contour; they are most common in postpubertal black women. Other types of non-neoplastic breast masses in children include simple cysts and galactoceles. A breast ultrasound can determine whether a breast mass is solid or cystic. Solid breast masses in postpubertal women are usually excised, as they are a source of concern for the child and parent, they rarely regress, and they may enlarge. Breast masses in prepubertal girls are usually observed, to avoid injury to the breast bud. Carcinoma of the breast is rare in children; to date, 60 cases have been reported in the English literature. Other types of malignancies that may affect the breast include rhabdomyosarcoma, leukemia, and lymphoma.

Congenital Chest Wall Deformities

Pectus excavatum is the most common anterior chest wall deformity in children. It is characterized by depression of the sternum with posterior angulation of the lower costal cartilages (Fig. 56-3). In some, the sternum is rotated, leading to a mixed deformity with posterior angulation of the costal cartilages on one side and anterior angulation on the other. Open and minimally invasive techniques are suitable for repair. The open technique involves an inframammary incision, elevation of the pectoralis muscle from the sternum, resection of the costal cartilages, anterior angulation of the sternum by osteotomy, and optional placement of a substernal metallic strut to hold the sternum in place; the strut is removed through a small incision 1 to 2 years later. The minimally invasive technique involves insertion of a 180-degree semicircular stainless steel bar across the anterior mediastinum under thoracoscopic guidance (Nuss procedure). Turning the bar elevates the sternum into the anatomically normal position; the bar is removed 2 to 3 years later. Overall, the operative times for the minimally invasive technique are shorter, and the cosmetic results appear superior compared with the open technique; however, the length of hospital stay, narcotic

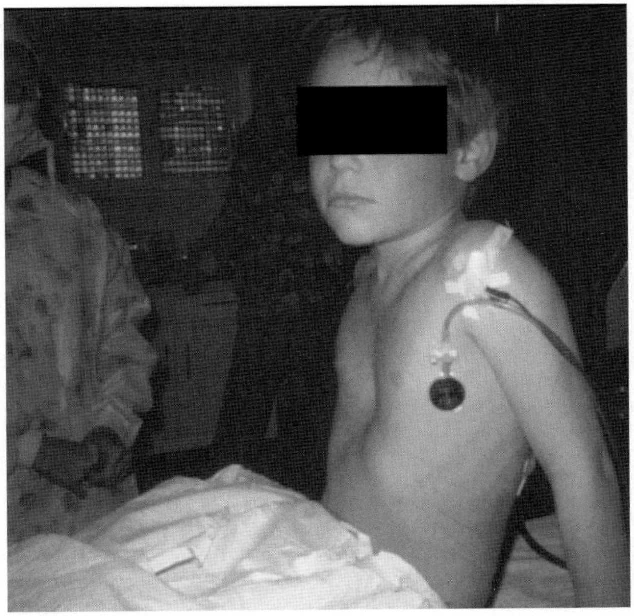

FIGURE 56–3 Pectus excavatum.

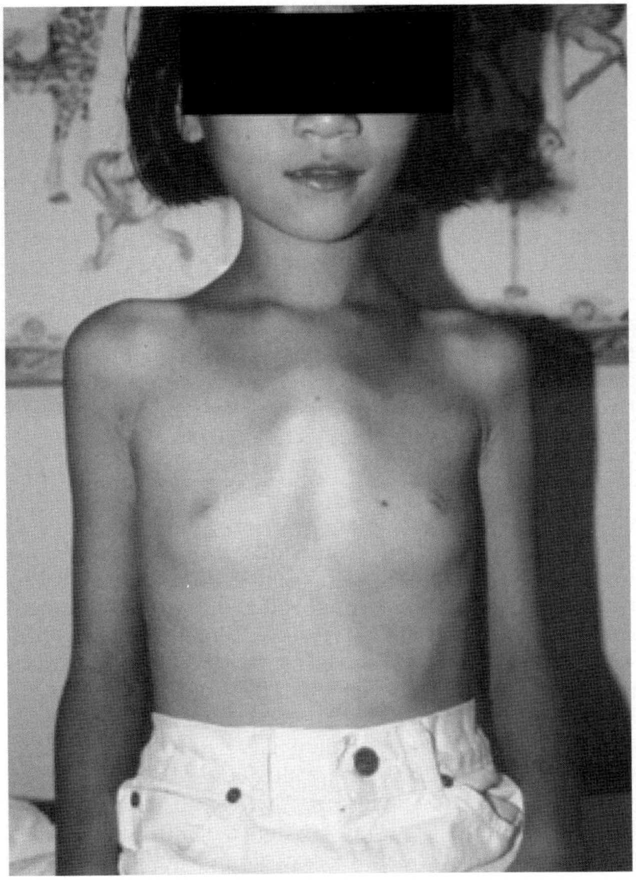

FIGURE 56–4 Pectus carinatum.

requirement for pain control, and the rate of reoperation are higher in children undergoing the Nuss procedure.

Pectus carinatum is a protrusion deformity of the anterior chest wall (Fig. 56-4). It is caused by relative overgrowth of the costal cartilages along one or both sides of the sternum and may therefore be either symmetrical or asymmetrical in appearance. Pectus carinatum is more frequent in boys and is 5 times less common than pectus excavatum. It is rarely associated with significant physiologic derangements in cardiopulmonary function; thus repair is principally for cosmetic reasons. Operative repair is similar to the open repair for pectus excavatum, requiring costal cartilage resection and sternal osteotomy; a minimally invasive procedure has not been described. The nonoperative repair uses custom-fitted compressive orthotics to mold the growing bone and cartilage.

PEARLS FOR ROUNDS

Infants are obligate nose breathers; obstruction of one or both nasal airways by a nasogastric, endotracheal, or feeding tube (or a combination of these) may impair breathing.

Anterior cervical lymphadenopathy is usually viral or bacterial; posterior cervical lymphadenopathy is less common and more often associated with systemic disease or neoplasia.

Infants with a posterolateral congenital diaphragmatic hernia are at risk for persistent pulmonary hypertension of the newborn (PPHN), as a result of *bilateral* pulmonary hypoplasia.

PPHN is potentiated by hypoxia, acidosis, and hypothermia; it increases right-to-left shunting and exacerbates hypoxia and acidosis; prevention is the key.

Congenital Diaphragmatic Hernia

The three forms of congenital diaphragmatic hernia (CDH) are defined by the location of the diaphragmatic defect and its associated clinical features. The most common and most life-threatening congenital diaphragmatic hernia is a posterolateral (foramen of Bochdalek) hernia. This defect is usually large, thereby permitting much of the bowel, spleen, and often liver to migrate into the chest and impair normal lung development. The result is bilateral pulmonary hypoplasia, which is characterized by a decrease in bronchiolar branching and the formation of a hypoplastic pulmonary arterial tree composed of highly pressure-sensitive and extremely vasoreactive pulmonary vessels. The term *congenital diaphragmatic hernia* typically refers to the posterolateral form, which is the focus of this section. The other two sites of herniation are the substernal space (foramen of Morgagni, where the internal mammary artery passes through the diaphragm) and the esophageal hiatus. These hernias are usually clinically silent and may not be discovered until later life.

Ninety percent of posterolateral CDHs occur on the left side, presumably because of the relative protection provided by the liver on the right side. Although the majority of cases are sporadic, the possibility of an underlying genetic defect is supported by familial occurrence. The overall incidence is one in 2500 live births, and one third will have one or more associated congenital anomalies. Cardiac anomalies are the most common, of which hypoplastic heart is the most frequent. Gastrointestinal, genitourinary, CNS, and skeletal anomalies also are observed.

Clinical Presentation and Diagnosis

A CDH may be suspected on a prenatal ultrasound if polyhydramnios, mediastinal shift, and absence of an intraabdominal stomach are present. A definitive diagnosis is possible if viscera are visualized within the fetal thorax. At this point, referral should be made to a center experienced in the management of CDH. In selected cases at specialized centers, fetal tracheal occlusion may be offered to augment in utero lung growth. In the absence of prenatal diagnosis, a CDH should be suspected clinically in any newborn with respiratory distress, absent breath sounds on the involved side, and a scaphoid abdomen. The diagnosis can usually be confirmed with a chest radiograph demonstrating bowel gas in the involved hemithorax, along with shift of the mediastinum (Fig. 56-5). The infant can be then be categorized into a high-, intermediate-, or low-risk group of disease severity, based on the birth weight and 5-minute Apgar score. This information is valuable in planning initial treatment, managing resources, and educating parents.

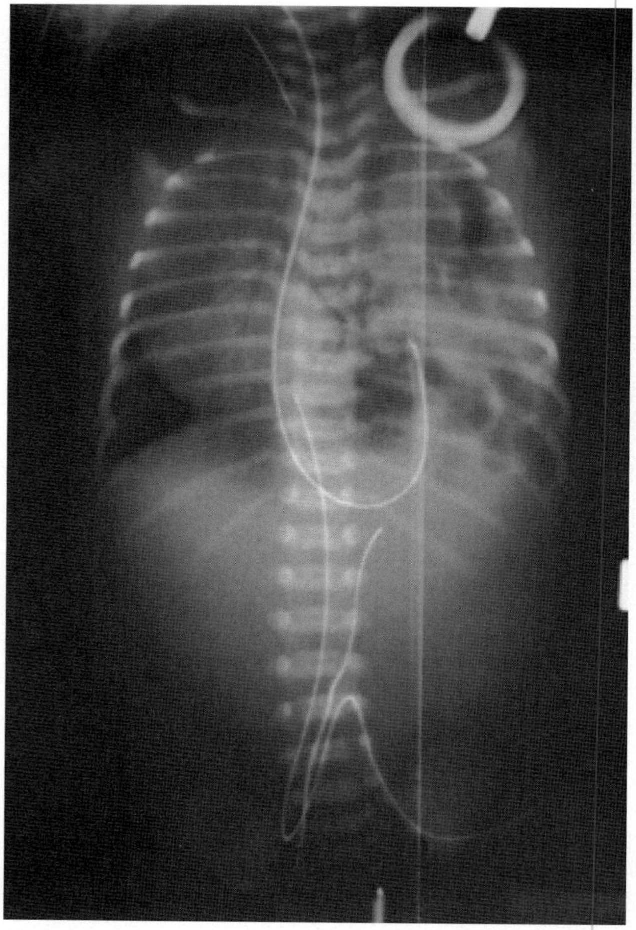

FIGURE 56–5 Left-sided congenital diaphragmatic hernia. Note the distended bowel loops in the left chest, deviation of the trachea and mediastinum to the right, and the location of the heart in the right chest, all of which result in bilateral pulmonary hypoplasia.

Treatment and Prognosis

Infants with a CDH are at risk for persistent pulmonary hypertension of the newborn (PPHN), due to impaired gas exchange and abnormal pulmonary vasoreactivity. PPHN is potentiated by hypoxia, acidosis, and hypothermia. Any of these factors can significantly increase pulmonary hypertension, causing an increase in right-to-left shunting, worsening hypoxia and acidosis, and progressive clinical deterioration. The severity of respiratory symptoms at the time of birth will depend on the degree of pulmonary hypoplasia and how the infant is managed. Most important, one must strive to prevent the onset of pulmonary hypertension and minimize the amount of lung injury caused by ventilatory support of the hypoplastic lungs. The infant should be kept warm, given 100% FiO_2 and a nasogastric tube inserted to decompress the intrathoracic gut, thereby limiting mediastinal shift and compression of the contralateral lung. Noninvasive preductal (right arm) and postductal (either foot) O_2 saturations should be monitored and an umbilical artery catheter placed. Permissive hypercapnia with spontaneous ventilation is preferred, to limit the amount of barotrauma. The goal is to maintain the preductal O_2 saturation above 85% to 90% and the pH greater than 7.25. If these goals cannot be met, the infant should be placed on continuous positive airway pressure or intubated, in an effort to promote respiratory alkalosis and relaxation of the pulmonary vasculature, thereby minimizing right-to-left shunting. Volume and vasopressors may be required to support the systemic circulation. If the infant has persistent hypoxemia and worsening acidemia, a trial of nitric oxide inhalational therapy with or without alternative modes of ventilation (such as high-frequency oscillatory or jet ventilation or both) my be undertaken.

Patients for whom these modes of therapy fail and who are thought to have sufficient lung parenchyma for survival are candidates for extracorporeal life support (ECLS).

ECLS, also known as extracorporeal membrane oxygenation or ECMO, is a form of cardiopulmonary bypass that allows lung rest and recovery from PPHN, without the adverse effects of severe ventilator-induced barotrauma. ECLS is typically offered to infants with severe respiratory distress who have a gestational age of older than 34 weeks or a birth weight greater than 2000 g, minimal or no intracranial hemorrhage (≤ grade I intraventricular hemorrhage), no significant coagulopathy, a reversible lung injury, and no major cardiac lesions, who, by historical criteria, have a greater than 80% predicted mortality. Venoarterial bypass is achieved by placing large catheters in the right internal jugular vein and right common carotid artery. Alternatively, infants with preserved cardiac function may be supported with venovenous bypass by using a double-lumen cannula via the internal jugular vein. The venovenous approach is preferable, for it spares the common carotid artery and enhances oxygen delivery to both the lungs and coronary circulation. ECLS improves survival of CDH by 10% to 20% and, if necessary, is usually implemented before surgical repair.

Operative repair is performed through a subcostal incision. The viscera are reduced into the abdomen, and the rolled margin of the diaphragm dissected free of the chest wall. Small defects are closed primarily. Larger defects are closed with a prosthetic or native tissue patch. If the abdominal wall cannot be closed, now that all of the viscera are in the abdominal cavity, a silicone sheet may be used to contain the herniated bowel in much the same way that an omphalocele may be managed.

Numerous studies at individual institutions have outlined the potential benefits of various treatment strategies in the management of CDH, including ECLS, delayed repair, and lower levels of ventilatory support. The overall survival rate for CDH is about 70%. Long-term follow-up data on infants with CDH has highlighted neurodevelopmental problems, pulmonary morbidity, gastroesophageal reflux, nutritional deficiencies, and skeletal anomalies.

Pulmonary Cysts

Bronchogenic cysts, congenital cystic adenomatoid malformations (CCAMs), pulmonary sequestrations, and congenital lobar emphysema represent a spectrum of congenital malformations of the lung.

Bronchogenic Cyst

Bronchogenic cysts probably arise from abnormal budding of the tracheobronchial tree during airway development. They are occasionally found in the lower neck, but more commonly in the mediastinum (two-thirds) or lung parenchyma (one-third). They are simple cysts surrounded by tissues similar to those of a normal bronchus, including cartilage, smooth muscle, and mucous glands.

Clinical Presentation and Diagnosis

In many cases, an abnormal connection is found between the cyst and the tracheobronchial tree, making infection of the cyst, with attendant fever and cough, a common presentation. In other cases, compression of the airway by the cyst may be present, causing wheezing, stridor, or dyspnea. Associated abnormalities are rare. Diagnosis may be suspected on a prenatal ultrasound showing a simple intrathoracic cyst. More commonly, the diagnosis is made in infancy or childhood when a chest radiograph—obtained as part of a fever workup—shows a round cyst containing air, fluid, or an air/fluid level (Fig. 56-6). A CT scan will confirm the diagnosis.

Treatment and Prognosis

Large bronchogenic cysts diagnosed in utero may be aspirated under ultrasound guidance to relieve mediastinal compression. Such cysts should later be excised—even if asymptomatic, based on the evidence that bronchogenic cysts can later become symptomatic and undergo malignant degeneration. Infected cysts should be managed with intravenous antibiotics and later resected. Extrapulmonary cysts may be approached thoracoscopically. Intrapulmonary cysts usually require partial or total lobectomy and are therefore managed with an open technique.

Congenital Cystic Adenomatoid Malformation

CCAMs are thought to be caused by disordered development of the terminal bronchioles in an isolated segment of lung. CCAMs are therefore composed of many inter-

PEARLS FOR THE OR

An infant's airway is small, easily traumatized, and highly prone to edema formation; significant loss of lumen diameter is accompanied by stridor and tachypnea.

Thyroglossal duct cyst excision includes excision of the central portion of the hyoid bone, to assure that all ductal remnants are removed.

Breast masses in prepubescent girls are usually observed, to avoid injury to the breast bud; those in postpubescent women are usually excised to obtain a diagnosis and allay fear.

Repair of pectus excavatum is primarily cosmetic; it greatly enhances self-image and has been shown to improve exercise tolerance.

When repairing a posterolateral congenital diaphragmatic hernia, remember that the diaphragmatic defect represents incomplete development of the third muscle layer of the chest wall; dissect the margin with care, and patch the diaphragm often.

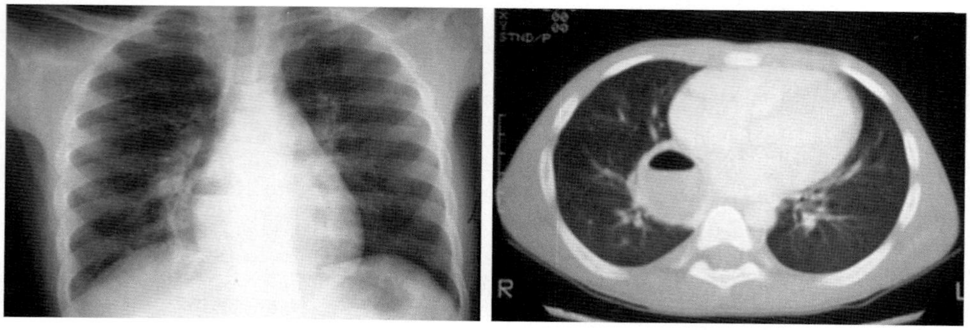

FIGURE 56–6 Infected bronchogenic cyst, visible on the chest radiograph as an air/fluid level along the right heart border. Chest computed tomography confirms the diagnosis and provides additional anatomic detail.

communicating cysts of variable size, rendering a lesion that ranges from multicystic to nearly solid.

Clinical Presentation and Diagnosis

CCAMs are first seen in a variety of ways, depending on their type, size, and location. Nearly half of those diagnosed in utero will have associated polyhydramnios, because of esophageal compression and impaired fetal swallowing. Infants who are diagnosed postnatally will typically have some form of respiratory distress, including tachypnea, retractions, or cyanosis. Older children usually initially have infectious complications, such as recurrent pneumonia at the same site. Typical radiographic findings include an air-filled or partially opacified, multicystic mass, with or without mediastinal shift. A CT scan of the chest may be helpful in differentiating a CCAM from a bronchogenic cyst or congenital lobar emphysema.

Treatment and Prognosis

Fetal intervention, including cyst aspiration, shunt placement, and open resection have been effective in highly selected cases. CCAMs that are diagnosed in infancy and childhood are removed at that time to resolve or avoid the detrimental effects of respiratory compromise and recurrent infection. This approach is supported by the reported association between CCAMs and rhabdomyosarcoma and other malignant tumors in young children. Partial or anatomic lobectomy is the operative procedure of choice, and outcome is generally very good, except when there is preexisting pulmonary hypoplasia.

Pulmonary Sequestration

A pulmonary sequestration is defined as anomalous lung tissue that receives its blood supply from a systemic artery. This tissue is thought to arise from abnormal bronchial budding during early foregut development. It may be described as *intralobar* or *extralobar*, depending on whether the lesion is contained within the normal lung or invested with a distinct pleural layer of its own. Intralobar sequestrations are more common, and the majority are located in the posterobasal segment of a lower lobe. An abnormal communication with the tracheobronchial tree is common. Failure to recognize that the blood supply arises from the aorta can lead to catastrophic intraoperative bleeding at the time of resection. Venous drainage is via a pulmonary vein or the systemic circulation.

Clinical Presentation and Diagnosis

Pulmonary sequestrations usually initially appear with recurrent pulmonary infections and related symptoms. The chest radiograph may show opacification in one of the posterior basal segments of the lung, or it may be nondiagnostic, depending on the size and location of the lesion. CT, ultrasonography, magnetic resonance imaging, or a combination of these may be helpful in defining the abnormal lung tissue. The latter is most help, for magnetic resonance angiography may accurately define the blood supply of the lesion.

Treatment and Prognosis

Pulmonary sequestrations are resected to alleviate symptoms and avoid future infectious complications. Extralobar sequestrations may be approached thoracoscopically, whereas intralobar sequestrations are approached by using an open technique, as they usually require a formal lobectomy. The arterial blood supply must be carefully identified and controlled, and any abnormal bronchiole connection carefully controlled. Recovery is typically uneventful.

Congenital Lobar Emphysema

Congenital lobar emphysema is a condition in which overdistention and air trapping are found in an affected lobe with resultant compression of the remaining normal lung tissue. It is caused by deficient cartilaginous support or bronchial obstruction in a conducting airway, leading to a ball-valve bronchial obstruction that allows inflation during inspiration but obstruction of the bronchus and therefore air trapping during exhalation.

Clinical Presentation and Diagnosis

Most patients are normal at birth, but several days to weeks later, they have respiratory symptoms that can range from mild tachypnea or wheezing to severe dyspnea with cyanosis. Overdistention of the affected lobe leads to compression and atelectasis of the ipsilateral normal lung. Further distention can compress and shift the mediastinum, adversely affecting the opposite lung. A chest radiograph will demonstrate hyperlucency of the overdistended lobe. The differential diagnosis includes pneumothorax, CCAM, and foreign-body aspiration. The latter is unlikely in infants younger than 6 months and usually affects the lower lobes.

Treatment and Prognosis

Lobectomy is indicated for symptomatic cases. The prognosis is excellent.

Suggested Reading

Friedberg J: Clinical diagnosis of neck lumps: A practical guide. Pediatr Ann 17:620–628, 1988.

Greenholz SK: Congenital diaphragmatic hernia: An overview. Semin Pediatr Surg 5:216–223, 1996.

Hebra A, Swoveland B, Egbert M, et al: Outcome analysis of minimally invasive repair of pectus excavatum: Review of 251 cases. J Pediatr Surg 35:252–258, 2000.

Nobuhara KK, Wilson JM: Pathophysiology of congenital diaphragmatic hernia. Semin Pediatr Surg 5:234–242, 1996.

Nuchtern JG, Harberg FJ: Congenital lung cysts. Semin Pediatr Surg 3:233–243, 1994.

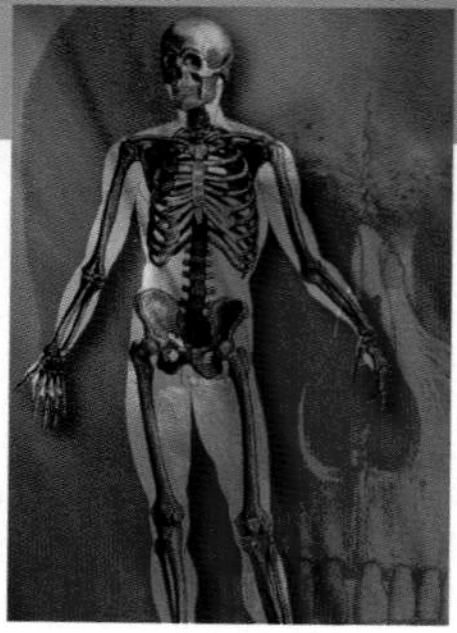

Chapter 57

Pediatric Gastrointestinal, Abdominal Wall, Inguinal, and Scrotal Disorders

STEVEN L. MOULTON, MD

Embryology

The fetal gastrointestinal tract is composed of the foregut, midgut, and hindgut. The foregut gives rise to the esophagus, trachea, stomach, and proximal duodenum. It is present in most embryos by day 20 of gestation and is lined by epithelial cells derived from embryonic mesoderm. During week 8 of gestation, the lumen of the **esophagus** is obliterated by proliferating epithelial cells. By week 10 of gestation, recanalization of the esophageal lumen occurs as the muscular layers of the esophagus form and provide mechanical support to the developing tube. If growth of the esophageal muscular or mesenchymal coat outpaces cellular division of the epithelial lining, the epithelium may become stretched and interrupted, leading to pure esophageal atresia. By week 16 of gestation, the structural components of the esophagus are in place, and neuronal development is sufficiently organized for swallowing to begin.

The respiratory tract first appears as a ventral diverticulum of the foregut on day 26 of gestation. The primitive **trachea** quickly elongates and splits into two lung buds that descend caudally into the mesenchyme, ventral to the developing esophagus. At this point, the trachea and esophagus are separated by the tracheoesophageal septum. Their closest association is at the level of the carina, which is the level at which most tracheoesophageal fistulae (TEFs) form. It is hypothesized that this close association, along with developmental mistiming or abnormal cell-to-cell signaling, can lead to segmental coalescence of the trachea and esophagus and the formation of any one of several tracheoesophageal anomalies. The most common type of tracheoesophageal malformations is proximal esophageal atresia with a distal tracheoesophageal fistula (Fig. 57-1).

The **stomach** develops from the lower end of the foregut during week 5 of gestation. As the stomach grows, it undergoes 90 degrees of counterclockwise rotation, positioning the left vagus nerve anteriorly. In general, congenital anomalies of the stomach are rare. Gastric outlet obstruction may be caused by an antral web or pyloric atresia. Congenital microgastria results from impairment of normal foregut development; the small stomach leads to gastroesophageal reflux, postprandial vomiting, malnutrition, and recurrent aspiration pneumonia. Gastric volvulus is a rare event caused by abnormal fixation of the stomach; it is associated with congenital diaphragmatic hernia and other anatomic disorders that impair gastric fixation.

The **duodenum** is derived from fusion of the distal foregut with the proximal midgut at the level of the ampulla of Vater. The blood supply to the duodenum is therefore derived from the celiac axis and branches of the superior mesenteric artery. The lumen of the duodenum is transiently obliterated by rapid epithelial cell growth between weeks 5 to 8 of gestation, just as occurs in the esophagus and stomach. Failure to completely recanalize the duodenum can lead to formation of a duodenal web or duodenal atresia and subsequent duodenal obstruction. Other causes of duodenal obstruction include annular pancreas and malrotation. Annular pancreas is produced when the ventral pancreatic bud fails to rotate properly to the right—behind the duodenum—to become incorporated into the dorsal bud; instead, it rotates to the left, effectively constricting the lumen of the duodenum. Malrotation refers to a wide spectrum of disorders caused by abnormal intraabdominal fixation of the intestinal tract.

Normal intestinal rotation occurs between weeks 8 and 10 of gestation. During this period, the c-loop of the duodenum becomes fixed, along with the pancreas, in the retroperitoneum. By week 10 of gestation, the duodenum has undergone 270 degrees of counterclockwise rotation around the axis of the superior mesenteric artery. This process fixes the retroperitoneal fourth portion of the duodenum behind the stomach in the left upper quadrant at the ligament of Treitz. Concurrent 270-degree counterclockwise rotation of the cecocolic loop fixes the cecum in the right lower quadrant, thereby splaying out the base of the small bowel mesentery from the left upper quadrant to the right lower quadrant. This arrangement minimizes the chances of the small bowel twisting on and kinking its blood supply (midgut volvulus). Once normal rotation is complete, the stage is set for elongation and return of the remaining midgut from the extraembryonic coelom to the peritoneal cavity. Errors in proper intestinal rotation are generally categorized as malrotation and nonrotation of the gut. These

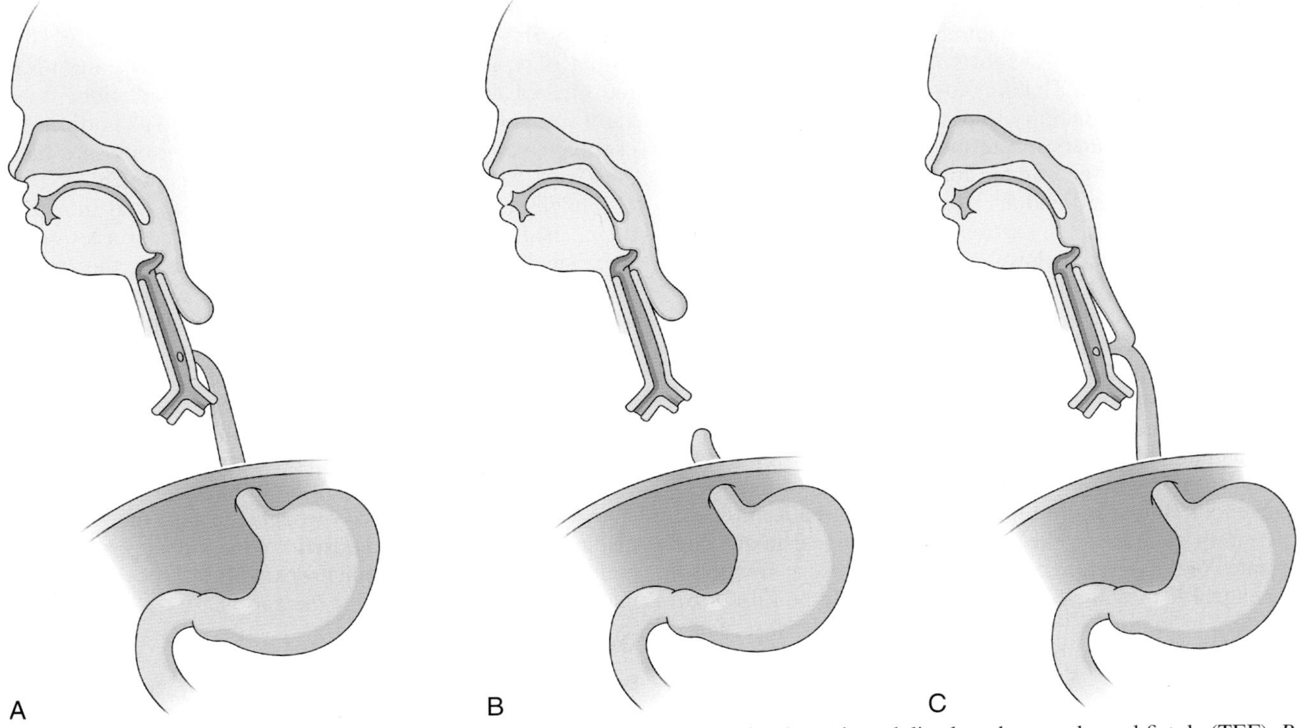

FIGURE 57–1 The three most common types of esophageal atresia. *A*, Proximal atresia and distal tracheoesophageal fistula (TEF). *B*, Esophageal atresia without TEF. *C*, TEF without esophageal atresia (H-type defect). (Adapted from Rowe MI, O'Neil JA Jr, Grosfeld JL, et al: Congenital abnormalities of the esophagus. In Essentials of Pediatric Surgery. Philadelphia, Mosby, 1995, p 398.)

potentially life-threatening anomalies are discussed in more detail later.

The hindgut is derived from the primitive endoderm of the yolk sac. Division of the hindgut by multiple septae, followed by fusion of the hindgut with ectodermal tissue from the anal pit, gives rise to the **genitourinary system**, **rectum,** and **anus**. Failure of proper development of the hindgut can result in a variety of urogenital and anorectal anomalies, including imperforate anus, cloaca, bladder exstrophy, and cloacal exstrophy.

Alimentary Tract Obstruction in the Newborn

Polyhydramnios on a prenatal ultrasound should raise suspicion of underlying obstruction of the gastrointestinal tract. Perinatal vomiting and abdominal distention also are abnormal and always require investigation. An important first consideration is whether the vomiting is bilious or nonbilious, as this will determine whether the site of possible obstruction is proximal or distal to the ampulla of Vater, and thereby categorize the possible causes. It also is important to determine the frequency and force of the emesis because, in general, the higher the obstruction, the earlier and more forceful the vomiting. For example, a newborn with an antral gastric web or proximal duodenal atresia will usually have forceful, *nonbilious* vomiting. In contrast, a newborn with malrotation and midgut volvulus or jejunoileal atresia will have less frequent and less forceful *bilious* vomiting. These anomalies and other common causes of alimentary tract obstruction in the newborn are discussed later.

Esophageal Atresia and Tracheoesophageal Fistula

The incidence of esophageal atresia with or without tracheoesophageal fistula is approximately 1 in 4000 live births. More than 50% of affected newborns have associated anomalies involving one or more organ systems. This constellation of congenital anomalies is referred to as the VACTERL association and includes *V*ertebral, *A*norectal, *C*ardiac, *T*racheo*E*sophageal, *R*enal and *L*imb anomalies.

Clinical Presentation and Diagnosis

Newborns with esophageal atresia constantly drool as they are unable to swallow their oral secretions. These secretions collect in the blind-ending upper esophageal pouch and may spill over into the airway, causing the baby to choke and cough. If the anomaly is unrecognized, the infant may experience episodes of cyanosis and respiratory distress with attempts to feed. The diagnosis of esophageal atresia is supported by the inability to pass a nasogastric tube into the stomach. An anteroposterior chest radiograph will often reveal a blind-ending air column in the upper thorax (representing the blind-ending esophagus), and may or may not demonstrate air in the gastrointestinal tract. The absence of gastrointestinal air below the diaphragm suggests pure esophageal atresia. If air is present below the diaphragm, then a fistulous communication must exist between the trachea and the esophagus. If the diagnosis of esophageal atresia remains in doubt, a small amount (0.5 mL) of water-soluble contrast material can be injected via a feeding tube into the proximal esophageal pouch.

Immediate management of the neonate with esophageal atresia with or without tracheoesophageal fistula includes intravenous fluids, antibiotics, and insertion of a Replogle-type sump catheter in the proximal esophageal pouch to aspirate oral secretions. If the infant has a tracheoesophageal fistula, the head of the bed should be raised to minimize reflux of gastric contents into the airway. A renal ultrasound should be obtained to evaluate for the presence of renal anomalies. An echocardiogram is important to evaluate for cardiac anomalies and to determine the anatomic position of the aortic arch. A normal aortic arch ascends to the right and descends down the left side of the vertebral column. An abnormal left-sided arch will descend on the right and prevent access to the esophagus and trachea via a standard right thoracotomy. The absence of significant associated anomalies affords early surgery with primary repair. Extremely preterm infants and those with significant comorbidities or major associated anomalies may benefit from a staged repair, beginning with a gastrostomy tube to decompress the stomach and minimize the risks associated with reflux of gastric secretions into the airway. Division of the fistula alone without performing an esophageal anastomosis may be necessary in extreme situations.

Congenital TEF without esophageal atresia is often referred to as an *H-type* fistula. Infants with this esophageal anomaly usually are first seen with coughing or choking during feeding. Occasionally, this anomaly will be missed during infancy and discovered in childhood, after several bouts of pneumonia or workup for a chronic cough. The fistula may not be evident on a routine esophagogram. A more reliable technique involves the use of video esophagography and the injection of contrast material through an esophageal catheter that is slowly withdrawn from the esophagus. Alternatively, bronchoscopy with esophagoscopy may confirm the diagnosis.

Treatment and Prognosis

Repair of esophageal atresia/tracheoesophageal fistula is usually performed via a right thoracotomy in the fourth intercostal space by using a retropleural approach. More recently, this procedure has been done thoracoscopically. The fistula is typically located in the membranous portion of the trachea at the level of the tracheal bifurcation. It is carefully isolated and divided, leaving a small portion of esophagus on the trachea, to achieve a secure closure that does not narrow the airway. The upper pouch of the esophagus is dissected free of the trachea, well into the upper mediastinum, to gain adequate length for a tension-free, single-layer repair. Additional length on the upper pouch can be gained by performing one or more circular myotomies or by using traction sutures. If the infant has pure esophageal atresia, a gastrostomy should be performed to enable bolus gastric feeds over a period of several months, to enlarge the stomach, and to allow the ends of the esophagus to grow. Further studies will determine if the esophageal gap has sufficiently narrowed to permit primary repair. If a primary repair is not feasible, the greater curvature of the stomach can be tabularized, brought up into the posterior mediastinum, and anastomosed to the upper esophageal pouch. Alternatively, a jejunal or colon interposition graft may be constructed to bridge the gap.

Duodenal Atresia and Stenosis

Duodenal obstruction may be complete (atresia) or incomplete (stenosis). It should be suspected when the nonspecific finding of polyhydramnios is made on a prenatal ultrasound. Duodenal atresia is commonly associated with other congenital anomalies including a variety of congenital cardiac, renal, and gastrointestinal defects (such as esophageal atresia, TEF, and imperforate anus). Infants with duodenal atresia are often premature, and about one third have Down syndrome.

Clinical Presentation and Diagnosis

In the majority of cases, the site of duodenal obstruction is distal to the ampulla of Vater. These infants have bilious vomiting within hours of birth and feeding, whereas those with proximal duodenal obstruction have nonbilious vomiting. Plain abdominal radiographs may demonstrate a classic "double bubble" sign, which results from gaseous distention of both the stomach and proximal duodenum (Fig. 57-2). If atresia is present, no distal air will appear in the bowel, whereas if stenosis is present, some air will be seen distal to the dilated duodenum. Contrast studies are usually not necessary to confirm the diagnosis, as swallowed air is an excellent contrast agent.

Treatment and Prognosis

A nasogastric tube is placed to decompress the stomach, and the infant is resuscitated with intravenous fluids. Operative repair of duodenal atresia is performed through a right upper quadrant transverse incision. Typical findings include a dilated duodenum and small-caliber distal bowel. Mobilization of the duodenum reveals the site of atresia or

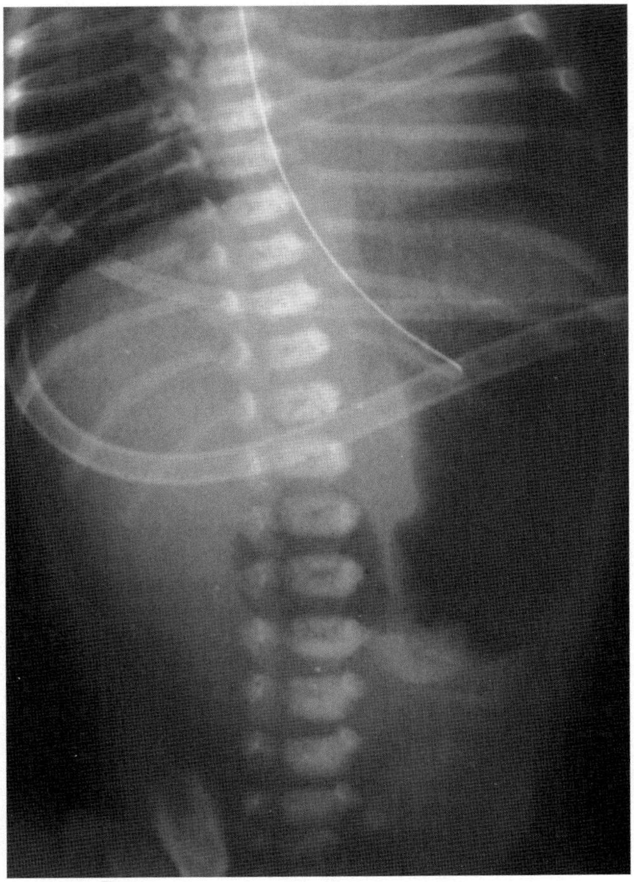

FIGURE 57–2 Two-day-old infant with bilious vomiting. Upright abdominal film shows classic double-bubble sign of duodenal atresia.

stenosis and its relation to the biliary ampullae, common bile duct, and mesenteric vessels. Abrupt transition from a hypertrophied and dilated proximal duodenum to a bowel wall of normal thickness suggests the presence of a duodenal web. Webs can be excised through an anti-mesenteric duodenotomy, being careful to preserve the medial portion of the web containing the ampulla. The most common repair, however, is a diamond-shaped side-to-side duodenoduodenostomy between the dilated proximal and the smaller-caliber distal duodenum. A central venous catheter is inserted for postoperative parenteral nutrition. A nasogastric or gastrostomy tube is necessary to decompress the stomach and proximal duodenum for 2 to 3 weeks after surgery, until the caliber of the proximal duodenum diminishes and normal peristaltic activity can resume. Once feeds are started, they are slowly increased until the distal bowel enlarges sufficiently to accommodate full feeds.

Jejunoileal Atresia and Stenosis

Jejunoileal atresia and stenosis are thought to result from intrauterine mesenteric ischemia and necrosis with subsequent resorption of the affected segment or segments. Ischemia may occur at any time during gestation, but is most often thought to occur later in fetal development as a result of intrauterine fetal intussusception, midgut volvulus, thromboembolic occlusion, or, in the case of omphalocele or gastroschisis, incarceration or kinking of the bowel at the level of the abdominal-wall defect. Atretic segments are most commonly found in the proximal jejunum or distal ileum and are limited to a single segment in approximately 90% of cases. Jejunoileal atresia is classified into four types, of which type 1 is the most common (Fig. 57-3).

Clinical Presentation and Diagnosis

Neonates with jejunoileal atresia usually have bilious vomiting, progressive abdominal distention, and failure to pass meconium. Infants with intestinal stenosis are more difficult to diagnose, as they typically have intermittent episodes of incomplete obstruction; eventually failure to thrive or complete obstruction develops. The gas pattern on a plain abdominal radiograph is often helpful in determining the approximate location of a small bowel atresia. In general terms, the lower the obstruction, the greater the number of distended loops and air/fluid levels. A barium enema is helpful in determining the presence or absence of an associated colonic or rectal atresia. Colonic atresia is uncommon and overall comprises about 10% of all cases of intestinal atresia.

Treatment and Prognosis

It is important to decompress the stomach and upper small bowel with a Replogle tube and correct any underlying metabolic derangements before proceeding with operative repair. A transverse upper abdominal incision provides excellent surgical exposure. Inspection to assure proper rotation of the bowel is carried out. The small bowel is exteriorized, and the entire bowel is carefully inspected from the ligament of Treitz to the sigmoid colon to determine the site and type of obstruction and to exclude other areas of atresia or stenosis. To ensure distal patency, a red rubber catheter is used to gently fill the distal small bowel and colon with normal saline. If isolated jejunal atresia is encountered, the dilated portion of jejunum should be resected (if short) or tapered (if long). When ileal atresia is found, resection should be limited to the most severely dilated segment to prevent malabsorption. In colonic atresia, resection may be more liberal. In most cases, an end-to-end or end-to-side anastomosis is favored.

Infants with jejunoileal atresia and sufficient bowel length generally have an uneventful recovery. Those with a small bowel length of less than 70 cm will carry the diagnosis of short-bowel syndrome (SBS) and require a more gradual

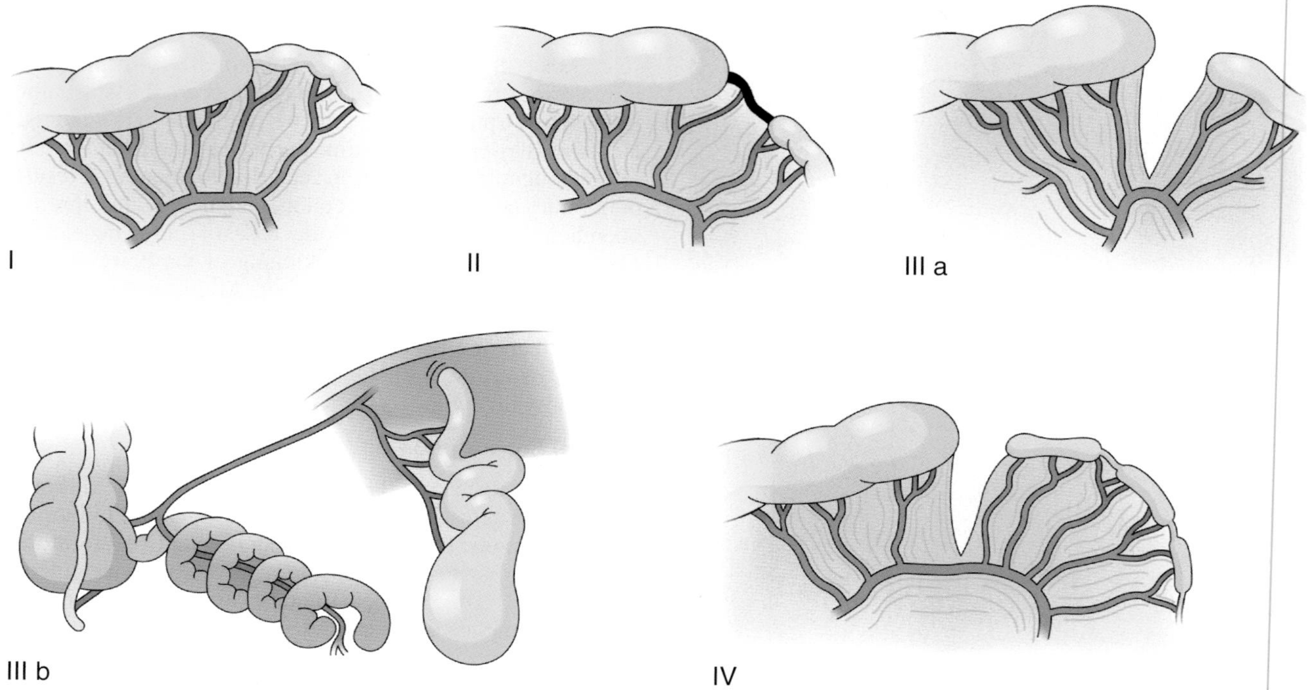

FIGURE 57–3 Classification of jejunoileal atresia. Type I, mucosal (membranous) atresia with intact bowel wall and mesentery. Type II, blind ends are separated by a fibrous cord. Type IIIa, blind ends are separated by a V-shaped (gap) mesenteric defect. Type IIIb, apple-peel atresia. Type IV, multiple atresias (string of sausages). (Adapted from Rowe MI, O'Neil JA Jr, Grosfeld JL, et al: Intestinal atresia and stenosis. In Essentials of Pediatric Surgery. Philadelphia, Mosby, 1995, p 511.)

transition to full enteral feeds. This may take months to years, depending on the length of the small bowel, and generally requires supplemental parenteral nutrition. Loperamide may be used to slow intestinal transit and therefore increase the nutritional mucosal contact time. Cholestyramine binds intraluminal bile salts and may be used to decrease their irritative effects on the colonic mucosa. Infants with loss of the terminal ileum should be given supplemental vitamin B_{12} and folic acid to prevent megaloblastic anemia.

Meconium Ileus

Meconium is a moist, sticky, green particulate matter composed of gastrointestinal secretions and other luminal debris that normally resides in the distal colon and rectum before birth. Meconium ileus refers to luminal obstruction of the distal small bowel caused by inspissated meconium. It occurs in about 15% of newborns with cystic fibrosis, which is an autosomal recessive disorder that primarily affects the white population. Cystic fibrosis is caused by a wide variety of mutations in the gene that encodes the cystic fibrosis transmembrane conductance regulator (CFTR) protein. The CFTR is a chloride-channel protein that affects luminal fluid balance in the respiratory, gastrointestinal, biliary, pancreatic, and reproductive systems.

Presentation and Diagnosis

In infants with uncomplicated meconium ileus, signs and symptoms of intestinal obstruction develop within the first 24 hours of life, usually beginning with abdominal distention, followed by clear and then bilious emesis. A family history of cystic fibrosis is found in about 20% of patients. Plain films of the abdomen show dilated loops of bowel without air/fluid levels and, in some cases, a *soap-bubble* or *ground-glass* appearance in the right lower quadrant (Neuhauser's sign), where air has mixed with the thick intraluminal meconium. The differential diagnosis includes ileal atresia, meconium plug syndrome (see later), Hirschsprung's disease, small left colon syndrome, and colonic atresia. A contrast enema will usually differentiate these diagnoses from meconium ileus, which demonstrates an unused colon (microcolon) with inspissated pellets of meconium in the distal ileum.

Infants with complicated meconium ileus have a more dramatic clinical presentation because of complications that stem from in utero obstruction of the distal small bowel. The heavy meconium-filled small bowel may twist just proximal to the site of obstruction, causing a volvulus and bowel ischemia. The ischemic bowel may perforate and spill meconium throughout the fetal peritoneal cavity

(meconium peritonitis), or the perforation may be localized by the surrounding loops of bowel, leading to the formation of a meconium pseudocyst. In some cases, the ischemic portion of bowel may undergo necrosis and resorption in utero, resulting in atresia of the bowel. Newborns with meconium peritonitis or a giant meconium pseudocyst will have abdominal distention at birth and bile-stained gastric aspirates. Plain films of the abdomen will show dilated loops of bowel and diffuse or localized intraperitoneal calcification. If the site of perforation has not sealed, ascites and evidence of intraperitoneal air or an air-filled pseudocyst may be present.

Treatment and Prognosis

Newborns with uncomplicated meconium ileus are managed with a hyperosmolar diatrizoate meglumine (Cystografin) enema, which acts by drawing fluid into the lumen of the bowel to loosen the inspissated material and allow it to pass. Infants that fail two or three therapeutic enemas and all neonates with complicated meconium ileus require a laparotomy. In the absence of perforation, it is the author's preference to inject Cystografin directly into the lumen of the ileum by using a 3-mL syringe and a 30-gauge needle. Within minutes the inspissated meconium can usually be manipulated into the colon and flushed out through the rectum by using a red rubber catheter in the stump of the appendix. If this fails, an antimesenteric enterotomy in the mid to distal ileum can be used to loosen and flush the meconium into the colon. Infants with atresia or perforation usually tolerate restoration of bowel continuity. In some cases, however, a proximal stoma may be the safer choice.

Survival rates average around 85% for uncomplicated meconium ileus; the rate is lower for those with complicated meconium ileus. Those with cystic fibrosis who survive must endure an incurable, life-limiting condition marked by chronic pulmonary disease, recurrent pulmonary infection, exocrine pancreatic insufficiency, and general ill-health. Intensive therapeutic regimens have extended the median life expectancy of a child born with cystic fibrosis to 40 years. Gene therapy holds promise as a means to treat the underlying genetic defect.

Meconium Plug Syndrome

Meconium plug syndrome is a relatively common cause of functional colonic obstruction in neonates. It is uncommonly associated with cystic fibrosis. Affected infants are often premature but otherwise normal, and the disorder is thought to be related to their immature myenteric nervous system. Stasis and excessive water absorption produce meconium plugs that obstruct the colon.

Presentation and Diagnosis

The clinical presentation is that of a distal bowel obstruction and was described earlier. A gentle rectal examination will reveal inspissated meconium and may be therapeutic. A contrast enema will be diagnostic and therapeutic, as it will dilate the colon, hydrate the meconium, and afford passage of the material.

Treatment and Prognosis

The diagnosis of meconium plug syndrome should be followed by a diagnostic sweat test to rule out cystic fibrosis. In addition, a suction rectal biopsy should be performed to evaluate for Hirschsprung's disease.

Hirschsprung's Disease

Hirschsprung's disease is a motility disorder that is characterized by the absence of ganglion cells in the rectum or more proximal bowel. It is thought to result from a halt in the rostrocaudal migration of enteric neurons during embryonic development. Aganglionosis is limited to the rectosigmoid colon in about 80% of patients. In 10% of patients, the level of aganglionosis is proximal to the splenic flexure, and in the remaining 10%, the entire colon is aganglionic. In rare cases, the entire length of the gastrointestinal tract is affected, a condition that is usually fatal. Hirschsprung's disease occurs in approximately 1 in 5000 live births and has a male-to-female preponderance of 4:1. Seven percent of patients have an affected family member, and the risk of familial occurrence is related to the length of the aganglionic segment: the longer the segment, the greater the risk. Hirschsprung's disease is commonly associated with other anomalies, including Down syndrome (3% to 5%), and a variety of congenital cardiac anomalies.

Clinical Presentation and Diagnosis

The clinical presentation of Hirschsprung's disease varies with the age of the child. Neonates usually present with bilious emesis, abdominal distention, and delayed or diminished stool frequency. A cardinal sign is delayed passage of meconium beyond the first 48 hours of life. The physical examination is notable for mild to moderate abdominal distention and visible loops of bowel beneath the abdominal wall. Infants who are not diagnosed in the perinatal period may appear later with a history of constipation and poor weight gain. The parent or caregiver may express concern about the child's abdominal distention and malodorous stools. Older children will have a history of chronic constipation and may be grossly distended. They have a tight anal sphincter, and withdrawal of a finger from the anus is usually followed by forceful discharge of gas and stool.

Hirschsprung's enterocolitis or toxic megacolon is a dreaded complication of undiagnosed Hirschsprung's disease. It may develop at any age and usually appears with increasing abdominal distention, borborygmus, and foul-smelling diarrhea. The disease may progress to include fever, vomiting, abdominal pain, and explosive watery diarrhea. The dehydration that follows is compounded by mucosal slough and a massive loss of protein-rich fluid into

the dilated bowel. The clinical course may progress to vascular collapse and an early septic death unless the patient is aggressively fluid resuscitated. Although the etiology of Hirschsprung's enterocolitis is thought to be related to stasis, the identification of *Clostridium difficile* toxin in the stools of a large number of these patients and the often prompt response to enteric vancomycin are important observations.

A contrast enema is diagnostic of Hirschsprung's disease in 80% of cases and is the radiographic study of choice. If positive, it will demonstrate the beginning of the aganglionic segment as a transition between dilated proximal colon and a segment of narrow distal colon or rectum. The transition zone is best seen if the colon is not evacuated before the study. In the presence of enterocolitis, a contrast enema may show mucosal spiculation in the affected region, submucosal dissection of contrast material, or perforation. Rectal manometry is another test that may be helpful in the diagnosis of Hirschsprung's disease. In normal individuals, rectal distention with a balloon-tipped catheter causes reflexive relaxation of the internal anal sphincter. Individuals with Hirschsprung's disease have a high resting pressure in the internal anal sphincter, which does not relax with rectal distention.

The diagnosis of Hirschsprung's disease is confirmed by obtaining a rectal biopsy 2 cm proximal to the dentate line in infants and 3 cm in older children. This may be performed at the bedside or in the clinic without anesthesia and must include the submucosa. Histologic analysis in patients with Hirschsprung's disease shows hypertrophied nerve trunks and the absence of ganglion cells in Auerbach's intermyenteric plexus and Meissner's submucosal plexus. Acetylcholinesterase staining shows a marked increase in stain uptake by the hypertrophied neurofibrils. If a sufficient tissue sample cannot be obtained by suction biopsy, a thicker, transrectal biopsy should be performed under general anesthesia.

Treatment and Prognosis

Three operations for Hirschsprung's disease are historically described in the literature: the Swenson, Duhamel, and Soave endorectal pull-throughs. All three have traditionally been preceded by a leveling colostomy, an operation during which the transition zone between ganglionic and aganglionic bowel is histologically identified. A functional, diverting colostomy is performed at the most distal portion of the colon where normal ganglion cells are seen. A functional colostomy allows the child to stool and grow until a definitive pull-through procedure is performed, usually between ages 6 and 12 months. At the time of that procedure, the colostomy is taken down, the aganglionic rectosigmoid colon is excised, and the normally innervated bowel is brought down and secured to the anus within 1 cm of the anal verge. The coloanal anastomosis is often protected by a loop ileostomy, which is closed 8 to 12 weeks after the endorectal pull-through.

Although operative mortality and functional results have improved over the past several decades, more recent efforts have focused on single-stage, transanal repairs in the newborn period. The transanal endorectal pull-through for short-segment disease avoids an abdominal incision and yields a functional result that is comparable to those of other established procedures. A laparoscopic-assisted abdominoperineal approach is used in patients with longer-segment disease, in whom division of the colonic mesentery and takedown of the splenic flexure may be necessary to gain sufficient length for the normally innervated colon to reach the perineum. Infants who undergo either procedure are usually fed on postoperative day 1 and discharged home on postoperative day 2 or 3. These procedures eliminate the need for a diverting colostomy and allow the infant to stool at a very young age. The cosmetic results are superior and the functional results quite favorable. Early results have shown nearly all patients to be continent of stool; however, several have required reoperation or developed early enterocolitis or both.

Imperforate Anus

During normal development, the rectum descends to the perineum within a funnel-shaped muscle complex. The upper portion of this funnel-shaped structure is known as the *levator muscle*, and the lowermost part is the *external sphincter*. These striated muscles are under voluntary control. When contracted, they elevate and pull the rectum forward to compress and occlude the lower anorectal canal, thereby preserving fecal continence and dignity. The *internal sphincter* is composed of circular, involuntary smooth muscle fibers within the lowermost anorectal bowel wall; the internal sphincter maintains closure of the anal canal except during defecation.

Imperforate anus refers to the absence of a normal anal opening. It is associated with incomplete descent of the rectum and hypoplasia of both the funnel-shaped muscle complex described earlier and the internal anal sphincter. Imperforate anus occurs within the spectrum of a wide variety of anorectal malformations, which are classified according to gender and whether a colostomy is indicated in early management (Box 57-1). About 10% of defects in boys are supralevator, meaning the rectum terminates above the level of the levator muscles. High defects such as this have severe muscle underdevelopment, sacral anomalies, impaired sensory and neuromuscular innervation, and a low likelihood of fecal continence after surgical repair. In the other 90% of male cases, the rectum terminates somewhere between the levator muscles and the perineum, often as a rectourethral fistula. Fistulous communications between the rectum and the genitourinary tract occur in girls as well. About one third of girls with an imperforate anus will have a rectovestibular fistula. An even greater number (40%) will have a cloacal malformation. A cloaca is an anorectal malformation in which the rectum joins with the vagina

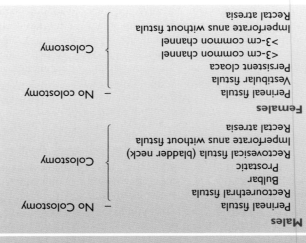

BOX 57–1 Classification of Anorectal Malformations

Type	Management
Males	
Perineal fistula	No Colostomy
Rectourethral fistula	Colostomy
Bulbar	Colostomy
Prostatic	Colostomy
Rectovesical fistula (bladder neck)	Colostomy
Imperforate anus without fistula	Colostomy
Rectal atresia	Colostomy
Females	
Perineal fistula	No colostomy
Vestibular fistula	Colostomy
Persistent cloaca	Colostomy
<3-cm common channel	Colostomy
>3-cm common channel	Colostomy
Imperforate anus without fistula	Colostomy
Rectal atresia	Colostomy

and urethra to form a common channel, which may be short (<3 cm) or long (>3 cm). Male and female patients can have an imperforate anus without a fistula.

The reported incidence of anorectal malformations is 1 per 5000 live births, and, in general, boys are more commonly affected and tend to have higher defects. Imperforate anus is associated with a wide variety of congenital malformations and several syndromes, including Down syndrome and the VACTERL association. Genitourinary anomalies are seen in about 50% of patients, and, in general, the higher the defect, the more frequently it is associated with a severe urologic problem. Cloaca, which occurs in approximately 1 of 50,000 births, is an example of a high anorectal malformation with a severe genitourinary anomaly. Cloacal exstrophy is the most complex anomaly associated with imperforate anus; these babies have an omphalocele and an exstrophic bladder, within which an open cecum and a blind-ending colon are found.

Clinical Presentation and Diagnosis

Initial management centers on determining the level of the anorectal malformation and any associated anomalies. A nasogastric tube is passed to decompress the stomach and rule out esophageal atresia. The genitalia and perineum are carefully inspected for evidence of a low fistula, which may appear as a whitish or dark-stained subcuticular tract along the perineal raphe or the lower scrotal raphe. A high or intermediate fistula would be suspected in a male infant if he has a cleft scrotum or an atypical hypospadius. If no fistula is evident and the perineum and genitalia are otherwise normal, a piece of gauze should be placed at the tip of the penis to collect any meconium that may pass with the urine. This finding would be evidence of a rectourethral or rectovesical fistula and indicate the need for a colostomy. Similarly, a female infant with an imperforate anus and a normal perineum should be observed for passage of meconium via a vestibular or higher vaginal fistula. If the vulvae are small and no hymen is present, it is likely that the infant has a cloacal anomaly. In this case, the urethra would not be visible, and the infant would pass both urine and meconium via a single orifice.

In most cases, the decision to create a colostomy should be delayed until the infant is 18 to 24 hours old. During this time, the distal rectum will distend and promote identification of a perineal fistula. If none is evident and the infant has not passed meconium via the penis or vagina, a lateral film of the infant in the prone position with a marker on the perineum should be obtained. If this film shows the air-filled rectum to be located within 1 cm of the perineum, the patient is considered to have a low defect and can be treated during the newborn period with an anoplasty. If the rectum is more than 1 cm from the perineum, the patient requires a colostomy. Until then, a chest radiograph should be obtained to look for evidence of upper vertebral and rib anomalies. A supine film of the abdomen and pelvis may reveal an anomaly of the lumbosacral spine and, depending on the degree of sacral agenesis, provide some initial prognostic guidance. An echocardiogram will determine if the infant has an associated cardiac anomaly, whereas an ultrasound examination of the abdomen will screen for renal and uterine anomalies. Anomalies of the limbs, particularly radial anomalies of the forearm, may be assessed clinically and radiographically to look for further evidence of the VACTERL association. Before discharge or in the early follow-up period, a voiding cystourethrogram should be performed to detect possible vesicoureteral reflux. In addition, because spinal cord anomalies are common and can be found even in patients who have normal plain films and low defects, spinal ultrasonography or magnetic resonance imaging should be performed in all neonates with an imperforate anus to rule out occult spinal pathology such as a tethered cord or a lipoma of the cord.

Treatment and Prognosis

Newborns with low anorectal anomalies such as an anterior anus or a rectoperineal fistula are generally managed with a perineal anoplasty in the first few days of life. In contrast, newborns with intermediate and high lesions are best treated with a completely divided left-lower-quadrant colostomy between the descending and sigmoid colons. This procedure will divert the fecal stream in preparation for a posterior sagittal repair. Before that repair is undertaken, it is highly desirable to obtain a distal colostogram. This study consists of injecting a water-soluble contrast material (e.g., Hypaque) into the distal stoma under fluoroscopic control to determine the length of the distal rectal segment and the site at which it terminates in the bladder or urethra. Enough pressure should be used to fill the bladder gently. Then when the baby passes urine, a voiding cystourethrogram will be obtained. If the

baby has a cloaca, an additional contrast study should be performed through the single orifice. This study will demonstrate the anatomic relation of all three structures that constitute the cloaca.

A posterior sagittal anorectoplasty is the gold standard for the repair of imperforate anus and its associated anorectal and genitourinary malformations. The operation is performed with the infant in the prone position. A midline incision is made from the coccyx to the perineum, and dissection is carried deeply between the sphincter muscles to the posterior wall of the rectum. The posterior rectal wall is opened, and the anterior urinary fistula (if present) divided. The urinary fistula is closed with absorbable suture. The rectum is carefully separated from the urogenital tract and mobilized down to the perineum. The perineum is reconstructed by using a muscle stimulator to place the rectum accurately within the pelvic muscle complex and the parasagittal fibers of the external sphincter. Laparoscopic-assisted anorectal pull-through for the repair of high imperforate anus is a minimally invasive technique that allows minimal perineal dissection and accurate placement of the rectum within the levator ani and external anal sphincter muscle complex. Several advantages of this technique include excellent visualization of the rectal fistula and surrounding structures, accurate placement of the bowel through the anatomic midline and levator sling, and minimally invasive abdominal and perineal wounds. Cloacal anomalies are best managed with total urogenital mobilization in combination with a posterior sagittal anorectoplasty.

Fecal incontinence is a common problem after the repair of intermediate and high anorectal anomalies, and these patients can generally be categorized into two groups. Those with incontinence and constipation are typically managed with daily large enemas through either the anus or a Malone appendicostomy. Patients with incontinence and a tendency toward diarrhea are usually instructed on a bowel-management program. The long-term prognosis for fecal continence varies, depending on the type and level of malformation, the associated vertebral defects, and the motivation of the patient and parents.

Necrotizing Enterocolitis

Necrotizing enterocolitis (NEC) is a life-threatening gastrointestinal infection most commonly seen in preterm infants. Its pathogenesis is related to the presence of gut bacteria, which breach the mucosal layer by either transmucosal passage or invasion through areas of mucosal damage. Bacterial killing within the bowel wall is ineffective, perhaps because of deficiencies in both specific and nonspecific immune mechanisms. As greater numbers of bacteria invade the wall of the intestine, a wide variety of inflammatory mediators are released. These coordinate the inward migration of many cellular elements, which cause further tissue destruction and greater exposure to invading bacteria. Failure to control the infection can lead to full-thickness necrosis, intestinal perforation, and sepsis. The overall incidence of NEC is 1 to 3 per 1000 live births. Risk factors include prematurity, birth weight less than 1500 g, and a history of enteral feeding. Eighty percent of affected infants are younger than 34 weeks' gestational age and weigh less than 2000 g at birth.

Clinical Presentation and Diagnosis

NEC is often heralded by nonspecific clinical findings of physiologic instability, such as lethargy, temperature instability, apnea, and bradycardia. More specific symptoms include feeding intolerance and vomiting. Physical findings may include abdominal tenderness, distention, visible bowel loops, and guaiac-positive stools. Late findings suggestive of an underlying bowel perforation include a bluish discoloration of the abdomen (caused by intraperitoneal meconium or blood or both), localized edema and erythema of the abdominal wall (caused by an underlying phlegmon or walled-off abscess), or a mobile mass (caused by an interloop abscess).

The white blood cell count is generally low, and thrombocytopenia nearly always present, probably due to sepsis and sequestration of these cellular elements at sites of bowel infection and necrosis. A metabolic acidosis also is common and is believed to be a result of hypovolemia with third-spacing of fluid into the peritoneal cavity. Plain films of the abdomen, including the standard anteroposterior and left lateral decubitus (or cross-table lateral) views, are important in diagnosis and close follow-up of any infant with suspected or definite NEC. Radiographs should be carefully evaluated for pneumatosis intestinalis, portal vein gas, pneumoperitoneum, a persistently dilated loop, or a combination of these (Fig. 57-4). Pneumatosis represents subserosal hydrogen gas produced by the invading bacteria

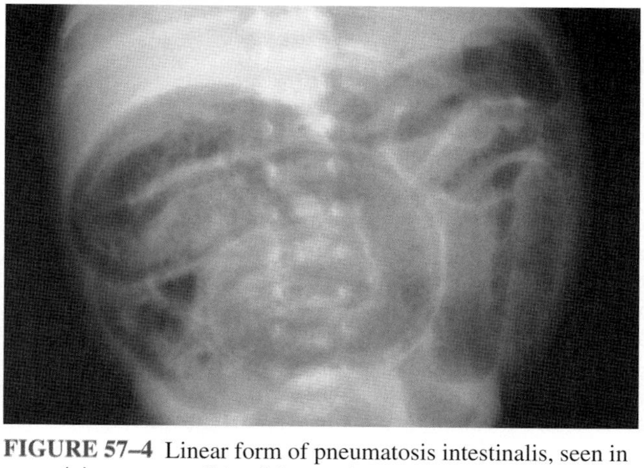

FIGURE 57–4 Linear form of pneumatosis intestinalis, seen in necrotizing enterocolitis of the newborn.

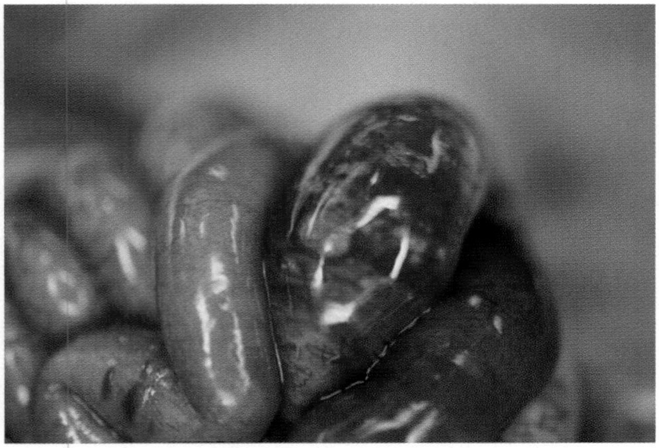

FIGURE 57–5 Subserosal hydrogen bubbles, representing the cystic form of pneumatosis intestinalis in necrotizing enterocolitis of the newborn.

(Fig. 57-5). This gas can track into the mesenteric veins and be transported to the liver, where it is temporarily trapped in the portal system and visible by radiograph. Portal vein gas is a particularly ominous sign, for it is associated with paninvolvement of the gut by NEC. A persistently dilated, air-filled loop of bowel on successive films of the abdomen suggests a focal ileus due to an adjacent phlegmon or walled-off abscess. Pneumoperitoneum is an obvious sign of bowel perforation.

Treatment and Prognosis

In 1978, Bell introduced a three-stage system to classify the various clinical and radiographic findings associated with NEC. Stage I infants have features suggestive of NEC, stage II patients have NEC, and stage III patients have advanced NEC with evidence of bowel necrosis. A modified version of Bell's classification is presented in Table 57-1. All infants with suspected or definite NEC are managed with gastric decompression, IV-fluid therapy, and broad-spectrum antibiotics. Stage I and stage II patients are initially managed nonoperatively with close clinical monitoring, frequent blood-gas determinations, serum platelet and white blood cell counts, as well as serial abdominal radiographs every 6 to 8 hours to allow early detection of clinical deterioration. Most infants with mild or suspected NEC (Bell stage I) will improve within 48 to 72 hours, after which the nasogastric tube is removed and antibiotics continued for a total of 5 to 7 days; feeds are slowly reintroduced and then advanced as tolerated. Bell stage II patients, along with Bell stage I patients for whom reintroduction of feeds fails but who remain clinically stable, are treated with gastric decompression and IV antibiotics for 2 weeks before feeds are restarted.

TABLE 57–1 Modified Bell's Staging Criteria for Necrotizing Enterocolitis

Stage	Clinical Findings	Radiographic Findings
I. Suspect NEC	Mild abdominal distention, poor feeding, vomiting	Mild ileus
II. Definite NEC	Above, plus marked abdominal distention GI bleeding	Significant ileus, pneumatosis, portal vein gas
III. Advanced NEC	Above, plus deterioration of vital signs, septic shock	Above, plus pneumoperitoneum, fixed loop

GI, gastrointestinal.

Infants with advanced or progressive NEC are quite ill, nearly all requiring aggressive fluid resuscitation, inotropes, and ventilatory support. The principles of surgery include careful handling of the premature gut, resection of only necrotic or perforated bowel, and preservation of the ileocecal valve, if possible. Resection and primary anastomosis can be performed safely in carefully selected patients. Multiple anastomoses and questionably viable bowel should be protected by a proximal stoma brought out through a separate incision. Leaving questionably viable bowel in situ with plans for re-exploration in 24 to 48 hours can help to distinguish viable from nonviable bowel and preserve intestinal length.

The overall mortality rate is about 25%. The major causes of morbidity include sepsis, stricture formation, and SBS. Strictures are more common in medically treated infants with NEC, and for this reason, some authors advocate a routine contrast enema before feeds are restarted. Strictures are more common in the colon (70%) and are usually heralded by abdominal distention, obstipation, bloody stools, or a combination of these. If a stricture is suspected, gastric decompression should be followed by a contrast study and appropriate surgery. SBS is the malabsorptive state that follows extensive resection of the small bowel, resulting in the loss of absorptive surface area and interference with a number of intestinal reflexes and feedback loops. The most important of these is a loss of absorption of vitamin B_{12}, folic acid, bile salts, and fat-soluble vitamins by the ileum.

Hypertrophic Pyloric Stenosis

Hypertrophic pyloric stenosis is a common cause of nonbilious vomiting in early infancy, characterized by gastric outlet obstruction due to hypertrophy and hyperplasia of the circular muscle of the pylorus. The incidence is about 1 per 500 live births. Pyloric stenosis is four times more

common in boys than in girls and tends to run in families, suggesting a sex-modified, polygenic inheritance.

Clinical Presentation and Diagnosis

Infants in whom pyloric stenosis develops appear well during the first 1 or 2 weeks of life. Regurgitation of food and nonbilious vomiting usually begin during weeks 3 to 5 of life, often prompting one or more formula changes. As the disease progresses over the next few days, the vomiting becomes more forceful and eventually projectile. The infant, however, remains hungry after vomiting and otherwise appears well. In the absence of intervention, the infant will eventually become dehydrated and lethargic. The physical examination is often notable for dry mucous membranes, visible gastric peristaltic waves in the left upper quadrant, and a palpable pylorus or "olive." Examination of the abdomen may be facilitated by elevating the lower extremities (to relax the abdominal musculature) and giving the infant a pacifier or a small amount of 5% dextrose in water. The examiner should stand on the left side of the infant and, with the fingers of the left hand, gently palpate the epigastrium from right to left, beginning just beneath the liver edge. The object is to catch the enlarged pylorus between the examiner's fingers and the infant's spine. Failure to palpate the pylorus warrants further study, as the presentation can mimic that of pylorospasm and gastroesophageal reflux. Other causes of nonbilious emesis in infancy include poor feeding technique, gastroenteritis, malrotation, a duodenal or antral web, or an enteric duplication cyst of the pyloric channel.

The most commonly used ultrasonographic criteria for pyloric stenosis are a muscle thickness of 4 mm or more and a channel length of at least 16 mm (Fig. 57-6). When ultrasonography is not available or if the pylorus is obscured by gas in the overlying bowel, a barium upper gastrointestinal (UGI) study should be performed. Positive findings on a UGI study include a narrow, elongated pyloric channel (string sign) and indentation of the gastric antrum by the hypertrophied pyloric muscle (Fig. 57-7). Any barium remaining in the stomach after completion of the UGI study should be evacuated with a nasogastric tube to avoid perioperative aspiration.

Nowadays, it is uncommon to see an infant with hypertrophic pyloric stenosis who has significant metabolic derangements or dehydration or both. The process begins with recurrent vomiting causing loss of chloride and hydrogen ions, leading to a metabolic alkalosis and hypochloremia. The initial response of the kidney is to maintain blood pH by reabsorbing hydrogen ions at the expense of sodium, potassium, and hydroxide (OH^-) ions. Continued vomiting depletes the intravascular volume, leading to sodium resorption and a marked loss of potassium (via an aldosterone-mediated mechanism) at the expense of an increasing pH. The resulting hypokalemia leads to hydrogen ion excretion and a paradoxical aciduria.

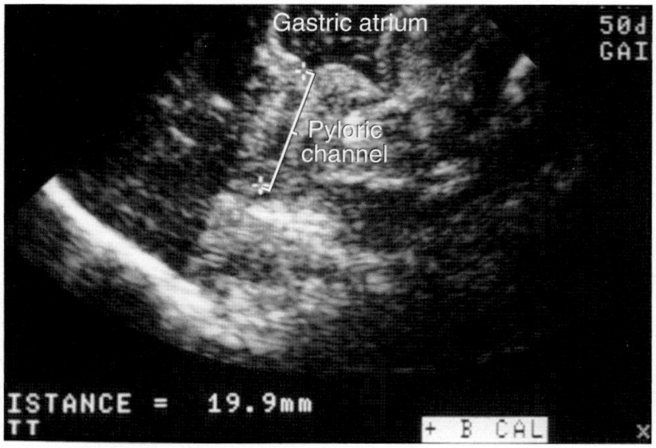

FIGURE 57–6 Ultrasound image of hypertrophic pyloric stenosis in a 4-week-old infant. The channel length is 19.9 mm.

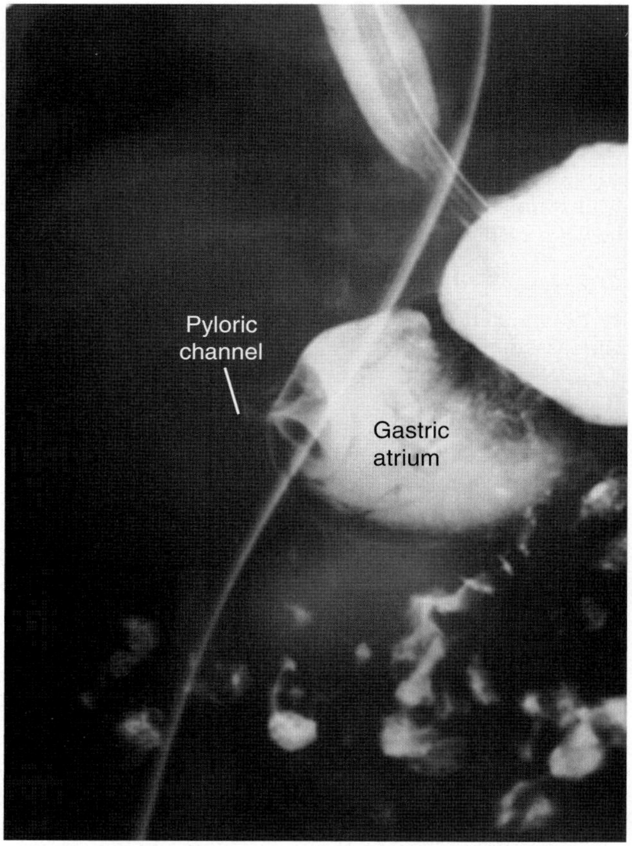

FIGURE 57–7 Upper gastrointestinal study illustrating a thin, elongated pyloric channel. The shoulders of the pyloric muscle can be seen pouting into the antrum of the stomach. A small amount of contrast material has moved distally into the duodenum and jejunum.

Severely dehydrated infants should be resuscitated with normal saline (20 mL/kg), after which 5% dextrose in normal saline (D5NS at 175 to 185 mL/kg/day) should be given until urine output is established; potassium (KCl, 10 mEq/500 mL) may then be added to the maintenance fluid. Infants who are not severely dehydrated should be managed with 5% dextrose in half-normal saline (D50.45NS with KCl 10 mEq/500 mL at 150 to 175 mL/kg/day). Resuscitation sufficient to proceed to the operating room is characterized by a urine output of 1 to 2 mL/kg/hr, normal sodium and potassium levels, and a bicarbonate (HCO_3^-) level of less than 30.

Treatment and Prognosis

The standard operation for pyloric stenosis is Ramstedt's pyloromyotomy. The operation is performed through a transverse right upper quadrant incision, circumumbilical incision, or laparoscopically. With an open technique, the pylorus is delivered or carefully held within the abdomen, and a longitudinal incision made with a scalpel along the length of the pylorus. The pyloric muscle fibers are split with a hemostat or pyloric spreader until the mucosa of the pyloric channel bulges through the myotomy. Care must be taken to avoid entry into the duodenum at the distal margin of the incision. The most common complication is wound infection. Other complications include wound dehiscence, incisional hernia, inadequate myotomy, and perforation. The rate of perforation with either open or laparoscopic techniques is generally 1% or less in most pediatric centers. If a mucosal perforation is detected, it should be repaired directly and a new pyloromyotomy performed along the inferior margin of the pylorus.

Malrotation and Midgut Volvulus

Malrotation is a congenital anomaly that encompasses a wide spectrum of abnormalities related to rotation and fixation of the midgut. Rotational anomalies occur when the proximal and distal loops of the midgut fail to undergo their expected 270-degree counterclockwise rotations during return of the midgut to the abdomen between weeks 10 and 12 of gestation. In essence, the proximal or duodenal loop rotates 270 degrees from a fixed point at the pylorus, to pass *behind* the superior mesenteric artery to the left upper quadrant, where it is attached in the retroperitoneum at the ligament of Treitz. Concomitantly, the distal or cecocolic loop crosses in front of the superior mesenteric artery, to locate the ileocecal junction in the right lower quadrant, where it is fixed to the retroperitoneum by lateral attachments along the ascending colon. These rotational events occur independently, so that failure of the ligament of Treitz to achieve its normal position is not necessarily associated with cecocolic malrotation and vice versa. Clinically significant malrotation occurs when the duodenal loop is *fixed to the right of the spine*, whereas the cecocolic loop rotates only 180 degrees to pass in front of the superior mesenteric artery, without descending to the right lower quadrant. This leaves the two points of fixation of the small bowel mesentery almost superimposed on one another at the base of the superior mesenteric artery. The resultant narrow base of the small bowel mesentery is at risk for twisting on itself, causing acute or chronic small-bowel ischemia. Malrotation is commonly associated with Ladd's bands, which are lateral attachments of the cecum that course across and can obstruct the underlying duodenum. This anatomic arrangement contrasts with the normal pattern of fixation, which is a broad diagonal base of mesentery that extends from the left upper quadrant to the right lower quadrant. The incidence of malrotation is about one per 500 cases, and it can be a natural consequence of several congenital anomalies, particularly omphalocele, gastroschisis, and congenital diaphragmatic hernia. Although most patients are first seen in the neonatal period, many others remain asymptomatic well into adult life.

Clinical Presentation and Diagnosis

Malrotation can become evident in a variety of ways, depending on the occurrence of midgut volvulus, the degree of duodenal obstruction, or both. The most common presentation is acute midgut volvulus. This can occur at any time in a susceptible individual's lifetime but is most common in the first month of life. The typical patient is an otherwise healthy infant who has sudden onset of bilious vomiting followed by abdominal distention. Bilious vomiting is a common presenting symptom in older children and adults as well; however, they have the additional complaint of acute abdominal pain that is out of proportion to their abdominal examination. The initial abdominal examination in all age groups may be completely normal, lulling the practitioner

PEARLS FOR ROUNDS

Know the differences in presentation, diagnosis, and management of pure esophageal atresia versus esophageal atresia with tracheoesophageal fistula.

Bilious vomiting always deserves attention; bilious vomiting in a newborn requires investigation.

Do not attribute the symptoms of abdominal pain, anorexia, nausea, and vomiting to gastroenteritis without first asking yourself, "Could this be appendicitis?"

Neonatal jaundice beyond age 2 weeks must be investigated, especially if the direct bilirubin level (conjugated fraction) is greater than 1 mg/dL.

Be able to list several different types of the most common omphalomesenteric duct malformation.

into dismissing the importance of the initial history of bilious vomiting. Unfortunately, a delay in diagnosis may be followed by progressive bowel ischemia, peritonitis, hypovolemic shock, and death due to massive intestinal infarction.

The important point is to consider the possibility of malrotation whenever a patient is seen with a history of bilious vomiting. Laboratory studies in the setting of malrotation with an acute volvulus will reveal a metabolic acidosis with a low serum bicarbonate (HCO_3^-) level. Plain films may reveal air in the stomach and duodenum with a paucity of distal bowel gas (caused by partial duodenal obstruction) or dilated bowel loops (caused by distal obstruction). The one exception is the newborn whose plain films may reveal a classic double bubble sign, caused by malrotation plus Ladd's bands or a duodenal web. If the diagnosis of malrotation is suspected but unconfirmed, an upper gastrointestinal contrast study should be done. In the setting of malrotation with midgut volvulus, this will show (1) dilation of the proximal duodenum tapering to a conical or beak shape; (2) a spiral or corkscrew appearance of the distal duodenum; (3) absence of the ligament of Treitz; and (4) the duodenum and proximal jejunum to the right of the spine.

Treatment and Prognosis

When the diagnosis of malrotation with midgut volvulus is made, resuscitation and laparotomy are performed in rapid succession to minimize the duration of intestinal ischemia. The abdomen is entered through a transverse right upper quadrant incision. The volvulus appears as a convoluted jumble of dilated, compromised bowel with a visible twist at the base of its mesentery. One or more *counterclockwise* twists may be necessary to reduce the volvulus. The anatomic situation is then clarified, and if the entire bowel appears viable, a Ladd's procedure is performed. This entails division of Ladd's bands between the cecum and the duodenum. The underlying visceral peritoneum over the superior mesenteric artery—medial to the duodenum—is then incised to splay out the base of the mesentery. The duodenum is freed up and inspected for an area of narrowing or stenosis; saline may be injected through a transpyloric catheter to confirm duodenal patency in a newborn. The duodenum is led down the right gutter, the small bowel is laid sequentially right to left in the midabdomen, and the cecum and descending colon are placed on the left side of the abdomen so that the bowel is nonrotated. Last, an appendectomy is performed to avoid future diagnostic confusion.

When an abnormality of rotation is discovered intraoperatively or incidentally during diagnostic evaluation for another problem that requires a laparotomy, correction of the malrotation should be carried out at the time of surgery. Similarly, if malrotation is discovered incidentally at the time of evaluation for a condition not requiring surgery, most surgeons recommend correction of the malrotation, regardless of the patient's age or symptoms. This recommendation is meant to avoid the unpredictable, catastrophic complication of midgut volvulus. An elective Ladd's procedure is easily performed with minimal morbidity by using either open or laparoscopic techniques.

Intussusception

Intussusception occurs when a portion of bowel invaginates into a contiguous segment of small or large bowel, causing a bowel obstruction. *Ileocolic* intussusception is the most common type of intussusception in infancy, and it usually occurs between ages 5 and 10 months. This peculiar age distribution, with few cases among infants in the first 3 months of life and a decline in incidence after the first year of life, is seen in many childhood infectious diseases and suggests an infectious etiology. In the setting of infection, enlarged mesenteric lymph nodes alongside the terminal ileum or lymphoid aggregates within the bowel wall are thought to serve as lead points, effectively causing the infantile bowel to intussuscept into itself. These cases are considered idiopathic, because no specific pathologic lead point (other than enlarged lymph nodes) can be identified. Idiopathic intussusception predominates in children younger than 2 years, and several different viruses have been implicated in its pathogenesis, as has a recently introduced and since withdrawn rotavirus vaccine. Children who are older than 2 years are more likely to have an *ileoileal* intussusception and an identifiable lead point, such as a Meckel's diverticulum, an enteric duplication cyst, pancreatic rest, or hemangioma. Ileocolic and ileoileal intussusception also occur after abdominal trauma and various abdominal operations.

Clinical Presentation and Diagnosis

The classic presentation is that of a healthy, well-nourished infant in whom episodic abdominal pain develops, characterized by screaming, irritability, and drawing the knees to the chest. Between these episodes, the infant may appear well and unaffected. Efforts to feed and comfort the child may lead to vomiting—first gastric and then bilious material—as intestinal obstruction progresses. Blood and mucus from the ischemic bowel may mix and pass with the stool, giving it a "currant jelly" appearance. The infant eventually becomes dehydrated and lethargic. Unfortunately, this typical presentation and sequence of events is often incomplete; some infants may be first seen with irritability alone, whereas others are simply lethargic. The intussusception may be palpated anywhere in the abdomen, but most commonly in the epigastrium as a sausage-shaped mass. With time, abdominal distention, tenderness, and eventually peritonitis will develop if a delay in diagnosis occurs.

Plain films of the abdomen should include a left lateral decubitus film with the right side up; if air is present in the ascending colon, an ileocolic intussusception is unlikely.

Late films may reveal a developing small bowel obstruction. In either case, an intravenous line should be established and appropriate fluid resuscitation begun before any attempt at hydrostatic or air enema reduction.

Treatment and Prognosis

About 60% to 70% of ileocolic intussusceptions can be reduced by barium or air-contrast enema. The former is performed under fluoroscopic control with the enema bag raised no more than 3 feet above the patient, to avoid overdistending and perforating the colon. Air-contrast enemas are performed under ultrasound guidance, and the pressure must be carefully controlled. If nonoperative attempts to reduce the intussusception are unsuccessful or perforation occurs, or if the infant has peritonitis indicative of perforation, then operative reduction is indicated. The procedure is carried out through a transverse right lower quadrant incision, as the intussusception has usually been reduced to this position by a preceding enema. The cecum is mobilized and the intussusception reduced by squeezing the proximal bowel out of the distal bowel in a retrograde fashion. Complete reduction of an ileocolic intussusception can be confirmed by identifying Treves' fold (a membranous fold along the inferior margin of the terminal ileum, where the ileum joins the cecum). If necrosis of the small bowel is encountered, a segmental resection with primary anastomosis is performed. The appendix is removed to avoid future confusion related to the right lower quadrant incision.

The recurrence rate after nonoperative reduction of an ileocolic intussusception is about 10% and may occur within days or months of the initial episode. If the child is young, a repeated hydrostatic or air-contrast reduction is acceptable. Operative reduction with the first recurrence is usually recommended in older children (older than 2 years), as they have a higher incidence of specific lead points causing intussusception.

Biliary Tract Disorders

Developmental anomalies of the bile ducts take many forms. The two most important anomalies are biliary atresia and choledochal cyst, both of which affect bile transport between the liver and the duodenum.

Biliary Atresia

Biliary atresia is characterized by luminal obstruction of a portion or all of the extrahepatic bile ducts. It is thought to be an acquired condition, because approximately 40% of patients pass normal meconium at birth, and about 60% pass obviously yellow feces for a short period thereafter. The incidence of biliary atresia is about 1 in 10,000 live births. The underlying cause is unknown, but several hypotheses exist, including in utero viral infections, ischemia, ductal plate malformation, and pancreaticobiliary malunion. Histopathologic studies of the extrahepatic bile ducts demonstrate a dynamic, sclerosing, obliterative process with various stages of inflammation, which may be a cause or a result of progressive ductal destruction. The extrahepatic ducts communicate with the intrahepatic ducts through an arborizing network of tiny, patent biliary channels at the porta hepatis. Patency of this arborizing biliary network is lost over time. By age 4 months, these structures are completely replaced by fibrous tissue, effectively nullifying any possibility of establishing bile drainage from the liver parenchyma.

Clinical Presentation and Diagnosis

Neonatal jaundice is usually physiologic, self-limited, and characterized by an indirect (unconjugated) hyperbilirubinemia. Common causes include impaired processing of unconjugated bilirubin by the immature liver and hemolysis, the latter due to Rh or ABO incompatibilities. Jaundice that persists beyond age 2 weeks is no longer physiologic and should be investigated, especially if the direct bilirubin level (conjugated fraction) is greater than 1 mg/dL. The differential diagnosis of hyperbilirubinemia in infancy includes infectious, metabolic, genetic, cholestatic, and obstructive disorders (Box 57-2).

Many infants with biliary atresia appear healthy at birth. Neonatal jaundice appears and then persists along with scleral icterus, light yellow stools, and hepatomegaly. Slight up and down fluctuations in the serum bilirubin levels may lull the practitioner to inaction. The urine turns brown as the serum bilirubin increases and splenomegaly develops. Normal growth and development in the first few months are followed by growth retardation, anemia, and malnutrition, due to severe liver dysfunction and malabsorption of fat and fat-soluble vitamins. In the absence of surgical intervention, the majority of patients will die of hepatic failure, esophageal variceal bleeding, infection, or a combination of these, before their second birthday.

BOX 57-2 Disorders Associated with Infantile Hyperbilirubinemia

Infection

Hepatitis (B or C), sepsis, syphilis, toxoplasmosis, cytomegalovirus, rubella

Metabolic or Genetic

α-1-Antitrypsin deficiency, galactosemia, cystic fibrosis, tyrosinemia, Gaucher's disease

Endocrine

Hypothyroidism, hypopituitarism

Extrahepatic Biliary Pathology

Biliary atresia, choledochal cyst, inspissated bile syndrome

Intrahepatic Biliary Pathology

Bile duct hypoplasia

The diagnosis of biliary atresia should be pursued with haste whenever considered, because prognosis worsens with increasing age at operation. The initial workup involves checking for bile in the nasogastric aspirate and looking at the color of the stool; green or brown stool suggests a patent biliary system. Several serum studies should be sent, including liver-function tests; additional investigations that are useful in the diagnosis of biliary atresia are listed in Box 57-3. An ultrasound study should be obtained to search for other causes of neonatal jaundice such as extrahepatic biliary dilatation or a choledochal cyst. In the setting of biliary atresia, ultrasonography will show increased echogenicity of the liver and a small, shrunken gallbladder that does not contract with feeding. Hepatobiliary scintigraphy, after pretreatment with phenobarbital to promote hepatic excretion, will demonstrate rapid isotope uptake by the liver and no excretion in the presence of biliary atresia. In contrast, hepatocellular causes of jaundice are characterized by delayed isotope uptake due to parenchymal disease and patency of the extrahepatic biliary system, as evidenced by excretion of the radionucleotide into the duodenum. Last, a percutaneous liver biopsy may be considered, provided the patient's coagulation status is normal or corrected. Histologic findings of portal fibrosis and bile duct proliferation are pathognomonic for biliary atresia.

BOX 57–3 Useful Investigations in the Diagnosis of Biliary Atresia

Hematology
- Complete blood count

Liver-function Tests
- Serum lipoprotein-X (>300 mg/dL suggest biliary atresia)
- γ-Glutaryl transpeptidase (>300 IU/L is consistent with biliary atresia)

Screening Tests for Infectious, Metabolic, and Genetic Disorders
- Blood and urine cultures
- Sweat chloride determination
- Thyroxin and thyroid-stimulating hormone
- TORCH screen
- VDRL titers
- Metabolic screen for aminoacidemia, α-1-antitrypsin

Imaging Studies
- Ultrasonography
- Hepatobiliary radionucleotide imaging
- Percutaneous liver biopsy

TORCH, toxoplasmosis, rubella, cytomegalovirus, herpes simplex, human immunodeficiency virus; VDRL, Venereal Disease Research Laboratory.

Treatment and Prognosis

An exploratory laparotomy, liver biopsy, and intraoperative cholangiography should be performed if the diagnosis of biliary atresia is suspected. The procedure is begun through a small right upper quadrant incision. The liver is typically firm and nodular with a green-brown color; a biopsy is taken for frozen and permanent sections. Cholangiography is carried out via the fundus of the gallbladder, unless this is shrunken or atretic. If cholangiography visualizes the extrahepatic bile ducts from the intrahepatic ducts to the duodenum, the diagnosis of biliary atresia is excluded. If biliary atresia is confirmed, the incision is enlarged and full exploration of the extrahepatic biliary system carried out. The atretic common hepatic duct is dissected to the hilum of the liver, where it broadens to form a cone of fibrous tissue. Within this cone are the patent, arborizing bile ductules described earlier. The cone is sharply transected flush with the surface of the liver and the specimen submitted for frozen-section analysis. If the bile ductules are smaller than 100 μm in diameter, the porta hepatis should be reexcised farther proximally. On demonstrating bile ductules of sufficient caliber, a Kasai procedure (hepatic portoenterostomy) is performed by anastomosing a Roux-en-Y loop of jejunum to the perimeter of the transected fibrous cone.

Cholangitis due to impaired drainage of the hypoplastic biliary system is the most frequent and serious complication after hepatic portoenterostomy. Cholangitis is initially seen with fever, leukocytosis, elevated transaminase levels and an increase in the serum bilirubin level. Maintenance of bile flow and prevention of infection are promoted through the use of chloretics, steroids, and antibiotics. Other complications include portal hypertension and fat malabsorption. The former can lead to variceal bleeding, hypersplenism, and ascites. Fat malabsorption and fat-soluble vitamin deficiencies may result from insufficient bile flow. The routine use of formulas with medium-chain triglycerides can prevent fatty acid deficiency. Careful monitoring of fat-soluble vitamin levels and appropriate supplementation can minimize the risks of blindness (vitamin A), rickets (vitamin D), bleeding diatheses (vitamin K), anemia, and poor wound healing (vitamin E).

The Kasai procedure has proven to be a durable and life-saving operation for many children. In general, one third of all who undergo a Kasai procedure for biliary atresia will have a good long-term result. Another one third will achieve bile flow but go on to progressive hepatic failure requiring liver transplantation. The other one third of patients will never establish bile flow and will therefore be early candidates for transplantation. These results serve to emphasize the importance of early diagnosis and treatment.

Choledochal Cyst

Choledochal cyst is a rare congenital disease encompassing various forms of intra- and extrahepatic dilatation of the biliary duct system (Fig. 57-8). The etiology of choledochal cyst formation is believed to be related to pancreaticobiliary

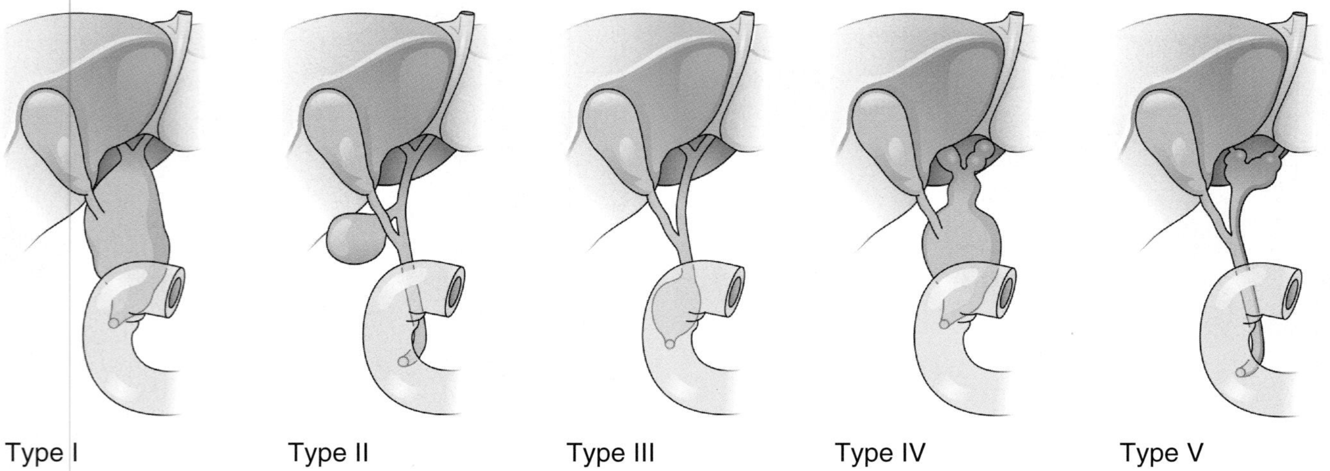

FIGURE 57–8 The five general forms of choledochal cyst that can be found by cholangiography, as originally described by Todani. (Adapted from Rowe MI, O'Neil JA Jr, Grosfeld JL, et al: Choledochal cyst. In Essentials of Pediatric Surgery. Philadelphia, Mosby, 1995, p 640.)

malunion, wherein the pancreatic duct inserts abnormally high (above the ampulla) into the common bile duct. Reflux of pancreatic enzymes into the common bile duct is thought to cause dissolution and aneurysmal dilatation of the bile duct walls. This theory is supported by numerous cholangiograms in affected patients and further supported by the high amylase content of choledochal cyst fluid.

Clinical Presentation and Diagnosis

The clinical manifestations of choledochal cyst vary according to the age of the patient at presentation. Neonates and young infants usually have obstructive jaundice, vomiting, acholic stools, and an abdominal mass. Older children, teenagers, and adults may exhibit one or more features of the classic triad of abdominal pain, jaundice, and a right upper quadrant abdominal mass. Fever and vomiting may occur with cholangitis.

Ultrasonography is an excellent screening method for the diagnosis of choledochal cyst. To confirm the diagnosis and delineate the ductal anatomy, the patient should undergo endoscopic retrograde cholangiopancreatography or magnetic resonance cholangiopancreatography (MRCP). MRCP is preferable in many cases, as it is highly accurate, noninvasive, and can be performed in the presence of pancreatitis. MRCP is especially helpful in the setting of distal ductal obstruction or stenosis. It also can help in planning operative resection by defining the proximal transition point between the normal hepatic duct and cystic dilatation and may avoid the need for intraoperative cholangiography.

Treatment and Prognosis

Cyst excision with a Roux-en-Y choledochojejunostomy is the treatment of choice. In years past, simple drainage of the cyst into either the duodenum or a Roux-en-Y limb of jejunum was recommended. These procedures are no longer performed because of the high rate of recurrent pancreatitis and the high risk of carcinoma developing in the cyst.

Abdominal Wall Defects

Neonatal abdominal wall defects include gastroschisis, exomphalos (omphalocele and hernia into the umbilical cord), prune-belly syndrome, various degrees of exstrophy (bladder and cloacal), and residual embryonic remnants of the umbilicus.

PEARLS FOR THE OR

Most postoperative problems begin in the operating room. Corollary: Antibiotics cannot compensate for poor technique.

"If the operation is difficult, you are not doing it correctly." —Robert Gross

Always establish distal patency when operating for bowel atresia or stenosis.

Sharp dissection and the use of "cutting" as opposed to "cautery" current cause less tissue trauma, which leads to better cosmetic results.

Know how a congenital inguinal hernia differs from an adult inguinal hernia — and how the repair differs.

Be able to list five reasons for surgical correction of an undescended testicle.

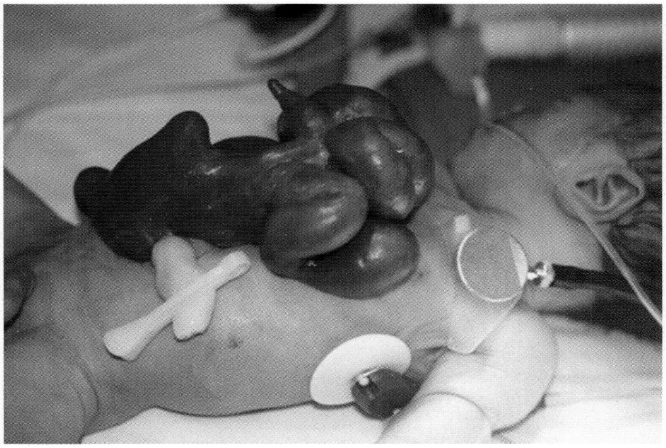

FIGURE 57–9 Gastroschisis. Note the matted bowel, the appendix, and the normal skin at the base of the umbilicus

Gastroschisis and Omphalocele

Gastroschisis and omphalocele represent two distinct embryonic anomalies of anterior abdominal-wall closure. The abdominal-wall defect in gastroschisis is usually to the right of the umbilicus and probably is related to atrophy of the right umbilical vein. The viscera protrude through the defect into the amniotic space and are bathed in amniotic fluid, which leads to the development of a thick, fibrinous inflammatory peel that covers the bowel (Fig. 57-9). This inflammatory peel is associated with prolonged hypomotility and absorptive problems.

During the sixth week of development, the midgut elongates and herniates into the umbilical cord. Failure of the intestines to return fully to the abdomen during week 10 yields an abdominal-wall defect with a translucent saclike covering called an omphalocele (Fig. 57-10). The umbilical vessels insert near the apex of the sac, which is covered by amnion and internally lined by peritoneum. Between 50% and 70% of infants with an omphalocele have other associated congenital anomalies, some of which are severe and incompatible with long-term survival. The common associated anomalies include structural cardiac, renal, limb, and facial anomalies; the lethal associated anomalies include trisomies 13, 18, and 21. When the sac is ruptured, it may be difficult to distinguish gastroschisis and omphalocele. Gastroschisis and omphalocele occur in approximately 1 per 5000 births, affecting boys and girls equally, with a high frequency of prematurity.

Clinical Presentation and Diagnosis

Gastroschisis and omphalocele can be detected and differentiated by prenatal ultrasonography. The principal clinical and pathologic features of these two anomalies are summarized in Table 57-2. The major differences are the presence or absence of a membrane-covered sac, the relation

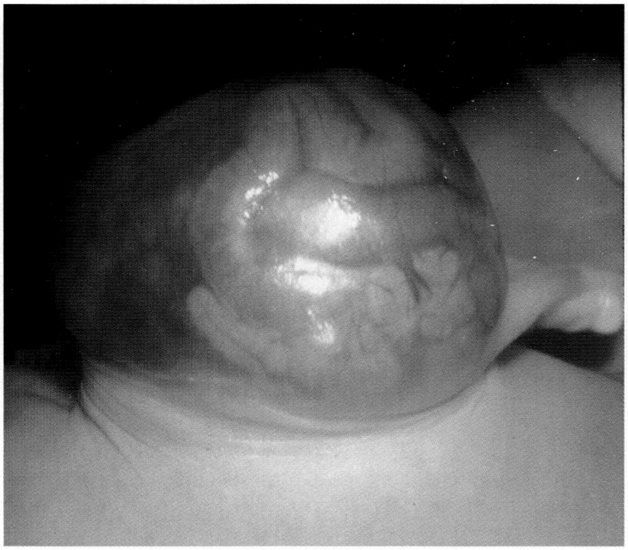

FIGURE 57–10 Omphalocele. Note the liver and small bowel tightly packed but viable; the base of the umbilicus is covered with amnion.

of the abdominal wall defect with the umbilicus, and the occurrence of the anomaly in isolation or in association with other congenital anomalies.

Treatment and Prognosis

Most infants with gastroschisis or omphalocele are delivered vaginally. Cesarean section delivery may be considered for infants with especially large omphaloceles, to avoid injury to the exteriorized liver. On delivery, the lower half of the infant's body is placed in a transparent bowel bag to help maintain sterility, prevent dehydration, and limit heat loss from the herniated viscera. This maneuver does not impede access to the head for airway control or access to the arms

TABLE 57–2 Differences between Gastroschisis and Omphalocele

	Gastroschisis	Omphalocele
Associated anomalies	10% (intestinal atresia)	50% (structural and chromosomal)
Sac covering abdominal contents	No	Yes
Normal base of umbilicus	Yes	No
Liver exteriorized	No	Often
Intestinal dysfunction (hypomotility and malabsorption)	Yes	No

for insertion of an intravenous catheter. A nasogastric tube is inserted to limit bowel distention, and prophylactic broad-spectrum antibiotics are administered. The initial fluid requirements of an infant with gastroschisis or a ruptured omphalocele are 2 to 3 times normal, averaging about 175 mL/kg/day of D5LR.

Infants with gastroschisis are usually brought directly to the operating room, whereas those with unruptured omphaloceles are first stabilized and evaluated for associated anomalies. Primary closure is the goal. This may not be possible if the abdominal wall defect is large, the bowel is distended, or the peritoneal cavity is small. Bowel that cannot be reduced into the abdomen is placed in a Silastic (Dow Corning, Midland, MI) silo and reduced into the abdomen at the bedside over a period of 3 to 6 days. If the infant has an associated bowel atresia, a temporary enterostomy is constructed at the time of the initial operation. Once the viscera are completely reduced, the Silastic is removed, and the fascia closed. Alternatively, for infants with large unruptured omphaloceles, the membrane may be sequentially ligated and the contents of the sac reduced into the abdomen. Still others recommend use of an escharotic agent, such as topical silver sulfadiazine, followed by delayed closure.

Prognosis for the newborn with gastroschisis is determined primarily by the condition of the exteriorized bowel and whether an associated bowel atresia is found, which occurs in about 10% of affected infants and may go unrecognized at the time of abdominal wall closure because of marked thickening and matting of the bowel wall. If the patient remains obstructed for more than 4 to 5 weeks, a contrast study should be obtained to determine whether the infant has a missed atresia or distal intraluminal web. Outcome for children with omphalocele is related to the presence of associated chromosomal and structural anomalies and the size of the defect.

Bladder and Cloacal Exstrophy

Bladder exstrophy refers to "eversion" of the posterior wall of the bladder through a defect in the anterior abdominal wall. This anomaly occurs as a result of failed closure of the anterior abdominal wall at the ventral end of the cloacal membrane (*cloaca* is a term that refers to the dilated portion of the hindgut that is the primordium of the urinary bladder and the rectum). The incidence of bladder exstrophy is 1 in 10,000 to 1 in 40,000 live births. Associated anomalies include other genitourinary abnormalities, epispadias, and splaying of the pubic bones with incomplete formation of the pelvic floor and muscles of urinary continence.

Cloacal exstrophy is the rarest and most severe form of the exstrophy complex. The posterior wall of the bladder and a large portion of the hindgut protrude outward through a large anterior abdominal wall and perineal defect. The incidence of cloacal exstrophy is low and is estimated at 1 in 300,000 live births. Associated anomalies include omphalocele, imperforate anus, pubic diastasis, spinal abnormalities such as myelomeningocele, renal abnormalities such as agenesis or ectopia, and absent genitalia. These patients require extensive reconstructive surgery. Urinary continence is achieved by catheterization of a compliant reservoir constructed of bladder and bowel. Bowel continence is achieved with an intestinal stoma or a colonic pull-through, supplemented with enema washouts.

Disorders of the Umbilicus

Omphalomesenteric Duct Malformations

The omphalomesenteric (or vitelline) duct allows nourishment to pass from the yolk sac to the fetal gut during the initial weeks of fetal development (Fig. 57-11). As the placental circulation develops, the duct regresses and usually becomes obliterated between weeks 5 and 7 of gestation. Incomplete regression can lead to five different congenital anomalies, depending on which portion of the omphalomesenteric duct remains.

1. A **patent omphalomesenteric duct** refers to persistence of the duct between the midgut and the

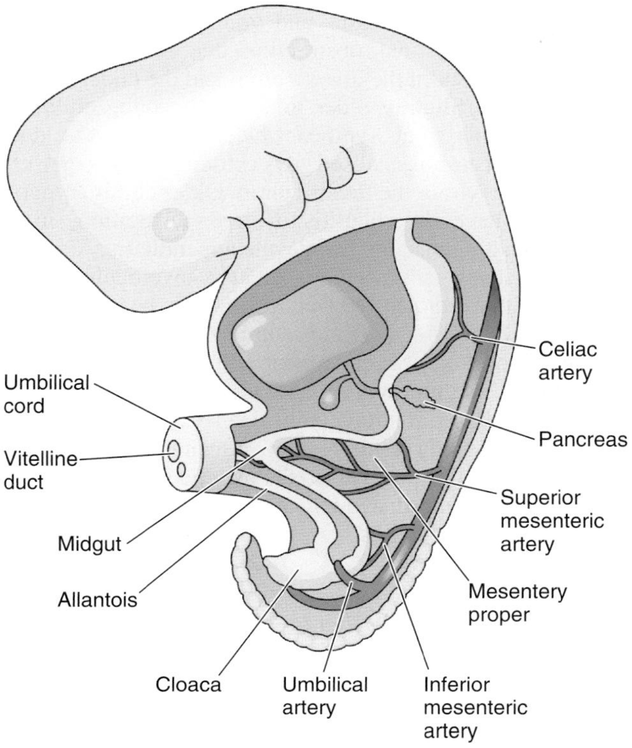

FIGURE 57–11 Umbilicus in a 5-mm embryo (week 5) demonstrating communication between the yolk sac and the alimentary tract. The allantois communicates with the cloaca.

umbilicus. This rather dramatic anomaly allows gas and feces to be extruded from the umbilicus.

2. An **umbilical sinus** is seen when the duct becomes obliterated at the intestinal end but remains patent at the umbilicus.
3. An **omphalomesenteric duct cyst** is a mucosa-lined remnant that does not communicate with the small bowel or umbilicus.
4. Complete obliteration of the mucosal lining may occur, yet a residual **fibrous cord** extends from the distal ileum or tip of a Meckel's diverticulum, to the underside of the umbilicus. This type of cord can act as a point of fixation to the anterior abdominal wall, about which a volvulus or internal hernia may occur, causing an acute small-bowel obstruction.
5. Last, a **Meckel's diverticulum** is a saclike remnant of the original duct that arises from the antimesenteric border of the distal ileum.

Meckel's Diverticulum

The most common omphalomesenteric duct malformation is a Meckel's diverticulum, which is present in 1% to 3% of the population.

Clinical Presentation and Diagnosis

Most symptoms develop during childhood and vary directly with patient age. Newborns and young infants typically present with intestinal obstruction due to a persistent fibrous cord between the diverticulum and the underside of the umbilicus. Slightly older infants and young children may have painless but significant bleeding per rectum due to peptic ulceration caused by ectopic, acid-secreting gastric tissue within the diverticulum. Older children more commonly have diverticulitis or free perforation, in a manner indistinguishable from acute appendicitis.

The diagnosis of a bleeding Meckel's diverticulum may be made with a radiolabeled technetium scan, because of the high affinity of ^{99m}Tc-pertechnetate to the mucus-secreting gastric mucosal cells. Pretreatment with pentagastrin and a histamine H_2 inhibitor will enhance uptake of the radiotracer and should be used if strong clinical suspicion exists after a negative initial study result. A positive scan is noted in about 90% of cases; false-positive results may be seen in cases of intussusception, intestinal duplication, arteriovenous malformation, and hydronephrosis.

Treatment and Prognosis

Laparoscopy is the preferred operative approach. Fibrous bands are easily divided, allowing the entire small bowel to be examined. If a diverticulum is present, it is usually located on the antimesenteric border of the bowel. Occasionally, the diverticulum may be folded over and kinked by a congenital band or an inflammatory adhesion. These bands or adhesions should be divided along with the vitelline vessels to expose the base of the diverticulum. If the diverticulum has a narrow and intact base, it may be divided with an endoscopic stapler. If, however, the base of the diverticulum is wide, thickened (suggesting the presence of ectopic tissue), or if inflammation or ischemia is present involving the adjacent ileum, a minimally invasive intestinal resection should be carried out through an umbilical incision.

Controversy still exists over whether to remove an incidental Meckel's diverticulum. Those in favor state that it is nearly impossible to determine by inspection or palpation whether a diverticulum contains heterotopic tissue, and even more difficult to determine which diverticula will lead to complications. Those against incidental Meckel's diverticulectomy cite the operative risks of wound infection, anastomotic leak, and intestinal obstruction from adhesion formation. These risks must be weighed against the roughly 5% lifetime probability of complications from an incidentally discovered Meckel's diverticulum. Fortunately, several factors associated with symptomatic diverticula have been identified. Resection is recommended if the diverticulum is longer than 2 cm, the patient is younger than 40 years, or heterotopic mucosa is suspected. Resection of an omphalomesenteric duct remnant also should be carried out in patients with an unexplained history of abdominal pain. Conversely, resection should not be performed during repair of gastroschisis, in asymptomatic patients who are at increased risk for infection, or in older asymptomatic patients.

Urachal Remnants

The urachus is an early embryonic tubular connection between the dome of the developing bladder and the allantois. It usually regresses in the fetal period to form the medial vesicoumbilical ligament. If obliteration does not occur, a **patent urachus** or an **urachal cyst** may remain between the dome of the bladder and the umbilicus. Other types of urachal remnants include urachal sinus and vesicourachal diverticulum.

Clinical Presentation and Diagnosis

A patent urachus usually is seen shortly after birth with a discharge of urine from the umbilicus. The diagnosis can be confirmed with a fistulogram, which should be followed by a voiding cystourethrogram to rule out lower urinary tract obstruction as a potential cause for the anomaly. An urachal cyst may be diagnosed by prenatal ultrasound; however, most children are seen initially with lower midline abdominal pain and infection. Physical examination is notable for fever and abdominal tenderness, which may be accompanied by erythema of the infraumbilical abdominal wall. An abdominal ultrasound will reveal an edematous, cystic structure within the lower midline abdominal wall.

Treatment and Prognosis

Early excision is recommended to prevent recurrent urinary tract infection, stone formation, and malignant degeneration.

An extraperitoneal dissection is followed by complete excision with a cuff of normal bladder tissue. If the child has an infected urachal cyst and sepsis, due to cyst rupture and peritonitis, primary incision and drainage followed by a secondary operation under sterile conditions may be preferred.

Inguinal and Scrotal Disorders

Undescended Testis

An undescended testicle is found in 3% to 4% of newborn boys and is more common in preterm infants. True undescent is pathologic beyond age 6 months and is found in approximately 1% of boys. Most undescended testes are unilateral (80%), and their abnormal position is attributed to one or more isolated mechanical events that may interfere with normal descent. In a smaller percentage of cases, they are bilateral (20%), a situation commonly attributed to hormonal imbalance.

Clinical Presentation and Diagnosis

Many children who are referred for evaluation of an undescended testicle have, in fact, a retractile testicle. This is a testicle that typically resides in the low inguinal canal or high scrotum, but that, on occasion, may be observed in the midscrotum while the child is asleep, at rest, or in a warm bath. Retractile testes are usually bilateral, and each hemiscrotum is well formed. If the testicle can be manipulated into the scrotum, completely released, and regrasped in the scrotum by the examining hand without further manipulation, one is dealing with a retractile testicle. In this case, the parents should be reassured and told that as the child matures and the testicle enlarges, gravity will overcome the "overactive" cremasteric muscle. If, conversely, the child is 6 months old and one must repeatedly manipulate the testicle to bring it into the scrotum, and it does not remain there when released, it is undescended and will require surgical correction. The five principal reasons for surgical correction of an undescended testicle are (1) preservation of fertility, (2) risk of trauma to the undescended testicle, (3) repair of an associated hernia, (4) cosmesis, and (5) the risk of testicular cancer.

Male fertility in the setting of an uncorrected unilateral undescended testicle ranges between 40% and 65%. In comparison, fertility in corrected unilateral undescended testicle repaired before age 6 years is about 80% to 90%. The lower fertility rate associated with an undescended testicle is attributed to the higher-temperature environment of the nonscrotal testis. Morphologic and histologic changes in the undescended testis include loss of testicular volume and progressive germ cell depletion starting at age 6 months. Germ cells may be completely absent beginning at age 18 months. Orchidopexy is therefore recommended before age 15 to 18 months.

A testis that lies in the inguinal canal is at risk for crush injury, as it is relatively immobile and underlain by ligaments and bone. About 90% of inguinal testes have an associated patent processus vaginalis, which predisposes to hernia formation. Operative placement of the testis into the scrotum reduces the risk of crush injury, corrects the associated hernia, and alleviates the psychological concerns of having only one testicle visible in the scrotum. Orchidopexy does not, however, protect against the eightfold to 10-fold increased incidence of testicular malignancy in patients with a history of cryptorchidism. Moreover, the rate of testicular malignancy in patients with a history of cryptorchidism appears minimally affected by the timing of orchidopexy. Thus orchidopexy is performed to facilitate examination of the testicle and allow early detection in the event a tumor develops.

In infants with bilateral *nonpalpable* testes, a human chorionic gonadotropin (hCG) stimulation test should be performed to determine whether any testicular tissue is present. If the serum testosterone level does not increase markedly in response to hCG administration, no testicular tissue exists. Children with bilateral, *palpable* undescended testes are more likely to have a hormonal deficiency or an underlying anatomic problem as a cause for testicular maldescent than are those with a unilateral undescended testicle.

Treatment and Prognosis

Orchidopexy for a palpable, undescended testicle is performed through a groin incision. The abnormal attachment of the gubernaculum is divided and the hernia sac carefully freed from the cord structures. Traction on the hernia sac allows the surgeon to bluntly dissect the vessels and vas deferens free of the overlying peritoneum, well up into the retroperitoneal space. The ability to bring the testicle into the scrotum is now limited by the length of the testicular artery. When the artery is particularly short, the testicle, its vascular pedicle, and the vas deferens are passed beneath the epigastric vessels, to take a medial lie and run directly into the scrotum.

The diagnosis of unilateral anorchia can be made only by direct visualization of blind-ending vessels and a blind-ending vas deferens. Management of a unilateral nonpalpable testis therefore begins with laparoscopy and not an imaging study. If the testicle is absent by these criteria, no further therapy is indicated. If the testicle is atrophic, it should be removed. If it is intraabdominal, but adjacent to the internal ring, a standard orchidopexy is performed. If, however, the testicle is more than 1 cm from the internal ring, the testicular vessels should be clipped and divided in preparation for a second-stage orchidopexy. In the interim, the testicle will develop a new blood supply via collaterals along the vas deferens. These collaterals will be sufficiently robust in 3 to 4 months to allow the testicle to be safely brought down into the scrotum.

Testicular Torsion

Testicular torsion refers to twisting of the testicle and cord structures, leading to acute disruption of blood flow to the testis and epididymis. Extravaginal (high-cord) torsion occurs predominantly in the perinatal period and refers to twisting of the extravaginal spermatic cord. Intravaginal torsion occurs predominantly in older children and is related to anomalous testicular suspension within the tunica vaginalis. Normally, the epididymal-testicular complex is fixed posteriorly within the tunica. Failure of proper fixation allows the testicle to twist on its blood supply. This anatomic anomaly in older children is referred to as the "bell-clapper" deformity.

Clinical Presentation and Diagnosis

Testicular torsion may occur several weeks to months before birth and appear in the newborn as unilateral cryptorchidism. Alternatively, testicular torsion may occur in the perinatal period and be evident during the newborn examination as a swollen testicle within an edematous and discolored hemiscrotum. In this case, because unilateral torsion may be followed shortly thereafter by bilateral torsion (so-called sequential torsion), emergency scrotal exploration with a contralateral orchidopexy is indicated. Adolescent boys with testicular torsion typically are seen late, after several hours of acute debilitating scrotal pain. The examiner should inquire about a history of trauma and sexual activity. Almost invariably, the child will have been at rest or been performing some low-level activity when he experienced sudden onset of unilateral testicular pain. Examination of the scrotum is notable for an enlarged, tender, and elevated testicle. The epididymis, which is usually posterior, may be medial or lateral, and the cremasteric reflex is absent.

Urinalysis is usually normal in the setting of testicular torsion. Scrotal ultrasound is useful in determining whether the entire testicle and epididymis are swollen (torsion), or just the epididymis (epididymitis). These findings may be complemented by Doppler ultrasonography, which is highly accurate in assessing testicular blood flow in adolescent but not in prepubertal boys. Young children with clinical and ultrasonographic findings consistent with testicular torsion should be surgically explored. Children who are considered unlikely to have testicular torsion by clinical criteria but in whom a definitive diagnosis of torsion of the appendix, testis, or epididymitis cannot be made should undergo a radioisotope scan to confirm normal blood flow to the testicles.

Treatment and Prognosis

Exploration for extravaginal testicular torsion in the perinatal period is performed through an ipsilateral inguinal incision to evaluate the cord and testicle; orchidopexy on the opposite side is performed through a contralateral scrotal incision. Older children are explored through a midline scrotal incision, which provides access to both hemiscrotums. The torsed testicle is detorsed in the direction one would open a book: counterclockwise on the right side and clockwise on the left. The ischemic testicle is placed in a warm, saline-soaked sponge while a contralateral orchidopexy with permanent suture is performed. The affected testicle is then reexamined, and if unsalvageable, it is removed. If the color of the affected testicle improves or it bleeds when incised, it may be salvaged. Orchidopexy is performed and the parents informed of the possibility that the testicle may survive or atrophy.

Suggested Reading

Albanese CT, Rowe MI: Necrotizing enterocololitis. Semin Pediatr Surg 4:200–206, 1995.

Masaki N, Ohi R: Biliary atresia. Semin Pediatr Surg 9:177–186, 2000.

Meijers C, Molenaar J. Congenital malformations of the enteric nervous system, including Hirschsprung's disease. In Freeman NV, Burge DM, Griffiths DM, Malone PSJ (eds): Surgery of the Newborn. New York, Churchill Livingstone, 1994, pp 159–170.

Peña A: Anorectal malformations. Semin Pediatr Surg 4:35–47, 1995.

Sigalet DL: Short bowel syndrome in infants and children: An overview. Semin Pediatr Surg 10:49–55, 2001.

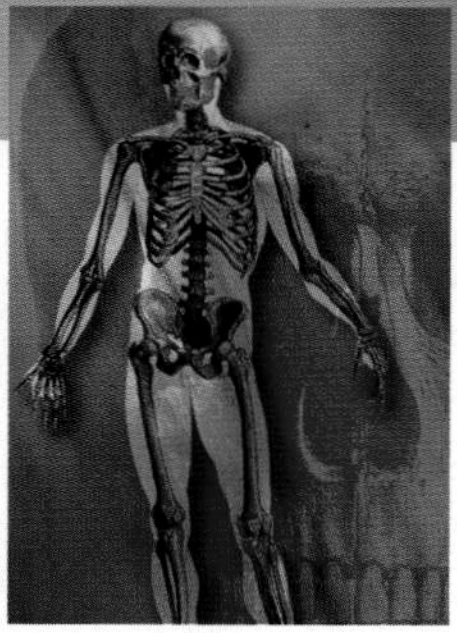

Chapter 58
Vascular Anomalies, Tumors, and Twins

STEVEN L. MOULTON, MD

Vascular Anomalies

Vascular anomalies include hemangiomas, vascular malformations, lymphatic malformations, and combined lesions. These lesions can be distinguished by their clinical presentation, radiologic evaluation, and pathologic findings. In general, they are frequently misdiagnosed and inappropriately managed. Greater understanding of the genetic and molecular mechanisms that underlie the development of vascular anomalies will likely lead to new therapeutic interventions in vascular biology, including new insight into the management of many other diseases, such as cancer, arthritis, and atherosclerosis.

Hemangiomas

Hemangiomas are the most common tumor of infancy. They are estimated to occur in 1 to 3 per 100 live births and are three times more common in girls, suggesting a hormonal influence. Hemangiomas are true endothelial cell tumors, characterized by benign proliferation of capillary endothelium beginning at about age 3 weeks. Maturation and subsequent involution of hemangiomas in childhood leads to flattening of the endothelial cells, vascular thrombosis, and deposition of collagen and adipose tissue. Their etiology is unknown. Recent genetic analysis reveals that hemangiomas are monoclonal in origin, even when multiple lesions are present. This suggests that proliferation of hemangioma endothelial cells may involve defects in endothelial cell regulation, growth, differentiation, or a combination of these.

Clinical Presentation and Diagnosis

Hemangiomas usually appear within the first few weeks of life as a red skin lesion or "stork bite," which gradually enlarges and causes a mass effect on surrounding normal structures. Superficial hemangiomas are raised, crimson, slightly nodular lesions with a rubbery texture (Fig. 58-1). Deeper lesions in the dermis or subcutaneous tissue may have a blue hue with normal overlying skin. Rapid growth is typically seen between ages 8 and 18 months, during which time basic fibroblast growth factor is markedly elevated in the urine (a distinguishing feature not seen in patients with vascular malformations). This phase of rapid growth is followed by a prolonged period of involution, such that about 50% of hemangiomas will resolve by age 5 years and up to 70% by 7 years (Fig. 58-2). Hemangiomas can impinge on important orifices, such as the airway, mouth, urethral meatus, and anus, or may impair the visual axis or encroach on an external auditory canal. Large hemangiomas of the torso may extend into the mediastinum or retroperitoneum, causing heart failure and a platelet-trapping thrombocytopenia (Kasabach-Merritt phenomenon). Large hemangiomas are associated with hypothyroidism because of expression of high levels of type 3 iodothyronine deiodinase activity in the hemangioma tissue. This means that children with large hemangiomas should be monitored for hypothyroidism and treated, if it is present, to prevent irreversible developmental delay, mental retardation, and other neurologic sequelae. The anatomic distribution of large hemangiomas is best determined by magnetic resonance imaging (MRI), which also can be used to distinguish one type of vascular anomaly from another.

Treatment and Prognosis

Most hemangiomas are small, self-resolving, and require no treatment. Those that impair the airway, an orifice, the visual axis, or an external auditory canal require treatment. Other indications for treatment include bleeding, ulceration with intractable pain, and a high potential for significant

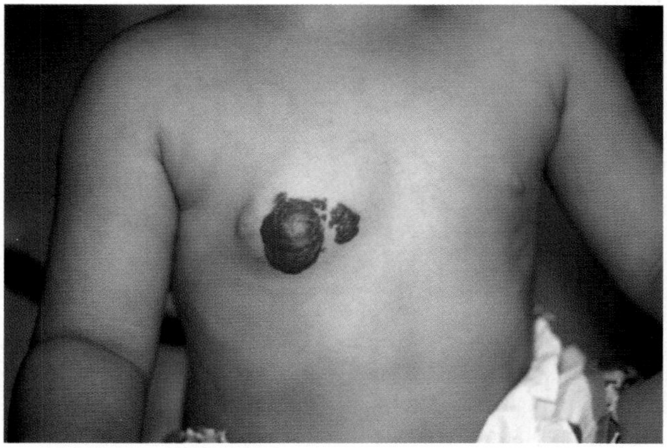

FIGURE 58–1 A 2-year-old girl with a "proliferative phase" right breast hemangioma. Note the inferolateral displacement of the nipple areolar complex.

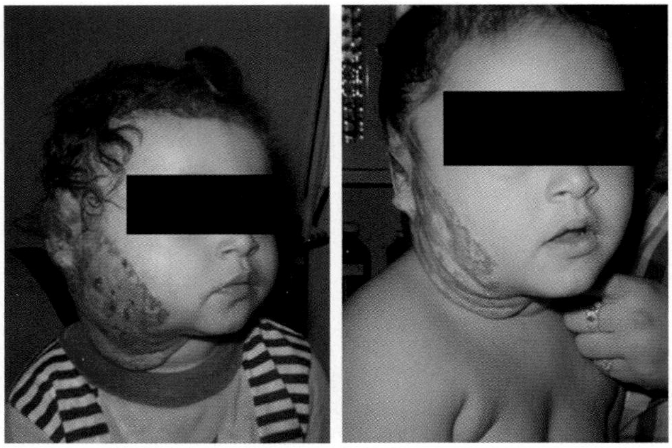

FIGURE 58–2 Natural history of a hemangioma involving the right cheek, ear, and neck. *A*, A 3-year-old; note uniform coalescence and flattening of lesion. *B*, Same patient age 5 years; note islands of normal-appearing skin within the midportion of the lesion.

facial disfigurement. Pharmacologic antiangiogenic therapy is initiated with corticosteroids. Nonresponders with life-threatening lesions are treated with interferon α 2a. Hemangiomas that affect the airway can be further managed with bronchoscopic endoluminal laser therapy. Lasers also are used to ablate proliferative cutaneous hemangiomas, although this is still controversial. Surgery is reserved for excision of redundant or fibrofatty tissue that may remain after incomplete regression of a hemangioma. In the future, we can expect the introduction of more specific and more potent antiangiogenic agents for the treatment of hemangiomas. These agents, if used early during the proliferative phase, may alter the natural history of hemangiomas, thereby preventing facial disfigurement and the emotional trauma that so often accompanies these anomalies.

Vascular Malformations

Vascular malformations are developmental errors of vascular morphogenesis. They are composed of malformed, often tortuous vessels with a quiescent endothelium. They can be subcategorized according to channel morphology and the flow characteristics of the lesion.

Clinical Presentation and Diagnosis

All vascular malformations are present at birth, and most are asymptomatic (Fig. 58-3). Slow-flow (venous and lymphatic) lesions may rarely appear with pain because of engorgement or focal intralesional thrombosis. Fast-flow (arterial and arteriovenous) lesions may occur with pain, high-output cardiac failure, or bleeding. A capillary vascular malformation of the face (also known as a port-wine stain) is a classic example of a slow-flow lesion. This flat, vascular lesion is usually a pale pink color in early life. If often conforms to the distribution of the trigeminal nerve and

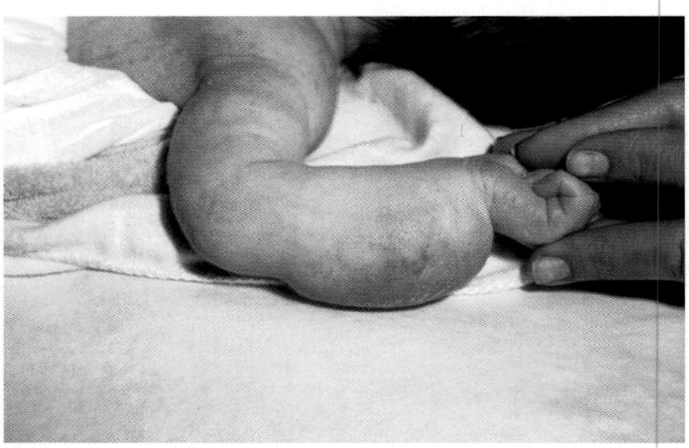

FIGURE 58–3 A 3-week-old neonate with a vascular malformation of right forearm. Note the overlying normal skin and the bluish discoloration of the lesion beneath.

grows in proportion to the child's growth. This lesion will not improve with time, but may darken and develop a cutaneous nodularity. For these reasons, it is essential that a correct diagnosis be made in early life, so that appropriate and timely therapy can be instituted before the parents develop false hope that the lesion will spontaneously regress.

Treatment and Prognosis

Antiendothelial therapy is not effective in the treatment of vascular malformations, probably because of the normal endothelial cell turnover that characterizes these lesions. The treatment options depend on the type and extent of the malformation. Capillary vascular malformations are best managed with a pulsed yellow-dye laser. Lasers operate on the principle that oxyhemoglobin selectively absorbs certain wavelengths of light. Blood that flows through the lesion transforms the light into heat energy, resulting in either coagulation or rupture of the endothelium. Minimal injury occurs to the overlying skin if proper dosing is used; however, multiple treatment sessions are usually necessary, and complete resolution of the malformation is not always possible. Venous vascular malformations include bulky, subcutaneous lesions of the face or body, early onset of varicose veins, and Klippel-Trenaunay syndrome (an extensive vascular and lymphatic malformation that typically involves a lower extremity). They are best managed with compression garments, although sclerotherapy, laser therapy, and surgical debulking can provide significant palliation and sometimes be curative.

Lymphatic Malformations

Lymphatic malformations are also known as cystic hygromas (if they involve the head and neck) or lymphangiomas (if they involve the trunk and extremities). They are caused by hypoplastic lymphatic channels or failure of the lymphatic system to communicate properly with the venous system.

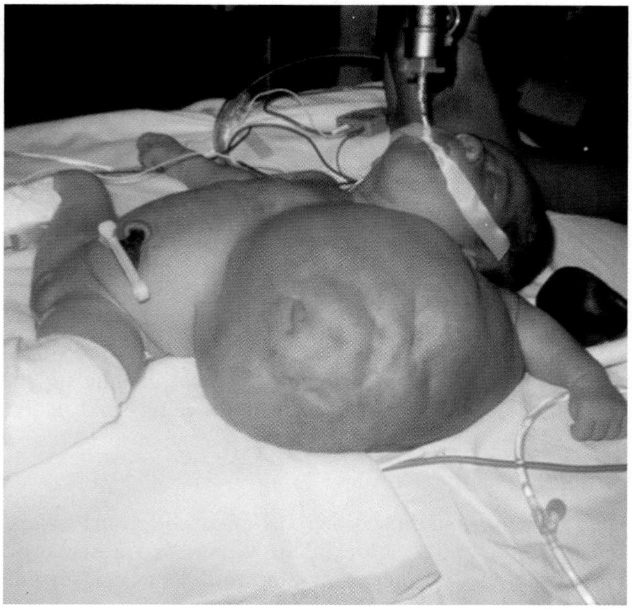

FIGURE 58–4 A newborn girl with a lymphatic malformation involving the left axilla, upper arm, and chest wall.

Clinical Presentation and Diagnosis

Lymphatic malformations are usually present at birth, and most are evident by the second year of life. They are usually asymptomatic, slowly growing lesions that appear as a flesh-colored, soft tissue mass with a spongy texture because of many small, fluid-filled cysts. Lymphatic malformations commonly occur at the confluence of major lymphatic channels. The most common locations are the posterior and anterior triangles of the neck, from which they may extend to involve the oral cavity, tongue, and submental regions. Other common locations include the axilla, trunk and extremities (Fig. 58-4).

A strong correlation is found between the prenatal diagnosis of a cervical lymphatic malformation and Turner's syndrome (>50%), Noonan's syndrome, and several chromosomal anomalies (trisomies 13, 18, and 21). Prenatal diagnosis should therefore be followed by cytogenetic analysis to determine fetal karyotype and provide counseling regarding the pregnancy. Infants with a prenatal diagnosis of a cervical lymphatic malformation who are carried to term should be delivered at a tertiary center, where preparations to deal with dystocia and postnatal dyspnea (due to airway impingement by the malformation) can be made.

Lymphatic malformations of the extremities most commonly affect the lower limbs and typically appear with lymphedema, which is an unremitting, painless swelling of the involved extremity. Lymphedema may present at birth (*lymphedema congenita*) or may begin later in life. *Lymphedema praecox* is an uncommon condition that chiefly affects girls, with onset around the time of puberty. When lymphedema begins after age 35 years, it is termed *lymphedema tarda*. These various lymphedema conditions probably represent a spectrum of lymphatic hypoplasia of the extremities, with the more severe malformations seen at an earlier age. In some patients, the edema may remain localized to the feet or ankles, whereas others may experience progression of the edema up the extremity, such that the extremity swells to many times its normal size. As the process progresses, the swelling becomes permanent because of fibrosis of the involved skin and subcutaneous tissue.

Treatment and Prognosis

Because lymphatic malformations tend to infiltrate and surround important normal structures, operative resection is challenging and often incomplete. Infants and children with cervical or axillary lymphatic malformations should undergo a chest radiograph and often an MRI scan to determine the extent of the lesion before any attempt at resection. Early operative therapy is recommended for lesions near the airway. Smaller lesions well away from the airway may be observed and surgery delayed. In some cases, such as asymptomatic lymphatic malformations of the mediastinum, which surround important structures and may be difficult to access, surgery may not be recommended. All patients with untreated lesions should, however, be counseled regarding their life-long risk for intralesional infection, hemorrhage, and rapid expansion. Percutaneous intralesional sclerotherapy with OK-432 (a lyophilized product of *Streptococcus pyogenes*) and bleomycin (0.6 mg/kg/dose) have been shown to cause acute inflammation and subsequent involution of small macrocystic lymphangiomas, leading to subsequent cure without invasive surgical intervention.

Pediatric Tumors

Wilms' Tumor

Wilms' tumor (nephroblastoma) is the most common malignant renal tumor of childhood. It constitutes 6% of all childhood tumors and has an incidence of 8 cases per million children per year in the United States.

Clinical Presentation and Diagnosis

Wilms' tumor usually is first seen between ages 1 and 5 years and is most commonly seen in 3- and 4-year-old children, with boys and girls are equally affected. The most common presenting sign is an asymptomatic abdominal mass. Hypertension may be present because of the production of renin by tumor cells. Hematuria is usually microscopic but may become gross after an episode of trauma. Wilms' tumor is associated with several congenital anomalies, especially ocular and genitourinary malformations (e.g., hypospadias and cryptorchidism).

A complete blood count is performed to check for the presence or absence of polycythemia, which may result from excessive secretion of erythropoietin by the tumor. A urinalysis is obtained along with blood chemistries, liver-function tests, and coagulation studies. It is advisable to check tumor markers such as serum α-fetoprotein (AFP), human chorionic gonadotropin (HCG), and the urinary excretion of vanillylmandelic acid (VMA) and homovanillic acid (HVA), because intrarenal neuroblastomas and teratomas are well described.

An abdominal computed tomography (CT) scan is obtained to evaluate the tumor and its relation to surrounding structures. The contralateral kidney is carefully evaluated, as 5% of Wilms' tumors are bilateral at presentation, and detection of a contralateral tumor alters the primary therapy. A chest CT is important to evaluate for the presence of lung metastases, and duplex imaging or magnetic resonance venography of the inferior vena cava is performed to evaluate for the presence of intracaval tumor extension via a renal vein.

Treatment and Prognosis

Operative therapy begins with a thorough exploration of the abdomen, to include careful evaluation of the liver, hilar and perirenal lymph nodes, and the contralateral kidney. Palpation of the renal veins and inferior vena cava is performed to exclude intravascular tumor extension. If the tumor is confined to one kidney, a radical nephroureterectomy is performed. Biopsy alone is performed if the tumor is deemed unresectable or a second tumor is found in the contralateral kidney. Unresectable tumors are pretreated with chemotherapy to reduce tumor bulk before definitive tumor resection. Synchronous bilateral tumors are biopsied at the initial operation, unless all tumors from both kidneys can be removed and sufficient renal tissue preserved for normal renal function. Patients with bilateral disease who are biopsied undergo one or two courses of chemotherapy followed by reimaging and possible radiation therapy, before complete excision of tumor from both kidneys.

The National Wilms' Tumor Study Group and International Society of Pediatric Oncology have conducted several large multi-institutional studies over the past several years, and these two groups are largely responsible for the improved survival and reduced morbidity associated with the treatment of Wilms' tumor. The overall survival rate of children with unilateral, favorable-histology Wilms' tumor is now more than 90% at 4 years. Risk factors for the local recurrence of Wilms' tumor include anaplastic (unfavorable) histology, positive para-aortic nodes, tumor rupture, liver metastases (as opposed to lung metastases), and early relapse (<15 months from diagnosis). Current research is focusing on the prognostic importance of certain associated gene alterations (e.g., deletion of 11p13 and 11p15), in an effort to identify a subset of patients with Wilms' tumor who do poorly and are therefore candidates for more intensive chemotherapy.

Neuroblastoma

Neuroblastoma is the second most common solid tumor in childhood (after brain tumors). About 600 new cases are diagnosed annually in the United States, and more than half the patients are younger than 2 years. Neuroblastoma arises from sympathetic neuroblasts; the most common location is the adrenal medulla. Neuroblastoma may, however, develop in any of the paraspinal ganglia of the sympathetic chain from the neck to the pelvis and in the pelvic organ of Zuckerkandl.

Clinical Presentation and Diagnosis

The clinical manifestations of neuroblastoma vary, depending on the location of the tumor, the presence of metastases, and whether the tumor produces any of several biologically active proteins. The typical patient is an ill-appearing toddler with a fixed, asymptomatic abdominal mass. A recent history of weight loss or general failure to thrive may be noted. Hypertension may be present because of catecholamine production by the tumor. Excess catecholamines may also cause flushing, sweating, and irritability. Tumors that arise in the upper mediastinum may involve the stellate ganglion and cause Horner's syndrome (meiosis, ptosis, and anhidrosis). Others may invade one or more neuroforamina, leading to spinal cord compression and paraparesis or paraplegia. Intractable, watery diarrhea and hypokalemia may be caused by excess tumor production of vasoactive intestinal polypeptide.

The diagnostic work-up for neuroblastoma parallels that for Wilms' tumor outlined earlier. A complete blood count, blood chemistries, liver-function tests, and coagulation studies are determined before any intervention. The initial blood work should include three important serum markers of neuroblastoma: ferritin, lactate dehydrogenase, and neuron-specific enolase (NSE). Serum ferritin is probably the most important tumor marker in terms of prognosis, and a level greater than 142 ng/mL indicates a poor outcome; similarly, pretreatment serum levels of lactate dehydrogenase greater than 1000 μg/mL and NSE greater than 30 ng/mL are associated with a poor outcome. A spot urine collection is obtained and analyzed for a variety of vasoactive substances, including catecholamines and their byproducts (e.g., HVA, VMA, metanephrines, and dopamine). Neuroblastoma can therefore be classified in the family of amine precursor–uptake decarboxylase (APUD) tumors.

An important imaging difference between Wilms' tumor and neuroblastoma is the finding of stippled calcification on CT scans in 80% of neuroblastoma cases. The CT will provide information about the primary tumor including location, vascular encasement, and the status of regional lymph nodes; lung, hepatic, and bony metastases also may be visualized. An MRI scan may give additional information about blood vessel involvement and help to determine resectability in difficult cases. An isotopic bone scan and a meta-iodylbenzylguanidine (MIBG) scan are required to assess the bone and bone marrow for distant disease. The bone scan will evaluate bone cortex, which is the most common site of metastatic disease and a negative prognostic indicator. The MIBG scan, together with a bone marrow aspirate, will screen for medullary bone involvement.

Treatment and Prognosis

The mainstay of therapy is complete surgical resection, as this is the most important indicator of long-term survival. Intermediate- and high-risk patients with advanced neuroblastoma are managed with an initial biopsy followed by intense preoperative chemotherapy with or without radiotherapy. This treatment strategy leads to shrinkage and fibrosis of the tumor, which facilitates tumor removal and reduces postoperative complications, ultimately leading to improved patient survival. Nevertheless, resection can be difficult and tedious as these tumors are quite vascular and invasive. They often surround and are adherent to important retroperitoneal vessels such as the celiac axis, superior mesenteric artery, inferior vena cava, and aorta. Tissue from the resected specimen is evaluated according to the Shimada classification, which divides the tumor into age-related favorable and unfavorable histologic categories.

In general, clinical stage I, II, and IVs (s = special) patients are categorized as low risk if their tumor has favorable biologic and histologic markers and is completely resected. These patients require less-intensive or no chemotherapy and have a 3-year survival rate of greater than 90%. Intermediate-risk patients are usually stage III or IV; these patients receive chemotherapy and are then reassessed for tumor resection. If the tumor is still thought to be unresectable, more chemotherapy is given before definitive resection. Intermediate patients undergoing resection have a 3-year survival rate of 30% to 50%. High-risk patients with unresponsive tumors or recurrent disease or both have a 3-year survival rate of less than 20%. Patients in this group may benefit from intensive cytoablative chemotherapy, followed by autologous bone marrow transplantation.

Hepatic Tumors

Tumors of the liver are the third most common abdominal malignancy in childhood, following neuroblastoma and Wilms' tumor. Three fourths of hepatic tumors in children are malignant, and hepatoblastoma is more common than hepatocellular carcinoma. Hemangiomas are the most common benign tumors of the liver in children.

Clinical Presentation and Diagnosis

Hepatoblastoma is more common in boys than in girls and typically develops in children age 1 to 3 years. Hepatocellular carcinoma (HCC) is usually seen in individuals with preexisting liver disease, such as neonatal hepatitis, biliary atresia, or hepatitis B. Most patients with hepatic tumors present with an asymptomatic abdominal mass. Less common signs and symptoms include anorexia, weight loss, and abdominal pain. Those with HCC may have an associated fever and thrombocytopenia.

The diagnostic workup for hepatoblastoma and HCC centers on identifying the extent of the tumor, its relation to the major hepatic vessels, its resectability, and tissue type. Abdominal ultrasonography is the most effective initial imaging study. Color flow Doppler is used to evaluate patency and involvement of the hepatic veins or inferior vena cava or both. CT and MRI are helpful in assessing the feasibility of resection and identifying pulmonary metastases. AFP is an important serum maker in diagnosis and especially follow-up for hepatoblastoma and HCC, because elevated levels are a reliable indicator of persistent or recurrent disease.

Treatment and Prognosis

Complete surgical resection provides the best chance for long-term survival. This usually entails a hepatic lobectomy or trisegmentectomy, either of which is generally well tolerated, as the liver has a tremendous regenerative capacity. Adjuvant, cisplatin-based combination chemotherapy is used for all stages of hepatoblastoma and HCC; however, hepatoblastoma is a much more chemosensitive tumor. The 5-year survival rate for children with hepatoblastoma is more than 50%, whereas the rate for those with HCC is less than 30%.

Rhabdomyosarcoma

Rhabdomyosarcoma is the most common soft tissue sarcoma of infancy and childhood. It has an incidence of approximately 4 cases per million children per year in the United States, yielding approximately 250 new cases per year. It originates from primitive mesenchymal cells and can therefore develop anywhere in the body. The most common sites are the head and neck, followed by the genitourinary system and the extremities. Rhabdomyosarcoma is a fairly aggressive tumor that invades locally and metastasizes by hematogenous and lymphatic spread.

Clinical Presentation and Diagnosis

The signs and symptoms of rhabdomyosarcoma depend on the location and size of the tumor, as well as the presence or absence of metastatic disease. Head and neck tumors are divided into orbital, parameningeal, and nonparameningeal sites. Parameningeal tumors (nasopharynx, sinuses, and middle ear) are often associated with cranial bone erosion and may have cranial nerve palsies or nasopharyngeal symptoms (e.g., a change in voice, nasal discharge, or epistaxis). Nonparameningeal tumors (other head and neck sites) may appear with hoarseness, occasional bleeding, or a mass. Rhabdomyosarcoma of the chest, abdominal wall, or an extremity usually is initially seen as an asymptomatic mass, which may be firm and relatively immobile. In contrast, tumors of the genitourinary tract typically occur with hematuria, urinary obstruction, or an abdominal mass. Those that are paratesticular may be seen as a painless swelling in the scrotum or inguinal canal and can be confused with a hernia, hydrocele, or varicocele. Diagnostic evaluation of a mass suggestive of rhabdomyosarcoma involves an MRI of the tumor and its nodal basin, followed by an excisional or incisional biopsy, depending on the size and location of the tumor.

Treatment and Prognosis

Rhabdomyosarcoma is managed with multimodal therapy, including surgery, radiation therapy, and chemotherapy. Total excision of the tumor is preferable if it will not result in unacceptable deformity. Regional lymph nodes that are clinically or radiographically suggestive of metastatic disease should be sampled with biopsy at the time of the initial procedure. If gross or microscopic tumor remains after excision and adequate surrounding tissue is present, then reexcision is advised. Combination chemotherapy together with radiation therapy is given to achieve local control of residual microscopic or macroscopic disease and also is used to treat positive regional nodes. The survival rate of patients with rhabdomyosarcoma depends on the type, site, and stage of the tumor at the time of diagnosis. In general, those with tumors arising in locations that produce symptoms have a better prognosis than do those with tumors arising in deep, poorly confined areas. This observation reflects the fact that the extent of disease (stage) at diagnosis is the most important prognostic factor.

Teratoma

Teratoma is derived from the Greek word, *teraton*, meaning "monster." The term is fitting, as these tumors are derived from pluripotent cells capable of producing a wide variety of tissue types, including hair and rudimentary teeth, that are foreign to the anatomic sites in which they may arise. The most common locations in children are the sacrococcygeal region and the ovary; other sites include the neck, anterior mediastinum, retroperitoneum, testicle, and central nervous system. Teratomas are classified as benign (70%), immature (15%), or malignant (15%). Those that are malignant may secrete AFP or β-hCG. Serum AFP or β-hCG levels (or both) should be measured preoperatively and, if elevated, monitored after completion of therapy as they can be useful indicators of success or relapse. The clinical features of some of the more commonly occurring teratomas are considered later.

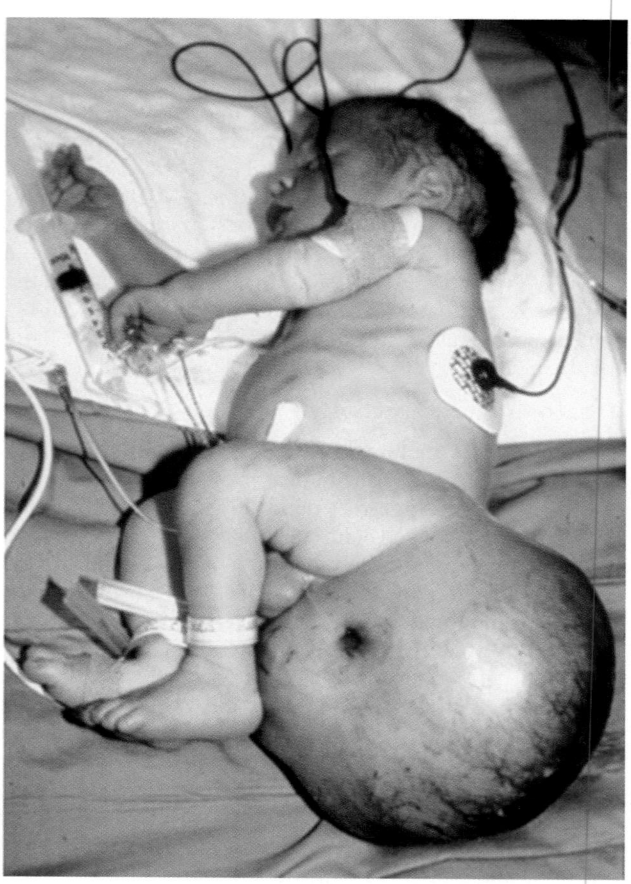

FIGURE 58–5 A newborn boy with large sacrococcygeal teratoma. Note displacement of the anus.

Clinical Presentation and Diagnosis

Sacrococcygeal teratoma is the most common type of teratoma in neonates. Many are diagnosed in utero, and most are apparent at the time of delivery as a posterior midline mass between the coccyx and the anus (Fig. 58-5). These tumors can be quite large and may extend deep into the infant's pelvis. In some cases, the external component of the tumor may be relatively small, and its presence suggested by a slight fullness with a patchy discoloration of the skin over the coccyx. A careful rectal examination with the examining finger directed posteriorly will help to determine the size and extent of the tumor. Serum studies should be sent for AFP and β-hCG. An MRI study will help to differentiate a sacrococcygeal teratoma from a rectal duplication or low meningocele.

Ovarian teratomas are the most common ovarian tumors in childhood. Girls usually have a pelvic mass or torsion, the

PEARLS FOR ROUNDS

Hemangiomas are true endothelial cell tumors, whereas vascular malformations represent errors in vascular development.

In general, 50% of hemangiomas will resolve by age 5 years and up to 70% by age 7 years.

Wilms' tumor is the most common renal tumor of childhood.

Rhabdomyosarcoma is a soft tissue tumor that can arise just about anywhere; early biopsy is warranted, because stage at diagnosis is the most important prognostic factor.

Thyroid nodules in children should undergo histologic evaluation, as 20% are malignant.

latter being heralded by the acute onset of lower abdominal pain; a careful rectal examination may detect the tumor. Plain films of the abdomen will show displacement of the bowel-gas pattern, and 50% will have evidence of calcification in the tumor. Ultrasonography will help to determine whether the lesion is solid or cystic and should include examination of the opposite ovary, as 15% will have bilateral involvement. A CT scan may detect liver metastases or retroperitoneal lymph node involvement or both in malignant cases.

Testicular teratoma is the most common testicular tumor in childhood. It usually appears between ages 1 and 3 years as painless testicular enlargement. The ipsilateral scrotum is likewise enlarged, and the testicle may be dark in appearance. The tumor itself is hard and has an irregular contour. It is easily differentiated from a hydrocele of the tunica vaginalis, which is smooth, uniform in contour, and translucent. Ultrasonography will typically reveal a solid or multicystic intratesticular tumor.

Treatment and Prognosis

Surgical resection is the treatment of choice for all teratomas. Sacrococcygeal teratomas require complete excision, including excision of the coccyx, to minimize the risk of recurrence. This should be done shortly after diagnosis, because the incidence of malignancy increases from 10% in neonates to about 70% in children older than 4 months. Sacrococcygeal teratomas with immature elements require careful follow-up, as these tumors appear capable of dedifferentiating into frankly malignant tumors if incompletely resected. Malignant tumors are treated with chemotherapy, yielding a 4-year survival of 90%.

Ovarian teratomas (both solid and cystic lesions) in the pediatric age group have an approximate 10% to 24% risk of being malignant. For this reason, and the fact that benign and malignant ovarian teratomas are clinically indistinguishable, all pediatric ovarian tumors and large ovarian cysts should be approached with an open technique and handled as if a malignancy were present. Ascites should be sent for cytology, and if no ascites is present, peritoneal washings should be obtained. If the tumor has a well-defined capsule with a compressed rim of normal ovarian tissue, enucleation of the tumor may be attempted, and the specimen sent for frozen-section analysis. If the frozen section shows malignancy, the remainder of the ovary should be removed. If no obvious demarcation exists between the tumor and the ovary on initial inspection, oophorectomy with or without salpingectomy (depending on whether the tube is adherent to the tumor) should be carried out directly. The peritoneum and omentum should then be inspected and the latter removed if abnormal or adherent to any intraabdominal sites. Last, the para-aortic and paracaval lymph nodes, as well as the contralateral ovary, should be carefully inspected with a biopsy of any abnormal areas.

Testicular tumors and teratomas are handled in a similar manner. The operative approach is through an inguinal incision, which allows the spermatic cord to be isolated and temporarily occluded with a vessel loop. The external inguinal ring is opened, and the tumor-bearing testicle delivered and inspected. The field is draped off, a biopsy of the tumor performed, and the specimen sent for a frozen section. If the tumor is malignant, a radical orchiectomy is performed by ligating and dividing the spermatic cord at the level of the internal ring. The inguinal nodes are inspected with a biopsy of any suggestive nodes.

The outcome of children with teratomas and other germ cell tumors has significantly improved over the last two decades. Stage I gonadal and extragonadal malignant tumors and all immature teratomas are now treated with surgery and close observation, whereas higher-stage tumors receive platinum-based chemotherapy. This therapy has been modified over the past several years based on large clinical studies carried out by the Children's Cancer Group and the Pediatric Oncology Group. The current survival rates for low-stage (I–II) and higher-stage (III–IV) gonadal tumors are 100% and 95%, respectively. In comparison, survival rates for extragonadal malignant germ cell tumors are approximately 90% (stages I–II) and 75% (stages III–IV).

Thyroid Cancer

Exposure to radiation is the most important known risk factor for the development of thyroid cancer. Another important risk factor is a history of successful treatment for a previous childhood malignancy. The incidence of thyroid cancer is between 1 and 2 cases per million children per year, and girls are more commonly affected than are boys. Thyroid tumors are categorized as papillary (most common, contain psammoma bodies), follicular (may have capsular or vascular invasion), medullary (arise from C-cells, multicentric, and tend to invade locally), and anaplastic (rare, invasive, and metastatic).

Clinical Presentation and Diagnosis

Children with thyroid cancer typically are first seen with a solitary thyroid nodule, a thyroid mass, or a metastatic lymph node. Because thyroid nodules are uncommon in children, they should raise suspicion of malignancy. A complete physical examination is performed, paying careful attention to the anterior triangles of the neck and any enlarged cervical lymph nodes. The suggestive mass should be evaluated with ultrasonography to determine its location in the neck and whether it is solid or cystic. This information will allow the practitioner to develop a differential diagnosis, which, if the lesion is solid, includes thyroid adenoma, thyroid carcinoma, ectopic thyroid, or an enlarged lymph node. If the lesion is cystic, it could be a thyroid or branchial cleft cyst, thyroglossal duct remnant, or cystic hygroma. If thyroid cancer is possible, a chest radiograph should be obtained to screen for lung metastases. A serum thyroid-stimulating hormone level should be checked to identify the rare patient with unsuspected thyrotoxicosis due to an autonomously functioning nodule.

Treatment and Prognosis

About 20% of thyroid nodules in children are malignant. Given this high rate of malignancy, and the fact that the role of fine-needle aspiration (FNA) cytology in the evaluation and management of thyroid nodules in children is still being defined, most pediatric surgeons recommend surgical resection of all thyroid lesions in children younger than 13 years. Adolescent patients with thyroid nodules are more cooperative and, like their adult counterparts, may be safely evaluated with FNA. The cytologic interpretation of the FNA sample will indicate that the nodule is benign, malignant, or suggestive of malignancy. Benign nodules can be monitored with serial physical examinations and ultrasound studies. Surgical resection should be performed if the nodule is malignant or suggestive of malignancy, or if a benign nodule is found to increase in size.

Surgical management consists of lobectomy with isthmusectomy or subtotal or total thyroidectomy, depending on the location and histology of the lesion. If the lesion is confined to one lobe of the thyroid and the histology is unknown, a lobectomy with isthmusectomy should be performed and the contralateral lobe left intact. If the final pathology is positive for malignancy, a completion thyroidectomy should be carried out within 6 to 8 days. If the lesion is known to be malignant based on the clinical presentation and FNA results, a total thyroidectomy is recommended. This is especially important with a history of radiation exposure or planned adjuvant radioiodine therapy (for locally advanced disease). The use of radioiodine after total thyroidectomy allows the patient to be scanned and treated for metastatic disease. If one or both recurrent laryngeal nerves are involved by tumor, they should be carefully dissected, and any residual disease treated with ^{131}I. The most common surgical complications are temporary hypoparathyroidism and injury to one or both recurrent nerves. Factors associated with a poor prognosis include: tumor larger than 2 cm diameter, psammoma bodies, nondiploid DNA, and anaplasia. Adjunctive therapy consists of thyroid suppression, local radiation therapy, and radioiodine therapy for metastatic disease. Patients should be monitored for recurrence with serum thyroglobulin levels and radioisotope scans. The overall 10-year survival rate for children with differentiated thyroid carcinoma and distant metastases at diagnosis, who receive adjuvant ^{131}I therapy, is essentially 100%.

PEARLS FOR THE OR

Lymphatic malformations tend to infiltrate and surround important normal structures; proper knowledge of surgical anatomy will help to preserve these structures.

When operating on a Wilms' tumor, explore the contralateral kidney for evidence of bilateral disease before proceeding to nephroureterectomy.

Preoperative chemotherapy for neuroblastoma facilitates tumor excision, reduces postoperative complications, and improves patient survival.

Benign and malignant ovarian teratomas are clinically indistinguishable and should be managed with an open technique.

Conjoined Twins

The incidence of conjoined twins is 1 in 200,000 live births, with a female-to-male ratio of 3:1. Conjoined twins are generally thought to develop when a single fertilized ovum fails to undergo complete division around days 15 to 17 of gestation. They may be diagnosed by prenatal ultrasound as early as 12 weeks of gestation, and by 20 weeks of gestation, the extent of the conjoined area may be viewed with sufficient accuracy to determine which viscera are shared. If the twins share a multichamber heart, they usually have a poor prognosis and termination of the pregnancy is recommended.

Clinical Presentation and Diagnosis

Delivery is followed by resuscitation, stabilization, and a thorough diagnostic workup to define the anatomy of the union. The workup may be carried out over a 4- to 6-month period and includes a wide variety of investigations, depending on the site at which the twins are joined. Thoracopagus ("thoraco" meaning chest, and the Greek word "pagos" meaning fixed) is the most common type of conjoined twin; it accounts for 40% of reported cases. Omphalopagus (umbilicus) is the next most common type, followed by pyopagus (sacrum/buttocks), ischiopagus (pelvis), and craniopagus (cranium).

Treatment and Prognosis

Detailed plans are made for separation if this is considered to be a viable option. Separation may involve a number of surgical subspecialists, including pediatric general, cardiac, orthopedic, and plastic surgeons. Two completely different anesthesia teams will be necessary (one for each twin), as proper fluid and electrolyte management is critical to avoid overhydration. Sepsis is a major cause of morbidity and mortality, particularly when separation leads to large skin defects. Unfortunately, despite careful planning and meticulous attention to detail, late postoperative deaths are common.

Suggested Reading

Fishman SJ, Mulliken JB: Hemangiomas and vascular malformations of infancy and childhood. Pediat Clin North Am 40:1177–1200, 1993.

Haase GM, Perez C, Atkinson JB: Current aspects of biology, risk assessment, and treatment of neuroblastoma. Semin Surg Oncol 16:91–104, 1999.

La Quaglia MP: Surgical management of neuroblastoma. Semin Pediatr Surg 10:132–139, 2001.

Nelville HL, Andrassy RJ, Lobe TE, et al: Preoperative staging, prognostic factors and outcome for extremity rhabdomyosarcoma: A preliminary report from the Intergroup Rhabdomyosarcoma Study IV (1991–1997). J Pediatr Surg 35:317–321, 2000.

Skinner MA: Cancer of the thyroid gland in infants and children. Semin Pediatr Surg 10:119–126, 2001.

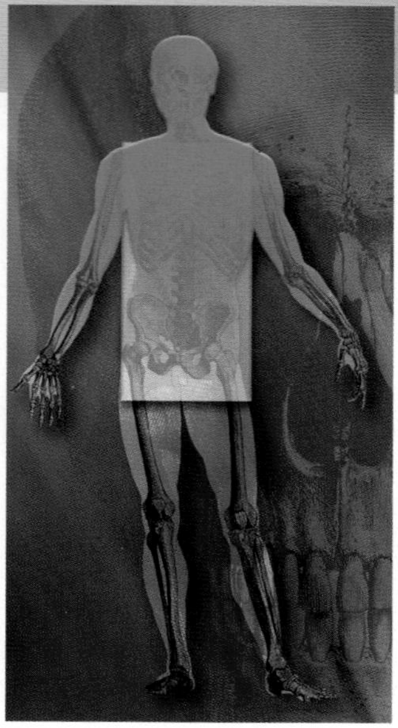

SECTION XV

PLASTIC SURGERY

Chapter 59

Surgical Techniques and Wound Management

C. STARCK JOHNSON, MD, and ELOF ERIKSSON, MD, PhD

A plastic surgeon is trained in managing all kinds of skin defects and deformities; congenital and acquired head and neck deformities; tumors of the skin, head, and neck; hand surgery; breast surgery; microsurgery; and laser surgery. Many of these problems are solved in collaboration with members of other specialties, particularly pediatrics, otorhinolaryngology, orthopedics, cardiothoracic surgery, vascular surgery, general surgery, urology, and dermatology. With a larger population of all patients undergoing various reconstructive and tumor-ablative procedures, the need for reconstruction of the skin and other structures is increasing.

Plastic surgeons have also been and are in the forefront of developing new surgical procedures such as transplantation, craniofacial surgery, advanced tissue-transfer procedures such as musculocutaneous flaps and free flaps, cosmetic surgery procedures, and many others.

Surgical Technique

Surgical procedures are, by nature, traumatic, and it is the obligation of every surgeon to minimize the trauma that is inflicted. It is very important not to use crushing instruments or to let tissues desiccate from exposure. It is equally important to minimize the amount of tissue that is destroyed by electrocautery, ligatures, or sutures. Dissection with electrocautery is usually recommended for muscle but not for fat and dermis. It is equally important to apply the same principle for the treatment of open wounds. Toxic solutions such as peroxide should be completely avoided. Dressings that provide a moist healing environment should be chosen over dry ones.

Skin Incisions and Excisions

Incisions should be placed inconspicuously, ideally so that neither the patient nor anyone else can see them. When this is not possible, they should be placed in the relaxed skin-tension lines, which are generally the same as wrinkle lines, which in most places are perpendicular to the direction of the underlying muscle. All incisions should be made as short as possible. When designing skin excisions, it is important to place the scar in or parallel to the relaxed skin-tension lines. It also is important to design the excision so that eversion of the skin edges is created. This is particularly true for the helix of the ear, the alar rim, and the eyelid margin. It also is possible to make the scars from excisions curved by giving the two sides of an excision a different degree of convexity.

Open Wounds

Acute Wounds

It is important to diagnose an acute open wound. Does it involve the skin only or is an injury to underlying muscles, nerves, blood vessels, bones, or tendons also present? A fracture can usually be ruled out on plain radiographs.

Once a diagnosis of the wound has been established, the timing of closure as well as the expertise needed for closure is determined. Most wounds that are not too contaminated and that are less than 8 hours old can be closed without an excessive risk of wound infection. It is important to determine if wound closure requires only an emergency room physician or if, for instance, the expertise of a plastic, general, or orthopedic surgeon is required. It is equally important to determine whether the wound closure can be carried out in the emergency room or if the patient needs to go to the operating room.

Chronic Wounds

Open wounds are usually referred to as chronic if they have been present for more than 1 month. It is very important to diagnose a chronic wound correctly. We prefer first to rule out systemic causes such as diabetes. After this, we move to rule out regional causes such as arterial or venous disease. Then, the possibility of a local etiology such as trauma is explored. It is equally important to establish whether necrotic tissue exists in the wound or if evidence of infection is present. Up to one third of chronic wounds have a sensitivity reaction to the topical treatment that they are receiving.

Débridement and Irrigation

Wound débridement usually is carried out with a scalpel under local or general anesthesia. All necrotic tissue is removed, and, in addition, tissue that has questionable viability and is significantly contaminated should be removed. In general, débridement should be conservative on the face and comparatively radical elsewhere. In the face, all tissues are very well vascularized, and facial skin is very hard to replace with skin of similar texture and color. In major traumatic injuries in which contamination is significant and viability is hard to assess, serial débridement is an acceptable treatment. The wound is débrided and irrigated on admission, and after this, it is packed in with sterile saline gauze. The wound is reexplored and redébrided 48 hours later and if necessary repacked and redébrided after another 48 hours. Usually, wound closure can be achieved within 96 hours. This method of serial exploration and débridement is more time consuming but may allow salvage of precious tissue that would otherwise need to be débrided.

Copious débridement with saline, or better, Ringer's lactate, is recommended before closure of any open wound. In a very important study by Condie and Ferguson (1964), it was found that copious irrigation with a pulsatile jet can remove all contaminants except for pus. In a small wound, a minimum of 500 mL of saline or Ringer's lactate is used, and, in a large wound, frequently several thousand milliliters of irrigation fluid is used. Pulsatile jet lavage is preferable, but in a small wound, a similar effect can be achieved with a large syringe with a flexible catheter.

Wound Closure

An open wound should be closed as soon as possible. It is generally agreed that less complicated methods for wound closure are preferable. The so-called reconstructive ladder (Fig. 59-1) is a commonly accepted progressive algorithm with which to choose a technique for wound closure. The first choice is always a linear closure, if necessary with undermining of adjacent skin. (It should be noted that the term *primary closure* describes only the timing of closure ([i.e., closure of the wound close to the time of wounding or surgical operation])). The most notable exception to this rule is pressure sores, in which a flap procedure is usually used. If a linear closure were to be done in the case of a pressure sore, it would likely leave a suture line under tension immediately over a bony prominence. Using a flap not only can reduce

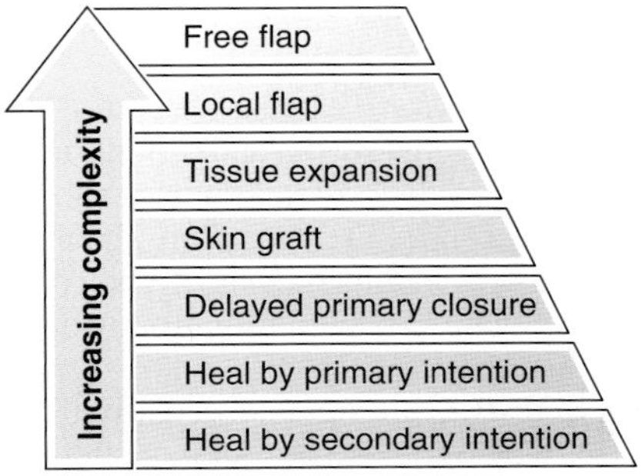

FIGURE 59–1 The reconstructive ladder.

the tension, but it usually also can allow placing the suture line away from the bony prominence.

In general, all anatomic layers of wounds, such as muscle, fascia, dermis, and epidermis, should be closed. Subcutaneous fat has minimal holding strength, and sutures are usually not placed in this layer. In skin wounds, the dermal closure contributes most of the strength.

Example: Venous Ulcer

Pathophysiology

Loss of valve competency in the deep or superficial venous systems or both leads to venous hypertension. Venous hypertension leads to the extravasation of proteinaceous fluid and erythrocytes into the extracellular space. Fibrin is deposited around the capillaries, and diffusion of oxygen and nutrients, as well as waste removal, is diminished. Chronic inflammation ensues, and the tissue eventually becomes fibrotic and hyperpigmented, called *lipodermatosclerosis*. The tissue is poorly vascularized, and the wound-healing processes are compromised. Moreover, it is easily traumatized.

Differential Diagnosis

Systemic causes of venous ulcers include metabolic disease (diabetes, gout, etc.), vasculitis (lupus erythematosus, rheumatoid arthritis, periarteritis nodosa, and allergic vasculitis), and hematologic disease (sickle cell anemia, thalassemia, polycythemia vera, and leukemia). Local causes of venous ulcers are dermatitis, neoplasm, infectious disease (bacterial, fungal, tuberculosis, and syphilis), and insect bites (brown recluse spider and sandfly.)

Workup and Evaluation

History. A careful history of onset, location, size, depth, drainage (fluid, pus, blood) should be taken. Activity, sock, and shoe wear should be noted. Is a history of previous ulcers noted, and if so, what was the treatment, and how successful was it? The medical history should include specific questions about previous leg operations (vein stripping, vein harvest for coronary bypass), claudication, rest pain, diabetes, chronic venous insufficiency, collagen vascular disease, and sickle cell anemia.

Physical Examination. The legs should be examined for evidence of venous stasis and lipodermatosclerosis. Doralis pedis and tibialis posterior pulses should be evaluated. Capillary refill and skin temperature should be checked. A careful neurologic examination should be performed. The ulcer should be evaluated with attention to location, size, depth, and drainage.

Laboratory Tests. Culture and sensitivities of wound fluid (quantitative cultures are best, but often impractical) must be performed. The vascular anatomy and competency can be evaluated with arterial and venous Doppler studies, ankle/brachial indices, pulse-volume recordings, and photoplethysmography. If the bone is involved, plain films should be obtained. In long-standing ulcers, biopsy should be done to rule out malignancy.

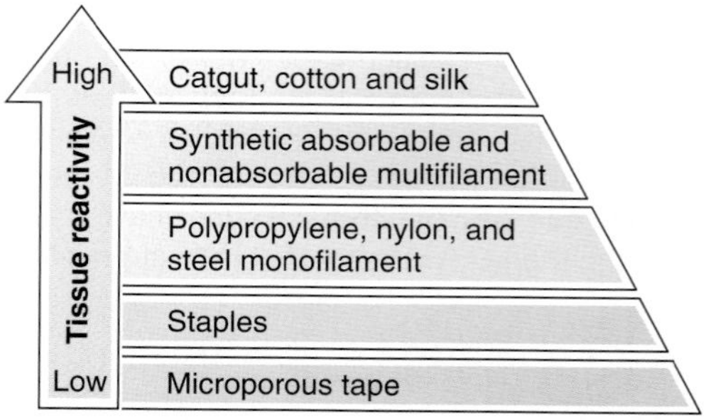

FIGURE 59–2 Wound-closure materials and continuum of tissue reactivity. Any wound-closure material in live tissue may be regarded as a foreign body, and as such can provoke an inflammatory response. Note that natural suture materials cause the greatest reaction, and microporous tape causes the least amount of reaction.

Treatment Alternatives

Conservative. The ulcer should be débrided, and a moist dressing should be applied. A compression wrap or garment should then be applied over the moist dressing. These dressings should be changed every week. Any infection should be treated with appropriate antibiotic coverage. Approximately 30% to 40% of venous ulcers will respond to conservative treatment within 4 months.

Surgical. Surgical options include varicose vein stripping (for superficial venous drainage problems), subfascial perforator ligation, valvuloplasty, vein-segment transposition and transplantation, and subfascial excision of ulcer and scar tissue. If coverage is needed, skin grafts, fasciocutaneous flaps, or muscle flaps with skin grafts can be used.

Wound-closure Materials

A wound is usually held together with sutures, staples, tape, or glue. Sutures are often described as either absorbable or nonabsorbable; they are made of natural and synthetic fibers and, depending on their composition, can provoke an inflammatory response (Fig. 59-2). Catgut used as plain catgut or chromic gut is harvested from ovine or bovine gut and is thus a natural absorbable suture. Common synthetic absorbable sutures include polyglactin-910 (Vicryl), polyglycolic acid (Dexon), polyglecaprone 25 (Monocryl), and polydioxanone (PDS). Important characteristics are the type of suture, the tensile strength of the suture, the time of absorption, the inflammatory/immune response, and how easy it is to handle the suture. In principle, an absorbable suture should maintain its tensile strength for at least as long as it takes for the coapted tissues to regain close to normal tensile strength across the wound. Plain catgut has usually lost most of its tensile strength within a week. At the other end of the spectrum, PDS usually maintains significant tensile strength at 4 weeks.

Nonabsorbable sutures can be natural or synthetic, and the suture can be composed of one or many filaments. In general, monofilament synthetic sutures such as nylon and polypropylene are preferred.

In tying a suture, the principle is to provide as many knots as it takes to give the knot the same breaking strength as the suture. This varies between three and six knots for various suture materials if the knot is tied in a two-handed fashion. When tied in a one-handed fashion, the knot is not as strong, and it takes approximately twice as many knots to achieve the same strength. The sutures should be left in place until the wound has sufficient breaking strength from the healing process to be able to withstand the various stresses of motion or trauma. Transepidermal sutures tend to leave significant scars if left in place for more than several days, and they are usually removed very early if a strong dermal closure has been achieved. Table 59-1 shows preferred suture types and the approximate time of suture removal if transepidermal sutures are used.

Commonly used needles are curved and usually attached to the suture. The authors usually prefer a needle with a cutting tip with a 3/8 circle curve. The exception is vascular sutures, which have a tapered tip. Staples are inferior to sutures in terms of precision, induction of scar, and ease of removal. They are generally used in large reconstructive procedures, such as in burn patients, when they are justified by the time savings. Surgical tape is usually used in combination with dermal absorbable sutures. It distributes tension over a large area and leaves no suture marks. It is important not to place the surgical tape under too much tension, which can cause blistering. Surgical glue is being used increasingly in small acute wounds with little tension because it can often be used without anesthesia. At this point, the holding strength is significantly less than that of sutures.

Skin Grafts

A skin graft is a piece of skin that is harvested from one area and then moved to another area and sutured in place to cover

TABLE 59–1 Preferred Suture Types and Approximate Time of Suture Removal if Transepidermal Sutures Are Used

Body Region	Percutaneous	Deep (Dermal)	Removal/Days
Scalp	4-0/5-0 Monofilament*	3-0/4-0 Polyglecaprone, polydioxanone	6–8
Ear	6-0 Monofilament	—	10–14
Eyelid	6-0/7-0 Monofilament	—	3–4
Eyebrow	5-0/6-0 Monofilament	5-0 Polyglecaprone, polydioxanone	3–5
Nose	6-0 Monofilament	5-0 Polyglecaprone, polydioxanone	3–5
Lip	6-0/7-0 Monofilament	5-0 Polyglecaprone, polydioxanone	3–4
Oral mucosa	5-0 Absorbable	—	—
Other parts of face	6-0/7-0 Monofilament	5-0 Polyglecaprone, polydioxanone	3–4
Chest/Abdomen	4-0/5-0 Monofilament	3-0 Polyglecaprone, polydioxanone	8–10
Back	5-0 Monofilament	3-0 Polyglecaprone, polydioxanone	12–14
Extremities	4-0/5-0 Monofilament	4-0 Polyglecaprone, polydioxanone	12–14
Hand	5-0 Monofilament	5-0 Polyglecaprone, polydioxanone	10–14
Foot/Sole	3-0/4-0 Monofilament	4-0 Polyglecaprone, polydioxanone	12–14
Penis	5-0/6-0 Monofilament	—	8–10

* Nylon or Proline.

a skin defect. A full-thickness skin graft (Fig. 59-3) is taken from an inconspicuous area, and the donor site can usually be closed in a linear fashion. It contains all layers of skin and is much thicker than a partial-thickness skin graft, which contains the epidermis and only a portion of the dermis. Skin grafts are harvested with a Dermatome (Fig. 59-4). The skin in the donor site regenerates from remaining deep hair follicles and sebaceous glands. Partial-thickness skin grafts are usually taken from the upper thigh or the buttock (Fig. 59-5), but in the case of a major burn, one may need to harvest skin grafts from any remaining intact portion of skin. A partial-thickness skin graft is often meshed to allow malleability, drainage, and expansion of the graft. Exceptions are the face, neck, hands, and forearm, where the waffled appearance of a meshed skin graft is usually not acceptable. For a facial defect, a full-thickness skin graft is preferred and is usually harvested from the preauricular, postauricular, or upper-eyelid skin. If a partial-thickness skin graft has to be used on the face, the upper inner arm is often the preferred donor site. In full-thickness skin grafts and nonmeshed partial-thickness skin grafts, multiple small perforations are made with a no. 11 scalpel to provide drainage. A so-called tie-over dressing also is used to immobilize the skin graft and to create moderate pressure over the skin graft. A partial-thickness skin-graft donor site should be covered with a controlled hydration dressing such as a polyurethane, hydrocolloid, or hydrogel.

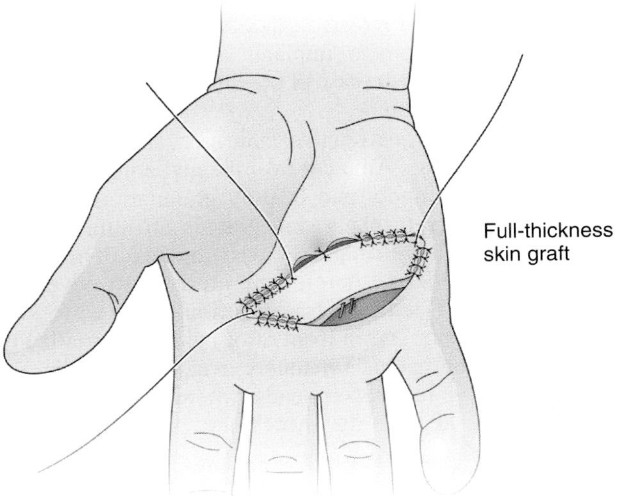

FIGURE 59–3 Full-thickness grafts are used for areas of wear and tear and weight-bearing. A full-thickness graft contains all of the layers of the skin including blood vessels. The blood vessels will begin growing from the recipient area into the transplanted skin within 36 hours.

PEARLS FOR ROUNDS

It is important to determine whether wound closure requires only an emergency room physician or whether the expertise of a plastic, general, or orthopedic surgeon is required. It is equally important to determine whether the wound closure can be carried out in the emergency room or the patient needs to go to the operating room.

Open wounds are usually referred to as chronic if they have been present for more than 1 month.

A wound is usually held together with sutures, staples, tape, or glue.

A healing wound will contract in three dimensions, resulting in a shortening of the scar.

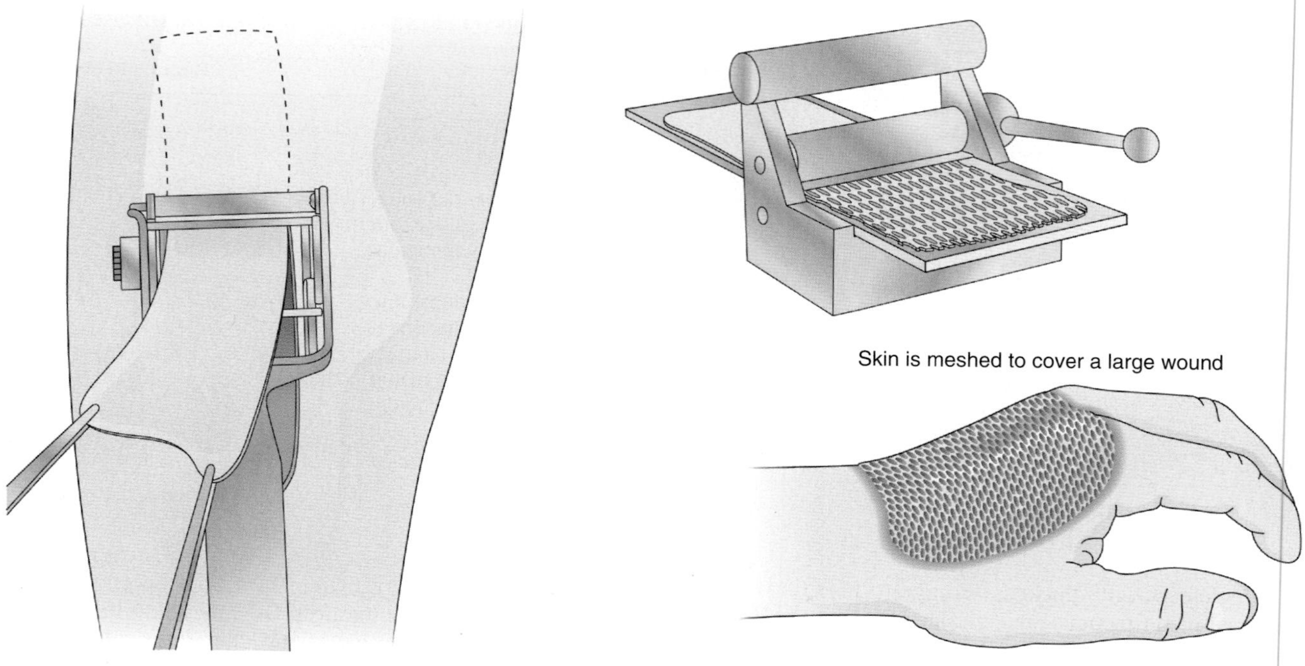

FIGURE 59–4 Skin graft technique. A skin graft is a surgical procedure in which a piece of skin is transplanted from one area to another. Often skin will be taken from unaffected areas on the injured person and used to cover a defect, such as a burn. If the area of the skin defect is especially large, the harvested skin may be meshed to stretch it into a larger patch. If the defect involves a great loss of tissue, a full-thickness graft—a flap of skin with underlying muscle and blood vessels—may be required. Taking the graft from the injured person makes rejection of the tissue unlikely.

Flaps

A flap is a segment or unit of tissue with its own blood supply; it has been partially or completely isolated from the surrounding tissue. When a flap is used for reconstructive purposes, it will carry its own blood supply, which, in a pedicled flap, comes in through its base, and, in a free flap, is provided by microvascular anastomoses to recipient vessels at the reconstructive site. By contrast, a skin graft does not have a blood supply of its own and relies completely on ingrowth of new vessels from the recipient bed. In reconstructive surgery, a flap may consist of skin with subcutaneous fat only, or it may include muscle, bone, tendon, nerve, fascia, or any combination of these tissues. The pedicle of the flap usually contains the dominant artery with accompanying veins and nerve. If a flap does not have a dominant pedicle bringing in its blood supply, it is referred to as a random flap. Flaps also may be classified according to their design, such as advancement flaps, rotation flaps, or transposition flaps. For advancement and rotation flaps, the donor site can usually be closed in a linear fashion, whereas the transposition flap often requires a skin graft for closure.

In general, the reconstructive ladder (see Fig 59-1) is the guide for the choice of reconstructive procedure. However, in some situations, a flap is the first reconstructive choice. Included in these indications are exposed bone without periosteum, exposed radiated blood vessels, exposed brain, an exposed nonbiologic implant, or an open joint. As mentioned earlier, in the case of pressure sores, a flap closure is usually the first choice.

Sometimes a strong relative indication exists for reconstruction with a flap. An ulcer over the malleolus may have adequate blood supply and healthy granulation tissue to support a skin graft, but a skin graft is too thin and not durable enough to withstand the wear and tear of activities of daily living. It is, therefore, preferable to cover the malleolus itself with a transposition flap with skin grafting of a donor site in front of or behind the malleolus itself. The same is true for ulcers over, for instance, the calcaneus or the metatarsal heads, where a thin skin graft will provide neither the necessary padding nor the durability.

Z- and W-Plasties

A healing wound will contract in three dimensions, resulting in a shortening of the scar. The contraction in a transverse dimension is usually of no consequence because of the short

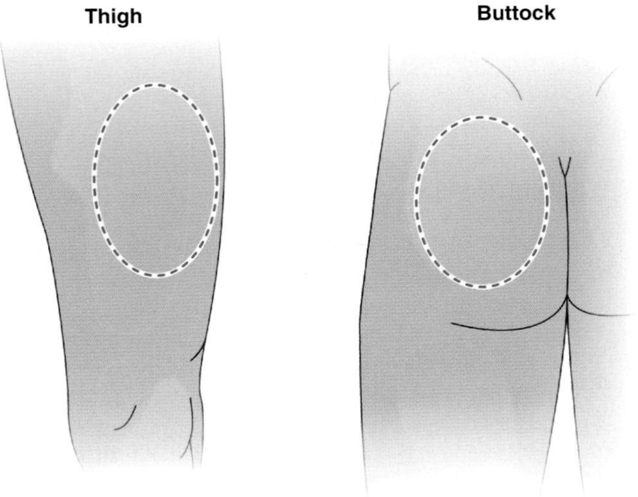

FIGURE 59–5 Common sites for skin-graft harvesting. The skin covers the entire body and acts as a protective barrier. Skin grafts may be recommended for extensive wounds, burns, and specific surgeries that may require skin grafts for healing to occur. The most common sites of harvest for skin grafts are the buttocks and inner thigh, areas that are usually hidden and therefore cosmetically less important.

distance of the scar. In the vertical dimension, eversion of the skin edges by design can usually reduce or eliminate the results of contraction. The major problem with wound contraction is usually in the longitudinal direction of the wound. Often a 10% to 20% shortening of the scar occurs in relation to the surrounding skin. This can be of major functional impact, particularly if the scar crosses the flexor surface of a joint. It also can be quite disfiguring if it crosses, for instance, one of the skin creases of the face. In such cases, the scars can be lengthened with a Z-plasty or broken up into smaller components by a W-plasty. For reconstructive procedures in the trunk and extremities, some type of Z-plasty is usually preferred (Fig. 59-6). The same is true for the facial areas surrounding the eye, the mouth, and where a crease exists. However, over the bony prominences such as the chin, the zygoma, and most of the forehead, W-plasties are usually preferred. If the limbs of a W-plasty are shorter than 5 mm, they add a diffuseness of the scar, which usually decreases its conspicuousness.

Microsurgery

Microsurgery implies that the surgical procedure is done under an operating microscope. The human eye can see objects that are slightly smaller than 100 μm (an optical angle of approximately 1 minute). It is usually practical to use an operating microscope when performing reconstructive procedures on structures that are smaller than 3 to 4 mm. The common dictum is that microsurgery requires four components: magnification, microinstruments, microsutures, and acquired microsurgical skills. An epi-illuminating double-headed operating microscope with a focal length of approximately 200 mm and with magnification ranging from ×4 to ×40 and with foot-operated position, focus, and zoom is usually required. At the upper end of the size spectrum, high-magnification loupes will often suffice. Microsutures are usually made of monofilament nylon with suture sizes 8-0 to 11-0. The authors prefer a suture size between 50 and 70 μm and a needle of approximately 100 μm in diameter. For review, please see Weiss and Pribaz.

Cleft Lip and Palate

Cleft lip (Fig. 59-7) and palate (Fig. 59-8) are relatively common defects that occur in more than 1 of 1000 live births. The incidence of isolated cleft palate is approximately half as high. In 14% of the cases, multiple malformations accompany the cleft lip and palate. If one sibling or parent has cleft lip or palate or both, the statistical likelihood that the next child will have cleft lip/palate is 4%. If two

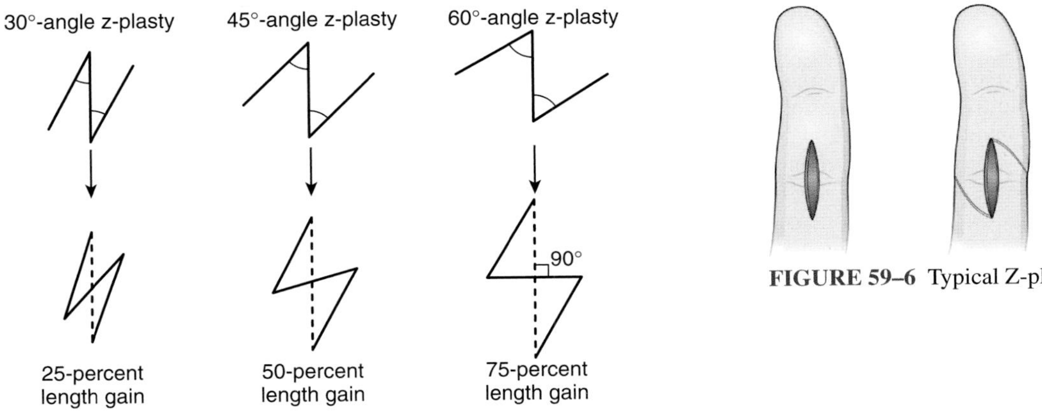

FIGURE 59–6 Typical Z-plasties.

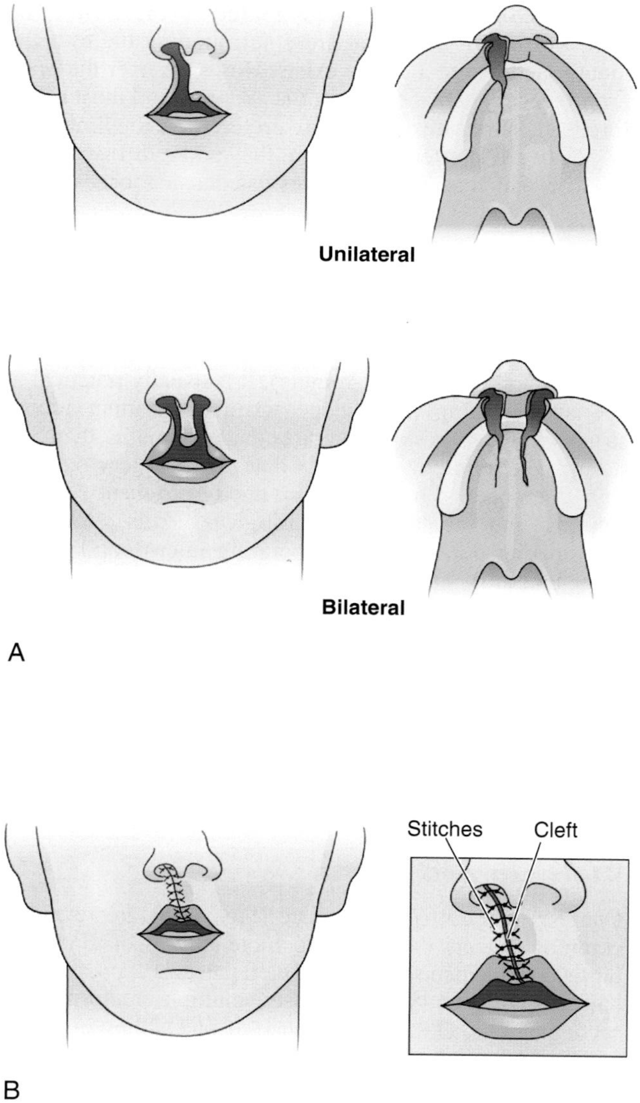

FIGURE 59–7 *A*, Cleft lip. *B*, Cleft lip repair.

primary relatives have cleft lip/palate, the next child has 17% risk of cleft lip/palate. The reconstruction of cleft lip (see Fig. 59-7) and palate (see Fig. 59-8) is done in several stages. Usually, the cleft lip is repaired at age 3 months or earlier, and the cleft palate, at age 6 months or earlier. Bone grafting of deficient alveolar bone is done at the time of the mixed dentition, usually between ages 9 and 10 years. If for some reason the repair of the palate is delayed, then a palatal obturator is usually used to allow early development of speech. Most methods that are used for repair of the unilateral or bilateral cleft lip are based on the descriptions by Millard. Several different techniques are used for repair of the palate, most commonly by pedicle flaps or V to Y advancement flaps. Cleft lip/palate patients should be referred to a center that has not only plastic surgery expertise, but also a dedicated team that can deal with speech and hearing as well as other problems that occur in these patients. Even if every plastic surgeon and some oral surgeons and otorhinolaryngologists have training in cleft lip and palate repair, the optimal treatment of these children is too important to be left to a surgeon who does only an occasional cleft repair. Most children have only one chance in their lifetime to have the best possible primary repair of the cleft.

PEARLS FOR THE OR

Incisions should be placed inconspicuously so that neither the patient nor anyone else can see them. When this is not possible, they should be placed in the relaxed skin-tension lines, which are generally the same as wrinkle lines.

When designing skin excisions, it is important to place the scar in or parallel to the relaxed skin-tension lines. It also is important to design the excision so that eversion of the skin edges is created.

Wound débridement is usually carried out with a scalpel under local or general anesthesia. All necrotic tissue is removed, and, in addition, tissue that has questionable viability and is significantly contaminated should be removed.

In general, all anatomic layers of wounds, such as muscle, fascia, dermis, and epidermis, should be closed. Subcutaneous fat has minimal holding strength, and sutures are usually not placed in this layer.

In skin wounds, the dermal closure contributes most of the strength.

Craniofacial Surgery

In craniofacial surgery, a bicoronal incision (usually from one ear to the other) is done, and the skin and periosteum are widely undermined. Osteotomies are then made, which allow the desired movement of the part of the craniofacial skeleton that is corrected. Bone grafts or alloplastic implant material is then used, together with fixation plates and screws, to provide stable fixation for the bone segments in the new place as well as for the bone grafts and alloplastic implants. Early craniofacial surgery was mainly directed toward congenital deformities such as Apert's and Crouzon's syndromes, but the surgical principles have been adapted to the treatment of fractures, reconstruction after tumor ablation, and aesthetic surgery.

The Facial Nerve

The facial nerve has an intracranial part, an intratemporal part, as well as an extratemporal part. Of most interest are

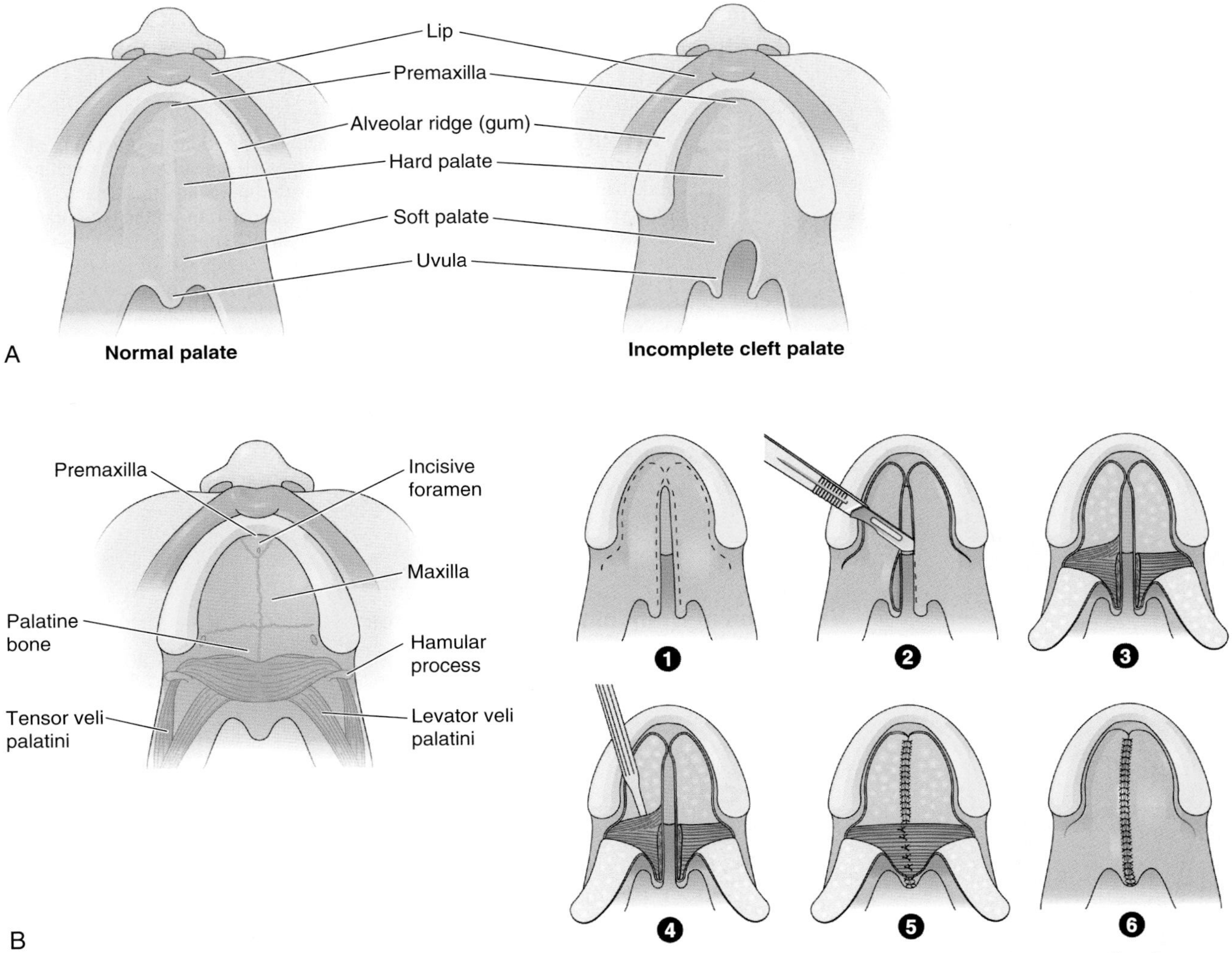

FIGURE 59–8 *A*, Cleft palate. *B*, Closure of cleft palate with push-back palatoplasty. 1, Two mucoperiosteal flaps are outlined. 2, Flaps are elevated off the hard palate. 3 and 4, The abnormal levator muscle insertion to the hard palate is identified and cut free. 5, The nasal lining is closed as a separate layer, and the levator muscle reapproximated. 6, The palatal mucoperiosteal flaps are closed in a V-Y fashion.

the motor branches to the five muscles of facial expression: the temporal, the zygomatic, the buccal, the marginal mandibular, and the cervical (Fig. 59-9). The anatomy varies greatly, but the branch(es) can usually be found in approximately the same area . It is very important to diagnose the etiology as well as precise location of facial nerve palsy because it can vary from the central distribution seen after a stroke to the total motor paralysis seen from acoustic neuromas or Bell's palsy to a partial injury from, for instance, trauma to the face.

Most injuries that the medical student or emergency room resident are going to deal with are either from penetrating trauma to the face or from Bell's palsy. In general, traumatic injuries to the motor branches distal to the stylomastoid foramen should be explored and repaired with microsurgical technique. The chance of significant return of motor function is great. If loss of a segment of nerve occurs, a nerve graft is usually indicated. For late reconstruction, a combination of static methods using pieces of fascia to suspend the corner of the mouth and the eye are used in combination with methods to reinnervate the facial nerve and transplantation or transfer of muscles. Overall, the results from corrective surgery of facial nerve palsy are excellent for symmetry at rest and often acceptable in situations of facial expression.

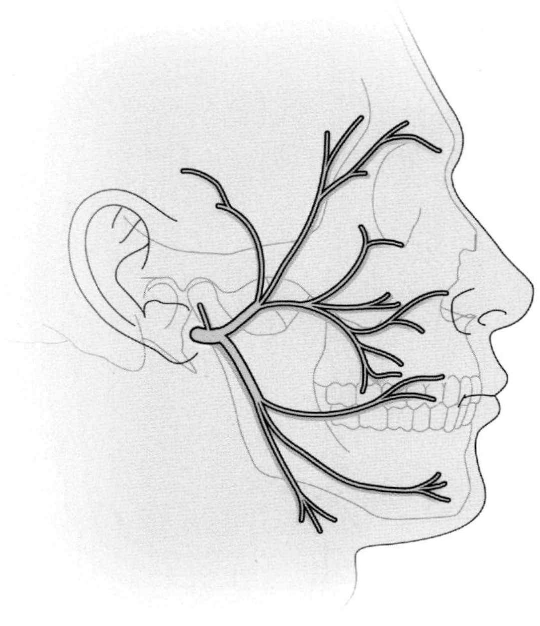

A

FIGURE 59–9 *A*, Innervation of the face. *B*, Variations in branching of the facial nerve. Major types and percentages of a facial nerve branching and anastomoses. In 13%, major divisions (temporal and facial) are independent; in 11%, anastomoses occur between rami of the temporal division; in 22%, connections occur between adjacent rami from the major divisions; in 21%, anastomoses representing a composite of those in the 11% and 22% categories occur; in 12%, proximal anastomoses occur within the temporal component, as well as distal interconnection between the latter and the cervical component; in 9%, two anastomotic rami connect the buccal division of the cervical to the zygomatic part of the temporal; in 5%, a transverse ramus, from the trunk of the nerve, contributes to the buccal ramus formed by anastomosis between the two major divisions; in 7%, richly plexiform communications occur, especially within the temporal portion of the nerve.

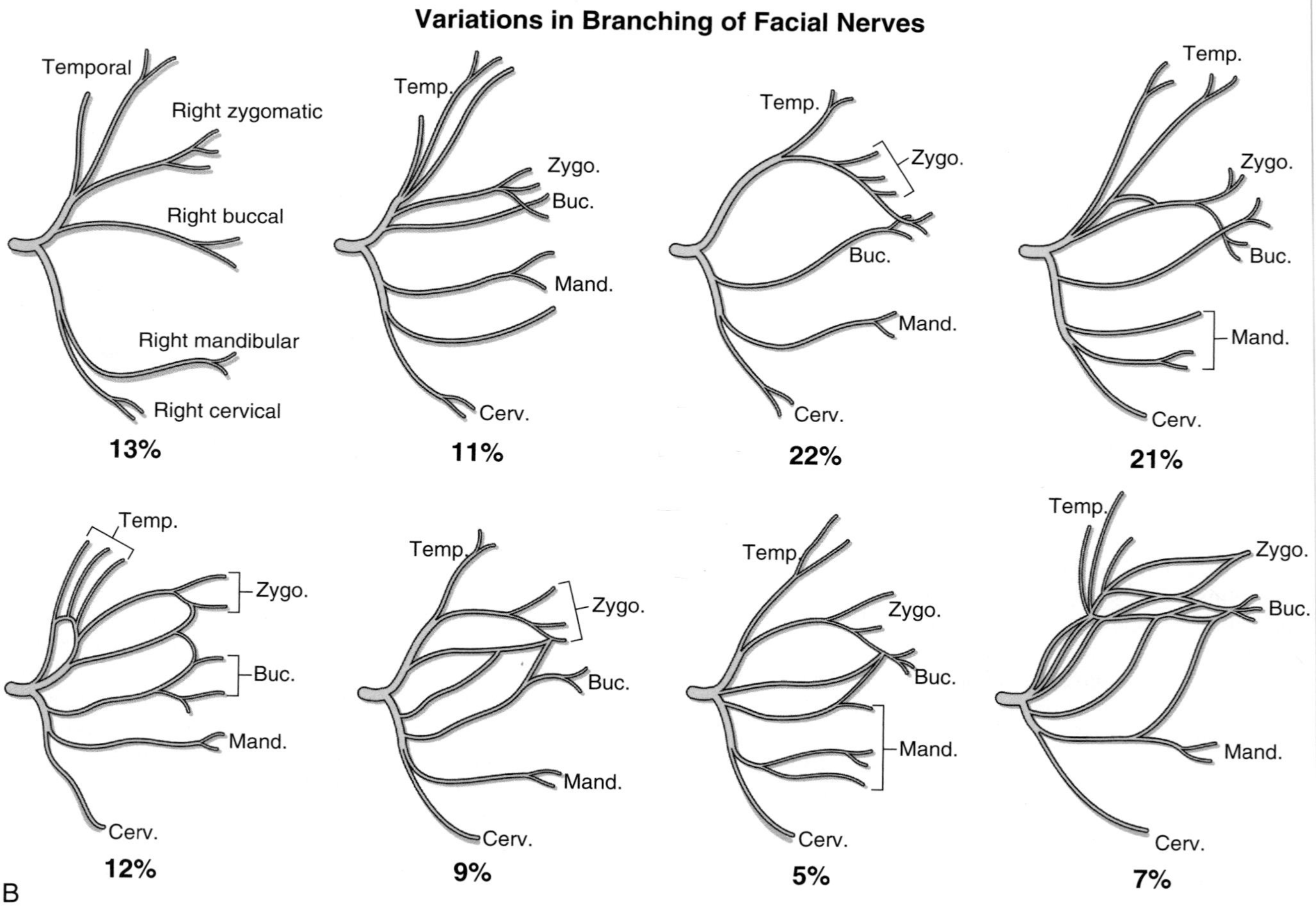

B

Implants and Biomaterials

Biomaterials are defined as "synthetic and treated materials that are employed for the fabrication of implantable devices that are to replace or augment tissue or organ function" (Spector). To predict the clinical performance of implants, it is very important to understand the properties of the biomaterials used in these implants and the development from inert devices to active biomaterials. Quite frequently, absorbable biomaterials are used as part of a tissue-engineering strategy. They also can be used for the delivery of various molecules, including proteins and genes. Both in skeletal-fixation devices and in tissue engineering, absorbable biomaterials are being used more frequently. Various metals and their alloys are often used for skeletal fixation systems as well as for implant materials in joints and other areas. Titanium and vitallium cause less tissue reaction, whereas the alloys are usually considerably stronger. Corrosion and microfragmentation are the main problems. Of synthetic materials, polymethylmethacrylate, polyethylene, and silicone are well tolerated by the body and are frequently used in plastic surgery. Breast implants containing silicone gel have recently been scrutinized, and it appears that silicone in a gel or elastomere does not induce any systemic illness. Ceramics are inert materials that can be used for skeletal augmentation or as joint implants. Absorbable polymers are frequently used in skeletal-fixation devices and seem to be both performing predictably and well tolerated by the body. It is clear that every implanted biomaterial will result in a foreign-body reaction of varying intensity. A great variability exists in the individual response to a certain implant.

Laser Surgery

Light amplification by stimulated emission of radiation (laser) has been used in devices since 1960. Currently, a large number of different lasers are all made in the same fashion, but the wavelength, the intensity, and the duration of the laser light will vary. A laser consists of an energy source, a gas or solid-state lasing medium, and a laser cavity. The majority of the lasers that are being used have a light in the visible spectrum (400 to 700 nanometers). The laser energy is delivered as a continuous wave, a pulsed wave, or a Q-switched wave. (The Q-switch renders one of the resonating mirrors nonreflective for periods of time.) The thermal effect of the laser is determined by the energy density, pulse duration, and the heat conduction of the tissue. The CO_2 laser (10,600 nm), which has a maximal heat absorption in water, is the most commonly used laser in plastic surgery for incisions, excisions, and surface treatment of wrinkled skin.

Suggested Reading

Millard D: Cleft Craft: The Evolution of its Surgery. Boston, Little, Brown, 1976.

Spector M: Biomaterials. In Achauer B (ed): Plastic Surgery: Indications, Operations and Outcomes. Vol. 19. St. Louis, Mosby, 2000, pp 239–260.

Weiss D, Pribaz J: Microsurgery. In Achauer B (ed): Plastic Surgery: Indications, Operations and Outcomes. Vol. 14. St. Louis, Mosby, 2000, pp 163–181.

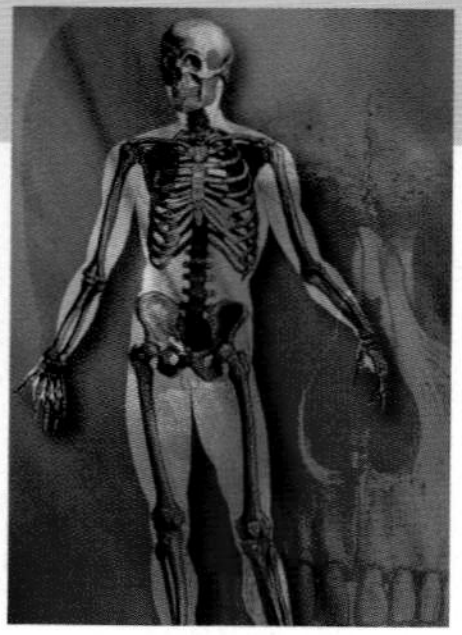

Chapter 60
Reconstructive and Aesthetic Breast Surgery

C. STARCK JOHNSON, MD, and ELOF ERIKSSON, MD

Macromastia

Breast size is determined by the combined volume of glandular tissue and fat. In a woman with a normal or less than normal amount of body fat and macromastia, most of the breast will consist of glandular tissue. In a woman who is significantly overweight and has macromastia, it is likely that the proportionately larger portion of the breast will consist of fat. The symptoms of macromastia, such as pain and fatigue in the shoulders and cervical and upper thoracic spine, are usually directly related to the size and weight of the breasts. Occasionally, neurologic symptoms also exist in the arms from the pressure on the brachial plexus. Frequently, grooving of the skin in the shoulders appears from the pressure of the bra straps (Box 60-1).

Breast reduction procedures aim to maintain circulation and sensation to the nipple and possibly also some lactating function. The authors prefer the inferior-medial pyramid technique for most patients who require a large breast reduction. This technique has been modified from the original description by Robbins and by Curtis and Goldwyn. The nipple is located at the top of the pyramid, which is based in the medial and inferior portion of the breast. Circulation and sensation to the nipple, as well as preservation of intact glandular and ductal units (Fig. 60-1), are as good as or better than those with other methods. However, as with most other breast-reduction techniques, the scars are quite conspicuous. For small- to medium-size reductions, many plastic surgeons therefore prefer to use a so-called vertical technique (Fig. 60-2), which limits the medial and lateral scars.

For reduction of extremely large breasts with a preoperative suprasternal notch-to-nipple distance of at least 40 cm, the authors prefer a nipple-grafting technique. With this technique, the risk of tissue necrosis or infection is less. It also is possible to create a small breast. However, particularly in the dark-skinned patient, a significant risk exists of conspicuous hypopigmentation of the areola. Most studies of breast-reduction procedures show patient satisfaction rates between 95% and 98%. Dissatisfaction is usually associated with scarring.

Gynecomastia

Gynecomastia refers to enlarged male breasts. Quite common in adolescence, gynecomastia after adolescence frequently results in a request for surgical reduction. When gynecomastia is unilateral, particularly if it is nodular to palpation, a biopsy should be performed to rule out breast cancer. Frequently, gynecomastia also is due to increased production or decreased breakdown of estrogen due to abnormal liver function.

In most cases of gynecomastia, the reduction can be performed with a combination of liposuction and glandular resection through a 1- to 2-cm inferior transareolar incision (Fig. 60-3). If more than approximately 500 g is removed from each breast, more extensive incisions or skin excision may need to be done.

Augmentation Mammoplasty

The breast implants that are currently used have a shell of a silicone elastomer and contain normal saline. The surface may be smooth or textured. Textured implants do not move in the tissue cavity where they are placed, and some studies have shown that they result in a softer breast than do the smooth implants. A large number of credible studies have shown that implants containing silicone gel do not cause any of the alleged systemic diseases, and it is expected that implants containing silicone gel will be fully approved by the Food and Drug Administration in the future.

In most patients, a submuscular implant is preferred (Fig. 60-4). A submammary, peripheral transareolar or axillary incision can be used. With saline-containing implants, it must be only approximately 2.5 cm long.

It is important to discuss the informed consent at length with these patients. Discussion should include problems related to the implant, capsular contracture, cancer detection, possible changes in nipple sensation, and the possibility of infection, hematoma, and postoperative pain.

Face

Facial reconstruction, other than that involving the nose and the eyelids, is usually indicated for trauma or tumor

BOX 60-1 Managing the Patient with Macromastia

Pathophysiology

It is believed that macromastia results from an increased sensitivity to hormonal stimulation of breast tissue. There appears to be a hereditary component of macromastia, as women with large breasts often have a family history. Macromastia may appear during menarche, or it may be the result of pregnancy, with failure of the breast to reduce in size substantially after delivery and nursing. Macromastia is often caused by obesity, in which case, the majority of the breast is made up of adipose rather than glandular tissue.

Differential Diagnosis

The differential diagnosis for macromastia is straightforward. A tumor would be unilateral, and the breast shape would be irregular. Pregnancy will cause enlargement of the breast, but the breast size should decrease with cessation of lactation.

Workup and Evaluation

History

A patient with macromastia may complain of fatigue and pain in the cervical and upper thoracic spine and the shoulder. The patient may experience breast pain, which may be premenstrual or independent of menstruation. Other symptoms include shoulder grooving by brassieres and maceration and infection of the inframammary regions.

Patients may complain of their breast getting in the way during normal activities, especially sports, and they may have difficulty finding ready-made clothes that fit. Patients may report a feeling of embarrassment or even disgust related to the breast.

Physical Examination

In a patient with macromastia, the surgeon should look for shoulder grooving and examine the patients for inframammary maceration or infection. The patient's weight should be noted, as well as the overall body habitus. Attention should also be apid to posture. The suprasternal notch-to-nipple distance is usually >30 cm.

Laboratory Studies

Laboratory studies are ordered per preoperative routine for age group. Type and crossmatch of blood is not necessary.

Imaging

A preoperative mammogram is indicated in women older than 40 years.

Treatment Alternatives

The only conservative approach to macromastia is weight loss. A decrease in overall weight of 20 kg roughly corresponds to an average reduction is breast weight of 400 g.

For breast reduction, the inferior pedicle, or inferior pyramid, is the most popular technique. Here the nipple sits at the apex of an inferiorly based pyramid. This technique allows preservations of circulation and sensation to the nipple, as well as preservation of intact glandular and ductal structures, but it does leave prominent scars. On small reductions, the lateral and medial components of the scar can be reduced. The inferior-pyramid technique can be used safely for breasts in which the suprasternal notch-to-nipple distance is <40 cm. If more, nipple grafting is preferred. The nipple-grafting technique has the disadvantage that nipple sensation and the ability to lactate will be completely lost, and sometimes hypopigmentation of the nipple or the areola occurs.

and sometimes for congenital deformities. In most cases, the first choice of reconstructive procedure is a local flap. If the defect is larger, a full-thickness skin graft or a regional flap or free flap may be indicated. These procedures are frequently combined with reconstruction of facial skeleton, nerves, sometimes muscle, and internal lining in the nasal oropharyngeal cavities.

Aesthetic facial procedures usually aim to reduce facial wrinkling and make the surface of the facial skin smoother. These procedures are sometimes combined with augmentation of the bony skeleton, either the chin or the zygomas. Traditional face-lift procedures, which are still commonly used, involve incisions in the hairline and around the ear, where the facial skin is elevated, pulled back, extra skin is excised, and the incisions closed (Fig. 60-5). However, other procedures, such as those involving the CO_2 laser and chemical peels, are quite common. In general, face-lifting procedures are used with a large excess of facial or neck skin, whereas the laser and peeled procedures are usually the first choice when facial wrinkling with less excess of skin is found, particularly in the neck. When the skin has been elevated, the underlying muscles and fascia are plicated in a posterior and superior direction. More recent methods allow the face-lift to be done in a partially subperiosteal plane, which increases the opportunities to move the facial fat. However, these procedures do have a higher complication rate from bleeding and nerve injury.

Nasal Surgery

Nasal Reconstruction

The two nasal functions that involve plastic surgery are the maintenance of the nasal airway and the appearance of the nose. The nose has an external lining of skin and an internal lining of mucosa. The nose is given its shape mainly by the nasal skeleton, consisting of bone and cartilage. If part of the nose is lost because of congenital absence, trauma, or tumor resection, it should be reconstructed with similar tissue. Sometimes this is not an option, and the mucosa may

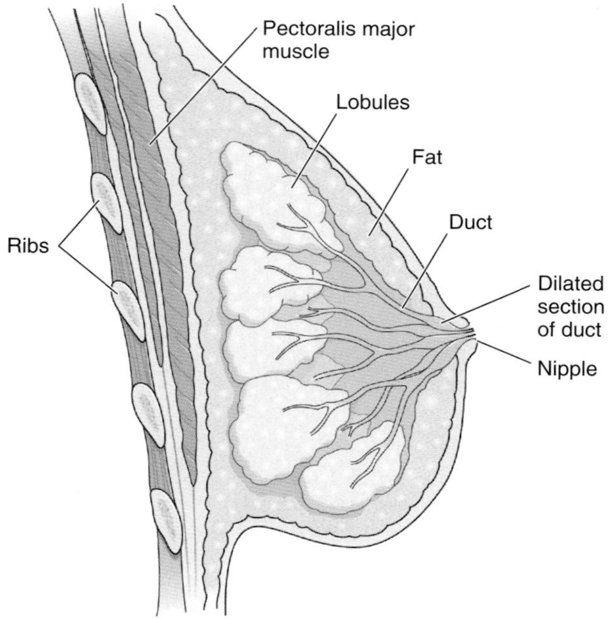

FIGURE 60–1 Most breast-reduction techniques attempt to maintain circulation and sensation to the nipple, as well as preservation of intact glandular and ductal units.

have to be reconstructed with skin, and cartilage replaced with bone. It appears that the nonmobile part of the nose will accept alloplastic materials, but only autogenous materials will provide relatively problem-free reconstruction of the mobile part of the nose. Large defects of the nose are usually reconstructed in subunits. It is usually not attempted to reconstruct small defects as subunits. For large nasal defects, the skin is usually reconstructed with a forehead flap over a nasal skeleton made from bone grafts. Usually, local turnover flaps are used for inside lining. Some patients do not want to go through the trouble of a nasal reconstruction and may then have a reconstruction with conventional prosthetics or osseointegrated prosthetics.

Rhinoplasty

Rhinoplasty can improve the shape, size, and general appearance of the nose. It can change the shape of the tip or bridge, narrow the span of the nostrils, or change the angle between the nose and upper lip. It also can relieve breathing problems.

Most principles and techniques used in the aesthetic rhinoplasty operation have developed from principles used in reconstructive nasal surgery. Either an intranasal incision through the mucosa or an extranasal approach through an incision in the columella can be used for access to the nasal skeleton. In general, the external approach provides better visibility and more predictable results. Preoperative imaging is frequently used to establish a goal for the aesthetic rhinoplasty. An excellent review of the aesthetic rhinoplasty operation has been provided by Tebbetts.

Eyelid Surgery

The eyelid anatomy is very well defined, and it is imperative that the various anatomic structures be carefully identified during reconstruction. Reconstructive procedures may include the tarsal plate, the canthal ligaments, the skin, and

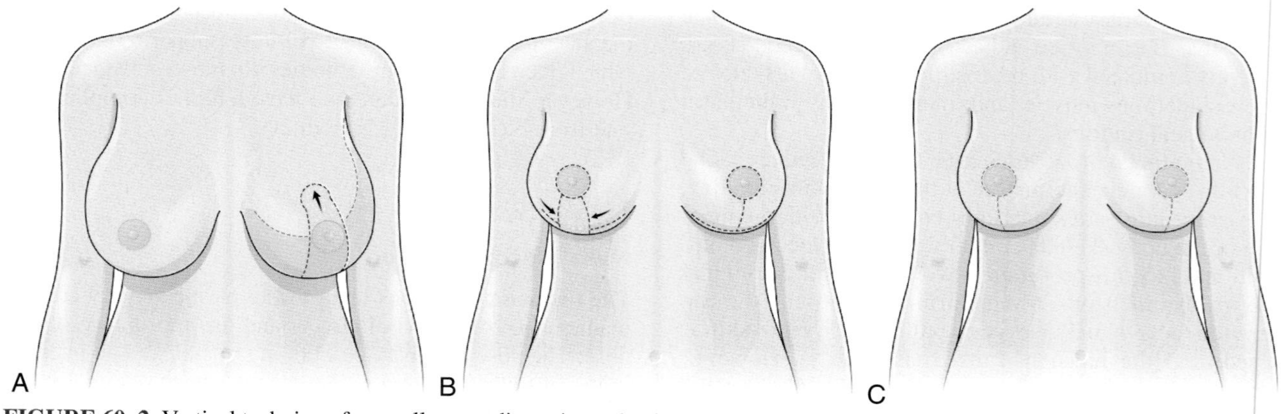

FIGURE 60–2 Vertical technique for small- to medium-size reductions. *A*, Incisions outline the area of skin, breast tissue, and fat to be removed and the new position for the nipple. *B*, Skin formerly located above the nipple is brought down and together to reshape the breast. Sutures close the incisions, giving the breast its new contour. *C*, Scars around the areola, below it, and in the crease under the breast are permanent, but can be easily concealed by clothing.

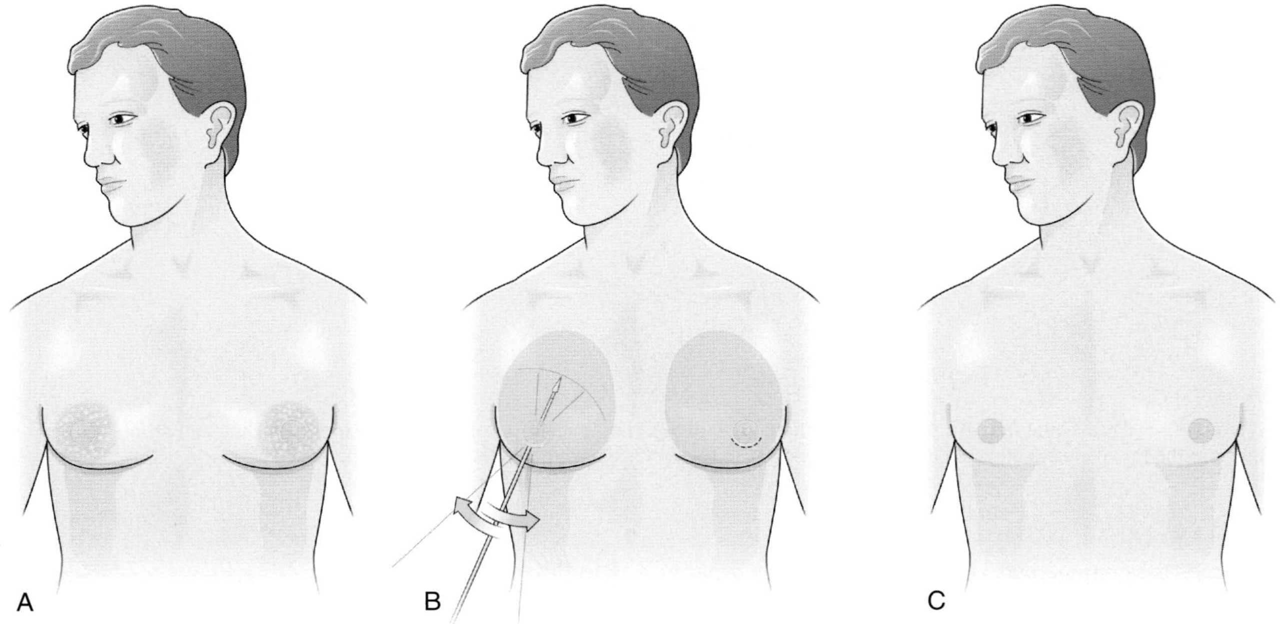

FIGURE 60–3 In gynecomastia, reduction can be performed with a combination of liposuction and glandular resection through a 1- to 2-cm inferior transareolar incision. *A*, Glandular tissue must be cut out, usually through a small incision near the edge of the areola. *B*, Fatty tissue can be removed by liposuction. A small, hollow tube is inserted through a tiny incision, leaving a nearly imperceptible scar. *C*, After surgery for gynecomastia, the patient has a more masculine chest contour.

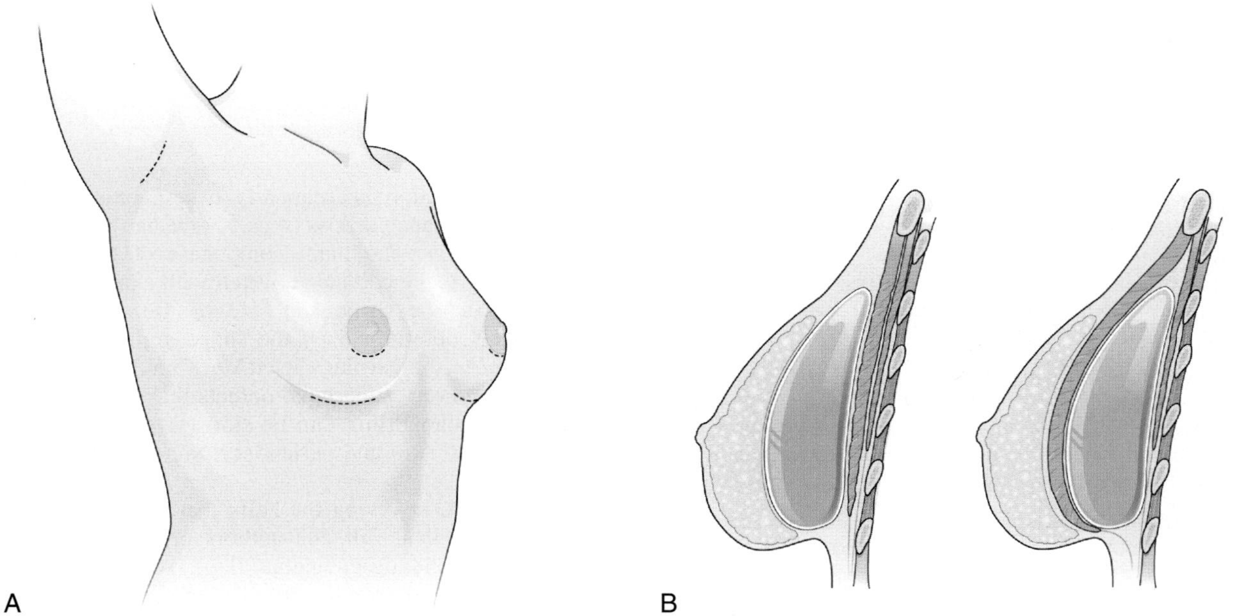

FIGURE 60–4 Augmentation mammoplasty. Breast augmentation is usually done to balance a difference in breast size, to improve body contour, or as a reconstructive technique after surgery. *A*, Incisions are made to keep scars as inconspicuous as possible, in the breast crease, around the nipple, or in the armpit. Breast tissue and skin are lifted to create a pocket for each implant. *B*, The breast implant may be inserted directly under the breast tissue or beneath the chest-wall muscle.

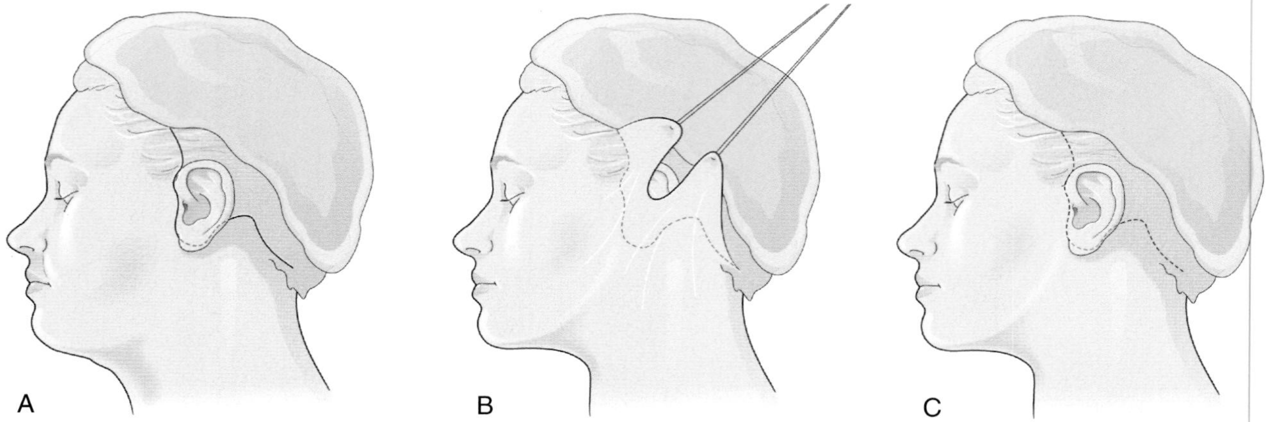

FIGURE 60–5 Traditional face-lift procedures, which are still commonly used, involve incisions in the hairline and around the ear (*A*), where the facial skin is elevated and pulled back (*B*), extra skin is excised, and the incisions are closed (*C*).

sometimes the conjunctiva. The lacrimal system is usually reconstructed, whereas the orbicularis muscle is not.

Lacerations are closed in an anatomic fashion, with attempts to evert the skin edges at the eyelid margin. For skin defects in the eyelid, the authors usually prefer full-thickness skin grafts from the opposite upper eyelid. Most full-thickness defects are in the lower eyelid, and if they need to be reconstructed with a flap, a tarsoconjunctival flap from the upper eyelid is usually the first choice. When the lacrimal ducts have been transected, they should be repaired with microscopic magnification, if at all possible.

PEARLS FOR ROUNDS

Macromastia results from an increased sensitivity to hormonal stimulation of breast tissue that may be hereditary, because women with large breasts often have a family history.

Macromastia may appear during menarche, or it may be the result of pregnancy, with failure of the breasts to reduce in size substantially after delivery and nursing. Macromastia is often caused by obesity, in which case, the majority of the breast is made up of adipose rather than glandular tissue.

The goal with breast-reduction procedures is to reduce the size of the breasts and at the same time to maintain circulation and sensation to the nipple and possibly also some lactating function.

Most studies of breast-reduction procedures show patient satisfaction rates between 95% and 98%. Dissatisfaction is usually associated with scarring.

Blepharoplasty

The blepharoplasty operation usually involves removal of skin and a strip of muscle. Fat also is removed in the medial and middle position in the upper eyelid and in the medial, middle, and lateral positions in the lower eyelid. If insufficient elasticity is found in the lower eyelid to keep it in a normal position, an eyelid-tightening procedure may be done. The scar in the upper eyelid is placed in the supratarsal crease and in the lower eyelid immediately below the lashes. The outcomes of eyelid reconstructive and aesthetic procedures are quite predictable, usually resulting in a high patient satisfaction rate.

Ear Surgery

Ear reconstruction is frequently necessary because of a congenital absence or loss of part of the ear from trauma or tumor ablation. The main component of the auricle or external ear is the cartilage covered with skin on both sides (Fig. 60-6). The shape and size of the ear are almost completely determined by the shape and size of the ear cartilage. As the cartilage itself does not carry any blood supply, only very superficial defects that involve skin and not the perichondrium can be skin grafted. If tissue loss includes both skin and perichondrium, a local or regional flap is used.

For defects involving the helix that include less than 2 cm of the helical rim, the authors prefer reconstruction with sliding chondrocutaneous flaps (Antia). This results in an ear that is shorter in vertical height, but that generally looks normal. If this smaller ear is designed to protrude more than the opposite ear, the overall impression (or illusion) will be that the ears are similar. For larger defects, the skin must be reconstructed with local flaps, and the ear

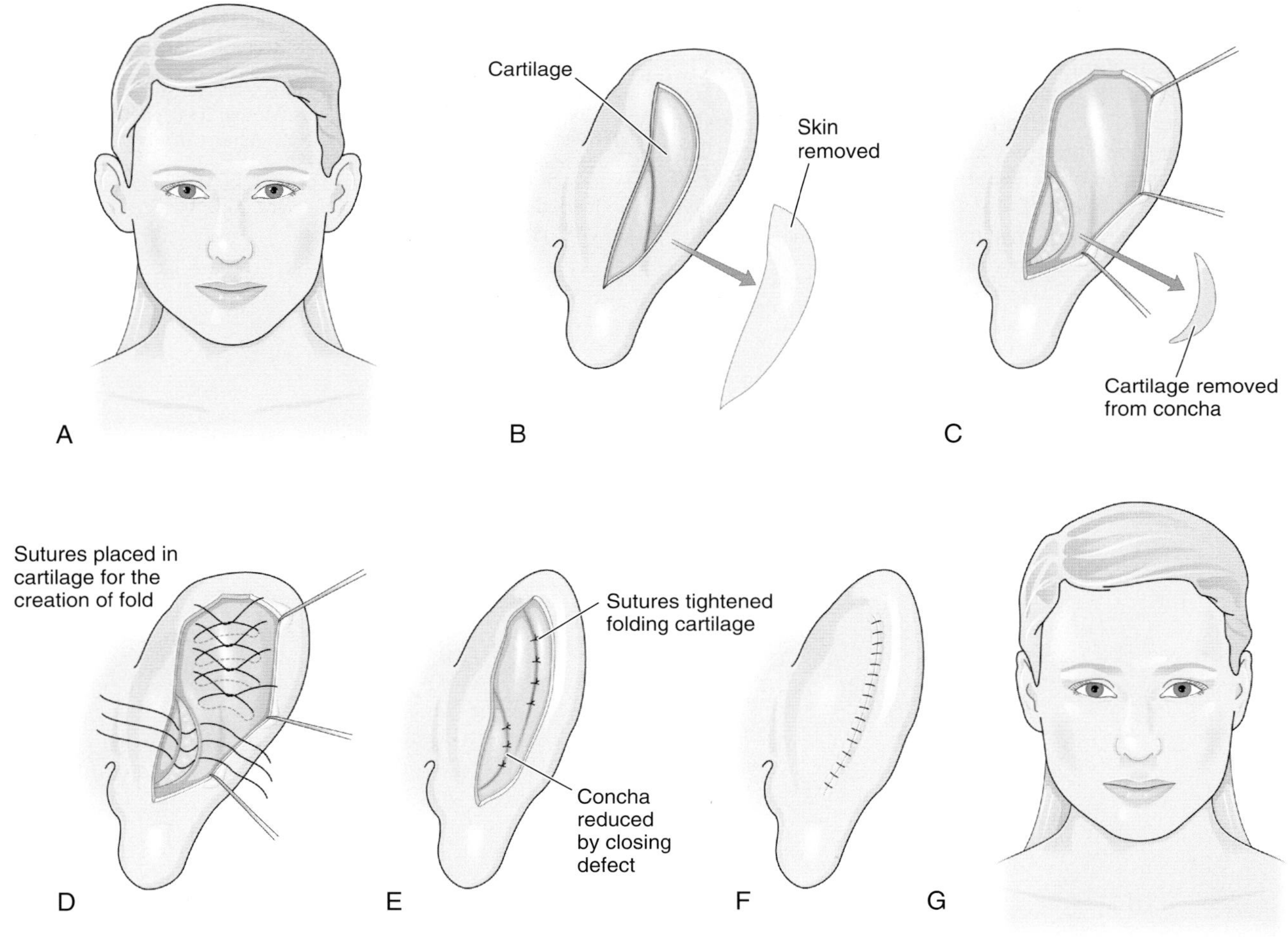

FIGURE 60–6 Ear reconstruction. *A*, Ears that appear to stick out or are overly large can be helped by ear surgery. *B*, An incision is made in the back of the ear so cartilage can be sculpted or folded. *C–G*, Creating a fold in the cartilage makes the ear lie flatter against the head and appear more normal.

PEARLS FOR THE OR

For small- to medium-size breast reductions, many plastic surgeons prefer to use a "vertical" technique, which limits the medial and lateral scars.

For reduction of extremely large breasts with a preoperative suprasternal notch-to-nipple distance of at least 40 cm, a nipple-grafting technique is commonly used, which reduces the risk of tissue necrosis or infection.

The breast implants that are currently used have a shell of a silicone elastomer and contain normal saline. In most patients, a submuscular implant is preferred. A submammary, peripheral transareolar or axillary incision can be used. With saline-containing implants, it must be only approximately 2.5 cm long.

framework, with a cartilage graft from either the opposite ear or rib cartilage. In cases in which the skin surrounding the area is missing, such as after full-thickness burns, the cartilage framework can be covered with a temporalis fascia flap and skin graft. In certain patients with complete loss of the ear, prosthetic reconstruction is a viable option, particularly when osseointegrated implants are used for anchoring of the prosthesis. Implants allow the patient to go swimming or participate in sports without the constant risk that the prosthesis will fall off.

Prominent ears are frequently corrected for psychological or aesthetic reasons or both. Most ears are prominent because of either a large concha or absence of the antihelical fold. The concha can be reduced by an excision of conchal cartilage, and many ways exist to create a new antihelix. These procedures are all done from an incision on the posterior side of the ear. The authors prefer the open otoplasty technique originally described by Nordzell. With this technique, a peripheral rim of cartilage is left intact, and through a posterior incision through skin and cartilage, the anterior side of the ear is exposed. The fold is then created by dermabrading the anterior surface of the area of the antihelical fold. This method seems to have more versatility and is faster to use than methods that require sutures to create the fold.

Suggested Reading

Nordzell B: Open otoplasty. Plast Reconstr Surg 106:1466–1472, 2000.

Spector M: Biomaterials. In Achauer B (ed): Plastic Surgery: Indications, Operations and Outcomes. St. Louis, Mosby, 2000, pp 239–260.

Tebbets J: Primary Rhinoplasties: New Approaches to the Logic and Techniques. St. Louis, Mosby, 1998.

Weiss D, Pribaz J: Microsurgery. In Achauer B (ed): Plastic Surgery: Indications, Operations and Outcomes, Vol. 14. St. Louis, Mosby, 2000, pp 163–181.

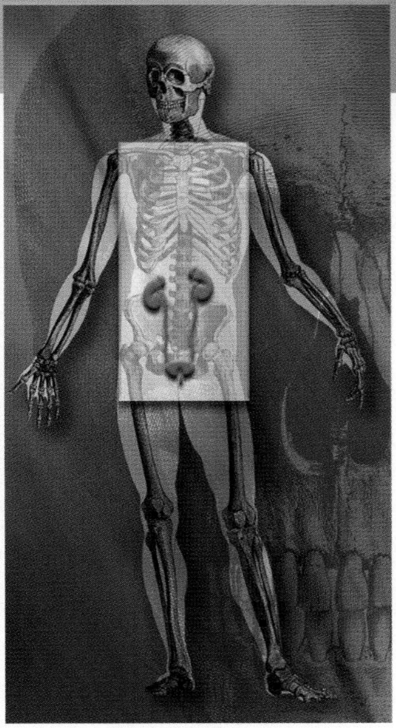

SECTION XVI

UROLOGY

Chapter 61

Anatomy and Oncology

PAUL K. PIETROW, MD, MICHAEL S. COOKSON, MD, and JOSEPH A. SMITH, JR, MD

Anatomy

Kidneys and Ureters

The kidneys lie along the borders of the psoas muscles and are obliquely positioned in the retroperitoneum. The kidneys and associated adrenal glands are surrounded by perirenal fat that is enclosed in Gerota's fascia. The right kidney lies in close proximity to the liver, the duodenum, the adrenal, and the hepatic flexure of the right colon. On the left, the kidney borders the tail of the pancreas, the left adrenal, and the splenic flexure of the colon (Fig. 61-1)

The blood supply to each kidney is usually through a single renal artery, with variations present in up to 40% of cases. The renal artery lies posterior to the renal vein and anterior to the renal pelvis. The right renal vein is short and enters the lateral aspect of the inferior vena cava (IVC). The left renal vein is longer and crosses anterior to the aorta to reach the IVC. It receives branches from the ipsilateral adrenal, gonad, and a lumbar vein before entering the IVC.

The renal collecting system includes the calyces, the renal pelvis, and the ureter. Eight to 12 minor calyces unite to form 2 or 3 major calyces, which in turn join the renal pelvis. The ureter is 22 to 30 cm in length and is divided into three segments. The upper ureter extends from the renal pelvis to the upper border of the sacrum, the middle ureter overlies the sacrum, and the lower ureter extends to the bladder. The renal calyces, pelvis, and upper ureter derive their blood supply from the renal arteries. The gonadal arteries supply the midureter, and branches from the common iliac, internal iliac, and vesical arteries supply the lower ureter.

The Bladder and Urethra

The bladder lies just behind the pubic symphysis and is considered a pelvic organ, although in childhood, it has a greater intraabdominal location. The superior portion of the bladder is covered with peritoneum. The median umbilical ligament, the remnant of the urachus, attaches the bladder to the anterior abdominal wall at the umbilicus. Condensations of the transversalis fascia (endopelvic fascia) also support the bladder.

The blood supply to the bladder consists of the superior, middle, and inferior vesical arteries, which arise from the hypogastric artery. In females, additional branches originate from the vaginal and uterine arteries. The bladder is surrounded by a rich plexus of veins that drain into Santorinis plexus superiorly and the pudendal plexus inferiorly. The two venous systems interconnect and also communicate with the dorsal vein of the penis and clitoris. Lymph node drainage from the bladder occurs via the external iliac, hypogastric, and sacral lymphatics.

The bladder receives innervation from both sympathetic and parasympathetic autonomic nerves. The sympathetic preganglionic nuclei are in the first and second lumbar segments and the 12th thoracic spinal cord segment. The sympathetic outflow proceeds through the inferior hypogastric plexus. Parasympathetic nuclei are in the second, third, and fourth sacral segments of the spinal cord and travel with the pelvic splanchnic nerves to innervate the bladder.

The male urethra is approximately 20 cm in length and is divided into an anterior and posterior portion by the urogenital diaphragm. The posterior component includes the membranous and prostatic urethra, and the anterior component includes the bulbar and penile urethra. The blood supply to the urethra is via the internal pudendal artery. The female urethra is about 4 cm in length and lies behind the pubic bone. The blood supply to the female urethra is derived from the inferior vesical, vaginal, and internal pudendal arteries.

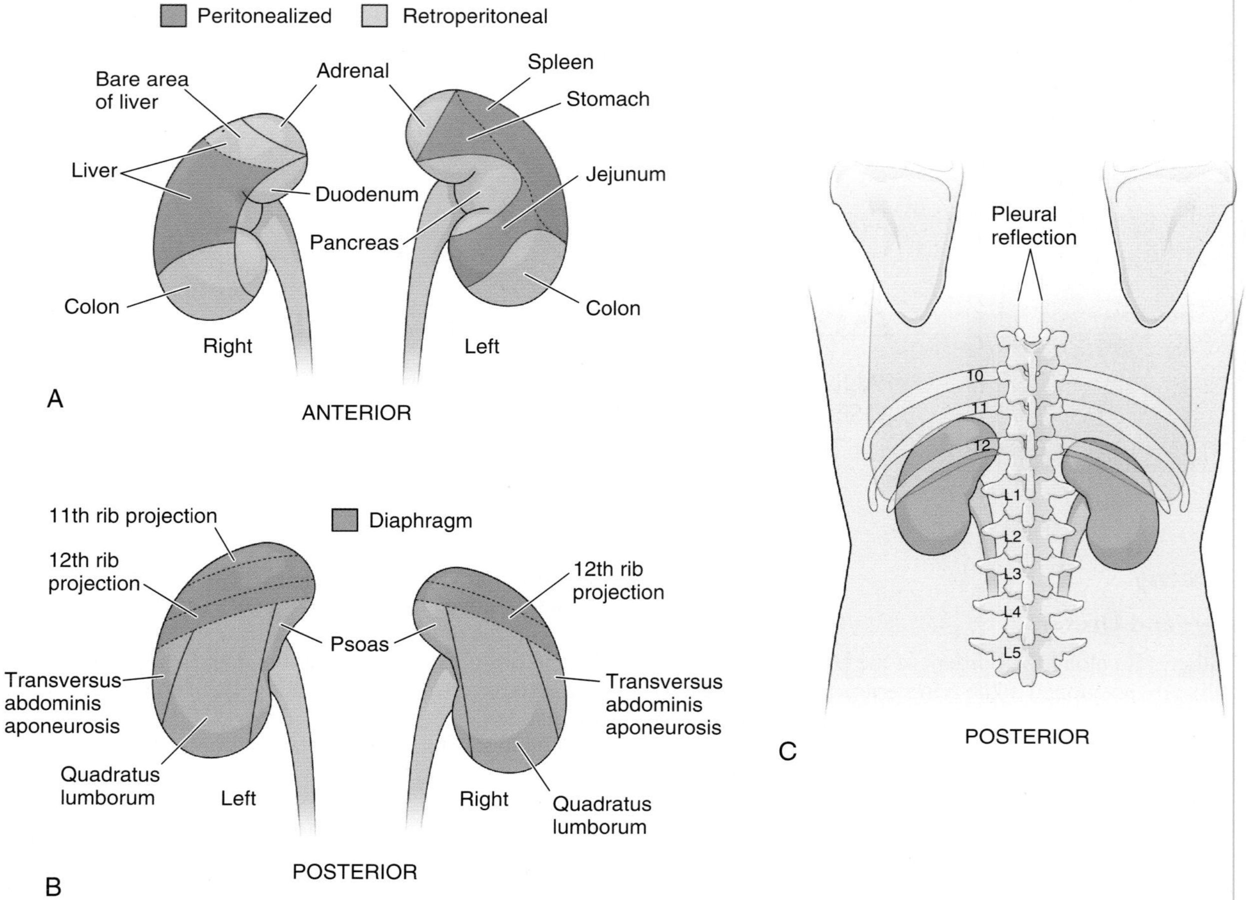

FIGURE 61–1 Anatomic relation of the kidneys to (*A*) the intraabdominal organs, (*B*) the muscles of the posterior body wall, and (*C*) the pleural reflections. (Adapted from Walsh PC, Retik AB, Vaughan ED Jr, Wein AJ (eds): Campbell's Urology, 8th ed, Vol 1. Philadelphia, Saunders, 2002.)

Prostate

The normal prostate gland weighs about 20 g and is located just distal to the bladder neck. It is supported anteriorly by the puboprostatic ligaments and inferiorly by the urogenital diaphragm. Incorporated within the prostate gland is an abundant amount of smooth muscle. This musculature represents the smooth involuntary sphincter of the male urethra.

The prostate gland is divided into discrete zones. The transition zone normally accounts for 5% to 10% of the glandular tissue of the prostate. The peripheral zone makes up the bulk of the prostatic tissue (70%) and covers the posterior and lateral aspects of the gland.

The prostatic artery originates from the inferior vesical artery and enters the gland posterolaterally. A large dorsal vein complex is located on the anterior surface of the prostate, and venous drainage of the prostate is abundant through this periprostatic plexus. Lymphatic drainage is primarily to the obturator and internal iliac nodes.

The Penis

The penis comprises spongy tissue: the paired corpora cavernosa and the solitary corpus spongiosum. The cavernosa are enclosed by the fibrous tunica albuginea, which helps provide rigidity during erection. Distal to the pubic symphysis, the cavernosa are divided by an incomplete septum. More proximally, they separate and fuse to the ischial rami. The corpus spongiosum is positioned ventrally with its distal portion expanding to form the glans penis. The main blood supply of the penis is the penile artery, the terminal branch of the internal iliac artery. Venous drainage from the penis is via the deep dorsal veins to the periprostatic venous plexus.

PEARLS FOR THE OR

The left renal vein has three branches (gonadal, lumbar, adrenal); the right has none.

A radical orchiectomy is performed through an inguinal incision to avoid violating the lymphatic drainage of the scrotum.

Unilateral hydronephrosis in the face of bladder cancer implies muscle-invasive disease.

Santorini's plexus is a network of veins on the dorsum of the prostate.

The neurovascular bundles sit next to the prostate at the 5 and 7 o'clock positions. They provide important input in the initiation and maintenance of an erection.

The dorsal nerves provide sensation to the penis. These nerves follow the course of the dorsal arteries and richly supply the glans. The cavernous nerves ramify in the erectile tissue to supply sympathetic and parasympathetic innervation from the pelvic plexuses.

The Testes

As the testes descend from their embryologic intra-abdominal position, they acquire fascial coverings from all of the layers of the abdominal wall. These comprise the external spermatic fascia, the cremasteric muscle, and the internal spermatic fascia. The parietal and visceral tunica vaginalis surround the testis with a mesothelium-lined pouch that is derived from peritoneum. The testis is fixed to the scrotal wall at its lower pole by the gubernaculum.

The testes are 4 to 5 cm in length, 3 cm wide, and 2.5 cm in depth and have a volume of 30 mL. The epididymis attaches to the posterolateral aspect of the testis. The long seminiferous tubules of the testis drain into the head of the epididymis (Fig. 61-2). The epididymal duct travels 6 m within its fibrous sheath before it thickens to become the vas deferens. The main blood supply to the testicle is the internal spermatic artery, which arises from the aorta. Lymphatic drainage returns to the retroperitoneum, its embryologic origin.

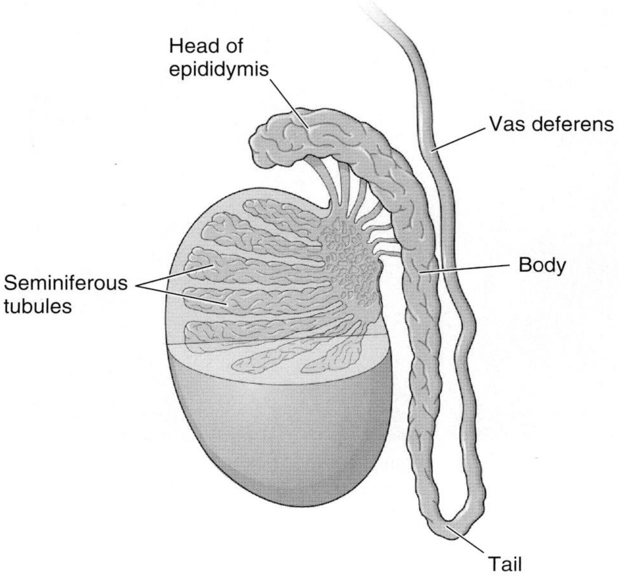

FIGURE 61–2 Cross section of the testis, epididymis, and vas deferens. (Adapted from Walsh PC, Retik AB, Vaughan ED Jr, Wein AJ (eds): Campbell's Urology, 8th ed, Vol 1. Philadelphia, Saunders, 2002.)

Oncology

Renal Cell Carcinoma

Pathophysiology

Malignancies of the kidney account for 3% of all adult cancers. The typical age range is between 40 and 60 years, although there have been reports of patients in their early 20s. The majority of cases are unilateral and sporadic. An association is found with von Hippel–Lindau disease and renal cell carcinoma, as in nearly all patients with this disorder, multiple, bilateral lesions will develop. Renal cell carcinomas arise from the proximal convoluted tubules. The most consistent chromosomal changes in renal cell carcinoma are deletions and translocations of the short arm of chromosome 3 (3p). No clear environmental factors are involved in sporadic renal cell carcinoma, although weak correlation with cigarette smoking has been found.

Differential Diagnosis

Renal cell carcinoma is the most common malignancy arising from the renal parenchyma. Simple renal cysts, however, are the most frequently encountered renal mass lesion (70% of all cases and found in roughly one third of all adults). These should be easily identified with basic radiologic studies. Whereas most simple cystic lesions are asymptomatic and require no intervention, some are complex (septations, wall thickening, calcifications, or a combination of these) and require further investigation to rule out malignancy (Fig. 61-3).

Angiomyolipoma is a benign tumor comprising fatty, muscular, and vascular elements (Fig. 61-4). These tumors may be isolated or occur in association with tuberous sclerosis. The lesions can grow to become quite large, increasing the risk of spontaneous hemorrhage within the retroperitoneum. Asymptomatic lesions smaller than 4 to 5 cm are generally observed with periodic imaging. Patients with an acute bleeding episode may require embolization.

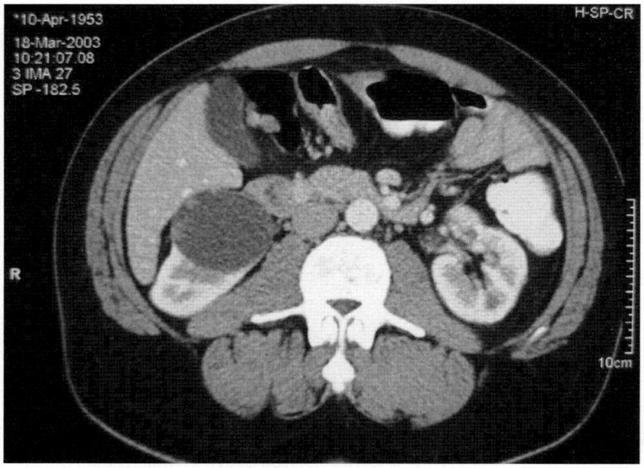

FIGURE 61–3 Computed tomography scan of a complex renal cyst. Note the sporadic thickening of the inner lining of the wall. This was pathologically proven to be renal cell carcinoma.

Symptomatic lesions or those larger than 4 to 5 cm may require surgical excision.

Oncocytomas are benign renal tumors characterized by eosinophilic granular cells. Despite some subtle computed tomography (CT) scan differences, these lesions are difficult to distinguish from renal cell carcinoma and are malignant until proven otherwise on pathologic examination.

Lymphoma can involve the kidney but is almost always part of a metastatic process. The presence of diffuse retroperitoneal lymph nodes as well as renal mass should help distinguish this disease. The kidney is a frequent site of metastatic deposits from solid tumors. These tumors are usually small and multiple and are often discovered only on autopsy. Lung cancer is the most common solid tumor to metastasize to the kidney, although ovarian, bowel, and breast sources also are quite common.

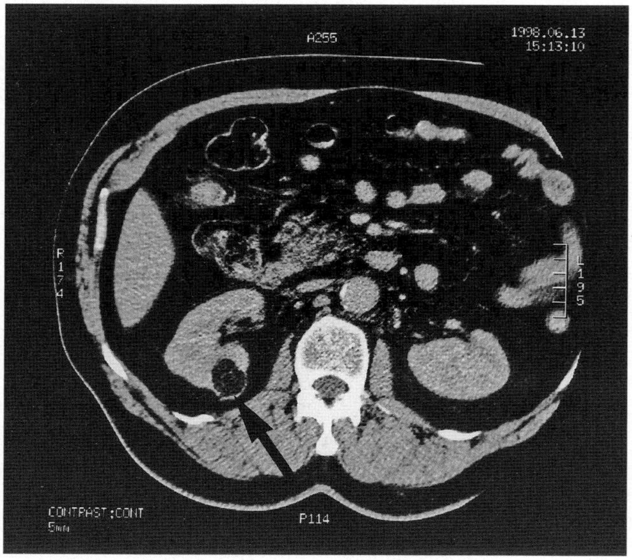

FIGURE 61–4 Computed tomography (CT) scan demonstrating an angiomyolipoma of the right kidney. Notice that the lesion has the same CT density as that of the surrounding perirenal fat, confirming the diagnosis.

Evaluation

Patients frequently are first seen with nonspecific complaints of back pain, weakness, weight loss, or fever. Hematuria (usually microscopic) is the single most common sign, occurring in 29% to 60% of cases. Of note, the classic triad of hematuria, flank pain, and a palpable abdominal mass is reported only in roughly 10% of cases. This tumor is often discovered incidentally. Renal cell carcinoma may be associated with a variety of paraneoplastic syndromes.

A complete blood count and electrolyte panel are usually obtained during preoperative evaluation. Of special interest is assessment of baseline renal function. Liver enzymes and alkaline phosphatase are measured to search for metastatic disease. A chest radiograph (posteroanterior [PA]/lateral) also is included.

CT with and without contrast has become the standard tool to evaluate complex cystic and solid renal masses. The vast majority of renal cell carcinomas exhibit at least a 20-Hounsfield unit enhancement with intravenous contrast (Fig. 61-5). Magnetic resonance imaging (MRI) can be used to confirm tumor extension into the renal vein or IVC.

The tumor, node, and metastases (TNM) staging system is currently the most commonly used (Box 61-1) system to define the extent of disease. Renal cell carcinoma metastasizes most frequently to lungs, bone, and brain.

Treatment

Treatment for renal cell carcinoma has traditionally been radical nephrectomy, which includes resection of the kidney, perinephric fat, and Gerota's fascia. Partial nephrectomy (nephron-sparing surgery) is indicated for patients with a solitary kidney or multiple tumors or those with von Hippel-Lindau disease, who are expected to have multiple recurrences. In addition, it has been proven to be as safe and effective as radical surgery for low-stage renal tumors that are smaller than 4 cm. Many surgical approaches to the kidney exist, and the choice should be based on a variety of factors including tumor size, extent, location, body habitus, and surgeon preference. Successful laparoscopic techniques also have been proven (Fig. 61-6). The renal vessels should be controlled before manipulation and dissection, and the renal artery is ligated before division of the renal vein. In cases of vena cava involvement, the venous system is controlled superiorly and inferiorly, and the tumor thrombus is removed.

Renal cell carcinoma does not respond well to radiation therapy, although painful bony metastases may respond to palliative treatment. In addition, this tumor is very resistant

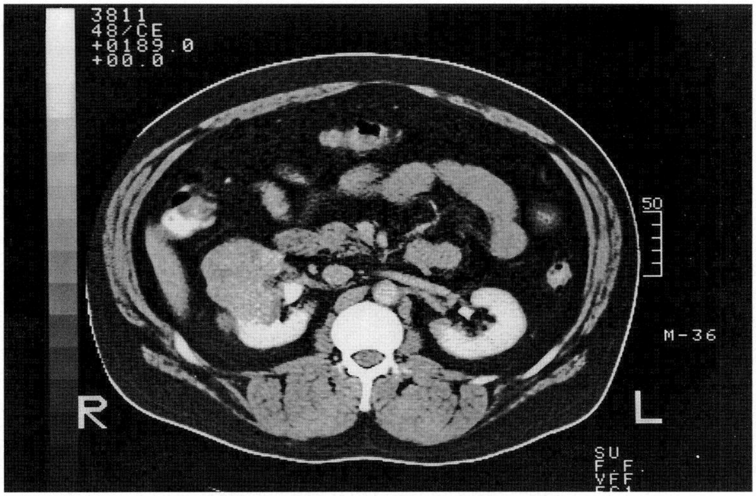

FIGURE 61–5 Large renal mass arising from the anterior aspect of the right kidney. The fact that it enhances with the administration of intravenous contrast makes it highly suggestive of renal cell carcinoma.

BOX 61–1 Kidney TNM Classification

T: Primary Tumor

TX Primary tumor cannot be assessed
T0 No evidence of primary tumor
T1 Tumor $\leq$7 cm or in greatest dimension, limited to the kidney
  T1a Tumor $\leq$4 cm in greatest dimension, limited to the kidney
  T1b Tumor >4 cm but $\leq$7 cm in greatest dimension, limited to the kidney
T2 Tumor >7 cm in greatest dimension, limited to the kidney
T3 Tumor extends into major veins or invades adrenal gland or perinephric tissues but not beyond Gerota's fascia
  T3a Tumor directly invades adrenal gland or perirenal and/or renal sinus fat but not beyond Gerota's fascia
  T3b Tumor grossly extends into the renal vein or its segmental (muscle-containing) branches, or vena cava below the diaphragm
  T3c Tumor grossly extends into vena cava above diaphragm or invades the wall of the vena cava
T4 Tumor invades beyond Gerota's fascia

N: Regional Lymph Nodes

NX Regional lymph nodes cannot be assessed
N0 No regional lymph node metastases
N1 Metastases in a single regional lymph node
N2 Metastases in more than one regional lymph node

M: Distant Metastasis

MX Distant metastasis cannot be assessed
M0 No distant metastasis
M1 Distant metastasis

From American Joint Committee on Cancer: AJCC Cancer Staging Manual, 6th ed. New York, Springer-Verlag, 2002, with permission.

to chemotherapy. Most recent protocols have used immunotherapy, particularly with interleukin-2 and interferons. Although occasional sustained, complete responses do occur, most series report partial response rates in the 10% to 20% range.

Adenocarcinoma of the Prostate

Pathophysiology

Carcinoma of the prostate is the most common solid-organ cancer in men in the United States and the second leading cause of cancer death. The vast majority of these tumors

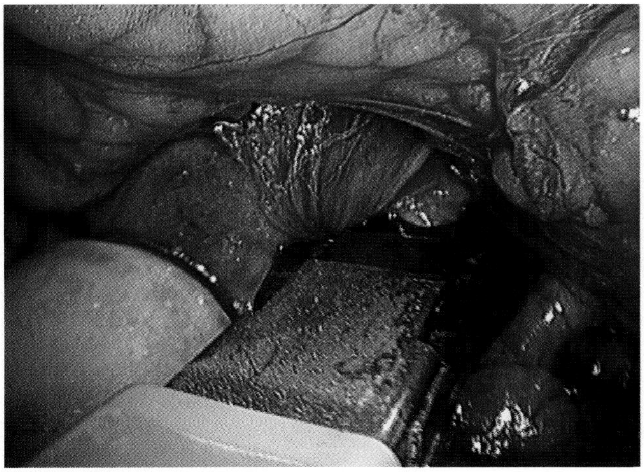

FIGURE 61–6 Intraoperative photograph of a right radical nephrectomy. An automatic clip applier is being used to control the renal artery. Note the renal vein to the left of the instrument.

are adenocarcinoma. African-American men have a higher incidence of prostate cancer and also tend to have more-aggressive, higher-stage disease. The incidence of this cancer increases with age. Adenocarcinoma of the prostate has two major clinical courses. The first is an indolent, asymptomatic cancer that is found incidentally at autopsy. The second presents a true threat to the patient's life expectancy. It can be difficult at times to predict the biologic behavior of any individual tumor.

Most patients are diagnosed after screening reveals a prostate specific antigen (PSA) value above the upper limit of normal of 4.0 ng/mL. Digital rectal examination (DRE) also can reveal irregularities of the normally smooth posterior contour. Either of these findings can prompt performance of a biopsy. A low fraction of PSA that is unbound in serum (<24%) can suggest the presence of cancer. Equally worrisome is a PSA increase of more than 0.75 ng/mL/year.

Differential Diagnosis

Elevations in PSA may be caused by prostate cancer, benign prostatic hyperplasia (BPH), prostatitis, cystitis, the presence of a Foley catheter, and even urinary retention. Irregularities of the DRE can be caused by carcinoma of the prostate or the bladder, previous inflammation, or prostatic cysts. The prostate is occasionally invaded by hematologic malignancies, pelvic tumors, colorectal cancer, or by direct extension from a bladder mass.

Evaluation

The vast majority of men with low-stage prostate cancer have no disease-related symptoms. Although some patients may describe obstructive-type voiding symptoms, this is usually caused by BPH in this age group. Patients with advanced disease may have pelvic pain, ureteral obstruction, or bone pain from distant metastasis.

The physical examination should focus on the consistency of the prostate gland on DRE. Advanced carcinoma feels hard and nodular and may have extension into surrounding tissues. Early cancer has a normal consistency or may demonstrate diffuse enlargement from associated (but unrelated) BPH. The rest of the examination searches for metastatic disease. Patients occasionally have the neurologic signs and symptoms of spinal cord compression from metastases, such as lower extremity weakness, decreased sensation, or bowel and bladder dysfunction.

Transrectal ultrasonography (TRUS) is used to image the gland and provide accurate measures of prostate size. Prostate cancers are typically found in the peripheral zone of the gland and sometimes appear as hypoechoic lesions (Fig. 61-7). TRUS is very helpful when used to guide needle biopsies of the gland. A CT scan is used to search for pelvic lymphadenopathy or evidence of metastatic disease when the PSA is greater than 20 ng/mL. A radionuclide bone scan may be useful when the PSA is more than 10 ng/mL or the tumor has a high grade.

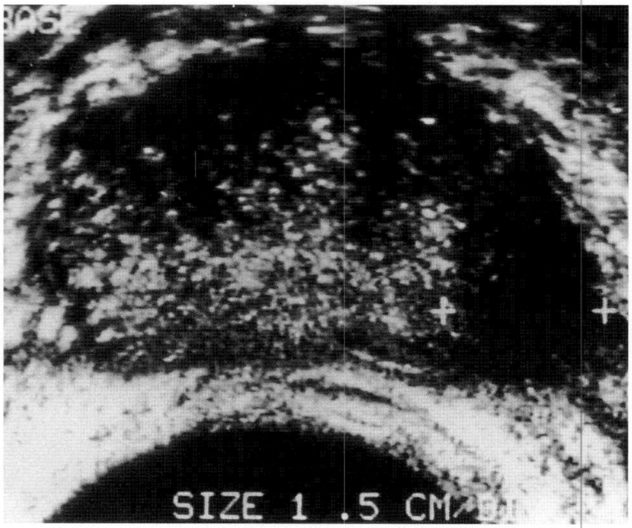

FIGURE 61–7 Transurethral ultrasound image of the prostate. Note the hypoechoic lesion (*marks*) in the left peripheral zone of the prostate. Such lesions are suggestive of tumor.

The TNM system has become the most widely used to stage prostate adenocarcinoma (Box 61-2). In addition, tumors are graded according to the Gleason scoring system, which assigns a number (1 to 5) to the predominant cancer as well as to the next most predominant grade. These two numbers are then totaled to provide the Gleason sum or score. Tumors with a score of 2 to 4 are considered well differentiated (least aggressive), whereas those with a score of 8 to 10 are poorly differentiated (most aggressive). The majority of patients initially have a score between 5 and 7 (moderately differentiated).

Treatment

The optimal treatment for localized prostate cancer remains controversial. For men with a life expectancy of less than 10 years, observation alone (termed *watchful waiting*) may be appropriate. Prostate cancer manifests partial androgen dependency, which has been used to treat advanced disease. The main source of serum testosterone can be removed by surgical castration (bilateral orchiectomy) or, more commonly, by medical therapy. Oral estrogens are effective but are associated with an unacceptable rate of cardiovascular side effects. Luteinizing hormone–releasing hormone (LHRH) analogues effectively suppress testosterone to the castrate range within 1 month of administration. LHRH analogues frequently cause vasomotor hot flashes. Loss of libido and impotence are a common consequence of either orchiectomy or LHRH agents. The adrenal glands may provide up to 10% of the circulating androgens. Studies examining the effects of blockade of these hormones with oral antiandrogen agents have been mixed.

BOX 61-2 Prostate TNM Classification

T: Primary Tumor

TX Primary tumor cannot be assessed
T0 No evidence of primary tumor
T1 Clinically inapparent tumor neither palpable nor visible by imaging
- T1a Tumor incidental histologic finding in ≤5% of tissue resected
- T1b Tumor incidental histologic finding in >5 % of tissue resected
- T1c Tumor identified by needle biopsy (e.g., because of elevated PSA)

T2 Tumor confined within prostate*
- T2a Tumor involves one-half of one lobe or less
- T2b Tumor involves more than one-half of one lobe but not both lobes
- T2c Tumor involves both lobes

T3 Tumor extends through the prostatic capsule†
- T3a Extracapsular extension (unilateral or bilateral)
- T3b Tumor invades seminal vesicle(s)

T4 Tumor is fixed or invades adjacent structures other than seminal vesicles: bladder neck, external sphincter, rectum, levator muscles, and/or pelvic wall

N: Regional Lymph Nodes

NX Regional lymph nodes were not assessed
N0 No regional lymph node metastasis
N1 Metastasis in regional lymph node

M: Distant Metastasis

MX Distant metastasis cannot be assessed (not evaluated by any modality)
M0 No distant metastasis
M1 Distant metastasis
- M1a Nonregional lymph node(s)
- M1b Bone(s)
- M1c Other site(s) with or without bone disease‡

PSA, prostate specific antigen
*Tumor found in one or both lobes by needle biopsy, but not palpable or reliably visible by imaging, is classified as T1c.
†Invasion into the prostatic apex or into (but not beyond) the prostatic capsule is classified not as T3, but as T2.
‡When more than one site of metastasis is present, the most advanced category is used. M1c is most advanced
From American Joint Committee on Cancer: AJCC Cancer Staging Manual, 6th ed. New York, Springer-Verlag, 2002, with permission.

Surgical removal of the prostate (radical prostatectomy) or external-beam radiation therapy (XRT) are the most commonly used treatments for clinically localized prostate cancer. Ten-year survival statistics for both treatments demonstrate solid results, but valid randomized comparisons are lacking. Brachytherapy, using percutaneous interstitial implantation of either iodine 125 or palladium 103, also is used, with acceptable outcomes. Cryotherapy (i.e., freezing of the prostate) is being investigated, but results published to date are inferior.

The retropubic approach to the prostate is generally preferred, as it allows the surgeon to perform a pelvic lymphadenectomy at the same setting, whereas the perineal approach requires a separate incision or laparoscopic dissection. Both approaches allow the preservation of the posterolateral neurovascular bundles, which can maintain potency if spared bilaterally.

Serum PSA should decrease to an undetectable range after radical prostatectomy as all PSA-producing cells ideally are removed. After radiation therapy, superior results are achieved in patients in whom the PSA level decreases to less than 0.5 ng/mL. Three consecutive increases in serum PSA are synonymous with tumor recurrence after XRT. Hormonal therapy can be used to treat patients with PSA recurrence, the timing of which is highly controversial.

Hormonal therapy can reduce PSA to undetectable levels in up to 80% to 90% of patients with advanced metastatic disease. The duration of response is typically 18 to 24 months in these patients, after which time, the cancer cells become hormone independent and resume their growth. Survival after this point is typically 12 to 18 months. No reliable therapies can alter survival at this point, although trials are under way. XRT may palliate discrete osseous metastases.

Transitional Cell Carcinoma of the Bladder

Pathophysiology

Carcinoma of the bladder is the fifth most common malignancy in the United States. The male-to-female ratio is 3:1. Cigarette smokers carry a four times greater risk. In addition, industrial exposures have been identified, including aniline dyes used in the textile industry. Acrolein, which is a by-product of cyclophosphamide, has been implicated. Carcinomas from these industrial or iatrogenic exposures can take up to 20 to 30 years to express themselves.

Nearly 90% of bladder malignancies arise from the transitional epithelium that lines the urinary system. Of these urothelial carcinomas, 70% are papillary (Fig. 61-8), 10% are sessile, and 20% are mixed. The TNM staging system (Box 61-3) is used to describe the extent of disease. Low grade, stage Ta lesions are at low risk for disease progression and are associated with a high survival rate. Because of a field-exposure effect, a high relapse rate of 50% to 70% exists for superficial disease. Approximately 15% to 20% of superficial carcinomas will progress to muscle-invasive disease. Muscle invasion portends a worse prognosis. Nearly all patients with metastatic disease are dead within 2 years.

Carcinoma in situ (CIS) arises from the lining of the bladder (Fig. 61-9). CIS is commonly multifocal and is often found with invasive disease. Up to 20% of patients with presumed CIS will have microscopic muscle invasion at the time of cystectomy. CIS treated with transurethral resection alone will progress to muscle invasion in 40% to 83% of cases.

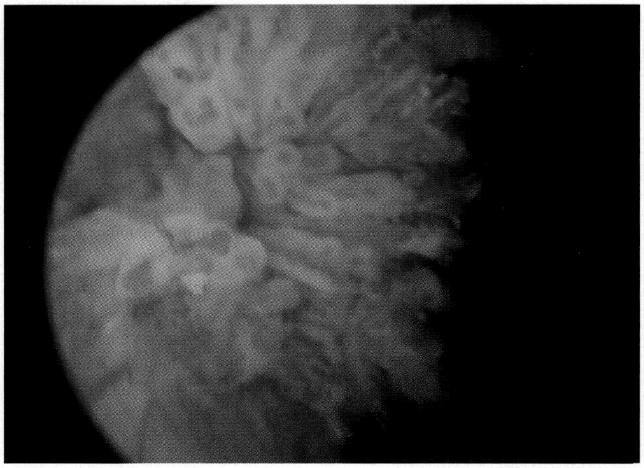

FIGURE 61–8 Cystoscopic view of a papillary transitional cell carcinoma of the bladder.

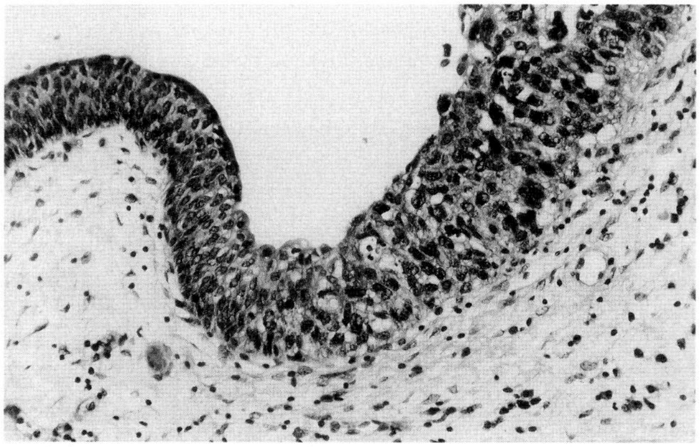

FIGURE 61–9 Microscopic image of carcinoma in situ of the bladder (*center* and *right*). These cells demonstrate loss of epithelial polarization, hyperchromasia, and mitoses. (Courtesy of Dr. Scott Shappell, Department of Pathology, Vanderbilt University Medical Center, Nashville, Tennessee.)

BOX 61–3 Urinary Bladder TNM Classification

T: Primary Tumor

The suffix (m) should be added to the appropriate T category to indicate multiple tumors. The suffix (is) may be added to any T to indicate presence of associated carcinoma in situ

TX	Primary tumor cannot be assessed
T0	No evidence of primary tumor
Ta	Noninvasive papillary carcinoma
Tis	Carcinoma in situ: "flat tumor"
T1	Tumor invades subepithelial connective tissue
T2	Tumor invades muscle
	T2a Tumor invades superficial muscle (inner half)
	T2b Tumor invades deep muscle (outer half)
T3	Tumor invades perivesical tissue
	T3a Microscopically
	T3b Macroscopically (extravesical mass)
T4	Tumor invades any of the following: prostate, uterus, vagina, pelvic wall, abdominal wall
	T4a Tumor invades prostate, uterus, vagina
	T4b Tumor invades pelvic wall, abdominal wall

N: Regional Lymph Nodes

NX	Regional lymph nodes cannot be assessed
N0	No regional lymph node metastasis
N1	Metastasis in a single lymph node, ≤2 cm in greatest dimension
N2	Metastasis in a single lymph node, >2 cm but ≤5 cm in greatest dimension; or multiple lymph nodes, none >5 cm in greatest dimension
N3	Metastasis in a lymph node, >5 cm in greatest dimension

M: Distant Metastasis

MX	Distant metastasis cannot be assessed
M0	No distant metastasis
M1	Distant metastasis

From American Joint Committee on Cancer: AJCC Cancer Staging Manual, 6th ed. New York, Springer-Verlag, 2002, with permission.

Differential Diagnosis

Adenocarcinoma accounts for fewer than 2% of all bladder cancers and may arise from a urachal remnant. It is often associated with cystitis glandularis or with bladder exstrophy. Most adenocarcinomas are invasive, with a poor 5-year survival rate. Urachal tumors are located in the dome of the bladder and sometimes appear with bloody discharge from the umbilicus.

Squamous cell carcinoma accounts for about 6% of bladder cancers in the United States but more than 75% of bladder cancers in Egypt. Squamous cell cancers are frequently associated with chronic bladder inflammation from foreign objects such as a Foley catheter or a bladder stone. Four fifths of squamous cell cancer in Egypt is caused by infection with the parasite *Schistosoma haematobium*.

Evaluation

Total, painless, gross hematuria is the most common presenting symptom. Patients frequently report an intermittent pattern of hematuria and many have been empirically treated with antibiotic therapy. Patients with higher-stage disease may report flank pain from obstruction of a ureter or lower-extremity edema from bulky pelvic lymphadenopathy. Urinary frequency, urgency, or dysuria (irritative symptoms) can be found with CIS or invasive tumors.

The physical examination searches for disease spread. Lymph nodes are palpated for signs of enlargement. A careful bimanual examination is performed to assess the mobility of the bladder. Those patients with a fixed bladder are suspect for having locally advanced disease. All patients require a transurethral resection or biopsy to provide a tissue diagnosis. A sample of the underlying bladder muscle as well as the tumor itself is required to evaluate the tumor stage fully. Random biopsies of apparently normal-appearing urothelium also should be sent, because CIS can have a wide array of presentations.

Urine is sent for cytologic evaluation, as many high-grade tumors and most cases of CIS will shed malignant cells. Accuracy, however, is highly operator dependent. Several urine markers are under study, but none has been more effective than cytology with cystoscopy.

Patients with muscle-invasive tumors or recurrent high-grade disease should be evaluated for metastasis. An elevated alkaline phosphatase raises suspicions of bone metastasis, whereas abnormal liver-function tests are concerning for hepatic involvement. Radiologic imaging includes a chest radiograph and a CT scan of the abdomen and pelvis. An intravenous pyelogram (IVP) or even a retrograde pyelogram is necessary to evaluate the renal pelvis and ureters and clear them of disease. Radionuclide bone scan or plain films may be required to search for bony spread.

Treatment

The optimal management of bladder carcinoma depends on tumor stage and grade. Nearly all superficial tumors can be completely resected transurethrally. All patients with previously resected disease should undergo surveillance with quarterly cystoscopy for the first year, with lengthening intervals as long as the patient is free of recurrence. Periodic IVP should be performed as well, because at least a 3% to 5% risk of late disease exists in the upper urinary tracts.

Recurrent superficial disease, T1 lesions, high-grade superficial tumors, or CIS are excellent candidates for intravesical therapy. The most commonly used drug is bacille Calmette-Guérin (BCG), an attenuated strain of *Mycobacterium bovis* frequently used as a tuberculosis vaccine. When placed within the bladder, BCG incites an intense immune response and has been proven to reduce time to disease recurrence and progression in both papillary tumors and CIS. It is typically given once a week for a total of 6 weeks. Studies have shown that maintenance BCG may further improve overall response rates. BCG often induces irritative symptoms of the bladder and may even trigger low-grade fevers. Systemic sepsis, or BCG-osis, can occur and is a medical emergency. Various chemotherapeutic agents also have been used intravesically with results that generally lag behind those with BCG. These include mitomycin C, thiotepa, and doxorubicin (Adriamycin).

Muscle-invasive cancers (T2 and higher) and aggressively recurrent superficial tumors are candidates for radical cystectomy. This entails removal of the bladder, prostate, perivesical fat, and pelvic lymph nodes. The anterior vaginal wall and uterus and ovaries are typically removed in women. Attempts at bladder-sparing surgery are generally reserved for highly selected tumors or patients not medically fit for radical surgery. On removal of the bladder, it is necessary to perform a urinary diversion. The standard is to create a conduit to the skin from a loop of ileum or colon. A stoma is created, and the patient is then required to wear a collection appliance. Continent diversions also can be developed out of detubularized bowel. Catheterizable diversions use the right colon as a reservoir and a limb of ileum to the skin. Increasingly, an orthotopic neobladder is created from detubularized ileum and is then anastomosed to the urethra. This allows the patient to void spontaneously per urethra and almost always avoids the need for self-catheterization. Quality-of-life studies have shown that these continent diversions can improve patient satisfaction.

Five-year survival rates are approximately 60% to 80% after cystectomy for T2 bladder cancers. For T3 tumors, the 5-year survival decreases to 37% to 61%, whereas patients with node-positive disease have a 5-year survival of less than 30%.

Radiation therapy alone is not effective. In addition, neoadjuvant XRT followed by salvage cystectomy is frequently associated with increased rates of complications.

Chemotherapy is generally offered to patients at high risk for failure (pathologic stage T3b, T4, and N1/2 disease) in the adjuvant setting or for those patients first seen with advanced disease. The standard regimen has been methotrexate, vinblastine, doxorubicin (Adriamycin), and cisplatin (MVAC). Durable complete response rates have been less than 15%, prompting investigation of a variety of new chemotherapeutic agents including gemcitabine, taxol, and ifosfamide.

Carcinoma of the Testis

Pathophysiology

Carcinoma of the testis occurs infrequently, but represents the most common malignancy among males aged 15 to 35 years. Germ cell tumors compose more than 95% of these lesions and are further divided into seminomatous and nonseminomatous neoplasms (NSGCT). Within nonseminomatous tumors, many tissue types may exist and may secrete a variety of tumor markers. In up to 40% of cases, germ cell tumors occur with mixed histology.

Whites have the highest incidence of this disease with a 5:1 ratio over African-Americans. Familial clusterings have been reported. A history of cryptorchidism can increase the relative risk for this disorder by 40 times. Orchidopexy performed early in life may reduce the risk of germ cell cancer and, at the very least, allows easier surveillance of this testis.

Differential Diagnosis

Benign cystic masses may occur in the scrotum and can be confused for a testis neoplasm. Cystic dilatation of the head of the epididymis, a spermatocele, should be easily palpable as distinct from the testis itself. These lesions should transilluminate. Hydroceles, a fluid collection within the tunica vaginalis surrounding the testis, should also be easily distinguished by transillumination. Rapid development or infection of these lesions can make the physical diagnosis difficult. Transcrotal ultrasonography helps in these situations.

Infections of the epididymis or testis also can mimic a solid lesion. The acute onset of an infection as well as a positive response to antibiotics and anti-inflammatory agents should help distinguish this cause. All of these patients should have a follow-up examination to ensure that the testis is indeed normal. Any remaining doubts should be cleared with an ultrasound.

Leydig cell tumors make up between 1% and 3% of all testis tumors. Although most occur between ages 20 and 60 years, approximately one fourth have been reported before puberty. Leydig cell tumors have an excellent prognosis after radical inguinal orchiectomy. Lymphoma may involve the testis and is the most common tumor found in men older than 50 years. Bilateral involvement carries a worse prognosis, as does relapsing disease.

Evaluation

A painless testicular mass is a primary testicular tumor until proven otherwise. However, many patients initially have diffuse testicular pain or swelling. Because infectious epididymo-orchitis is more common than tumor, a trial of antibiotics is often undertaken. If testicular discomfort or the findings or both do not revert to normal within 2 to 4 weeks, testicular ultrasonography is indicated. Patients with advanced disease may complain of abdominal or back discomfort, shortness of breath, gastrointestinal disturbance, or even neurologic deficits.

The physical examination should center on evaluation of the scrotal contents as well as a search for distant disease. The testis is palpated for size, consistency, tenderness, and evidence of fixation. The spermatic cord also should be palpated for evidence of abnormal thickening. The contralateral testis should always be examined. The abdominal examination is usually benign. Signs of a pleural effusion should be sought, and the supraclavicular nodes should be palpated.

Testis cancer is associated with predictable tumor markers. α-Fetoprotein (AFP) may be elevated with embryonal carcinoma, teratocarcinoma, or yolk sac tumors. It is never found with pure seminoma. β-Human chorionic gonadotropin (β-hCG) can be elevated with embryonal carcinoma, choriocarcinoma, and with 5% to 10% of patients with pure seminoma. Lactate dehydrogenase (LDH) also can be high but is nonspecific. LDH correlates well with level of tumor burden and is particularly useful when monitoring patients with advanced seminoma. AFP has a serum half-life of 5 to 7 days, whereas that of β-hCG is 24 to 36 hours. All patients should have levels of AFP, β-hCG, and LDH determined before radical orchiectomy. Failure of these markers to decline at appropriate rates after surgery implies residual metastatic disease.

All patients require a chest radiograph to rule out pulmonary metastases. In addition, a CT scan of the abdomen and pelvis is performed to search for retroperitoneal disease (Fig. 61-10). However, 20% to 30% of patients with a

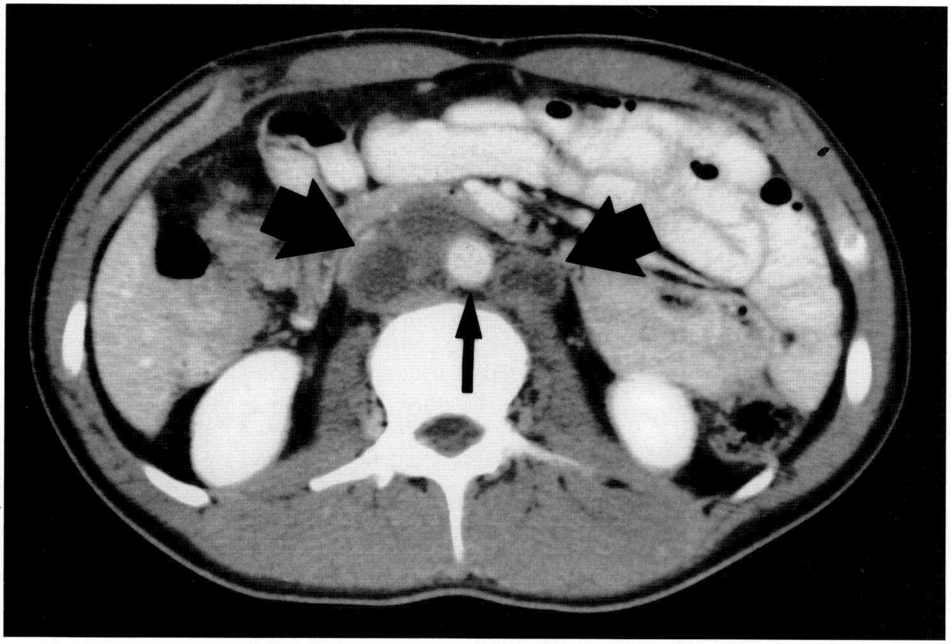

FIGURE 61–10 Computed tomography scan revealing bulky retroperitoneal adenopathy (*wide arrows*) surrounding the aorta (*thin arrow*).

BOX 61–4 Testis TNM Classification

T: Primary Tumor

Tumor stage is generally determined after orchiectomy, at which time, a pathologic stage is assigned

- pTX Primary tumor cannot be assessed (if no radical orchiectomy has been performed, TX is used)
- pT0 No evidence of primary tumor (e.g., histologic scar in testis)
- pTis Intratubular germ cell neoplasia (carcinoma in situ)
- pT1 Tumor limited to the testis and epididymis without vascular/lymphatic invasion; tumor may invade into the tunica albuginea but not the tunica vaginalis
- pT2 Tumor limited to testis and epididymis with vascular/lymphatic invasion, or tumor extending through tunica albuginea with involvement of the tunica vaginalis
- pT3 Tumor invades the spermatic cord with or without vascular/lymphatic invasion
- pT4 Tumor invades the scrotum with or without vascular/lymphatic invasion

N: Regional Lymph Nodes: clinical

- NX Regional lymph nodes cannot be assessed
- N0 No regional lymph node metastasis
- N1 Metastasis with a lymph node mass ≤2 cm in greatest dimension; or multiple lymph nodes, none >2 cm in greatest dimension
- N2 Metastasis with a lymph node mass >2 cm but ≤5 cm in greatest dimension; or multiple lymph nodes, any one mass >2 cm but ≤5 cm in greatest dimension
- N3 Metastasis with a lymph node mass >5 cm in greatest dimension

N: Regional Lymph Nodes: pathologic

- NX Regional lymph nodes cannot be assessed
- N0 No regional lymph node metastasis
- N1 Metastasis with a lymph node mass ≤2 cm in greatest dimension and five nodes or fewer positive, none >2 cm in greatest dimension
- N2 Metastasis with a lymph node mass >2 cm but ≤5 cm in greatest dimension; or more than five nodes positive, none >5 cm; or evidence of extranodal extension of tumor
- N3 Metastasis with a lymph node mass >5 cm in greatest dimension

M: Distant Metastasis

- MX Distant metastasis cannot be assessed
- M0 No distant metastasis
- M1 Distant metastasis
  - M1a Nonregional nodal or pulmonary metastasis
  - M1b Distant metastasis other than to nonregional lymph nodes and lung

S: Serum Tumor Markers

(N indicates the upper limit of normal for the LDH assay)

- SX Serum marker studies not available or not performed
- S0 Serum marker study levels within normal limits

	LDH		hCG (mIU/mL)		AFP (ng/mL)
S1	<1.5 × N	and	<5000	and	<1000
S2	1.5–10 × N	or	5000–50,000	or	1000–10,000
S3	>10 × N	or	>50,000	or	>10,000

LDH, lactate dehydrogenase; hCG, human chorionic gonadotropin; AFP, α-fetoprotein.
From American Joint Committee on Cancer: AJCC Cancer Staging Manual, 6th ed. New York, Springer-Verlag, 2000, with permission.

negative CT may still have occult metastatic nodes. Head CT is indicated for patients with diffuse disease or for suggestive neurologic signs or symptoms. The cancer can be properly staged according to the TNM system (Box 61-4).

Treatment

Therapy for any testis suspected of having carcinoma begins with a radical inguinal orchiectomy. The approach is made as if performing an inguinal hernia repair. The spermatic cord is clamped early in the dissection, and the testis is delivered up out of the scrotum and into the wound. The spermatic cord is divided at the level of the internal inguinal ring. Testicles suggestive of carcinoma are not approached through the scrotum, as this could alter the otherwise predictable lymphatic drainage.

Therapy for seminomas versus nonseminomatous germ cell tumors (NSGCT) has noticeable differences. Low-stage seminoma (I, IIA/B) is often treated with low-dose external radiation to the retroperitoneum and ipsilateral pelvic

PEARLS FOR ROUNDS

Normal prostate specific antigen is defined as less than 4 ng/mL, but the definition of normal can vary according to age.

The peripheral zone of the prostate is responsible for most prostate cancer.

The most common cause of bladder cancer is smoking.

Bladder cancer most often is first seen as gross, painless hematuria.

Only 10% of patients initially have the classic triad of renal cell cancer (flank pain, abdominal mass, hematuria).

Urge incontinence caused by bladder obstruction may not resolve after surgery to relieve the blockage in up to 25% of patients.

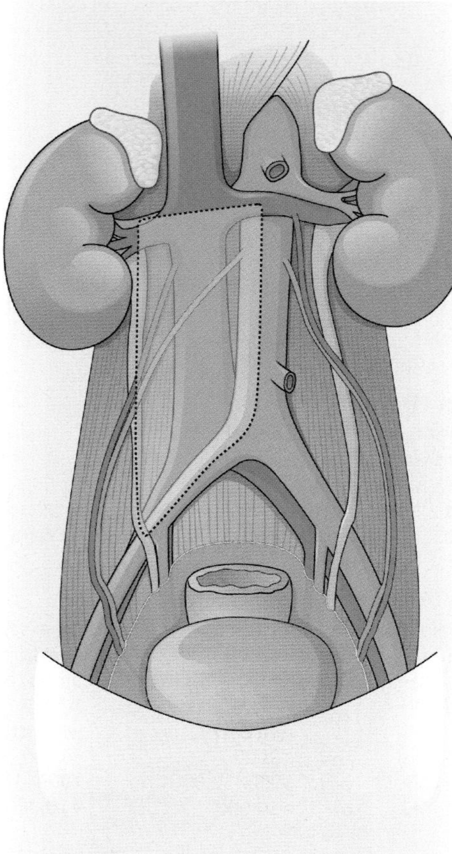

FIGURE 61–11 Nerve-sparing template for right retroperitoneal lymph node dissection. (Adapted from Foster RS, Donohue JP: Nerve-sparing RPLND. AUA Update Series, Lesson 15, Vol XII. Houston, Texas, American Urological Association, 1993, with permission.)

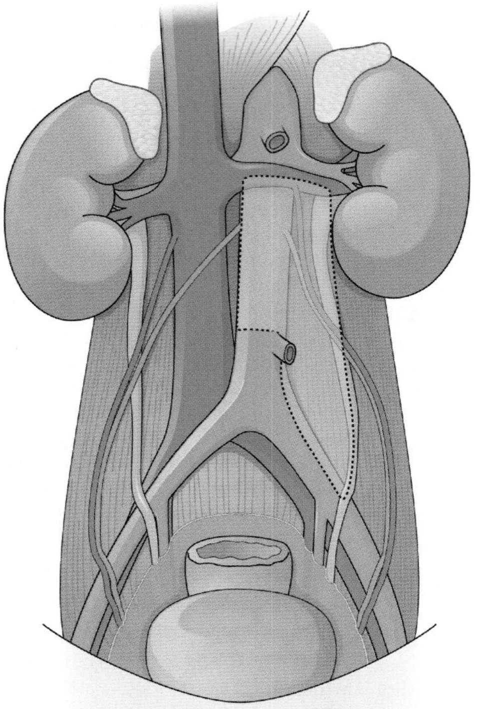

FIGURE 61–12 Nerve-sparing template for left retroperitoneal lymph node dissection. (Adapted from Foster RS, Donohue JP: Nerve-sparing RPLND. AUA Update Series, Lesson 15, Vol XII. Houston, Texas, American Urological Association, 1993, with permission.)

nodes. Relapse is uncommon and is typically salvaged with chemotherapy.

Therapy for low-stage NSGCT is controversial. Relapse for stage I tumors is 30% and can be higher if the pathology showed lymphovascular invasion, a preponderance of embryonal cells, or invasion into the spermatic cord. Reliable patients without these poor prognostic findings can be followed up on a surveillance protocol with the plan for chemotherapy or retroperitoneal lymph node dissection (RPLND) in the event of a recurrence. Surveillance entails monthly chest radiographs and tumor markers as well as CT scan every 2 to 3 months during the first year. This schedule is lengthened in ensuing years. Alternatively, these same patients could undergo a nerve-sparing RPLND. This operation involves a midline incision from the xiphoid process to the umbilicus. The colon is reflected, and the lymph nodes within the primary drop zones are dissected. Modified templates (Figs. 61-11 and 61-12) spare the sympathetic outflow below the inferior mesenteric artery. Antegrade ejaculation can be preserved in more than 90% of cases. Cure rates are in the 90% to 95% range.

Patients with stage IIA NSGCT are usually offered RPLND, with relapse rates less than 20%. Patients with high-risk findings on their RPLND specimen can be offered two cycles of adjuvant chemotherapy to avoid the increased toxicity of a full course at the time of recurrence.

Patients with bulky stage II or stage III germ cell tumors (seminoma or NSGCT) are treated with chemotherapy. The most common regimen uses bleomycin, etoposide, and cisplatin in three or four cycles. Bleomycin is associated with pulmonary toxicity, whereas etoposide can induce myelosuppression. Platinum agents have the potential for neurotoxicity.

Adjuvant RPLND is indicated for residual masses after chemotherapy. These masses can have residual tumor, teratoma, or fibrotic scar. Patients whose tumor markers fail to normalize after chemotherapy are best served with salvage chemotherapy rather than RPLND. Salvage regimens typically include vinblastine, ifosfamide, and cisplatin. Response rates to this therapy can be as low as 25%.

Suggested Reading

Grossfeld G, Wolf JS Jr, Litwan M, et al: Asymptomatic microscopic hematuria in adults: Summary of the AUA best practice policy recommendations. Am Fam Physician 63(6):1145–1154, 2001.

Hernandez J, Thompson IM: Diagnosis and treatment of prostate cancer. Med Clin North Am 88(2):267–279, 2004.

Leach GE, Dmochowski RR, Appell RA, et al: Female Stress Urinary Incontinence Clinical Guidelines Panel summary report on surgical management of female stress urinary incontinence. J Urol 158(3 Pt 1):875–880, 1997.

Shelley MD, Burgon K, Mason MD: Treatment of testicular germ-cell cancer: A Cochrane evidence-based systematic review. Cancer Treat Rev 28(5):237–253, 2002.

Smith JA Jr, Labasky RF, Cockett ATK, et al: Bladder Cancer Clinical Guidelines Panel summary report on the management of nonmuscle invasive bladder cancer (stages Ta, T1 and TIS). J Urol 162(5):1697, 1999.

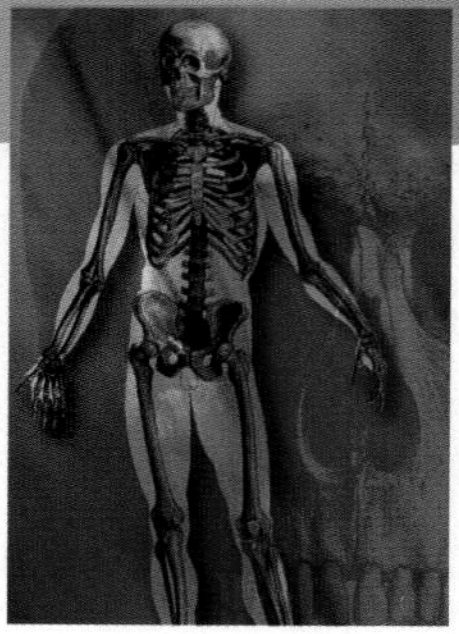

Chapter 62

Urinary Tract Dysfunction

PAUL K. PIETROW, MD, MICHAEL S. COOKSON, MD, and
JOSEPH A. SMITH, JR, MD

Benign Prostatic Hyperplasia

Pathophysiology

Benign prostatic hyperplasia (BPH) is a very common condition and involves the hyperplastic growth of tissue within the prostate gland. Anatomic research has shown that the majority of this hyperplasia occurs in the transitional zone of the gland that surrounds the urethra as it traverses the prostate. Histologic evidence of BPH occurs in nearly 50% of men by age 50 years, and the incidence approaches 90% in men aged 90 years and older. However, not in every patient with histologic evidence of BPH will clinical symptoms develop. The growth, maturation, and eventual hyperplasia of the prostate gland are under the influence of testosterone, which is converted to the more potent dihydrotestosterone (DHT) by the enzyme 5-α reductase.

Enlargement of the prostate may result in a relative bladder-outflow obstruction because of its position surrounding the urethra. In addition, a dynamic component of obstruction is caused by stromal tissue rich in α-adrenergic receptors. This factor makes it difficult to predict the degree of symptoms based purely on the size of the patient's prostate.

No apparent causal association exists between BPH and other pathologic conditions of the prostate. The natural history of BPH is variable. Significant spontaneous symptomatic improvement is not uncommon, and many patients report waxing and waning of symptoms. Some patients go on to experience extremely poor flow rates or even urinary retention.

Differential Diagnosis

Several pathologic processes can lead to enlargement of the prostate. Adenocarcinoma of the prostate can cause marked irregularities in the gland and can lead to obstructive symptoms if diagnosed late. In addition, transitional cell carcinoma of the bladder can involve the prostate gland. Lymphoma and rectal cancers have been reported to involve the prostatic parenchyma.

Strictures of the bladder neck or of the urethra can cause significant obstruction and thereby mimic BPH. Historically, sexually transmitted diseases of the genitourinary system have been the greatest source of these strictures, with *Neiserria gonococcus* the prime culprit.

More frequently, these strictures are iatrogenic, from previous cystoscopy or transurethral resection of the prostate or bladder. Trauma of any kind, even from a misplaced or difficult Foley catheterization, can lead to stricture anywhere along the passage.

Weakness of the detrusor muscle can cause a diminished urinary stream reminiscent of obstructive disease. This is often secondary to poor neurologic input to the bladder. The autonomic nerves to the bladder may be injured during pelvic surgery, pelvic fracture, spinal cord injury, or even systemic illnesses such as diabetes mellitus. In addition, the detrusor may not be able to contract effectively after the release of long-standing obstruction.

Evaluation

Classic obstructive symptoms are hesitancy in initiating voiding, a decrease in the force of the urinary stream, terminal dribbling, intermittency, a feeling of incomplete bladder emptying, or a combination of these. Irritative voiding symptoms such as frequency, urgency, and nocturia also are common. The symptoms have a gradual onset and may progress to the point of acute urinary retention. Symptoms may be quantified by a validated questionnaire termed the International Prostate Symptom Score, which can be used to monitor a patient's response to therapy. Perhaps the most important question asks how bothersome these symptoms are to the patient. A few patients initially have silent prostatism, which may have very few symptoms, but chronic high-grade obstruction. This leads to severe trabeculation of the bladder and potential renal damage.

Patients may have a history of recurrent urinary tract infections from urinary stasis, episodes of hematuria, bladder stones, or even a urinary stream that occasionally stops abruptly and with great discomfort (stranguria). A history of previous treatment should be sought, including medications (over-the-counter and prescription) and surgical management.

Digital rectal examination (DRE) of the prostate may demonstrate palpable enlargement of the gland. BPH characteristically has a smooth contour and a soft consistency. A careful DRE should search for any nodule or pelvic fixation, which would be suggestive of malignancy. Palpation of the suprapubic region occasionally reveals an enlarged bladder, indicative of incomplete emptying. Dipstick or microscopic examination of the urine may reveal signs of an infection. Serum measurements of creatinine are not routinely needed. PSA should be measured.

Measurement of the patient's urine flow rate may show a weakened stream (usually <15 mL/sec in symptomatic patients). An abnormal amount of urine in the bladder after voiding can be demonstrated either by direct catheterization or by ultrasonography over the suprapubic region.

Contrast studies are not routinely indicated in the evaluation of BPH, but intravenous pyelograms (IVPs) obtained for other reasons may show "J-hooking" of the distal ureters as they are pushed cephalad into the bladder by a large prostate lobe. Transrectal ultrasonography of the prostate may be used to measure the volume of the prostate when planning for certain types of therapy or for performing prostate biopsy to rule out malignant involvement.

Sophisticated assessment of detrusor strength, bladder compliance, and coordination between the bladder and sphincter may be obtained with a urodynamic evaluation. This study is indicated for those patients with suspected neurologic disorders or those with symptoms that are out of proportion with the rest of the history and physical. Cystoscopy is not needed for the diagnosis, but is indicated when the patient has had hematuria, a previous transurethral resection of the prostate (TURP) or other manipulation, or when a significant risk for urethral stricture disease exists.

Treatment

In the majority of patients, treatment decisions are based on the level of bother that BPH creates. Goal-directed therapy is therefore applied after careful discussion of the risks and benefits of the various therapeutic options. Watchful waiting is a reasonable alternative for those patients with minimal bother. This patient may be followed up periodically or asked to return when treatment is desired.

Medical treatment for BPH has largely replaced surgery as first-line therapy. Medical management uses agents that block α_1-adrenergic receptors that are found in high concentration in the prostatic urethra and bladder neck. These "α blockers" can bring about the relaxation of this periurethral stroma and allow easier voiding. These agents also exert effects on the bladder and within the central nervous system. Nonselective α blockers (terazosin and doxazosin) require titration to effective doses. Agents that target α_{1a}-receptors (tamsulosin and alfuzosin) may induce less postural hypotension and do not require titration. All agents are reasonably well tolerated and show their effects within several days of initiation.

Finasteride is a 5-α-reductase inhibitor that blocks the conversion of testosterone to DHT. Long-term therapy with this agent can bring about reductions in prostate size and may improve urinary flow rates. Subset analysis of large clinical trials demonstrates that this drug is most effective for patients with large (>50 g) prostates. It may take up to 6 months of therapy before the maximal benefit of this agent is realized. Importantly, finasteride has been shown to decrease serum PSA values by nearly 50%. Screening PSA values should therefore be doubled when taking this drug. Finasteride is well tolerated with very few side effects, although a small percentage of patients notice sexual dysfunction such as decreased libido or impotence.

Surgical removal of obstructing prostate tissue has become less common with the advent of medical therapy for BPH but still remains the gold standard. Surgery can be performed via an open or transurethral route. An open surgical approach is usually chosen for patients with a very large (>80 g) prostate. The prostate is approached through a lower midline abdominal incision, and the enlarged adenomatous tissue is enucleated by sharp dissection with scissors and blunt finger dissection through either the bladder (suprapubic prostatectomy) or the prostatic capsule (simple retropubic prostatectomy).

TURP is the most common approach to remove obstructing tissue (Fig. 62-1). During a TURP, a modified endoscope is used to visualize the prostate lobes while an electrocautery loop is used to resect to the level of the prostatic capsule. Alternatively, a transurethral incision of the prostate (TUIP) can be performed in patients with smaller glands. Most patients remain in the hospital for 1 or 2 nights after TURP and are discharged voiding spontaneously. The risk of incontinence is low (1% to 2%), and treatment-related impotence occurs in fewer than 5% of patients. In properly selected patients, treatment results are excellent, and usually a substantial increase in urinary flow rate occurs.

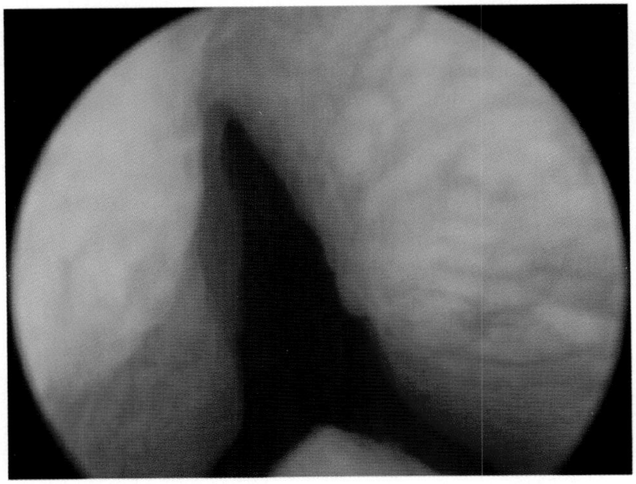

FIGURE 62–1 Large prostate lobes seen during cystoscopy. These lateral lobes are removed during transurethral resection of the prostate.

PEARLS FOR THE OR

Post-transurethral resection syndrome manifests as MS changes/seizures, bradycardia, and hypotension. It is caused by hyponatremia due to the absorption of irrigation fluids.

The distal limit of resection during a transurethral prostatectomy is the verumontanum, which estimates the position of the voluntary urethral sphincter.

Brisk hemorrhage during a sling operation is usually caused by injury to the perivesical venous plexus.

The potential space between the bladder and the pubis is called the space of Retzius.

In recent years there has been an increasing push for even less invasive methods to destroy prostatic tissue. Most methods are performed in an outpatient surgery center or within the physician's office. Transurethral microwave thermotherapy (TUMT) uses a urethral catheter with a small microwave unit at the tip. Energy, in the form of heat, is applied to the prostate, and the treated tissue later sloughs or is absorbed. Urinary flow rates are not as high as those after TURP, but symptom scores have been shown to improve substantially. The durability of this procedure, however, is as yet unproven.

Incontinence

Pathophysiology

Micturition, the voluntary act of voiding, is a complex event requiring coordination between the central nervous system, the somatic and autonomic nervous systems, the bladder musculature (the detrusor), and the external sphincter. The two basic phases of normal micturition are storage and emptying. During the storage phase, the bladder can accommodate increasing urine volumes by increasing the tone of the internal and external sphincters and by inhibiting any activity of the detrusor. This is brought about mainly by innervation from the sympathetic nervous system (T11 to L2). The emptying phase entails the relaxation of the sphincters and the bladder neck and then the active contraction of the detrusor. This phase is predominantly under the control of parasympathetic innervation (S2-S4). Somatic innervation of the external sphincter via the pudendal nerve (S2) also helps with urine storage and control. The cerebral cortex and the brainstem exert voluntary control by integration at the pons.

Urinary incontinence is the involuntary loss of urine. As the complex physiology of normal micturition implies, no single explanation exists for voiding dysfunction. Any process that interferes with the nervous system and its pathways can lead to voiding dysfunction or incontinence or both. To this end, trauma, pelvic or urinary tract surgery, neuromuscular disorders, diabetes, and cerebrovascular accidents are all common causes of incontinence.

Many older women are prone to incontinence because of changes in their pelvic anatomy. In the normal position, the bladder neck and internal sphincter sit within the intraabdominal compartment. Any increase in intraabdominal pressure is transmitted not only to the bladder but to the bladder neck and sphincter as well. Therefore the bladder pressure does not exceed the sphincter pressure, and continence is maintained. With pelvic descensus, the sphincter and bladder neck lie outside of the intraabdominal compartment, and any increase in pressure can then overcome the resistance of the sphincter (Fig. 62-2). This is referred to as stress urinary incontinence (SUI). Previous pelvic surgery and a history of multiple vaginal deliveries can predispose a woman to this very common problem.

Differential Diagnosis

Incontinence is classified by the symptoms associated with the leakage of urine and can be divided into four categories: continuous, stress, urge, and overflow urinary incontinence.

Continuous incontinence is usually caused by an abnormal connection between the urinary stream and the outside world, thereby bypassing the normal control of the sphincter

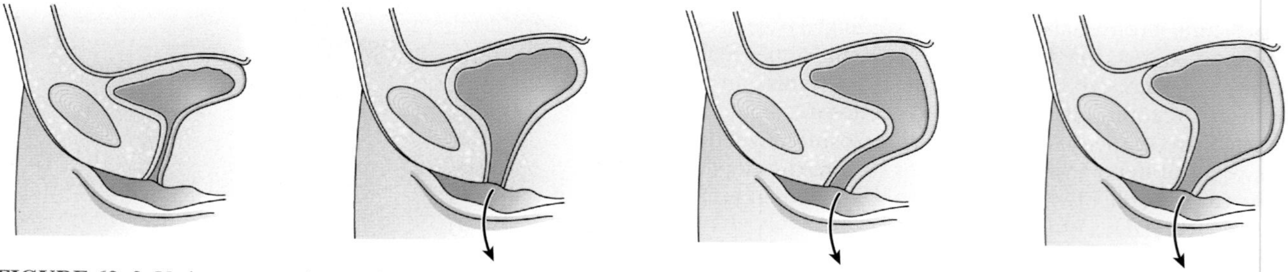

FIGURE 62–2 Various types of stress-induced urethral descent. In each scenario, portions of the urethra or bladder neck or both drop deeper into the pelvis, thereby allowing the loss of urine per urethra. (Adapted from Walsh PC, Retik AB, Vaughan ED Jr, Wein AJ (eds): Campbell's Urology, 8th ed, Vol 2. Philadelphia, Saunders, 2002, p 1035.)

and bladder neck. Fistulae between the vagina and the ureters, bladder, or urethra are all possible and are usually iatrogenic. Ectopic ureters in females may cause the ureter to empty into the vagina or the vestibule of the introitus.

Stress incontinence is caused by the relaxation of the pelvic suspensory ligaments and muscles. Multiple gestation, pelvic surgery, hysterectomy, and obesity are all common causes of SUI. SUI may develop in men after radical prostatectomy or after an overaggressive TURP.

Urge incontinence is the precipitate loss of urine proceeded by a strong urge to void. During an episode of urge incontinence, an involuntary contraction of the detrusor overpowers the sphincter. These uninhibited contractions can be the result of a neurologic lesion, such as from multiple sclerosis, or secondary to bladder irritation from cystitis, tumor, or a stone. In a large number of patients, no cause has been found. The uninhibited contractions also can be precipitated by a change in position or by increased intraabdominal pressure, making the clinical differentiation between stress incontinence and detrusor instability quite difficult.

Overflow urinary incontinence is the result of a chronically distended bladder that never empties. As a result, the bladder eventually fills to the point that no more urine can be accommodated, and small amounts dribble out through the urethra. Bladder-neck obstruction from severe BPH or prostate cancer can cause overflow incontinence, as can tight stricture disease. In addition, neurologic lesions that cause bladder atony (neurogenic bladder) are common (e.g., diabetic autonomic neuropathy, altered mental status, medications, or spinal cord injury).

Evaluation

An accurate and detailed history is crucial to the evaluation of incontinence. Each patient should be queried as to the amount of leakage, its frequency, the presence or absence of urgency, associated symptoms, and fluid habits. Women should provide an obstetric history. A complete list of medications is vital, and this must include over-the-counter agents. A history of pelvic surgery or previous anti-incontinence surgery is important. A total number of pads used per day should be obtained, as this information can be used to monitor response to therapy. Finally, the patient should detail what treatments have already been tried.

The physical examination includes special attention to the abdomen, back, pelvis, and rectum. Perianal sensation, anal sphincter tone, as well as lower extremity motor and sensory function and reflexes should be evaluated. A pelvic examination should be performed, searching for pelvic prolapse. The vaginal tissues should be inspected, and their levels of estrogenization should be assessed. Women with suspected stress incontinence should be examined in the lithotomy position with a full bladder. About 80% of patients with stress incontinence will leak in this position with coughing (Marshall's test); an additional 10% will leak when their pelvis is raised by 45 degrees. A Bonney test is performed by transvaginally elevating the bladder neck to its proper anatomic position and having the patient cough.

All patients should have a urinalysis performed to search for infection or hematuria. Suggestive specimens should be sent for culture or cytology. Patients with long-standing obstruction and overflow incontinence should have serum measurement of blood urea nitrogen and creatinine. A measurement of the postvoid residual urine should be performed.

Patients with complex voiding histories, symptoms suggestive of detrusor instability, or incontinence refractory to medications are candidates for sophisticated urodynamic evaluation. In this study, a small catheter is inserted into the bladder, a pressure gauge is placed in the rectum, and surface electrodes are placed over the perineum to detect external sphincter activity. The bladder is slowly filled with saline or contrast material until the patient feels full, and the patient is then instructed to void (Fig. 62-3). Premature contractions of the bladder should be apparent on the tracing, as should any episodes of incontinence. The patient is routinely asked to perform Valsalva maneuvers during filling, and a leak-point pressure should be obtained.

Cystoscopy is not routinely performed unless a search for malignancy or a source of hematuria is indicated. Radiologic studies are not routinely ordered but play a crucial role in the diagnosis of continuous incontinence. IVP or cystogram or both may be required to demonstrate the presence of a fistula.

Treatment

The treatment of incontinence varies and is directed at the underlying cause. Continuous incontinence almost always requires surgical repair of the abnormal connection between the urinary stream and the outside world. Vesicovaginal fistula can be repaired via a vaginal or a transvesical approach. In either case, it is important to secure several water-tight layers of closure over the defect. An interposition graft may be necessary, especially for large defects or in irradiated tissue. Peritoneum, small bowel, labial fat pad, or even muscle grafts have been described. Most fistula repairs have a reasonable success rate, but the patient should be warned that postoperative recurrence is still a potential complication.

Urge incontinence is best treated with attempts to quiet the unstable bladder. Anticholinergic medications such as propantheline, oxybutynin, or tolterodine can suppress detrusor instability to some degree in the majority of cases. Common side effects include dry mouth and constipation. Patients with glaucoma also should be careful when using these drugs. Occasional patients have medication-refractory instability and severe enough symptoms to warrant surgical therapy. One possibility is to augment the bladder with detubularized small bowel in an attempt to disrupt the

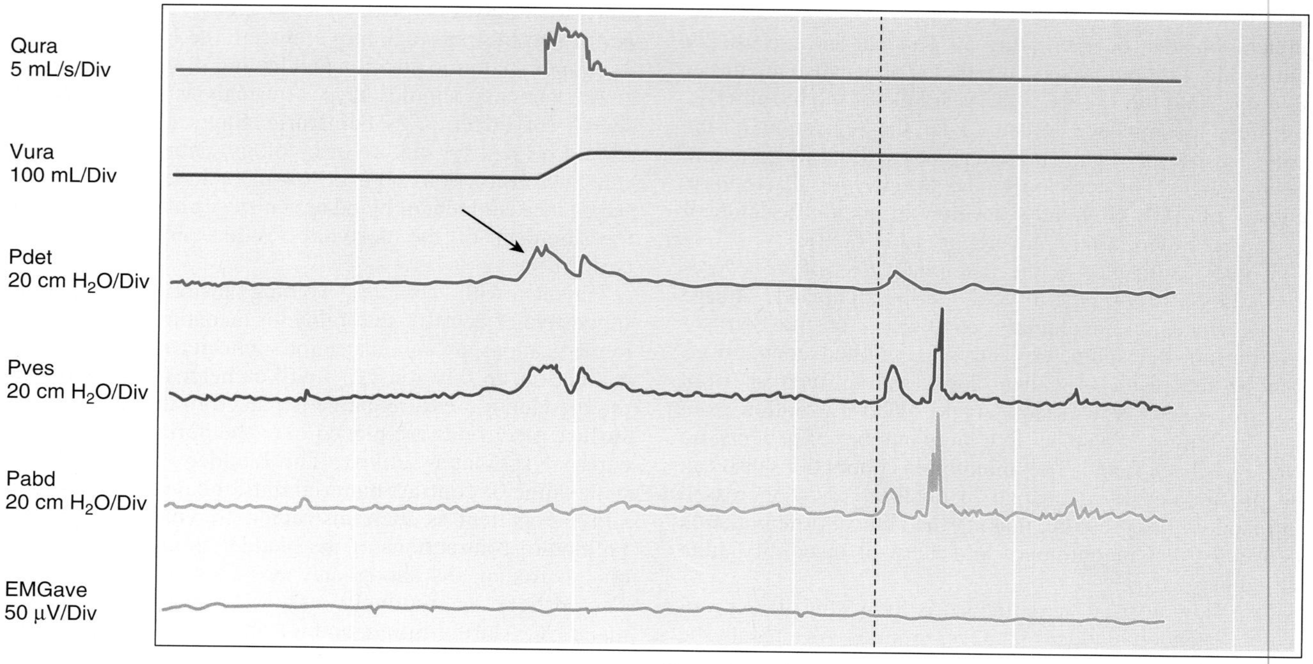

FIGURE 62–3 Urodynamic testing of a 51-year-old woman with urge incontinence. Notice how the premature contraction (*arrow*) demonstrated on the detrusor pressure line (P_{det}) causes leakage of urine that is measured on the urine flow line (Q_{ura}). V_{ura}, volume of urine voided; P_{det}, detrusor pressure as calculated from the subtraction of the measured abdominal pressure (P_{abd}) from the measured vesicle pressure (P_{ves}); EMG_{ave}, electrical activity of the external sphincter

pathologic detrusor. Not all patients are able to void spontaneously after this procedure and become dependent on intermittent self-catheterization. The use of electrostimulation of the sacral nerve roots is becoming increasingly popular.

Mild SUI may respond to simple pelvic floor–strengthening maneuvers known as Kegel exercises. Postmenopausal women without contraindications to hormonal replacement therapy should undergo attempts to re-estrogenize the vaginal epithelium. Moderate SUI may respond to medical therapy with agents such as the tricyclic antidepressant imipramine. Low-dose imipramine has anticholinergic effects that can quiet the bladder as well as α-adrenergic agonist activities that can stimulate contraction of the bladder neck.

Surgical management of SUI attempts to restore the bladder neck and urethra to the proper anatomic position. The Marshall-Marchetti-Krantz procedure uses an anterior abdominal approach to anchor the bladder neck and proximal urethra to the underside of the pubic symphysis. The Burch procedure also uses an abdominal approach to suspend the paravaginal tissues from Cooper's ligament. Both of these procedures carry a risk of producing an acute angulation of the urethra, thereby causing urinary retention. In addition, the open abdominal approach has a longer recovery period.

Alternatively, the bladder neck and urethra can be supported by using a combined vaginal and suprapubic

PEARLS FOR ROUNDS

Sling operations have the highest-rated long-term success for the treatment of stress urinary incontinence.

The size of a man's prostate is not a good predictor of the amount of urinary symptoms that he may have.

Benign prostatic enlargement and stress urinary incontinence are diseases of "patient preference" (i.e., the severity of bother usually determines the level of management).

Strong indications for a transurethral prostatectomy include **g**ross hematuria, **r**ecurrent urinary tract infections, urinary **r**etention, **r**enal insufficiency due to bladder dysfunction, and bladder **s**tones (GRRRS).

Urge incontinence caused by bladder obstruction may not resolve after surgery to relieve the blockage in up to 25% of patients.

approach. A "sling" of autologous or donor material can be passed around the urethra. This provides a backboard for the urethra to press against during episodes of increased intraabdominal pressure. With the aid of long needle guides, sutures connected to the sling material are passed behind the pubic symphysis and up into a suprapubic incision. The suspension sutures are then tied over the anterior rectus fascia with only mild tension. Success rates of greater than 90% have been achieved with these procedures, although most studies have follow-up less than 5 years.

Overflow incontinence is treated by removing the outlet obstruction or circumventing the atonic bladder. A TURP can be performed to remove obstructing prostate tissue. Bladder atony is a more difficult problem, however, as no effective way exists of making the detrusor squeeze in a coordinated fashion. Placement of an indwelling Foley catheter can allow the bladder to drain but is associated with a significant risk of recurrent urinary tract infections. Self-catheterization performed every 4 to 6 hours is a better solution and has been proven to be safe and effective since its introduction in the 1970s. Note that patients who have had relief of long-standing obstruction may never regain full function of the detrusor.

Suggested Reading

AUA Practice Guidelines Committee: AUA guideline on management of benign prostatic hyperplasia (2003). Chapter 1: Diagnosis and treatment recommendations. J Urol 170(2 Pt 1):530–547, 2003.

Holroyd-Leduc JM, Straus SE: Management of urinary incontinence in women: scientific review. JAMA 291(8):986–995, 2004.

Larson TR: Rationale and assessment of minimally invasive approaches to benign prostatic hyperplasia therapy. Urology 59(2 suppl 1):12–16, 2002.

Leach GE, Dmochowski RR, Appell RA, et al: Female Stress Urinary Incontinence Clinical Guidelines Panel summary report on surgical management of female stress urinary incontinence. J Urol 158(3 Pt 1):875–880, 1997.

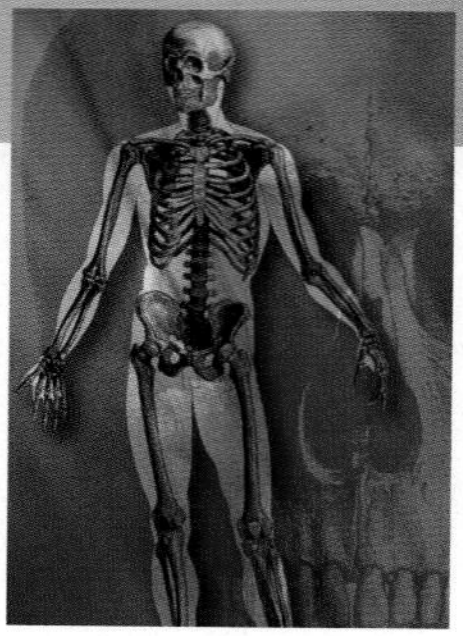

Chapter 63
Urinary Tract Lithiasis and Infections

PAUL K. PIETROW, MD, MICHAEL S. COOKSON, MD, and
JOSEPH A. SMITH JR, MD

Urinary Lithiasis

Pathophysiology

Urinary lithiasis is a ubiquitous problem that affects 2% to 3% of people in the Unites States at any one time. The peak incidence occurs in male patients age 20 to 40 years. Nephrolithiasis is frequently recurrent. Without treatment, the typical patient has a 10% risk of recurrence at 1 year, 35% within 5 years, and nearly 50% at 10 years.

The process of stone development is complex and multifactorial. A shortened list of identified risk factors includes a high animal-protein diet, extremes of calcium ingestion, decreased fluid intake, a sedentary lifestyle, and excess oxalate consumption (found in such common foods as iced tea, chocolate, and greens). These patients tend to form the most common type of stone, composed of calcium oxalate. Calcium phosphate stones should prompt an evaluation for distal renal tubular acidosis (type I) or primary hyperparathyroidism. Uric acid stones can be found in patients with excessive dietary consumption of purines. Cystinuria is caused by an autosomal recessive trait that interferes with amino acid transport within the kidney. Patients with recurrent urinary tract infections are at risk of developing struvite stones, which are composed of magnesium, ammonium, and phosphate. In addition, many compounds have been reported to precipitate within the urinary collecting system. These include medications such as triamterene or the protease inhibitors used to treat human immunodeficiency virus disease.

The actual mechanics of stone formation are not completely understood but seem to involve the precipitation of these various compounds to form a crystal. This crystal either builds on itself or perhaps coalesces with other crystals to form a larger stone. Various disorders of renal or gastrointestinal metabolism also are involved in stone formation. Diminished release of citrate into the urine, hypocitraturia, reduces the levels of this known stone inhibitor.

Differential Diagnosis

Calcific densities within the renal collecting system are most frequently due to urinary lithiasis. However, transitional cell carcinoma of the renal pelvis or ureter may occasionally calcify and have the appearance of a stone. In addition, calcified renal masses or complex cysts should be distinguished from true stones.

Not all stones are radiopaque on conventional plain films; filling defects within the renal collecting system may sometimes require further evaluation before treatment. Blood clots, renal papillary necrosis, or even fragments of retained stents may be found.

Evaluation

Patients frequently are first seen by their physicians with renal colic, which is the abrupt onset of sharp, cramping pain in the flank with possible radiation to the groin or genitalia. They are often unable to find any comfortable position and often report accompanying nausea and vomiting. As the stone moves down the ureter toward the bladder, many patients report the increased sensation of urinary frequency and urgency. Patients with complete obstruction of the ureter or renal pelvis also may be febrile or show systemic signs of infection. Not all stones are symptomatic, however, and silent stones can cause considerable injury to a kidney before being discovered. It is not uncommon for stones to cause vague abdominal or back discomfort. These patients require a high index of suspicion to find their stones.

The physical examination should focus on a careful palpation of the abdomen in search of a mass or evidence of a grossly hydronephrotic kidney. Costovertebral angle tenderness may be indicative of infection within the kidney but is highly nonspecific.

A random urine specimen should be sent for analysis to look for evidence of infection and measurement of pH. Microscopic hematuria is frequently present in these specimens but is not a requirement for diagnosis. Serum chemistries are frequently determined to assess overall renal function. This is especially necessary before the administration of intravenous (IV) contrast for an imaging study. Measurement of serum calcium can help screen for hyperparathyroidism.

Complex metabolic studies can be carried out but are usually reserved for patients with recurrent nephrolithiasis. This includes measurement of basic serum electrolytes as well as of magnesium, calcium, phosphate, uric acid, and

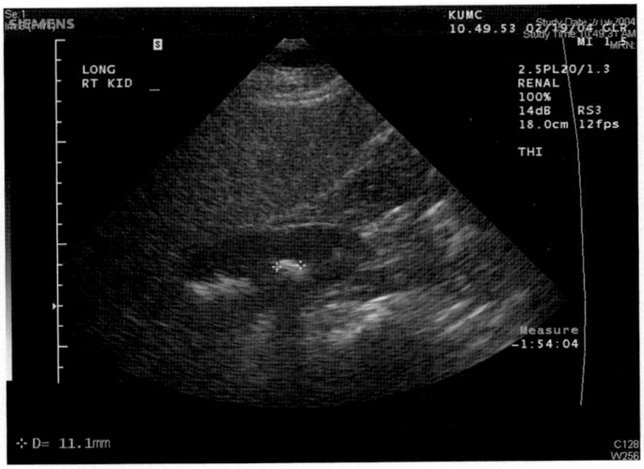

FIGURE 63–1 Ultrasound image of a right renal calculus (*marks*). Notice the hyperechoic lesion and the acoustic "shadow" that it casts.

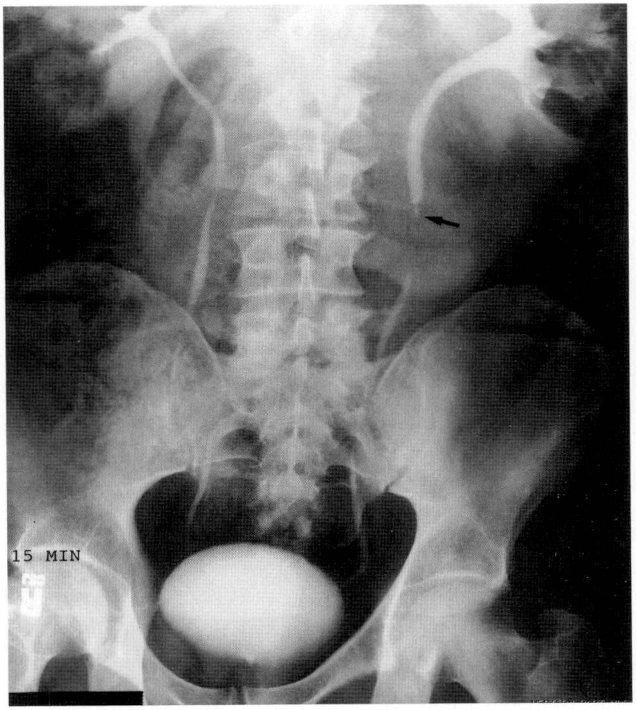

FIGURE 63–2 Intravenous pyelogram demonstrating a partially obstructing calculus within the left midureter (*arrow*).

parathyroid hormone. A 24-hour collection of urine can be obtained, and measurements of urinary sodium, calcium, citrate, magnesium, oxalate, uric acid, cysteine, and creatinine are made. Total urine volume is important as a gauge of the patient's fluid-intake habits. Urine pH also is routinely measured.

Renal stones may be imaged with ultrasound and show an intense hyperechoic lesion. They typically cast an acoustic shadow behind them (Fig. 63-1). Plain films such as a kidneys/ureters/bladder (KUB) film may be used to screen for renal stones because approximately 90% of all stones are radiopaque. An IV pyelogram will fill the collecting system with filtered contrast and can pinpoint the level of obstruction from a stone or other pathologic process (Fig. 63-2). Spiral computed tomography (CT) scan (without IV contrast) has become increasingly popular in the evaluation of renal colic and has the added advantage of being able to help diagnose other intraabdominal pathologic processes. Because CT scan images are based on density, all stones including radiolucent stones can be visualized by this method (Fig. 63-3).

Treatment

Therapy for urinary calculi is dependent on the size, location, and composition of the stone. Additionally, the level of patient discomfort and the presence or absence of associated infection will influence treatment. Patients with intractable pain or the inability to tolerate oral intake may require hospital admission for the administration of IV fluids and parenteral narcotics. Those patients with evidence of infection and obstruction often require immediate attention to relieve the obstruction. This can be done with a percutaneous nephrostomy tube or with a ureteral stent. Definitive treatment of the stone is performed after the patient defervesces. In general, stones smaller than 4 mm have a greater than 90% chance of spontaneous passage, whereas stones larger than 6 mm have an increasingly lower chance of passage. The three most common sites of stone impaction include the ureteropelvic junction, the pelvic brim as the ureter passes over the iliac vessels, and the ureterovesical junction (Fig. 63-4).

Stones composed of uric acid can sometimes be treated with alkalinization of the urine through oral therapy. These stones eventually dissolve. In addition, recurrence of these stones can be prevented with the use of citrate-containing alkalinizing agents. Long-term therapy with allopurinol can decrease the level of uric acid in the urine. D-Penicillamine or Thiola (α-mercaptopropionylglycine) can be used for the prophylaxis of cystine stones. However, both agents are frequently poorly tolerated by patients because of adverse side effects.

Hypercalciuria may be treated with low doses of hydrochlorothiazide, which limits calcium excretion in the urine. Patients with hypocitraturia are given potassium citrate to improve levels of this stone inhibitor. All patients are encouraged to increase their fluid intake to several liters per day as well as to adhere to a moderate-calcium, low-salt, low-purine diet.

Extracorporeal shock wave lithotripsy (ESWL) machines generate a shock wave outside the body and focus this

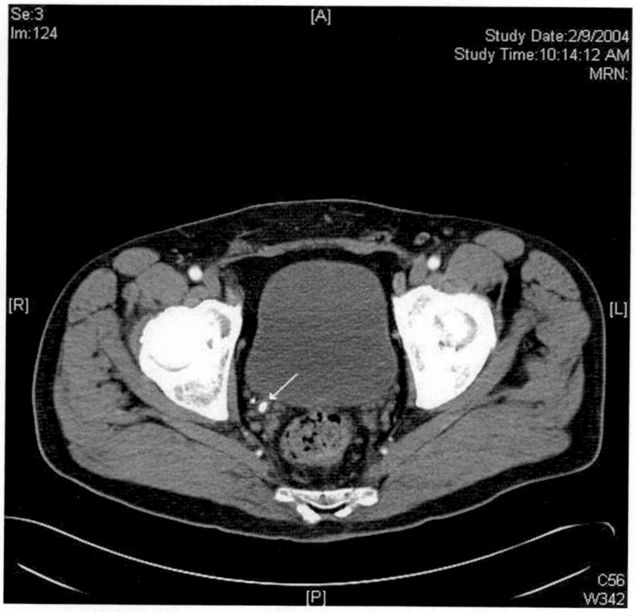

FIGURE 63–3 Computed tomography image of a calculus within the distal right ureter (*arrow*). Notice that the stone has a dense (white) appearance. The other small densities are within nearby veins (phleboliths).

energy on the calculus. This energy causes fragmentation of the calculus. Renal stones as large as 2 cm are frequently treated with ESWL, as are smaller ureteral stones. Stone-free rates decrease as the stone increases in size. Larger renal stones frequently require repeated ESWL for complete clearance. ESWL is contraindicated in pregnancy, coagulopathy, uncontrolled hypertension, or active infection. The effects of ESWL energy on the human ovary are unclear, and many centers will not treat distal ureteral stones in women of child-bearing age.

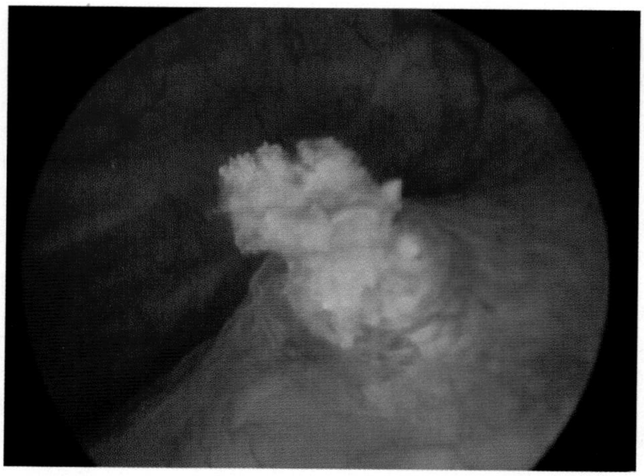

FIGURE 63–4 Cystoscopic view of a calculus lodged within the ureter just before entry into the bladder.

PEARLS FOR THE OR

The most common type of urinary stone is composed of calcium oxalate.

Urinary calculi are most likely to cause obstruction at the ureteropelvic junction, the pelvic brim, or the ureterovesical junction.

Extracorporeal shock wave lithotripsy is contraindicated in the face of active infection, coagulopathy, and pregnancy.

The holmium laser has a depth of penetration of 0.5 to 1.0 mm.

Percutaneous kidney stone surgery is usually reserved for stones larger than 2 cm.

Flexible or rigid ureteroscopes also can be used to clear stones within the urinary tract. Flexible ureteroscopes are particularly helpful for reaching stones above the pelvic brim, whereas shorter rigid scopes are frequently used for distal stones. Ureteroscopes have a working channel that allows the passage of intracorporeal lithotriptors (laser, pneumatic, or electrohydraulic). This allows the destruction of the stone in situ, leaving sand and gravel to be passed by the patient (Fig. 63-5). Success rates are generally higher in the distal ureter, but improved equipment has increased the stone-free rates for even proximal calculi.

Renal stones larger than 2 cm or stones in a lower-pole calyx often require a percutaneous approach to the collecting system, referred to as a percutaneous nephrostolithotomy (PCNL). PCNL requires placement of a guide-wire through the renal parenchyma and down the ureter. The tract is dilated, and a 30F sheath is placed into the collecting system. A nephroscope is then passed down this sheath, and the stone is fragmented with an ultrasonic or pneumatic lithotripter. Large-volume calculi ("staghorn") may require multiple procedures for complete clearance. Open surgical treatment, once the mainstay of stone management, is now performed in only very rare cases. Nephrectomy may be performed in a poorly functioning kidney with a large stone burden.

Prostatitis

Pathophysiology

The term *prostatitis* implies an inflammatory or infectious process within the prostatic parenchyma. In clinical practice, however, this term is often loosely applied to true bacterial infections of this gland as well as nonspecific or chronic pain or both of the perineum and deep pelvis.

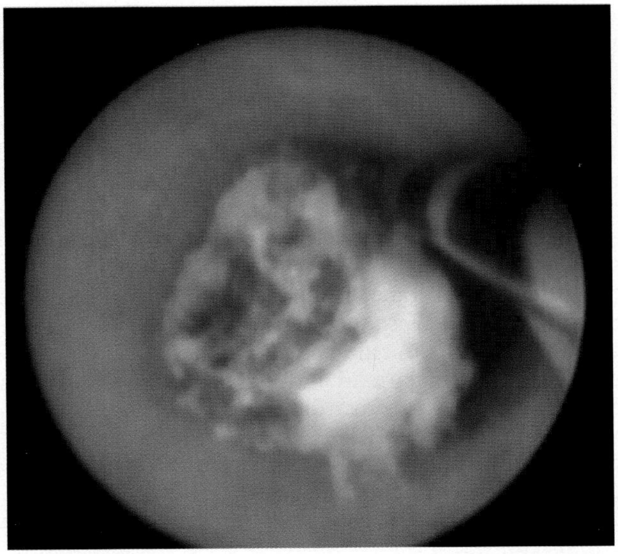

FIGURE 63–5 Endoscopic view of a calculus within the lumen of a ureter. The laser fiber (entering at 6 o'clock) uses highly focused energy to destroy the stone in situ.

Attempts to understand this disorder have involved the creation of a classification system with four separate categories: (1) acute bacterial prostatitis (ABP), (2) chronic bacterial prostatitis (CBP), (3) nonbacterial prostatitis (NBP), and (4) prostatodynia.

Acute bacterial infection of the prostate is uncommon and accounts for less than 5% of all cases of prostatitis. The majority of cases are caused by gram-negative organisms, especially strains of *Escherichia coli*. Gram-positive bacteria rarely cause acute prostatitis, although strains of *Enterococcus* have been implicated. Bacteria are thought to access the prostatic acinar glands via the reflux of infected urine into the prostatic ducts.

CBP may result from persistent or recurrent infection with the same causative organisms. Calcifications within the prostate gland may become colonized with bacteria and act as a nidus for persistent reinfection. NBP and prostatodynia are the least well understood entities. NBP indicates that expressed secretions from the prostate gland will demonstrate leukocytes but will fail to grow any organism when cultured. Reflux of urine into prostatic ducts may play a role in NBP. Attempts to implicate difficult-to-culture organisms such as *Chlamydia, Trachomatis, Mycoplasma,* or *Ureaplasma* species have met with mixed success. The etiology of prostatodynia is elusive. Theories including pelvic floor tension, myalgia, and bladder neck/urethral spasm have been studied by using urodynamic evaluation, but no consistent causes have been identified.

PEARLS FOR ROUNDS

Only uric acid calculi can be dissolved with oral medication (creating urinary alkalinization).

Of urinary stones, 90% are radiopaque.

The risk of kidney stone recurrence can be reduced by striving to produce 2 L of urine per day and maintaining a low-salt and low-animal-protein diet.

Acute bacterial infection makes up a small component of all men diagnosed with "prostatitis."

Roughly 50% of patients will have a repeated stone episode within the next 10 years.

Differential Diagnosis

Any infection of the lower urinary tract may be confused for prostatitis. Disorders of the anus or rectum may occasionally refer pain to the deep pelvis. Patients with deep pelvic pain and excessive irritative symptoms such as urgency, frequency, or dysuria may have malignancy within the bladder or prostate. This is especially true of carcinoma in situ of the bladder. Patients with distal ureteral calculi and especially with bladder stones also may have the same nonspecific pelvic complaints that are common with NBP or prostatodynia.

Evaluation

Symptoms of ABP include fever, chills, malaise, and myalgia. Local symptoms of frequency, urgency, low back pain, and bladder-outlet obstruction also are common. Physical examination may demonstrate high temperature, abdominal pain, distention, or a combination of these. Digital rectal examination reveals an exquisitely tender, warm, swollen prostate. Severe pain and even bacteremia can result from vigorous massage of the acutely infected prostate.

The clinical features of CBP are not as specific as those of acute prostatitis. Primary complaints consist of genitourinary pain, dysuria, clear discharge, recurrent urinary tract infections, and sometimes sexual dysfunction. Patients with NBP or prostatodynia have complaints similar to those with CBP, including genitourinary pain, painful ejaculations, and back pain. Physical examination is usually unremarkable and nonspecific, but some men have significantly tender prostates on digital rectal examination.

All patients should have a urinalysis and have a urine specimen sent for culture. Urine cytology also may be requested if any suspicion of bladder malignancy exists. Cultures of prostatic fluid can be obtained from expressed prostatic secretions. They are collected after vigorous prostatic massage. Seminal cultures are rarely helpful.

The occasional patient may require transrectal ultrasonography (TRUS) of the prostate to rule out the possibility of abscess or malignancy. In addition, TRUS-guided biopsies of the gland may then be taken, if indicated. Patients with complex urinary symptoms may benefit from urodynamics, which evaluate the performance of the detrusor muscle and the external sphincter during urine storage and active voiding.

Treatment

Acute prostatitis is potentially life threatening. Broad-spectrum parenteral antibiotics are indicated with specific attention to covering gram-negative organisms of the urinary tract. Fluoroquinolone antibiotics are particularly helpful, as these have been shown to achieve high concentrations within prostatic tissue. Urethral instrumentation should be avoided, and patients with acute retention may even require placement of a suprapubic cystotomy tube.

Once the acute episode of bacteremia has resolved, the patient should be continued on an oral antibiotic such as ciprofloxacin or trimethoprim-sulfamethoxazole for 3 to 4 weeks to prevent the acute infection from becoming chronic.

CBP is frequently treated with a 3- to 4-week course of these same oral antibiotics. Adjunctive measures such as nonsteroidal anti-inflammatory agents, hot Sitz baths, and a cushioned seat also are used to promote resolution of the prostatic inflammation.

Patients with NBP or prostatodynia are frequently given an empiric trial of antibiotics. Prolonged, repeated courses of these agents are rarely helpful if the patient fails to have any response. Some clinicians have recommended a 2-week trial of doxycycline, minocycline, or erythromycin to treat uncommon organisms such as *Ureaplasma* or *Chlamydia trachomatis*.

Transurethral resection of the prostate should be reserved for patients with proven chronic bacterial prostatitis and prostatic calculi. In addition, a subset of elderly men with recurrent infections despite antibiotic suppression may have associated bladder-outlet obstruction and could benefit from surgery.

Attempts to relax the bladder neck with α-blockers have been found to increase the urinary flow rate and decrease symptom scores in some patients with NBP and prostatodynia, and an empiric trial of these agents is often used. Some patients with prostatodynia have the inability to relax the muscles of their pelvic floor. A subset of these patients may benefit from biofeedback training or even low doses of a benzodiazepine such as diazepam.

Suggested Reading

Delvecchio FC, Preminger GM: Medical management of stone disease. Curr Opin Urol 13(3):229–233, 2003.

Fuchs GJ, Yurkanin JP: Endoscopic surgery for renal calculi. Curr Opin Urol 13(3):243–247, 2003.

Hua VN, Schaeffer AJ: Acute and chronic prostatitis. Med Clin North Am 88(2):483–494, 2004.

Pak CY: Medical prevention of renal stone disease. Nephron 81(suppl 1):60–65, 1999.

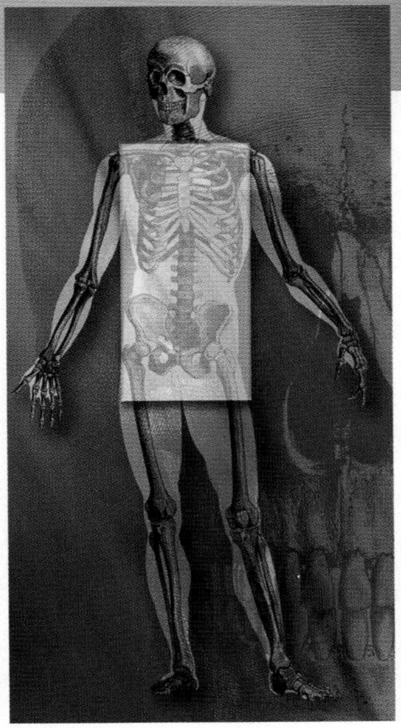

SECTION XVII

SPECIAL TOPICS

Chapter 64

Anesthesia

KEITH P. LEWIS, MD, and GLYNNE D. STANLEY, MBChB

Recent Trends in Anesthesiology

Over the past few decades, significant changes have occurred in anesthesiology and surgery. Same-day surgery and laparoscopic and minimally invasive techniques, in conjunction with the demands of an aging patient population, have all contributed to major advances in the development and delivery of anesthesia services. Surgeries are performed on older and critically ill patients, necessitating careful and thorough preoperative evaluation by the anesthesiologist. The anesthesiologist is being regarded as the **perioperative physician**.

This chapter begins with a brief review of anesthesia methods, agents, and monitoring techniques and then focuses on the major preoperative, intraoperative, and postoperative issues pertaining to the surgical patient.

Methods of Anesthesia

Patients may be managed with (1) **general anesthesia,** which involves the use of parenteral or inhalational anesthetics; (2) **regional anesthesia,** such as **spinal anesthesia, epidural, or nerve-block techniques** involving the use of local anesthetics; (3) a **combination of general and regional anesthesia**; or (4) **monitored anesthesia care,** which involves the titration of intravenous (IV) agents to provide sedation/analgesia while maintaining spontaneous ventilation or **straight local anesthesia** by the surgeon.

Parenteral Hypnotic Drugs

Drugs that produce sleep are referred to as hypnotics. These agents are typically given intravenously to produce unconsciousness before intubation or placement of a laryngeal mask airway. The following hypnotics are commonly used.

Thiopental is a barbiturate that has a rapid redistribution from the brain to inactive tissue (skeletal muscle) and is associated with early awakening. Adverse effects include myocardial depression, hypotension, and apnea in certain patients.

Propofol is a nonbarbiturate that has a rapid onset of action and is associated with a quick recovery and clearness of mind in the postoperative period. With the advent of same-day surgery and the need for early patient discharge, these characteristics make propofol a popular agent. Adverse effects include pain on injection, cardiovascular depression, vasodilatation, and apnea.

Etomidate is a nonbarbiturate that causes rapid unconsciousness and tends to be used in emergency situations in patients with cardiovascular instability or coronary artery disease. Adverse effects include myoclonic movements and adrenocortical suppression. In the severely hypovolemic patient, hypotension may still occur with the administration of etomidate or any other induction agent.

Ketamine is a phencyclidine derivative that causes dissociative anesthesia, which is characterized by profound amnesia and analgesia. With a dissociative technique, the drug is administered parenterally and the patients are detached from their circumstance, maintaining their airway without intubation in certain circumstances. They may tolerate a procedure without other agents. They may just stare into space. Unlike other hypnotic drugs, ketamine has intrinsic analgesic activity. Ketamine generally maintains hemodynamic stability by increasing sympathetic tone. It may produce tachycardia, which can limit its usefulness in patients with coronary artery disease. Adverse effects include cardiovascular stimulation, tachycardia, decreased seizure threshold, increased intracranial pressure, and delirium during recovery. The delirium can be treated with a benzodiazepine.

Midazolam is a water-soluble benzodiazepine that has anxiolytic and anticonvulsant properties at lower doses and acts as a hypnotic at higher doses. Midazolam can produce anterograde amnesia. Obstetric patients given midazolam who are undergoing cesarean section may not remember the delivery of the child. A specific reversal agent called flumazenil is available for accidental overdose.

Inhalational Anesthetic Agents

Inhalational agents can be used for the induction of anesthesia (typically in pediatrics) via face mask or for the maintenance of anesthesia throughout a surgical procedure. The exact mechanism of action of these agents is still not fully understood. As a general rule, lipid solubility correlates with potency, whereas blood solubility correlates inversely with the speed of onset.

To compare the potency of inhalational agents, the concept of **minimal alveolar concentration** (MAC) is used. The MAC is the anesthesia concentration at 1 atmosphere of pressure that will inhibit reflex movement in 50% of subjects who are exposed to a noxious stimulus. It is important to stress that patients will be asleep and unaware of their surroundings at concentrations well below the MAC (often at 25% to 30% of the MAC value). The concentration at which 50% of patients fall asleep and 50% remain awake is sometimes referred to as either the "sleep MAC" or the "awake MAC."

Inhalational agents can be classified as halogenated or nonhalogenated based on their chemical structure.

Halogenated Inhalational Agents

The halogenated agents have different MAC (Table 64-1) values and are summarized here:

Halothane is the oldest of the halogenated drugs and has the lowest MAC. It has a sweet odor, is good for mask induction of anesthesia, and is a potent bronchodilator. Halothane has 20% hepatic metabolism and is converted to substances that may cause a hypersensitivity reaction and hepatitis with fever, eosinophilia, arthralgia, and rash.

Isoflurane is a commonly used agent with a pungent odor and 0.2% hepatic metabolism. Its use is sometimes associated with coronary steal syndrome, in which coronary blood flow is diverted from potential ischemic to normal coronary arteries.

TABLE 64–1 Minimum Alveolar Concentration (MAC) of Halogenated Inhalational Anesthetics

Anesthetic	MAC (% vol/vol)
Halothane	0.75
Isoflurane	1.17
Enflurane	1.63
Sevoflurane	1.80
Desflurane	6.60

Enflurane has a pungent odor, 2% hepatic metabolism, and the potential to induce seizure activity in susceptible patients.

Sevoflurane is nonpungent and nonirritating to the airways and is ideal for mask induction. It has minimal metabolism and is associated with a rapid onset and rapid recovery.

Desflurane is the agent with the highest MAC. It has a pungent odor and is irritating for the airways with minimal metabolism. It is administered via a special vaporizer, and its rapid onset and rapid awakening are major advantages.

Nonhalogenated Inhalational Agents

The only nonhalogenated anesthetic used today is **nitrous oxide.** This gas is often combined with other inhalational agents to maintain general anesthesia. Nitrous oxide has a rapid onset of action and exerts an analgesic action. It has 35 times the blood solubility of nitrogen. When nitrous oxide enters a closed space (such as an obstructed bowel, pneumothorax, or as a result of air embolism), it will markedly expand this space with potentially dangerous effects. Surgeons often request no nitrous oxide during abdominal cases to avoid bowel distention. When patients awaken from general anesthesia, nitrous oxide diffuses rapidly into the alveoli and displaces oxygen. This is termed **diffusion hypoxia** and is prevented by the use of supplemental oxygen in the immediate postoperative period.

Muscle Relaxants

Muscle relaxants produce skeletal muscle relaxation that facilitates surgical exposure and tracheal intubation, allowing a lower concentration of other anesthetics. One major risk of using muscle relaxants, without using an adequate amount of narcotic or inhalational agent, is the risk that patient may remain awake, aware, and paralyzed during the operation. **Awareness** is extremely rare, but when it occurs, it can have significant psychological and medicolegal consequences. Muscle relaxants are classified as depolarizing or nondepolarizing agents, based on their mechanism of action.

Depolarizing Muscle Relaxants

The only **depolarizing muscle** relaxant that is currently available for clinical use is **succinylcholine.** It has a rapid onset (15 to 30 seconds) and a brief duration of action (3 to 5 minutes). In patients with a full stomach requiring surgery, succinylcholine is often used for a rapid-sequence induction (see Intraoperative Management).

Succinylcholine depolarizes the postsynaptic membrane by mimicking the action of acetylcholine. The drug initially causes transient muscle contractions called **fasciculations,** which are followed by a relaxation phase. It is metabolized by plasma cholinesterase and has no specific antagonist for reversal.

PEARLS FOR ROUNDS

Special problems in patients with morbid obesity
- Obstructive sleep apnea
- Difficult intravenous access
- Rapid desaturation during intubation
- Risk of aspiration
- Difficult oxygenation/ventilation
- Difficult intubation
- Risk of positioning/nerve injury
- Multiple comorbidities
- Specialized postoperative monitoring
- Injury to staff

The side effects of succinylcholine include bradycardia (especially in pediatric patients), hyperkalemia, arrhythmias, increased intraocular and intracranial pressure, malignant hyperthermia (in susceptible patients), and postoperative myalgias. Neck, shoulder, and abdominal myalgias can be quite debilitating, especially in the context of same-day surgery procedures.

Nondepolarizing Muscle Relaxants

The nondepolarizing agents attach to the neuromuscular receptor, where they compete with acetylcholine, producing activation. More than 70% of receptors must be occupied for skeletal muscle relaxation to occur. The onset of action may take several minutes. The actions of nondepolarizing agents can be reversed by the use of a reversal agent.

Based on their duration of action, the nondepolarizing agents are classified as short, intermediate, or long acting. Careful attention to the cardiovascular side effects and differences in metabolism will allow selection of the best agent for each patient.

Short Acting. Mivacurium has a rapid onset, is metabolized by plasma cholinesterase, and may not require pharmacologic reversal.

Intermediate Acting. Atracurium, cisatracurium, vecuronium, and **rocuronium** are examples. Atracurium is associated with spontaneous in vivo degradation (Hoffman elimination) at all doses and is associated with histamine release at high doses. Cisatracurium is similar to atracurium but has a slower onset and minimal histamine release. Vecuronium undergoes renal excretion and has minimal cardiovascular effects. Rocuronium has a rapid onset and also has minimal cardiovascular effects. Avoidance of tachycardia or significant bradycardia is crucial in patients with coronary artery disease.

Long Acting. Pancuronium, pipecuronium, and **doxacurium** are examples. Pancuronium is the most commonly used of the three. It can produce tachycardia due to vagolytic activity and is dependent on renal excretion for elimination. Pipecuronium and doxacurium are similar to pancuronium but are not associated with cardiovascular side effects.

Agents That Reverse Neuromuscular Blockade

Although the actions of succinylcholine cannot be reversed pharmacologically, the actions of nondepolarizing muscle relaxants can be reversed by the administration of **neostigmine** when neuromuscular function begins to return. Neostigmine acts by causing the accumulation of acetylcholine at the neuromuscular junction, competitively displacing the nondepolarizing agent from the receptor.

Bradycardia, miosis, hypersalivation, and hyperperistalsis can occur if neostigmine is used alone for reversal. This cholinergic stimulus can be undesirable in patients with fresh bowel anastomosis, which theoretically could be disrupted. To prevent these undesirable effects, an anticholinergic agent such as **atropine** or **glycopyrrolate** must be administered concurrently, often in the same syringe in equal volumes to neostigmine. Glycopyrrolate is favored because it does not cross the blood/brain barrier and is devoid of the central cholinergic side effects seen with atropine. Another less frequently used reversal agent is edrophonium.

Local Anesthetics

Mechanism of Action

Local anesthetics decrease sodium permeability in nerve fibers, producing a decrease in depolarization so the critical threshold potential is not achieved. As a result, the action potential is not generated, resulting in blockade of nerve conduction.

Local anesthetics contain a tertiary amine and a benzene ring with an intermediate chain in between, which can be either an ester or an amide group. The tertiary amine is hydrophilic, whereas the benzene ring is lipophilic. The ionized form of the local anesthetic binds to the nerve membrane while the unionized form permeates the lipophilic nerve sheath.

Local anesthetics are more potent in basic as opposed to acidic tissue. Infected tissue is acidic, which prevents penetration of the local anesthetics through the nerve sheath, because it will exist in the ionized form. When the surgeon uses local anesthesia to incise and drain an abscess, it may be difficult to anesthetize the tissue. Other factors such as nerve size are important, with the concentration necessary to block the nerve directly corresponding to the physical size of the nerve. Myelinated nerves are blocked by lower concentrations of local anesthesia than are unmyelinated fibers. The addition of local vasoconstrictors (i.e., epinephrine) will reduce the systemic uptake, enhancing the duration of the local anesthetic, minimizing the chance of systematic toxicity.

The Use of Local Anesthetics

The use of local anesthetics by surgeons is extremely common and, in selected cases, allows operations without the involvement of the anesthesiologist. Local anesthetics also are used routinely by the anesthesiologist for nerve blocks of the extremities as well as spinal and epidural anesthesia. They can be applied topically to the skin or mucous membranes or injected by diffuse infiltration or as a specific nerve block. With the latter, the local anesthetic agent is injected in the immediate proximity of the nerve to produce a distal block. Local anesthesia can be used as a supplement to general anesthesia for intraoperative and postoperative analgesia.

Local Anesthesia Agents

The most commonly used **amide** agents are **lidocaine, bupivacaine, mepivacaine** and **etidocaine**. **Ester** local anesthetics include **cocaine, chloroprocaine, procaine, benzocaine,** and **tetracaine**. The amides are hepatically metabolized, whereas the esters are metabolized by pseudocholinesterase in the plasma. Allergic reactions are much more likely with ester agents due to metabolism to paraminobenzoic acid (PABA).

When choosing a local anesthetic, one must pay particular attention to the drug concentration, the volume administered, and the use of vasoconstrictors or other additives. Typically, surgeons use lidocaine and bupivacaine in a variety of concentrations with and without epinephrine. Lidocaine is used for its short to medium duration, whereas bupivacaine is selected for its longer action. Other agents are often selected by anesthesiologists for complex nerve blocks and spinal and epidural anesthesia. The newer agents such as ropivacaine and levobupivacaine offer a larger margin of safety, particularly in reference to cardiac toxicity.

Local anesthetics are administered to provide analgesia and, in certain circumstances, produce muscle relaxation, which is the case with spinal, epidural, and certain blocks of the extremities. When dosing local anesthetics, one must pay close attention to the maximal dose not to be exceeded to avoid systemic toxicity (Table 64-2).

TABLE 64–2 Recommended Maximum Local Anesthetic Infiltration Doses

Local Anesthetic	Dose (mg/kg)
Lidocaine	4.5
Lidocaine with epinephrine 1:200,000	7
Mepivacaine	4.5
Mepivacaine with epinephrine 1:200,000	7
Bupivacaine	1–2

Infiltration Field Block

Injection of local anesthesia by infiltration can cause burning and pain before onset of anesthesia. A small needle (25 to 27 gauge), slow injection of the drug, and decreasing the acidity of the solution can minimize pain on injection. Sodium bicarbonate can be added to lidocaine before injection (1 mL of 8.4% $NaHCO_3$) to every 10 mL of lidocaine solution. Infiltration techniques are useful for excision of typical "lumps and bumps." For liposuction, a **tumescent technique** can be performed. This technique couples the installation of warm normal saline with a very dilute concentration of lidocaine (0.05% to 0.1%) with epinephrine and sodium bicarbonate. Larger-than-normal total doses of lidocaine (more than 55 mg/kg) with epinephrine can be administered.

Extremity Blockade

The **Bier block** is an intravenous regional anesthesia technique in which the arm is drained of venous blood by elevation and compression and then filled with a dilute solution of lidocaine via a distal vein. A tourniquet is applied before the local anesthetic injection, allowing surgery lasting about 1 hour. Early deflation of the tourniquet (i.e., at 15 minutes) can be dangerous because of the risk of lidocaine toxicity with the rapid IV circulation. This technique is useful for upper extremity and distal lower extremity procedures. The anesthesia rapidly subsides when the tourniquet is deflated.

Specific nerves can be blocked, such as the median and ulnar nerve for hand surgery. The brachial plexus can be blocked by a variety of techniques such as the intrascalene, supraclavicular, and axillary approaches, based on the site of the surgery (i.e., shoulder vs. wrist). A nerve stimulator can facilitate locating the nerve to minimize the risk of a "spotty" blockade. Intercostal nerve blocks are popular to facilitate thoracic procedures or treat pain of secondary rib fracture to avoid pneumonia.

Spinal Anesthesia

Spinal anesthesia is performed by injecting a small amount of local anesthetic into the subarachnoid space. Typical insertion of the spinal needle occurs at the lumbar 3 to 4 interspace. The spinal cord typically ends at the L2 interspace. Advantages of spinal anesthesia include rapid onset, profound blockade, and ease of access to the spinal space, as opposed to epidural anesthesia (Table 64-3).

Epidural Anesthesia

Epidural anesthesia can be applied at any point along the vertebral column by a variety of techniques that allow proper identification of the epidural space. In contrast to spinal anesthesia, epidural onset is more gradual, and a longer duration can be achieved by the insertion of an epidural catheter for a continuous drug infusion or intermittent

TABLE 64–3 Comparison of Spinal Anesthesia and Epidural Anesthesia

Characteristic	Spinal Anesthesia	Epidural Anesthesia
Technical difficulties	Fewer	More
Needle size used	Smaller (25- to 30-gauge)	Larger (17-gauge)
Anesthetic used	Same	Same
Hemodynamic changes	Rapid	Gradual
Duration	Fixed	Titratable
Postoperative pain control	Requires intrathecal opioids	Retention of epidural catheter provides long-term analgesia
Risk of headache	Higher	Lower
Risk of epidural hematoma	Lower	Higher
Costs	Lower	Higher

boluses. Because the dura is not intentionally punctured with an epidural technique, the potential for spinal headache is low. Failure rates are higher with epidural than with spinal because of the variability in identification of the epidural space.

Systemic Toxicity

The most serious complications associated with local anesthetics are related to inadvertent intravenous injection. The systemic toxicity is directly related to the concentration of the drug in the blood. Important factors in the development of systemic toxicity include the volume and concentration of drug injected, as well as the site of injection. Vascularity of the injection site is critical, with intercostal blocks producing the highest systemic level because of the high vascularity of the area. Systemic uptake and absorption can be limited by adding vasoconstrictors such as phenylephrine or epinephrine. The vasoconstrictors will limit the peak blood level and slow the time necessary to achieve a high level. Vasoconstrictors such as epinephrine can produce hypertension, tachycardia, arrhythmias, chest pain and digital ischemia. To minimize side effects of the vasoconstrictors, it is recommended to limit the concentration of epinephrine to no more than 1:200,000. Vasoconstrictors should not be used in distal digital or penile procedures to avoid potential ischemia and necrosis.

Cardiotoxicity

Local anesthetics all produce vasodilatation, with the exception of ropivacaine. In addition, smooth muscle relaxation and direct myocardial depression may occur. Cardiotoxicity is more likely in critically ill patients with hypoxia, acidosis, hypercarbia, and systemic hypotension. Of all the local anesthetics, bupivacaine is the most dangerous in reference to cardiotoxicity, producing myocardial depression and arrhythmias, which can be difficult to treat. The cardiotoxicity of lidocaine does not produce the same degree of reentrant arrhythmias and ventricular fibrillation as seen with bupivacaine.

Central Nervous System Toxicity

Avoidance of IV injection and strict adherence to maximal dosing guidelines will help minimize the risk of central nervous system (CNS) toxicity that can occur with *all* local anesthetics. The early symptoms of CNS toxicity include dizziness, tinnitus, and lightheadedness that can lead to disorientation. As CNS toxicity progresses, unconsciousness, seizures, and respiratory arrest can result. Supportive care with airway protection and medications like midazolam and pentothal can be helpful.

Allergic Reactions

The ester local anesthetics are metabolized to PABA, which can produce allergic reactions. Methylparaben and metabisulfite are used as preservatives in many local anesthetic solutions and also can be metabolized to PABA, producing allergic reactions.

Combinations of Agents

Quite often surgeons will mix two different local anesthetic drugs together. The combination will take advantage of the rapid onset of one agent and the long duration of the second drug, resulting in postoperative analgesia. This technique minimizes the risk of toxicity because it is not additive. A surgeon may use lidocaine first for an inguinal hernia repair and before closure inject bupivacaine in strategic areas for postoperative analgesia.

Monitoring Techniques

Basic Techniques

The American Society of Anesthesiologists has established basic standards for monitoring patients undergoing general anesthesia. For all patients, **electrocardiography** and the **monitoring of blood pressure, pulse,** and **body temperature** are indicated. A **precordial esophageal stethoscope** allows assessment of ventilation, cardiac sounds, and heart rate throughout the surgical procedure and is used routinely in pediatric anesthesia.

Many anesthesia mishaps that occurred in the past were related to inadequate oxygenation resulting from a misplaced endotracheal tube or a disconnected ventilator. These problems are now easily detected early by **pulse oximetry,** which provides real-time measurement of blood oxygen saturation, and by **end-tidal carbon dioxide ($ETCO_2$) monitoring,** which allows continuous assessment of pulmonary ventilation during surgery. A sudden decrease in the $ETCO_2$ level suggests a ventilator disconnection or pulmonary embolus, whereas an increase in the $ETCO_2$ level may indicate hypoventilation or herald the onset of malignant hyperthermia. Although pulse oximetry assesses oxygenation status, hypercarbia can occur without changes in O_2 saturation.

Many additional monitoring techniques are available to minimize cardiac risk and to avoid postoperative complications.

Arterial cannulation. Cannulation of the radial or femoral artery allows continuous monitoring of blood pressure, allowing rapid intervention when adverse changes in pressure occur. In addition, arterial blood gas samples can assess coagulation status, acid-base balance, and electrolyte concentrations.

Central venous cannulation. The monitoring of central venous pressure and pulmonary artery pressure is particularly helpful for managing patients with cardiovascular disease and cases associated with significant hemodynamic alterations. Cardiac ischemia may produce changes in pulmonary artery pressure before electrocardiogram (ECG) changes, allowing earlier intervention. Special pulmonary artery catheters allow continuous assessment of mixed venous oxygen saturation (SVO_2). A decrease in SVO_2 may signal light anesthesia or cardiac dysfunction, causing increased tissue oxygen extraction, whereas an increase in SVO_2 suggests sepsis or shunting that causes reduced oxygen extraction.

Transesophageal echocardiography. The intraoperative use of transesophageal echocardiography (TEE) allows continuous assessment of cardiac filling and function. Valvular lesions, wall-motion abnormalities, and cardiac filling status can be continuously assessed by TEE. Wall-motion abnormalities on TEE, due to ischemia, may show up before changes in the pulmonary artery pressures or the ECG.

Electroencephalography. Electroencephalographic monitoring may reveal brain ischemia during certain high-risk procedures, such as carotid endarterectomy or deep hypothermic circulatory arrest. Early detection of abnormal patterns will allow therapeutic interventions (such as increasing the systolic blood pressure) to try to minimize the risk of ischemic injury.

Bispectral index monitoring. This summation electroencephalographic index provides continuous data on the depth of anesthesia to ensure that the patient is appropriately asleep, while allowing optimization of anesthetic depth. With the advent of the new short-acting anesthetic agents and "light anesthesia" techniques, use of the bispectral index (BIS) has increased.

Somatosensory evoked potential. Monitoring of the *s*omato*s*ensory *e*voked *p*otential (SSEP) provides information on spinal cord integrity. During scoliosis surgery, a change in the SSEP pattern may signal excessive spinal cord manipulation, which could be remedied intraoperatively to avoid postoperative weakness or paralysis.

Intubation Equipment

The Laryngoscope

Standard laryngoscopes consist of a handle that houses a battery, which actives the blade, which has a light source to aid in visualization of the vocal cords for endotracheal intubation. The same handle can be used to attach different blades as necessary. Different shapes and sizes of blades are available, and the two most common are the curved (MacIntosh) and straight (Miller) blades (Fig. 64-1). The curved blade is placed between the base of the tongue and the pharyngeal epiglottic surface. In contrast, the straight blade is inserted beneath the laryngeal surface of the epiglottis. With both blades to gain access to the glottic opening, the blade is moved forward and upward in the axis of the laryngoscope blade. Easier visualization of the glottic opening can be facilitated by pushing downward or by producing lateral movement of the thyroid cartilage, by using the right hand on the external surface of the patient's neck. With both techniques, one should avoid levering the blade to avoid damage to the teeth (i.e., dislodged tooth) or gums.

In theory, the straight blade gives better exposure of the glottic opening. The curved blade is less traumatic to the epiglottis and also gives more space to advance the endotracheal tube. Blades are used based on personal preference and training of the anesthesiologist.

Endotracheal Tubes

Endotracheal tubes (ETTs) are sized based on the internal diameter of the tube. The tube is marked on the outside with numbers corresponding to the number of centimeters from the tracheal tip of the tube (Table 64-4). Typically, the distance from the lips to the tracheal tip is monitored to avoid too distal or inadequate insertion through the glottic opening. Tubes are available in 0.5-mm internal diameter increments. Typical adults will require a no. 7 or 8 ETT. ETTs have an inflatable cuff at the distal part of the tube to allow a tight seal against the tracheal mucosa when inflated with air. In adults, the cuff allows the delivery of positive-pressure ventilation. In children, the seal may be adequate

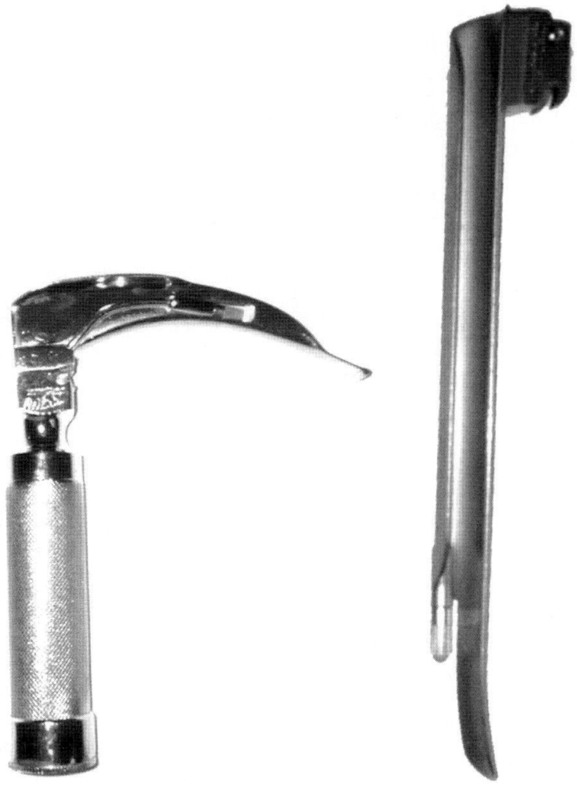

A B

FIGURE 64–1 *A*, MacIntosh blade. *B*, Miller blade.

without the need for an inflatable cuff. Pediatric tubes are supplied with and without cuffs. ETTs are available in low- and high-pressure cuffs. High-pressure cuffs can cause ischemia to the tracheal mucosa because of the high pressure necessary to inflate the cuff to produce a seal. Low-pressure cuffs more adequately conform to the shape of the trachea at much lower pressures, which decreases the chance of tracheal injury. When the pressure on the tracheal wall is in excess of capillary arteriolar pressure (32 mmHg), tracheal mucosal ischemia may occur.

TABLE 64–4 Endotracheal Tube Size and Length Characteristics

Age	Internal Diameter (mm)	Distance from Lip to Tip of ETT Midtracheal (cm)
Premature	2.5	10
1–6 mo	3.5	11
2 yr	4.5	13
6 yr	5.5	15–16
10 yr	7.0	17–18
≥ 14 yr	8.0–9.0	20–22
Adult	7.0–8.0	20–22

ETT, endotracheal tube.

Endotracheal Tube Placement

With the laryngoscope described, the tongue is displaced to allow exposure of the glottic opening. The ETT is passed by using the right hand by advancing the ETT down the right side of the mouth. The tube should be gently passed through the whitish vocal cords until the endotracheal cuff disappears. The cuff is inflated, and breath sounds are assessed visually and by auscultation for bilateral breath sounds. The cuff should be positioned halfway between the vocal cords and the carina. For the typical adult patient, the tube should be 20 to 22 cm at the corner of the mouth. The tube is carefully taped in place to avoid movement or dislodgement during the case. One should be able to palpate the cuff during inflation just above the suprasternal notch. Movements, such as head flexion, can advance a tube previously taped in place into the right mainstem bronchus, which can produce oxygen desaturation and hypoxemia. Typically, head flexion advances the tube and extension can pull the tube out of the trachea. Constant vigilance is pivotal to avoid accidental extubation. In addition to oral endotracheal intubation, nasotracheal intubation can be used.

Fiberoptic Intubation

In patients with known difficult or unanticipated difficult glottic visualization, a flexible bronchoscope can be used. The airway is anesthetized by using topical anesthesia with the patient typically maintaining spontaneous ventilation. First, the ETT is passed through the nose or the oropharynx, and the fiberoptic bronchoscope is passed through the endotracheal tube. The bronchoscope is advanced through the vocal cords, and then the ETT is passed over the bronchoscope, which serves as a stylet. A standard bronchoscope can be used with a no. 8 ETT, whereas a pediatric bronchoscope will allow a 5-mm internal diameter ETT. In cases in which the exact position of the ETT is critical, the bronchoscope can be used for visual confirmation.

Special Equipment

Problems that involve airway management have been minimized by the establishment of a standardized algorithm for dealing with difficult intubation and by the increased use of the laryngeal mask airway (LMA). In patients who cannot be intubated or ventilated with standard techniques, the LMA may come in handy.

Laryngeal mask airway. The LMA is a device that surrounds the glottic opening and provides effective ventilation without directly passing through the vocal cords (Fig. 64-2). Special LMAs allow passage of an ETT through the LMA apparatus (intubating LMA). In addition, LMAs are available that can produce a

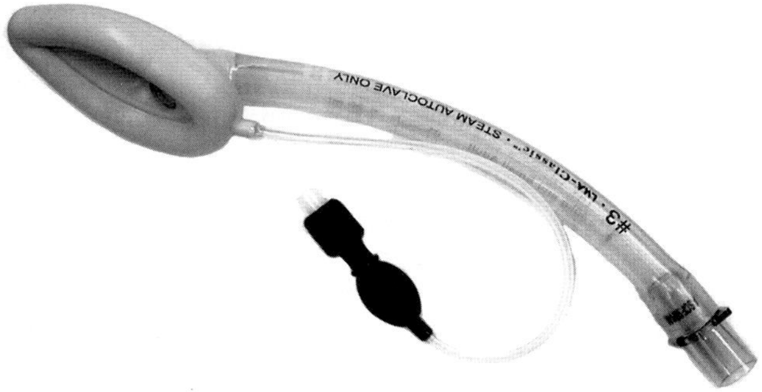

FIGURE 64–2 Laryngeal mask airway.

seal, minimizing the risk of aspiration of gastric contents and allowing passage of an orogastric tube to deflate the stomach.

Eschmann stylet. This device is a flexible rod that is placed between the vocal cords. The ETT is slid over the device. It is useful when it is difficult to get the ETT to pass through the vocal cords, even though they can be seen directly.

Retrograde wire. This wire is introduced through the cricoid membrane and is directed cephalad, so it comes out the mouth. The ETT is then slid over the wire into the trachea.

Light wand. This device is placed through the mouth. The lights in the room are dimmed so the wand tip (which has a bright light) can be viewed on the surface of the neck. The wand is maneuvered until the light is seen shining through the cricothyroid membrane. The ETT is then passed over the wand.

PEARLS FOR THE OR

Malignant hyperthermia
Causes
- Succinylcholine
- Inhalation agents

Symptoms
- Tachycardia
- Arrhythmias
- Acidosis
- Increased oxygen consumption
- Hypercarbia
- Tachypnea
- Cyanosis or mottling
- Hyperkalemia
- Hyperpyrexia
- Muscle rigidity
- Death if untreated or undiagnosed

Treatment
- Dantrolene is the drug of choice.
- Stop the inhalation agent.

TABLE 64–5 American Society of Anesthesiologists (ASA) System for Classifying Health Status and Assessing Risks Associated with Anesthesia

Risk Category*	Preoperative Health Status
ASA 1	Generally healthy patient with no underlying systemic disease
ASA 2	Patient with mild to moderate systemic disease (e.g., hypertension, anemia, or non–insulin-dependent diabetes mellitus)
ASA 3	Patient with multisystem organ disease (e.g., insulin-dependent diabetes mellitus combined with hypertension or obesity
ASA 4	Patient with severe or life-threatening systemic disease (e.g., active congestive heart failure or unstable angina)
ASA 5	Moribund patient with little chance of survival (e.g., ruptured abdominal aneurysm)

* A brain-dead organ donor is sometimes classified as ASA 6. An E is added to the risk categories for emergency cases.

Preoperative Risk Assessment

Risk Classification

The American Society of Anesthesiologists (ASA) has developed a classification system in which patients are assigned preoperatively to one of five anesthesia risk categories based on their health status (Table 64-5). Patients in category 1 have the lowest risk, and those in category 5 have the highest risk. Patients undergoing an emergency operation (such as surgery for bowel obstruction or perforated appendix) are believed to be at additional risk, regardless of their classification status, and are given an emergency (E) status. A patient with diabetes, congestive heart failure (CHF), and renal failure with a perforated colon would be classified as an ASA IV E.

Preoperative Evaluation

Airway Assessment

The airway must be carefully evaluated before anesthesia is administered. Even if regional (spinal or epidural) or MAC anesthesia is planned, intubation with an ETT may be required during the procedure for unanticipated circumstances. To predict preoperatively whether intubation is likely to be difficult, the clinician should ask the patient to sit upright, open the mouth as widely as possible, and maximally protrude the tongue. The airway can then be classified on the basis of the structures seen. In a **class I airway,** visible structures include the soft palate, fauces, uvula, and tonsillar pillars. In **class II,** the soft palate, fauces, and uvula can be seen. In **class III,** only the soft palate and base of the uvula are visible. In **class IV,** the soft palate is not visible at all. Intubation is likely to be

BOX 64–1 Risk Factors Associated with Difficult Intubation

Decreased mouth opening (less than three finger breadths)
Prominent upper incisors or receding lower jaw
Decreased thyroid-to-mentum distance (less than three finger breadths)
Decreased neck extension or short neck
Morbid obesity
Pregnancy (especially with preeclampsia accompanied by pharyngeal soft tissue swelling and glottic edema)

easiest in class I airways and most difficult in class IV, particularly if other risk factors associated with difficult intubation are present (Box 64-1). Morbidly obese patients offer significant airway and other risks to the surgeon and anesthesiologists.

Preoperative Screening

"Routine testing" does not exist in the current healthcare market. New guidelines have significantly reduced the amount of preoperative laboratory testing. Elderly patients undergoing cataract surgery have similar outcomes with and without preoperative testing. In the past, all patients underwent extensive testing, with multiple laboratory values, ECG, and chest radiographs before surgery. Now each center has its own guidelines for testing/assessment, but the primary purpose of the Preadmission Screening Center is to prepare patients for surgery from a medical standpoint and to provide preoperative education and teaching.

Preoperative Medications

Diuretics are typically stopped before surgery. Some drugs like digoxin may be continued for atrial fibrillation but stopped if given for CHF. Digoxin toxicity can be difficult to treat and dangerous if it occurs intraoperatively. Drugs that interfere with platelet function, such as nonsteroidal anti-inflammatory agents, are typically stopped 10 days or more before the date of surgery because of concerns about platelet dysfunction and bleeding.

In the past, monoamine oxidase (MAO) inhibitors were stopped 2 weeks before surgery, but they are now continued until the time of surgery. Narcotics such as meperidine should not be used concurrent with MAO inhibitors, because the drug interaction can produce hypertension, CNS excitation, delirium, seizures, and death.

Insulin is typically given in half the usual preoperative dose in conjunction with the establishment of a glucose-containing IV.

Most anesthesiologists continue all cardiac medications on the day of surgery and give them with a small sip of water. Rebound hypertension is a potential complication associated with the rapid withdrawal of α-adrenergic receptor and calcium channel blockers. The angiotensin-converting enzyme inhibitors may complement the protective effects of β-blockers but occasionally cause severe hypotension in the context of general anesthesia.

Cardiac Evaluation

Abnormal murmurs and heart sounds should be evaluated, because valvular heart disease may have major ramifications for the choice and delivery of an anesthetic. In patients with severe aortic stenosis, hypotension on induction of anesthesia may result in endocardial hypoperfusion, with a decrease in blood pressure that may be impossible to treat because of the stiff, thickened left ventricular wall. For these patients, spinal anesthesia may be contraindicated, because the decrease in systemic vascular resistance and preload associated with spinal anesthesia may produce life-threatening hypotension. In contrast, patients with severe mitral regurgitation can benefit from vasodilatation, which favors forward blood flow, reduces end-diastolic volume, and avoids pulmonary edema. The key to management of patients with severe mitral regurgitation undergoing surgery is to keep them *f*ast (heart rate), *f*orward (decrease afterload), and *f*ull (volume status)—the three Fs.

Various noninvasive and invasive cardiac tests are available to assess the patient's cardiac status, including exercise testing, ejection-fraction analysis, dobutamine stress echocardiography, and dipyridamole thallium imaging. Coronary angiography is clearly the gold standard, but it does have its own inherent risks. Regardless of the test used, the anesthesiologist must know preoperatively if the patient is at increased cardiac risk. If the patient has well-controlled hypertension, normal results on dobutamine stress echocardiography, and an ejection fraction of 60%, the cardiac risk is mild to intermediate. If the ejection fraction is 30% and reperfusion changes are well documented on thallium imaging or dobutamine echocardiography, then the risk is high. Patients at high risk should probably undergo cardiac catheterization and possible coronary stent placement or even coronary artery bypass surgery in certain selected cases before high-risk procedures such as peripheral revascularization. Many patients who are not candidates for management with drug-eluting stents or coronary artery surgery should be optimized on medical management before entering the operating room (OR). Those patients at extremely high risk may require perioperative β-blockers, invasive monitoring, and postoperative ICU monitoring.

Perioperative Myocardial Infarction

The incidence of concurrent coronary artery disease is the highest in patients with vascular disease (70%), and their major perioperative complications are cardiac in origin. The relation between perioperative myocardial infarction (PMI), ischemic cardiac events, and adverse cardiac

BOX 64–2 Factors Most Commonly Associated with Adverse Cardiac Outcomes in Surgical Patients

Active angina pectoris
Congestive heart failure
Diabetes mellitus
Diastolic hypertension (blood pressure >110 mmHg)
Recent myocardial infarction
Renal insufficiency
Smoking

outcome is still not entirely clear. It is generally believed that avoidance of intraoperative tachycardia and hypotension are two important measures to minimize cardiac ischemia and PMI (Box 64-2)

In the older anesthesia series, the majority of PMIs were transmural and associated with a high mortality rate (>50%). With the availability of serial cardiac isoenzymes, non–Q wave MIs are now more frequently detected and are associated with a lower mortality rate. In the late 1990s, investigators reported that, in a large series of patients undergoing peripheral vascular surgery for a femoral/distal bypass graft, the overall incidence of PMI was approximately 4.5%, and the associated rate of deaths occurring secondary to MI was less than 10%.

The incidence of PMI in various groups undergoing surgery is summarized in Table 64-6. Most perioperative MIs occur on postoperative day 3 or 4. The risk of **reinfarction** in patients with previous MIs depends on the amount of time that has elapsed since the most recent MI (Table 64-7). The risk is highest in those whose most recent MI occurred less than 3 months earlier.

In patients who sustained an MI in the past, the overall risk of reinfarction has been reported to be about 7%. With all the new techniques available in the catheterization laboratory to manage lesions, the risk of reinfarction may be much lower than previously quoted. β-Blockade in the perioperative period is often initiated to reduce risk. ICU monitoring and use of pulmonary artery catheters has not been shown to decrease the rate of reinfarction directly.

TABLE 64–6 Comparison of Risks for Perioperative Myocardial Infarction (MI) in Various Patient Populations

Patient Population	Risk of Perioperative MI
Entire population	<1%
Patients with a history of successful coronary revascularization	0–1.2%
Patients with known coronary artery disease	1%–2%
Patients with peripheral vascular disease	1%–15%
Patients with previous MI	5%–8%

TABLE 64–7 Risk of Reinfarction after an Initial Myocardial Infarction (MI)

Time from Initial MI	Risk of Reinfarction
1–3 mo	15%–36%
3–6 mo	15%
>6 mo	1%–5%

Pulmonary Assessment

In all patients undergoing any type of anesthesia, careful preoperative auscultation of the lungs is critical for detecting wheezing or other pulmonary abnormalities and to establish a baseline for further comparison. New-onset wheezing may represent an allergic reaction to the preoperative antibiotic or may be the first sign of CHF. Baseline arterial blood gas measurements and pulmonary function tests should be performed preoperatively to optimize the pulmonary status of high-risk patients. Aggressive preoperative bronchodilators and even corticosteroids may help minimize the risk of postoperative pulmonary complications, including wheezing, atelectasis, and pneumonia. Smoking should preferably be stopped 6 weeks before an elective operation.

Renal Assessment

For patients with renal problems, a baseline serum creatinine level should be determined. Because contrast dye can be used for preoperative angiography, this can lead to a significant deterioration in renal function if not recognized before surgery. If diabetes mellitus is present, it should be tightly controlled preoperatively. Elevated intraoperative serum glucose levels may lead to adverse neurologic sequelae and increase the risk of wound infection. Renal failure and diabetes put the patient at significant risk and must be tightly controlled.

Medical History

Allergic reactions may result from exposure to anesthetic agents, antibiotics, contrast agents, latex, or other substances. Regardless of the cause, these reactions represent a major risk during anesthesia and surgery. Manifestations of a severe allergic reaction include the following: intraoperative hypotension, bronchospasm, and urticaria. Any previous allergy must be carefully evaluated and documented in the chart.

Pseudocholinesterase deficiency has an incidence of about 1 in 3500. The use of succinylcholine will result in the need for prolonged ventilation in patients with pseudocholinesterase deficiency. Succinylcholine has a normal half-life of 3 to 5 minutes, but it may leave patients with this deficiency paralyzed for hours. If a family history of pseudocholinesterase deficiency is known, the patient should be assessed preoperatively for enzyme activity and anesthetized with a muscle relaxant that does not rely on cholinesterase for metabolism. In addition to having a genetic component, it may be triggered by pregnancy, end-stage liver disease, or alkylating antineoplastic agents.

Neuromuscular disorders must be carefully assessed, because normal doses of muscle relaxants used intraoperatively can produce prolonged and exaggerated paralysis. Patients with myasthenia gravis may not need muscle relaxants at all during surgery. Young male patients with Duchenne muscular dystrophy may develop profound hyperkalemia that leads to cardiac arrest if they are given succinylcholine. The relatively occult nature and the late presentation of Duchenne muscular dystrophy often preclude preoperative diagnosis of this life-threatening condition.

Malignant hyperthermia is a familial condition that has an incidence of about 1 in 35,000 individuals. Malignant hyperthermia results from uncoupled calcium transport in the muscle at the subcellular level. It represents a hypermetabolic state with a variety of manifestations including acidosis, arrhythmias, cyanosis/mottling, hypercarbia, hyperkalemia, hyperpyrexia, increased oxygen consumption, muscle rigidity, tachycardia, and tachypnea. Acidosis can be profound, and death will occur if the condition is undiagnosed or not treated appropriately. The agents responsible for triggering malignant hyperthermia include **succinylcholine** and **all inhalational agents** used for general anesthesia. Unfortunately, a previous uneventful exposure to these agents does not guarantee future safety. If malignant hyperthermia occurs in the OR or recovery setting, it must be diagnosed early and treated aggressively. **Dantrolene** is the drug of choice and must be started immediately, with the surgery quickly halted to allow the aggressive interventions necessary to save the patient's life (Box 64-3).

Preoperative Optimization

The concept of performing preoperative "tune-ups" on certain high-risk patients in the ICU setting before the OR remains controversial. Some experts recommend the preoperative insertion of a pulmonary artery catheter to generate Starling curves to optimize cardiac output. Others believe that preoperative tune-ups have their own significant risks, including pneumothorax associated with line placement and myocardial ischemia caused by overzealous use of inotropes. The initiation of intraoperative central monitoring, after hemodynamic decompensation has occurred in the OR in high-risk patients, is probably not the ideal approach. Certain studies have demonstrated worse outcomes when compared with preoperative optimization.

Most clinicians line the patient up immediately before the OR.

BOX 64-3 Steps in the Management of Malignant Hyperthermia

1. Stop the administration of inhalational agents.
2. Call for help.
3. Administer 100% oxygen.
4. Stop surgery as soon as possible.
5. Begin intravenous treatment with dantrolene and chilled sodium chloride.
6. Institute measures for surface cooling and begin cold lavage of body cavities.
7. Continuously assess the acid base status.
8. Provide systematic treatment for arrhythmias.
9. Complete the surgery as soon as possible.
10. Continue invasive monitoring for 24 to 48 hours.
11. Assess the need for mannitol treatment to promote diuresis.

Intraoperative Management

Nothing-by-mouth Status

Recommendations concerning eating and drinking before surgery are being changed in many medical centers. Guidelines are becoming more liberal, allowing ingestion of clear liquids (such as water) up to 4 hours before surgery. Typically patients have nothing by mouth (NPO) after midnight, regardless of the time of their surgery.

An acid-neutralizing drug such as Bicitra is frequently given before anesthesia induction in patients with risk factors for aspiration, including obesity, pregnancy, and hiatal hernia. However, it is important to note that the efficacy of Bicitra and other prophylactic antacids has recently been called into question.

In general, if the patient has eaten and the scheduled surgical procedure is not an emergency procedure, surgery should be delayed for 6 to 8 hours. If the surgery must be performed immediately or the patient has risk factors for aspiration, then a **rapid-sequence induction** can be performed. This involves preoxygenation with 100% oxygen to denitrogenate the lungs, cricoid pressure to guard against esophageal regurgitation, and simultaneous injection of the induction agent and succinylcholine. There is *no* assisted ventilation of the lungs. After muscle fasciculations occur, the trachea is intubated with a styletted ETT (to facilitate ease of tube placement), and the endotracheal cuff is inflated. The lungs are rapidly assessed for bilateral breath sounds. The expired breaths are examined for ET_{CO_2} to confirm that the tracheal tube has been properly placed. Cricoid pressure is released once the ETT is confirmed not to be in the esophagus. A gastric tube (oral or nasal) should be inserted to empty the stomach after the airway is secured.

If the patient begins to vomit before the insertion of the ETT, the bed is immediately placed in Trendelenburg position and the patient is placed on his or her side. The oropharynx is suctioned, and the airway is secured thereafter. The lungs are then ventilated with 100% oxygen, and bronchoscopy is carried out to determine whether aspiration of food or other particulate matter has resulted. If aspiration has occurred, bronchoscopic lavage is performed to remove any foreign matter. At this point, elective surgery may have to be postponed if aspiration is evident. It may take 6 to 8 hours for the pulmonary damage to become evident, and, in some cases, the development of respiratory distress syndrome may occur thereafter. The risk of aspiration with anesthesia is 1 in 2131.

The Difficult Airway

It is not always possible to predict which patients will be "easy intubations." The safest way to deal with a potentially difficult airway is to perform a **fiberoptic intubation** while the patient is still awake and breathing spontaneously. If a patient becomes unconscious, the tongue drops back, and time becomes a critical issue if you cannot oxygenate or ventilate, with the potential for hypoxic brain injury and even death. For awake fiberoptic intubation, the nasal, oropharyngeal, and glottic structures can be anesthetized by using a combination of vasoconstrictors and topical anesthesia administered by local spray, nebulization, or both. The superior laryngeal nerves, which supply the supraglottic structures, may be infiltrated with a local anesthetic, and local anesthetic can be injected directly through the cricothyroid membrane to anesthetize the lower airway to prevent coughing and gagging. The ETT is then guided into the trachea over a flexible bronchoscope by either the nasal or the oral route. All measures should be taken to be gentle and cautious to avoid bleeding and tissue edema. Suction and supplemental oxygen can be administered via the side arm of the bronchoscope. Local anesthetics also can be injected through the bronchoscope to spray the vocal cords and trachea directly and thereby facilitate ETT placement. Sedation for awake intubation must be titrated carefully, and the premature use of muscle relaxants should generally be avoided. Once the airway is secured, hypnotics and muscle relaxants can be safely given. Keeping the patient breathing spontaneously is crucial until the airway is secured.

Safety Profile of Different Anesthesia Techniques

Patients often question which method of anesthesia is the safest or best for their procedure. The bottom line is that there is no definitive best answer. Each technique has certain advantages and disadvantages associated with its use (Table 64-8; see also Table 64-3).

TABLE 64–8 Advantages and Disadvantages of Four Methods of Anesthesia

Method	Advantages	Disadvantages
General anesthesia	Airway can be secured; the patient is asleep; surgery can be performed on any site of the body; anesthesia can be sustained for as long as necessary; and muscle relaxants can be administered if needed	Intubation may be difficult; the patient is unable to communicate problems; clotting cascade is activated; hemodynamic changes occur with induction and emergence from anesthesia; patient is at risk of awareness during neuromuscular blockade; the procedure may damage the teeth or oropharynx; and postoperative nausea and vomiting may occur
Spinal anesthesia	Spinal block lowers the risk of pulmonary embolism and increases blood flow to the lower extremities; anesthesia is localized to the surgical site; the patient is awake and can advise of problems (e.g., shortness of breath and chest pain); and preemptive analgesia or intrathecal opioids can be administered	Airway is not secured; duration of block cannot be titrated; block may be spotty; blood pressure may decrease rapidly with onset of block; heart rate may decrease; the patient may become agitated; and side effects include spinal headache, urinary retention, paresthesias, and cauda equina syndrome
Epidural anesthesia	Epidural block has a positive effect on coagulation; hemodynamically stable; provides postoperative analgesia; anesthesia is localized to the surgical site; the duration can be titrated; and the patient is awake and can communicate problems	Airway is not secured; epidural block may fail; epidural catheter may migrate and cause adverse neurologic effects; postoperative care is labor intensive; and side effects include hypotension, nausea, pruritus, urinary retention, paresthesias, and epidural hematoma
Monitored anesthesia care	Anesthesia can be titrated to effect; the patient is awake and can communicate problems; minimally invasive; few side effects, and frequently allows early discharge	Airway is not secured; anesthesia may be inadequate; sedation may become excessive, requiring intubation; surgical options are limited; and interaction of operating room and teaching staff may be limited by the procedure

Claims have been made that spinal anesthesia can improve blood flow in the lower extremities and that epidural anesthesia can have positive effects in preventing arterial graft thrombosis in patients undergoing distal revascularization procedures. Older patients with hip fractures may have improved 30-day survival with spinal as opposed to general anesthesia. In contrast, general anesthesia is known to produce a hypercoagulable state with decreased fibrinolytic activity.

In the past, spinal anesthesia was associated with a much higher incidence of **postdural puncture headache** (PDPH). This was attributed to the large diameter (18 to 20 gauge) of the spinal needle and, to a lesser extent, to the shape of the needles used. Contemporary needles are much smaller (25 to 30 gauge) and have specially designed "pencil points" that separate the dural membrane rather than puncturing it. Reducing the amount of cerebrospinal fluid (CSF) leakage seems to be the major factor in lowering the incidence of PDPH. PDPH is often debilitating, with nausea, severe headache, tinnitus, and photophobia, often resulting in the patient lying flat in bed because of the postural nature of the PDPH. Treatment includes conservative management with bed rest, IV fluids, analgesia, and caffeinated products. If the headaches persist despite conservative measures, an **epidural blood patch** may be administered if other diagnoses are excluded (i.e., meningitis). The technique includes identifying the epidural space in the area of the previous dural puncture with an epidural needle. Venous blood (25 to 50 mL) is withdrawn from the patient's arm by using sterile technique and then injected via the epidural needle until the patient experiences pressure in the lower-back buttocks (typically 15 to 25 mL). If successful, the patient will experience immediate relief of symptoms. The blood patch can be repeated 24 to 48 hours later if needed.

Side effects of epidural anesthesia include hypotension, nausea, urinary retention, and pruritus. In addition, the epidural catheter can migrate into the CSF, producing spinal anesthesia. If the catheter migrates into an epidural vein, it may cause CNS effects ranging from agitation and confusion to grand mal seizures secondary to local anesthetic toxicity.

Since the introduction of a low-molecular-weight form of heparin called enoxaparin, the incidence of epidural hematoma after regional anesthesia has increased dramatically. This complication can produce paralysis, even if decompressive spinal surgery is performed immediately. If an epidural block becomes unusually dense in the postoperative period, the epidural infusion should be stopped immediately, and an investigation to rule out epidural hematoma should occur. If any doubt exists about the distribution, duration, or characteristics of an epidural block, then spinal computed tomography or magnetic resonance imaging must be performed to rule out hematoma. A motor block that is profound and out of proportion to the sensory anesthesia may be the only indication that this complication has occurred.

Combined Anesthesia Techniques

Some experts have suggested that for high-risk patients, it may be more beneficial to use a combination of general and epidural anesthesia, as opposed to general anesthesia alone. For example, for a patient requiring pancreatectomy, general anesthesia may be used in combination with an epidural nerve block. If a combined technique is used, the epidural nerve block is established before the surgical incision. Some pain theorists believe that the incision or other incoming noxious stimuli can actually "rev up" the pain pathways and that this can perpetuate and exaggerate the pain experience. With starting the epidural anesthesia before the skin incision, the afferent arm of the pain loop will be blocked. The epidural catheter could be left in place for 72 hours postoperatively, resulting in excellent analgesia while allowing deep breathing, coughing, and even early ambulation, in certain situations. A combined technique offers the advantages of securing the airway and allowing a lower dosage of inhalational agent to be used, because the epidural nerve block can produce surgical anesthesia by itself. The combination of techniques makes it possible for the patient to be awake and comfortable at the end of surgery and can reduce the incidence of nausea and vomiting associated with general anesthesia alone.

Extubation Criteria

Before extubation takes place, the patient should be awake and capable of exhibiting protective airway reflexes and should exhibit stable vital signs. The patient's ability to raise the head from the operating table and to grip the anesthesiologist's hand purposefully on command is an indication that it is safe to consider extubation in the OR. In addition, the muscle relaxant should be adequately reversed. Most important, the patient must exhibit adequate respiratory rate, tidal volume, and inspiratory pressure.

Reasons to delay extubation include the presence of residual anesthesia (inhalation agents), hemodynamic instability (bleeding, decreased or increased blood pressure), poor oxygenation, morbid obesity, hypothermia, old age, and neuromuscular disease. When in doubt, it is better for the patient to remain intubated and enter the recovery room with the tube in place, where blood gas analysis can occur and respiratory mechanics be obtained.

Postoperative Nausea and Vomiting

Nausea and vomiting occur commonly after anesthesia and surgery. Because nausea is one of the symptoms of myocardial ischemia, the possibility of ischemia should always be considered if nausea and vomiting occur in high-risk cardiac patients. The most commonly used antiemetics include **metoclopramide, scopolamine,** and **ondansetron.** Metoclopramide increases the lower esophageal sphincter tone and promotes gastric emptying. Ondansetron is a serotonin-receptor antagonist that is highly effective but is much more costly than the other agents. Scopolamine is an anticholinergic agent (like atropine) that is applied preoperatively as a transdermal patch and left in place postoperatively. Some patients experience annoying CNS side effects (dysphoria). Droperidol, a butyrophenone, was used frequently in the past as an antiemetic, but cases of torsades de pointes have limited its usefulness. Other antiemetics that may be used include **prochlorperazine, diphenhydramine,** and **propofol** in small doses. A nasogastric tube inserted intraoperatively may decrease the postoperative nausea if it is placed on active suction.

Postoperative Management

Temperature Regulation

Studies have shown that intra- and postoperative hypothermia is associated with an increased incidence of infection and bleeding. Basic methods for maintaining the patient's temperature in the OR include warming the IV fluids, warming and humidifying inspired gases, increasing the room temperature, and using a warming blanket. Preventing loss of temperature is the key, because rewarming hypothermia patients postoperatively is slow and can result in significant postanesthesia care unit (PACU) delays.

Pain Management

In many cases, intravenous **patient-controlled analgesia** (PCA) is used to manage postoperative pain. A loading dose of an appropriate narcotic is given, and then the patient is able to self-administer small doses of the narcotic to maintain a level of comfort. PCA is delivered via an infusion pump that is connected to a release button and timing device. A maximal dose and lockout interval is predetermined to prevent accidental overdose. During the lockout interval (which typically lasts for 6 to 10 minutes), pushing the button will not result in release of the narcotic. Although it is possible to combine the use of PCA with a continuous background infusion of the narcotic, this increases the risk of respiratory depression. The most commonly used agents for PCA are **morphine, hydromorphine,** and **fentanyl.** The effectiveness of meperidine for postoperative analgesia has been recently questioned. In a patient with renal failure, meperidine use should be avoided because the drug may accumulate in the body, causing agitation and, in some cases, seizures.

Depending on the type of surgery and the characteristics of the patient, postoperative pain can be managed with **local anesthetics, narcotics,** or a **combination of both. Lidocaine** is typically used to initiate an epidural block, and then an infusion of **bupivacaine** or another long-acting agent is started. Lipid-soluble opioids, such as **fentanyl,** have a relatively rapid onset and tend to spread minimally throughout the CSF, whereas more water-soluble drugs, such as **morphine,** have a slower onset and spread to a greater degree throughout the CSF. When neuraxial narcotics are used, the potential for sedation and delayed respiratory depression is always present. Although the respiratory depression may occur as late as 12 hours after the epidural dose is administered (i.e., morphine), the problem is usually heralded by a gradual increase in somnolence, so with careful monitoring, the remedial action can be taken (i.e., slow infusion rate/narcotic antagonist) to avoid significant morbidity. The pruritus associated with epidural anesthesia is often mild, but it may require treatment with antihistamines, naloxone, and even propofol.

When local anesthetics are used in high concentrations, they can produce hypotension and significant motor block. These side effects can be minimized by using a dilute concentration, such as 0.0625% bupivacaine, instead of a 0.2% or 0.5% concentration. The use of an opioid drug in combination with a low concentration of a local anesthetic can increase the analgesic effect.

Summary

With the rapid changes occurring in surgical techniques and more frequent use of minimally invasive approaches, many patients are being discharged home the day of surgery or early the next morning. Administration of an oral anti-inflammatory agent (cyclo-oxygenase [COX] inhibitors), 650 mg of acetaminophen, and a narcotic like oxycontin by mouth with a sip of water before the surgical incision in orthopedic surgery can dramatically reduce postoperative pain. Use of SAFE (*s*hort-*a*cting *f*ast *e*mergence) drugs, such as propofol, remifentanil, and rapidly metabolized muscle relaxants, will allow rapid wake-up and short PACU stays for many ambulatory patients. *T*otal *i*ntra*v*enous *a*nesthesia (TIVA) without the use of inhalational agents may minimize postoperative nausea and vomiting. Aggressive use of blocks directly by the surgeon or the anesthesiologist will help minimize postoperative pain and suffering. Combination of general anesthesia with epidural anesthesia continued into the postoperative period will provide excellent anesthesia for complex abdominal surgeries such as a Whipple or aortobifemoral bypass graft. When used in conjunction with a depth-of-anesthesia monitor, the dose of TIVA can be carefully titrated to avoid overdose, prevent awareness, and ensure short wake-up times. Patients entering the ORs of the future will likely be older and sicker than ever before. Constant vigilance and attention to detail is central to all anesthetic plans.

Suggested Reading

American Society of Anesthesiologists Task Force on Management of the Difficult Airway: Practice guidelines for management of the difficult airway. Anesthesiology 78:597–603, 1993.

Berlauk JF, Abrams JH, Gilmour IJ, et al: Preoperative optimization of cardiovascular hemodynamics improves outcome in peripheral vascular surgery: A prospective, randomized clinical trial. Ann Surg 214:289–299, 1991.

Engelhardt T, Webster NR: Pulmonary aspiration of gastric contents in anaesthesia. Br J Anaesth 83:453–460, 1999.

Goldman L, Caldera DL, Nussbaum SR, et al: Multifactorial index of cardiac risk in noncardiac surgical procedures. N Engl J Med 297:845–850, 1997.

Roizen MF: Cost-effective preoperative laboratory testing. JAMA 271:319–320, 1994.

Samsoon GLT, Young JRB: Difficult tracheal intubation: A retrospective study. Anesthesia 42:487–490, 1997.

Sieber FE: The neurological implications of diabetic hyperglycemia during surgical procedures at increased risk for brain ischemia. J Clin Anesth 74:540–544, 1997.

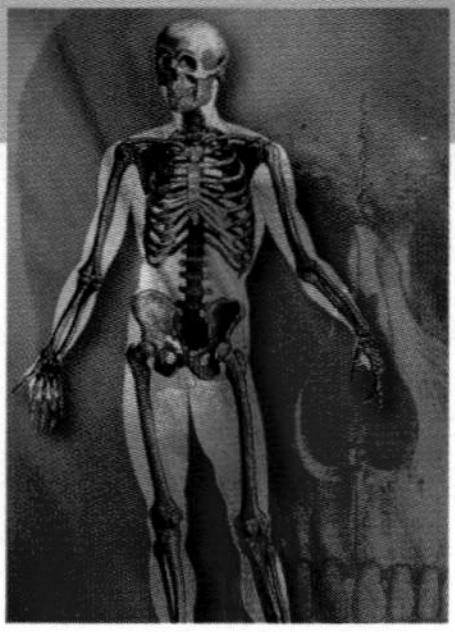

Chapter 65
Dermatologic Surgery

DENNIS LEE, MD, MARINA I. FELDMAN, MD, MBA, and
GARY S. ROGERS, MD

Dermatologic surgery is perhaps the youngest of surgical disciplines. It entails and incorporates features from a variety of surgical fields including plastic surgery, otolaryngology, and aspects of orthopedic surgery and surgical oncology. Dermatologic surgery specializes in the treatment of diseases of the skin, subcutis, and soft tissues. The mainstay of this specialty is the management of skin cancer and reconstruction of surgical defects after extirpation of malignancies. Dermatologic surgery also encompasses a variety of esthetic procedures.

A fundamental knowledge of the skin and subcutaneous tissues combined with knowledge of surgical principles, tissue dynamics, and physiology is necessary to be a skillful dermatologic surgeon. In addition, one also must be facile, with understanding of tumors of the skin. Finally, aesthetic surgery requires knowledge of the pathophysiology of cutaneous photoaging as well as the dynamics of soft tissue manipulation. This chapter is divided into three sections: (1) principles of skin surgery, anesthesia, regional anatomy, tissue biomechanics, and surgical techniques; (2) common skin cancers and their treatment; and (3) esthetic procedures of the skin such as dermabrasion, liposuction, laser treatments, and botulinum toxin injection.

Principles of Skin Surgery

Local and Regional Anesthesia for Skin Surgery

Field block or ring block is a type of infiltrative anesthetic technique that places the anesthetic agent circumferentially around the lesion to be excised. It is commonly used to avoid cyst rupture in cyst removal. Other blocks include those for the digits, the ears, and the penis.

Nerve blocks involve the injection of anesthetic agents into peripheral nerves. Advantages include less toxicity due to the small amounts required for a nerve block, greater surface area reached, and lack of distortion of the surgical site.

Excisional Surgery

Fusiform (Elliptical) Excision

This is the most commonly designed excision in cutaneous surgery; it ensures wound closure with minimal tension. The excision should be fusiform, or football shaped, with a 3:1 ratio of long axis to short axis and with apex angles of 30 degrees. The long axis should be parallel to the relaxed skin-tension lines (RSTLs) to have a good cosmetic appearance. The skin specimen should be excised in uniform thickness with straight perpendicular edges (not beveled). Undermining the ends of the ellipse will help flatten the tips.

Primary Closure

Primary closure is defined as closure by sutures at the time of the excision.

Second-intention Healing

Generally, all wounds can heal by second intention, given enough time to preclude any preexisting medical diseases that cause poor wound healing, such as diabetes, peripheral vascular disease, renal failure, and malnutrition. Second-intention healing can provide excellent cosmetic results in certain anatomic locations, particularly those that are concave, such as the medial canthus, alar groove, conchal bowl, and temple. Interestingly, the scalp, which is a convex structure, heals well by second intention. Second-intention healing should not be considered in areas adjacent to fixed structures such as the eyelid or lip, because wound contraction can distort these structures.

Grafts

The two types of skin grafts are full-thickness skin grafts and split-thickness skin grafts (Table 65-1). They are used in surgical sites with large defects whose wound edges cannot close by approximation with low tension. Complications may include graft failure due to smoking or hematoma formation.

Regional Tissue Transfer

Skin flaps are composites of skin and subcutaneous tissue that have been transferred to another location along with the blood supply. The three main types of flaps are advancement, rotation, and transposition. The location and tissue movement of the surgical defect determines the choice of the flap to be used.

TABLE 65–1 Two Types of Skin Grafts

	Full Thickness	Split Thickness
Composition	Epidermis + full dermis	Epidermis + varied dermis
Donor sites	Preauricular, postauricular, or supraclavicular	Inner upper arm, upper thigh
Advantage	Better texture match to recipient site with no indentation	Supply for large defect

- Advancement flaps are created by incisions releasing adjacent tissue, which is advanced over the defect. It is useful in areas where tissue must be moved in a single direction, and loose tissue is available in that direction. It may be used in the eyebrow area, forehead, preauricular area, upper lip, and the helix of the ear
- Rotation flaps are created by the rotation of skin about a pivot point into the defect. They may be used for defects of the cheek, lip, nose, forehead, or scalp.
- Transposition flaps are created by transposing loose adjacent tissue over a normal island of skin to cover the defect. Transposition flaps are best used for midcheek, temple, upper nose, and chin defects.

Criteria for skin flap design include where the loose skin is available, which flap will cause the least tension, how the scar can be placed in cosmetic-unit junctions or along the RSTLs, and which flap will allow optimal color match and texture and thickness of skin.

Skin Cancer

Basal and Squamous Cell Carcinomas

Basal and squamous cell carcinoma are malignancies of keratinocytes that arise within the epidermal layer of the skin. Over time they may invade into the dermis and subcutaneous tissues. On invasion, squamous cell carcinoma (SCC) may develop the potential for metastasis. Basal cell carcinoma (BCC) rarely metastasizes. Far more common than metastasis is the ability for these cancers to be locally invasive and destructive of the skin and surrounding tissues.

Epidemiology of Squamous and Basal Cell Carcinoma

It is estimated that, in the United States, 250,000 cases of SCC and more than 1.25 million cases of BCC were diagnosed in 2004. These tumors are most commonly seen in parts of the world where light-skinned individuals receive extensive amounts of intense sunlight. This indicates that ultraviolet light exposure and skin type (skin coloring) are the most important factors in developing skin cancer. The incidence of SCC and BCC in the United States is highest in the southern rather than in the northern parts of the country. It also has been shown that the incidence of skin cancer is higher in Australia and New Zealand than in England, although all of these countries have high densities of Celtic people.

In light-skinned people, most SCC and BCC occur in anatomic areas that have prolonged exposure to sunlight. This is not true in darker-skinned individuals.

Clinical Manifestations of Squamous Cell Carcinoma

Squamous cell carcinoma (Fig. 65-1) arises within the keratinocytes. Thus the development of intraepidermal SCC, also called *carcinoma in situ,* is the first and earliest form of SCC. The anatomic location of the growth, as well as the inciting factor (sunlight, arsenic, coal tar), determines the name given to the disease; for example, in situ SCC on the glans penis is referred to as *erythroplasia of Queyrat,* and when it arises from arsenic ingestion, it is referred to as an *arsenical keratosis.* Carcinoma in situ often remains within the epidermis for extended periods but can progress to invasive carcinoma in an unpredictable manner.

The clinical manifestations of SCC can include a cutaneous horn, which is a protruding wartlike structure in which the carcinoma is often present at the base of the horn (see Fig. 65-1). Arsenical keratoses usually develop on the palms (Figs. 65-2 and 65-3) and soles and again are often confined to the epidermis. These lesions are often 2 to 4 mm in diameter, are hard, and have a yellowish hue and a rough surface.

Bowen's disease is perhaps the most common form of intraepidermal SCC. It can occur on any anatomic site. Most

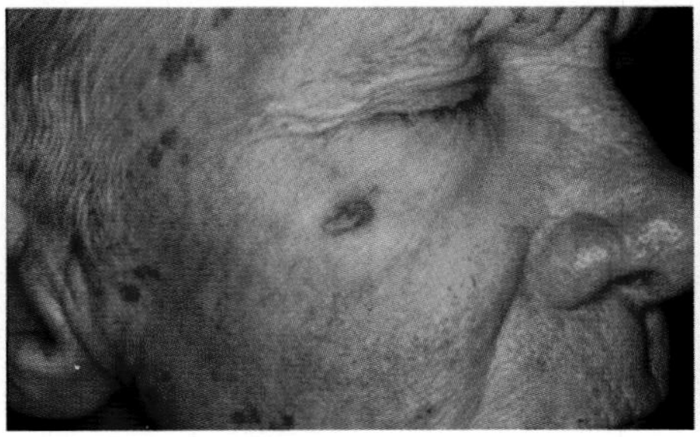

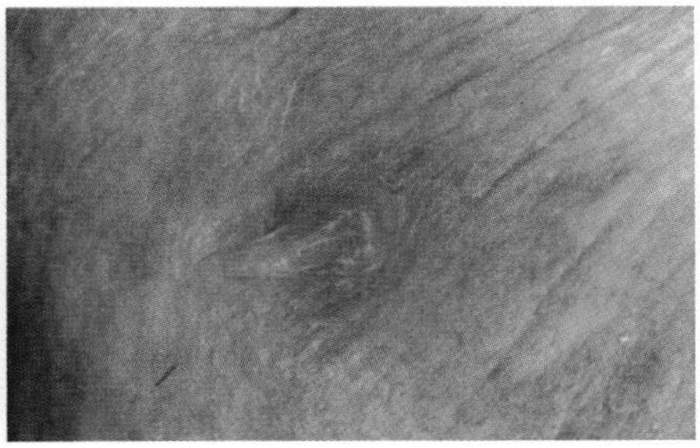

FIGURE 65–1 Squamous cell carcinoma.

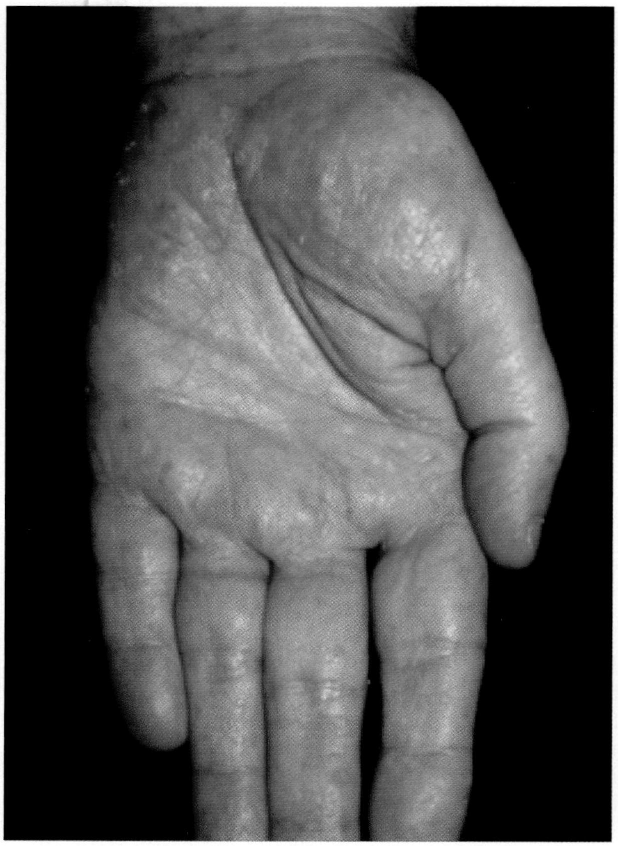

FIGURE 65–2 Arsenical keratoses.

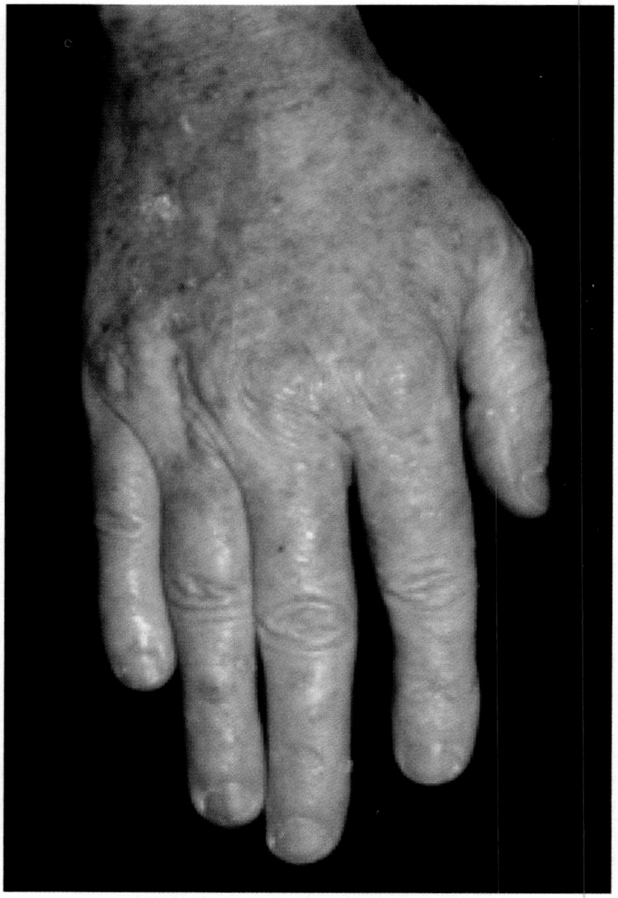

FIGURE 65–3 Arsenical keratoses.

commonly, it will appear as a 5-mm to 2-cm erythematous, thin, and scaly plaque (Fig. 65-4). These tumors usually remain in situ for many years before developing into invasive SCCs.

Invasive SCCs are tumors that usually develop from carcinoma in situ (Fig. 65-5). Roughly 12% of SCCs arise from preexisting solar keratoses (cutaneous in situ keratinocytic dysplasia). Bowen's disease progresses to invasive SCC roughly 5% of the time.

The risk of aggressive biologic behavior of invasive SCC is often a function of the precursor lesion. It is rare for invasive SCC to become metastatic when it arises from an actinic keratosis (in situ dysplasia); however, invasive SCC that arises in a scar or site of prior radiation can have a relatively high risk of metastasis.

The clinical appearance of invasive SCC is variable. Most commonly it is first seen as a red, eroded, and friable nodule. Often, a raised border exists on these lesions. On occasion, dense keratinaceous debris is found. Before metastasis, these tumors also can be highly destructive. Most worrisome is the phenomenon of neural invasion, especially on the head and neck. Extension along the peripheral nerves to the ganglion can often result in direct invasion of the skull. When SCC arises on the lip, it may arise from leukoplakia, which is a result of smoking

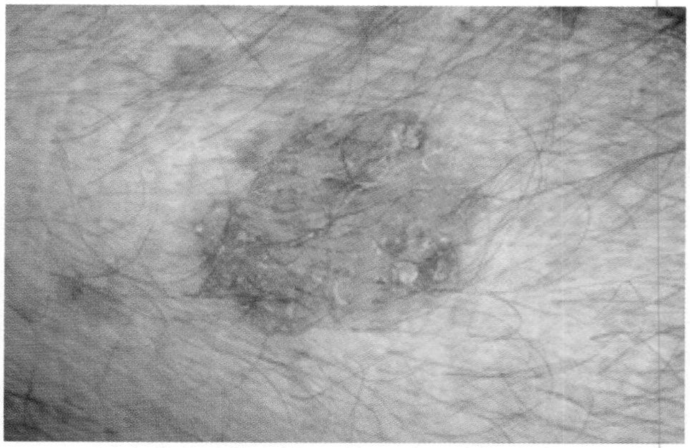

FIGURE 65–4 Bowen's disease.

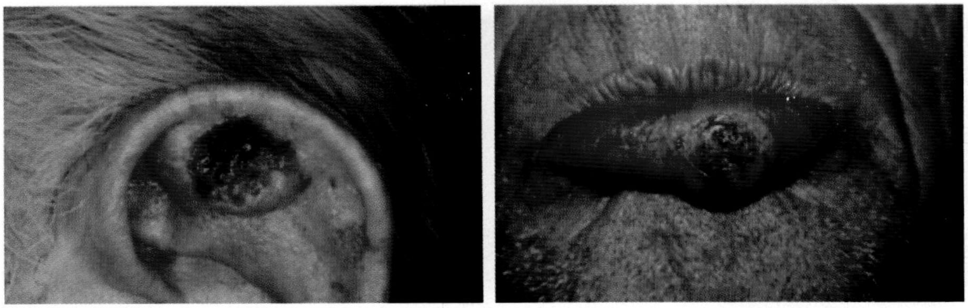

FIGURE 65–5 The clinical appearance of invasive squamous cell carcinoma.

or sun exposure. SCC, when sun related, is almost always located on the lower lip. Approximately 90% of the carcinomas of the lip occur on the lower lip. These lesions usually appear as a single nodule or an ulceration. The surrounding skin often exhibits extensive actinic cheilitis: in situ dysplasia of the lip skin. SCC of the lip is more dangerous than when it arises on the skin, as rapid invasion and metastasis more often occur.

The risk of metastasis is a function of the tumor size, extent of invasion, and degree of differentiation of the cancer cells. Clearly, anaplastic and poorly differentiated tumors are the most worrisome. This is often and most commonly seen when the tumors arise in chronic sinus tracts, burn scars, or in sites of radiation damage.

Clinical Manifestations of Basal Cell Carcinoma

BCC of the skin arises, as the name implies, from the basal layer of the epidermis. The cells are large and hyperchromatic. BCC can often arise at the base of epidermal appendages such as hair follicles. This can permit deep extension of the tumor. Although metastasis from BCC is very rare, deep extension by the cancer and destruction of surrounding tissues and organs (e.g., orbital invasion and perineural spread) can cause severe morbidity.

Clinical types of BCC include the following.

- Nodular BCC appears as an ulcerated pink, shiny nodule (Fig. 65-6). This is often referred to as the "rodent ulcer" appearance of BCC. Histologically, these tumors are composed of large islands of tumor cells, often with central necrosis.
- Superficial BCC appears as a simple red patch (Fig. 65-7). Occasionally it can be eroded and scaly and resemble Bowen's disease. Histologically, the tumor cells are confined to the epidermis.
- Micronodular BCC is often similar in appearance to nodular BCC; these tumors have a greater propensity for subclinical extension. Therefore the recurrence rate with standard modalities (destruction, excision, and radiotherapy) is high. Mohs micrographic surgery is often used to ensure complete extirpation of the tumor.
- Morpheaform or infiltrating BCC often appears as a flat white to pinkish patch (Fig. 65-8). This can be easily confused with a scar. Morpheaform BCC is associated with very widespread subclinical extension, often several centimeters beyond the clinical edge of the skin lesion. Histologically, multiple fine nests of basaloid cells often track in an "indian file" pattern of chords within a dense fibrotic stroma.
- Metatypical BCCs have clinical features and the biologic behavior somewhere between BCC and SCC. Histologically, both basaloid cells and keratin pearls can be admixed. These tumors are often best described as BCC with features of SCC.

Therapy

The treatment of SCC and BCC is quite variable. Multiple factors, including size, prior treatment, anatomic location, and depth of invasion must be considered. The treatment modalities encompass surgical excision (conventional and

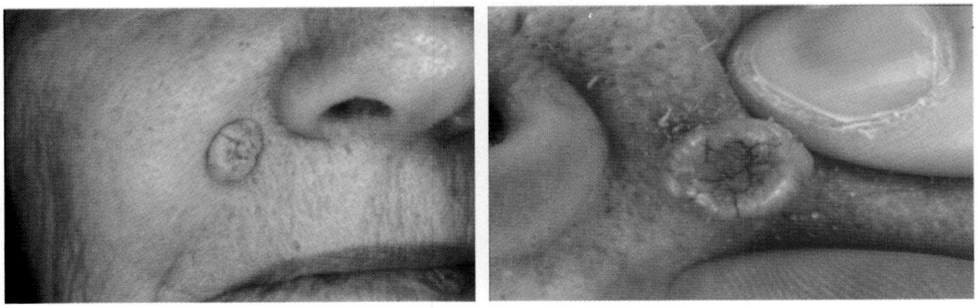

FIGURE 65–6 Nodular basal cell carcinoma.

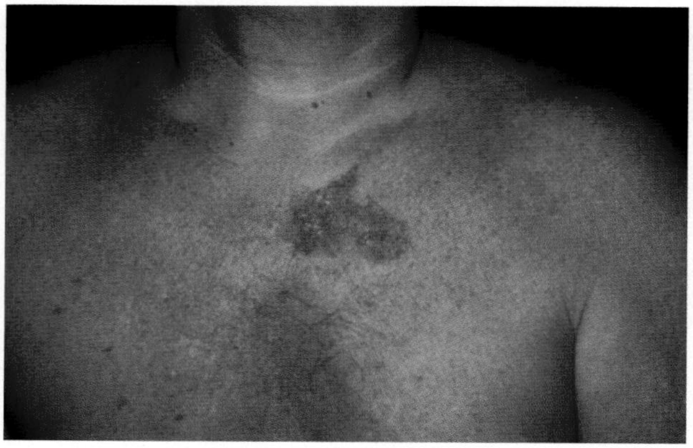

FIGURE 65–7 Superficial basal cell carcinoma.

Mohs technique), radiation therapy, and a destructive modality (cryotherapy or electrodessication and curettage).

Before any decision making regarding treatment of these lesions, a careful examination of the regional adjoining lymph nodes is essential. The presence of metastasis will clearly alter the treatment plan. The most common site of metastasis of SCC is first to the regional adjoining lymph nodes, followed by metastasis to the lung.

The histology of the tumor must be considered before embarking on any therapeutic modality. For the most part, intraepidermal (in situ carcinomas) can be readily managed by means of a destructive modality. This includes electrosurgery, simple curettage, or cryosurgery.

Invasive SCC or BCC is ideally managed by surgical excision either by conventional excision with permanent sections, excision with frozen sections, or by means of Mohs micrographic technique.

PEARLS FOR ROUNDS

Skin cancer is the most common cancer in America. Annualized, more than one person an hour dies of skin cancer in the United States each year.

More skin cancers are diagnosed in the United States each year than all other cancers of all anatomic sites combined

Of patients diagnosed with a skin cancer, in 40%, a second, unrelated skin cancer will develop within the next 5 years.

Mohs surgery is the treatment of choice for nonmelanoma skin cancers in cosmetically sensitive areas, for which other therapies (e.g., standard excision) have failed, that have aggressive histologies (e.g., morpheaform), or that have a high risk of metastasis.

The ABCDs of melanoma stand for **a**symmetry, **b**order irregularity, changing **c**olor or two or more colors, and large or changing **d**iameter.

Ester anesthetics should not be used in patients with allergies to PAST: **pa**ra-aminobenzoic acid, **s**ulfur drugs, and **t**hiazide diuretics.

Amide anesthetics (bupivacaine, mepivacaine) have an "i" before "-caine."

Concave areas (such as alar groove, medial canthus) heal well by secondary intention. The scalp, which is convex, also heals well by secondary intention and is the exception to this rule.

Mohs micrographic surgery is usually reserved for tumors with aggressive histologic features, recurrent tumors, or those located in critical anatomic sites on the central face. The technique was originally described by Fredrick Mohs, MD, a general surgeon at the University of Wisconsin in Madison. It entails removal of the tumor with precise margin control to ensure complete extirpation of the malignancy.

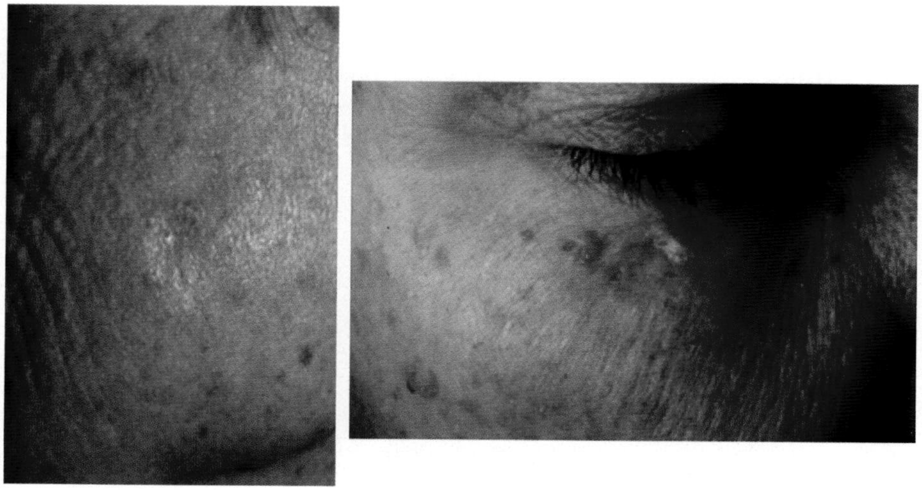

FIGURE 65–8 Metatypical basal cell carcinoma.

Compared with conventional frozen or permanent sections, which examine less than 1% of the true surgical margin, Mohs surgery examines 100% of the resection margins.

Originally described in the 1950s, the technique involved a chemical fixative applied to the tumor and peritumoral tissues on the patient (fixed tissue technique). The tissue was then resected and the margins analyzed. If residual tumor was identified, the precise mapping technique permitted localization of the tumor "roots," and additional tissue was resected and analyzed. This was continued (additional stages) until all residual cancer cells were successfully removed. Today, the fixed tissue technique is rarely used. Instead, the fresh tissue technique is used. This entails resection of the cancer without the fixative paste being applied to the skin. The tumor is excised with conventional surgical technique, by using extremely conservative margins (often less than 1 mm). The excised tissue is processed, in a manner analogous to that of frozen sections, by specially trained technicians to permit histologic examination of 100% of the resection margins. If residual tumor is identified, the area of tumor extension is marked on a "map" that corresponds to the surgical wound and additional tissue in that area is resected. The cycle then repeats. Multiple stages are often required to resect the cancer. Once the malignancy is fully resected, reconstructive surgery of the wound can commence if necessary. The entire Mohs procedure and reconstruction are usually accomplished in one sitting under local anesthesia.

Radiation therapy is best reserved for three circumstances: (1) large lesions that cannot be surgically resected, (2) for use in patients who cannot undergo surgery, and (3) an adjunct to surgical care.

Malignant Melanoma

Malignant melanoma is one of the most serious health problems in the United States today. The incidence of melanoma is increasing faster than that of any other cancer, with the exception of lung cancer in young women. Patients are commonly worried about pigmented lesions on the skin, and this is an increasing component of the physician's daily practice. For this reason, it is critical that the practicing physician be competent in the early recognition of melanoma, its diagnosis, and its treatment.

Multiple possible reasons can be found for the increasing incidence of melanoma. Most commonly, it is thought to be due to the increased incidence of sun exposure on a recreational basis. Unlike that of BCC and SCC, the etiology of melanoma may be more closely tied to blistering and peeling sunburns during adolescence. SCC and BCC are most commonly thought to be related to the total amount of lifetime sun exposure. Therefore whereas SCC and BCC have their peak incidence after age 60 years, malignant melanoma often strikes individuals in their most productive years of life: in their 30s, 40s, and 50s.

Epidemiology

Melanoma currently represents 1% of all cancers by incidence (excluding nonmelanoma skin cancer). The overall incidence in the United States is 4.5 per 100,000 population per year in whites and 0.6 per 100,000 in dark-skinned races. The sex ratio is roughly even. The incidence of melanoma is dependent on latitude: The northern United States, as assessed by the Detroit Cancer Center, has an incidence of 3.1 per 100,000 population, whereas in the southern United States (Dallas), the incidence is 7.2.

The improving prognosis associated with melanoma is likely due to earlier detection rather than to improvements in treatment modalities. In terms of anatomic distribution, the most frequent site of melanoma in male patients is on the back, followed by chest and upper extremities. In female patients, the most common incidence is on the lower extremities, followed by the back, upper extremities, and head and neck. The most frequent site of melanoma in blacks and Asians is on the soles, followed by mucous membranes, palms, and nail beds.

Methods for Early Recognition of Melanoma

Clinical Presentation and Evaluation. The early recognition of melanoma is critical in terms of maximizing the patient's prognosis. A four-step approach to the early recognition of melanoma, loosely described as the ABCDs, has been provided by the American Academy of Dermatology. Although no feature by itself can diagnose a melanoma, when taken together, a lesion exhibiting these features should be sampled by biopsy (Figs. 65-9 and 65-10).

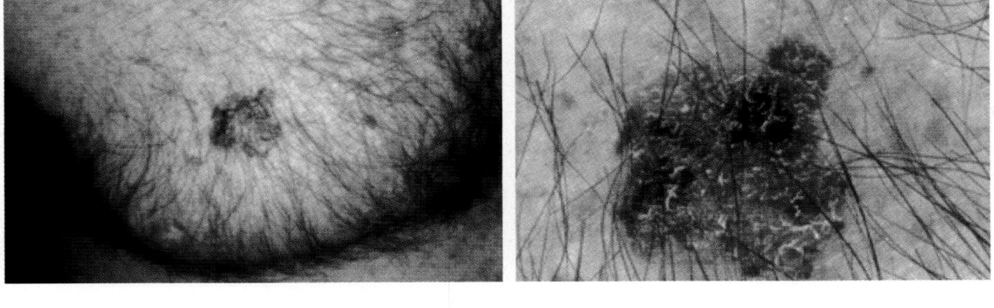

FIGURE 65–9 These melanoma lesions are asymmetrical and exhibit irregular borders.

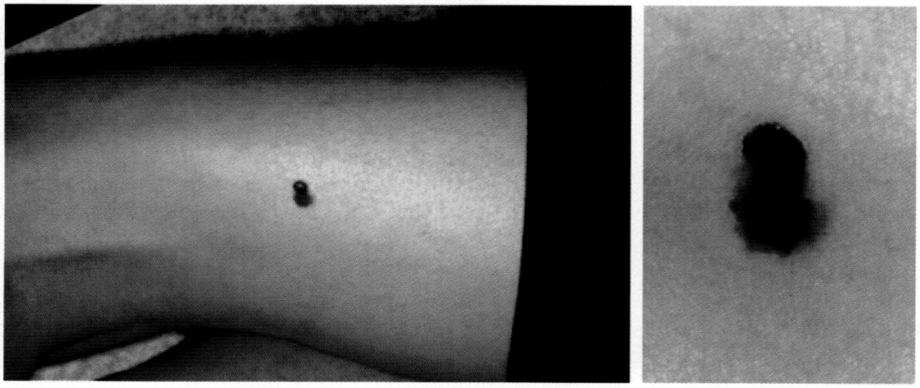

FIGURE 65-10 Color changes of melanoma.

- **A** stands for asymmetry. If the lesion cannot be bisected with both halves having similar morphology, the lesion is defined as asymmetrical.
- **B** stands for border irregularity. If the borders of the lesion are notched, variegated, or have a bleeding of pigment into the surrounding skin, this would be considered border irregularity.
- **C** stands for color. Play of color is critical in the early recognition of melanoma. Although the classic color changes ascribed to melanoma are red, white, and blue, the early recognition of melanoma is more critical with subtle nuances of color, such as variegation in hues of brown, black, and fawn color. The play of color of the lesion is one of the most critical features in the early diagnosis of melanoma.
- **D** stands for diameter. In general, if the lesion is larger than the diameter of a pencil eraser, it is worthy of being considered for biopsy. Although melanoma often can start very small, 6 mm is thought to be the threshold at which a pathological diagnosis can be rendered.

The ABCDs taken together are most important in the early diagnosis of melanoma. In addition, a mole that has changed morphology over a period of time increases the probability of its being melanoma. Several newer technologies are being developed with digital imaging to better assess changing moles over time.

Dysplastic and Congenital Pigmented Lesions. It is believed that any melanocyte has the potential for malignant conversion. However, controversy exists on the risk of conversion of congenital nevi and dysplastic nevi into melanoma.

Dr. Wallace Clark first described dysplastic nevi in the 1970s in kindred of families with a high incidence of melanoma. Much controversy ensued when Dr. Clark described these moles as being "dysplastic" (originally called *BK moles*), as the definition of dysplasia can be misleading. The most recent data suggest that the dysplastic nevus syndrome can be divided into two categories: sporadic and familial. Several investigators have shown convincing data that patients with sporadic dysplastic nevi may have a no higher risk for melanoma than the average population. However, patients with the familial dysplastic nevus syndrome, now referred to as the *familial atypical mole and melanoma syndrome*, may have a several hundred–fold higher risk of developing melanoma at one point in their lifetimes. These patients often have hundreds of atypical moles scattered on the trunk and proximal extremities.

Much work must be done to better ascertain the risk of malignant conversion in patients with dysplastic nevi, as it is thought that almost one third of the U.S. population has at least one mole that could be classified as dysplastic.

Congenital nevi are defined as moles present at birth. The incidence of congenital nevi is thought to be between 0.6% and 1.2% of the U.S. population. Although it is well known that the risk of melanoma developing in a large congenital nevus may approach 6%, the data on small congenital nevi, those smaller than 1.5 cm in diameter, are far less convincing. Several investigators argue that the risk of malignant conversion of small congenital nevi is no larger than that in the average population. Other data indicate that a slightly higher incidence of malignant conversion may occur in small congenital nevi as well.

The problem with treating congenital nevi is that large lesions can be deeply invested in the underlying muscle. When they arise on the back, they can extend into the spinal canal. Therefore it is sometimes impossible to resect fully a giant congenital nevus. The management of patients with these lesions is often best handled by a center that specializes in the treatment of pigmented lesions. The decision to resect such a lesion must weigh factors such as ease of observation for change, cosmetic disfigurement, and psychological factors such as anxiety in the patient and family members.

Treatment of Cutaneous Melanoma

The diagnosis of melanoma is made by histopathologic interpretation of the excised specimen. When a patient is first seen with a pigmented skin lesion that is suggestive of melanoma, a biopsy should not be delayed and must be performed in the office setting as soon as possible. Ideally, the biopsy of a suggestive lesion should remove the entire clinical lesion but only a minimal amount of the surrounding healthy tissues. Many problems have arisen when the surgeon, in an attempt to provide both diagnosis and cure, has attempted to resect widely a pigmented lesion suggestive of melanoma. In some cases, large disfiguring scars have been created in lesions that turned out not to be melanoma; in other settings, the operation revealed melanoma but the resection margins were insufficient based on the tumor histopathology. It is therefore best to separate the biopsy procedure from the definitive treatment.

The definitive treatment should be performed only after the appropriate diagnostic tests have been completed. When the physician is presented with a patient with a suggestive pigmented lesion, an excisional biopsy (with 1- to 2-mm margins) is the ideal specimen for diagnosis. Shave biopsies and curettings can often cut through the tumor and interfere with correct prognostic interpretation. Ideally, the long axis of the excisional biopsy should be parallel to lymphatic drainage. This will simplify the therapeutic resection should the lesion indeed reveal melanoma. Once the diagnosis of melanoma has been established, it is important to evaluate the patient for evidence of metastasis by both physical examination and a limited panel of diagnostic tests. Furthermore, because melanoma can have a familial pattern, all first-degree relatives of the patient newly diagnosed with melanoma should be examined.

A thorough physical examination should be performed on the patient with melanoma. Special attention should be paid to the regional draining lymph nodes, as in excess of 50% of patients who have metastases will have their first site of metastasis as the regional draining lymph node. The order of frequency of metastasis beyond the draining lymph nodes includes lungs, followed by brain and liver metastases.

The use of laboratory testing for aiding in melanoma staging also is controversial. In general, the level of staging of diagnostic testing should be tied to the probability of discovering metastatic disease. In general, a chest radiograph and serum lactate dehydrogenase (LDH) are sufficient for patients with tumors of intermediate risk. Clearly, patients with high risk for metastases may benefit from a head magnetic resonance imaging (MRI), chest computed tomography (CT), and serum LDH and creatine phosphokinase. Nuclear medicine scans have not been found to be helpful in the laboratory evaluation of patients with melanoma.

The primary means of treating malignant melanoma is surgical resection. A National Institutes of Health consensus conference was held to determine the appropriate resection margins for different stages of melanoma disease. In general, most surgical resections for melanoma can be performed under local anesthesia in an outpatient setting. For in situ tumors (Clark level I), surgical resection with a 5-mm margin of healthy tissue down to the subcutaneous fat is sufficient. Tumors that invade up to 2 mm in depth should be resected with a 1-cm margin of healthy tissue down to but not including the underlying muscular fascia. Tumors greater than 2 mm in depth should be resected with a 2-cm margin of healthy surrounding tissue down to the underlying muscular fascia.

The use of Mohs micrographic surgery for melanoma is currently in an investigational stage. The advantages of applying the Mohs technique would be to provide an improved local recurrence rate and to do so in a tissue-conserving manner. For this reason, Mohs should be considered only when the tumor is in a critical anatomic site (e.g., nose, eyelid, or lip). In these cases, the resection margin can often be reduced to 3 to 6 mm.

In patients who have tumors between 1 and 4 mm in thickness, sentinel node biopsy is rapidly being accepted into medical practice. This technique is replacing elective regional lymph node dissection as the first-line management for those patients. The technique allows the surgeon to map precisely the regional draining lymphatics with a nuclear medicine scan. Radioactive technetium colloid is injected around the biopsy site. The regional lymphatics are mapped out, and, often under local anesthetic, the first draining node (i.e., the sentinel node) can be mapped. It is then a relatively simple and straightforward task to excise this one lymph node. If this node is free of tumor, the patient can be spared a full elective lymph node dissection. In the event that the tumor has, in a microscopic manner, invaded this sentinel node, the patient is then an ideal candidate for therapeutic lymph node dissection of the entire basin. The sentinel node technique is a diagnostic and staging method to determine better which patients would benefit from removal of the regional draining lymphatics and undergo adjuvant immunotherapy.

Unfortunately, once melanoma has spread beyond the skin and regional lymph nodes, the prognosis becomes far more dire. In general, resection of lung and brain metastases does not improve survival. The overall survival for a patient with a lung or brain metastasis is usually less than 6 months, regardless of therapeutic intervention. Great progress has now been made in terms of melanoma vaccines to treat patients with metastatic disease, as has biochemotherapy with the spectrum of interferons and interleukins.

Finally, it is important to reiterate that early detection and early surgical treatment are the mainstays of treatment for this disease.

Merkel Cell Carcinoma

Merkel cell carcinoma (MCC) is a rare and potentially aggressive neuroendocrine cancer of skin. The tumor usually arises within the dermis and has been shown to have immunohistochemical markers of neuroepithelial differentiation. MCCs most commonly arise on the head and neck region, followed by upper and lower limbs, but in some reports, they have been found in the nasal mucosa, lips, and vulvar region. Wide local resection with 3-cm margins and adjuvant radiotherapy is often recommended in patients with MCC. However, recently, Mohs surgery has been shown to result in better local control than excision (31.7% vs. 8.13%).

Dermatofibrosarcoma Protuberans

Dermatofibrosarcoma protuberans consists of large nodular lesions located mainly on the trunk and typically diagnosed in 30- to 50-year-old individuals. The nodular lesions become more painful as they enlarge and often ulcerate and become infected. Histologically the lesions contain atypical spindle cells, probably of fibroblast origin, located around a core of collagen tissue. Immunohistochemical stain of some reveals CD34 expression. Because of local recurrences, complete surgical excision is recommended and is generally curative. However, a study from Lisbon, Portugal, showed no difference in the recurrence rates between a group that underwent surgical excision and a group that underwent Mohs micrographic surgery.

Lentigo Maligna Melanoma

Lentigo maligna (LM) and lentigo malignant melanoma are the slowest-growing forms of malignant melanoma and have the least potential to metastasize. LM usually begins as a flat, tan or brown, irregularly shaped patch on the face of elderly patients. Both normal and malignant melanocytes are present, and the patch usually expands slowly over the course of years within the epidermis (LM) before it invades the dermis (lentigo maligna melanoma). Standard excision margins are often inadequate for LM. In light of this, as well as of the fact that LMs often occur on cosmetically sensitive areas (i.e., the face), efforts have been made to use Mohs micrographic surgery to ensure clean margins with maximal tissue conservation.

Aesthetic Surgery of the Skin

Laser Surgery of the Skin

The development of laser technology has revolutionized the treatment of vascular lesions, pigmented lesions, actinically damaged skin, and even hypertrichosis and hirsuitism. The word "laser" is an acronym that stands for *light amplification by stimulated emission of radiation*

Laser Physics and Tissue Interaction

Laser light has four properties that give it unopposed advantages in dermatologic surgery. First, it has a uniquely uniform wavelength, as determined by the lasing medium within the machine. Second, it is coherent (i.e., the waves of light are in phase in both time and space). Third, the light is collimated (i.e., focused to travel across long distances with little dissipation or spreading. Finally, the light beam can be of extremely high energy.

Chromophores are agents within the skin that absorb certain wavelengths of light. Knowing the peak absorbances of different chromophores (e.g., melanin) allows targeting of discrete skin elements without damaging others.

Laser Treatment of Vascular Lesions

The peak absorbance of hemoglobin is associated with a yellow-light wavelength of 585 to 595 nm, thereby making pulsed-dye laser (595 nm) an excellent modality for treating vascular lesions.

Epidermal cooling with a cryogen spray before each pulse or water-cooled devices makes the procedure more comfortable and minimizes the damage to the epidermis, reducing the chance of blistering and hypo- or hyperpigmentation. For most lesions, especially those that require multiple treatments for resolution, laser leaves the patient with purpura, which persists for 4 to 14 days. Darker-skinned patients also risk temporary hypopigmentation, as much of the light energy also can be absorbed by the pigment lying over blood vessels.

For patients with facial telangiectasias, the krypton, copper bromide, and potassium-titanyl-phosphate (KTP) lasers also are available. These modalities all have a rapid train of pulses that allows the physician to trace along the target vessel. Success and adverse effects are dependent on technique; however, purpura associated with pulsed-dye laser is generally minimal to nonexistent.

Pigmented Lesion Lasers and Tattoo Treatment

The peak absorbance of melanin occurs at wavelengths of more than 600 nm, making the 694-nm ruby or 755-nm alexandrite lasers best for targeting pigmented lesions and tattoo pigment. In 1987, the Q-switched ruby laser with a high rate of energy delivery with a short pulse duration (delivering megawatt and gigawatt intensities within nanoseconds) demonstrated selective destruction of melanosomes and tattoo particles, which are spared by longer pulse durations. Pigment that resides in the dermis, such as the darkening within some surgical or traumatic scars, is often too deep to be destroyed effectively by the lasers available today. Unable to differentiate between lesional and constitutive (baseline normal for an individual) pigment, laser causes temporary hypopigmentation until natural turnover of the sloughed pigmented skin cells.

It is imperative to assess clinically, and if necessary histologically, any pigmented lesion before subjecting it to a laser treatment. Benign lentigines (age or sun spots) or ephelides (freckles) are frequent targets of these lasers, and some of these may actually be premalignant or malignant lesions, LM and lentigo maligna melanoma, respectively. In addition to lentigines and ephelides, café-au-lait spots, nevus spilus, Becker's nevi, as well as the deeper pigment of nevus of Ito and Ota can be significantly cleared by the ruby or alexandrite laser.

In terms of tattoo removal, amateur tattoos respond best to treatment, whereas professional tattoos are more difficult to eradicate. Black and dark blue inks have the best resolution. Those with red, yellow, light blue, and green colors occasionally cannot be removed completely. Side effects of tattoo treatment include texture changes, hyper or hypopigmentation, and, rarely, scarring.

Laser Hair Removal

With the advent of lasers specifically designed for hair removal, many follicles can be targeted simultaneously without the risk of an invasive needle stick necessitated by electrolysis. Multiple treatments are necessary, as only a percentage of hairs at any given time are in the anagen (growth) phase, a phase during which hairs are most amenable to destruction by laser.

Melanin in the hair itself is the target for hair-removal lasers. Thus the best candidates have light skin color and dark hair color to avoid competing epidermal pigment. Patients of Mediterranean, Middle Eastern, Hispanic, and Asian descent can often be successfully treated, but blondes are not candidates for laser hair removal. Patients with a tan have an increased incidence of side effects.

Long pulse durations are used to allow slow heat build-up within the hair follicles while sparing destruction of the smaller melanosomes. Epidermal cooling assists in sparing the skin from blistering and hyper- or hypopigmentation. No infections, scarring, or long-term complications occurred in 900 patients treated with three laser hair-removal systems over a period of 2 years, as reported by Nanni and Alster. However, the long-term efficacy of the available laser hair-removal systems will be better understood as longer follow-up data become available.

Cosmetic Laser Resurfacing

The development of pulsed or scanned CO_2 lasers now allows photodamaged skin to be removed in a more precise manner. Water in the skin absorbs energy in the infrared spectrum; thus the erbium:YAG (2940 nm) and CO_2 lasers (10,600 nm) are used for skin resurfacing. Water absorbs this energy, leading to vaporization of tissue fluid with debris left behind. Beneath the zone of vaporization, a zone of thermal damage may later slough.

Also when the superficial dermis and epithelium regenerate, a more youthful appearance is achieved, with decreased numbers and depths of rhytids (wrinkles). Acne, some surgical scars, and fine-to-deep wrinkles may significantly improve. Perioral and periocular regions as well as sagging skin folds on the cheeks respond well, whereas lines resulting from muscle motion (e.g., forehead or glabellar furrows and the nasolabial fold) tend to reform on repeated muscle motion. Isolated areas such as the perioral area or cheeks are best treated with local anesthesia, including nerve blocks and topical preparations. Full-face treatment is often conducted under intravenous sedation or general anesthesia.

With the use of CO_2 laser, usually a 1- to 2-week period is required for re-epithelialization, while skin is weeping and crusted, and 4 to 6 weeks of bright erythema. Possible adverse sequelae include hyper- and hypopigmentation, infections, prolonged erythema, and scarring. The risk of scarring and keloid formation is greatly increased if the patient has had oral isotretinoin treatment for acne within a year of resurfacing.

With the erbium:YAG laser, the recuperation time is decreased because it ablates thinner layers of tissue without the underlying thermal damage; however, this prevents efficient capillary coagulation, leading to a bloodier field, and prevents some of the collagen injury and subsequent tightening. The erbium:YAG is thus a better modality for treating finer lines and photodamage. It is often used to feather out areas adjacent to CO_2 laser–treated skin.

All patients should receive prophylaxis against herpes simplex virus, and some physicians routinely prescribe pre- and postoperative oral antibiotics. Prompt attention to any complications may avert permanent disfigurement.

Changes in technology are rapid within the laser industry; thus new methods of treatment that are more efficacious, safe, and cost-effective are emerging all the time. However, new technology is never a replacement for the excellent hands-on training and judgment required to operate these machines and treat patients safely.

Botulinum Toxin

BOTOX is botulinum toxin, a purified neurotoxin complex produced from fermentation of *Clostridium botulinum*. In 1992, dermatologist Alastair Caruthers and his wife, J. Caruthers (ophthalmologist), were the first to introduce and study the cosmetic use of botulinum toxin. Since then, BOTOX has been shown to be safe and effective in treating rhytids caused by facial expressions. It has now gained popularity and is widely used by dermatologic surgeons in combination with other cosmetic procedures.

Botulinum toxin blocks neuromuscular transmission by binding to receptor sites on motor nerve terminals, entering the nerve terminals, and inhibiting the release of acetylcholine. A botulinum toxin injection produces partial chemical denervation of the muscle, resulting in a decreased response in muscle to facial mimicking. Some reinnervation of the muscle may occur, thus slowly reversing the effect of BOTOX injection. The injections are therefore indicated for the temporary improvement in the appearance of moderate to severe glabellar lines in adults and are of more benefit in patients age 65 years or younger.

In 1997, Schnider and colleagues introduced the use of BOTOX in treating focal axillary and palmar hyperhidrosis. BOTOX is postulated to cause chemical denervation of the apocrine sweat glands, blocking stress-induced and spontaneous discharge of the glands.

PEARLS FOR THE OR

Before infiltrating the surgical area with anesthesia, mark out the skin-tension lines and cosmetic units of the face.

When injecting local anesthesia, direct the needle into areas that are already anesthetized, and then advance the needle in the subcutis to the area that must be anesthetized.

When suturing on a scalp with dark brown/black hair, use polypropylene (Prolene) suture, which is blue, rather than nylon sutures, and leave long tails. This will make it easier to find and remove the stitches on the day of suture removal.

When suturing a flap in place, do not put many deep stitches at the tip of the flap. This can strangulate this critical area of the flap and lead to tip necrosis.

When sewing a graft/flap in a difficult-to-reach location (e.g., conchal bowl), consider using dissolvable sutures to spare the patient and staff from trying to remove the sutures later on.

An elliptical excision should have a 3:1 ratio of the long axis to the short axis and apex angles of 30 degrees.

Tension on the wound edges is the number one killer of flaps (flap necrosis).

BOTOX injections are contraindicated in individuals with known hypersensitivity to any ingredient in the formulation or in those with a neuromuscular disorder. These groups of patients are at increased risk for significant systemic effects such as dysphagia, respiratory compromise, and sudden death. Because of the possibility of development of immunogenicity to BOTOX, it is recommended that the injections occur at intervals no less than every 3 months. As always, careful screening of patients for the procedure and use of correct technique of administration decrease the chances of side effects and yield the best results.

Liposuction

Suction lipectomy has its origins in the 1970s work of the Fischers in Italy and Ilouz and Fournier in France and is now the most commonly performed cosmetic surgical procedure, with almost 300,000 cases performed in 1996 alone. The majority of these procedures are performed in surgical centers or office-based operating suites; only a minority are performed in a hospital-based setting.

Use of "tumescent anesthesia" in 1980s (i.e., infusion of a large volume of dilute lidocaine and epinephrine into a fatty compartment until a swelling or tumescence was achieved) has decreased blood loss, bruising, and postoperative soreness while allowing greater surgical accuracy and minimizing postsurgical irregularities and the need for intravenous sedation or general anesthesia.

Electric vacuum suction pumps attached to liposuction cannulas are often used for the procedure. Cannulas are available with a huge variety of aperture styles, tip shapes, lengths, widths, and composition. Good technique is imperative in obtaining a smooth result. Preoperative photographs are invaluable in monitoring the patient after surgery and as a reference during the surgical procedure.

Preoperatively patients are evaluated for general health, history of weight gain and loss, surgical history and bleeding disorders, medications, and their goals in seeking liposuction. Obese individuals are generally poor candidates for liposuction, unless they have discrete objectives. Patients must be informed that liposuction is a means not of weight loss but of body contouring. Diet and exercise are imperative to maintain results. Patients should be warned that cellulite texture will likely not improve with surgery.

Far more common than serious adverse medical sequelae are aesthetic complications. Asymmetry and irregular skin contour may be minimized by good technique and the use of the thinner cannulas made possible by the tumescent technique. In the interest of managing patient expectations, it is re-emphasized that results from liposuction are not fully appreciated until 6 months after the procedure. This allows time for full skin contracture, softening of induration in the treatment areas, resolution of residual numbness in overlying skin, and fading of scars at incision sites. At the 6-month follow-up, any areas of asymmetry, irregularity, or incomplete contour correction can be identified and discussed, and a touch-up procedure planned if necessary.

Dermabrasion

The abrasive technique for removal of superficially lying lesions was first introduced by Kromayer in 1930. Since then, it has been used for removal of rhynophyma, shallow acne scars, and fine rhytids. Dermabrasion is performed by manual operation of a high-speed rotary drill on a handheld power tool that abrades and removes skin-surface irregularities. The area to be treated is cooled first with ice packs and then frozen with a dichlorotetrafluoroethane (Freon) stream. Care should be taken to protect the eyes and the hair of the patient. Dermabraded skin heals as a superficial partial-thickness burn. The wound is left open and treated with an antibiotic ointment. Although infections are rare, herpes simplex virus infections of abraded area have been reported, and so acyclovir prophylaxis is now recommended to prevent compromise of the procedure. Because pigmentary changes and mild irritation may occur, it is preferable to limit sunlight exposure for several months and cosmetics for several weeks after the procedure to minimize these risks.

Acknowledgment: We thank Daniel Loo, MD, Professor of Dermatology, Boston University School of Medicine, Boston, Massachusetts, for providing all of the figures for this chapter.

Suggested Reading

Caruthers A, Caruthers JA: Treatment of glabellar frown lines with *C. botulinum*-A exotoxin. J Dermatol Surg Oncol 18:17–21, 1992.

Do D, Krejci-Papa N, Rogers GS: Surgical excision for skin cancer. In Rigel D, Friedman R, Dzubow L (eds): Cancer of the Skin. Philadelphia, Elsevier, 2005.

Holmkvist KA, Rogers GS: Treatment of perioral rhytides: A comparison of dermabrasion and superpulsed carbon dioxide laser. Arch Dermatol 136(6):725–731, 2000.

Jackson T: Local Flaps in Head and Neck Reconstruction. St. Louis, Quality Medical Publishing, 2002.

Salasche S, Bernstein G, Senkarik M: Surgical Anatomy of the Skin. Norwalk, Conn, Appleton & Lange, 1998.

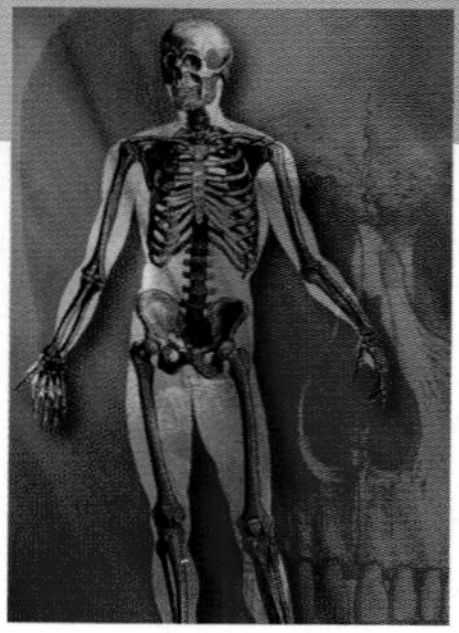

Chapter 66

Minimal-Access Surgery

NATHANIEL J. SOPER, MD, and VALERIE J. HALPIN, MD

Applications for Minimal-Access Surgery

The terms *minimal-access surgery and minimally invasive surgery* refer to operations in which the incisions are much smaller than those involved in traditional ("open") surgery and in which video endoscopic imaging techniques are commonly used.

Laparoscopic techniques were first described as early as 1901. The modern era of minimally invasive surgery began in the 1980s, with the introduction of the miniature video camera and transmitting equipment that allowed an entire operating team to view surgical procedures on a video screen. Since the introduction of laparoscopic cholecystectomy in the 1980s, this technique has become the gold standard for treating symptomatic cholelithiasis. Other laparoscopic procedures are now being performed with increasing frequency, and many minimal-access techniques are undergoing scrutiny in prospective randomized trials. As new technology has continued to evolve and find additional applications, surgeons and patients alike have rapidly embraced it because its use is generally associated with shorter hospitalizations, less postoperative pain, faster recuperation, and decreased costs.

Diagnostic Laparoscopy

Laparoscopy is becoming an increasingly valuable tool for evaluating a variety of intraabdominal and other disorders.

Elective applications include the assessment of chronic abdominal pain, abdominal masses, liver disease, ascites, inguinal hernias, and ventral hernias. Laparoscopy is frequently useful in the diagnosis and staging of malignant neoplasms. The magnified view can often identify small metastatic peritoneal implants that cannot be detected by computed tomography, magnetic resonance imaging, or ultrasonography. It also can help assess tumor response to neoadjuvant chemotherapy or radiation therapy. In some cases, laparoscopy can replace "second-look" laparotomy.

Emergency applications of laparoscopy include the evaluation of acute abdominal pain and peritonitis. Diagnostic laparoscopy is especially useful in assessing acute abdominal pain in young women, whose gynecologic problems are frequently confused with acute appendicitis. In these women, the procedure has been estimated to reduce the rate of unnecessary laparotomies by one third. In medically compromised patients in intensive care settings, laparoscopy can be used to exclude acute biliary tract disease or ischemic bowel disease and thereby avoid nontherapeutic laparotomies. In some medical centers, laparoscopy has occasionally been used to evaluate tangential gunshot wounds and stab wounds to the abdomen; however, this use remains controversial, because the introduction of air into the peritoneal cavity may lead to severe hypotension in the presence of hypovolemia.

Therapeutic Laparoscopy

As mentioned earlier, **laparoscopic cholecystectomy** is now considered the gold standard for removing a diseased gallbladder. While the patient is undergoing this procedure, the common bile duct also can be explored and assessed. **Laparoscopic tubal ligation** is another well-accepted minimally invasive procedure.

Laparoscopic appendectomy is less well accepted than laparoscopic cholecystectomy, because it may not be more cost-effective or less painful than a standard appendectomy. However, laparoscopic appendectomy does have a place in the armamentarium of the general surgeon and is particularly appropriate for patients who are obese, women of childbearing age, and patients whose diagnosis is unclear.

Laparoscopic inguinal herniorrhaphy, which can be performed transabdominally or by using totally extraperitoneal access to place prosthetic mesh in the preperitoneal space, has ardent enthusiasts and opponents. The procedure seems ideally suited for patients with bilateral or recurrent hernias.

In patients with gastroesophageal reflux disease (GERD), studies have shown that open Nissen fundoplication is more effective than medical management. Although few patients are willing to undergo a major open abdominal or thoracic operation for the treatment of GERD, many more have expressed their willingness to undergo **laparoscopic fundoplication** or **other laparoscopic antireflux procedures.** Initial reports indicate that laparoscopic fundoplication yields results similar to those of the open procedure, yet is associated with decreased postoperative pain and a shorter hospital stay. At this time, long-term studies are ongoing to verify the effectiveness of minimally invasive surgery for patients with GERD.

Laparoscopic colon resection in patients with benign colon disease has been reported to decrease the length of the hospital stay and shorten the duration of postoperative ileus but to cost about the same amount as open colectomy. Randomized trials are currently under way to assess the role of laparoscopic colectomy for the treatment of malignant disease. The largest U.S. trial recently showed laparoscopic-assisted colectomy to be as oncologically successful as open colectomy.

The surgical management of morbid obesity has rapidly expanded in the last decade with the introduction of **laparoscopic gastric bypass**. This procedure has been shown to reduce wound complications, decrease postoperative pain, and improve respiratory function, all resulting in shorter hospital stays and improved recovery. Weight loss is equivalent to that with the open procedure. Other restrictive bariatric procedures include **laparoscopic vertical banded gastroplasty** and **laparoscopic adjustable gastric banding**. These procedures are less technically challenging; however, they have not been shown to reliably produce the same degree of weight loss in the U.S. population.

The surgical removal of solid organs, including **laparoscopic splenectomy, laparoscopic adrenalectomy**, and **laparoscopic nephrectomy,** is becoming the standard of care at institutions where the expertise is available.

A variety of **other minimal-access procedures** are undergoing investigation. These include minimally invasive types of vagotomy, esophagocardiomyotomy, biliary bypass, saphenous vein harvest, pelvic lymph node dissection, salpingo-oophorectomy, hysterectomy, and bladder-neck suspension. Minimally invasive parathyroidectomy with directed single-gland exploration is now possible with the use of preoperative sestamibi scanning and intraoperative rapid parathyroid hormone assay. Anecdotal reports have reported pancreatic pseudocyst-gastrostomy, pancreatic resection, gastrectomy, rectal prolapse repair, thyroidectomy, hepatic resection, coronary artery bypass graft, and cardiac valve repair.

General Guidelines for Minimal-Access Surgery

Evaluation and Selection of Patients

Candidates for minimal-access surgery should undergo a thorough and careful preoperative history and evaluation, because they must be able to tolerate not only a laparoscopic procedure but also an open procedure if conversion to one becomes necessary.

As surgeons gain more experience, the **contraindications to laparoscopic surgery** are decreasing. The following remain absolute contraindications to laparoscopic abdominal procedures: advanced generalized peritonitis, hypovolemic shock, massive abdominal distention with clinical evidence of bowel obstruction, uncorrected coagulopathy, and inability of the patient to tolerate a formal laparotomy. Relative contraindications include prior abdominal or pelvic surgery, previous generalized peritonitis, obesity, advanced cardiopulmonary disease, and pregnancy.

Preoperative Management of Patients

In most patients undergoing elective abdominal surgery, general anesthesia is the anesthesia of choice, because it allows for the greatest control of ventilation and abdominal muscle relaxation.

Patients should be instructed to take nothing by mouth at least 8 hours before the procedure begins. Antibiotics and a histamine H_2-receptor antagonist are given by the intravenous route preoperatively. Compression stockings and sequential compression devices are applied to the lower extremities to prevent deep venous thrombosis. Consideration should be given to tube decompression of the stomach and bladder. A Foley catheter in the bladder may be appropriate for some procedures.

Choice of Equipment and Techniques

Laparoscopic operations require the presence of gas in the peritoneal cavity (pneumoperitoneum). Various gases can be used, and either a closed technique or an open technique can be used to create the pneumoperitoneum, as described later.

Currently, the vast majority of laparoscopic operations involve the insufflation of **carbon dioxide.** However, because of the potential for hypercapnia, acidosis, cardiac arrhythmias, and other detrimental effects caused by transperitoneal absorption of CO_2, other insufflating gases have been used experimentally for creating the pneumoperitoneum. These include **nitrous oxide, helium,** and **argon,** each of which has other potential drawbacks, such as combustibility, insolubility, or expense.

Any gas insufflated into the peritoneal cavity can affect the normal physiology by elevating the diaphragm or reducing venous return via compression of the vena cava. Thus some surgeons use miniaturized retracting devices to elevate the abdominal wall manually to create a working space. However, the devices are generally cumbersome, and the exposure is usually not as good as that afforded by creating a pneumoperitoneum.

A spring-loaded Veress needle (Fig. 66-1) and trocar are used in the closed technique for creating the pneumoperitoneum. Many instruments commonly used in open surgery have been modified to facilitate laparoscopic procedures. These include clip appliers, linear cutting staplers, argon-beam coagulators, and various monopolar and bipolar cautery devices. For coagulation and division of vascular pedicles and small vessels (vessels smaller than 4 mm), ultrasound energy may be used in the form of harmonic shears (LaparoSonic Coagulating Shears, Ethicon-

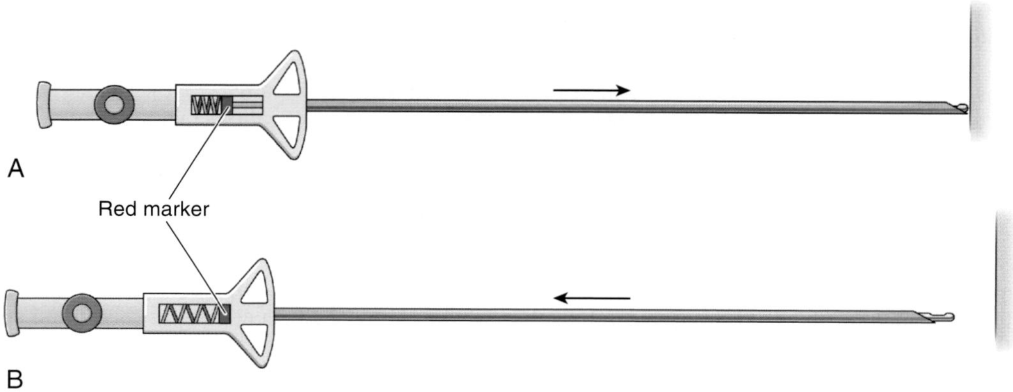

FIGURE 66–1 Testing the retractable tip of a disposable Veress needle. *A*, The blunt tip retracts as it contacts resistance (e.g., a knife handle or abdominal fascia). *B*, When the needle is pulled away from the point of resistance, the blunt tip springs forward and protrudes in front of the sharp edge of the needle. (Modified from Soper NJ, Odem RR, Clayman RV, McDougall EM (eds): Essentials of Laparoscopy. St. Louis, Quality Medical Publishing, 1994, with permission.)

Endosurgery, Inc., Cincinnati, OH). With any device transmitting potentially harmful energy into the closed space of a pneumoperitoneum, great care must be taken to prevent danger to surrounding tissues.

Procedures Involved in Abdominal Laparoscopic Operations

Creating a CO_2 Pneumoperitoneum and Initial Port

The initial step in laparoscopy is creation of a pneumoperitoneum. This can be done with a closed or open technique.

Closed Technique

The steps in the closed technique are as follows:

1. The Veress needle is carefully examined to ensure that the spring mechanism is intact (see Fig. 66-1) and that the lumen flushes easily.
2. The lower abdominal fascia is grasped and elevated to protect the intraabdominal organs. The Veress needle is inserted at a right angle to the abdominal wall, toward the pelvis, but angled away from the aortic bifurcation and the iliac vessels. The surgeon should hear two or three clicks as the needle passes through the fascia and the peritoneum.
3. The needle position is checked by aspiration with a syringe that is partially filled with saline solution. From 3 to 5 mL of the solution is injected into the needle. If blood, urine, or intestinal contents are aspirated, the needle should be removed and reinserted. If resistance is met, the syringe is most likely located in the abdominal muscle or the omentum and should be repositioned. If no resistance is met, the syringe is aspirated again. A drop test is performed by removing the plunger from the syringe and observing the saline meniscus. The saline solution should flow rapidly by gravity into the peritoneal cavity. Elevating the abdominal wall will create negative intraabdominal pressure and enhance the flow of the solution.
4. Once the surgeon is satisfied that the needle is in the proper location, the CO_2 line from the insufflator is attached to the needle for insufflation. The initial abdominal pressure should be less than 10 mmHg, and the abdomen should be slowly insufflated to a pressure between 10 and 15 mmHg. If the initial abdominal pressure is high, the Veress needle should be rotated to ensure that it is not abutting omentum, bowel, or abdominal wall. If the pressure remains high, the needle should be removed and reinserted. On insufflation, the abdomen should expand symmetrically and be tympanitic to percussion.
5. When the abdomen is distended with a pressure of 12 to 15 mmHg, the Veress needle is removed, and a trocar is inserted. To allow passage of the full circumference of the trocar sheath, a skin incision is made at an appropriate site (either at the umbilical crease or at another site, depending on the procedure).
6. While the abdominal wall is stabilized manually or by use of towel clips, the trocar is passed blindly into the abdomen, initially in the direction perpendicular to the skin and then in the direction of the operating field (Fig. 66-2).
7. After the sharp inner trocar enters the peritoneum, the trocar is removed, and the outer sheath is secured in place. This forms the first port.

Open Technique

In the open technique, the first port is placed into the peritoneal cavity under direct vision. This reduces the risks

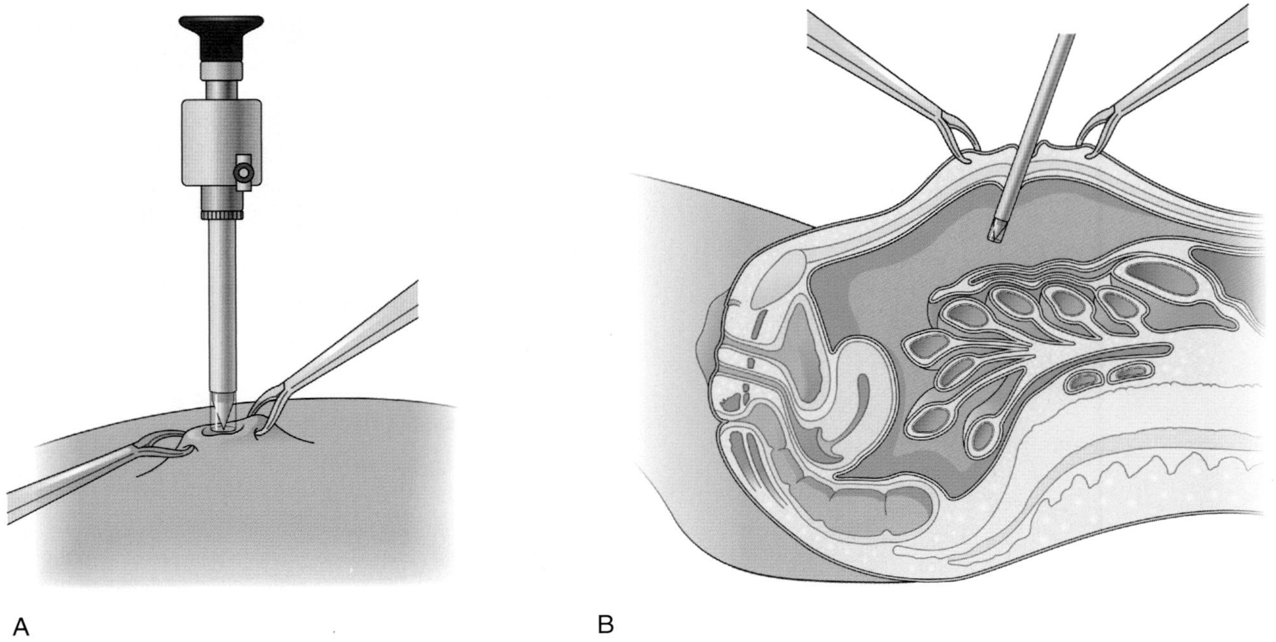

FIGURE 66–2 Trocar insertion. *A*, Towel clips placed near the edges of the umbilical incision are used to stabilize the abdominal wall during trocar insertion. *B*, Upward traction on the towel clips maintains the distance between the abdominal wall and the underlying structures during trocar insertion. (Modified from Jones DB, Wu JS, Soper NJ (eds): Laparoscopic Surgery: Principles and Procedures. St. Louis, Quality Medical Publishing, 1997, with permission.)

of blood vessel, bowel, and bladder injuries that are associated with the blind placement of the Veress needle and first trocar described in step 6. Many surgeons prefer to use the open technique routinely when the umbilicus is used for insertion of the initial port. It is particularly useful in patients with previous abdominal surgery, pregnancy, or evidence of bowel distention. The steps in the open technique are as follows:

1. The appropriate location for the incision is determined, and a 1.5- to 2.0-cm incision is made. The location depends on the procedure being performed. For laparoscopic cholecystectomy, the initial trocar is placed at the umbilical ring with either a vertical or a semicircular incision. In laparoscopic procedures at the gastroesophageal junction, the trocar is placed left and superior to the umbilicus.
2. Blunt dissection of the subcutaneous tissue is performed to expose the fascia. A Kocher clamp is placed on the linea alba, and traction is exerted upward. A 1–cm vertical incision is made in the linea alba. The two lateral edges are grasped with Kocher clamps and elevated.
3. A Kelly clamp is inserted into the incision and pushed through the peritoneum. As the clamp is withdrawn from the peritoneum, its jaws are spread to enlarge the peritoneal opening. A finger is inserted into the opening to confirm that it is intraperitoneal and to sweep away any adhesions.
4. Stay sutures are placed into the superior and inferior aspects of the fascial incision. A blunt-tipped (Hasson) trocar is placed under direct vision through the opening into the peritoneum. The stay sutures are pulled up tightly around the suture wings of the cannula to ensure an airtight seal and prevent the escape of CO_2 around the trocar (Fig. 66-3).
5. The CO_2 insufflator is attached to the trocar, and the abdomen is insufflated to a pressure of 15 mmHg.

Placing Additional Ports

One trocar is commonly used for diagnostic laparoscopy, but additional trocars are required for therapeutic laparoscopy. The appropriate location of additional ports must be determined. All additional ports should be placed under direct video monitoring. The location of each port depends on the procedure being performed. Ideally, operating trocars should be placed at a 30- to 60-degree angle with the axis of the videoscopic line of vision and operative site to form an equilateral triangle or a diamond. The angle between two operating ports should be 60 to 120 degrees. The distance from the port to the operative site should be about half the total length of the instrument being used for dissection. Because most instruments are 30 to 40 cm in

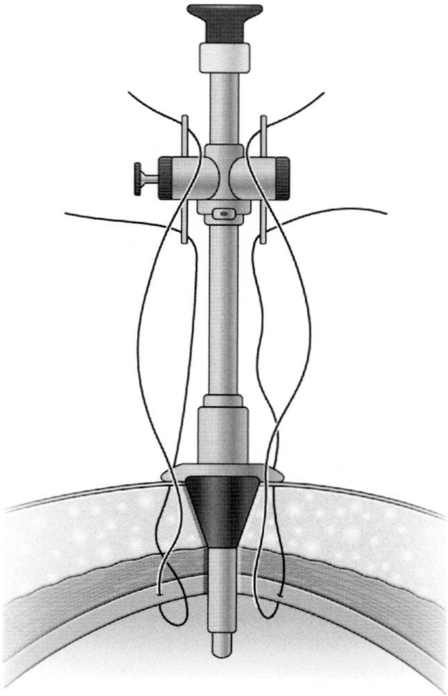

FIGURE 66–3 Securing the Hasson cannula to the abdominal fascia. The fascial stay sutures are tightly wound around the suture wings on the outer sheath. This secures the sheath in place and seals the fasciotomy and peritoneotomy. (Modified from Jones DB, Wu JS, Soper NJ (eds): Laparoscopic Surgery: Principles and Procedures. St. Louis, Quality Medical Publishing, 1997, with permission.)

PEARLS FOR ROUNDS

In comparison with open surgery, laparoscopic surgery is usually associated with smaller incisions, shorter hospitalizations, less postoperative pain, faster recuperation, and decreased costs.

Diagnostic laparoscopy is especially useful for the evaluation of abdominal pain in women of childbearing age or in patients whose diagnosis is unclear.

Laparoscopic techniques have reduced the threshold for surgical referral for several common diseases, including symptomatic cholelithiasis and gastroesophageal reflux disease.

Laparoscopic cholecystectomy is now the gold standard for removing a diseased gallbladder.

Laparoscopic inguinal herniorrhaphy may be performed transabdominally or completely extraperitoneally.

Contraindications to laparoscopic abdominal procedures include advanced generalized peritonitis, hypovolemic shock, massive abdominal distention with clinical evidence of bowel obstruction, uncorrected coagulopathy, and inability of the patient to tolerate a formal laparotomy.

The CO_2 pneumoperitoneum may cause hypercapnia, acidosis, and cardiac arrhythmias, especially in patients with cardiopulmonary diseases.

Alternatives to the CO_2 pneumoperitoneum should be considered in high-risk patients.

Improper trocar placement during laparoscopic surgery can result in major vascular injury, intestinal injury, or air embolism.

length, this translates into 15 cm from port to operating site. This gives the least distortion at the tip while allowing maximal movement at the fulcrum (the port site).

The site of the port is checked before the trocar is inserted. The abdominal wall is indented manually and the site is identified with the video camera. The abdominal wall is transilluminated to locate any superficial vessels to be avoided. If the surgeon is unsure about the appropriate location for port placement, a Veress needle may be passed, and its location and angle of approach to the operative field viewed.

The skin and peritoneum are infiltrated with a local anesthetic, and a small stab incision is made with a size 11 blade. The trocar is grasped in the palm of the surgeon's hand, with the middle finger extending down the trocar sheath to act as a brake against the abdominal wall. The trocar is introduced in a direct line with the planned surgical field to point naturally in the operative direction. This minimizes the pressure placed on the sheath during the procedure and maximizes the surgeon's touch and feel for dissection and tissue palpation.

Under direct video monitoring, the trocar is inserted with slow, steady pressure through the abdominal wall. Care is taken to avoid injuring the abdominal viscera as the obturator tip and sheath are guided into the peritoneal cavity. If difficulty is found in passing the trocar, the abdominal wall can be grasped with towel clips on either side of the trocar and elevated to increase the distance between the wall and the abdominal viscera.

Recognizing and Managing Complications

In minimal-access surgery, the three most significant complications are **major vascular injury, intestinal injury,** and **air embolism.** The first two injuries are usually associated with puncture by the Veress needle or the first trocar. Air embolism occurs with inadvertent placement of a Veress needle into a major vessel and insufflation with CO_2.

A major vascular injury should be suspected if sudden hemodynamic compromise develops during a laparoscopic procedure. If a major vessel is injured, the abdomen should be opened immediately and the injury repaired.

The magnitude of intestinal injuries varies. A visceral injury that is small and sealed may require only observation.

If a trocar lacerates the bowel, suture repair by laparoscopy or laparotomy is required.

If air embolism occurs, the abdomen should be desufflated and the patient placed in Trendelenburg position with the left side down. Placement of a central venous catheter allows aspiration of the gas from the right side of the heart, where it can block blood flow through the pulmonary valve.

Exiting the Abdomen

After the laparoscopic procedure is completed, the abdomen is surveyed to detect hemorrhage or visceral injury. The operative site is irrigated and examined to ensure that hemostasis has been obtained. The peritoneum is scanned from the pelvis to the upper quadrants to exclude any previously unrecognized injuries.

The ports and laparoscope are carefully removed. The valve on the laparoscope sheath is opened to allow the pneumoperitoneum to evacuate, and then the sheath is removed. The entry-site incisions are irrigated and inspected for hemostasis. For postoperative pain control, the subcutaneous and muscle layers are infiltrated with 0.25% to 0.50% bupivacaine. At port sites that are 5 mm or smaller, the skin is approximated with Steristrips. At port sites larger than 5 mm, the fascia can be closed by direct suturing after the port is removed or by placing full-thickness sutures under laparoscopic guidance (Fig. 66-4). The skin is then closed with subcuticular sutures and Steristrips.

Suturing and Knot Tying

Suturing and knot tying are critical skills for surgeons to master before attempting advanced laparoscopic procedures.

Extracorporeal Knot Tying

Extracorporeal knots are knots that are tied outside the abdominal cavity and then advanced into the operative field with a knot pusher. Square knots and sliding-loop knots are the most frequently used types. Preformed knots are available, but with practice, surgeons can quickly make their own extracorporeal knots. Extracorporeal knot-tying techniques can be used to ligate vessels, approximate tissue, reconstruct organs, and suture anastomoses. These techniques are recommended for tissue that will tolerate extra suture being drawn through it.

Three disadvantages limit the application of extracorporeal knot tying. First, at least 32 cm of suture material is required, and this long suture may saw through delicate tissue as it is withdrawn and the knot is formed. Second, the tissue may tear during advancement of the knot pusher. To avoid disruption, the knot pusher should be envisioned as an extension of the surgeon's finger. The knot should be pushed down to the tissue without pulling up on the suture. Third, an air leak will occur whenever suture material is introduced or withdrawn through the reducer sheath. Any ongoing air leak can be reduced by an assistant sealing the reducer orifice with a fingertip during extracorporeal knot tying.

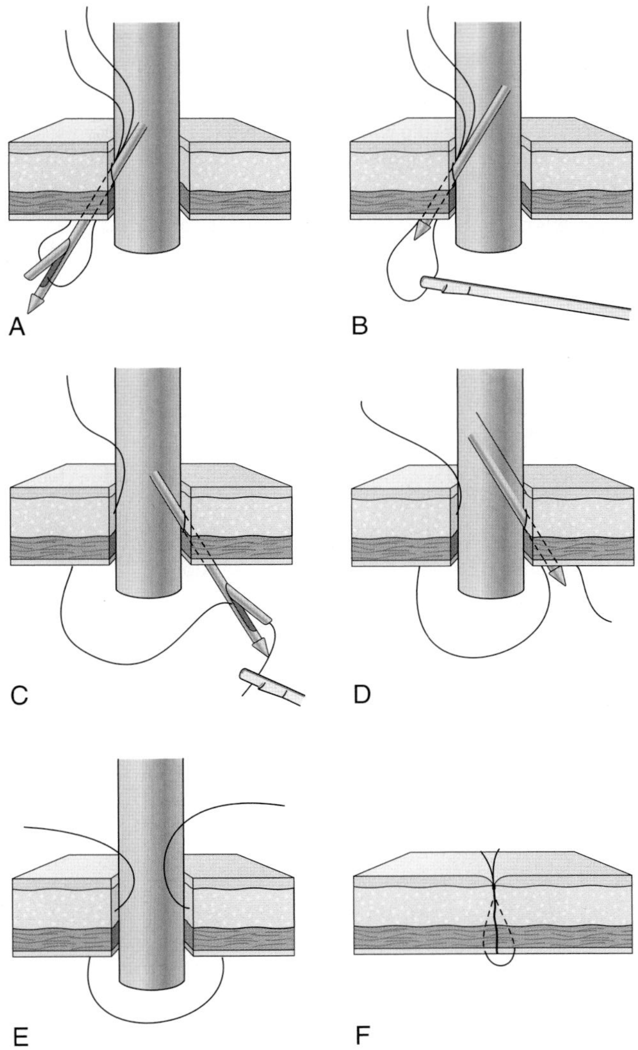

FIGURE 66–4 Laparoscope-assisted fascial closure. *A*, The suture material is grasped with a needle-nosed forceps. Under direct laparoscopic vision and with adequate pneumoperitoneum, the fascial closure device and suture are inserted into subcutaneous tissue directly adjacent to the trocar cannula. All tissue layers are incorporated as entry is made into the peritoneal cavity. The suture is then released. *B*, The suture is grasped, and one tail of it is pulled into the abdomen. The closure device is then removed. *C*, The closure device is reinserted, again under direct vision but on the opposite side of the trocar cannula. All tissue layers are incorporated. The suture is grasped and retrieved. *D*, The closure device is removed as the suture is held securely with the forceps. *E*, After sutures have been placed in all of the desired sites, the trocar cannula is removed. *F*, The suture is knotted deeply to the skin edges. (Modified from Soper NJ, Halpin VJ, Meyers BF: Minimally invasive surgery: Laparoscopic and thoracoscopic techniques. In Baker RJ, Fischer JE (eds): Mastery of Surgery, Vol. 1. Philadelphia, Lippincott, 2001, with permission.)

PEARLS FOR THE OR

Before laparoscopy is begun, all electronic equipment should be checked.

Before a Veress needle is inserted, it should be examined to ensure that the spring mechanism is intact and that the lumen flushes easily.

The risk of blood vessel, bowel, and bladder injuries is lower with open trocar insertion than with closed trocar insertion.

The locations for trocar placement depend on the procedure being performed. The appropriate location for a secondary port can be verified by sounding it out with a Veress needle.

All secondary trocars should be placed under direct laparoscopic vision.

Extracorporeal knot-tying techniques are useful on tissue that will tolerate extra suture material being drawn through it.

To avoid tissue tearing during extracorporeal knot tying, the knot pusher should be treated as an extension of the surgeon's finger.

Intracorporeal knot-tying techniques are appropriate for delicate tissues.

During intracorporeal suturing, the suture tail should be kept short and next to the knot to facilitate knot tying.

Extracorporeal Sliding Knots. Sliding knots can be used to tie off a pedicle, such as a blood vessel, cystic duct, or appendiceal base. They also can be used to close openings in cystic structures and to prevent spillage, such as spillage from a ruptured gallbladder.

Examples of preformed sliding knots are the Endoloop (Ethicon, Inc., New Brunswick, NJ) and the Surgitie (U.S. Surgical Corporation, Norwalk, CT). The preformed loop is introduced after backloading into a 3-mm reducer sleeve. A grasping forceps is passed through the loop and stabilizes the pedicle of tissue (Fig. 66-5). The loop is slipped off the grasping instrument and encircles the pedicle. When the proximal plastic end of the push-bar apparatus is snapped, the suture material is pulled, and the loop closes snugly around the pedicle. Finally, the suture is cut, leaving a 5-mm tail.

The key to proper loop ligature placement is to place the tip of the knot pusher exactly where the knot should finally rest.

Extracorporeal Square Knots. An extracorporeal square knot is the simplest and most secure knot to tie through a laparoscope.

After the tissue is sutured, both ends of the suture material are exteriorized through the same port. The square knot is created by separately advancing two half-hitches with a knot pusher (Fig. 66-6). Attention is taken to throw the second half-hitch in the direction opposite to that of the first half-hitch to create a square knot. If both half-hitches are thrown in the same direction, this will form a slipknot, rather than a square knot.

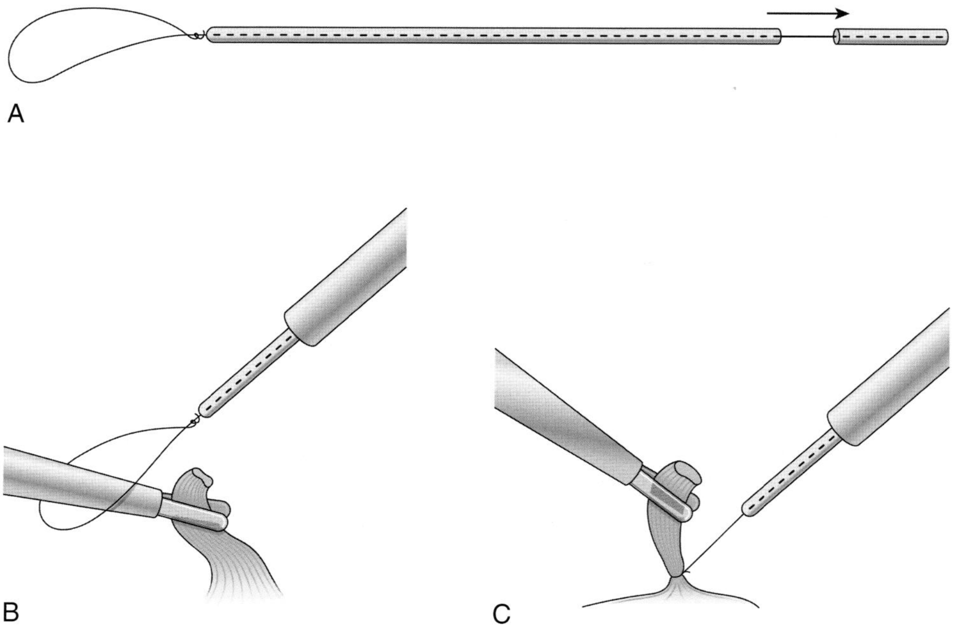

FIGURE 66–5 Loop ligature placement. *A*, The preformed loop ligature is used to tie off a pedicle. *B*, The grasping instrument is encircled before the pedicle is elevated. *C*, The loop is slipped down to the proper position and tightened. (Modified from Jones DB, Wu JS, Soper NJ (eds): Laparoscopic Surgery: Principles and Procedures. St. Louis, Quality Medical Publishing, 1997, with permission.)

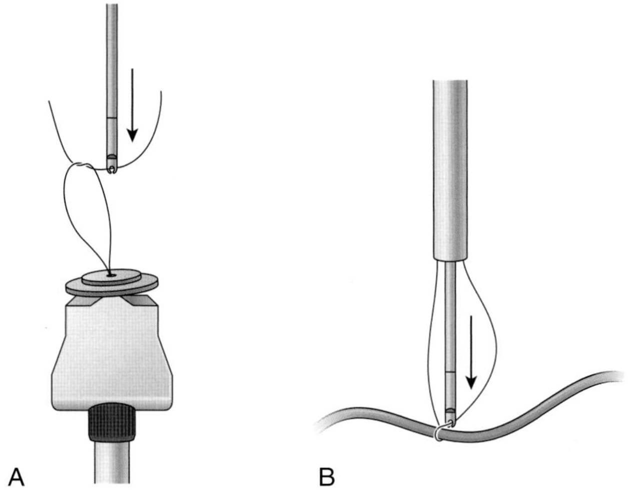

FIGURE 66–6 Use of a knot pusher. *A*, The knot pusher is placed on the end of the suture material. Both ends of the suture are held by the nondominant hand of the surgeon so neither end re-enters the trocar. *B*, The knot is pushed down and tightened around the vessel. (Modified from Soper NJ, Odem RR, Clayman RV, McDougall EM (eds): Essentials of Laparoscopy. St. Louis, Quality Medical Publishing, 1994, with permission.)

To advance the square knot, both half-hitches can first be converted into a sliding slipknot configuration by lightly pulling above and below the knot on the same side. With the slipknot, the throws can be easily advanced with the knot pusher to the desired tension. Pulling the two limbs of the suture material in opposite directions will again form the locking square-knot configuration. The surgeon can reconvert a square knot to a slipknot and back again intracorporeally until the knot is cinched down.

In laparoscopic surgery, as in open surgery, additional half-hitches are formed and advanced to complete the knot.

Intracorporeal Knot Tying

Intracorporeal suturing techniques are preferred for delicate tissues, such as the intestine or bile duct, or for completing a running suture line. Working within the abdomen avoids the seesaw effect and tugging on tissues that occur during extracorporeal knot tying as long segments of suture material are carried through tissue and out the same port. The disadvantage of intracorporeal suturing is the degree of difficulty. Under 15-fold magnification, all movements are exaggerated. The surgeon is required to be intentional and precise; otherwise, considerable operative time is lost.

For an **intracorporeal square knot,** the length of the suture material should be 8 to 12 cm. A shorter or longer length will make it hard to loop around the instruments. After a bite of tissue is incorporated in the suture, the suture tail is best kept short and strategically placed next to the knot, where it can be readily grasped (Fig. 66-7).

Several ways exist to loop a suture around an instrument. To begin, two loops are fashioned around one instrument, similar to a traditional twice-thrown surgeon's knot. Double winding for the first half-knot allows a certain amount of locking. Whether the suture is looped once or twice, the wrapped instrument holds the short end of the suture and carries it through the loop. Grasping the tail as near to the tip as possible will facilitate passing the suture through the loop. Looping the long end about the instrument begins the second half-hitch, but in this instance, the wrap is made in the opposite direction to square the knot. As before, the

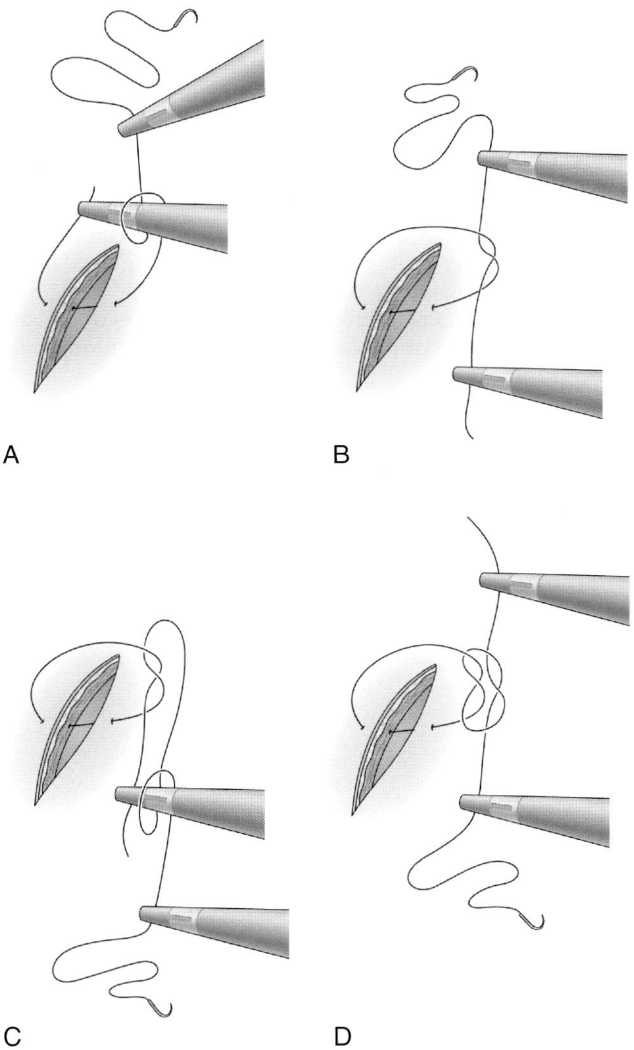

FIGURE 66–7 Intracorporeal instrument tie. *A*, Initial loop. *B*, First half-hitch. *C*, Second loop, with loop in opposite direction. *D*, Square knot. (Modified from Jones DB, Wu JS, Soper NJ (eds): Laparoscopic Surgery: Principles and Procedures. St. Louis, Quality Medical Publishing, 1997, with permission.)

instrument wrapped with suture material grasps the short end of the suture and pulls it through the loop. Alternating the direction of further loops ensures that the knots will be squared.

An alternative method for forming loops is to use a triple-twist knot. With the needle held at its tip, the needle holder is rotated 360 degrees four times as the suture wraps around the instrument shaft. The needle is then dropped. Next, the needle holder grasps the tail of the suture and passes it through the loops. The throw is completed in the usual fashion by pulling the ends of the suture apart to form a surgeon's knot. Additional ties are thrown for greater knot security.

It is sometimes difficult to maneuver instruments within a given port angle. In this situation, the suture material may be positioned to form a loop upon itself while it is lying on adjacent tissue. A grasping instrument is then used to pick up the suture where it crosses itself, or the loop may remain lying on the tissue surface. A second instrument is inserted through the loop and grasps the short tail of the suture to complete the throw. The second half-hitch is similarly formed, but in the opposite direction. This technique is particularly easy with the depth perception gained from three-dimensional laparoscopes.

Numerous other techniques have been described and illustrated in standard texts for laparoscopic suturing, and multiple designs of needle holders and grasping instruments are marketed. Surgeons must practice the various techniques in an inanimate setting until they become facile enough to apply them in clinical practice.

Suggested Reading

Apelgren KN, Cowan BD, Metcalf AM, Scott-Conner CE: Laparoscopic appendectomy and the management of gynecologic pathologic conditions found at laparoscopy for presumed appendicitis. Surg Clin North Am 76:469–482, 1996.

Callery MP, Strasberg SM, Soper NJ: Complications of laparoscopic general surgery. Gastrointest Endosc Clin North Am 6:423–444, 1996.

Conlon KC, Dougherty E, Klimstra DS, et al: The value of minimal access surgery in the staging of patients with potentially resectable peripancreatic malignancy. Ann Surg 223:134–140, 1996.

Gadacz TR: Update on laparoscopic cholecystectomy, including a clinical pathway. Surg Clin North Am 80:1127–1143, 2000.

Hartley JE, Monson JRT: The role of laparoscopy in the multimodality treatment of colorectal cancer. Surg Clin North Am 82:1019–1033, 2002.

Jones DB, Wu JS, Soper NJ, eds: Laparoscopic Surgery: Principles and Procedures. St. Louis, Quality Medical Publishing, 1997.

Nguyen NT, Wolfe BM: Laparoscopic Bariatric Surgery. Adv Surg 36:39–63, 2002.

Soper NJ: Laparoscopic management of hiatal hernia and gastroesophageal reflux. Curr Prob Surg 36:765–838, 1999.

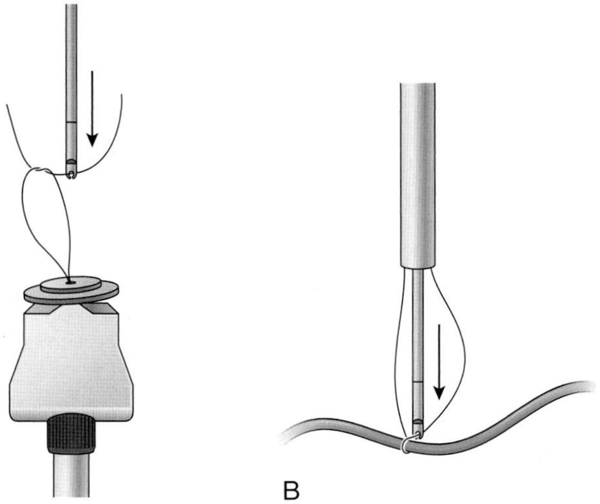

A B

FIGURE 66–6 Use of a knot pusher. *A*, The knot pusher is placed on the end of the suture material. Both ends of the suture are held by the nondominant hand of the surgeon so neither end re-enters the trocar. *B*, The knot is pushed down and tightened around the vessel. (Modified from Soper NJ, Odem RR, Clayman RV, McDougall EM (eds): Essentials of Laparoscopy. St. Louis, Quality Medical Publishing, 1994, with permission.)

To advance the square knot, both half-hitches can first be converted into a sliding slipknot configuration by lightly pulling above and below the knot on the same side. With the slipknot, the throws can be easily advanced with the knot pusher to the desired tension. Pulling the two limbs of the suture material in opposite directions will again form the locking square-knot configuration. The surgeon can reconvert a square knot to a slipknot and back again intracorporeally until the knot is cinched down.

In laparoscopic surgery, as in open surgery, additional half-hitches are formed and advanced to complete the knot.

Intracorporeal Knot Tying

Intracorporeal suturing techniques are preferred for delicate tissues, such as the intestine or bile duct, or for completing a running suture line. Working within the abdomen avoids the seesaw effect and tugging on tissues that occur during extracorporeal knot tying as long segments of suture material are carried through tissue and out the same port. The disadvantage of intracorporeal suturing is the degree of difficulty. Under 15-fold magnification, all movements are exaggerated. The surgeon is required to be intentional and precise; otherwise, considerable operative time is lost.

For an **intracorporeal square knot,** the length of the suture material should be 8 to 12 cm. A shorter or longer length will make it hard to loop around the instruments. After a bite of tissue is incorporated in the suture, the suture tail is best kept short and strategically placed next to the knot, where it can be readily grasped (Fig. 66-7).

Several ways exist to loop a suture around an instrument. To begin, two loops are fashioned around one instrument, similar to a traditional twice-thrown surgeon's knot. Double winding for the first half-knot allows a certain amount of locking. Whether the suture is looped once or twice, the wrapped instrument holds the short end of the suture and carries it through the loop. Grasping the tail as near to the tip as possible will facilitate passing the suture through the loop. Looping the long end about the instrument begins the second half-hitch, but in this instance, the wrap is made in the opposite direction to square the knot. As before, the

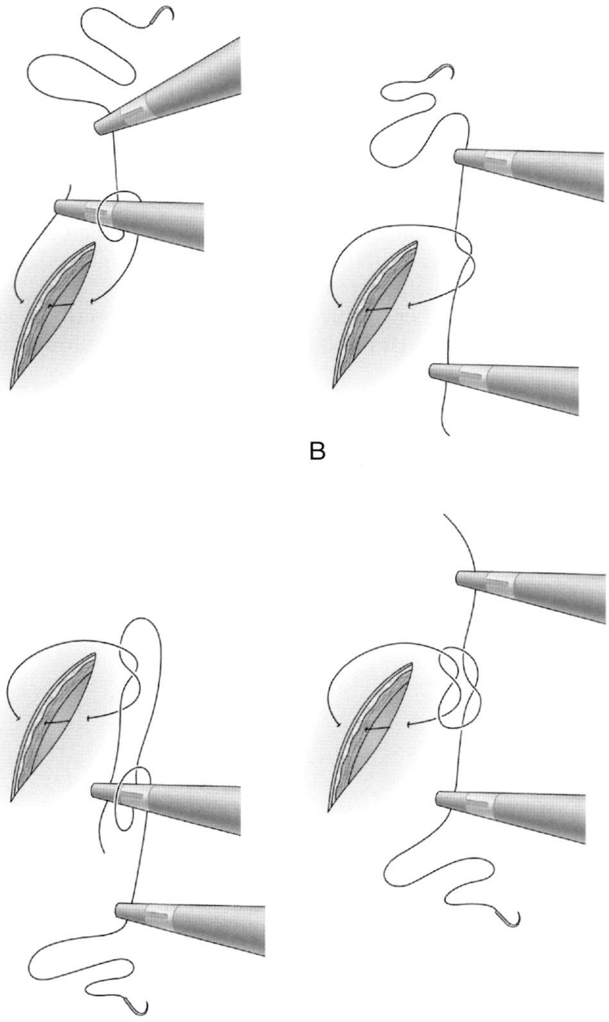

A B C D

FIGURE 66–7 Intracorporeal instrument tie. *A*, Initial loop. *B*, First half-hitch. *C*, Second loop, with loop in opposite direction. *D*, Square knot. (Modified from Jones DB, Wu JS, Soper NJ (eds): Laparoscopic Surgery: Principles and Procedures. St. Louis, Quality Medical Publishing, 1997, with permission.)

instrument wrapped with suture material grasps the short end of the suture and pulls it through the loop. Alternating the direction of further loops ensures that the knots will be squared.

An alternative method for forming loops is to use a triple-twist knot. With the needle held at its tip, the needle holder is rotated 360 degrees four times as the suture wraps around the instrument shaft. The needle is then dropped. Next, the needle holder grasps the tail of the suture and passes it through the loops. The throw is completed in the usual fashion by pulling the ends of the suture apart to form a surgeon's knot. Additional ties are thrown for greater knot security.

It is sometimes difficult to maneuver instruments within a given port angle. In this situation, the suture material may be positioned to form a loop upon itself while it is lying on adjacent tissue. A grasping instrument is then used to pick up the suture where it crosses itself, or the loop may remain lying on the tissue surface. A second instrument is inserted through the loop and grasps the short tail of the suture to complete the throw. The second half-hitch is similarly formed, but in the opposite direction. This technique is particularly easy with the depth perception gained from three-dimensional laparoscopes.

Numerous other techniques have been described and illustrated in standard texts for laparoscopic suturing, and multiple designs of needle holders and grasping instruments are marketed. Surgeons must practice the various techniques in an inanimate setting until they become facile enough to apply them in clinical practice.

Suggested Reading

Apelgren KN, Cowan BD, Metcalf AM, Scott-Conner CE: Laparoscopic appendectomy and the management of gynecologic pathologic conditions found at laparoscopy for presumed appendicitis. Surg Clin North Am 76:469–482, 1996.

Callery MP, Strasberg SM, Soper NJ: Complications of laparoscopic general surgery. Gastrointest Endosc Clin North Am 6:423–444, 1996.

Conlon KC, Dougherty E, Klimstra DS, et al: The value of minimal access surgery in the staging of patients with potentially resectable peripancreatic malignancy. Ann Surg 223:134–140, 1996.

Gadacz TR: Update on laparoscopic cholecystectomy, including a clinical pathway. Surg Clin North Am 80:1127–1143, 2000.

Hartley JE, Monson JRT: The role of laparoscopy in the multimodality treatment of colorectal cancer. Surg Clin North Am 82:1019–1033, 2002.

Jones DB, Wu JS, Soper NJ, eds: Laparoscopic Surgery: Principles and Procedures. St. Louis, Quality Medical Publishing, 1997.

Nguyen NT, Wolfe BM: Laparoscopic Bariatric Surgery. Adv Surg 36:39–63, 2002.

Soper NJ: Laparoscopic management of hiatal hernia and gastroesophageal reflux. Curr Prob Surg 36:765–838, 1999.

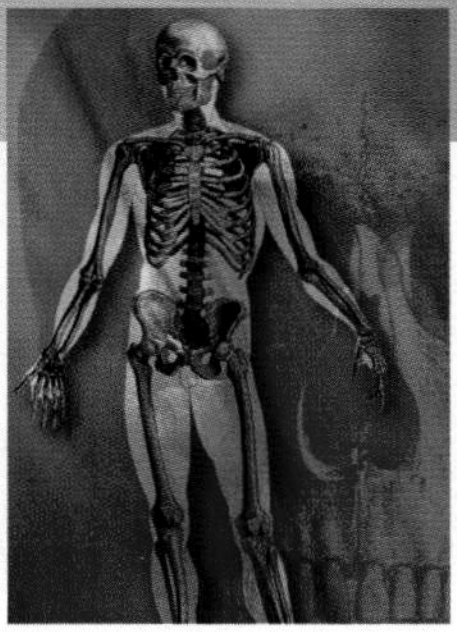

Chapter 67
Transplantation

THOMAS M. FISHBEIN, MD, and SANG I. CHO, MD

The Immunobiology of Transplantation

Transplantation of an organ between genetically disparate individuals leads to an immune response because of specific recognition of antigenic differences between donor and recipient. The cumulative effect of these immune responses leads to immune rejection and ultimately loss of the organ transplant. The immunologic nature of tissue rejection was well documented more than 50 years ago by Medawar and colleagues. Since then, our understanding of immune responses has developed considerably, and we have a better understanding of the molecular and cellular events that result in graft rejection.

Recent discoveries and better understanding of transplant immunobiology have led to the development of a number of novel immunosuppressive agents. These new immunosuppressive agents provide more effective control of immune rejection and have improved short- and long-term transplant survival, as documented over the past decade.

This section includes a brief description of the current state of knowledge on allogeneic recognition, the histocompatibility complex, T-cell receptors and activation, the role of cytokines, and tolerance induction.

Allogeneic Recognition

The recognition of transplantation antigen by T cells is referred to as *allogeneic recognition*, which has two distinct pathways.

The Direct Pathway

T-cell receptors (TCRs) directly recognize intact allogeneic major histocompatibility complex (MHC) molecules. This pathway generates primary cytotoxic $CD8^+$ T-cell responses and causes allograft rejection.

The Indirect Pathway

$CD4^+$ TCRs recognize donor MHC allopeptides after processing and presentation by self–antigen-presenting cells (APCs). The recipient APCs internalize the exogenous foreign protein shed from the graft, process the peptides for presentation to T cells, and provide the requisite signals for T-cell activation. Once the antigen-specific TCRs on the surface of $CD4^+$ T cells are triggered, a series of intracellular events is initiated, culminating in the synthesis of an array of new protein molecules leading to an interleukin-2 (IL-2)–induced alloimmune response.

The Histocompatibility Complex

An array of inherited proteins on cell surfaces initiates transplant immune responses and rejection. The genes that encode for these proteins—the histocompatibility genes—are located on different chromosomes in each species and are responsible for the host's recognition of the graft as either self or foreign. This complex of genes is present in all vertebrates, and in humans, they are located on the short arm of chromosome 6. Because of their central role in antigen recognition and immune response, this group of genes has been defined as the MHC.

Incompatibility between donor and recipient MHC antigens leads to allograft rejection. The observation of rejection and graft-versus-host disease in recipients of organs or bone marrow from MHC-identical siblings, however, implies that a protein structure other than MHC can be recognized by T cells and can result in initiation of immune responses. Indeed, such peptides are referred to as minor histocompatibility antigens. Minor histocompatibility antigens can initiate rejection in patients who receive allografts from human leukocyte antigen (HLA)-identical donors.

The MHC genes in humans encode polymorphic cell-surface molecules known as HLAs. HLA gene products are inherited in a mendelian codominant fashion. At least six separate genes are involved in the HLA system. Phenotypically, each is represented by two codominant alleles, one from the paternal gamete and one from the maternal gamete. Thus a single strand of parental chromosome containing alleles of the HLA system is called a haplotype, and every person has two haplotypes. The HLA system is further divided into class I and class II antigens, according to the cellular distribution, chemical and crystallographic structure, and immunologic function of these antigens.

HLA class I antigens (HLA-A, -B, and -C) are found on virtually all cell surfaces. These molecules are composed of one highly polymorphic peptide (α chain) and a monomorphic β_2-microglobulin (β chain). Antigens associated with class I molecules are recognized by $CD8^+$ T cells.

In contrast to class I antigens, class II antigens (HLA-DR, -DP, -DQ) have a more restricted cell distribution, and are generally expressed by APCs such as B cells, monocytes, macrophages, dendritic cells of lymphoid organs, renal mesangial cells, Kupffer's cells, and alveolar type 2 lining cells. Class II molecules are composed of two MHC-encoded and noncovalently associated polymorphic chains (α and β). Class II molecules play a central role in the initiation of immune response to transplantation antigen. Recognition of foreign class II antigens activates CD4+ T cells and stimulates generation of cytokines.

Lymphocyte Cross-matching and Panel Reactive Antibodies

The lymphocyte cross-match detects preformed anti-HLA antibodies in the serum of the transplant recipient directed against T and B lymphocytes of the potential donor. Kidney transplantation in the presence of a positive T-cell cross-match leads to hyperacute rejection. Liver grafts tolerate a positive T-cell cross-match better than do other organs and rarely develop hyperacute rejection. The significance of a positive B-cell cross-match remains controversial. A positive B-cell cross-match does not cause hyperacute rejection but may lead to inferior 1-year graft survival.

The microlymphocytotoxicity test is the most commonly used assay for lymphocyte cross-matching. To increase the sensitivity of the standard cross-match, more sensitive techniques have been developed to detect antibodies that may be missed in the standard microlymphocytotoxicity test. Flow cytometry cross-match and antiglobulin cross-match detect very low levels of anti-HLA antibody.

The microlymphocytotoxicity test also is used to screen for preformed anti-HLA antibodies against T cells from a panel of donors selected to represent the HLA specificities. The anti-HLA antibodies thus detected are called panel reactive antibodies (PRAs). The higher a patient's percentage of PRAs, the more difficult it is to find a cross-match–negative cadaveric donor.

The T-cell Receptor/CD3 Complex and T-Cell Activation

The TCR is a heterodimer that consists of two polypeptide chains, α and β chains, linked to each other by disulfide bonds. Both chains have variable (V) and constant (C) regions. The V regions of the TCR are responsible for antigen binding. Although the TCR allows T cells to recognize MHC-bearing antigen, the initiation of intracellular signaling depends on an additional complex of peptides known as the CD3 complex (Fig. 67-1). The CD3 complex consists of at least five peptide chains. When the TCR binds the antigen, the CD3 complex undergoes a conformational change that activates an intracellular signaling pathway, involving tyrosine kinase. This antigen-induced signal transduction by the TCR-CD3 complex is

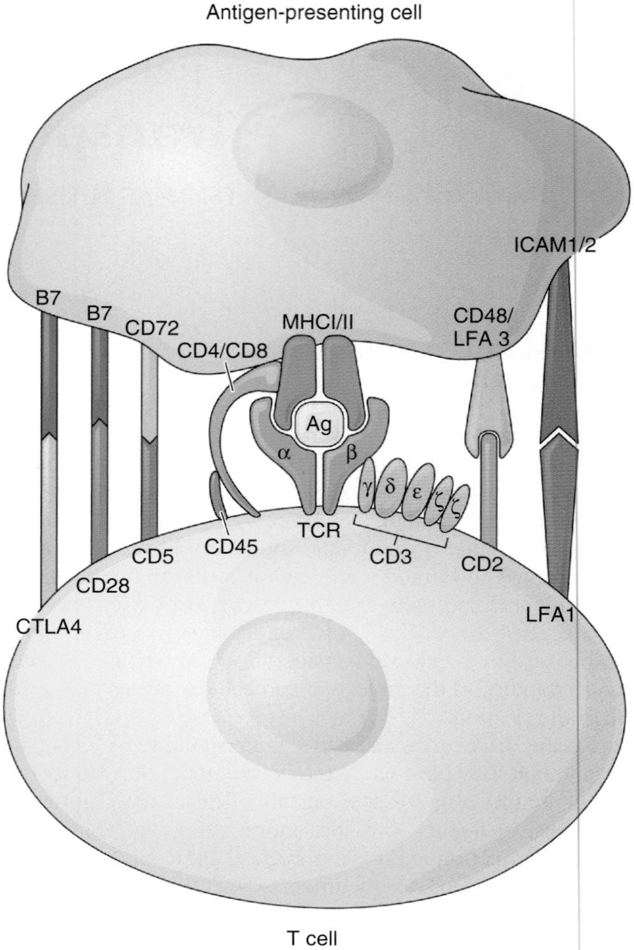

FIGURE 67–1 T-cell receptor/CD3 complex with accessory molecules on the antigen-presenting cells and T cells.

referred to as signal one of the process of lymphocyte activation. This first signal is essential but not sufficient for activation of T cells. The second signal, antigen independent, must be provided through accessory molecules.

Accessory molecules are nonpolymorphic membrane proteins and are identical on all T cells of a species. They are often involved in adhesion reactions. Accessory molecules stabilize the interaction between cytotoxic T cells and target cells by binding to specific ligands on target-cells surfaces; in addition, they provide an antigen-independent second signal for T-cell activation and enhance antigen recognition by increasing the affinity between the TCR and the MHC-bearing antigen. CD4 and CD8 molecules expressed on the surface of T cells, for example, are accessory molecules that enhance the interaction between the TCR and MHC-bearing antigen. CD4 molecules bind to class II MHC molecules and facilitate TCR-CD3 complex–mediated signal transduction in class II–restricted cells. CD8 molecules bind to class I MHC molecules and facilitate interaction between class I–restricted T cells and target cells.

Other T-cell membrane proteins, such as CD2, CD28, lymphocyte function–associated antigen 1 (LFA-1), and very late activation molecule (VLA) are cell-adhesion molecules of the integrin superfamily. By binding to various ligands, such as LFA-3, B7, intercellular adhesion molecule (ICAM)1 and 2, vascular cell adhesion molecule 1 (VCAM1), and fibronectin, they provide additional co-stimulation signals to T-cell activation and proliferation.

The dual activation of T cells, by the TCR/CD3 complex and accessory molecules, triggers $CD4^+$ T cells to activate IL-2–receptor gene expression, augmenting the entire cascade of T-cell activation. If a TCR is triggered without an accompanying second signal, the T cell is driven into an anergic state.

After alloantigen recognition, the antigen-specific TCR allows appearance of newly phosphorylated tyrosine residues mediated by phosphotyrosine kinase. This process, in turn, activates an enzyme called phosphatidyl inositol phospholipase, leading to signaling events such as production of the second messenger inositol 1,4,5, triphosphate (IP3) and diacylglycerol (DAG). IP3 stimulates the release of ionized calcium from intracellular stores, and DAG, in the presence of increased intracytoplasmic calcium, activates protein kinase C. Cytoplasmic calcium forms a complex with the calcium-dependent regulatory protein calmodulin. These calcium-calmodulin complexes activate other kinases, such as calcineurin. Calcineurin plays a critical role in the activation of IL-2 gene transcription. As a consequence of calcineurin activation, nuclear factor of activated T cells (NF-AT) is generated, and IL-2 gene transcription is enhanced.

Cytokines

Cytokines are soluble antigen-nonspecific proteins, synthesized by a variety of cells (e.g., T cells and monocytes) in response to antigenic stimulation. Cytokines initiate their action by binding to their specific receptors on the surfaces of target cells. They induce humoral and cellular responses including activation, proliferation, and differentiation of T and B cells, macrophages, and hematopoietic cells. Cytokines also play a nonspecific inflammatory role as mediators of the constitutional responses to antigenic stimulation.

In the initiation of the immune response, several cytokines, including tumor necrosis factor (TNF) and interferon-γ (IFN-γ), direct the maturation of T cells toward the Th1 subsets, whereas other cytokines, such as transforming growth factor-β (TGF-β), direct the maturation of T cells toward Th2 subsets. Cytokines synthesized by Th1 cells are generally involved with enhancement of the cellular immune response. These proteins (IL-2, IFN-γ, and IL-12) upregulate MHC expression and increase inflammation and target-cell injury. They also increase expression of adhesion molecules of endothelial and epithelial cells of the graft and facilitate natural killer (NK) cell and macrophage mediated cytotoxicity. Another set of cytokines, synthesized by Th2 cells, are generally involved with downregulation of the cellular and humoral immune responses. These proteins are IL-4, IL-5, IL-10, and IL-3.

Tolerance Induction

Tolerance, a state of immune acceptance, is a situation in which the immune response to the transplant antigen is absent without any immunosuppressive therapy. This phenomenon must be specific to the donor antigen. Grafts of additional donor-specific tissue, including skin, are accepted without a need for immunosuppression, while the host maintains a normal immunologic response to third-party antigen, and grafts from another source will be rejected.

During lymphocyte ontogeny, the immune system eliminates autoreactive clones of lymphocytes and preserves the clones that recognize foreign antigens in the context of self. Self-tolerance is thus initiated during development in the thymus and maintained in the periphery. Mechanisms involved in the induction of tolerance in adults are deletion, anergy, suppression, immune ignorance, and microchimerism. These mechanisms offer possible avenues for the manipulation of the human immune system and tolerance induction in transplantation.

Promising approaches for tolerance induction include (1) blocking the second signal necessary for T-cell activation (co-stimulatory blockade); (2) preferentially activating Th2 cells to increase production of Th2 cytokines, while selectively inhibiting Th1 cells to decrease IL-2 and IFN-γ production; and (3) using modified donor MHC with suppressogenic rather than immunogenic properties to redirect the immune response toward tolerance.

Immunosuppressive Agents

In recent years, a number of new agents have been approved by the Food and Drug Administration (FDA) for use in organ-transplant recipients. In addition, other new agents are undergoing clinical trials or preclinical investigation. Clinical applications of immunosuppressive agents that are approved by the FDA are described in this section.

The availability of multiple alternative immunosuppressive agents allows tailoring of immunosuppression to the needs of the individual patient, based on his or her immune activity and vulnerability to toxic effects.

Induction Immunosuppression

Early post-transplant renal dysfunction, also known as delayed graft function (DGF), has been common after cadaver-donor kidney transplantation and is associated with inferior short- and long-term graft survival. The mainstay of current immunosuppressive therapy involves calcineurin inhibitors, which are nephrotoxic. Therefore sequential induction therapy was developed, wherein antilymphocyte antibody given during the period of graft dysfunction allows delayed administration of the nephrotoxic calcineurin inhibitor, after renal recovery from DGF.

For induction immunosuppression, either a polyclonal antibody to human T cells (antithymocyte globulin [ATG]), or a monoclonal antibody to $CD3^+$ T cells (OKT_3) is used. Recently a humanized anti–IL-2–receptor antibody also was approved by the FDA and is used for induction in many centers. These are described in more detail later. Induction immunosuppression is used in combination with maintenance immunosuppression for 7 to 14 days, after which maintenance immunosuppression is continued.

Polyclonal Antibodies

Polyclonal antibodies to human lymphocytes are produced by immunizing either horses or rabbits with human lymphoid tissue, mainly human thymocytes, and then collecting the immune sera to obtain the γ-globulin fraction. The immune sera are then purified to eliminate unwanted antibodies such as anti–red cell, platelet, and stroma antibodies.

Two polyclonal antibody formulations are available for clinical use. One is ATGAM (horse ATG) and the other is thymoglobulin (rabbit ATG). After ATG administration, circulating lymphocytes and T-cell counts decrease dramatically, probably because of lymphocyte lysis or phagocytosis by the reticuloendothelial system. ATG is usually used as part of induction immunosuppression or as treatment for steroid-resistant acute rejection. When ATG is used for steroid-resistant rejection, more than 90% of episodes are successfully controlled.

Common side effects of ATG are fever, chills, and arthralgia due to infusion of foreign protein. Thrombocytopenia and leukopenia due to antiplatelet or antileukocyte antibodies also are common. Serum sickness or anaphylaxis is occasionally observed. The incidence of opportunistic infections such as cytomegalovirus (CMV) increases with ATG treatment.

Monoclonal Antibodies

OKT3

OKT3 is a monoclonal antibody directed against the CD3 antigen complex found on all mature T cells. OKT3 binds to the CD3 complex of human T cells and causes endocytosis of the TCR and its loss from the cell surface. The T cells become ineffectual and within an hour are opsonized and removed from the circulation into the reticuloendothelial system.

OKT3 depletes $CD3^+$ T cells as well as other T cells with other surface markers (CD4, CD8, CD11). Within a few days, T cells carrying CD4, CD8, and CD11 reappear in the circulation, but without CD3, and they are ineffective. These are called modulated cells. $CD3^+$ T cells may reappear in the circulation later in the course of OKT3 treatment because of the production of neutralizing antibodies.

In the original U.S. multicenter study, acute rejection episodes were reversed in 94% of patients treated with OKT3 compared with 75% of those treated with intravenous (IV) methylprednisolone. Because of the profound T-cell depletion and subsequent risk of opportunistic infection, OKT3 is reserved for treatment of steroid-resistant rejection in many centers.

OKT3 is administered as a daily IV dose for 10 to 14 days. Side effects are most common during the first 2 days of treatment and include fever and chills, rigors, dyspnea, wheeze, and pulmonary edema. These side effects, termed cytokine-release syndrome, are caused by sudden release of T cell–derived cytokines such as tumor necrosis factor (TNF), IL-2, and IFN-γ into circulation. Symptoms are usually attenuated by maintaining a euvolemic state and by pretreatment with high dose of intravenous methylprednisolone.

Anti-Tac Antibodies

Anti-Tac antibody binds to the P55 subunit of the IL-2 receptor and blocks the formation of the high affinity chain of the receptor and subsequent activation of T cells by IL-2. Two formulations of anti-Tac antibody, daclizumab (Zenapax) and basiliximab (Simulect), are available for clinical use.

Daclizumab is a humanized monoclonal antibody that binds to the α chain of the human IL-2 receptor. In a multicenter study, daclizumab reduced acute rejection significantly when it was used as a part of triple immunosuppression. Adverse side effects have been rarely observed with daclizumab.

Basiliximab is a chimeric, mouse-human monoclonal antibody that binds to the high-affinity α chain of the IL-2 receptor. This specific binding of basiliximab to IL-2

PEARLS FOR ROUNDS

The most common technical complication associated with kidney transplantation is lymphocele. (A collection of lymphatic fluid surrounding the graft may cause renal compression, hydronephrosis, and elevated creatinine levels.)

Cytomegalovirus infection after a transplant usually causes fever and malaise and commonly occurs approximately 6 weeks after transplant. It also may be associated with tissue-invasive disease, such as gastroenteritis or hepatitis.

Spontaneous bacterial peritonitis occurs in patients with chronic liver disease, is the result of severe protein-synthesis dysfunction, and indicates an inability to opsonize bacteria. Of these patients, 50% die within 6 months of this diagnosis if not given a transplant.

receptor competitively inhibits IL-2–mediated activation of T cells. In the U.S. multicenter trial, acute rejection of kidney transplants was significantly reduced when basiliximab was used in conjunction with cyclosporine and steroids. Basiliximab is well tolerated; adverse effects are rarely observed.

Maintenance Immunosuppression

A variety of maintenance immunosuppression protocols are used by transplant centers. Double therapy uses two drugs—usually a calcineurin inhibitor and steroids. Triple therapy uses a three-drug combination—usually, a calcineurin inhibitor, steroids, and an antimetabolic agent (mycophenolate mofetil or azathioprine). The effectiveness of mycophenolate mofetil has made it the preferred agent over azathioprine at many transplant centers.

Corticosteroids

Corticosteroids, the first immunosuppressive agents used in organ transplantation, still play an important role in immunosuppressive therapy, particularly as the first line of antirejection treatment. Corticosteroids inhibit the expression of several cytokines (e.g., IL-1, -2, -3, and -6; TNF-α; and IFN-γ). The blockade of IL-1 and IL-6 expression by APCs is particularly important, as these cytokines provide critical signals for IL-2 expression by activated T cells. Corticosteroids also cause a lymphopenia by redistribution of lymphocytes from the vascular compartment to lymphoid tissue. Furthermore, they inhibit macrophage migration.

Side effects of corticosteroids are multiple. They are common at higher doses; with lower doses, side effects can be dramatically reduced. With improved maintenance immunosuppression afforded by new drugs such as mycophenolate mofetil, tacrolimus, and sirolimus, the ability to safely discontinue long-term maintenance steroids is increasing.

Azathioprine

Azathioprine (Imuran) was the mainstay of immunosuppression for transplant recipients until cyclosporine, a calcineurin inhibitor, was approved by the FDA in 1983. Azathioprine, a purine analogue, inhibits purine nucleotide synthesis. Today it is generally used as part of triple therapy for the prevention of acute rejection. With FDA approval of mycophenolate mofetil, however, azathioprine is less commonly used. The common side effects of azathioprine are mainly bone marrow suppression with leukopenia, thrombocytopenia, and macrocytic anemia. Azathioprine also causes occasional hepatic dysfunction and alopecia.

Mycophenolate Mofetil

Mycophenolate mofetil (Cellcept) was approved by the FDA for maintenance immunosuppression in 1995. The active compound, mycophenolic acid (MPA), inhibits inosine monophosphate dehydrogenase (IMPDH), the rate-limiting enzyme for de novo purine synthesis in T and B cells. Mycophenolate mofetil also blocks the proliferation of T and B cells, inhibits antibody formation and cytotoxic T-cell generation and downregulates the expression of adhesion molecules on lymphocytes.

Three large randomized studies in kidney recipients demonstrated a significant reduction in acute rejection with mycophenolate mofetil compared with azathioprine or placebo. The common side effects of mycophenolate mofetil are gastrointestinal (nausea, vomiting, and diarrhea), bone marrow suppression (leukopenia), and an increased incidence of tissue-invasive CMV infection.

Cyclosporine

The original cyclosporine formulation (Sandimmune), approved by the FDA in 1983, contributed to a significant reduction in acute rejection and improvement of patient and graft survival in all types of solid organ transplants. A microemulsion formulation of cyclosporine (Neoral) was introduced in 1995; it provides better bioavailability, less interpatient and intrapatient variability, and absorption is less bile-salt dependent. With Neoral, bioavailability is increased by 15% to 30%.

Cyclosporine forms a complex with its cytoplasmic receptor protein (cyclophilin) and then binds to calcineurin. The normal function of calcineurin is to dephosphorylate certain nuclear regulatory proteins, such as NF-AT, and facilitate their passage through the nuclear membrane. Inhibition of calcineurin therefore impairs the expression of several critical T-cell activation genes, including those for IL-2 and its receptor. Cyclosporine also enhances the expression of transforming growth factor (TGF-β), which also inhibits IL-2 and the generation of cytotoxic T cells. Increased expression of TGF-β is implicated in the development of interstitial fibrosis, the main feature of cyclosporine-induced nephrotoxicity.

Monitoring of cyclosporine blood levels is essential, because its metabolism varies in individuals and between patients. Trough levels are usually measured, and correlate well with the therapeutic window of cyclosporine. Cyclosporine levels can be measured with high-performance liquid chromatography assay (HPLC), radioimmunoassay (RIA), or TDX fluorescence polarization assay (FPIA). FPIA is most popular and widely used because it is a simple and rapid assay.

Side effects of cyclosporine include nephrotoxicity, neurotoxicity, hepatotoxicity, hypertrichosis, gingival hyperplasia, hyperlipidemia, glucose intolerance, tremor, hyperuricemia and gout, hyperkalemia, hypomagnesemia, thromboembolism, and thrombotic microangiopathy. Nephrotoxicity, the most important side effect, is dose dependent. Cyclosporine decreases renal blood flow and glomerular filtration rate because of reversible vasoconstriction of the afferent arteriole. It also increases renal interstitial fibrosis.

Tacrolimus

Tacrolimus (Prograf), formerly known as FK506, is a macrolide antibiotic compound isolated from *Streptomyces tsukubaensis.* It shares many characteristics with cyclosporine. Tacrolimus is at least tenfold more potent than cyclosporine on a weight basis, however.

Tacrolimus blocks T-cell activation by mechanisms similar to those of cyclosporine. Unlike that of cyclosporine, small-bowel absorption of tacrolimus is independent of bile salts. Like cyclosporine, it binds to a specific intracytoplasmic-binding protein (FKBP), and this complex blocks the action of calcineurin and impairs the release of IL-2 and its receptor.

The U.S. trials in cadaveric kidney transplantation, in which tacrolimus was compared with cyclosporine, showed significant reduction in acute rejection with tacrolimus. Both U.S. and European randomized trials in liver transplantation revealed lower rejection rates as well, although no improvement in patient or graft-survival rates.

The side effects of tacrolimus are similar to those described with cyclosporine. The incidence of nephrotoxicity is similar. Slightly higher rates of neurotoxicity and new-onset diabetes mellitus are reported with tacrolimus, whereas the incidences of hyperlipidemia, hirsutism, and gingival hyperplasia are significantly lower with tacrolimus.

Sirolimus

Sirolimus (Rapamune), formerly known as Rapamycin, is a macrolide antibiotic compound that has demonstrated potent immunosuppressive activity and been associated with prolonged allograft survival in animal models. Its mechanism of action is different from that of tacrolimus and cyclosporine. Sirolimus binds to a cytoplasmic binding protein, FKBP, to form sirolimus-FKBP complex. This complex does not block calcineurin; rather, it engages a protein-designated mammalian target of rapamycin (mTOR). This protein complex, in turn, impairs the capacity of cytokines to trigger T cells to enter the cell-division cycle. Sirolimus may act synergistically with cyclosporine. The common side effects of sirolimus are thrombocytopenia and hyperlipidemia. Sirolimus in commonly used in conjunction with a calcineurin inhibitor.

Treatment for Acute Rejection

Management of acute rejection requires rapid and accurate diagnosis and prompt initiation of treatment. Currently, corticosteroids and antilymphocyte preparations are the main components of antirejection treatment. Because the intensified immunosuppression used to treat acute rejection impairs host defenses, it also increases the risk of opportunistic infection. Thus it is generally advisable to confirm the diagnosis of rejection by allograft biopsy. Nevertheless, initial episodes of acute rejection, in cases in which the diagnosis appears clear clinically and other causes are ruled out, may be treated with antirejection drugs without biopsy confirmation.

Mild acute cellular rejection (grade I) is usually treated with a high dose of steroid, although practices vary according to the organ transplanted and center-specific practices. Moderate to severe acute rejection (grades II and III) are treated initially with OKT3 in some centers. Intravenous methylprednisolone has been used as a first choice of treatment in many centers. Among the anti-lymphocyte antibodies, a 10- to 14-day course of OKT3 is commonly used for the treatment of steroid-resistant acute rejection or severe acute rejection. OKT3 is effective in reversing acute rejection in 94% of such renal transplant patients. Monitoring of lymphocyte subsets has been used with OKT3 treatment for acute rejection to confirm efficacy and to modify the dose according to the clearance of lymphocytes from the peripheral circulation.

Kidney Transplantation

Vascular surgical techniques requisite for organ transplantation were originally developed by Alexis Carrell and C.C. Guthrie at the turn of the 20th century. The first successful human kidney transplant was performed between identical twins and reported by Merrill and Murray in 1956. Introduction of the antimetabolite agent azathioprine, by Schwartz and colleagues, and the addition of corticosteroids set the stage for current immunosuppression and allowed widespread application of kidney transplantation for patients with end-stage renal disease. Immunosuppressive techniques were further refined with the introduction of cyclosporine, tacrolimus, mycophenolate mofetil, serolimus, and polyclonal and monoclonal antibodies.

Medicare began coverage of the cost of kidney transplantation in 1972 after the End Stage Renal Disease Act was passed. In 2002, 14,523 kidney transplants were performed in the United States—8287 with cadaver kidneys and 6236 with living-donor kidneys. Since 1993, the number of cadaver-donor and living related–donor transplants has remained unchanged. However, a 37.5% increase per year has occurred in the number of living unrelated kidney transplants since 1993. As of November 2003, 59,892 patients were waiting for cadaver-donor kidneys in the United States.

Indications for Kidney Transplantation

Kidney transplantation is the treatment of choice for the majority of patients with end-stage renal disease. Kidney transplantation improves quality of life and increases life expectancy. Nearly all patients are considered candidates for kidney transplantation. Exclusion criteria appear in Table 67-1. Potential transplant candidates must be

TABLE 67–1 Exclusion Criteria for Kidney Transplantation

Absolute Contraindication	Relative Contraindication
Uncontrolled malignant tumor	Severe cardiovascular disease
Active systemic infection	Obesity
Other end-stage organ diseases (cardiac, pulmonary, vascular, hepatic)	Prior malignant tumor
Active autoimmune diseases	Chronic obstructive lung disease
Active AIDS	Uncontrolled urinary tract infection
Active IV drug use	Primary renal diseases with high postoperative recurrence rate
Life expectancy <5 yr	History of medical noncompliance
	Psychosis
	Inadequate social support
	Decreased mental capacity

AIDS, acquired immunodeficiency syndrome; IV, intravenous.

systematically screened for dental, cardiopulmonary, vascular, genitourinary, and gastrointestinal disease.

Because many transplant candidates are older than 55 years and diabetes mellitus is a common cause of renal failure, the transplant candidate usually requires an extensive cardiac evaluation including a history and physical examination, electrocardiogram, chest radiograph, echocardiogram and, if indicated, stress tests. Patients with significant coronary artery disease may require coronary arteriography followed by pretransplant coronary artery angioplasty or bypass surgery. Patients with an active infection should not be transplanted until the infection is cleared, to decrease the likelihood of life-threatening postoperative sepsis.

Donor Evaluation and Nephrectomy

The primary goal of the living-donor evaluation is to ensure the safety and well-being of the donor. Contraindications for living-donor donation are ABO incompatibility, positive lymphocytotoxic cross match, age younger than 18 years, active malignancy, infection, hypertension, diabetes mellitus, proteinuria, renal disease or reduced renal function, increased medical risk for surgery, and inability to give informed consent.

The best MHC match is an identical twin. The next best match is a MHC-identical (two-haploid identical) sibling, followed by a one-haploid identical sibling or parent. If a suitable blood relative is not found, consideration is given to living unrelated kidney donation, especially from a spouse.

The open living-donor nephrectomy is usually performed through an oblique flank incision through the bed of the 12th rib. The muscle layers are divided, and the retroperitoneum is entered. Gerota's fascia is incised, and the kidney is mobilized. The ureter is identified and mobilized down over the iliac artery, at which level the ureter is divided. The periureteral fatty tissue is included with ureteral dissection to ensure an adequate blood supply to the ureter. The majority of living-donor nephrectomy is now being performed laparoscopically.

More recently, the laparoscopic approach to donor nephrectomy has emerged as a less-invasive alternative method for removing the kidney for the purpose of kidney transplant. Benefits to the patient undergoing live-donor transplantation include decreased blood loss, shorter hospital stay, faster recovery, reduced patient morbidity, and improved cosmetic result. Most patients are discharged by the second postoperative day. The number of live-donor nephrectomies being performed in the United States has increased because of the availability of the laparoscopic approach, and this is thought to be due to the clear advantages to the donor patient. Instead of the standard flank incision, the operation is done through two to three small laparoscopic trocar sites and a small incision where the kidney is removed. The procedure can be done by using the hand-assisted technique, in which the surgeon's hand is inserted through a very small 7-cm incision through which the kidney is eventually removed intact. As with the open approach, the left kidney is preferred for laparoscopic donor nephrectomy because of the longer length of the left renal vein. Unlike a standard flank approach in which the kidney is removed without entering the peritoneal cavity, the laparoscopic donor nephrectomy is performed through a transperitoneal approach. Once the hand port and trocar sites are inserted, the colon is reflected medially to enter the retroperitoneum. The renal artery and vein are identified and dissected free. The ureter is dissected free down to the left iliac artery. The rest of the kidney is then mobilized and eventually removed by dividing the renal artery, renal vein, and ureter.

Cadaveric Donor Evaluation and Nephrectomy

Kidneys can be used from cadaveric donors between the ages of 1 and 70 years. After a patient has been declared brain dead and consent for organ donation has been obtained from the next of kin, the cadaver donor is properly supported to maintain adequate hydration, normal blood pressure, and adequate organ perfusion. In addition to a detailed history and physical examination, blood samples are taken for evaluation of renal function (serum creatinine, blood urea nitrogen, and serum electrolytes), hepatic function (serum bilirubin, alanine aminotransferase, and prothrombin time) and pancreatic function (serum glucose and amylase). In addition, the donor is screened for hepatitis B and C, human immunodeficiency virus, human T-lymphocyte virus (HTLV)-1, and cytomegalovirus (CMV). The donor's cause of death, length of time of cardiac or pulmonary arrest, severity and duration of hypotension, vasoactive drugs, alcohol use, drug abuse, and social and medical history also are reviewed, and consideration is given to risk factors for organ dysfunction or disease transmission through transplantation.

Optimal conditions for kidney donation exist when the donor has normal renal function; no history of renal disease, hypertension, or diabetes mellitus; no malignancy except primary central nervous system (CNS) tumor; and no sepsis. Cadaver-donor nephrectomy is usually done as a part of a multiorgan-procurement procedure. This is described in detail under the section on liver transplantation.

Kidney Preservation

Kidneys may be preserved for no more than 24 to 48 hours, to allow enough time for tissue typing and cross-match, selection and preparation of a recipient for kidney transplantation, and sharing of organs around the country. Good preservation permits immediate function of the kidney after transplant and reduces patient morbidity, hospital stay, and hospital cost. It may also improve long-term graft survival. Kidneys are preserved either by a simple cold storage by using University of Wisconsin (UW) solution (Table 67-2) or by machine perfusion.

For simple cold storage, kidneys are flushed with UW solution and immersed in this solution at 4°C until transplanted. UW solution has a high concentration of potassium, low sodium concentration, and high osmolarity. Addition of lactobionic acid, raffinose, and hydroxyethyl starch suppresses cellular swelling observed in hypothermic (4°C) kidney preservation.

For machine perfusion, kidneys are placed on the perfusion pump, and continuous intra-arterial perfusion is maintained by using a hydroxyethyl starch–based perfusate. Machine perfusion provides a constant supply of energy substrates and oxygen for aerobic metabolism of kidneys; in addition, it removes metabolic end products.

TABLE 67–2 Composition of UW Solution

Component	Concentration
K lactobionate	100 mmol/L
KOH	100 mmol/L
Raffinose	30 mmol/L
KH_2PO_4	25 mmol/L
NaOH	20 mmol/L
Adenosine	5 mmol/L
$MgSO_4$	5 mmol/L
Glutathione	3 mmol/L
Allopurinol	1 mmol/L
Pentafraction (hydroxyethyl starch)	50 g/L
Penicillin	200,000 U/L
Insulin	40 U/L
Dexamethasone	16 mg/L

pH 7.4; sodium, 25 ± 5 mEq/L; potassium, 125 ± 5 mEq/L; osmolarity, 310 ± 10 mOsm
UW, University of Wisconsin.

Significant reductions in the incidence of delayed graft function have been reported by several investigators when kidneys were preserved by machine perfusion.

Surgical Techniques

The kidney-transplant procedure is usually performed under general anesthesia. After anesthesia is induced, a Foley catheter (18 to 20F) is placed in the bladder, and an antibiotic solution is instilled to distend the bladder, facilitating identification of the bladder for ureteral implantation. The incision is placed on either iliac area, extending from the pubic tubercle to the superior medial area of the anterior superior iliac spine. The extra peritoneal space is entered by dividing the external oblique, internal oblique, and transversalis muscles. The epigastric artery and veins are usually divided, as well as the round ligament. The spermatic cord is usually preserved and retracted medially. The external iliac artery and vein are dissected from the common iliac bifurcation to the inguinal ligament. The internal iliac artery is rarely used for arterial anastomosis, to preserve pelvic circulation.

The arterial anastomosis is established end-to-side between the external iliac artery and the renal artery for living-donor transplants, or with a Carrell patch (aortic patch) for cadaver-donor transplants. The internal iliac artery also may be used for end-to-end anastomosis to the renal artery in some instances. The end-to-side venous drainage is established between the external iliac vein and the renal vein.

Ureteral implantation is generally accomplished by using the technique of ureteroneocystostomy. Intravesical ureteroneocystostomy (Leadbetter-Politano technique) requires opening the bladder and creating a submucosal tunnel through the posterior bladder wall. The spatulated ureter is then sutured to the bladder mucosa in a posterior and lateral portion of the bladder. Extravesical uretero-neocystostomy (Liche technique) requires making a small opening in the anterior and superior aspect of the bladder. The ureter is sutured to the bladder mucosa, and bladder muscle is reapproximated over the ureteral anastomosis, creating an antireflux mechanism. In rare circumstances, ureteropyelostomy between the recipient ureter and the donor renal pelvis is used, when the donor ureter is not adequate for ureteral implantation. The kidney is placed in the iliac fossa and stabilized by peritoneum. The Foley catheter is left in place for several days to protect the ureteral implantation site.

Rejection of Kidney Transplants

Allograft rejection remains the most common cause of transplant failure. Three types of transplant rejection are well documented (hyperacute, acute, and chronic rejection).

Hyperacute Rejection

Hyperacute rejection is mediated by preformed anti-HLA antibody of the recipient against the graft and occurs soon after transplantation. The graft is infiltrated with polymorphonuclear leukocytes and platelets. This is soon followed by intragraft vascular thrombosis and graft failure. Preformed anti-HLA antibodies are usually generated by pretransplant blood transfusion, pregnancy, and previous transplantation. Hyperacute rejection can be avoided by using sensitive pretransplant cross-matching tests. No successful treatment exists for hyperacute rejection. Plasmapheresis or immunoabsorption offers limited short-term benefit.

Acute Rejection

Acute rejection accounts for 85% of all rejection episodes. It is mediated primarily by T cells and occurs during the first 6 months after transplantation. Clinical signs and symptoms of acute rejection, such as weight gain, oliguria, fever, malaise, and graft tenderness, are less reliable under current immunosuppressive protocols. Therefore the diagnosis of acute rejection is based on laboratory data, renal imaging studies, and renal biopsy. Biopsy findings are graded according to the Banff schema (Table 67-3). Acute rejection is easily reversible in the majority of cases, as described earlier in the section of immunosuppression.

Chronic Rejection

Chronic rejection leads to slow deterioration of graft function over months to years. A slow progressive increase in serum creatinine is accompanied by proteinuria. Graft biopsy shows arterial smooth muscle–cell proliferation with luminal narrowing, tubular atrophy, interstitial fibrosis, and glomerular sclerosis. Chronic rejection is caused by immunologic and nonimmunologic mechanisms. The immunologic mechanism is mediated by B and T cells, with antidonor humoral immunity playing a critical role. Nonimmunologic mechanisms include chronic hyperperfusion, hyperlipidemia with atherosclerosis, and drug-induced nephrotoxicity.

TABLE 67–3 Banff Schema for Graft Rejection

Banff Classification	Biopsy Findings
Normal	No mononuclear cells in tubules, no interstitial inflammation, no arteritis, glomerulitis, or tubular atrophy
Grade I	Significant interstitial mononuclear tubulitis (>4 mononuclear cells/tubule)
Grade IIA	Mild to moderate intimal arteritis
Grade IIB	Severe intimal arteritis involving >25% of the luminal area
Grade III	Transmural arteritis, arterial fibrinoid necrosis, and necrosis of medial smooth muscle cells
Chronic rejection (Grades 0,I,II,III)	Interstitial fibrosis, tubular atrophy, glomerular sclerosis, and myointimal hyperplasia

Surgical Complications

Vascular Complications

The most common vascular complications include renal artery stenosis or thrombosis and renal vein thrombosis. Renal artery stenosis occurs in 2% to 10% of patients, as early as a few days or as late as many years after transplantation. The stenosis may be related to technical imperfections with the anastomosis, recipient iliac artery atherosclerosis, or intimal injury causing myointimal hyperplasia. Renal artery stenosis is suspected in transplant patients with refractory hypertension, deteriorating renal function under treatment with an angiotensin-converting enzyme inhibitor, a change in the intensity of systolic bruit over the transplanted kidney, or a combination of these. Diagnosis is suggested with magnetic resonance (MR) angiography and confirmed with conventional arteriography. Percutaneous transluminal angioplasty (PTA), the initial treatment of choice, is successful in 60% to 85% of patients. A restenosis rate of 30% has been reported with PTA, however. When PTA fails, surgical correction is accomplished usually with saphenous vein bypass between the iliac artery and the renal artery distal to the stenosis.

Renal artery thrombosis is rare and usually occurs in the immediate post-transplant period. It is usually caused by technical complications of the anastomosis or by kinking and torsion of the renal artery. Hyperacute rejection or irreversible acute rejection also can cause renal artery thrombosis. Thrombosis may first be seen as a sudden cessation of urine output by a previously functioning transplant. Diagnosis is made by nonvisualization of the kidney on radioisotope renal scan or arteriography. Immediate surgical thrombectomy is mandatory for salvage of the allograft. Delayed correction of renal perfusion results in eventual graft nephrectomy in the majority of cases.

Renal vein thrombosis is caused by technical complications related to the renal vein anastomosis, thrombosis of the iliac vein, or irreversible acute rejection. Graft tenderness and swelling with hematuria are signs of renal vein thrombosis. A radioisotope renal scan shows poor or absent perfusion to the allograft. Early exploration with renal vein thrombectomy is necessary. In the majority of cases, however, the allografts are no longer viable because of prolonged venous hypertension and hemorrhagic infarct, and nephrectomy is necessary.

Urologic Complications

Urinary tract complications—urine leak or obstruction—occur in 2% to 10% of patients; ischemia of the donor ureter is the usual cause. Preservation of the blood supply to the donor ureter during donor nephrectomy is important in preventing these complications. Urine leaks occur commonly at the ureterovesical anastomotic site; this is usually caused by technical failure of the anastomosis or necrosis of the distal ureter. Rarely, urine leaks occur in the renal transplant collecting system, caused by ischemic necrosis of the renal pelvis. Decreased urine output associated with fluid discharge from the wound suggests urine leak. Ultrasound study shows perirenal fluid collection, and radioisotope renal scan documents extravasation of radioisotope outside of renal collecting system. Diagnosis is usually made by cystography and retrograde or antegrade pyelography. Percutaneous stenting provides temporary control of urine leaks. Surgical repair of ureterovesical anastomosis is usually necessary. When urine leaks are caused by significant ureteral necrosis, pyeloureterostomy using the recipient ureter is indicated.

Ureteral obstruction occurs in fewer than 5% of patients. Ureteral ischemia leading to fibrosis and stricture formation is the common cause. Symptoms are usually absent, and the diagnosis is made during the investigation of an increasing serum creatinine level. Renal ultrasound study demonstrates dilated renal calices. Percutaneous antegrade pyelogram demonstrates the site of obstruction, usually the ureterovesical anastomotic site. Stenting with balloon dilation of the stricture by antegrade or retrograde approach is successful in more than 50% of patients. For long or recurrent stricture, pyeloureterostomy using the recipient ureter is usually indicated.

Lymphocele

Lymphocele, lymphatic fluid collection between the lower pole of the kidney and the bladder, is not uncommon after kidney transplantation, with a reported incidence of 1% to 18%. Disrupted iliac lymphatics or renal hilar lymphatics are believed to be the source of these collections. Most lymphoceles are asymptomatic and discovered by routine ultrasonographic examination. Only symptomatic lymphoceles require therapy. Lymphoceles can impair renal function by compressing the urinary collecting system, causing hydronephrosis. Percutaneous external drainage provides a temporary decompression, although recurrence is frequently observed. Definitive therapy is provided by internal drainage, creating an opening between the lymphocele and the peritoneal cavity. Internal drainage of a lymphocele also can be created laparoscopically. Because evidence of most technical complications of renal transplantation can be diagnosed with duplex ultrasonography, this has become the initial diagnostic investigation to evaluate post-transplant renal dysfunction.

Liver Transplantation

Orthotopic liver transplantation, currently the only successful therapy for end-stage liver failure, has been developed over the last 30 years after experimental work pioneered by Dr. Thomas Starzl, who attempted the first human liver transplant in 1963. Before liver transplantation was possible, patients with end-stage liver disease inevitably progressed to lethal complications of either portal hypertension or liver synthetic dysfunction.

In the majority of liver transplant operations, the native liver is removed and replaced with either a whole or partial graft in the position of the native liver. This liver allograft is able to provide adequate drainage of the portal blood supply, as well as to support the complex metabolic needs of the body. The development of liver transplantation has had a widespread impact on our understanding of such diverse physiologic processes as hepatic regeneration, immunosuppression and transplantation tolerance, ischemia and reperfusion, and hemostasis/coagulation.

The success of liver transplantation has steadily improved over the last two decades, with 1-year patient and graft survival rates in the United States of 85% and 80%, respectively, and 5-year patient and graft survival rates of 75% and 65%, respectively. Continued success has led to the application of liver transplantation to an increasingly broad population, leading to a worsening disparity between the supply of transplantable organs and the number of candidates on the waiting list. As of November 2003, data from the United Network for Organ Sharing showed that more than 18,000 patients were waiting for liver transplantation in the United States alone, whereas 5,040 liver transplants were performed in 2002. In direct response to the shortage of organs, complex surgical techniques make it possible to split a single liver for transplantation into two recipients (split-liver transplantation) or to transplant a portion of a liver that has been removed from a living donor (living-donor transplantation).

Indications

Liver diseases generally fall into three categories: cholestatic, hepatocellular, or metabolic. Each of these types of disease can lead to end-stage liver failure, although the clinical manifestations may vary among disease categories or among individual patients. Cholestatic diseases are characterized by intracellular accumulation of bile salts, which leads to the development of secondary hepatocellular injury and biliary cirrhosis. In affected patients, jaundice, pruritis, hepatomegaly, and ascites usually develop as portal hypertension ensues. The development of synthetic dysfunction, heralded by protein malnutrition, muscle wasting, and secondary infection (e.g., spontaneous bacterial peritonitis) occurs late in the course of disease. In contrast, hepatocellular diseases such as viral hepatitis lead to cirrhosis and signs of portal hypertension before the development of cholestasis and clinical jaundice.

Hepatitis C, first identified serologically in 1989, is currently the leading cause of cirrhosis and indication for liver transplantation in the United States. Reportedly, as many as 2.7 million people are chronically infected with the hepatitis C virus (HCV); these individuals are expected to account for a large proportionate increase in the number of deaths from liver-related diseases in the future. We hope that routine screening of banked blood for HCV will limit new exposures, although the disease remains common among alcoholics and intravenous drug users.

Among children, cholestatic and metabolic diseases are more common causes of end-stage liver disease than are hepatocellular diseases. Extrahepatic biliary atresia is the most common indication for liver transplantation among pediatric patients in the United States today. Wilson's disease, fulminant liver failure, and hemochromatosis also are common indications. In children with end-stage cirrhosis, clinical signs and symptoms develop similar to those seen in adult patients, whereas children with metabolic diseases due to hepatocyte-based enzyme deficiencies have end-organ damage related to their underlying metabolic disease. For example, patients with primary hereditary oxalosis display normal liver synthetic function, and portal hypertension does not develop, but they have end-stage renal disease due to oxalate stone deposition in the kidneys, and cardiomyopathy due to oxalate deposition in the myocardium. Liver replacement restores normal enzyme function and prevents end-organ damage. For some metabolic diseases, it is hoped that hepatocyte transplantation or gene-replacement therapies will someday replace the need for vascularized organ transplantation. Although preliminary evidence indicates that this may be achieved in the future, such approaches are still experimental, and whole-organ liver transplantation remains the standard care for most of these diseases to date.

Donor Evaluation and Management

The evaluation of organs from a cadaveric multiorgan donor is usually the first step toward a successful transplant. Because the large majority of liver transplants in the United States are done with cadaveric organs, this section deals with evaluation of these organs only. Donors of cadaver organs have generally had irreversible CNS damage and brain death. Conditions for donor retrieval are optimal when brain death has not been accompanied by damage to other organ systems, as is usually the case with isolated head injury or CNS bleeding (e.g., subarachnoid hemorrhage). The transplant physician's goal is to maintain the normal physiologic state of the cadaveric donor until the organs can be removed. This goal often involves the coordination of teams retrieving organs for patients at different transplant centers.

As the donor progresses from irreversible CNS damage to brain death, and after brain death has been confirmed, various physiological insults may require correction in the intensive care unit for the cadaveric organs to remain viable. Diabetes insipidus often ensues after brain death and leads to brisk diuresis of nonconcentrated urine. This can be controlled by administration of vasopressin and adequate hydration. Dehydration leads to poor end-organ perfusion and may result in poor allograft function or primary nonfunction (in which the transplanted liver does not function adequately to sustain life). The brain also releases tissue plasminogen activator after brain insult, resulting in coagulopathy.

Many other donor-related risk factors have been implicated as causes of poor allograft function, although few have been rigorously proven. Moderate or severe macrovesicular steatosis in the allograft has been reliably associated with poor outcome after transplantation, likely in part because of the inability of the lipophobic preservation solution to enter and preserve fat-laden hepatocytes. Other donor-related factors that may play a role in poor allograft function include hypernatremia, acidosis, ethanol use, high-dose pressor use for hypotension, sepsis, and hypoxia. Liver chemistries, particularly the level of alanine aminotransferase (which is not produced by other organs), may reflect ischemic insult. Ultimately, assessment of each donor must be multifactorial and aimed at judging the physiologic condition of the organ to be procured.

Multiorgan Procurement

The donor operation commences with a long midline incision from the sternal notch to the symphysis pubis. This incision allows wide exposure of the intra-abdominal and thoracic organs. The liver is mobilized from the stomach by dividing the lesser omentum and the left gastric artery. Care must be taken first to ensure that no accessory or replaced left hepatic branch arises from the left gastric artery. If this is present, the origin of the left gastric artery from the celiac artery must be preserved, with the branch entering the liver to supply the left lobe. The bile duct is identified and transected, allowing bile production to be assessed. The gastroduodenal artery is then divided, allowing the hepatic artery to be separated from the duodenum and pancreas. Supraceliac aortic exposure and control is then obtained at the level of the diaphragm. The right colon and distal small bowel are mobilized and eviscerated onto the chest wall by dividing their peritoneal attachments. This maneuver exposes the abdominal aorta, inferior vena cava, left renal vein, and both kidneys. The greater omentum is divided, allowing access to the pancreas, and the inferior mesenteric vein is divided. The base of the small-bowel mesentery is encircled and divided, disconnecting the intestinal tract from the pancreas and liver. The infrahepatic vena cava also is visualized just above the entrance of the renal veins. The abdominal aorta may now be cannulated at its bifurcation with a large-bore aortic cannula for later infusion of cold UW solution for the core cooling of liver, kidneys, pancreas, and intestine (see Table 67-2). If thoracic organs are being procured for transplantation, they will be preserved with cardioplegia specific to the practice of that transplant center.

When all teams are prepared, the intrapericardial or infrarenal inferior vena cava is vented to prevent venous hypertension, and core cooling is begun, exsanguinating the donor blood and perfusing the organs with preservation solution. Systemic heparinization is given to prevent microthrombi, and surface cooling is accomplished with a frozen slush solution. The liver, pancreas, and spleen are then removed en bloc after division of the ligamentous attachments of the liver and division of the vena cava above the renal veins. Division of the portal vein and splenic artery in a 4°C ice bath complete the separation of the pancreas from the liver, both of which can be used for transplantation in different patients. The two kidneys are then removed en bloc, with segments of aorta and vena cava, the renal arteries and veins, and ureters. Care is taken during mobilization of the ureters to avoid skeletonizing them, which may compromise ureteral blood supply. The en bloc specimen is then brought to the back table, where each kidney is separated from the other by dividing the aorta and vena cava anteriorly and posteriorly. Excessive fatty tissues are removed, and the kidneys and other abdominal organs are preserved at 4°C until the time of transplantation.

Liver Transplant Techniques

Liver transplantation is generally performed in patients with severe portal hypertension and coagulopathy and is therefore a technically challenging procedure. A thorough understanding of liver anatomy and the various biliary and arterial anomalies is critical to technical success. The three phases of the liver transplant procedure are referred to as preanhepatic, anhepatic, and postanhepatic. The preanhepatic phase, during which the native liver is removed, requires division of the ligamentous attachments, hepatic artery, and any anomalous branches of the common bile duct; and dissection of the portal vein. The suprahepatic and infrahepatic vena cava also must be exposed, dissected, and encircled. This allows total vascular isolation of the organ, followed by its removal. Because the vena cava carries the blood returning to the heart from the lower body and abdominal viscera, clamping this vessel to allow hepatectomy may result in hemodynamic instability. When this is the case, venovenous bypass may provide venous return, providing stability during the hepatectomy and anhepatic phase of the transplant. Blood is removed through portal venous and infrahepatic vena caval cannulas and continuously returned to the heart via the axillary vein. A centrifugal pump, which does not require systemic heparinization, is used as part of the circuit in these severely coagulopathic patients.

The anhepatic phase of a liver transplant consists of implantation of the new liver. Four vascular anastomoses are required to place the liver in an orthotopic (native) position. The suprahepatic vena cava, the infrahepatic vena cava, the portal vein, and the hepatic arteries must all be reconstructed. Many variations of liver-transplant technique exist, but end-to-end anastomoses of these vessels are standard. A common variation of orthotopic implantation is the piggyback technique. In this procedure, the entire native liver is removed from the native vena cava after ligating all short hepatic veins. In this way, the native vena cava is preserved, with intact lower-body venous return to the heart. Clamps are placed only on the hepatic veins and the portal vein when the native liver is removed. The suprahepatic vena cava of the donor liver is anastomosed end-to-end to the cloaca of the native hepatic veins, and the donor infrahepatic cava is ligated. Maintenance of native caval flow usually obviates hypotension during the anhepatic phase of the procedure.

When the new organ is in position, with vascular anastomosis completed, the liver is reperfused, and the hyperkalemic preservation solution must be removed to avoid cardiac arrest. The solution may be vented through the infrahepatic caval anastomosis before reinstitution of outflow through the suprahepatic vena cava. Despite this maneuver, reperfusion may still result in a syndrome of hemodynamic instability, coagulopathy, and acidosis. If the liver functions promptly, clotting factors will soon be produced, limiting coagulopathy. If allograft function is poor, severe coagulopathy may ensue, with tissue plasminogen activator and other anticoagulant factors being produced. This cascade of events marks a difficult postanhepatic phase of the transplant. When hemostasis is achieved, biliary reconstruction is required, via either direct choledochocholedochostomy or Roux-en-Y hepaticojejunostomy. Cholecystectomy is performed, as the gallbladder is denervated with liver procurement, and preservation results in a high rate of stone formation.

Surgical Anatomy of the Liver

To understand the complex advanced techniques of partial liver transplantation, a thorough understanding of hepatic vascular and biliary anatomy is essential. The liver has left and right surgical lobes defined by the plane between the gallbladder fossa and the suprahepatic vena cava. On either side of this plane runs an invaginated sheath of Glisson's capsule in which are a main left or right hepatic artery, a portal vein, and a hepatic duct branch. The biliary structures are nourished by a peribiliary arteriolar plexus of vessels deriving from the arterial branch to that lobe. The lobes are further divided, such that left lateral and medial sectors and right anterior and posterior sectors are formed. Again, these divisions reflect divisions of the accompanying vessels and biliary ducts. These sectors are further subdivided into eight total segments, each of which has an arterial, portal venous, and biliary radicle, and which is drained by a hepatic venous branch, as initially described by Couinaud (Fig. 67-2). Portal venous branches from the left portal vein run to the right within the falciform ligament to segment four and are called switchback branches for this

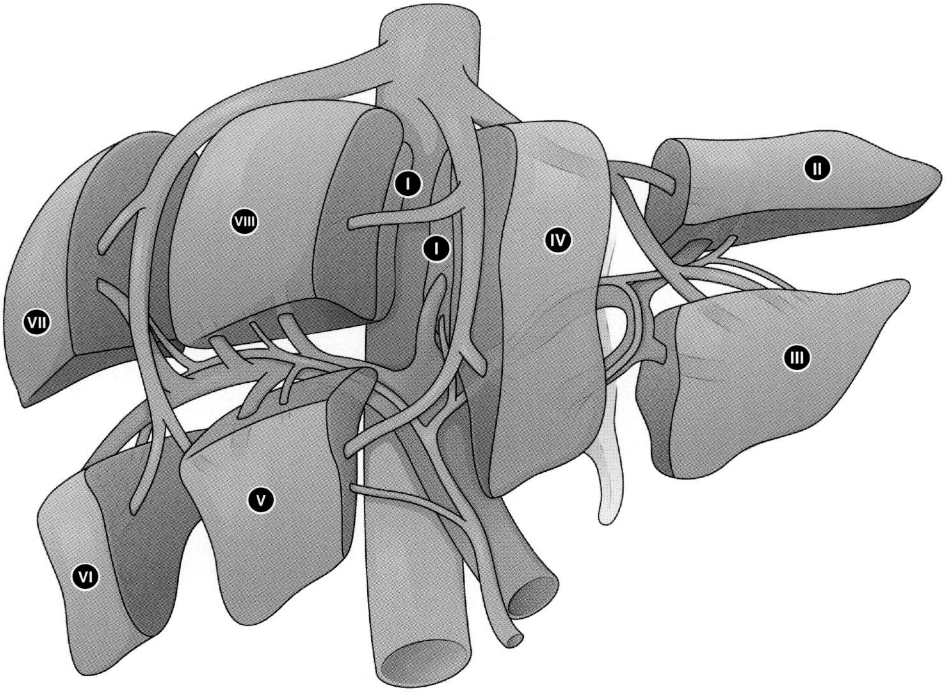

FIGURE 67–2 The segmental vascular anatomic basis for liver surgery, as originally described by Couinaud. The right lobe consists of segments V to VIII, the left lobe of segments II to IV, and the left lateral area of segments II and III.

reason. The three main hepatic veins, left, middle and right, are formed by confluence of segmental veins draining the right posterior, right anterior, and left lobes of the liver.

Reduced Liver, Split-Liver, and Living-Donor Transplantation

The lack of pediatric size-matched organ donors led to a high rate of death on the waiting list among small pediatric candidates for liver transplantation and served as the impetus for the development of partial liver-transplant procedures. Broelsch first described the successful use of the left lateral segment of the liver resected from a parent and transplanted into a child. This has become a standard technique in pediatric liver transplantation (Fig. 67-3).

In this procedure, the left hepatic artery, left branch of the portal vein, and left hepatic vein are dissected and removed with the lateral segment of a live donor's liver after division of caudate venous branches draining into the cava and division of portal branches feeding segment IV. More recently, such techniques have been extended to the use of a whole left or right lobe of a live donor's liver for transplantation in adults. Split-liver transplantation refers to a similar procedure, in which a left lateral segment resected from an adult cadaveric liver is transplanted into a child, and the right trisegment graft from the same liver is transplanted into another patient, usually an adult. These complex techniques require hepaticojejunostomy for reconstruction of the left or right lobe biliary ducts, as well as piggyback implantation of the partial liver graft with anastomosis of the donor hepatic vein directly to the recipient hepatic veins.

Liver Allograft Rejection

Liver allograft rejection occurs in some 30% to 70% of recipients, usually during the first 90 days after transplantation. Rejection may be classified as acute cellular rejection or chronic rejection. Vascular rejection may occur in rare cases in which a positive lymphocytotoxic cross-match exists, but vascular and hyperacute rejection, which are seen in renal transplantation, are fortunately rare in liver transplantation. The reason for the resistance of the liver to antibody-mediated rejection remains unclear. Acute cellular rejection may be further classified as mild, moderate, or severe, based on histology and clinical parameters. Acute cellular rejection is accompanied by a triad of lymphocytic infiltration, endothelialitis, and bile-duct damage. Treatment usually consists of a glucocorticoid bolus. Steroid-resistant rejection is typically treated with antibody preparations that eliminate activated T cells from the circulation, such as OKT3, which is directed against the CD3 receptor of mature T cells. Polyclonal antibody preparations, discussed in the section on immunosuppression, are equally efficacious. Although these agents are highly effective at treating the majority of acute rejection episodes, they carry a higher risk of infectious complications than does steroid treatment and are therefore reserved for second-line therapy.

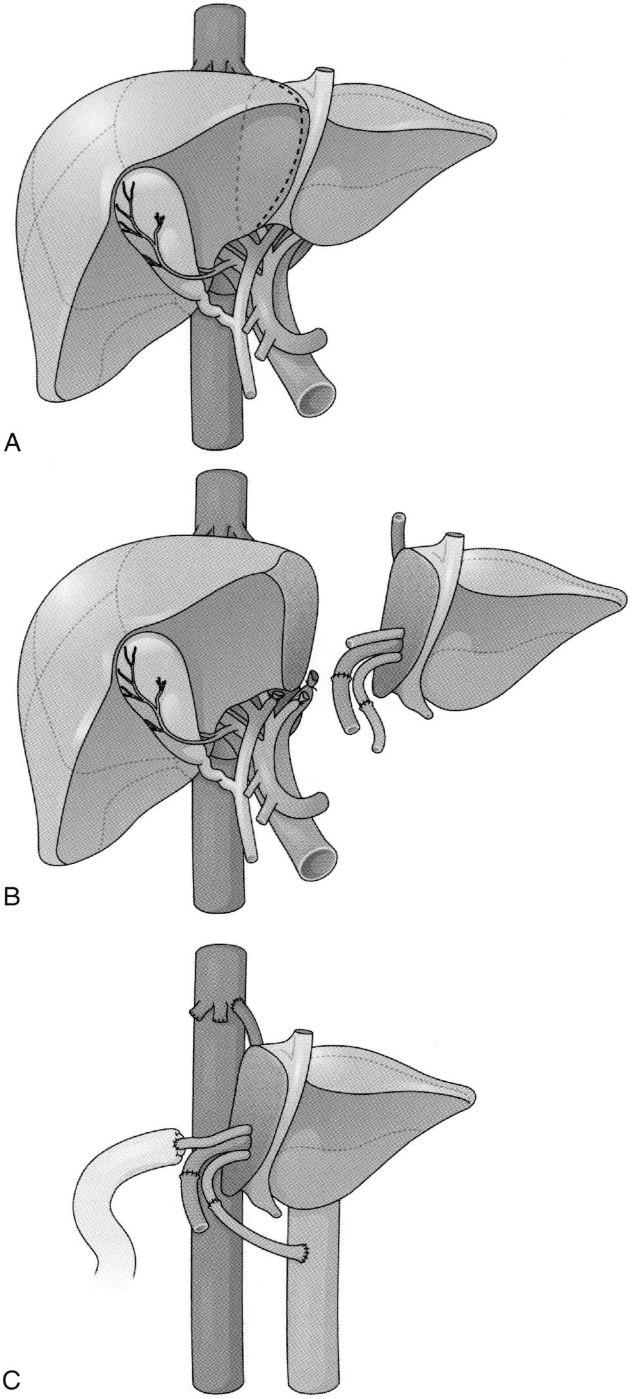

A

B

C

FIGURE 67–3 In living-donor liver transplantation, an anatomic segment of liver with associated vascular and biliary structures is removed for transplantation. Here, the left lateral segment is procured for transplantation into a child. *A*, The plane of trans-section. *B*, Vascular reconstruction. *C*, Biliary drainage via Roux-en-Y hepaticojejunostomy.

PEARLS FOR THE OR

A *replaced hepatic artery* refers to a branch that usually arises from the proximal 2 cm of the superior mesenteric artery. It travels posterolateral to the portal vein, supplying the right lobe. It is present in 15% of people.

The ureter of the renal allograft is usually cut short before anastomosis to the bladder because the blood supply to the upper two thirds of the ureter arises from the renal artery, and the lower third is supplied by arterial branches from the bladder. Thus only the proximal ureter has reliable arterialization after transplant.

The pancreas has a dual blood supply. The head of the pancreas receives blood via gastroduodenal and inferior pancreaticoduodenal arteries, whereas the body and tail depend on branches of the splenic artery.

Chronic rejection is a humoral and cell-mediated phenomenon of chronic small bile ductular damage resulting in progressive biliary fibrosis, known also as the vanishing bile duct syndrome. Chronic rejection may respond to sustained elevated blood levels of tacrolimus, but frequently requires liver retransplantation because of progressive cholestasis and cirrhosis. Chronic rejection appears in fewer than 5% to 10% of liver-transplant recipients at most experienced centers.

Complications

Vascular Complications

The most common vascular complication is hepatic artery thrombosis, which occurs after 2% to 8% of transplants. In the native condition, the bile ducts receive blood supply from the choledochal vessels running parallel to the duct and bringing blood from the pancreaticoduodenal arcade and gastroduodenal artery. Because these vessels are transected when the liver is removed for transplantation, the biliary tract of the transplanted liver is entirely dependent on the hepatic artery for arterial blood and oxygen supply. The radicles of the biliary tree are nourished by a periarteriolar biliary plexus deriving from the hepatic artery. If the hepatic artery thromboses after transplant, ischemia of the entire biliary tree results, leading to a variety of secondary biliary complications. In the first few days after transplantation, this can lead to ischemic breakdown of the biliary anastomosis and bile leak. It may appear as an elevation of the liver chemistries and can progress from liver necrosis to sepsis and death if not recognized early. When hepatic artery thrombosis occurs late, it may lead to diffuse stricturing of the intrahepatic bile ducts. This serious complication has led to the use of routine screening with Doppler ultrasonography in the early postoperative period at most centers. Optimal management is usually retransplantation, although occasionally, hepatic artery thrombosis will be asymptomatic or the artery can be revascularized by thrombectomy if recognized early.

Portal vein thrombosis may occur after liver transplantation, although rarely except in small pediatric cases or with preexisting portal vein thrombosis. This is usually a devastating complication resulting in acute liver failure and death, if not treated with urgent retransplantation. Occasionally, portal vein thrombosis also may be treated with early thrombectomy and revascularization. Rarely, stricture of the large suprehepatic caval anastomosis may occur, resulting in extremity edema and signs of recurrent portal hypertension such as bleeding or ascites formation. Because most of these complications can be evaluated with Doppler ultrasonography, this has become the standard first test in evaluation of the post-transplant patient with elevated liver chemistries.

Biliary Complications

Biliary strictures or leaks also may occur after liver transplantation in the absence of hepatic artery thrombosis. In such cases, the strictures are usually seen at the site of choledochocholedochostomy after liver transplantation. These strictures also are usually ischemic, as the distal donor duct is farthest from the arterial inflow (see section on liver surgical anatomy). Strictures may be diagnosed by elevation of the canalicular enzymes, the bilirubin and screening ultrasonography suggesting dilatation of the intrahepatic ducts. These findings should lead to confirmation of the diagnosis by endoscopic retrograde cholangiopancreatography (ERCP) or percutaneous transhepatic cholangiography, examinations that detail biliary anatomy. Standard management is usually conversion of biliary drainage to Roux-en-Y hepaticojejunostomy or revision of such an anastomosis. In poor-risk patients, balloon dilatation or biliary stent placement also may alleviate obstruction. Placement of T-tubes across the choledochocholedochostomy is standard at some centers, and removal of these tubes may lead to bile leak and chemical peritonitis. Endoscopic stent placement or papillotomy may be required in such instances; operation may be required if such measures are ineffective.

Infectious Complications

Infectious complications of liver transplantation are similar to those of other solid-organ transplants and may be predicted to some degree by the time frame after transplantation (Fig. 67-4). The intense immunosuppression necessary in the early post-transplant period may lead to the development of early bacterial or fungal sepsis. Prophylaxis against *Pneumocystis carinii* pneumonia is standard in most centers. CMV, an ordinarily innocuous organism, may cause systemic viremia after transplant, resulting in pneumonitis, hepatitis, or a syndrome of myalgias, fatigue, and fevers known as the CMV syndrome. CMV syndrome most often occurs during the second or third month after transplantation and is treated with antiviral therapy and decreased immunosuppression, as tolerated.

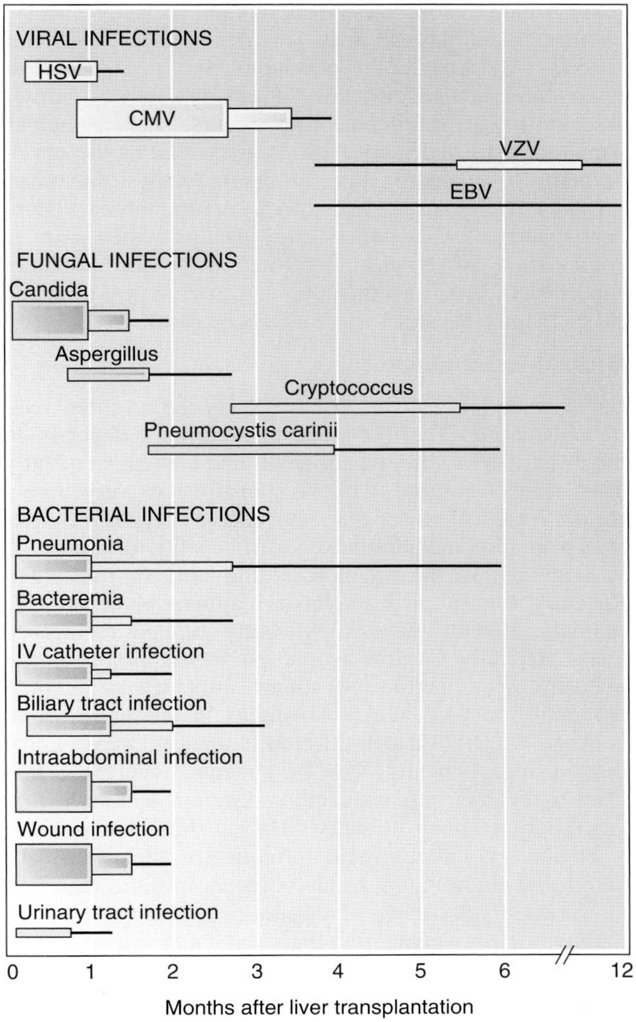

FIGURE 67–4 Time of presentation of infections commonly seen after liver transplantation. HSV, herpes simplex virus; CMV, cytomegalovirus; VZV, varicella-zoster virus; EBV, Epstein-Barr virus. (Modified from Emmanouilides C, Holt CD, Winston DJ: Infections after liver transplantation. In Busuttil RW, Klintmalm GB (eds): Transplantation of the Liver. Philadelphia, WB Saunders, 1996.)

Another pathogenic virus after transplantation is the Epstein-Barr virus (EBV). Proliferation of B cells, stimulated by this virus, is usually controlled by negative feedback of activated T cells. These T cells identify and eliminate B cells infected with the virus and harboring EBV DNA. However, under largely T cell–directed transplant immunosuppression, these proliferating B cells are not eliminated and instead may proliferate unchecked. This process may lead to the development of post-transplant lymphoproliferative disease. Similarly, other viruses associated with development of tumors, such as human papillomavirus and herpesviruses, may lead to the development of squamous skin cancers or Kaposi sarcomas, presumably because of the lack of immunoregulatory competence. These tumors are ideally treated with a combination of surgical removal, decreased immunosuppression, antiviral therapy, and sometimes systemic chemotherapy in refractory or advanced cases.

Disease Recurrence

Some underlying liver diseases may recur after liver transplantation. The likelihood of recurrence depends on the disease. The viral hepatitides B and C recur frequently after transplantation, whereas hepatitis A very rarely recurs. Risk factors for the recurrence of hepatitis B after transplantation includes presence of hepatitis B viral DNA or e-antigen in the recipient at the time of transplant. Recently, long-term prophylaxis regimens of hepatitis B immune globulin have significantly limited recurrence rates. Hepatitis C virus is present in the blood of the majority of hepatitis C patients after transplantation. Although the percentage of patients in whom recurrent hepatitis C cirrhosis will develop is unclear, we do know that in approximately 15% of patients, recurrence that leads to death or retransplantation develops within the first year after transplant. Primary biliary cirrhosis and primary sclerosing cholangitis recur infrequently after transplantation, but autoimmune hepatitis recurs in more than half of patients. All of these diseases may progress more rapidly after transplantation than in the native liver, where the course is usually insidious. Alcoholic liver disease also may recur after transplantation and is best prevented by cautious recipient selection, usually requiring a period of proven abstinence before transplantation. Fulminant hepatic failure of unknown etiology rarely recurs after transplantation.

Pancreas Transplantation

Juvenile-onset diabetes, or type 1 diabetes, is a deficiency in insulin production by the native pancreas, leading to altered glucose homeostasis. Two large multicenter studies demonstrated recently that tight control of the blood glucose levels with exogenous insulin administration in such patients improves long-term survival. However, abundant evidence indicates that long-term exogenous insulin use does not effectively prevent the development of secondary diabetic complications in a subset of the insulin-dependent diabetic population. This finding led to the development of pancreas transplantation as a means of returning glucose homeostasis to normal in such patients. Successful pancreas transplantation is currently the only therapy that can return a type 1 diabetic to normal glucose homeostasis.

Early animal studies and attempts at pancreas transplantation were pioneered at the University of Minnesota. Although these attempts were largely unsuccessful, they led to the standardization of techniques that allowed later success in humans. Later developments independently by Corry and Sollinger with urinary bladder drainage of the pancreatic secretions via a segment of duodenum accompanying the pancreas allograft improved the monitoring of rejection. Transplantation of the pancreas with a concomitantly transplanted kidney from the same donor resulted in further improvements in long-term graft survival. Great interest has developed in the transplantation of islet cells, which could provide the necessary insulin for glucose homeostasis without incurring the morbidity of whole-organ transplant surgery. This therapy is currently undergoing a multinational clinical trial.

Indications

Currently more than 1 million juvenile-onset diabetics live in the United States. In the majority of these patients, secondary complications of their disease will ultimately develop. Data from the United Network for Organ Sharing show that 4500 people currently await pancreas transplantation in the United States. Most of these patients have had renal insufficiency as a result of diabetes and will receive simultaneous kidney-pancreas transplants, although an increasing proportion are now receiving pancreas transplants after a kidney transplant or alone. Whole pancreas transplantation is currently indicated for the remediation of secondary complications of insulin-dependent diabetes. The most common of these has been renal failure requiring renal-replacement therapy. Although the risk of immunosuppression is already accepted for kidney transplantation, the only increased risk incurred with simultaneous kidney-pancreas transplantation is the potential for technical complications arising from placement of the pancreas graft. Such insulin-dependent diabetic patients have been demonstrated to fare worse after kidney transplantation than do other recipients of kidney transplants, because of the unchecked progression of diabetic vasculopathy. Some evidence suggests that simultaneous pancreas and kidney transplantation may slow or halt the progression of such chronic vasculopathic as well as neuropathic changes.

Patients who have undergone prior kidney transplantation and in whom recurrent diabetic glomerulopathy develops in the transplanted kidney may undergo pancreas transplantation in an effort to halt this progression to end-stage renal failure as well. This is known as pancreas after kidney transplantation. Candidates for isolated pancreas transplantation are those prone to hyperlabile diabetes despite adequate insulin therapy and patients with hypoglycemic unawareness, placing them at risk for diabetic coma.

Surgical Technique

The surgical anatomy of the pancreas involves a dual arterial blood supply arising from both the celiac and superior mesenteric arterial trees. The supply to the head of the pancreas comes from both the gastroduodenal artery above and the inferior pancreaticoduodenal artery from the superior mesenteric artery. The body and tail of the pancreas receive their blood supply from branches of the splenic artery. Whole-organ pancreas transplantation was made feasible with organs procured from simultaneous liver donors by the development of the iliac artery Y-graft technique. In this way, a single inflow vessel provides blood supply to the entire organ, which is usually placed in the pelvis, similar to kidney placement. Systemic venous drainage is typically provided through the proximal portal vein anastomosed to the common iliac vein. Alternatively, the portal vein may be anastomosed to the superior mesenteric vein to provide more physiologic portal drainage. Neither technique has proven to offer superior long-term function of the allograft.

The transplanted pancreas will continue to produce exocrine secretions, and these are currently drained through the intact ampulla into a short segment of duodenum transplanted in continuity with the pancreas. This duodenum may be anastomosed to the urinary bladder (bladder drainage), providing amylasuria, which may be monitored as a marker of pancreas allograft function. Alternatively, enteric drainage into the native jejunum through either Roux-en-Y anastomosis or side-to-side duodenojejunal anastomosis has recently gained favor. Bladder drainage has been associated with the long-term complications of recurrent dehydration, metabolic acidosis from loss of bicarbonate-rich pancreatic secretions in the urine, and bladder ulceration. Approximately 15% of patients receiving bladder drainage have required conversion to enteric drainage because of these or other complications. Other noteworthy complications of pancreas transplantation include postreperfusion pancreatitis, leak from the duodenal anastomosis, and standard post-transplant infectious complications of immunosuppression.

Results

Current results of pancreas transplantation are the best when the pancreas is transplanted simultaneously with a kidney. In this case, measurement of the serum creatinine level serves as a marker of possible rejection. Surrogate serum markers of pancreas rejection such as lipase, amylase, and pancreatic polypeptide have been investigated but have not proven routinely reliable. Current 1- and 5-year graft survival rates for this procedure are 79% and 61%. Graft survival refers to freedom from the need for any insulin in the recipient. Kidney allograft survival in pancreas recipients is similar to kidney-graft-alone survival rates. Recent advances have improved the outcome of pancreas after kidney and pancreas–alone transplantation. These include the use of percutaneous pancreas allograft biopsy and the routine use of tacrolimus for maintenance immunosuppression.

Intestinal Transplantation

End-stage intestinal failure has only recently been recognized as a clinical entity and can be defined as the inability to maintain nutrition or fluid and electrolyte balance because of loss of intestinal mucosal surface area or dysfunctional syndromes. This state is most commonly caused by the short-gut syndrome secondary to intestinal resection, but patients with motility disorders such as visceral myopathy, and those with malabsorption, also may require lifelong parenteral nutrition for the treatment of intestinal failure. Current management with parenteral nutrition can produce 60% to 75% 5-year survival rates. However, some patients experience life-threatening complications such as the development of recurrent catheter sepsis, major vessel thrombosis, or the development of cholestatic liver disease on parenteral nutrition. These patients can be salvaged and often returned to a near-normal lifestyle with intestinal transplantation. Because of the relative safety of nutritional management with parenteral nutrition, intestinal transplantation has generally been reserved for patients with life-threatening complications of parenteral nutrition.

Surgical Technique

The surgical technique of intestinal transplantation was first experimentally attempted in dogs by Alexis Carrell. Experimental reperfusion injury and preservation were studied by Owen Wangensteen 60 years later. However, the immunogenicity of the intestine did not allow successful human transplantation until the advent of tacrolimus in 1990. Currently, the clinical success of intestinal transplantation is improving, and this has become the standard treatment offered to patients with intestinal failure with life-threatening complications of parenteral nutrition.

The intestine can be transplanted alone or in combination with other organs, depending on accompanying organ disease in these often very debilitated patients. Intestinal allografts are currently most commonly placed in orthotopic position with infrarenal aortic inflow and caval venous drainage. Enteric continuity is reestablished proximally with some form of distal ileostomy, which allows surveillance endoscopic mucosal biopsies to evaluate the organ for possible rejection.

When advanced liver disease accompanies intestinal failure, a composite liver-intestine transplant is best performed. Rarely, diffuse visceral thrombosis or locally advanced benign tumors require removal of all abdominal gastrointestinal organs and multivisceral transplantation. Current results are best for isolated intestinal transplantation or liver-intestinal transplantation, with patient survival at 2 and 5 years of approximately 60% and 55% at experienced centers. Severe acute rejection with graft loss to rejection remains problematic. Additionally, the bacteria-laden graft has been a frequent source of sepsis associated with the need for enhanced immunosuppression during rejection crises. It is hoped that new immunosuppressive regimens and the addition of tolerance-induction protocols will improve results of intestinal and multiorgan transplantation procedures in the future. With continued improvement, intestinal transplantation before the development of secondary liver failure or severe debility should ultimately become the therapy of choice for patients with intestinal failure.

Suggested Reading

Abu-Elmagd K, Reyes J, Todo S, et al: Clinical intestinal transplantation: New perspectives and immunologic considerations. J Am Coll Surg 186:415–527, 1998.

Emre S, Schwartz, M, Miller C: The donor operation. In Busuttil R, Klintmalm G (eds): Transplantation of the Liver. Philadelphia, WB Saunders, 1996, pp .

First MR: An update on new immunosuppressive drugs undergoing preclinical and clinical trials: Potential applications in organ transplantation. Am J Kidney Dis 29:303, 1997.

Grant D: Intestinal transplantation: 1997 report of the international registry: Intestinal Transplant Registry. Transplantation 67(7): 1061–1064, 1999.

Gruessner RWG, Sutherland DER, Troppman C, et al: The surgical risk of pancreas transplantation in the cyclosporine era: An overview. J Am Coll Surg 185:128–144, 1997.

Suthanthiran M, Strom TB: Renal transplantation. N Engl J Med 331:36, 1994

Valente JF, Alexander JW: Immunobiology of renal transplantation. Surg Clin North Am 78:1, 1998.

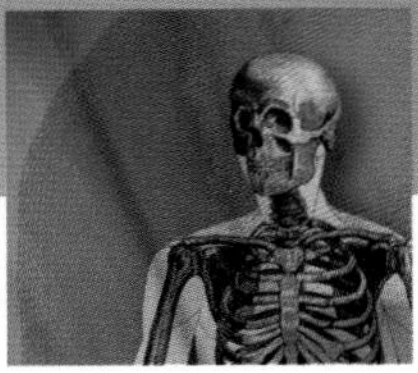

INDEX

Note: Page numbers followed by "b" indicate a box; those followed by "f" indicate a figure; and those followed by "t" indicate a table.

A

C

D

E

G

H

J

M

N

P

S

U

U